LIVING WITH METABOLIC SYNDROME

Naheed Ali, MD

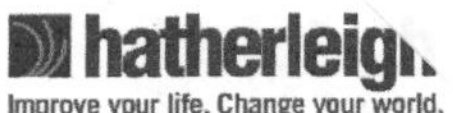

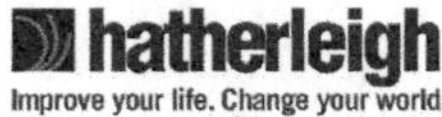

Hatherleigh Press is committed to preserving and protecting the natural resources of the earth. Environmentally responsible and sustainable practices are embraced within the company's mission statement.

Visit us at www.hatherleighpress.com and register online for free offers, discounts, special events, and more.

Living with Metabolic Syndrome

Library of Congress Cataloging-in-Publication Data is available.
ISBN: 978-1-57826-590-9

Living with Metabolic Syndrome is dedicated to my readers, to metabolic syndrome patients, and to all who provided inspiration and support for my research.

CONTENTS

Part III: Faces of Metabolic Syndrome

Part IV: Resolutions

Part V: Homestretch

Appendices

METABOLIC SYNDROME POST-DIAGNOSIS CHECKLIST

✓ Day 1: Learn the full definition of metabolic syndrome. See Preface and Chapter 1.

✓ Day 2: Learn about how blood sugar impacts metabolic syndrome. See Chapters 5 and 20.

✓ Day 3: Learn the symptoms of metabolic syndrome. See Chapter 8.

✓ Day 4: Understand your diagnosis. See Chapter 10.

✓ Day 5: Make a list of all your questions for future doctor visits. See Chapters 11 and 12.

✓ Day 6: Visit your endocrinologist. This specialist is described in Chapter 13.

✓ Day 7: Devise an initial diet plan. See Chapter 22 for some ideas.

✓ Day 8: Start a medication diary. See Chapter 24 for information on prescription drugs.

✓ Day 9: Find out if any surgery is necessary. See Chapter 25.

✓ Day 10: Seek out a support system. Use Chapter 29 as a guide.

PREFACE

METABOLIC SYNDROME is characterized by a combination of health problems that facilitate accumulation of excessive fats around the waist area, high triglycerides, low HDL cholesterol, and elevated blood pressure and sugar. In other words, this condition is a bundle of risk factors that work against the general well-being of the body. As evident from its sparse definition, the syndrome is primarily denoted by unhealthy lifestyle choices such as being physically inactive, as well as the intake of more calories than one can utilize.[1]

The word "syndrome" was derived from a Latin term that means "to run together." The risk factors that together jointly represent metabolic syndrome are: obesity, **hyperglycemia**, **atherosclerosis**, and **hypertension**. Other factors include insulin resistance, increase in uric acid, diabetes mellitus, abdominal obesity, over-clotting, and excessive parcels of cholesterol in the bloodstream.[2]

DEMOGRAPHICS AND FIGURES

Metabolic syndrome is widespread throughout the world and has been found to increase with age and higher BMI values. The occurrence of metabolic syndrome differs with race and ethnicity, and has shown different patterns for men and women. Studies estimate that 20–25 percent of world populations are affected by metabolic syndrome.[3]

A study conducted on a number of participants over 20 years of age showed that approximately 34 percent of adults have the risk factors often associated with metabolic syndrome. People in the age group of 40–59 years of age were about three times as likely to develop the syndrome. Men who were 60 years of age or older were more than four times as likely to have metabolic syndrome, whereas females in the same age group were six times as likely to develop it.[4]

IMPORTANCE OF A COMPREHENSIVE APPROACH

A comprehensive, in-depth approach to metabolic syndrome, such as the one followed in this book, is worthwhile due to the syndrome's nature as a collective illness. Metabolic syndrome is firmly a case of a number of symptoms occurring together. Treatment for a standalone symptom or diet modification designed to treat any one of the associated conditions isn't going to be successful long-term; correction of the syndrome requires a deliberation of all the factors at work, and a comprehensive treatment plan that addresses all of the working parts. Such a comprehensive approach combines drug treatment along with exercise and diet modification—much like the syndrome it seeks to treat, any single modus operandi of treatment might not prove to be useful for all people with metabolic syndrome.[5]

Before commencing with the chapters of this book, readers should note that, while the author's intention is to produce a book that is relatively easy to comprehend, there may be advanced terminology used on occasion where necessary. A glossary of terms has been provided in the back of the book on page 151.[6]

PART I

Groundwork

1

Real Meaning of Metabolic Syndrome

THE TERM "metabolism" comes from the Greek "metabole," meaning change. "Meta-" is a Greek prefix meaning "with, across, or after"; in chemistry, it denotes change, reaction, and alteration. The suffix "-ism" comes from the Greek term "isma," and is used to form nouns of action, state, condition, and doctrine. As a result, the combined meaning of the term metabolism is chemical occurrences, taking place within a living entity to sustain life. These processes include digestion and the transportation of nutrients into and in between cells.[7]

The Theologus Autodidactus by Ibn Al-Nafis in the 13th century is arguably the first recorded use of the word *metabolism*. In his work, Al-Nafis discussed the idea that the body and its parts are in a constant state of flux. The study of these processes continues today in biochemistry, which is the in-depth investigation of the chemical reactions needed to sustain the life of an organism.[8]

CLASSIFICATION AS SYNDROME

The term "syndrome" refers to a knot of symptoms that together constitute a single condition (as opposed to a disease, which is caused by pathogens). Microbes such as viruses aren't always the cause of a disorder, and *condition* is an eclectic medical term. Depending on how a diagnosis of syndrome is reached, different physicians may use various indicators (such as the amount of sugar molecules in **blood plasma** or the presence of diabetes).[9]

The main issue with a syndrome, or collection of symptoms, is that they will all attack the body at the same time, resulting in a number of conditions, or at least the potential for other conditions. Examples include potential heart problems, blood pressure spikes, and more often than not, type-2 diabetes. Some people also report feeling pain, especially in their extremities. All of these conditions are metabolic to some degree, and can affect the chemistry of the body as a whole while interrupting (or even rewriting) how it processes chemicals. Because these conditions are associated with one another, but aren't necessarily always present together, it's considered a general pattern of ill health, or "syndrome."[10]

However, a syndrome is a nebula of symptoms that are characteristic of a single medical condition. The word syndrome is used in medical genetics, for example Down syndrome, whereas **acquired immune deficiency syndrome (AIDS)** is an example of a non-genetic occurrence. The term is derived from the Greek "sundrome," which is the combination of "sun," meaning together, and "dramein," meaning to run. Avicenna, through his publication *The Canon of Medicine,* was the forerunner for the concept of a syndrome in the clinical context, and the idea was developed further by Thomas Sydenham in the 17th century.[11]

A syndrome differs from a disease in that the latter is caused by distinct pathogens, including viruses, bacteria, and fungi. A disease is often, but not always, contagious. The microbes cause dysfunction in the characteristic internal balance of your body—a process called homeostasis. A medical disorder, by contrast, is a disturbance in the normal functioning of organs. These can be mental disorders, genetic disorders, and emotional or behavioral complaints. The term *disorder* is typically used in medicine to identify problems not caused by infectious pathogens. By contrast, a medical condition is a broader term that refers to all illnesses, injuries, diseases, and disorders (absenting those that are mental in nature).[12]

CONNECTIONS TO METABOLISM

The name "metabolic syndrome" originates from its connection to the body's overall metabolism (or basically "the state of the body overall" when the original Latin is used), and is dependent on any number of factors (hence the "syndrome" part of the name). Like many other medical disorders, there are of course other names for metabolic syndrome. Some of these names include cardio-metabolic syndrome, insulin resistance syndrome, metabolic syndrome X, Reaven's syndrome (after Gerald Reaven), and syndrome X. The syndrome has been internationally referred to by the acronym CHAOS, which stands for **coronary artery disease**, **hypertension**, adult onset diabetes, obesity, and stroke. Historically, all of these refer back to the same disorder, even though some of them have been revised to fall under more specific types of medical illness.[13]

All in all, to gain a clear understanding of the terms *metabolism* and *syndrome*, it's helpful to examine their origins. You should also note that each of the above methods of determining whether something is a syndrome, disease, or a condition, is as accurate and legitimate as the next.

2

History of Metabolic Syndrome

IT HAS been observed that the likelihood of developing metabolic syndrome increases with age; meaning, as an individual grows older, his or her chances of acquiring the syndrome increase as well. In this chapter, we will follow the path of metabolic syndrome's role in history, from the discoveries of old to modern clinical findings. In doing so, we will also uncover the origins of other associated conditions, such as diabetes.

HISTORICAL SIGNIFICANCE OF OBESITY

It wasn't until the late 1950s that the term "metabolic syndrome" started circulating in full force within medical circles. The majority of the general public only came to know about the syndrome and the different risk factors associated with it in the 1970s.[14] In 1947, a French doctor named Jean Vague noted that obesity in the upper body tended to aggravate diseases related to what is now known as metabolic syndrome. Some of those diseases include diabetes, gout, **calculi**, and **atherosclerosis**. Although the individual symptoms had been noted to group together as early as 1927, Vague's discovery was the first real step. Until that time, no one had really consolidated the available information to come to a conclusion. Vague's handiwork consisted of models of how body fat was accumulated in different body types, specifically the difference between male and female bodies, with a special interest in obesity. As part of that work, he noticed that the obese had a number of symptoms in common. His initial research into this phenomenon would soon expand into the groundwork for future discussions about metabolic syndrome.[15]

HISTORICAL SIGNIFICANCE OF DIABETES

In 1977, Hermann Haller coined the phrase "metabolic syndrome" for when diabetes mellitus and an excess of fat, protein, and uric acid together increase the risk of heart disease, due to the risk of atherosclerosis. Haller essentially confirmed the discovery made by Vague when he associated the syndrome with too much liver fat, disproportionate uric acid in the blood, and diabetes mellitus. While Haller's research continues to be focused primarily on diseases of the kidney, he is also currently researching the ways in which protein accumulates in the urinary system.[16]

At about the same time, Pierre Singer added to all of this by noting that textbook diabetes (diabetes mellitus), gout, **hypertension**, and obesity usually occurred alongside excessive protein and fats in the bloodstream. Singer again used the term metabolic syndrome, and associated it with contributing antecedents to **myocardial infarction**, which is more commonly known as a heart attack. Singer noted that heart attacks led to a set of abnormalities, among them intolerance to glucose, hypertension, and excessive cholesterol and insulin in the bloodstream. Singer, known for his work in clinical nutrition and diabetes worldwide, linked the above conditions with aging, obesity, and heart disease. He boasts more than 30 years of metabolism-related research experience, primarily based in Israel. He's also soaked up the accolades for metabolic syndrome research throughout the past few decades.[17]

The next development came more than a decade later, when in 1988 during his renowned Banting Lecture, Gerald Reaven presented resistance to insulin as the primary cause of metabolic syndrome. In the modern world of medicine, metabolic syndrome is now defined as the constellation of abnormalities that culminates to type-2 diabetes as well as vascular irregularities wherein plaque buildup has occurred. As a member of the Stanford University academic family,

Reaven received numerous prizes for his scientific achievements related to the study of metabolic syndrome.[18]

The fundamental description of diabetes, which almost always accompanies metabolic syndrome, came from Aretaeus of Cappadocia, an ancient Greek physician, in the first century CE. This doctor discovered the high amount of urine being dispatched via the kidneys and named the condition diabetes. Aretaeus tried to decipher the condition but never completed a proper prognosis, which led him to determine that living with diabetes shortens lifespan, and that patients are blighted from living a supposedly painful life. The term mellitus, meaning sweet, was introduced by John Rollo in the late 1700s in order to differentiate this type of diabetes from the other types of insulin resistance.[19]

Avicenna (980-1037), originally hailing from medieval Persia, gave detailed information on diabetes mellitus in *The Canon of Medicine.* Avicenna saw diabetes as resulting from an abnormal appetite, as well as malfunctioning of sexual functions, and he drew distinctions between primary and secondary levels of diabetes.

HISTORICAL SIGNIFICANCE OF HIGH BLOOD PRESSURE

The history of high blood pressure, another condition considered a slice of the metabolic syndrome pie, began when William Harvey mapped the workings of the heart and blood vessels, and described the related system as blood circulation. In 1808, Thomas Young went on to propose hypertension as a disease, and a couple of decades later, Richard Bright confirmed the same. However, the mention of hypertension in clinical circles truly started in the year 1896, after Scipione Riva-Rocci invented the sphygmomanometer, the generic tool used to measure blood pressure. Further clinical milestones were reached, and people started understanding the condition more thoroughly. Before the use of pharmacological treatment of hypertension commenced, physicians of the 19th and 20th century used three treatment options.[20] The options included restriction of sodium, surgical ablation of some parts of the nervous system, as well as **pyrogen therapy**, which involved injecting patients with substances that induced fever so that blood pressure could safely decrease. More studies and experiments took place in the 1970s as captopril, an agent consumed orally, surfaced. Captopril then led to the development of other drugs used to modulate high blood pressure.[21]

HISTORICAL SIGNIFICANCE OF HEART DISEASE

People began concerning themselves seriously with heart disease in the early 20th century. Until the 1940s, heart disease had seldom occurred, but in the latter half of the century, experts declared the developing epidemic to be among the most serious the world had seen. During this period, cases of occluded or blocked blood vessels, strokes, and heart attacks were widely reported, and many individuals lost their lives. Studies began in earnest, and in 1948, a 30-year study commenced, involving more than 5,000 people, ranging in age from 30 to 62 years. No one in the study developed heart disease, and every two years they went for a comprehensive physical exam. The causes and main cures of heart disease remain unknown, but tools and treatments for combating the condition continue to evolve.[22]

HISTORICAL APPROACHES

Historically, the health of a metabolic syndrome patient has depended on the lifestyle he chooses. Living responsibly today is all about avoiding long-term illnesses in the years to come. Metabolic syndrome can be treated, and these specific remedies are tied to the history of the disease. Because of its connection to obesity, doctors initially treated metabolic syndrome with diet modifications, specifically a high-protein, low-calorie diet. As doctors gained more knowledge about the associated diseases, chemical treatments were developed, designed to deal with some of the more easily remediable conditions that have existed throughout history, such as diabetes.[23]

In addition, counseling is also a substantial part of the game plan in modern treatment regimens. Part of the protocol in treating metabolic syndrome is examining the reasons why the person pursued unhealthy lifestyle habits in the first place. All of these approaches are ways to review the syndrome, and to perhaps cure or at least ameliorate its effects in the person afflicted.[24]

3

Anatomy of Metabolic Syndrome

IT IS common for most doctors to study general medicine, and then specialize in the study of another subfield. A qualified doctor or a general practitioner may opt to be a surgeon, neurologist, pediatrician, dermatologist, cardiologist, neurologist, internist, or an **anesthesiologist**, in addition to their knowledge of the basic fundamentals. Likewise, studying metabolic syndrome from multiple angles is needed to fully appreciate each and every aspect of the disorder.[25]

To that end, the general study of anatomy is invaluable. Understanding how multiple systems within the body function and interact is necessary to knowing how various treatments for any given disorder will work. For example, one of the most prevalent diseases today is obesity, which, as has been stated, is known to be fused with metabolic syndrome. Because of the rise in the number of people who are experiencing this disease, more and more doctors are turning their attention to the different research studies on how obesity is caused, as well as how it can be prevented. These studies look at the role of human anatomy in addressing several metabolic symptoms, asking questions like: "How are the two different medical fields related? What is their importance in the fight against obesity? How can the two help each other understand and battle the rise in obesity cases?"[26]

LINK BETWEEN HUMAN ANATOMY AND METABOLIC SYNDROME

The study of human anatomy is the scientific study of the structure of the human body, including the organs, systems, and tissues. Metabolic syndrome is a disorder in the way that the body both stores and utilizes energy, and can be divided into five separate medical conditions, each of which acts in and effects specific parts of the body. An understanding of basic anatomy is crucial to understanding metabolic syndrome as a whole; after all, it truly is a disorder greater than the sum of its parts.

All of the following are key anatomic players in the health of those with metabolic syndrome:

- Cardiovascular anatomy: The heart is essentially the core of the cardiovascular system. It is also directly linked to the ill effects of obesity, as it can lead to fatal cardiovascular diseases such as stroke or heart failure. Similarly, high blood pressure due to obesity can lead to the malfunction of your heart. This is due to the fact that the heart can no longer pump the right amount of blood to the different parts of the body.[27]
- Digestive anatomy: Metabolic syndrome is a condition where otherwise healthy organs have difficulty properly using and storing energy. The digestive system is responsible for breaking down and digesting all the food that the body consumes, reducing food into its various nutrients so that the body can use them for energy. A poor digestive system is linked to issues with the metabolic system.[28]
- Adipose anatomy: Adipose tissues can be found beneath the human skin around the internal organs, in the bone marrow, as well as in the breast tissue. Their purpose is to provide insulation and protection from heat and cold. They also reserve **lipids** that can be burned and used as energy to protect the body from excess sugar. Adipose tissues are linked to metabolic syndrome because they are responsible for the proper storage

and use of the body's energy. If these tissues aren't properly utilized, they can multiply, thereby contributing to obesity.[29]

HOW ANATOMY CAN BE USED TO ADDRESS METABOLIC SYNDROME

To summarize: reviewing and studying the anatomy of the human body can help medical practitioners understand why metabolic syndrome occurs so frequently in the first place. The study of physical anatomy enables them to find the reasons behind the rampant cases of obesity. It can also help to find solutions, so that people who have the syndrome can find relief from their symptoms.[30]

Moreover, the study of the human body can help put the final nail in metabolic syndrome's coffin in the following ways:

- It can benefit surgeons during surgical procedures on an obese patient. One of the most common treatments for metabolic syndrome or obesity is through a gastric bypass surgery. Obese people, often desperate to glean treatment for their condition, resort to going under the knife. Other patients will have a gastric bypass surgery because their condition is already fatal in the long term. With the help of the knowledge of human anatomy, surgeons can easily navigate through the fat that has already coated the different organs of their patient. This way, they can perform the surgery with ease and increase the overall success rates of the procedure.[31]
- Understanding the relationship between anatomy and metabolic syndrome can help physical trainers and nutritionists to assist their clients in their desire to lose weight and get healthy. They learn how the body converts fat into muscle, as well as how the body can be taught to burn more fat and calories. This knowledge gives trainers and nutritionists an edge in creating effective fitness training and diet regimens for their clients.[32]
- It can also help pharmaceutical companies to develop the right medicines to fight metabolic syndrome. Pharmaceutical giants

> can use the framework of human anatomy in order to know how the digestive system works. They can use this information to engineer safe and reliable pharmaceutical products that help people improve their metabolic rates, while enabling them to burn more calories. In addition, they can formulate drugs that are more effective and efficient in downing high blood pressure, sugar levels, and LDL levels.[33]

While some may still be skeptical about the role of human anatomy in understanding metabolic syndrome, a firm grasp of the basics is crucial when it comes to expanding the frontiers of medical science. We must aim to continuously learn and search for answers; the human body is anatomically complex, and is capable of incredible adaptation. There will always be new anatomical disorders surfacing every once in a while that require medical professionals to revisit anatomy over and over again.[34]

4

Physiology of Metabolic Syndrome

PHYSIOLOGY REFERS to the savoir faire of mechanical, biochemical, and physical functions of the human body, as its tissues and organs. Physiology differs from anatomy by focusing on the function, rather than the structure of the body. Consequently, a firm understanding of physiology both complements and enhances one's ability to understand and address syndromes.[35]

Since metabolic syndrome can involve both minor and serious symptoms, knowledge of human physiology helps healthcare professionals such as nurses, doctors, dieticians, and others to prevent and manage the condition. This chapter will cover the ways in which understanding human physiology in relation to metabolic syndrome can assist not only healthcare practitioners but sufferers of the disorder in finding effective treatment and prevention methods.[36]

NERVOUS SYSTEM

When a person develops metabolic syndrome, one of the most affected systems is the nervous system. Metabolic syndrome disturbs the system in such a way that patients stop feeling their body parts correctly. The central nervous system is composed of the brain and the spinal cord. When the brain experiences a setback, just about every other organ in the body will feel the impact, because the nervous system normally communicates with other regions physiologically.

Once this process has been interrupted, normal activities such as regular exchange of sensory information can be distorted or disrupted.[37]

If the brain isn't responding properly, every other aspect including memory, thought process, and control systems diminish as well. Hearing, taste, smell, and vision can also become disrupted or reduced. The study of human physiology helps to unriddle the cause behind the malfunction of the above systems. The science also offers solutions for rectifying the damaged senses and organs. Human physiology connects every system, organ, and sense, which helps efforts to overcome medically significant obstacles.[38]

IMMUNE SYSTEM

Physiology as a science also covers the immune system of the human body, including white blood cells, lymph nodes, lymph channels, and the thymus. The immune system helps the body to hold its own while keeping diseases at bay. Metabolic syndrome interferes with the immune system, rendering it useless, or at least diminished, and incapable of protecting the body from illness or infection. Human physiology offers insight on how to treat and restore the immune system.[39] When the immune system is working at less than its best, even minor illnesses can result in severe damage or death. It is only by using the knowledge gained by the study of human physiology that medical professionals can attempt to come up with solutions. Furthermore, study of this science offers new insights to all those involved in the fight against metabolic syndrome.[40]

ENDOCRINE SYSTEM

Another key system in normal body function is the **endocrine system**. The endocrine system and its constituent parts are primarily glands; namely the adrenals, **pancreas**, gonads, parathyroid, and the pituitary glands. These glands produce unique hormones used by the body for normal growth. Metabolic syndrome often causes an imbalance with some of the hormones, to the point of exceeding the physiologically ideal level. At other times, the production of hormones may go well below the required level, causing an imbalance.

As far as physiology is concerned, an imbalance occurs due to factors such as stress and depression, among others. Human physiology therefore helps metabolic syndrome experts understand how to address hormonal imbalances in the body. For instance, the science may offer information on how to deal with stress and depression in a bid to better balance the hormones.[41]

DIGESTIVE SYSTEM

Physiology also provides unique insights into the digestive system, another system intimately involved in the study of metabolic syndrome. For the physiology of digestion, metabolic syndrome clients should note that the digestive process really begins first in the mouth, and therefore involves the mouth, teeth, esophagus, stomach, and intestines, in that digestive order. Peripheral organs in the system include the liver, gallbladder, and the salivary glands. The digestive system breaks down food and removes the unused residue from the body. Metabolic syndrome may affect the digestive systems, causing patients to encounter vomiting, diarrhea, loss of appetite, and so forth. The problems may not come all at once, either; hence, the need for understanding human physiology. When addressing digestion, human physiology offers knowledge for treating otherwise complex disorders in the digestive system, such as Crohn's disease or celiac disease (common to metabolic syndrome patients).[42]

RESPIRATORY SYSTEM

Respiratory physiology includes the nose, trachea (windpipe), lungs, and the pharynx (throat). A disorder in these organs can cause respiratory problems such as labored breathing, allergies, and increasing a person's chance of developing flu-like symptoms. The physiology of human breathing gives specialists a deeper understanding of how to avoid and manage problems with the respiratory system. In regards to metabolic syndrome, a major issue in one respiratory organ may affect the other related organs as a result, which demonstrates the importance of treating problems related to obesity early, such as chronic obstructive pulmonary disease (COPD) and sleep apnea.[43]

CIRCULATORY SYSTEM

The cardiovascular system, also known as the circulatory system, consists of the heart and all associated blood vessels. The physiological function of the heart is to pump blood from its chambers through the blood vessels, which circulate the oxygenated blood to all parts of the body. In addition to oxygen, blood carries nutrients, immune cells, and hormones to the areas where they are needed. In cases where metabolic syndrome affects the heart, many complications can develop. For instance, a problem with one of the major blood vessels, such as a serious blockage, may disrupt the entire process, preventing sufficient blood supply from reaching all the necessary organs. A problem with the arteries, such as clogging, burdens the heart and makes it vulnerable to diseases that can take advantage of its weakened state. Remember that even a single heart attack can cause death, almost instantaneously. Human physiology helps people to discover means of avoiding heart-related issues.[44]

INTEGUMENTARY SYSTEM

Physiology can also offer wisdom on how to deal with problems affecting the integumentary tissues. These tissues comprise all body coverings, such as the skin, hair, and nails. The system also consists of certain glands, such as sweat glands and **sebaceous glands**. A disorder in the integumentary system can affect you in more ways than one. For example, a patient may start experiencing hair loss, dryness of the skin, excessive sweating, and so forth. Such problems may appear normal at first, but if left unattended these issues may progress to severe levels resulting in a lot of suffering. Human physiology guides people to know how best to deal with the conditions that result from issues in the integumentary tissues.[45]

URINARY SYSTEM

Urinary organs, which include the kidneys, urethra, and bladder, can also be affected by problems related to metabolic syndrome. These organs serve to extract water from the blood, eventually converting it into urine. Urine transports many waste products, including unusable water itself, allowing the body to flush toxins from its system. All toxins can poison the body at some point if the urinary organs fail to flush them out.[46] A disorder in the urinary system may affect an organ such as the kidney, making it incapable of removing waste. Urinary difficulties known to be related to metabolic syndrome include bladder leakage, increased urinary frequency, intermittent emptying of the bladder, and increased frequency of urination at night. Human physiology offers methods of maintaining a thriving urinary system.

MUSCULOSKELETAL SYSTEM

Physiologically, the musculoskeletal system—bones and joint tissue—enhances one's mobility. Metabolic syndrome may affect either the bone structure or the muscles themselves. Therefore, understanding physiology offers guidelines on how to protect one's joints and sustain muscle mass.[47]

In summation, any approach to metabolic syndrome cannot be fully effective without a proper understanding of physiology. It outlines in detail the roles of the parts of the body and the possible health risks, and suggests ways of preventing the syndrome from occurring. Understanding physiology helps a person to avoid engaging in activities that negatively affect the body and heighten the chances of acquiring illness. People should therefore study human physiology for insight on prevention, control, and management of metabolic syndrome.[48]

5

Importance of Sugar Health

THESE ARE unhealthy times. Men and women wake up in the morning, grab a coffee, rush to work, snack on processed, fatty foods, munch again on sugar-rich doughnuts in the afternoon, and then rush back home with takeout. It isn't their fault; it's just how modern life works. With long commutes and heavy workloads, no one really has the time to shop for fresh ingredients, cook healthy food, and eat right. Is it any wonder that millions of people in the industrialized world suffer from one or more chronic conditions?

THE PANDEMIC OF THE FUTURE

These long-standing conditions include heart disease, high blood pressure, and, of course, diabetes. At last count, at least 340 million people worldwide suffer from sugar imbalance, and many millions have died from the side effects of clinically high blood pressure.[49] In fact, diabetes—one of the characteristics of metabolic syndrome—is one of the most prevalent disorders in the world. Diabetes is the seventh leading source of death in the U.S. alone. (Although these statistics are alarming, they're nothing compared to the statistics emerging about the little-known condition called metabolic syndrome.[50])

INFLUENCE OF SUGAR ON HEALTH

In the early 1980s, the use of high-fructose syrup (HFS) by the majority of companies was in full swing. Until that time, most processed food items contained sugar. However, companies started promoting high-fructose syrup as a healthy alternative to sugar, and people were swayed into accepting the substitute as the healthier choice. Putting all the marketing spins aside, both sugar and high-fructose syrup are much the same, at least in terms of their molecular structure.[51]

FRUCTOSE

Sugar (or sucrose) consists of a single glucose molecule fixed to a carbohydrate molecule of fructose. HFS, on the other hand, is almost twice as sweet as sugar due to its 55 percent fructose content and 45 percent glucose content.[52] Fructose is a form of natural sugar. It doesn't stimulate the exuding of insulin and it has a low **glycemic index**. Fructose is readily available in most foods such as baked pastries, corn starch, and many others. It is a source of calories, and its intake stimulates the increase of body fat construction by the liver. Fructose also does not debase the **ghrelin** hormone levels responsible for reduction of appetite. This in turn results in an increased yearning for and consumption of calories. It also means that one must consciously limit their intake of fructose to avoid over-consumption.[53]

Both of the above (sugar and HFS) break down inside the body the same way, and the physiological effects of these molecules constitute the primary reason why people experience obesity and other chronic health conditions. Glucose is immediately used by the body to yield energy, but fructose is different. Only the liver can metabolize fructose, as it holds the valuable transporter enzyme needed to get the job done. Most active individuals can consume a lot of sugar, which is customarily metabolized by the liver into a stored form called glycogen.[54]

ALL ABOUT GLYCOGEN

Glycogen is a storage molecule your body uses for sugar, which is kept in different parts of the liver. For most modern individuals, their livers are already drenched in it. Eating more sugar forces the liver to convert the excess into fat stored all over the body. In individuals with metabolic syndrome, your liver also becomes resistant to insulin due to the extra fructose, and refuses to understand the chemical messages delivered by insulin. Traditionally, it has been the task of insulin to convert or carry sugar to body cells where the latter molecule is scorched for energy. Fatty tissue, as it happens, is resistant to insulin; therefore, the **pancreas** has to produce more insulin to keep up with the steadily climbing amounts of glucose and fructose being produced in your body. The net result is that you gain weight and slowly progress toward active, full-blown diabetes.[55]

This results in a continually worsening scenario in which you eat more, become overweight, develop insulin resistance, and eventually bottom out into a sugar disorder. Of course, neither concentrated sugars nor HFS contain any of the vitamins, minerals or fibers that could heal or otherwise ameliorate metabolic syndrome, but they *do* displace essential elements in the diet. As people consciously consume more sugar in their diet, they further the progress of their own obesity and impaired metabolism.[56]

KEEPING YOUR SUGAR LEVELS IN HEALTHY RANGE

Although sugar maintenance in today's modern environment may seem like an insurmountable task, it's actually quite easy to do. It is possible to control one's sugar consumption, thereby alleviating metabolic syndrome as a result. The best way to regulate metabolic syndrome is by implementing a few guidelines, such as the following:[57]

- Control the intake of processed food as much as possible. For example, most people keep their fridges stocked with processed meat and snacks. To prevent obesity, researchers recommend switching over to as much fresh food as possible.[58]

- Restrict the consumption of processed carbohydrates. However, those with metabolic syndrome must keep in mind that good carbs and fiber are beneficial for health, as they balance out blood sugar levels considerably.[59]

- Moderation of meals and portion control is also advocated. Nutritionists recommend eating smaller meals three to six times a day on smaller plates to ensure that not as much food is consumed. To restrict obesity development in kids, it's also a good idea to wait 20–25 minutes before rationing second portions so that the nervous system can assess food intake and overall fullness.[60]

- You can increase the amount of fruit eaten in a single day. Fruit does contain fructose, but it's the healthy variation, which is beneficial and not as dangerous as processed corn syrup. Fresh fruit juice is also preferable to processed fruit juice.[61]

- Sugar itself should be limited in one's diet. It is recommended to use sugar substitutes such as aspartame, **acesulfame potassium**, **saccharin**, **sucralose**, and **neotame**. However, metabolic syndrome sufferers should make sure that these substitutes aren't being combined with processed carbohydrates.[62]

- Exercise is a fundamental part of controlling metabolic syndrome. Exercise burns up fat tissue, helps you to eat healthily (including proper sugar intake), and ensures that the body's organs remain healthy.[63]

- "Carb-counting" can be put into practice, which helps to ensure that body sugar is properly balanced. This way, you will be getting carbohydrates evenly throughout the day. It will also help if you select the right sort of carbs for each meal or snack.[64]

In the end, one's health really comes down to one's diet, in which sugar plays a crucial role. Obesity and physical inactivity also contribute to sugar imbalance, which, in essence, can lead to metabolic syndrome. Pursuing a more active lifestyle could therefore mark a significant upturn in health, particularly for those battling metabolic syndrome. A healthy diet along with an optimized exercise plan is the best way to ward off blood sugar-related health disorders such as diabetes. In fact, men and women over the age of 30 should actively implement a nutritionally balanced diet and supplement it with a form of exercise mentioned in Chapter 23.

At the end of the day, what is needed is a fundamental understanding of the causes of metabolic syndrome (such as sugar disorders), and an active understanding by all adults to improve their sugar health.[65]

6

Importance of Hormone Health

IT'S A sad truth that on any given day people don't care much about their bodies—until something starts to go wrong. One of the most underrated and underappreciated warning mechanisms in the human body are hormones. These chemical messengers are responsible for regulating a lot of the important processes in the human body, such as appetite, metabolism, sex drive, growth, and so on. There are many different types of hormones present in the human body, both male and female, such as estrogen, progesterone, testosterone, thyroid hormone, melatonin, serotonin, cortisol and adrenaline. An imbalance in hormone production is one of the catalysts that can cause metabolic syndrome to spiral out of tether.

Hormonal imbalance can present in one of two ways: overproduction and underproduction of hormones.[66] Maintaining standard levels of these hormones in the body is very important for the good health and well-being of an individual. Despite this, many metabolic syndrome sufferers may not know how to address their own hormone problems, let alone understand the overall importance of hormone health.[67]

CONNECTION BETWEEN HORMONES AND METABOLIC SYNDROME

As we saw in Chapter 2, one of the primary indicators of metabolic syndrome is insulin resistance. Insulin is a hormone dispensed by the pancreas which is used for digesting the carbohydrates in foods such as pasta, sugar, fruits, cereal, bread, rice, and so on. When the body shows signs of being unable to properly make use of insulin, chances are the individual has developed metabolic syndrome. People with insulin resistance will often fail at losing weight with conventional diets as their bodies don't burn fats and calories the way they should. The bottom line is that you will experience tremendous weight gain as fats clog your cells, which contributes to metabolic syndrome.[68]

Insulin isn't the only hormone connected with metabolic syndrome; in the case of females, the hormones responsible for fertility can become unbalanced, paving the way for polycystic ovary syndrome (PCOS) to set in. These hormones include follicle stimulating hormone (FSH) and estrogen. Polycystic ovarian syndrome is a hormonal anomaly, and it is closely associated with metabolic syndrome. People who face thyroid hormone snags are also likely to develop metabolic syndrome because of their inability to handle excess glucose and the high cholesterol levels in their arteries. Excess glucose and cholesterol will also reduce the rate of your metabolism.[69]

WHY MAINTAIN HORMONE HEALTH?

Since it has been well-established that hormones have a close connection with metabolic syndrome, it's only natural that one should take good care of their hormone levels and maintain good hormone health. Those with metabolic syndrome should therefore make an effort to become educated about the effective ways of maintaining wholesome hormone health. Both men and women can re-establish insulin balance in their bodies by upholding target hormone levels. Ideal target hormone levels vary among individuals, and an endocrinologist can determine whether your levels are appropriate. Medications can be provided by your doctor if hormone levels need to brought back to normal. Since insulin, when acting correctly in the bloodstream, can counteract the ill-effects of metabolic syndrome, the importance of maintaining good hormone health can't be stressed enough.[70]

"Looking good" and becoming more fit is just a matter of getting one's hormones in order. After all, hormones affect one's health in meaningful ways. With today's modern lifestyles, people by and large lead stressful and hectic lives, and so they rarely get time to take care of their hormones. Due to adverse lifestyle factors, individuals inadvertently cultivate metabolic syndrome within themselves. It's important to remember that even the slightest hormone imbalance can have significant effects on the numerous complex chemical processes of metabolism.[71]

RECOMMENDATIONS

Studies have shown that restoring hormone balance in the body, especially fat-storage hormones such as estrogen (which also serves as a sex hormone), is key in terms of losing unnecessary weight and ensuring that those extra pounds never return.[72]

While working to achieve good hormone health, some people may be required to take medications on a regular basis. However, this is only half the battle; while medication can help to overhaul an unbalanced **endocrine system**, the individuals must also take charge of their health and incorporate healthy lifestyle changes in order to maintain any positive changes to their hormone levels. Having a healthy hormonal balance is easy; you just need to take the right steps and above all, be consistent. The results are worth it; maintaining balanced levels of hormones such as thyroid, cortisol, progesterone and testosterone helps to keep the levels of insulin and glucose in check—which in turn works to prevent diabetes (one of the major constituents of metabolic syndrome).[73]

One of the best ways of restoring hormone health is to work with your doctor to determine the severity of the hormone imbalance and to undergo treatments such as **bio-identical hormone replacement** for restoring hormone health and balance. Yet these solutions are required in critical cases only; in the event of mild cases of metabolic syndrome, simply adopting a few significant lifestyle changes should do the trick.[74]

The best path to take for preserving or improving one's hormone health is also among the easiest—sleep. The best medicine for a wide variety of sicknesses, a good night's slumber is often all it takes to restore one's hormone levels. The ill effects of adverse dietary and lifestyle factors can be more-or-less compensated for through sleep; therefore, it's best for individuals with metabolic syndrome to avoid becoming a night owl or remaining sleep-deprived.[75]

Another first-rate tactic of improving one's hormone levels is to stay happy and maintain a healthy diet and lifestyle. As far as hormones and metabolic syndrome are concerned, eating healthy is the nub to successfully battling metabolic syndrome. Bringing in wholesome foods, rich in vitamins and essential nutrients, is a must when tackling metabolic syndrome. It's also smart to steer clear of processed foods or foods high in sodium, sugars and fats, because these can be a considerable contribution to obesity. Also, the practice of eating proteins and carbohydrates together can slow down the body's ability to create hormones such as serotonin; therefore, one should eat grains and proteins separately when possible.[76]

Patients with metabolic syndrome should also work to manage their stress levels, and should include periodic relaxation and rejuvenation activities throughout their day to counteract the build-up of stress. This is doubly important now, taking into account the pace of the modern lifestyle; frustrations, demands, deadlines and hassles can pile up on top of you before you know it. Therefore, it's recommended that you practice simple yet effective methods of shelving tension to ensure that being stressed doesn't become your normal way of life. You can deter stress by avoiding drugs, cigarettes, and alcohol. Meditation has also been proven to help. Baby steps like these make a huge difference when it comes to combatting the negative hormonal aspects of metabolic syndrome.[77]

7

Importance of a Healthy Circulatory System

IT'S VITAL that sufferers of metabolic syndrome maintain the overall health of their circulatory system. Doing so will help to keep your system safe from metabolic dysfunction. Metabolic syndrome affects most of the tissue involved in receiving and processing blood, and therefore can interfere with the normal work of body systems such as circulation. In this chapter, we'll explore the ways in which control of one's circulatory health can help to manage metabolic syndrome.[78]

LINKS TO IMMUNE SYSTEM

When a person is diagnosed with metabolic syndrome, their immune system—in which the circulatory system plays a vital role—is somewhat compromised, leaving them vulnerable to diseases. A healthy metabolism makes sure that the body has an adequate supply of white blood cells when an infection occurs. Therefore, it follows that an imbalance in one's metabolism leads to an imbalance in one's white blood cell count, as well as their overall effectiveness in fighting infection. To address this, one should prioritize consumption of foods containing the vital nutrients required by body tissues, such as proteins, carbohydrates, and vitamins. Apart from a proper diet, a metabolic syndrome patient can revitalize their immune system by doing regular exercises.[79]

You should also recognize that a healthy diet and physical exercises will further improve the circulatory system, which in turn enriches the immune system. Weakened immunity is a recipe for any number of opportunistic illnesses associated with metabolic syndrome to strike. Overall, maintaining a healthy immune system calls for the sort of combined approach mentioned in the previous chapters, such as eating healthy foods and maintaining exercise routines consistently.[80]

HORMONE BALANCE AND THE CIRCULATORY SYSTEM

A healthy circulatory system will also ensure that the body doesn't overproduce or under-produce hormones. Individuals with hormonal imbalances often require outside help when balancing hormone levels, such as resting, workouts, and therapy, among others. Hormonal imbalance can affect anyone, whether young or old, and regardless of gender.[81]

METABOLISM AND THE CIRCULATORY SYSTEM

A stable circulatory system increases the rate of metabolism, thus helping the body to burn fat fast. The foods we consume contain fat, which the body burns at a certain rate daily. However, sometimes the body will fail to burn all the fat—especially if a person consumes too much of it. A patient may also fail to exercise sufficiently, leading to an increase of fat. However, with an increase in metabolism, you can burn all the fat your body cannot utilize.[82]

Accumulation of body fat can result in a variety of disorders, such as weight gain, diabetes, heart disease, and so forth—all which are connected to circulatory system health. To increase the rate of metabolism, you can use homemade remedies such as eating foods that increase metabolic rate, like the following:

- green tea
- chilies
- spinach
- oatmeal
- avocado

- almonds
- cheese
- milk
- asparagus
- whey protein
- tofu

Herbal products have also been shown to enhance the rate of metabolism. You can also engage in physical activities.[83]

IMPROVEMENT OF CARDIOVASCULAR HEALTH

Furthermore, a healthy circulatory system results in and supports a healthy heart, which in turn influences all the systems, organs, and tissues in your body. Excess body fat can hinder the heart's ability to function, as fat may spread to the area close to the heart. Additionally, some fat may get into the arteries and veins carrying blood from the heart. The heart is then forced to do extra work, as it tries to forcefully pump blood through the molecular barriers the fat creates.[84]

This strain gradually exhausts the heart, and you will start to experience circulatory shock and heart attacks. As a major heart attack can cause instant death, patients should take steps to ensure good circulatory health *before* a problem takes shape. Disorders such as obesity don't occur in a day; they take time to develop. People should begin adopting healthy lifestyles as early as childhood to prevent these issues from ever gaining a foothold. Moreover, consumption of products such as tobacco, high amounts of alcohol, and fatty foods can all have a negative impact on one's heart. Failure to exercise regularly also hinders the functions of the circulatory system.[85]

IN RELATION TO CHRONIC ILLNESS

A healthy circulatory system also affects the body's ability to manage most long-term illnesses, such as diabetes. Illnesses will progress to chronic stages if the body's ability to fight them is diminished. Once the body has reached this level of exhaustion, even minor illnesses can begin damaging body tissues, cells, and organs, all of which are normally responsible for helping a patient in recovering from metabolic syndrome. If the immune system shuts down due to prolonged untreated illness, the "minor" illnesses will progress from minor to severe, and can become chronic diseases. For instance, a small problem such as an increased level of sugar can transform into diabetes, a condition that has no cure. [86]

In short, if people can prevent or address illnesses when they first occur, they can lower their odds of developing chronic illness. To that end, metabolic syndrome patients should begin by living a healthy lifestyle, and the moment a disorder presents, they should seek immediate medical attention. Lifestyle changes known to strengthen the immune system include quitting smoking and drinking, maintaining a healthy diet, and getting enough sleep. Additionally, going for regular medical examinations can also help in identifying problems in the circulatory system before it becomes a serious condition.[87]

IMPROVED RECOVERY FROM METABOLIC SYNDROME

In today's world, the consistent use of medication to treat preventable chronic conditions is common, and sometimes even expected. Yet, there are many who take barely any medication, and who do not require serious medical attention in their lives—all because they maintain a healthy circulatory system on their own. Such people prove how a healthy circulatory system keeps illnesses away as well as helps the body recover from illnesses naturally. The body *can* heal itself naturally—if all the organs function as required.[88]

MAINTAINING THE RIGHT BALANCE

Keeping the circulatory system in good health allows you to maintain an energy balance. This means that all the parts of the body are working to use the available energy properly and toward normal growth. Likewise, if energy usage is unbalanced or improperly directed, the healthy organs are forced to work twice as hard to compensate, and will become exhausted twice as quickly. For instance, when the body produces levels of insulin too high for it to make use of, the insulin will instead attack other parts of the body, such as the walls and the inner lining of the stomach. This in turn slows the functionality of the affected regions, eventually resulting in metabolic syndrome and energy imbalance. By contrast, a good energy balance and a high energy output leave the person with metabolic syndrome in good temperament and high spirits. Productivity goes up as well.[89]

Overall, there are many compelling reasons why a metabolic syndrome patient should work to maintain a healthy circulatory system. Eating a healthy diet and maintaining regular meal times for consistent energy usage is the best way to keep your circulatory health balanced and strong. Some people skip meals in the hopes of losing weight, but neglecting meals only compels the body to underutilize the fat it receives; in essence, skipping meals "tricks" your body into conserving calories for the perceived long haul ahead. Apart from eating well, you should also formulate a workout plan that toughens all facets of the body, including the circulatory system.[90]

RECOMMENDATIONS

Finally, simple exercise, such as jogging, running on the treadmill, biking, dancing, and so forth, can serve as basic remedies for metabolic syndrome. People with sedentary occupations, such as desk jobs, should schedule workouts, to take place three or four days a week. Going for regular medical checkups and staying informed about one's circulatory health will also pave the way to better health.[91]

PART II

Clinical Picture

8

Pathology of Metabolic Syndrome

THESE DAYS, many people struggle with metabolic syndrome—a situation wherein the patient suffers from a series of problems, including high blood pressure, high serum triglycerides, and increased abdominal fat, all of which can be detrimental. It's important to identify and understand the **pathology** of a syndrome, as there are certain warning signs that help to determine whether someone is at risk. While pathology normally involves the stringent study of diagnosis, the word will also be used to mean signs and symptoms of metabolic syndrome (for the purpose of this chapter).[92]

UNUSUAL HUNGER AND THIRST

It's normal for a person to become thirsty and hungry over time. However, when someone experiences inordinate dehydration and appetite, there could be an underlying symptom at fault. This is especially true when you suffer thirst or have a hankering for food without having exerted yourself. While it is natural to experience hunger and thirst after physical labor where the body has been exerted, experiencing thirst or hunger too often could be a sign of metabolic syndrome.[93]

OBESITY

Among the major signs often present in the conglomerate of

symptoms known as metabolic syndrome, obesity is often the first. If a person develops unusual weight gain, it can trigger an unhealthy body mass. Moreover, obesity is often the cause of a number of issues associated with high blood pressure and heart disease. Obesity (or fat cells specifically) works against the body's metabolism and opens the door to multiple health issues. Therefore, obese individuals are more likely to fall victim to the syndrome. Therefore, overweight individuals need to consult their doctor to find out whether they qualify as obese. Once someone undergoes unhealthy weight gain, especially along the abdominal area, he's more likely to have the syndrome.[94]

BLOOD PRESSURE

Inconsistent blood pressure is another symptom of the syndrome. Preserving a normal blood pressure is imperative for any person to live a healthy life. In fact, blood pressure numbers play a vital role in defining the overall health of an individual. Although individuals with normal blood pressure are not completely immune, they are often able to cope more easily with self-limiting diseases, as compared to those who have aberrant blood pressure. Although minor fluctuations in pressure aren't an issue, persistent imbalances can result in poor circulation and sluggish metabolism, each of which can be harmful to the sufferer in the long run.[95]

INSULIN RESISTANCE

Insulin resistance is yet another often-overlooked symptom of metabolic syndrome. In individuals with insulin resistance, cells don't react normally to insulin, and glucose can't enter into cells as easily. As a result, glucose levels in the bloodstream increase, regardless of the body's attempts to regulate the glucose by producing more insulin. When someone isn't able to generate adequate insulin to uphold the blood sugar levels within superlative range, it can ultimately result in diabetes.[96]

SLEEP APNEA

Sleep apnea is also considered to be a key indicator of metabolic syndrome. For those who are not familiar with the term, sleep apnea is a sleep disorder in which there are one or more pauses in breathing, or consistently shallow breaths while sleeping. The pauses can last anywhere from a few seconds to a few minutes. This type of disorder can drastically disrupt someone's sleep, resulting in substandard sleep quality. As a result, patients will commonly experience lethargy during the day. Sleep apnea has three main types, namely obstructive sleep apnea, central sleep apnea, and complex sleep apnea.[97]

Anyone can suffer from this kind of disorder, but it affects many metabolic syndrome patients who are overweight, and usually affects men. Apnea has several associated symptoms, but the common ones occur during sleep, including pauses while snoring, minor choking, and gasping. Sleep apnea is sometimes mistaken for snoring, and as a result is sometimes left undiagnosed. This can result in stroke, **hypertension**, or even heart failure. Though there are many who snore, sleep apnea can be recognized due to its aftereffects during the day.[98]

EYESIGHT TROUBLES

Most individuals experience weakening vision as they age; it is common to develop eyesight problems as the years go on, especially after reaching the age of 40. However, some persons who have metabolic syndrome experience blurred vision when they're much younger. Minor eyesight troubles are not necessarily a big issue, but blurry vision at an early age could be an indicator that the person may be afflicted with metabolic syndrome.[99]

DARKENING OF THE SKIN

Most parts of the human body have consistent skin color under normal circumstances, but in some cases the sufferer of this particular syndrome will have darkened skin, medically known as **hyperpigmentation**. Common areas of the body include areas under the arms. If the armpit areas of a person are increasingly dark, it's a likely sign of metabolic syndrome.[100]

FREQUENT URINATION

Everyone experiences the call of nature, and there's nothing unusual about it. However, frequent urination is rarely a good sign. Constant urination causes dehydration. When that happens, the metabolism slows, resulting in obesity.[101]

EFFECTS ON THE IMMUNE SYSTEM

The human body is capable of fighting diseases to a great extent. This is particularly true in the case of infections or sores that result due to some kind of injury. In some cases, a person needn't seek any treatment to recover from illness. However, in many cases minor treatments can play a key role in treating infections. When a person who has minor sores or infections isn't able to properly recover, the individual may be suffering from metabolic syndrome.[102]

OTHER SYMPTOMS

Dizziness, vertigo, and fainting are common experiences when it comes to metabolic syndrome; often, patients feel dizzy on account of something as simple as inclement weather conditions. Similarly, some persons feel faint after doing strenuous work. However, some individuals will faint after only a smidgen of work; a few folks even fall unconscious without any obvious reason. Any such weakness could be a noteworthy sign of the syndrome.[103]

Every so often, people fail to realize that they're dealing with metabolic syndrome until they observe severe symptoms of the condition. The simple reason is that most do not actually know the pathology of metabolic syndrome. Although the condition can be treated with advanced medications and surgery, an evaluation of the symptoms completed as early as possible is in your best interests. That's why it is advisable to keep an eye on one's general health before the disorder becomes serious.[104]

9

Causes and Risk Factors of Metabolic Syndrome

IT IS clear that the modern-day lifestyle and diet are contributing factors to metabolic syndrome. However, other factors, when taken together, can accelerate the pathological progress of the syndrome. Some of these factors include excess sugar, saturated fats, too many calories, unsatisfactory exercise, stress, and lack of sleep. In some instances, the medicine used for treating the condition can have negative effects, which may even lead to aggravating your metabolic syndrome.[105]

GENETICS

Genetics can also be a risk factor for metabolic syndrome. Plenty of people have a genetic component that makes them more prone to metabolic syndrome, despite the fact that metabolic syndrome is largely due to shortcomings in insulin regulation. Insulin resistance can be due to certain genes that are passed down through generations; thusly, relatives can have similar insulin control. Genetic mutations, however, can cause inconsistencies in insulin response. In cases like those of identical twins, the responses to insulin are almost identical.[106]

OBESITY

Obesity can be considered both a symptom and a potential cause of metabolic syndrome. This condition is normally indicated by a large waistline or a high BMI. By definition, obesity is the condition of having too much fat, not necessarily just being overweight. Excess fat around the stomach can cause metabolic syndrome. The condition is also known as visceral obesity, and it can lead to abnormalities such as **dyslipidemia**, glucose intolerance, and insulin resistance—all of which are often signs of metabolic syndrome. **Hyperinsulinemia**, another condition related to obesity and metabolic syndrome, is caused by an excess production of insulin due to insulin resistance.

Obesity results in many health issues. Among them is damage to the immune system. When the immune system fails, all the illnesses that the immune system formerly kept away will attack the body. Obesity is a source of both physical and emotional pain; living on medication for life really takes a toll on people, which is why doctors recommend that metabolic syndrome clients avoid obesity at all costs.[107]

EXCESS WEIGHT

Another major risk factor is excess weight (remember, obesity is excess *fat*, not excess weight). When a person gains excess weight, the expansion of the waist circumference can spread **adiposity**, and that in turn spearheads metabolic syndrome. The unhealthy lifestyle of an individual also increases the chances of acquiring the syndrome.[108]

CARBS

A substantial portion of the risk factors of developing metabolic syndrome arises from lifestyle and diet. Taking in smaller amounts of carbohydrates will help to reduce the chances of developing the condition. The logic behind this is that when you ingest more carbohydrates, extra calories are taken in, and thus, excess insulin is required to break down the glucose. For people who are insulin resistant, even more insulin must be produced to compensate for the resistance, and the result is hyperinsulinemia. The excess insulin will in turn stimulate liver cells to generate the triglycerides responsible for insulin resistance. This shows that high amounts of triglyceride will also increase the chances of having metabolic syndrome. In order to avoid this, people should consider consuming fewer carbohydrates, and avoid foods high in fat.[109]

GLYCEMIC INDEX

After finishing a meal, depending on the different nutrients consumed, glucose levels will vary. These levels are indicated by the glycemic index, which ranks foods by their ability to raise glucose levels. Simply put, the glycemic index is a numerical table for foods rich in carbohydrates. The index is based on the effect of food on the glucose levels following meals. Glycemic load is the ranking of that specific food based on the glycemic index and other factors. People with metabolic syndrome are encouraged to eat foods that have a low glycemic index, and should be using this index when preparing their meals and portion sizes. The overall diet should have a high glucose load, which is also suggestive of a low glycemic index. Calculating the glucose load involves multiplication of the carbohydrate weight in grams with the glycemic index, then dividing the number by 100.[110]

The higher the position of the food in the glycemic index, the higher the rate of digestion. A high rate of digestion will rapidly increase glucose levels, while foods with low glycemic index are digested and absorbed slowly, and thus, the rate of glucose increase is reduced. There's a direct relationship between a high glycemic index and insulin resistance, in that the higher the glycemic index of foods consumed, the higher the insulin resistance will be. High insulin levels can spark low levels of glucose, which will increase hunger, stress, and carbohydrate craving. In this way the glycemic index of food can indirectly cause metabolic syndrome. Metabolic syndrome sufferers should maintain a low-glycemic index diet in regards to sugar-related risk factors such as low blood sugar levels. It is a good idea to load up on proteins early in the morning in the form of egg whites, and to cut down on sugary sweets throughout the day.[111]

STRESS

Stress can also be considered as a risk factor associated with metabolic syndrome. Research studies carried out in recent years have indicated that a person living with chronic stress for a long time can develop metabolic syndrome, due to the physical effects stress can have on the body. Stress contributes by meddling with the balance of hormones in the body, which in turn causes levels of glucose and insulin to rise. When that happens, a person can begin to suffer from **visceral adiposity** (fat in the internal organs), resistance to insulin, **hypertension**, and unusual fat accrual in the blood. Ways to relieve stress include yoga, meditation, and anti-anxiety medications (made available by your physician).[112]

FIBER

Lack of fiber is another risk factor for metabolic syndrome. Fiber is commonly known to aid in bowel movement, but it also influences the absorption of other **micronutrients**. For example, fiber slows down absorption of carbohydrates and thus adjusts the glycemic index of the food consumed. High fiber content will also help in reducing insulin resistance, which is another risk factor of metabolic syndrome. Fiber also regulates the rate at which the person who has metabolic syndrome feels hungry, since it sharply reduces the rate of stomach emptying. Thus, you will ingest less food. It's important to pick out items with high fiber content to undercut the risk of developing the syndrome.[113]

TRANS-FATS

Foods high in trans-fats, such as cookies, doughnuts, muffins, crackers, and pies, decrease insulin sensitivity, even in small amounts. They also lead to a rise in glucose levels. In addition, they confuse the **lipid profile** by increasing **low-density lipoproteins** *(LDL)* and **high-density lipoprotein** *(HDL)* levels. Trans-fats have a variety of effects that exacerbate the symptoms of metabolic syndrome. They have been known to increase the chances of developing cardiovascular disease and **coronary artery disease**. The advantage is that they leave the body soon after the supply is cut off.[114]

SALT INTAKE

Excessive salt is notorious for increasing a patient's blood pressure, another factor in metabolic syndrome. The relationship between salt consumption and metabolic syndrome is complex, in that increased salt intake eventually leads to increased salt sensitivity. It's important to note that this increased sensitivity is brought about by common reactions to metabolic syndrome. Bottom line: Avoid excessive salt intake.[115]

LACK OF MICRONUTRIENTS

A dearth of **micronutrients**, such as minerals and vitamins, can also cause metabolic syndrome. An inadequate intake of minerals (such as calcium) may lead to an unwanted decrease in insulin sensitivity. Some of the nutrients also work to reduce cholesterol levels and control hypertension. Other minerals, such as magnesium and zinc, will also drop the resistance of insulin in the body. Vitamins such as B12 (cobalamin) and B3 (niacin) can reduce insulin sensitivity and reverse the negative effects of metabolic syndrome.[116]

SMOKING AND DRINKING

Smoking and overconsumption of alcohol can be responsible for insulin resistance, an increase in low-density proteins, and a lessening of high-density proteins. All of these changes are associated with metabolic syndrome and other diseases.[117]

SEDENTARY LIFESTYLE

As far as sedentary lifestyle is concerned with regards to metabolic syndrome, patients should note that these days, a growing number of people are substituting time spent online for time spent in social situations. Shopping, trading stock, meeting with friends; just about everything is now possible through the Internet. However, all this convenience has made people lazy, and sedentary lifestyles are on the rise. Unfortunately, inactivity can have any number of ill effects, such as metabolic syndrome. If you have metabolic syndrome, you can overcome sedentary practices by performing exercises and keeping yourself busy with hobbies.[118]

To conclude, it is important to know that high blood pressure, elevated blood sugar levels, and insulin resistance are the key risk factors associated with metabolic syndrome. Other contributing factors include obesity with increasing fat around the abdominal and thigh areas, together with elevated blood sugar levels, increased HDL levels, low LDL levels, inflammation, and a proclivity toward blood clotting. Although medical research is constantly being advanced, as of yet there is no definitive treatment for the disorder. However, it is generally agreed that metabolic syndrome is caused by scores of risk factors, some of which have yet to be discovered.[119]

10

Diagnosing Metabolic Syndrome

DUE TO the complex nature of the relationships between the various coexisting disorders that the syndrome represents, the process of diagnosing metabolic syndrome can be a herculean task. The whole condition can go overlooked due to the lack of noticeable, distinguishing symptoms. High cholesterol, for example, can easily go unnoticed without lab tests, as there are only a handful of obvious markers for this health issue. Many patients with metabolic syndrome will notice symptoms associated with obesity or diabetes first, without attributing these to the syndrome itself. In this way, certain signs of metabolic syndrome may be incorrectly attributed to be symptoms of obesity.[120]

DIAGNOSTIC ROADBLOCKS

Most of the diagnosable aspects of metabolic syndrome correspond to being at a heightened risk for heart disease, stroke, and diabetes, a risk that is increased exponentially when the symptoms are combined. The more metabolic risk factors an individual has, the more likely metabolic syndrome becomes, and the greater the risk of cardiovascular issues and other complications. Despite the difficulty of diagnosis, however, determining whether a person is suffering from metabolic syndrome is vital to reducing the effects the syndrome will have on one's health. The sooner the syndrome is diagnosed, the sooner treatment of the negative factors can commence. Therefore, it's important to confer with a doctor about scanning for metabolic syndrome when a person has one or more of the following risk factors, some of which are also considered symptoms:[121]

- Abdominal obesity
- Sedentary lifestyle
- Diabetes, or family history of the disease
- Insulin resistance

Risk of metabolic syndrome increases with age and is more common in Hispanic, Asian, and Aboriginal people. Persons of these origins should take special note of the risk factors and indicators of metabolic syndrome.[122]

DIAGNOSTIC CHECKLIST (AT A GLANCE)

From a diagnostic standpoint, metabolic syndrome is a disorder that can be defined by the conjunction of energy problems related to an increased risk for diabetes and heart disease. As metabolic syndrome involves a grouping of conditions, which can vary by individual, it can be a mare's nest to isolate. The presence of one correlated condition, after all, doesn't necessarily indicate metabolic syndrome. To simplify the process of diagnosis, a basic checklist of ailments related to metabolic syndrome has been developed (see Chapter 21). Diagnostic signifiers of metabolic syndrome include the following.[123]

LARGE WAIST CIRCUMFERENCE

Obesity is both an underlying cause and a symptom of metabolic syndrome. This most obvious diagnostic feature of the disorder is noted as a heaviness in the waist area (as opposed to the hip area, where typical non-obese patients would be widest). This factor of metabolic syndrome is a major cause of every other condition mentioned in the diagnostic worksheet. An individual is considered to have central obesity if their body mass index is greater than 30, or if the waist has a circumference greater than 34.6 inches/88 cm for females or 40 inches/102 cm for males. Diagnostic testing requires simple measurement around the waist, or calculation of body mass index using weight and height. Often, this aspect of metabolic syndrome is easily visible and can be caught early, as the obese patient normally presents with an "apple-shaped" figure.[124]

HIGH LEVELS OF TRIGLYCERIDES

While the body naturally creates triglycerides (fats in the blood), the levels may be increased when the amount of calories consumed is greater than nutritional requirements. Excess calories are stored as fat in the blood for later use. High triglyceride levels are usually harmless, but can upswing the risk for heart difficulties. Triglycerides at 150 milligrams per deciliter of blood may be indicative of metabolic syndrome. In order to determine triglyceride levels, pathologists will take a blood sample for use in clinical assessments.[125]

High-density lipoproteins (HDL), or "good" cholesterol, essentially carry "bad" or low-density cholesterol (LDL) back to the liver, where it's broken down for use in the body. Low levels of good cholesterol means high levels of bad cholesterol, which trigger buildup in blood vessels and reduce overall circulation. This all causes an increased risk of heart attack and stroke. For this diagnostic condition to be met, the HDL level would be below 50 mg/dL for men or 40 mg/dL for women. Similar to triglyceride levels, a blood test is required to determine both good and bad cholesterol levels. You may be asked to fast before the test, and in some cases temporarily discontinue taking prescription drugs that can increase cholesterol levels, such as birth control pills or **diuretics**.[126]

HYPERTENSION

Hypertension is a major risk factor for heart attack, stroke, and aneurism. It often accompanies both obesity and metabolic syndrome. To fulfill the requirements of a diagnosis of hypertension, your blood pressure would be equal to or higher than 130/85. The doctor will use a blood pressure cuff to assess your pressure level. This test is commonly performed during routine examinations by your primary care doctor.[127]

ELEVATED BLOOD SUGAR LEVELS

Elevated blood sugar levels are commonly associated with obesity and metabolic syndrome. A fasting blood glucose level of over 100 mg/dL is required to meet this criterion. Moreover, a previous diagnosis of type-2 (adult onset, or non-insulin dependent) diabetes is equal to this condition in terms of severity. As for diagnostic tests, a blood sample must be taken to determine fasting blood glucose levels. You'll need to refrain from eating anything for a few hours before the assessment takes place.[128]

The standards for diagnosis based on these factors vary slightly by organization. For instance, the European Group for the Study of Insulin Resistance (EGIR) requires insulin resistance within the top 25 percent, as well as two of the other conditions. Alternatively, the International Diabetes Foundation (IDF) requires central obesity and two of the other conditions. These standards often appear to reflect the specific interests of the organization. However, the general consensus of the scientific community is that in order to be confirmed as having metabolic syndrome, a patient must present with three out of the five aforesaid diagnostic benchmarks.[129]

It is likely that many individuals don't realize or consider the cumulative effects of individual diet and lifestyle decisions. It seems that a great deal of people don't (or won't) come face to face with these effects until the metabolic syndrome has already developed. However, diagnosis of metabolic syndrome can put individuals on the right track to improving their life. Mitigation of metabolic syndrome symptoms after correct diagnosis includes a more active lifestyle and a well-rounded diet with fewer fats and carbohydrates. This is essential for lessening the post-diagnosis effects of the syndrome and for conserving heart health.[130]

11

Role of Family Practice Physicians in Metabolic Syndrome

AFTER RECEIVING your diagnosis, you'll find yourself meeting frequently with your family practice physician or general practitioner. In addition to playing an important role in the fight against metabolic syndrome, these doctors also cater their services to patients suffering from a variety of illnesses, both from their homes or in a clinical setting. More to the point, this means that these physicians assist in the management and diagnosis of common conditions known to be associated with metabolic syndrome. The following chapter explains the role that family practice physicians play in regard to the syndrome and your treatment.[131]

PUTTING INTENSIVE TRAINING TO USE

Family physicians undergo intense training in obstetrics and pediatrics, which enables them to handle cases like pregnant patients suffering from metabolic syndrome. These experts work hand in hand with other clinical professionals to help patients deal with pregnancy and any likely issues associated with the pregnancy, up to the point of delivery.[132] The physicians help their pregnant clients to deliver their babies, while also providing the newborns with the necessary care.

Apart from the above roles, some family physicians are also involved with other services linked to their field of specialization. Some doctors will pursue coaching, while others teach students at various educational institutions. Other family physicians engage in research, working to discover more about the syndrome to improve treatments. Most of the corrective options used today came from meticulous research studies conducted by professionals. Still others work as occupational health officers, advising people on healthy habits, while some assume administrative roles heading various medical centers. Basically, family practice physicians may take any number of directions in the field of medicine, but they seek to solve the problem of metabolic syndrome when needed.[133]

A TYPICAL DAY FOR A FAMILY PRACTICE PHYSICIAN

Over the course of a single afternoon, a family practice doctor can attend to more than 20 metabolic syndrome sufferers. In addition to the breadth of information required in order to be certified as a family doctor, this quick pace ensures a similarly paced growth in experience in patient care. When interacting with their patients, the family physician refers to their medical records, examines the patients themselves, and conducts or orders tests as needed. Depending on the test results, the general practitioner can make referrals to a related specialist, start a treatment course, or provide medical counseling. When addressing metabolic syndrome, family physicians engage themselves at several stages of treatment. They'll be your first point of contact and work to obtain firsthand information regarding the condition that's challenging you. These visits serve as the foundation of your future treatment, so please don't hesitate to question your doctor about your condition and your treatment options, in order to make more informed decisions down the line.

OFFERING ANALYSIS

During their examination, family doctors will usually analyze you in order to see the extent of the damage caused by metabolic syndrome. At this point, they can offer helpful options and approaches you can take to begin feeling better. A proper diagnosis depends on an open and honest line of communication between you and your physician, so please don't hold anything back when receiving evaluation. Every useful piece of information then goes into the records, for use in long-term care (which metabolic syndrome requires).[134]

OFFERING ADVICE

As far as advice is concerned, family medicine doctors are well trained about metabolic syndrome, and can use that information to provide you with accurate and comprehensive counsel. Their advice will focus on responsible and healthy living in an attempt to manage your syndrome, while also discouraging you from pursuing any incorrect or unproven clinical techniques. Your doctor will also outline the possible clinical procedures that you can choose from, depending on the nature and extent of your symptoms. Your physician may also recommend an assortment of treatments based on your preference. In addition, family physicians can advise you on several rehabilitation packages, such as obesity behavioral medicine programs, doctor-supervised low-calorie diets, and strict blood pressure monitoring schedules, which can help you in dealing with your condition.[135]

MONITORING PROGRESS

Whether you start receiving therapy from home or at a clinic, you will require professional assistance to help keep your treatment on track. Different people respond differently to treatment; some may even fail to respond to approved treatments. Family physicians ensure that patients are administered the correct medication, submit findings to relevant specialists, and otherwise monitor the status of their patients. If you fail to show improvements after a stretch of treatment, your physician can also suggest and oversee a change in medication.[136]

Family doctors also help patients to deal with contributing factors to metabolic syndrome, in an attempt to control symptoms like high blood pressure. Hypertension (otherwise known as high blood pressure) doesn't really emanate from any specific source; other conditions force its occurrence. Patients who suffer from high blood pressure often start by experiencing other illnesses that later double back into hypertension. Some of these conditions include stress, clogged arteries and depression, among others. All of these conditions remain within the context of metabolic syndrome, and fall under the purview of family medical practice.[137]

CONSULTATION

When you first enter a clinic seeking consultation on metabolic syndrome, it will likely be a family physician who offers you consultation services. Patients turn to physicians for various reasons, such as prevention, management, and treatment of the condition. Due to the extensive knowledge that family physicians possess, this puts them in the best position to offer you helpful consultation. Family physicians are trained in ways to best direct patients, and can offer first-rate reviews and opinions. While rushing off to your physician the moment you suspect you have metabolic syndrome may not strictly be necessary, family physicians are in the best possible position to assuage concerns and treat any symptoms you might be experiencing.[138]

UNIQUENESS OF THE SPECIALTY

Family practice is different from other associated medical fields in a number of ways. For example, family practice does not involve many complex surgical procedures. More importantly, family practice involves interacting with their patients at a more personal level, as compared to other medical disciplines. Some fields just require the doctor to conduct tests and issue drugs; in family practice, the physician meets with their patients face to face, discussing their problems and going over potential solutions.[139]

Over the course of treating your metabolic syndrome, you're likely to interact with any number of physicians and specialists, performing examinations and running tests to determine the best methods of treatment. However, throughout the process, your family physician is your best resource in addressing your symptoms, deciding on treatment options, and offering counsel as needed. An extremely valuable resource, their role in the treatment of your metabolic syndrome cannot be overstated.

12

Role of Internists in Metabolic Syndrome

INTERNAL MEDICINE specialists (internists) are doctors who combine their clinical expertise with technical knowhow to diagnose, treat, and care for sick adults and teens. Most professionals study for five years to complete their preliminary medical education. After that, they complete their postgraduate education before specializing in internal medicine. It may take anywhere from three to 10 years for an internist to complete their education, after which they will frequently be called upon by other doctors to offer second opinions (due to their wider range of knowledge). However, over the last three years, more and more internists have begun taking the reins as primary care physicians (although this is partly due to an overall shortage of doctors). As a result, the onus of learning about the myriad symptoms related to metabolic syndrome falls upon them. This is to the overall benefit of those with metabolic syndrome, as a skilled medical professional can better help them oversee their health.[140]

INTERNISTS VS. METABOLIC SYNDROME

Ideally, virtually any physician can provide you with general health care; however, internists are particularly valuable for their insight and experience. This is especially true in cases of metabolic syndrome—because the condition is an insidious one, and it can creep up quite slowly. The symptoms are vague and most doctors fail to consider them as a group, resulting in a sneaky condition that suddenly flares up, becoming lasting diabetes (and other illnesses) over time.[141]

As a result, it is the sheer breadth of knowledge that internists possess that renders them best equipped to deal with your condition. They act as medical detectives, drawing on a greater base of knowledge to make a more accurate, descriptive diagnosis. Should you suspect metabolic syndrome as the cause of your symptoms, it's best to make sure you consult with a qualified internist right away. Before visiting the doctor, make sure to prepare a detailed medical history, including lab reports (such as complete blood count and sugar levels) all of which are useful in helping your physician to make an informed decision. The internist will then consider any tests that ought to be done, and will look for the biological markers that indicate metabolic syndrome, such as elevated concentrations of cholesterol.[142]

SCREENINGS AND TESTS USED BY INTERNISTS

As for things to expect at initial visits to an internist's office, you should know that internists follow screening guidelines to help find patients already suffering from metabolic syndrome. The most common screening guidelines and tests at first visits are as follows:[143]

- Ascertain risk factors: Men and women with a family history of diabetes and high blood pressure are more likely to develop metabolic syndrome. Individuals with associated conditions like fatty liver, polycystic ovaries, sleep apnea, gallstones, HIV, etc., may also develop the condition. There are many more risk factors that predispose a client to metabolic syndrome, and an internist will provide help during the screening appointment. Metabolic syndrome sufferers can mention whether they wish to be evaluated completely.[144]
- Diagnostic tests: A precise medical history is necessary to ascertain the patient's predisposition to metabolic syndrome. Your medical history in particular should record any family history of diabetes, high blood pressure, and cardiac conditions

that may have affected parents and close relatives. A complete medical check-up is also necessary, which should include fasting **lipid profiles**, glucose checks, and a complete **anthropometric** data record of height, weight, BMI, and waist circumference. You might also be checked for conditions such as hypertension, diabetes mellitus, and so forth to get your condition under control.[145]

- Medications typically prescribed by internists: For some patients, lifestyle changes, exercise, and dieting just aren't enough. For these patients, the internist may write prescriptions to control cholesterol such as statins, **fibrates**, or nicotinic acid. The internist might also order **diuretics** to control high blood pressure such as ACE inhibitors, or anti-diabetics used to control blood sugar levels. He'll decide which medications are best suited to control your underlying conditions.[146]

WHAT TO EXPECT FROM YOUR INTERNIST

An internist may have specific instructions to control your weight and sugar levels. He will also issue specific instructions for overpowering metabolic syndrome sooner. The syndrome is easy to control—provided an expert catches the symptoms as early as possible. The condition can show effects during childhood, as well as in teens and adults, resulting in a series of complications such as high blood pressure, increased inflammation, and clotting. These symptoms are often so vague that even internists can tend to take each symptom individually rather than all together as a syndrome. That being said, internists still play a critical role, especially during the illness' primary stages.[147]

13

Role of Endocrinologists in Metabolic Syndrome

ENDOCRINOLOGISTS ARE physicians with the special training and skills necessary to diagnose illnesses and disorders associated with the glands of the human body. These may be illnesses that affect the glands individually, or they may disturb other parts of the body as well. In this chapter, we will be outlining the role of endocrinologists in metabolic syndrome care.[148]

A VISIT TO THE ENDOCRINOLOGIST

An endocrinologist spends his time seeing patients who suffer from disorders of the **endocrine system**. After observing a patient, the endocrinologist will make a diagnosis of any illnesses that may be affecting the glands. He interprets symptoms as they may relate to hormones, and then decides upon the most effective treatment option. His ground plan must first seek to restore hormonal balance in some way or another.

Every now and then, an endocrinologist may need to review your laboratory results, and x-rays, as well as select medical procedures before coming to a conclusion on a case of metabolic syndrome. It is the role of the endocrinologist to effectively convey what would otherwise be a complex explanation of the inner workings of your glands and related hormones. On the whole, endocrinologists maintain a high level of discipline and patient confidentiality, ensuring that your evaluation and treatment proceeds quickly and efficiently in the right direction.[149]

HORMONE HELP

As a metabolic syndrome patient, you may sometimes face conditions that lead to you producing either an excess or a lack of a certain hormone or hormones. To deal with the problem, endocrinologists will assist you in identifying the cause behind the hormone irregularities. By doing so, your body can regain its balance, preventing further complications.[150]

DIABETES HELP

When dealing with diabetes, a common aspect of metabolic syndrome, endocrinologists will help you with accurate and specialized sugar management, a form of care that an internist or a family doctor usually can't offer. Endocrinologists can also guide and advise you on the various ways of living an active and healthy life, while still treating your diabetes. When people start living responsibly by engaging in healthy activities and follow the right diet as advised by an endocrinologist, they can prevent or manage diabetes. Some of the activities that patients should practice include frequent exercise, consuming proper nutrients, and avoiding foods that harm or weaken the body and fan the flames of illness. Diabetes, a chronic disease, requires a combination of preventative and management measures, as there are not many medications that can completely control diabetes.[151]

HELP AGAINST STUNTED GROWTH

Endocrinologists also assist children with the growth and development of both their brains and bodies. Stunted growth (or a complete lack of growth) occurs due to imbalances in the body. Young metabolic syndrome patients require their physiological functions to work normally and in harmony with one another, as failure to do so can lead to improper development. At this point, endocrinologists will investigate the reasons behind the imbalance by scheduling therapeutic meetings with the parents. After identifying the problem, endocrinologists will then advise younger patients accordingly, on how to live a life that enhances growth. To prevent hampered growth, parents should therefore take their children for regular medical checkups.[152]

TRAINING AND OCCUPATION

You should understand that the practice of endocrinology requires an advanced, interactive approach. An endocrinologist cannot diagnose a problem without proper input from you; the majority of **endocrine** ailments are not immediately visually apparent. That alone requires endocrinologists to develop communication skills, in addition to developing a dedicated and engaging bedside manner. In fact, endocrinologists undergo a special training program, requiring two to three years of additional study, before they are able to service outpatient and inpatient clients, including offering various regimens associated with metabolic syndrome. Even then, endocrinologists continue to study and advance their medical skill by participating in methodical conferences and research-based rounds to keep their training up to date.[153]

Ultimately, endocrinology requires a holistic approach, and as such requires a clear and honest exchange of information between the patient and the physician. Don't be afraid to engage your endocrinologist in conversation; many of the symptoms of hormone excess and deficiency can seem abstract, presenting as a lack or overabundance of energy. Discussing your day-to-day symptoms is crucial to providing your endocrinologist with the data he needs to make an accurate diagnosis.

14

Role of the Hospital in Metabolic Syndrome

THE ROLE that hospitals will typically play in your treatment revolves around providing accurate information regarding the general condition of metabolic syndrome, in addition to treating the syndrome itself. However, due to the extent of the issues associated with metabolic syndrome, as well as the number of confirmed cases, hospitals are currently overwhelmed—and the problem will only get worse if the syndrome continues to progress. The following chapter lays out some of the options that hospitals provide for your treatment.[154]

INFORMING THE MASSES

One of the most valuable services that hospitals can provide during your treatment is the maintenance of precise, well-kept records, so that you can engage in prevention at the individual level. With there being evidence that the factors that contribute to metabolic syndrome originate at birth, these records are invaluable for making proper diagnoses/treatment plans. Without the proper facts, individuals can suffer in silence and live with lifelong pain, increasing the rate of unnecessary mortality. Unfortunately, even with this information available, people often only consider metabolic syndrome *after* the condition has begun to affect them. Take advantage of the resource of hospital records to avoid the opportunistic illnesses known to accompany this syndrome, such as stress and depression.[155]

If you suspect that you or a loved one might be afflicted with metabolic syndrome, or if you are concerned about the symptoms you are experiencing, know that hospitals can also provide a wealth of information regarding warning signs and triggers related to the syndrome. Make use of this information in the fullest, to better serve your health and the health of others. In turn, hospitals should make a point to pass on this information in a way that both informs and engages their audience, including by hosting educational workshops and organizing symposiums.[156]

SCIENTIFIC RESEARCH

Hospitals can also provide additional treatment plans for metabolic syndrome sufferers, outside the normal battery of options. They do this by sponsoring research programs, which in turn work to develop new and revolutionary methods of combatting metabolic syndrome and its composite ailments. This research also focuses on the various malignant factors that contribute to the syndrome—related illnesses that tend to come to light more frequently than others.[157]

And, although they are currently limited by the amount of available data on the syndrome, hospitals also work with research programs to focus on finding the soundest therapies available. After all, without proper research on a disease, hospital-based prescriptions may not always work, particularly in elderly patients. In fact, elderly patients have died because of incorrectly prescribed medication. Information regarding the progress of these studies, and their findings, should be available from your area hospitals.[158]

THE ROLE OF THE PATIENT

If you suspect metabolic syndrome may be at work, you should seek medical examination early on. Swift treatment helps not only you, but also assists in the global effort to eradicate the syndrome. Studies have indicated that metabolic syndrome advances with age, with older people falling ill more often. These reports also recommend that young people keep a close eye on their health developments as they grow older. These recent studies have assisted seniors by making them aware of the dangers that their advanced age exposes them to, so that they can lead healthy lives.

MERGING WITH OTHER GROUPS

Hospitals also serve as an aggregate for the information and resources provided by a wealth of individuals and organizations, all of which have focused their attention on addressing this syndrome. For example, some of these organizations can provide you with alternative treatment options to fight your syndrome, such as natural remedies (herbs and other tools of reinvigoration). While these groups tend to show irregular results, you should be careful not to ignore their efforts, as they all work toward the larger scheme of metabolic syndrome research. Hospitals can network with these other resources to determine how best to perfect their practices. These types of shared efforts, both in formal and informal fields of medicine, can go a long way toward dealing a heavy blow to the syndrome.[159]

CREATING AWARENESS

In order to treat this syndrome with the seriousness it deserves, you will require a proper understanding of the dangers it poses. Awareness efforts by hospitals serve as a wakeup call, focusing on the hard truths about the syndrome. These efforts typically take the form of newspaper articles, health periodicals and health magazines, websites, and other available publications. The use of radios, televisions, and movies also helps in relaying the information to the people.[160]

COUNSELING

After receiving the test results showing that you have already developed metabolic syndrome, there is a likelihood that you will experience a series of traumatic stages colloquially known as the stages of grief—first comes disbelief, denial, or shock, continuing on as the reality of your situation dawns on you. During that period, opportunistic sicknesses can take advantage of a weakened body and attack certain vital systems, including the immune system, among others. Your area hospital should be able to provide adequate counseling services to help you move through this process, be they in-house or through an associated practice. Know that counseling takes time and calls for continued monitoring and emotional support, as this is key to preventing a relapse in your condition. If the services provided by your hospital are insufficient, there are numerous counseling services available that provide a holistic approach, ensuring that you feel valued and cared for by your medical professional team, as well as by society in general.[161] There are even professional counselors who can provide support and care to middle-aged patients, senior patients, men, and women separately. When working with these counselors, the key is to develop a personal connection, so that you can understand each other better.[162]

FURTHER RECOMMENDATIONS

To recap, hospitals can play a major role in dealing with your metabolic syndrome. Apart from offering treatment, they help you to prevent and manage your syndrome correctly. Above all, hospitals work toward inspiring people to abandon their sedentary lifestyles. Even though some people may still ignore the advice and guidance of professional caregivers, if the information spreads through society, the frequency of metabolic syndrome will truly diminish. Heed the advice of hospitals and primary care physicians to promote healthy living—the health conditions of tomorrow are entirely determined by the lifestyles of today.[163]

PART III

Faces of Metabolic Syndrome

15

In Relation to Abnormal Blood Pressure

INSULIN RESISTANCE and high blood pressure are viewed as "diseases of civilization," illnesses, which are only possible under the conditions of excess endemic to first-world culture. In the contemporary environment, thanks to the overconsumption of unhealthy food and inactive lifestyles, these disorders are at an all-time high. Reduced sensitivity to insulin is a sign of numerous pathological symptoms linked with hypertension.[164]

TRUE CONNECTION TO METABOLIC SYNDROME

As patients with metabolic syndrome generally suffer from blood pressure-related illnesses, heart diseases and metabolic syndrome share common symptoms, such as difficulties breaking down lipids and proteins, increased oxidative stress, glucose imbalance, **hypercoagulability**, as well as skin damage. Early research proposed the name "circulatory syndrome" to refine the metabolic syndrome concept by including aspects of cardiac diseases like renal impairment, arterial stiffness, and heart blockage. It has become apparent that insulin resistance (and the resulting actions of insulin-targeted body parts to make up for the defect) has an important role in the development and progress of metabolic syndrome.[165]

Medical research has shown that approximately 50 percent of hypertensive individuals have glucose intolerance, whereas as least

80 percent of patients with type-2 diabetes report high blood pressure. Besides the metabolic effects, insulin influences the relaxation of blood vessels (thus reducing blood pressure) by revitalizing the generation of certain dilating substances. Insulin also controls sodium restraint by stimulating sodium reabsorption in the kidneys, thus policing blood pressure levels.[166]

Research studies have showed that insulin resistance can develop not only in traditional insulin-responsive tissues, but also in heart tissues where insulin affects the risk of heart diseases and high blood pressure. This is generally connected with metabolic syndrome and high blood pressure, which confer a higher risk for type-2 diabetes as well as heart diseases.[167]

THE SCIENCE BEHIND IT ALL

The relationship between blood pressure level, insulin resistance, and subsequent **hyperinsulinemia** is well recognized. In untreated hypertensive patients, fasting as well as post-meal insulin levels are greater than normotensive controls (normal blood pressure levels), regardless of the body mass index. There is a direct relationship between insulin concentrations and blood pressure levels. Insulin resistance and hyperinsulinemia also can be found in rats with genetic **hypertension**. Interestingly, the relationship of insulin resistance and Stage-1 hypertension (blood pressure of 140-159/90-99) doesn't happen in Stage-2 hypertension (blood pressure of 160 or higher/100 or higher).[168]

This all implies a common genetic predisposition for essential hypertension and insulin resistance, an idea also backed by the finding of modified glucose metabolism in children with normal blood pressure who are born of hypertensive patients. The prevalent genetic landscape of insulin resistance and hypertension is also supported by the demystification of certain genetic defects in individuals with combinations of insulin resistance, obesity, **dyslipidemia** as well as blood pressure-related plights. These deficiencies consist of a "beta-3" gene mutation, which controls the reduction of fat, and the existence of two more mutated genes. One of these genes regulates insulin levels and blood pressure level, and the other governs the intake of food.[169]

Deficiency in CD36, a well-known molecule that moves fats, is also considered to be involved in the predisposition to insulin resistance and unsteady blood pressure. Besides genetic predisposition, metabolic syndrome is implicated in the development of abnormal blood pressure through irregularities in the counter-regulation of insulin. These include **ion exchange**, and improved activities of the sympathetic central nervous system and the kidney systems, along with the following:[170]

- Amplified oxidative stress
- Blood volume expansion
- Progressive kidney ailment
- Loose fat in the blood
- Sodium retention
- Left ventricular hypertrophy (swelling/increased volume)
- Shifts in blood sugar
- Over-reactive heart

For example, in healthy subjects, insulin evokes a net nervous system reflex, while at the same time countering the body's natural instinct to constrict the blood vessels in response. On the other hand, in high blood pressure patients, insulin induces nerve stimulation higher than those seen in usual subjects, while still nullifying vessel dilation. This whole mechanism is engaged in defective regulation of blood vessel constriction, which results in an upturn in blood pressure levels.[171]

As far as metabolic syndrome is concerned, its effects on blood pressure is complex, and in some ways uncertain. The effect isn't isolated, and makes up for the deterioration of pulse wave velocity (PWV), which denotes strain of the arteries and is associated with high cholesterol. Pulse wave velocity is also used to prevent potential cardiovascular events in patients with either high blood pressure or serious diabetes.[172]

Endless clinical and demographic evidence show a positive link between metabolic syndrome and high blood pressure. The cohabitation of insulin resistance and **hypertension** leads to a significant increase in the chance of getting cardiovascular disease as well as type-2 diabetes. For this reason, maintenance of healthy blood pressure can reduce or even prevent your risk of metabolic syndrome, opening the doors to a number of health benefits. Different patients require different time periods for the symptoms and byproducts of metabolic syndrome to stick out. When caught in advance, blood pressure can be kept down using medication. Although as yet we do not have a definitive cure for hypertension, patients can use medicines to keep the pressure at a manageable level and still lead a normal lifestyle.[173]

16

In Relation to Cholesterol Problems

ON DEVELOPING metabolic syndrome, patients experience taxing pain due to clogged arteries (from high cholesterol) in several parts of the body, which may spread further if left untreated. High cholesterol, in turn, can result in far-reaching medical difficulties in the following ways:[174]

CHOLESTEROL AND BODY FAT

Cholesterol is found mostly in fatty foods, and high levels of it may be caused by overconsumption of these foods. When a metabolic syndrome patient consumes foods with high levels of cholesterol, their body doesn't utilize all the saturated fat. Naturally, the organs require only a precise amount of fat every day; if the levels go up, that residual fat tends to stick around. Those fat cells are then shipped to the "storage compartments" of the body that store unneeded fat. Areas where fat accumulates include the waistline or the area encasing the belly.[175]

After some time, this fat starts to harm the body slowly. Energy requires muscles, not excess body fat. Therefore, those fat cells remain idle, acting as a breeding site for metabolic syndrome. Gradually, minor illnesses begin developing until a person begins noticing subtle symptoms such as headaches, stomach pains, and so forth.

Obesity can begin as early as childhood, especially if the child regularly consumes sugary and fatty foods. As compared to the normal weight gain, which simple exercises and proper diet can handle, obesity can take a long time to rectify. Cholesterol triggers obesity when all the unused cholesterol builds up within the body. Obesity has been strongly linked to metabolic syndrome. When people start adding weight and tread closer to obesity, they tend to continue eating due to stress and low self-esteem. People suddenly start craving sugary foods and junk foods for consolation. The rising cholesterol clings on as the waist circumference broadens. The disorder (high cholesterol) then transitions from weight gain to obesity, and even though some people reverse the situation, many live with obesity for the rest of their adulthood.[176]

CHOLESTEROL AND HIGH BLOOD SUGAR

Another action for which cholesterol is responsible is aggravation of high blood sugar, a component of metabolic syndrome. Cholesterol is often consumed with some amount of blood glucose, and when too much of that glucose is consumed, he suffers from imbalanced blood sugar levels. In most cases, such a situation occurs when a person avoids eating and drinking for some time. Skipping meals causes glucose levels to rise beyond the daily recommended amount. When high blood sugar occurs, the chances of acquiring heart disease go up as well.[177]

CHOLESTEROL AND HIGH BLOOD PRESSURE

Many metabolic syndrome sufferers live with high blood pressure without even knowing it. Although high blood pressure can occur due to many reasons, cholesterol is the No. 1 cause. High levels of cholesterol in the body clog the arteries, causing the heart to make extra effort to exhort blood past the barriers caused by cholesterol. That extra effort causes the blood to leave the heart at a higher rate than normal, thus raising the level of pressure.[178] This pressure eventually exhausts the heart, and if not attended in due time, the heart's beating capacity gradually slows (over a very long time, not suddenly). When the heart slows down, blood stops reaching other vital organs in the body, causing a severe paucity of metabolism. Inadequate blood in the system inhibits the functionality of the other body parts, thereby hindering growth and the ability of the body to fend off both mild and severe conditions. From there, all the opportunistic factors of metabolic syndrome attack almost instantly, and negative symptoms begin to materialize.[179]

TARGETING CHOLESTEROL

As for dealing with cholesterol as a metabolic syndrome sufferer, you should first note that cholesterol medication doesn't exactly cure metabolic syndrome, meaning that prevention remains the better option. Parents and caretakers should resist feeding their children fatty foods containing high levels of cholesterol. Such foods result in adverse health conditions in a child, and they may even cause premature death. Sugary soda and energy drinks offer no health benefits, and they can even fuel diseases. Secondly, individuals with metabolic syndrome should make sure they take only the recommended amount of cholesterol daily so that the body can utilize all of it before the next meal. Most foods come with labels that denote the amount of cholesterol per serving. Third, people should formulate a workout routine; most obese people spend too much time seated and avoiding simple endeavors such as walking. Power strolls in the mornings or evening help to suppress high cholesterol and metabolic syndrome.[180]

Physical workouts help the body to burn fat and use all the internal cholesterol, leaving none unused, avoiding opportunistic illnesses. People should use medications as prescribed by their doctor, as these elements affect the body's ability to process cholesterol and manage other factors of metabolic syndrome. These medications work by either dampening the severity of the cholesterol-related illness or by improving the ability of the body to protect itself from attacks. When all is said and done, high amounts of bad cholesterol can contribute to metabolic syndrome, and people should consume it in moderation. Patients can live safely by changing the way they live in terms of cholesterol limitation and physical activity.[181]

17

In Relation to Excess Body Fat

OF THE factors that influence metabolic syndrome, excess body fat contributes the most. The unneeded fat compounds all the other factors and almost acts as a flashpoint, from which all the other problems begin. For instance, risk factors such as high blood pressure, higher rates of blood clotting, and pro-inflammatory states all arise from obesity. These conditions occur once the metabolic syndrome patient begins to store excess fat in their body. Obesity contributes to metabolic syndrome in a multitude of ways.[182]

A LOOK INTO OBESITY

A metabolic syndrome patient should look to maintain a weight that is consistent with his height for the body to remain healthy. From a clinical standpoint, medical professionals estimate obesity by measuring the circumference of the abdominal area. Abdominal weight gain, specifically, contributes vastly to metabolic syndrome. The body stores belly fat around the **visceral organs** as well as in any other places it can find space to cram fat into. Fat in the visceral region contributes more to the risk factors of metabolic syndrome than fat in any other area of the body. An average person will develop obesity owing to reasons explained in this chapter.[183]

DIET AND OBESITY

Poor diet leads to weight gain, as body fat comes from the food we eat. Overeating predisposes you to weight gain, because you're not giving your body ample time to burn off the fat. Furthermore, all the food remaining in the system then goes to the fat storage areas of the body. Poor diet includes foods such as fatty foods, junk food, overconsumption of red meat, skipping meals, and many others. Skipping meals adds to body fat because the body takes the available fat in organs and stores it in bulk, in case a person doesn't eat the next scheduled meal. In a similar vein, when a person finally eats a meal after skipping the previously scheduled one, the stored fat remains unused. Gradually the stored fat snowballs, and after some time, it assumes the form of gut fat. Eating processed and highly refined foods also leads to obesity, because the body may fail to properly assimilate such foods. When digestion occurs, these foods remain in the system, causing a buildup of fat.[184]

INACTIVITY AND OBESITY

The human body requires frequent movement so that it can utilize the food it consumes. If a metabolic syndrome sufferer spends their entire day seated, most of that food remains unused. To induce body movement (one way to get rid of excess body fat), people should engage in exercises such as speed-walking and jogging. For instance, people who work at an office should try walking up the stairs instead of taking the elevator. Those at home can take the time to go for power walks or jogs. An inactive patient not only faces the risk of obesity, but many of the other risks bracketed with metabolic syndrome. The hazards involved include hypertension, problems with the glands, uneven growth of the body, and so on.[185]

UNHEALTHY LIVING

Unhealthy habits contribute to excess body fat in many ways. Consumption of products such as alcohol in high amounts leads to obesity. Alcohol pins down unneeded fat and carbohydrates, and because people don't normally work out after drinking, all that fat stays in the body. Regular alcohol consumption also accelerates heart problems. Most of the fat generated from alcohol over time remains in the body, especially around the belly and waistline.[186]

Another unhealthy lifestyle factor is the overuse of technology, because it encourages the body not to expend any energy at all. Using vehicles all the time, even when traveling only a short distance, falls in the category of neglectful living because the body doesn't get an opportunity to utilize stored fat. An unhealthy lifestyle comes with many disadvantages, not only to the personal health of an individual but also to his finances. Ways to avoid overdependence on technology include replacing virtual/social media interaction with physical interaction (actually meeting people face to face), and replacing video games with athletics. It's important to remember that some conditions such as heart diseases require you to take expensive prescription drugs and receive medical attention for the rest of your life. Such treatments don't come cheap.[187]

STRONG LINKS BETWEEN OBESITY AND METABOLIC SYNDROME

While blood pressure may normally stay at a certain level, with the accumulation of fat, the pressure goes up, hence the term "high blood pressure." In the process of determining whether a person suffers from metabolic syndrome, medical professionals use a simple strategy, examining negative factors such as increased circumference around the waist, high blood pressure, high levels of glucose, and elevated triglyceride levels. All of the above conditions transpire from a surplus of fat cells.[188]

After a person gains excess body fat, his resistance to insulin is increased. This ultimately leads to diabetes, another serious risk factor for metabolic syndrome. At this time, no medication can cure diabetes, meaning that obese people risk living with diabetes for the rest of their life if no action is taken. Obesity also affects hormonal imbalance, another risk factor of metabolic syndrome. Hormonal imbalance occurs due to many matters, but regardless of the cause, these imbalances poses real danger to anyone it affects.[189] These imbalances arise in two ways: low production of hormones or excessive production of hormones. Both over- and underproduction of hormones impact growth adversely.

Other problems associated with excess body fat include stress and chronic depression. Obese people may experience mental despair due to issues such as low self-esteem and lack of self-worth. When a person feels bad about himself, he stays away from others, and that in turn leads to stress. Ways to deal with stress include proper time management, avoidance of caffeine, and indulging in physical activity.[190]

Stress weakens the good things in life and accelerates bad habits, such as the frenetic use of alcohol, smoking, and illicit substance abuse. These then lead to obesity, as well as other conditions related to metabolic syndrome such as hypertension, and the cycle starts all over again. When all those problems come together, a metabolic syndrome sufferer starts aging at an astonishing rate, as their metabolism becomes dangerously imbalanced.[191]

Every individual must take it upon themselves to manage and control the level of fat in their body. Obesity brings a host of problems, but taking simple precautionary measures such as avoiding certain foods and exercising regularly makes a lot of difference in the long run. When an obese person acquires metabolic syndrome, it can also burden friends and loved ones. Hence, people should take care of their health not just for their own sake, but for the sake of the other people in their lives as well.[192]

18

In Relation to Heart Attacks

HEART ATTACKS can kill patients easily. A single attack can forestall the heart indefinitely. To avoid overworking the heart, patients can use several treatment options to unblock the arteries. Treatment varies from one person to the next, and some people manage to keep their blood pressure down for many years. For other patients, the problem may quickly get out of hand, especially if the condition develops to a severe case. Moreover, your age determines the chances of survival—younger people tend to respond to treatment faster and more effectively due to the strength of their hearts, as compared to older individuals. With proper diet and regular exercise, people can prevent heart attacks (or at least improve their chances of recovery).[193]

HEART ATTACKS AND BODY FAT

People with metabolic syndrome and heart disease often suffer from obesity or excess body fat. Excess body fat comes from overconsumption, especially if a person hasn't been eating the right food. The extra fat (which remains unused after the body processes all the food) remains in the body. That fat then begins attracting and fueling other illnesses—among them high blood pressure. Atypical cholesterol levels will be imminent, paving the way to **atherosclerosis** in the long run, as the heart is forced to work harder than normal. The resultant burden to the heart increases blood pressure. [194]

HEART ATTACKS AND BLOOD PRESSURE

When blood pressure rises, one of the problems that can occur is a heart attack. If the condition isn't helmed properly, the heart may fail completely due to the extra effort it makes to pump blood through the arteries. The heart requires some space for it to beat normally, and if fat smothers it, pumping decelerates, which can then cause a heart attack.[195]

HEART ATTACKS AND BLOOD SUGAR

The body requires several things to function normally, and among them is sugar. Whether abnormally low or high, a sugar imbalance has negative effects on the body as a whole. When the level of sugar in the blood goes up, the sugar strains the functioning of the heart, making it increasingly difficult to supply blood throughout the body. At this point, a person starts experiencing heart attacks, mildly at first, but as the levels of sugar continue to rise, more bouts can occur. Some medications do help in bringing the level of sugar in the blood down, making it easier for the heart to keep on pumping. If ignored, the sugar can stop the heart completely at the physiological level, especially if it penetrates into the major arteries. To avoid increasing the level of sugar in the blood, people should reduce their intake of refined sugars. Sugary drinks such as sodas and processed juices, as well as sugary foods like cakes may escalate the problem so individuals should avoid them completely if possible. Instead, people should consume natural juices and fruit, as such products offer other essential nutrients, known to be advantageous in keeping metabolic syndrome at bay.[196] Alternatively, metabolic syndrome sufferers looking to specifically avoid heart attacks should consume fat from items such as avocado and coconuts, as these foods contain certain types of beneficial fats.[197]

HEART ATTACKS AND FATTY FOODS

Patients who eat a lot of fatty foods face a high risk of heart attacks. When fat accumulates in the body, most of it remains unused because the body can only burn a certain amount. That fat then breeds other illnesses, and worse still can even incapacitate arteries in the form of caustic **lipids**. After the body's ability to store fat is exhausted, the remaining fat does irreparable damage. Blocked arteries hinder blood from flowing normally, thus putting strain on the heart.

A WELL-ROUNDED APPROACH

Heart attacks are risky to people of all ages. Some people may undergo several heart attacks in their lives, while others die from only one attack. Medications can help with obesity and metabolic syndrome, but the most effective preventive measure involves physical exercise. Exercise helps in corroding fat and strengthening the heart, thus reducing the risk of attacks. Secondly, engaging in workout sessions weekly (or daily if possible) speeds up the process of fat burning and keeps the heart rejuvenated at all times. Simple exercise and activities such as cycling help the heart to stay young and healthy.[198]

The heart behaves much the same as a car engine—every other body function depends on it, and just as cars require regular servicing, people need to undergo consistent medical examinations. The risk of heart attacks and other factors that contribute to metabolic syndrome can be prevented when identified in time.[199]

Metabolic syndrome clients can sidestep heart disease by adjusting their lifestyles. The activities a person does or doesn't engage in determine his overall health. For instance, living rashly and avoiding body movement and physical activity contribute to metabolic syndrome. Regular exercise is required for organs and muscles to function normally, but even simple workouts such as walking, jogging, riding a bicycle, running, and so forth play a major role in the health of the heart.[200]

19

In Relation to Sugar Imbalance

METABOLIC SYNDROME affects millions of Americans, but insulin resistance (one of the components of metabolic syndrome caused by an imbalance of sugar in the bloodstream) affects over 100 million people in the United States alone. That's just under one-third of the nation's current population. It's become such a predominant health problem that the health industry is predicting that this disorder will eventually bankrupt the entire health care system.[201]

THE INNER WORKINGS OF BLOOD SUGAR

Metabolic syndrome and insulin resistance are major factors in heart-related predicaments and diabetes, two of the most common causes of fatality in the civilized world. With the indisputable connections between metabolic syndrome, sugar imbalance, and thyroid dysfunctions, it's critically important to recognize where the relations are and how to spot them. To begin: metabolic syndrome is caused by **hyperglycemia**, which presents when a person consumes too many carbohydrates. Another way to look at metabolic syndrome would be to point to excessive carbohydrate intake or sugar disease. When a person retains too many carbohydrates, the **pancreas** begins to secrete insulin to direct the excess sugars from the bloodstream to certain cells where they are warehoused until needed to produce energy. Over time, the storage cells begin to lose their efficiency in responding to the excess insulin secreted. The pancreas continues to expend insulin in an effort to get the glucose into the cells, and that results in a sugar imbalance over time. Severe or chronic **hypoglycemia** can cause a plethora of life-threatening conditions, including seizures, coma, and even death.[202]

The body is designed to work properly—when all systems are functioning correctly. The human organism is programmed to recognize severe low blood sugar as a threat. When a person's blood sugar levels plunge dangerously low, the body triggers the adrenaline glands to secrete cortisol, which in turn alerts the liver to release glucose (which was stored in the form of glycogen). That will bring sugar levels back to normal. This continued production of cortisol can negatively impact the body because it's one of the hormones exerted by glands when the sympathetic nervous system, responsible for the "fight or flight" response, is alerted. This response includes increases in heart rate, lung action, and blood flow to skeletal muscles.[203]

As with all systems, each one affects the other and the human body isn't any different. The body, while incredible in its design, is only as good as the sum of its parts. When major hormone secretion systems deteriorate, then other systems begin to go as well. The damage that occurs can trigger thyroid dysfunction, which can cause metabolic syndrome in a variety of ways. The rate of glucose uptake slows, which cuts back the rate of glucose absorption in the midsection. This delays the response of insulin to elevated blood sugar, thus slowing the removal of insulin from the blood.[204]

OBESITY AND SUGAR IMBALANCE

One of the single most significant factors in the development of metabolic syndrome is obesity—specifically, abdominal obesity or "belly fat." Being overweight in this way will actually promote sugar imbalance in a person. Losing weight with the assistance of a physician or trained dietitian can dramatically rally the body's ability to use insulin properly. The goal is to determine the source of distress in a person's metabolism and correct it. Sugar imbalance directly affects the metabolism and will throw it into a blustery whirlwind if not treated correctly. If a patient feels that they're suffering from these symptoms, a visit to the doctor is an important first step.[205]

PHYSICIAN INVOLVEMENT

Doctors can run checks to determine exactly which hormones are out of balance and just how a patient's body is metabolizing sugars so that the balance can be adjusted accordingly. Whether a person suffers from high or low blood sugar, there's probably some degree of insulin resistance present. Although high blood sugar can cause insulin resistance, insulin resistance itself can cause low blood sugar. Known as reactive **hypoglycemia**, this begins when the body continues to secrete excess insulin in response to food intake that may or may not be appropriate. For example, a meal high in carbohydrates will cause blood sugar levels to fall below normal in response to the sugars ingested. Furthermore, a good doctor/patient relationship is imperative at this point, especially if there's any problem indicating a future clinical disorder. The doctor can assist you in making goals for dieting and maintaining a proper balance between the amount of sugars and starches so that the metabolism doesn't plummet out of its ideal range.[206]

When addressing the situation with the doctor, the key is to make sure that blood sugar stays within a healthy scope. There are two specific targets that the doctor will look to hit. The first is the fasting blood glucose level, which will measure a patient's blood sugar before eating or drinking anything. There's discussion among doctors as to what ranges should be considered normal, but for a fasting blood glucose, 75-95 mg/dl is generally considered normal. Some believe 100 to be the cutoff, citing evidence that blood sugar in the mid-90s is predictive of future diabetes years later. Eighty mg/dl is generally considered the limit on the low end, but there are many healthy people who have a fasting blood sugar in the 70s, especially if they are on a low-carb diet.[207]

The second target, and the most important, is called the post-prandial blood glucose. This is a test that measures your blood sugar a few hours after eating. This demonstrates exactly how your body is metabolizing food and secreting glucose, insulin, and cortisol, and in what amounts. This test has been created to serve as the most accurate in predicting potential diabetic issues. The normal post-prandial blood sugar count is 120 mg/dl. Most healthy people are under 100 mg/dl two hours after eating a full meal.[208]

IDEAL BLOOD SUGAR LEVELS

A person who is considered hypoglycemic needs to keep their blood sugar above 75 throughout the day. This is easily accomplished with a low to moderate carbohydrate diet, consumed in frequent, small amounts. By contrast, a patient who presents as hyperglycemic needs to keep their blood sugar below 120 mg/dl a couple of hours after each meal, usually by forgoing sugar consumption. To determine a healthy amount of carbs per day, consult with a physician and work together to finalize the appropriate amount of carbohydrates for you, determine the best way to monitor blood sugar, and set goals for you to regain control. Many people who do have issues with maintaining the right amount of sugars in their bloodstream purchase a blood glucose meter, which is a simple, cost-effective way to monitor blood glucose throughout the day. The doctor is also the best source of information for the best type of monitor and how many times per day to check blood sugar. Keeping a diary and staying in contact with one's physician are critical for keeping sugar metabolism at a healthy level.[209]

Understanding the connections between sugar imbalance and metabolic syndrome is also imperative. Once a patient realizes that the condition is developing, they can begin to take preventative measures to correct the situation. While it may seem obvious or simple, it does require attention to detail and meticulous restraint on the part of the patient.[210]

20

Types of Sugar Disorders

A SUGAR DISORDER, collectively called diabetes mellitus or diabetes, is a general term used to describe a spectrum of diseases that affect the metabolism. These disorders occur due to the body's inability to balance the levels of blood sugar over a long period. When sugar disorders occur, they cause ill effects in the human body, which explains why individuals who have metabolic syndrome suffer from different types of sugar disorders. Well-known sugar disorders include type-1 diabetes, type-2 diabetes, and gestational diabetes.[211]

TYPE-1 DIABETES

Type-1 diabetes comes about when there is an absence of beta cells. These cells produce insulin; as such, the loss of these cells is an indicator of insulin deficiency. During the early stages of type-1 diabetes, most patients don't even realize that they are suffering from it, because they outwardly appear in good health. In the early stages, responsiveness to insulin in patients suffering from this type of diabetes occurs largely as it does in a healthy person.[212]

Sadly, type-1 diabetes can also affect children, so parents should take their children for regular check-ups. As with all diseases, early detection of sugar disorders helps in the prevention of future complications. Besides the loss of beta cells, a person with metabolic syndrome can acquire type-1 diabetes genetically, inheriting it from their parents. To boot, type-1 diabetes can worsen with illnesses stemming from viral infections or diet.[213]

TYPE-2 DIABETES

Type-2 diabetes comes about when the body resists insulin. In some cases, the disorder could stem from low secretion of insulin. In cases where your organs secrete low amounts of insulin, and then begin to resist that small amount of insulin, the disorder can worsen dramatically. In other words, patients with this disorder can suffer from low insulin secretion, insulin resistance, or both. When it affects the future metabolic syndrome sufferer, type-2 diabetes steps up its attack by reducing the sensitivity to insulin itself. Some medications, as well as precautionary measures, can help in this situation. Furthermore, the causes of type-2 diabetes vary; some patients acquire it from the lifestyles they lead, including failure to eat a healthy diet, lack of physical exercises, stress, consumption of sugary foods, and consuming some types of fat, such as saturated fat and trans fats, increases the probability of suffering from sugar disorders.[214]

GESTATIONAL DIABETES

Gestational diabetes, the third type of sugar disorder, bears many similarities to type-2 diabetes. Gestational diabetes involves a combination of inadequate secretion of insulin and responsiveness of the body to insulin. As the namesake suggests, gestational diabetes affects pregnant women, and it may improve or disappear altogether following birth. Therefore, proper medication and constant supervision from a medical professional can treat gestational diabetes in full. Patients suffering from the disorder can control their appetite and monitor sugar intake. If a pregnant woman ignores the disease, she can potentially damage her health or that of her unborn child. If the fetus contracts the disease, it could also incur conditions such as malformation of the skeletal muscles, anomalies in the central nervous system, and in worst cases prenatal death.[215]

OTHER TYPES OF SUGAR DISORDERS

Aside from the above three categories of sugar disorders, metabolic syndrome patients can also become affected by other types such as pre-diabetes and **latent autoimmune diabetes**, as well as congenital diabetes, cystic diabetes, and steroid diabetes. Pre-diabetes occurs when the level of glucose in the blood rises above normal. Many patients live with pre-diabetes before it develops into type-2. Latent autoimmune diabetes affects adults and, if not trammeled early, will develop into type-1 diabetes. Congenital diabetes occurs because of genetic defects in the secretion of insulin. Cystic diabetes comes from conditions related to fibrosis, while steroid diabetes occurs from an addiction to high doses of steroids.[216]

SIGNS AND SYMPTOMS OF SUGAR DISORDERS

When someone develops a sugar disorder, the symptoms may take some time to manifest, and there will typically be discrepancies from patient to patient. Going for frequent medical check-ups is the best way an individual can detect the problem before it really takes root. Typically, symptoms include increased thirst, frequent urination, raised appetite and food cravings, headaches, fatigue, itchy skin, and slow healing of bruises. The above symptoms occur in the early stages of the disorders, and as they resemble symptoms of other diseases, a patient may fail to know the exact difficulties at hand; hence, the need for regular medical examinations. More serious symptoms include ulcers of the foot, kidney failure, and stroke. Therefore, it's better not to wait around until the sugar disorder is no longer controllable.[217]

MANAGEMENT AND PREVENTION OF SUGAR DISORDERS

If a metabolic syndrome sufferer makes the necessary changes in lifestyle and the disorder persists, the condition can still be managed via lifestyle changes, as mentioned earlier. While no medication can completely cure the many sugar disorders existing today; medication can still manage these diseases. With proper management, a patient can survive for many years. Management of sugar disorders starts with education and seeking advice when needed. With adequate information, people can better know how to spot the preliminary signs and symptoms of sugar disorders, as well as how to promote recovery early on.[218]

The person with metabolic syndrome should remember that normal body weight enhances the ability of the body to persevere against sugar disorders. As a result, healthy diet and exercise—in other words, keeping fit—supports immunity and enhances body functionality, thus enabling a person to respond to their body's health needs.[219]

Medications can help in management of sugar disorders, and many patients actually spend most of their lives using them. For instance, many diabetic patients use doses of insulin to help offset spikes in blood sugar levels. Patients should understand that they can live with these conditions and still enjoy full lives.[220]

Having completed this chapter, you should know that all the blood in the body moves through the heart, assisting in the normal functions of the limbs. When the level of sugar in the blood traveling through the arteries skyrockets, the heart develops complications. These present as organs that are dependent on the heart becoming unable to handle the excess amount of sugar. Heart disease, associated with blood sugar complications, can kill at the drop of a hat, with no medication or treatment currently available that can cure the condition. Consequently, many people die of heart related problems all over the globe. People should make sure that they keep their blood sugar at a level that doesn't exceed 100 milligrams per deciliter. The person who has metabolic syndrome should know that sugar disorders come with their fair share of adversities to overcome, for both patients and family members alike.[221]

21

Disorders Associated with Metabolic Syndrome

THE FOLLOWING sections cover some of the common medical disorders patients often complain of after fully developing metabolic syndrome.[222]

ULCERS

Patients with metabolic syndrome sometimes develop ulcers due to excess production of insulin. The organs may release more insulin than the body can handle, or they may even produce only a minuscule amount of insulin, which they then fail to utilize at all. The unused insulin then finds a way to force other molecules (known as insulin growth factors or IGFs) of the body to attack the walls of the stomach. When these substances meet the fragile walls of the digestive system, they perforate the linings, causing corrosive damage. That destruction then manifests itself as pain, and medical professionals deem the condition to be an ulcer.[223]

Ulcers can easily harm you, even leading to loss of appetite, as individuals with metabolic syndrome start to detest the taste and smell of food. When ulcers are combined with other diseases, the corrosive damage can intensify, leading you to experience a lot of pain. If detected early, a person can control the condition before it causes other illnesses, but people should take medication only under directions from a qualified medical professional.[224]

INFERTILITY

Metabolic syndrome can affect almost every part of the body, including the reproductive organs. These organs require the constant flow of blood and oxygen to function effectively, and metabolic syndrome interferes with that flow, causing a core imbalance and rendering the reproductive organs useless. The problems that can arise from infertility are numerous, with patients undergoing physical as well as emotional turmoil. Some medications do treat infertility, especially during the early stages, but doctors may still find it prudent to advise patients to pursue surgical alternatives. To avoid all those problems, people should go for medical check-ups regularly. Early identification of the problem prevents future complications such as stress, as well as the hormonal manifestations described earlier. Treatments can be provided by an endocrinologist (see Chapter 13).[225]

ALLERGIES

Allergies can be common among metabolic syndrome patients. The syndrome can damage several systems and bodily functions such as airways and the digestive system. When that happens, the body starts to resist specific types of food, aromas, and so forth. That negative reaction to certain foods marks the start of allergies. Allergies, like other medical woes, can start slow and progress, limiting what a person can eat, drink, and smell. Most people live with their allergies, but they can rectify the problem if they seek professional medical help. Actually, certain medications and lifestyle changes can keep allergies away forever. Avoiding things that aggravate allergies, maintaining a healthy lifestyle, and taking proper medication can suppress the intensity of allergies so that a person can live a normal life.[226]

FATIGUE

Getting tired after doing some kind of work isn't necessarily a sign of a serious problem. However, fatigue in the absence of mental or physical labor is cause for concern. Unusual fatigue could mean that the body's metabolism isn't running properly, which indicates that blood circulation has slowed down. A consistent feeling of being overtired often leads to sitting idle. That, in turn, can result in weight gain, especially along the abdominal zone, one of the foremost effects of metabolic syndrome.[227]

Metabolic syndrome restricts the functionality of several parts of the body. When these parts stop working or work slowly, the problem escalates. Healthy parts of the body then begin to overwork to compensate for lost production, which takes the form of continuous effort that no amount of slumber can relieve.[228] Fatigue can easily hinder your recovery, because it affects all the parts of the body, leaving a person immobilized. With intense fatigue, even appetite is reduced, to the extent that the patient can even succumb to internal starvation. Fatigue comes about due to continued inactivity of the body, as lack of movement leads to a build-up of body fat. That body fat then clogs and hinders other organs from functioning and eventually, fatigue strikes. The age or gender of a person doesn't matter; it affects everyone. Therefore, people should engage in various exercises, such as those discussed in Chapter 23, to avoid unnecessary fatigue.[229]

MENOPAUSE

Metabolic syndrome may cause early menopause in females, even before they reach the latter half of their life. This happens because the reproductive organs of women develop problems such that their ovaries can't fertilize eggs. Some medications and treatment plans can reverse the situation during the early stages, but if a woman marginalizes the problem for a long time, the condition can get out of hand, to the point that no medication can treat it. Therefore, women should adopt a healthy lifestyle to avoid injuring their reproductive organs, especially if they intend to have more children. Examples of lifestyle changes for female patients include proper nourishment of the body and becoming more physically active. Nevertheless, the best preventative measure would be to go for check-ups periodically.[230]

The transition to menopause itself often serves as a challenge unique to women suffering from metabolic syndrome. During the bodily changes that accompany menopause, women experience various hormonal changes. Apart from that, females go through stress during menopause as they begin adapting to the transformations in their bodies. Endocrinologists can come in and help women to deal with hormonal strain and the related hormonal imbalances caused by stress. But all of this additional stress can lead to other illnesses, such as high blood pressure—all the more reason why females who have metabolic syndrome should deal with the condition early on. The treatment offered by formal caregivers helps in the restoration of hormonal imbalances, leaving you happier and better empowered to adapt to menopause. By doing so, women develop a positive ethos and enjoy long and healthy lives thereafter.[231]

The issues described in this chapter as being associated with and influenced by metabolic syndrome often occur due to poor lifestyle choices. This means that people can prevent them before they strike. Living a sedentary lifestyle culminates in a number of conditions that medication may not be able to fully control. Some of the habits that cause metabolic syndrome include eating junk food, excessive consumption of alcohol, skipping meals, and failure to give the body time to rest. Apart from that, lack of physical exercises and spending long hours seated at work or at home also cause symptomatic problems associated with metabolic syndrome. Therefore, people should make the necessary changes in life to avoid the above (and other unwelcome) illnesses.[232]

PART IV

Resolutions

22

Natural Approaches

METABOLIC SYNDROME increases one's chances of diabetes, stroke, certain cancers, and coronary heart disease. Therefore, it is crucial to adopt a natural, effective plan that will help to avoid these life-threatening conditions. The major contributors to the onset of the disease include increased intake of simple sugars, lack of exercise, and an overall unhealthy lifestyle. The three primary conditions associated with metabolic syndrome include hypertension, obesity with high cholesterol, and resistance to insulin. These elements have yet to be effectively treated with traditional medicine. Taking a collective approach in treating the condition is more effective, an approach that includes the use of natural remedies. This approach for treating metabolic syndrome includes some basic lifestyle changes, nutritional interventions, or both. These two routes provide useful first-line options for a cost-effective approach to treating metabolic syndrome.[233]

DIET AND METABOLIC SYNDROME

To begin with, metabolic syndrome patients should consider eating foods such as the following:

- whole grains (such as buckwheat, barley, millet, rye, or wheat)
- foods rich in fiber (such as lima beans, broccoli, lentils, or split peas)
- protein-rich items (such as fish, eggs, yogurt, or poultry)

In addition, individuals should avoid consumption of sugary beverages, red meat, overconsumption of alcohol, and smoking. The best preventive measure for sugar disorders involves fine-tuning one's lifestyle so that all the parts of the body can function harmoniously, allowing the body to develop normally. When some organs stop operating, production and secretion of things such as insulin slows down or halts completely, thus compounding the chances of acquiring sugar disorders.[234]

FIBERS

Fibers are the parts of plants that can't be completely digested by the human body. They are categorized as being either soluble or insoluble fibers. Soluble fibers benefit you by altering your appetite, and lowering blood cholesterol levels and overall body weight. Beta-glucan is an example of a soluble fiber that can effectively lower the levels of blood glucose and cholesterol. It is commonly found in the cell walls of fungi, bacteria, and lichens. Some fibers suppress the appetite by providing a feeling of fullness, thus reducing calorie intake per meal. Other fibers, such as **phaseolamin**, will slow sugar absorption and hamper sugar cravings. Eating vegetables and foods with high fiber content, such as navy beans, garbanzo beans, and fiber-infused cereals, helps bring down low-density lipoproteins, while at the same time increasing the levels of high-density lipoproteins, otherwise known as "good" cholesterol. Soluble fibers are present in consumables such as oatmeal, lentils, and fruits such as oranges and strawberries, among others.[235]

FATTY ACIDS

Many patients with metabolic syndrome have a condition where their **eicosanoid** pathways lead to the production of pro-inflammatory and clot-promoting naturally occurring fatty acids, which in turn leads to undue blood clotting and excessive inflammation when a patient is affected by metabolic syndrome. This process occurs as a result of insufficient or imbalanced proportions of fatty acids, which otherwise help in thinning the blood, preventing excessive clotting, and reducing inflammation. One important fatty acid is omega-3, which is commonly found in fish. Wild Alaskan salmon, arctic char, and Atlantic mackerel have the highest omega-3 levels. This is why a patient suffering from metabolic syndrome is advised to consume fatty fish in large quantities. They can also take an omega-3 supplement in the form of a tablet. This will help in the management of the condition in an easy way without the side effects associated with pharmacological treatment.[236]

A lack of omega-3 oils can result in metabolic syndrome. Omega-6 oils, however, have the effect of reducing sensitivity to insulin. Having a higher proportion of omega-6 oils than omega-3 also increases the level of low-density lipoprotein, which is documented globally among clinical communities as the "bad" form of cholesterol. Consumption of relatively more omega-3 will partially replace the omega-6 acids. Omega-3 also revitalizes the level of high-density lipoprotein, the "good cholesterol." As a result, it reduces the risk of developing metabolic syndrome. Another advantage of omega-3 oils is that it lowers the chances of cardiovascular disease.[237]

ANTIOXIDANTS

Some of the risk factors of metabolic syndrome, such as large amounts of abdominal fat, can be handled by antioxidants. Antioxidants are useful in the elimination of free radicals in the body, which are produced through natural processes, such as the production of energy. These free radicals can cause cardiovascular disease, which the use of antioxidants can easily prevent. Antioxidants can also help in the management of oxidative stress and **glycation**—both common signs of metabolic disease. Coenzyme Q10, an example of an antioxidant, can help in the reduction of excess insulin in the body and blocks some causes of **coronary artery disease (CAD)**, such as cholesterol. Some antioxidants include alpha-lipoic acid, carotenoids which can be easily found in fruits and vegetables such as broccoli, spinach, carrots, papaya, and the like.[238]

The DASH plan helps to reduce sodium intake and overall body weight. The Dietary Approaches to Stop Hypertension (DASH) follows a healthy and balanced eating regimen founded on research analyses conducted by the National Heart, Lung, and Blood Institute (NHLBI). These studies have shown that DASH can bring hypertension to a standstill and encourages the development of blood lipids (fats in the blood circulation), thereby lowering the risk of cardiovascular disease. The DASH stratagem is not a fad diet, but rather focuses on easy to follow, simple recipes. It focuses on vegetables, fruits, and skim or low-fat dairy items; includes whole grains, seafood, poultry, beans, nuts, and vegetable oils; and restricts sodium, desserts, sugary drinks, and red meats. In terms of health benefits, DASH is low in saturated fats and trans-fats, and high in potassium, magnesium, fiber, and protein. The DASH eating program is lower in sodium than the emblematic American diet. The original DASH studies found evidence that a dieting regimen including 2300 milligrams (mg) of sodium per day suppressed high blood pressure, and a diet with only 1500 mg of sodium per day further decreased hypertension.[239]

FUNCTIONAL FOODS

Functional foods are meals that provide nutrition beyond the basic requirements of a balanced approach to diet. Natural supplements have the ability to contribute toward the prevention of some illnesses, such as cardiovascular disease and type-1 diabetes. Adding functional foods to a well-balanced diet will prevent further development of metabolic syndrome, and will do so from a natural standpoint. Some of these functional foods include fortified milk, fortified cereals, cream butter, and fortified juice. (Fortified in this case means invigorated with nutrients that are not there naturally.) All these foods benefit the body by providing valuable nutrients, while also providing nutritional supplements such as calcium, among others.[240]

HERBS

Herbs have been used for centuries for treating various types of ailments. They also constitute a major component of conventional medicine. Some of the plants found useful in handling metabolic syndrome include onions, lemon, and **ivy gourd**. These should be taken according to manufacturer labels and recommendations. They can be consumed in the form of foods or supplements. If all of these plants are taken in the correct proportions, they can help in balancing sugar absorption and blood pressure, and will also work to control depression, all of which helps in easing metabolic syndrome. While conventional medicine has noted side effects, some serious, herbs are a more natural approach to treating metabolic syndrome.[241]

LIFESTYLE CHANGES

As far as lifestyle changes are concerned, adopting new, healthy habits represents the most wide-ranging, easy, and effective way to fight off metabolic syndrome. Examples of lifestyle revamping include the cessation of drug abuse, smoking, reduction of caffeine intake, and doing away with simple sugars. All these will aggravate the syndrome and should be avoided in order to prevent it. Changes in behaviors such as food intake and eating patterns will also help to manage metabolic syndrome. Following the guidelines of the glycemic index will help you to know what to eat (supposing that one is suffering from the condition for a long period of time). Some dietary requirements include a variety of fruits and vegetables, whole grains and low-fat foods; and avoidance of trans-fats, salty foods, beverages with added sugars, and high-fat dairy products. In essence, lifestyle modifications relate to such changes as improved diet based on fruits and vegetables, quitting smoking, and reduced alcohol consumption. Patients should also be encouraged to remodel their day-to-day life to avoid any relapse of metabolic syndrome. "Remodeling" techniques include keeping a stress diary, a dietary log, a medication chart, and adjusting one's sleep schedule.[242]

VITAMIN D INTAKE

Studies have shown an inverse link between vitamin D3 insufficiency, cardiovascular disease and metabolic syndrome. This means that reduced exposure to the sun can also contribute to the condition. Low vitamin D3 has also been connected to parathyroid hormone, which is associated with the insulin resistance in the condition.

Research has also established that a patient who isn't exposed regularly to the sun will have higher cholesterol levels than a person who receives sufficient vitamin D3. The best sources of vitamin D include fish, milk, egg yolks, cream butter, liver, and other fortified foods such as cereals.[243]

23

Exercises for Metabolic Syndrome

METABOLIC SYNDROME is an increasingly common issue worldwide, a trend that is expected to mushroom as people continue their sedentary lifestyles. Luckily, the condition can be controlled, in part, by physical workouts. Studies have shown that exercise affords the most benefits for metabolic syndrome sufferers, as it can actually control the condition and prevent future medical dilemmas. Losing just 5 percent to 10 percent of one's body weight can influence metabolic syndrome considerably and quickly improve one's overall health.[244]

ADVANTAGES OF EXERCISE

Exercise helps improve blood circulation to all body parts, which helps in flushing out harmful waste through sweat. Apart from simple body movement, people can prevent metabolic syndrome (to a certain extent) by working out at a local gym or beginning a regular exercise program at home. The body requires a variety of movements and exercise types to develop normally, and a deficiency in this area can result in serious health damage in the long run. People should seek to practice an active lifestyle if they hope to remain free of the conditions associated with metabolic syndrome.[245]

Lack of exercise is also a risk factor, due to its effect on how the body processes extra calories. In addition, participating in exercise will increase one's insulin sensitivity, which will improve the regulation of glucose. Physical training stimulates the removal of fatty acids from the blood and bolsters liver efficiency, thereby enhancing insulin and glucose as well.[246]

Exercise can also increase blood flow in the body, reduce the risk of chronic conditions, prevent heart disease, and improve muscle tone. For those not sure of how to begin a workout regimen, a doctor or personal trainer can prescribe clinically approved exercise sequences for any number of situations. Metabolic syndrome sufferers may struggle to adopt or follow a workout regimen, and can often fall off the diet bandwagon, ending up heavier than when they started. For this reason, trainers will oftentimes start an obese patient on a simple program to promote initial weight loss to show early results and build confidence. However, weight loss theories vary from person to person, and there are those who claim that a graduated weight loss project may lead to motivational collapse. While the following sections emphasize a few of the top exercises recommended for metabolic syndrome, check with a licensed healthcare professional before starting any intensive workout program.[247]

RECOMMENDED EXERCISES

Among the most popular drills to help with metabolic syndrome are high-intensity workouts. These routines elicit a specific type of energy production in the body and are exceedingly specialized to ensure weight loss and fitness. Basically, these workouts consist of alternating periods of high-intensity workouts with low-intensity workouts. This ensures that you have alternating workout and rest periods, and it helps people stick to a rote workout. The high intensity intervals raise the heart rate while the recovery periods allow the heart to relax and prepare itself for another vigorous workout. The whole program usually has a few different routines to exercise different body parts at varying exercise levels.[248]

Although there are doctors who don't endorse high intensity workouts, the technique is very effective. Some routines take only 10–15 minutes each. The practice also reduces body cortisol levels, eases inflammation, and lets the exerciser lose weight evenly. The person's metabolism also continues to burn fat for up to 36 hours following a workout.[249]

Interval training is also very effective at triggering weight loss, resulting in a toned body. Clinical studies show that exercising at a moderate pace daily for 45 minutes to 90 minutes can lead to brisk weight loss. However, this also means it's necessary to implement mottled exercise habits. For example, trainers recommend at least two and a half hours of physical activity per week, consisting of 15-minute rounds, such as playing doubles tennis, two hours of jogging, two hours of **calisthenics**, and so forth. Other exercise routines that may be added to the overall regimen include swimming, dancing, skiing, and playing ball games. This varied regimen ensures that the routine doesn't get boring and people don't get lose motivation during the workout.[250]

Concerning combo techniques, doctors often recommend a variety of various forms of yoga to assist in managing mental stress, along with cardiovascular techniques to control body weight. A BMI of less than 25 is ideal for losing weight and getting toned. Studies have shown that a combination of vigorous activity along with dietary control and lifestyle changes can easily offer a preferential level of health. This is directly in contrast to any kind of moderate activity. For example, men and women who train vigorously for two to three hours weekly can lose much more weight than people who walk at temperate speeds for two to three hours daily.[251]

SETTING UP THE PERFECT WORKOUT ROUTINE

The following are some tips for constructing the perfect workout:

- Meet with a professional trainer to get expert help on how to set up a correct workout routine. High intensity exercises in particular are very strenuous on the body, and an improperly organized workout may cause muscle strains and tears that will take a long time to recover.[252]
- People should never go into any workouts cold—unless they have an appetite for muscle pains and soreness the next day. The

best way to warm up is to run through the same exercises you'll be doing during the routine, but at a very slow speed.[253]

- It is paramount to choose different exercises to use in the routine. For example, a lower body workout can be constructed by jogging in place, while adding lunges, squats, mountain climbers, and toe raisers to the routine. An upper body workout can be done by adding push-ups, shoulder presses, and lateral and anterior arm lifts to the workout pattern. It's also possible to add crunches, lateral crunches, shin slaps, and leg swings. You should perform each of these routines for three rounds, and then start a slower routine. This produces a high-low process that's best suited for toning muscles.[254]
- For those who are not inclined to exercise, it can be helpful to combine walking and running to mix up the variety of exercise even further. You can open the routine with a warm up, then intersperse their walking with a jog, or even a full-on run. Incorporating a range of exercise in this regard will ensure much faster weight loss and muscle toning.[255]
- Health experts frequently recommend the use of a timer with an alarm to make certain that the workout regimen is correctly completed. Depending on the type of routine, using a timer to pace the routine and spread it out over a period of time will ensure a fortified workout.[256]
- It is advisable to spread out recovery practices during the workout process. If your muscles are training for the first time, they may not be used to strenuous routines. Adding a recovery period between workouts leads to a better, safer workout experience. These can be as simple as skipping rope for 30 seconds after each workout routine.[257]
- One very important thing to remember is that exercise is often draining and it will make any dieter ravenously hungry. You should try to eat sensibly before and immediately after a work-

out. Trainers can provide an optimized nutritional schedule, or a nutritionist could be hired to aid in planning a diet. This is necessary, as most people tend to overeat just after their routine, negating all the benefits of their gym session. To counteract overeating, some dieticians suggest charging up with a light protein bar and then having a smoothie to provide energy replenishment, without adding unnecessary calories.[258]

Know that the disorder can be controlled with diet, exercise, and lifestyle changes. With a disciplined exercise blueprint, you can reduce the risk of type-2 diabetes enormously. However, it is also a good idea to check with a doctor and a physical trainer prior to getting on board with any extensive routine.[259]

24

Medicinal Approaches

IN TERMS of a pharmacological approach to metabolic syndrome, any discussion must begin with insulin. Artificial insulin has been a pharmacological windfall for diabetes patients, and it is often prescribed for patients with type-2 diabetes. Its main purpose is to control the levels of glucose or sugar in the blood, something that a person with diabetes (and oftentimes metabolic syndrome) is unable to do without medication. The hormone insulin aids in processing glucose or sugar from food, and moving it to the cells from the bloodstream. Glucose stored in the cells can then be turned into fuel for energy. Insulin prescribed to diabetics replaces the natural insulin in your organs and supports the uptake of sugars.[260]

MEDICINAL TREATMENT OF DIABETES

Insulin comes as a liquid shot, and is injected subcutaneously (under the skin) so that it can enter the bloodstream. It is usually prescribed once other recommended therapies such as a low-glucose diet or weight reduction fail. In some cases, the doctor might prescribe more than one form of insulin for you to use. Insulin carries certain side effects, such as headaches, hypoglycemia, skin itching, rashes, and symptoms similar to the flu. Mild symptoms include redness and minor bruising at the injection site.[261]

Oral medications for diabetes are meant to stimulate the pancreas into manufacturing insulin on its own, and are usually prescribed for patients with type-2 diabetes. Medications such as sulfonylureas work on the pancreas by blocking **adenosine triphosphate** (**ATP**) and potassium, reducing the penetrability of the beta cells to potassium. This results in the admission of calcium into the cells of the pancreas, which is then stimulated to increase the production of insulin. These medications may cause headaches, weight gain, abdominal pain, hypersensitivity, and long-term weight gain.[262]

MEDICINAL TREATMENT OF HYPERTENSION

Diuretics are customarily prescribed to jettison excess sodium from the blood of hypertensive patients with metabolic syndrome. These medications increase the amount of water and salt in the urine, allowing more of these substances to be eliminated naturally. Excess sodium in the blood can increase fluid buildup in the blood vessels, making it difficult for the body to pump blood. This, in turn, increases blood pressure. By reducing the level of sodium in the body, diuretics help lower blood pressure. These drugs also carry certain side effects, such as frequent urination, fatigue, weakness, **arrhythmias**, dizziness, muscle cramps, and electrolyte imbalances.[263]

Beta blockers (also known as beta-adrenergic blocking agents) help control high blood pressure by reducing the potency of epinephrine or adrenaline. Beta blockers slow heart rate so the beats are at a slower pace, thus reducing blood pressure. These capsules also improve blood flow by relaxing the blood vessels.[264] Aside from reducing blood pressure to a certain extent, beta blockers also help treat or prevent other conditions, including angina, irregular heart rhythm, migraines, heart attack, and heart failure. Side effects may be experienced by metabolic syndrome patients taking these medications, such as headaches, dizziness, cold hands, stomach upset, diarrhea, constipation, insomnia, depression, shortness of breath, or fatigue.[265]

Alpha blockers, on the other hand, relax specific muscles to keep small blood vessels open. This allows blood to flow more smoothly, thus easing blood pressure. This is done by keeping the norepinephrine and noradrenaline hormones from triggering the muscle walls of the veins and arteries, which causes contraction of blood vessels.

These medications are also used to treat other conditions involving the circulatory system, tumors of the adrenal gland, and enlarged prostate. Two common alpha blockers used to treat hypertension are doxazosin and prazosin.[266] Ironically, alpha blockers may result in low blood pressure for first-time users, a disorder that may also cause dizziness, especially when getting up after lying or sitting down. These side effects can be minimized by taking the first dose before bedtime. Alpha blockers may also cause headaches, increased or forceful heartbeat, nausea, and weight gain. They may also react with certain types of medications, including **calcium channel blockers**, beta blockers, and drugs to treat erectile dysfunction.[267]

MEDICINAL TREATMENT OF HEART DISEASE

When approaching heart disease pharmacologically, metabolic syndrome patients should keep in mind that angiotensin-converting-enzyme (ACE) inhibitors address the issue of narrow blood vessels by inhibiting the action of a chemical known as angiotensin II. This chemical triggers the contraction of the muscles surrounding the blood vessels, causing these vessels to tighten up. That in turn leads to raised blood pressure. By blocking the bustle of angiotensin II, ACE inhibitors help regulate blood pressure and allow the heart to pump blood more easily.[268]

Aside from heart disease and hypertension, ACE inhibitors are also prescribed to treat chronic kidney disease and diabetic kidney disease. They may also be prescribed to a patient after a heart attack. Some of the most common side effects include low blood pressure, dizziness, diarrhea, drowsiness, and dry cough. Some patients may also experience swelling of the eyes, tongue, or lips, and dysfunction of the kidneys.[269]

Aldosterone receptor antagonists are prescribed to reduce the risk of heart failure. These belong to a group of drugs known as diuretics, which aid the body in eliminating excess fluids. The antagonist drugs slow aldosterone, a hormone that controls the secretion of potassium. This action allows these medications to aid in lowering blood pressure and reducing heart congestion, thus protecting the heart. These drugs are very effective in treating advanced cases of heart failure.[270] Due to their effects, these antagonists increase the presence of potassium throughout your body and can affect the role of the kidneys. As a result, patients who take these medications are often advised to undergo blood tests regularly and to have their kidney function monitored. Older medications of this form may also cause breast tenderness or enlargement in men.[271]

Calcium channel blockers are used to treat high blood pressure and chest pain (angina). They work by preventing calcium from being absorbed by the cells in the walls of the blood vessels and in the heart. When this happens, blood vessels widen and relax, allowing blood to flow more smoothly. Calcium channel blockers can also help reduce heart rate, thus relieving chest pain and arrhythmias. Calcium channel blockers have certain side effects, including dizziness, nausea, fatigue, **edema** of the lower extremities, headache, rapid heartbeat, and skin rash. Some types of calcium channel blockers may also have adverse reactions when mixed with products containing grapefruit.[272]

MEDICINAL TREATMENT OF OBESITY AND ABDOMINAL FAT

Appetite suppressants used for treating obesity in metabolic syndrome patients are known as anorectics. They are classified as noradrenergic drugs and **selective serotonin reuptake inhibitors (SSRIs)**. Noradrenergic drugs quell the feeling of hunger and are taken before meals. These medications work by directing the adrenal glands to produce epinephrine and norepinephrine, two hormones that obstruct the hunger signal on its way from the brain to the rest of the body. As a result, a person doesn't feel as hungry as he normally would and will eat less.

Serotonin reuptake inhibitors, on the other hand, reduce the concentrations of serotonin—a chemical in the brain that affects food cravings—in the non-cellular, liquid part of the bloodstream. These drugs are called "reuptake inhibitors" because serotonin is normally a hormone that gets secreted by the same cells that later remove it from the body.[273]

These medications produce the feeling of fullness and satiety even if the stomach isn't physically full. In the end, individuals using these anti-obesity medications eat less and begin to lose weight over time. Appetite suppressants are generally taken orally. They may cause headaches, nausea, dizziness, dry mouth, fatigue, constipation, or stomach upset, especially during initial use. Additionally, these medications may cause serious side effects, such as chest aches, trouble breathing, changes in mood, swelling, and a throbbing heart (palpitations).[274]

Lipase inhibitors "take the edge off" of **lipases** when fat is ingested into the body. These medications reduce the total amount of fats absorbed by the gastrointestinal system and bind with fat in the intestines to prevent it from being absorbed into the bloodstream altogether. Some of the most common side effects of lipase inhibitors include abdominal cramping, incontinence, and abnormal bowel movements. Lipase inhibitors may also make it difficult for the body to absorb fat-soluble vitamins. Side effects tend to be minor and are temporary, although they may worsen with ingestion of fatty diets.[275]

In short, metabolic syndrome patients may already be on prescription drugs to control **hypertension** and diabetes. Everyone should be aware that certain medications in these groups like SSRIs sometimes cause weight gain instead of controlling it, an internecine reality of metabolic syndrome treatment. Note that these medication regimens are usually not needed, and can be replaced with other effective medications.[276]

25

Surgery and Metabolic Syndrome

MANY PATIENTS with severe metabolic syndrome elect to undergo bariatric surgery to streamline their condition. This involves surgically altering the stomach, intestine, or both to artificially create weight loss, particularly in the abdominal area of the body. Globally, thousands of bariatric surgical procedures are conducted on people with metabolic syndrome every year. Progression of the much safer **laparoscopic** strategies has made surgical treatment widely accepted. Laparoscopic manipulation is also called minimally invasive surgery.[277]

WHEN SURGERY IS NECESSARY

To be eligible for bariatric surgery, patients typically meet the following requirements:[278]

- Have a body mass index (BMI) of greater than 40 kg/m^2, or else a BMI in excess of 35 kg/m^2 with a severe terminal problem such as diabetes or a high-risk **lipid profile**
- Have tolerable operative risk
- Have unsuccessfully attempted almost all practical nonsurgical approaches to lose weight and control obesity-associated symptoms

While not all surgeons agree, there is some evidence to suggest that surgery is appropriate for sufferers with a BMI of 30 to 35, so long as long-term issues are limited.

Factors which may prohibit surgery often include:[279]

- A related psychiatric disorder
- Current alcohol or drug abuse
- Cancer which is not currently in remission
- Any other critical, life-threatening disorder

THE PROCESS

Most of the procedures are carried out using narrow tubes, which result in less pain and a reduced healing period, compared to those of open surgery. Conventionally, the surgery itself is categorized as malabsorptive or restrictive, referring to the intended mechanism of weight loss. Restrictive operations reduce stomach size, thus restricting the amount of the food held there. Malabsorptive surgery builds a direct connection between the small intestine and the stomach. This partially blocks off absorption of nutrients and calories. Even so, other elements seem to promote weight loss. For instance, roux-en-y gastric bypass (abbreviated RYGB and generally categorized as malabsorptive) and sleeve gastrectomy (typically classified as restrictive) both lead to metabolic or hormonal changes that support fullness, as well as weight loss and hormonal alterations.[280] Examples include an increase in insulin release that speeds up the regression of your diabetes.

ROUX-EN-Y GASTRIC BYPASS SURGERY

After RYGB or sleeve gastrectomy, levels of certain hormones such as "peptide-yy" and **glucagon-like peptide-1** are amplified, possibly resulting in satiety, weight loss, and remission of sugar levels. Improved insulin sensitivity is noticeable immediately following surgery, and it is only a short time before substantial weight loss is observed, thus suggesting that **neurohormonal** (neurological and hormonal) factors are dominant in reduction of diabetes.[281]

Roux-en-y gastric bypass surgery accounts for approximately 80 percent of weight loss procedures and is typically carried out laparoscopically. A portion of the inner abdomen is removed from the rest of the stomach, forming a belly pouch. Additionally, food bypasses a portion of the stomach and small intestine, where it is usually absorbed, minimizing the quantity of food and calories metabolized. The stomach pouch is affixed to the first part of the small intestine, reducing the rate of the stomach's emptying.[282]

The section of small intestine pegged with the bypassed stomach is also connected to the final part of the small intestine. This system enables **bile** acids as well as pancreatic enzymes to blend with gut contents, offsetting malabsorption and nutritional inadequacies. Roux-en-y gastric bypass is especially helpful in treating severe metabolic concerns and diabetes; remission rates are as much as 62 percent after six years.[283]

For most patients who have undergone RYGB, consuming high-fat and also high-sugar foods could cause "dumping syndrome," symptoms of which may include lightheadedness, abdominal pain, profound sweating, nausea, and diarrhea. Dumping syndrome could reduce the rate of metabolism of such foods.[284]

SLEEVE GASTRECTOMY

Historically, sleeve gastrectomy, another form of minimally invasive surgery, has been suggested only if patients are found to be at too high a risk for operations like RYGB. It may also be suggested for patients with a BMI over 60, even if another comparable procedure is performed. Even so, since sleeve gastrectomy brings about sustained weight loss, it has found increased use as the ideal treatment for long-term obesity. A portion of the stomach is taken out, creating a tubular stomach passage. There are no anatomic alterations to the small intestine, though there may be adjustable gastric banding. Even though weight loss surgery is conventionally categorized as a restrictive operation, it is also associated with **neurohormonal** fluctuations. The most severe problem is gastric leakage at the suture line, but that only makes up a piddling percentage of complications.[285]

ADJUSTABLE GASTRIC BANDING

Usage of adjustable gastric bands has largely subsided in America, though it is still a possible option. During this procedure, a band is placed around the top part of the stomach to split the stomach into a smaller upper pouch and a greater lower pouch. Usually, the band itself is attuned by injecting saline into it by means of a port that's positioned beneath the skin. Once saline is infused, the band broadens, limiting the top pouch of the belly. As a consequence, the pouch holds a lot less food, causing patients to eat more gradually, with fullness occurring earlier. This technique is normally carried out laparoscopically. Saline can also be removed from the band in case complications arise or the band is excessively limiting. Furthermore, weight loss with the band can vary and is linked to the frequency of follow-up. More consistent check-ups lead to better weight loss rates. Even though postoperative mortality happens much less often than in individuals who decide on RYGB, long term complications, and even the need for repeat surgeries are possible.[286]

BILIOPANCREATIC REDIRECTION

Biliopancreatic diversion is a procedure where a part of the gut is taken away, resulting in limitations in metabolism. The remaining portion empties into the duodenum. The duodenum is shortened and connected to the ileum, bypassing much of the small intestine, including the intersection (the sphincter of Oddi) through which bile (as well as pancreatic enzymes) enters. The point of all this is the declination of food absorption. This process is logistically challenging but can occasionally be carried out laparoscopically. Sadly, malabsorption and nutritional inadequacies can develop after the operation.[287]

VERTICAL BANDED GASTROPLASTY

Vertical banded gastroplasty isn't viewed highly as a medical alternative, because complication rates are high and the resultant weight loss is meager. For this process, a stapler is employed to split the stomach into a smaller upper pouch and a bigger lower pouch. A nonexpandable plastic band is positioned around the opening where the top pouch evacuates material into the lower pouch.[288]

PREOPERATIVE ASSESSMENT

For all of these surgeries, preoperative evaluation includes assessing and fixing possible complications as much as possible, evaluating readiness and capability to engage in lifestyle adjustment, and eliminating issues preventing post-operative healing. All patients need to be examined by a dietician to assess a postoperative diet as well as to determine their fitness to make required changes in lifestyle. Patients may also be inspected by a psychologist or other competent mental health care consultant to detect any complicating psychiatric disorder or any dependencies that disqualify surgery. They will also work to address upcoming postsurgical barriers. Preoperative evaluation isn't always necessary, but it might be recommended depending on clinical investigations and the approach taken to manage additional conditions.[289]

There are many types of surgical procedures used for treating metabolic syndrome and its associated conditions. Depending on your health and overall condition, diagnoses of metabolic syndrome may be accompanied by surgical recommendations. Patients are required to adhere to particular restrictions, and to visit their physician on a regular basis once surgery is complete.[290]

26

Addressing the Genetics

METABOLIC SYNDROME is among the fastest growing health-related problem for specific gene pools. Experts have determined that it poses as a major risk factor for various cardiovascular diseases as well as diabetes mellitus. Metabolic syndrome can be considered to be the interaction of both genetic and environmental factors with all major risk factors of the syndrome being strongly inherited. In a number of genes, the common genetic variations increase the predisposition to metabolic syndrome. These genetic variations interact with other genes and certain environmental factors to develop the disorder.[291]

The genes that code for optimal storage of fats and energy during fasting tend to contribute the most to the observable characteristics (phenotype) of metabolic syndrome. In certain people, variations of these genes influence the metabolism of fat, sugar, and other associated environmental reasons, increasing vulnerability to the syndrome. Moreover, three groups are said to be prone to metabolic syndrome: people who are diabetic, heart attack survivors, and hypertensive patients.[292]

ROLE OF GENETICS IN DIABETES

Metabolic syndrome experts believe that genetics plays a significant role in developing type-1 and type-2 diabetes, both universally accepted as chronic conditions that are increasingly affecting millions around the world. Generally, the risk of developing diabetes is affected by whether a person's parents or siblings have it. The possibilities of developing either of the diabetes types may differ accordingly. For instance, if both parents have type-1 diabetes, there is an increased risk of developing diabetes. With type-2 diabetes the average increase in the percentage of the risk is much higher, especially where both parents are forced to live with the disease.[293]

Some forms of diabetes such as the maturity-onset diabetes of the young (MODY), and those that bud from **mitochondrial** transfiguration of DNA, are directly inherited, meaning that genes are forwarded from one generation to another. If you have resounding genetic susceptibility, you have a higher risk of developing diabetes. However, there are other genes that provide a higher level of immune tolerance for those who are non-diabetic. Certain hereditary conditions such as those characterized by muscle decay, heart defects, or cataracts may develop diabetes.[294]

ROLE OF GENETICS IN HYPERTENSION

Hypertension is responsible for millions of deaths each year. Studies suggest that hypertension develops from a rather complex interrelation between genetics and environmental lifestyles, such as excessive alcohol intake, dietary sodium (salt) intake, and body weight. Several genes with hypertensive traits have been detected over the years, leading investigators to look for the true roles that genetics plays in hypertension. In fact, experts believe that there's much similarity in blood pressure within families (as opposed to amid families)—a hypothesis that hints at some level of inheritance. A small gene mutation can cause hereditary forms of blood pressure. These gene mutations affect blood pressure by altering the ability of the kidney to handle salt content.[295]

ROLE OF GENETICS IN HEART DISEASE

Genetic factors are considered to play some role in heart diseases, high blood pressure, as well as other cardiovascular problems. However, it's also possible that people with a history of heart disease share common environmental risk factors, which tend to increase their risks of contracting heart disease. If genetic factors are combined with an unhealthy lifestyle, the risk of heart disease intensifies. Genetic disorders such as **familial hypercholesterolemia**, which causes imbalanced levels of cholesterol, are associated with high risks of premature heart attacks. Such disorders usually present at birth. Therefore, early genetic examination of such disorders can help in reducing the risk of developing heart diseases.[296]

ROLE OF GENETICS IN BODY FAT

Recent scientific studies indicate that obesity has reached epidemic levels, especially in environments where there is physical inactivity as well as increased intake of high-calorie foods. A variation in people's responses to certain environments links genetics to the development of obesity. So, how does genetics influence fat content? Primarily, genes are responsible for meting out "instructions" on how to respond to certain environmental factors. Studies among twins, family members, and adopted families indicate that variation in weight is due to genetic factors. In most cases, obesity results from interaction among a number of genes and environmental factors.[297]

All in all, metabolic syndrome is a condition closely connected to the interaction between genetic and situational factors. Individuals predisposed to this disorder include diabetics, high blood pressure patients, and heart attack survivors. Studies have also linked genetics to other issues such as hypertension, diabetes, and obesity.[298]

27

Addressing the Mind

METABOLIC SYNDROME is a health disorder that occurs when a host of other ailments combine; however, what is often overlooked are the mental and emotional difficulties that can arise leading up to, and stemming from, this syndrome. Diseases, sicknesses and disabilities result in not only physical hardships, but also psychological and emotional stress. Individuals struggling with debilitating conditions are emotionally and mentally strained, which makes their overall outlook in life bleak. The feeling of being a lifelong patient can have a devastating effect on one's mental health which, if left untreated, can lead to hot-potato psychological concerns, depression, and an ultimate loss of interest in life.[299] This chapter will discuss some of the common mental woes that occur when an individual is battling metabolic syndrome.[300]

BIPOLAR DISORDER

Bipolar disorder is a condition that causes your mind to swing between bouts of depression to extreme bliss, and vice versa. A person with metabolic syndrome can wake up very happy in the morning, but after some time, their mood suddenly declines toward despondency. Neither you nor an outside observer can explain the sudden change of mood. Bipolar disorder removes all control of one's own emotions; moreover, metabolic syndrome exacerbates the temperament, and cases range from mild to severe.[301]

People with metabolic syndrome often suffer from sadness after they learn that medication can't cure them of their persistent medical issues. Patients will begin to dwell on events of the past and present, while trying to either avoid or plan out their future. During this period, some of the things people said or did before take hold of your mind. When reliving happy moments, for example, a bipolar patient will become overjoyed, and their mood will lighten up; however, as they try to avoid thinking of sad or painful times in their history, their mood will dramatically darken, leading to a period of depression. Bipolar patients will also experience irritability during those periods when they are rocking back and forth between happiness and sadness, often for no clear reason.[302] Managing bipolar tendencies can present a real challenge to family members and caretakers. Without proper knowledge and skill, mood swings can take an emotional toll on those who care for them, as well. Continuance of metabolic syndrome can trigger bipolar disorders as well, as the syndrome affects your self-esteem and confidence.[303]

SCHIZOPHRENIA

Schizophrenia is another disorder that's sometimes observed in people with metabolic syndrome. In general, this psychiatric illness makes it difficult for a person to differentiate between reality and fantasy. Schizophrenia also confuses one's emotional responses; patients find it difficult to determine proper reactions to situations, crying at funny moments and laughing at sad moments. These patients may also find it challenging to act within the confines of social norms, a condition that gives way to sheepishness. Schizophrenia can cause you to hallucinate, develop inaccurate beliefs and delusions, as well as foster confusion throughout. Most schizophrenics see the whole world as conspiring to be critical of them, making it increasingly difficult to relate with others. This is compounded in the case of metabolic syndrome sufferers by the persistent belief that they can no longer live a normal life.[304] Patients with schizophrenia and metabolic syndrome will find that the latter condition can severely aggravate the former.[305]

DEPRESSION

Most people experience depression now and again, and for a range of reasons. The reasons may include the loss of a loved one, loss of a job, family breakups, financial troubles, insecurity, and many more. Depression can lead to premature death, especially if a patient reaches a point where he is considering suicide. To combat depression, mental health professionals work against depression-related issues so that patients can constructively defend against their immediate and forthcoming problems. In some cases, clients with severe depression decide to terminate their lives, as opposed to living with the reality of the syndrome. Therefore, caretakers of patients suffering from metabolic syndrome should try to motivate and encourage depressed individuals to look at life constructively. Although drugs cannot cure depression, patients often do recover after accepting counseling and therapy.[306]

If depression occurs as a result of metabolic syndrome, the situation can quickly become serious. Depression causes a barrage of health conditions, such as hormonal imbalances. Patients with metabolic disorders normally face depression, especially after they see the test results. The head-scratching confusion, belligerence, dissension, and pain that come with the realization hit many patients hard; some don't recover fully. Depression, like many other disorders, can vary in intensity, but the effects can persist indefinitely. Metabolic disorder can spread throughout the body, with even the healthy parts acquiring complications with time. Such happenings can sometimes cause patients to lose hope or faith, and their bearing toward life transmutes wholly.[307]

ANXIETY

Medical research confirms that the medical connections between anxiety and metabolic syndrome don't exist, but patients may still experience extreme worry during treatment. Since psychiatric medicine is more than just a science, you should know that anxiety is a mental state whereby a person lives in constant fear. The apex of that fear results in a state whereby normal mental functions are hindered. When anxiety kicks in, patients avoid doing things they used to do, simply for fear of the unknown. Metabolic syndrome might aggravate anxiety indirectly, as patients begin to fear that they may not live long enough. When such thoughts start crossing their minds, their ambitions topple, as does their overall productivity. Anxious patients exhibit signs such as obsession, phobia, social anxiety, and inferiority complexes. Post-traumatic disorders also present in patients with long-term illnesses, as they keep replaying the traumas they went through in the past. Such thoughts make it increasingly difficult for people to carry on with their lives. As the metabolic disorder advances, apprehensive patients lose themselves more and more. However, people can manage and bring anxiety under control using therapy and counseling. A patient suffering from an anxiety disorder may require a person to serve as a confidant from time to time. Reassuring the patient, making him feel secure and valued, does help to counter anxiety.[308]

BEHAVIORAL DISORDERS

In general, a behavioral disorder is a mental disorder whereby a person starts acting and behaving strangely. The issue can begin during a person's early years, and most cases occur in response to a specific event in a person's life. In this case (when they realize they suffer from metabolic syndrome), they tend to display some unusual behavioral disorders such as obsessive-compulsive disorder (OCD) and attention deficit hyperactivity disorder (ADHD).[309]

RECOMMENDATIONS

As far as the management of mental disability is concerned, metabolic syndrome patients should make a note of the fact that people can help patients, by showing compassion and understanding. They need to come to understand that it isn't a battle they need to fight alone. Various techniques and approaches have worked before, and are still effective now. One way people can assist patients is by providing guidance and counseling. Mentally ill patients require counseling sessions that can free them from the negative effects of their dark thinking. Avoid dwelling too much on your situation to reduce the intensity of these problems. Secondly, people can engage patients with mental disorders in activities that occupy their minds and keep them busy. If you stay active all day, depression and anxiety may well be eased. Favorable methods to staying active include speed-walking, running, and low-intensity exercise routines.[310]

When a person who has metabolic syndrome feels accepted, he can live and manage whatever obstacles he may encounter. In cases where the situation persists, seeking authoritative medical assistance from professionals in the medical field is recommended. Such professionals include psychologists, counselors, as well as other professionals who provide alternative mental therapies such as art therapy, music therapy, and wilderness therapy.[311]

28

Addressing the Pain

THE COMBINED health conditions that make up metabolic syndrome cause pain throughout the affected systems in the body. This chapter discusses some of the more common pains associated with the syndrome, along with effective means of alleviating that pain.[312]

HEADACHES

Patients may experience piercing headaches from time to time, and while there aren't any concrete reasons behind headaches, no one experiences headaches and migraines without some cause. A hectic schedule, the stress of long-distance travel, even prolonged reading can result in a headache. Still, some people do experience headaches without any obvious cause; these headaches could be a sign of developing metabolic syndrome. When patients contract metabolic syndrome for the first time, the brain becomes aware that something isn't right. On detecting the problem, it hurls signals to the body in the form of headaches. The headache may start as severe, and may develop into a minor migraine later.[313]

Patients experience headaches when there are hormonal imbalances in the body. With hormonal disparity, the body doesn't function normally and this failure to operate eventually leads to pain. The headaches could range from mild, especially during the early stages, to severe, as metabolic syndrome advances. Patients are subjected to headaches because of conditions such as stress, hormonal imbalance, low supply of blood to the head, and so forth.

Initially, simple over-the-counter medications such as painkillers will normally eliminate the headaches, but as metabolic syndrome progresses, the medications will stop working. Therefore, without identifying the actual problem and its origin, headaches can progress, and in worst cases, they can cause mortality. In essence, people who have metabolic syndrome should seek medical attention whenever they experience painful, regular headaches.[314]

FIBROMYALGIA-RELATED PAIN

Fibromyalgia affects mostly women, and expresses itself through retroactive pain, insomnia, and fatigue. This condition is known to accompany metabolic syndrome, and it occurs due to either excess body fat or lack of physical activity. Lack of movement combined with overeating or consumption of unhealthy foods will cause obesity, and as that fat accumulates around the abdomen and the waist, fibromyalgia slowly develops. As the days go by and the woman continues her sedentary lifestyle, pain starts developing, from mild to intense. The pain then advances from forceful to chronic, and from there, she may live with the pain indefinitely, as the pain goes on to affect other, healthier regions. Pregabalin and milnacipran HCI are a couple of medication options for fibromyalgia-induced pain.[315]

STOMACH AND ABDOMINAL PAIN

Stomach pain affects both men and women suffering from metabolic syndrome. The pain clasps the belly region due to inflammations in the intestines. Some foods and drinks may perforate the intestines over time because of the food's chemical content. This inflammation can cause metabolic syndrome, and when the belly develops tenderness, the first symptom is pain. Initially, the pain may seem normal, and over-the-counter drugs may treat it. However, as the root of the problem lurks unmediated, the pain continues, advancing to a point where you cannot eat anymore. People who experience stomach pain as a result of metabolic syndrome need robust treatment plans that focus on the main cause of the pain itself.[316]

Individuals who have metabolic syndrome may experience abdominal pains at some point in their life, although research has yet to determine whether the syndrome is directly related to stomach pain. Abdominal or stomach pains lurk about as a result of some negative stimulus associated with certain foods or drinks, and the illness of the internal organ of the body. For instance, if you ingest a certain type of food that you are allergic to, or have a sensitivity to, this causes harm to the stomach, which is relayed through to the rest of the body as stomach pains. The negative connection between foods eaten and the internal organs of the body occurs due to an imbalance of the bodily functions. If a patient starts experiencing stomach pains frequently, he should seek immediate medical treatment. Using over-the-counter medications to treat the pain only leads to additional ill effects, as the drugs may not be addressing the underlying causes. In addition, the drugs may affect other tissues and cause irreparable damage to other body parts in the process.[317]

INSULIN-RELATED PAIN

Metabolic syndrome can cause either high or low production of insulin. When insulin increases, part of it remains unused. That excess insulin then damages the walls of the arteries, leaving you in pain. The body may begin to resist the insulin, and when that happens, all the insulin then starts damaging the other delicate tissues in the body. Excess insulin also affects the kidneys, as it leads to a loss in the excretion of salt by the kidneys. If the kidneys do not excrete the required amount of salt, that salt affects the kidneys and hinders its functionality and ability to flush waste out from the body. The waste and harmful toxins try to find a way out of the body, and by so doing, they affect the other healthy parts. The reaction between the toxins and the other body parts manifests itself through pain, which is how doctors detect problems in the kidneys. Kidney failure or similar complications cause a lot of pain as the accumulated toxin passes through as poisons, dealing irreparable damage. Ways to avoid these issues include stringent regulation of blood pressure, quitting smoking, and control of **lipids**. [318]

JOINT PAIN

People with metabolic syndrome often complain of pain in the joints, especially in the wrists, ankles, feet, and hands. Furthermore, serious pain in the joints which is painful enough to cause a patient difficulty when moving mostly occurs due to high levels of sugar in the blood, one of the factors common in metabolic syndrome sufferers. Joint pain can begin by affecting an individual limb, or it can start by affecting both hands and feet at the same time. People with these aches face difficulties when going about their daily lives. Gout and other illnesses start developing early, or as soon as a person starts consuming foods with high cholesterol. Moreover, patients can live with the disease for many years without their knowledge of it, only to see the pain suddenly jump in severity. Joint pains might subside after using some medications, but even after other symptoms go away, the pain often still lingers. You can address joint pain related to metabolic syndrome with salt soaks, lubrication of the joints with olive oil rubs, and non-weight–bearing exercises (such as swimming).[319]

CHEST PAIN

When a person develops metabolic syndrome, after some time he will experience chest pains and breathing trouble. Chest cramps sometimes occur from hypertension. When the pressure of the heart is bolstered, the body works overtime, trying to deal with the tension. Due to the extra exertion, patients start experiencing trouble breathing, and the extra respiratory effort creates pain in the chest as a result. At this point, you may even acquire asthmatic conditions.[320]

DEALING WITH PAIN AT ITS SOURCE

However, patients can deal with the pain and still enjoy life, regardless of the extent of the syndrome. Metabolic syndrome sufferers looking to live a pain-free life should immediately avoid consuming foods that aggravate the disorder. When they cease eating unhealthy foods, the progression of the condition is restricted and the drugs can work unhindered. Secondly, patients should halt their usage of substances that accelerate pain. For instance, if people stop smoking and drinking alcohol excessively, they can deal with the pains associated with the syndrome before engaging medical professionals. Thirdly, patients with excess body fat should engage in physical exercises regularly to control their weight. Maintaining a normal weight helps to prevent and curb pain. Fourthly, if the pain persists even after practicing healthy lifestyle habits, patients should take prescribed medications to address the pain. Nevertheless, sufferers must first undergo blood tests, x-rays (if bone damage is involved), and cardiac stress tests, so that they can use the correct pain drugs, best suited to their condition.[321]

To summarize, metabolic syndrome patients must understand that pain and metabolic syndrome go hand-in-hand, as the contributing factors of the syndrome affect the body. Metabolic syndrome shouldn't stop anyone from going on with life, and patients should remember that a good diet and regular exercise help in the general health of a person. In addition, regular medical examinations help when attempting to snip the syndrome in the bud.[322]

PART V
Homestretch

29

Collective Efforts

METABOLIC SYNDROME affects the lives of people all over the world. Both the sick and the otherwise affected require access to certain resources in order to manage their condition. Yet with modern advancements in technology and medicine, people today can prevent the syndrome. They simply require the necessary information and direction of resources, something that is best managed by the chief administrative body; in other words, the government. In this chapter, we examine the resources and services the government can provide to those seeking treatment for, or information on, metabolic syndrome.[323]

EDUCATING THE PUBLIC

Similar to hospitals, governments serve as overseers, directing the major resources that can help in the effective education of the public. In the past, people have suffered and died from metabolic syndrome simply because they didn't know about the condition. Modern governments can learn from this example and work to increase awareness of metabolic syndrome. This in turn leads to people practicing healthy lifestyles as they grow into maturity.[324]

There is also a lot that *you* can do in terms of increasing the government's role in treating and preventing metabolic syndrome. Write to your local and state representative, asking them to spread information, whether by setting up educational forums at a national level, or educating civic leaders and public officials on the syndrome and other health concerns. These officials can then pass on what they've learned to their constituencies. Publication of educational materials, such as journals, magazines, and so on can also help in educating all residents.[325]

In addition, governments can assist medical personnel and other professionals in the search for better methods of dealing with the syndrome. The medical field requires adequate financial support to conduct studies and investigate new theories, experiments that cannot be conducted without the right equipment. When it comes time to vote, and even during non-voting years, it is the role of the constituent to be vocal in support of medical research and adequate medical funding. In order to reap the benefits that a focused government can provide, patients must make their voices heard.

The government can also help its people by constructing sufficient medical facilities, designed to deal with the syndrome at different stages. Governments should also equip the existing centers with the necessary resources for them to manage the syndrome. Creating medical facilities close to the people can reverse the situation, as compared to situations with inadequate facilities, resources, and personnel.[326]

HOW CORPORATIONS CAN HELP

Corporations can also play a major role in the prevention and treatment of this syndrome. Firms can help their clients by offering helpful information on matters to do with metabolic syndrome, while other companies come up with various campaigns to promote awareness. Companies can also donate a portion of their revenue to sponsor research aimed at halting metabolic syndrome, including offering ongoing financial support to medical centers specializing in chronic illnesses.[327]

Truthfully, the best way that corporations can help in the fight against metabolic syndrome would be to stop selling or promoting those products listed in this book—high sugar, high calorie products. While it may be a financial liability at first, such a move could save the lives of millions of potential patients. The first step to incentivizing this type of radical business move begins with you—the consumer. Much like the role the patient must play when working with the government, metabolic syndrome sufferers must learn to speak through their shopping habits, to show corporations that they no longer desire to be fed these nutritionally deficient, ultimately harmful products.[328]

PATIENTS HELPING OTHER PATIENTS

You can also help other sufferers to manage their metabolic syndrome, and lead prosperous and healthy lives as a result. Metabolic syndrome patients often connect better with each other than they relate to others, which puts them in a better position to help each other. By simply conversing with another sufferer, you can assist one another immensely. That connection relieves stress, and holding frequent conversations can help you to express your inward feelings and difficulties. These conversations may take different forms; talk about anything you want to, and in general you'll leave happier than when you arrived.[329]

Individuals who have metabolic syndrome can rally one another by making others feel valued. Self-esteem and self-worth plays an integral role in our development as people. Compassion helps in raising self-esteem and self-worth, as human beings have an instinctive need to feel cherished. Acts of empathy truly do affect how a patient responds to certain treatments.[330]

Therapy also works wonders, thanks to the tireless efforts of mental health professionals and researchers. You can make use of group therapies to discuss the various issues affecting you. By so doing, you can begin to feel more immersed in each other's lives. Group therapies also assist in comparing how you feel and how the array of treatment options affects you. Try holding group therapies once or twice weekly as you work collectively, supplying important connections. For example, suggest an alternative remedy offering good results to other members of your group, who may not be aware of it. By networking in this way, you may soon find various new methods and techniques for dealing with the syndrome. Above all, we need to work together to fight metabolic syndrome on all fronts.[331]

30

Conclusion

IT IS important to understand that the problems associated with metabolic syndrome *can* be controlled, and that you *can* continue to enjoy a high quality of life. However, in order to do this, you must have confidence to handle the obstacles the syndrome presents, patience in undergoing medical and emotional treatments, and hope for the future, a trust that every "today" will deliver a better "tomorrow." Understanding the importance of having hope, patience, and confidence is really the core of living with metabolic syndrome.[332]

HAVING HOPE

When dealing with metabolic syndrome, it's necessary for both you and those who are close to you to cling on to hope. There are many areas where hope is needed for you to have a normal life despite their syndrome. Total recovery from metabolic syndrome may be difficult to achieve, but living a normal life even in the midst of such a debilitating condition is very much possible. Hope is a powerful mindset that helps patients suffering from the worst cases of metabolic syndrome to keep fighting and pull through.[333]

This syndrome is often a cause of obesity, and obese patients are sometimes subjected to negative remarks from their peers. While this ridicule may not physically harm you, your emotions are thoroughly affected by piercing insults. It's only through a solid frame of mind and hope that one can emotionally survive such an onslaught.[334]

HAVING CONFIDENCE

Acknowledging the importance of confidence will help people who have metabolic syndrome to overcome their ill-perceived sense of inferiority. Confidence can only be maintained if you have the will to live a normal life. That's why metabolic syndrome patients must leverage their confidence to overcome the barrier of shame that has enveloped them for the majority of their life.[335] One of the treatments prescribed to people suffering from metabolic syndrome is to stay optimistic. This can be done by conditioning the mind to see hope in every situation. The mind is a crucial part of a person's spirit, and utilizing its might can expedite the healing process of the body. The first point that a patient should accept is that a person's facade is not the sum of who they are as a person. The fear of looking unappealing to others shouldn't be a reason for limiting the scope of your life. The key idea here is to discard mainstream conceptualization, and to recall the beauty that's hidden away behind the mask of this disorder.[336]

Patients should also accept that it's nobody's "fault." Becoming obese because of this syndrome is not the result of ill behavior, but because of one's personal limitations. This kind of disorder should not be seen solely as the result of poor diet or a sedentary lifestyle. People should understand that beating yourself up isn't the solution. You must stand proud, striving to serve as an inspiration to others, someone from whom they can draw their strength.[337]

HAVING PATIENCE

It is important for patients to realize that victory over this condition cannot and will not arrive at their doorstep overnight. Patience is needed for both the patient and his medical team. It's only through patience that any treatment to augment the morale of the patient is successful. Patience is the result of understanding both the medical disorder and the emotions you'll be experiencing. On the part of the sufferer, patience with the healing process is necessary. You must also understand the difficulty of the situation and how those who are helping are also sacrificing for your benefit. This combination of understanding and selflessness toward sufferers and those who help them can only persevere with patience.[338]

Aside from the emotional part of the therapy used to treat people with metabolic syndrome, the medical side of the recovery process should not go unmentioned. The other problems caused by metabolic syndrome should be regularly examined by an expert physician, and patients should follow the advice to the best of their ability. It is necessary for metabolic syndrome sufferers to cooperate with doctors and to bow to the latter's advice and follow it religiously, even if it is difficult to do so. Some examples of general advice that should be followed include: maintaining a balanced diet, general improvement of lifestyle, and the inclusion of exercise in one's activities. In the end, those who have metabolic syndrome should recognize that when push comes to shove, "life is what you make it."[339]

APPENDIX A: GLOSSARY OF TERMS

acesulfame potassium: A substance similar to sugar that can be used as an alternative for sugar, and it is free from calories. It is also popularly called acesulfame K or Ace K.

acquired immune deficiency syndrome (AIDS): An immunity disorder caused by the human immunodeficiency virus (HIV) infection characterized by lowering the body's immunity and causing an increased susceptibility to opportunistic infections.

adenosine triphosphate (ATP): The currency for transfer of energy at the molecular level. Basically, it is a nucleoside triphosphate that acts as a coenzyme in a cell.

adiposity: Defined as the state of when one is obese.

alpha-lipoic acid: A naturally occurring fatty acid that is a derivative of octanoic acid. It plays a major role in cellular metabolism as well.

anesthesiologists: Specialists in the field of anesthesia and perioperative medicine.

anthropometric: Related to measurements of the human body in terms of sizes and proportions.

arrhythmias: An irregular heartbeat due to any disturbance in the normal rhythm.

atherosclerosis: The disease condition of arteries in which the inner walls get coated with a fatty material resulting the narrowing of the lumen within the arteries.

bile: A greenish-yellow alkaline fluid produced by the liver and stored in the gall bladder. It is released for the digestion of fats.

biliopancreatic diversion: A surgery by which one part of the stomach is cut off and removed and the remaining portion is connected with the lower part of small intestine.

bio-identical hormone replacement: A therapy in which hormones are used that are quite similar in structure to the natural hormones produced by the human body.

blood plasma: The pale yellow fluid part of the blood that forms 55 percent of the total volume of blood and carries the blood cells within.

calcium channel blockers: A class of medications designed to treat heart disease and high blood pressure. These drugs work by decreasing the movement of calcium into the cells of the blood vessels and the heart.

calculi: A hardened aggregation of minerals in the body, such as that of the gallbladder or kidney.

calisthenics: An exercise form that consists of a combination of exercises (especially rhythmic movements) carried out without the help of any machine or gadget.

coronary artery disease (CAD): One of the most common causes of heart attack as a plaque layer is formed on the inner walls of the arteries of the heart, causing a decrease in the size of the lumen and thereby diminish the blood flow to the heart.

edema: A swelling that is formed due to the trapping of fluid in the tissues within the body.

eicosanoid: A collective term that is used to describe prostaglandins and the related compounds.

endocrine: Related to endocrine glands that secrete hormones.

endocrine system: The collective term used to describe a set of endocrine glands that secrete hormones and deposit them directly in the blood through which it is carried to the target organ for which the hormone was released specifically.

diuretics: Substances that promote urine production within the kidneys.

dyslipidemia: A term used to describe any malfunctions in lipid metabolism, like deficiency or overproduction of lipoproteins.

familial hypercholesterolemia: A hereditary disorder associated with abnormally high levels of LDL (low-density lipoprotein) present in the blood putting the person at a greater risk of developing heart diseases.

fibrates: Substances derived from fibric acid that are effective against the reduction of levels of blood triglycerides.

ghrelin: A hormone produced by cells of the stomach wall and pancreas. It suppresses appetite.

glucagon-like peptide-1: An appetite suppressant derived from proglucagon gene and is secreted by intestinal L cell as a hormone from the gut.

glycation: The process in which a sugar molecule and a protein or a lipid molecule bind together with the help of covalent bonds in the absence of any enzymatic action.

glycemic index: A value that indicates the effect of a carbohydrate-containing food on the levels of blood glucose.

high-density lipoproteins: High density molecules that transport triglycerides, cholesterol, and other lipids (fats) between tissues.

hypercoagulability: The condition in which a person develops an increased predisposition for clotting of blood.

hyperinsulinemia: A state of the body when an abnormally high level of insulin is being produced by the pancreas to counter the condition of insulin resistance within the body.

hyperglycemia: An excess of blood sugar in the bloodstream, typically associated with diabetes mellitus.

hyperpigmentation: The condition in which the skin becomes dark due to the excess production of melanin.

hypertension: The state when a person's blood pressure is higher than the normal level.

hypoglycemia: A deficiency of blood sugar.

ion exchange: The exchange of ions, which are atoms or molecules with a net positive or negative electrical charge. Cells do this to produce energy, among other functions.

ivy gourd: A tropical plant, also called as Coccinia grandis, widely recognized for reducing high blood pressure and controlling diabetes.

laparoscopic: Also called keyhole surgery. It is a type of surgery that is performed through small incisions made at various distances away from the actual site of operation.

latent autoimmune diabetes: A form of diabetes that's quite similar to type 1 diabetes and is a slow progressive form of diabetes. The pancreas is unable to produce the sufficient quantity of insulin required due to the slow destruction of cells that produce insulin.

lipases: Enzymes that break down fats.

lipid profile: Panel of blood exams that screen for irregularities in lipids, such as cholesterol and triglycerides.

lipids: Organic compounds that do not dissolve in water but dissolve in alcohol or chloroform. They constitute fats, steroids, oils, waxes, cholesterol, and triglycerides.

lipoprotein: A compound formed by the union of lipid and protein and so it is called as a conjugate protein. It plays an important role in the transport of lipids within the circulation.

low-density lipoproteins: Low-density molecules that transport triglycerides, cholesterol, and other lipids (fats) between tissues. Low-density lipoproteins are known to cause high cholesterol levels.

micronutrients: Nutrients that are needed in very small quantities but that are extremely essential for normal physiological functions.

mitochondrial: Relating to the mitochondrion. Mitochondria are cell organelles that are the "power plants" of a cell due to their capacity to generate ATP molecules.

myocardial infarction: Also called a heart attack. It is the medical emergency in which cardiac ischemia develops due to a blood clot within the blood vessels of the heart resulting in the blocking of the blood supply to the part falling distal to the clot.

neotame: A synthetic sweetener known to be 7,000 to 13,000 times sweeter as compared to normal table sugar.

neurohormonal: Of neurohormones. A neurohormone is a hormone that is generated from neurosecretory cells (for example, cells of adrenal medulla) and transmitted to the circulation.

pancreas: A gland that has two major functions: digestive (as it secretes pancreatic juice) and endocrine (as it releases hormones like insulin and glucagon).

pathology: A branch of medicine that deals with the art and science of studying and diagnosing various diseases.

phaseolamin: Derived from kidney bean (Phaseolus vulgaris) and has an inhibitory effect on alpha-amylase. Hence, it can be used in various weight-reduction regimes.

pyrogen therapy: A therapy in which fever is induced with the aim of utilizing the therapeutic properties of hyperthermia of the whole body in the treatment of cancer.

saccharin: A popular sugar substitute used as a sweetener in foods and beverages.

sebaceous glands: Microscopic glands that lubricate and waterproof the skin.

selective serotonin reuptake inhibitors (SSRIs): A group of drugs used for the treatment of anxiety and depression disorders.

sucralose: A synthetic sweetener derived from sucrose, which is at least 500 times sweeter than normal sugar.

visceral adiposity: Fat deposition occurring within the peritoneum in between the internal organs that has been recognized as a risk factor for various metabolic disorders.

visceral organs: The internal organs of the body.

APPENDIX B
FOR FURTHER READING

Beck-Neilson H. The metabolic syndrome: Pharmacology and clinical aspects. New York: Springer; 2013.

Bell D, O'Keefe J Jr. Metabolic syndrome essentials. Burlington, MA: Jones &Barlett Learning; 2010.

Brand-Miller J, Foster-Powell K, Leeds A. The new glucose revolution: Pocket guide to the metabolic syndrome. Boston, MA: Da Capo Press; 2004.

Byrne CD, Wild SH. The metabolic syndrome. Hoboken, NJ: Wiley-Blackwell; 2011.

Challem J. Syndrome x: The complete nutritional program to prevent and reverse insulin resistance. Hoboken, NJ: Wiley; 2000.

Das UN. Metabolic syndrome pathophysiology: The role of essential fatty acids. Hoboken, NJ: Wiley-Blackwell; 2010.

Haynes AJ. The insulin factor: Can't lose weight? Can't concentrate? Can't resist sugar? Could syndrome x be your problem? London, UK: Thorsons; 2004.

Haynes AJ. The insulin resistance factor: A nutritionist's plan for reversing the effects of Syndrome X. San Francisco, CA: Conari Press; 2012.

Isaacs S, Vagnini F. Overcoming metabolic syndrome. Omaha, NE: Addicus Books; 2005.

Karst K. The metabolic syndrome program: How to lose weight, beat heart disease, stop insulin resistance and more. Hoboken, NJ: Wiley; 2006.

Mittal S. The metabolic syndrome in clinical practice. New York: Springer; 2007.

APPENDIX C ABOUT THE AUTHOR

Naheed Ali, M.D., Ph.D. is a medical writer, editor, and educator. A graduate of Adelphi University, Dr. Ali received his medical degree from Xavier University School of Medicine. His postgraduate work includes a certificate in Lifestyle Medicine and Nutrition from Harvard Medical School and a Ph.D. from the College of Natural Health. Dr. Ali is the author of ten books for patients and caregivers.

APPENDIX D: ENDNOTES

1 Alberti KG, Zimmet P, Shaw J. Metabolic syndrome—a new worldwide definition. A consensus statement from the International Diabetes Federation. Diabet Med. 2006 May;23(5):469-80.

2 Lilienfeld SO. Is psychopathy a syndrome? Commentary on Marcus, Fulton, and Edens. Personal Disord. 2013 Jan;4(1):85-6.

3 Stern MP, Williams K, González-Villalpando C, et al. Does the metabolic syndrome improve identification of individuals at risk of type 2 diabetes and/or cardiovascular disease? Diabetes Care. 2004 Nov;27(11):2676-81.

4 Ervin RB. Prevalence of metabolic syndrome among adults 20 years of age and over, by sex, age, race and ethnicity, and body mass index: United States, 2003-2006. Natl Health Stat Report. 2009 May 5;(13):1-7.

5 Bianchini JA, da Silva DF, Nardo CC, Carolino ID, Hernandes F, Nardo N Jr. Multidisciplinary therapy reduces risk factors for metabolic syndrome in obese adolescents. Eur J Pediatr. 2013 Feb;172(2):215-21. doi: 10.1007/s00431-012-1865-7.

6 Dandona P1, Aljada A, Chaudhuri A, et al. Metabolic syndrome: a comprehensive perspective based on interactions between obesity, diabetes, and inflammation. Circulation. 2005 Mar 22;111(11):1448-54.

7 Schuster S, Fell DA, Dandekar T. A general definition of metabolic pathways useful for systematic organization and analysis of complex metabolic networks. Nat Biotechnol. 2000 Mar;18(3):326-32.

8 Mahdi M. The TheologusAutodidactus of Ibn at-Nafis by Max Meyerhof, Joseph Schacht. JAOS. 1974;94(2):232-234.

9 SorichMJ, McKinnon RA, Miners JO, et al. The importance of

local chemical structure for chemical metabolism by human uridine 5'-diphosphate-glucuronosyltransferase. J Chem Inf Model. 2006 Nov-Dec;46(6):2692-7.

10 Cheung BM, Li C. Diabetes and hypertension: is there a common metabolic pathway? Curr Atheroscler Rep. 2012 Apr;14(2):160-6.

11 Nezhat C, Nezhat F, Nezhat C. Endometriosis: ancient disease, ancient treatments. Fertil Steril. 2012 Dec;98(6 Suppl):S1-62.

12 Datz C, Felder TK, Niederseer D, et al. Iron homeostasis in the metabolic syndrome. Eur J Clin Invest. 2013 Feb;43(2):215-24.

13 Sirdah MM, Al Laham NA, Abu Ghali AS. Prevalence of metabolic syndrome and associated socioeconomic and demographic factors among Palestinian adults (20-65 years) at the Gaza Strip. Diabetes Metab Syndr. 2011 Apr-Jun;5(2):93-7.

14 Hildrum B, Mykletun A, Hole T, et al. Age-specific prevalence of the metabolic syndrome defined by the International Diabetes Federation and the National Cholesterol Education Program: the Norwegian HUNT 2 study. BMC Public Health. 2007 Aug 29;7:220.

15 Vague J. The degree of masculine differentiation of obesities: a factor determining predisposition to diabetes, atherosclerosis, gout, and uric calculous disease. Am J Clin Nutr. 1956 Jan-Feb;4(1):20-34.

16 Haller H, Elger M, HentschelH, et al. Nephrogenesis is induced by partial nephrectomy in the elasmobranch Leucorajaerinacea. J Am SocNephrol. 2003 Jun;14(6):1506-18.

17 Singer P. Diagnosis of primary hyperlipoproteinemias [article in German]. Z Gesamte Inn Med. 1977 May 1;32(9):129-33.

18 Reaven GM. Banting lecture 1988. Role of insulin resistance in human disease. Diabetes. 1988 Dec;37(12):1595-607.

19 Lakhtakia R. The history of diabetes mellitus. Sultan Qaboos Univ Med J. 2013 Aug;13(3):368-70.

20 Moser M. Historical perspectives on the management of hypertension. J Clin Hypertens (Greenwich). 2006 Aug;8(8 Suppl 2):15-20.

21 Atkinson AB, Robertson JI. Captopril in the treatment of clinical hypertension and cardiac failure. Lancet. 1979 Oct 20;2(8147):836-9.

22 Mahmood SS, Levy D, Vasan RS. The Framingham Heart Study and the epidemiology of cardiovascular disease: a historical perspective. Lancet. 2014 Mar 15;383(9921):999-1008.

23 Sarafidis PA, Nilsson PM. The metabolic syndrome: a glance at its history. J Hypertens. 2006 Apr;24(4):621-6.

24 Sarafidis PA, Nilsson PM. The metabolic syndrome: a glance at its history. J Hypertens. 2006 Apr;24(4):621-6.

25 Bergman EM, Verheijen IW, Scherpbier AJ, et al. Influences on anatomical knowledge: The complete arguments. Clin Anat. 2014 Apr;27(3):296-303.

26 Sharma PK, Fidler JL, Schleck CD, et al. Mo1934 influence of obesity on GE junction anatomy and its reversibility following eight loss. Gastroenterology. 2013 May;144(5):S698–S699.

27 Pérez Pérez A, Ybarra Muñoz J, Blay Cortés V, et al. Obesity and cardiovascular disease. Public Health Nutr. 2007 Oct;10(10A):1156-63.

28 Litten-Brown JC, Corson AM, Clarke L. Porcine models for the metabolic syndrome, digestive and bone disorders: a general overview. Animal. 2010 Jun;4(6):899-920.

29 Greenberg AS, Obin MS. Obesity and the role of adipose tissue in inflammation and metabolism. Am J Clin Nutr. 2006 Feb;83(2):461S-465S.

30 Després JP. Is visceral obesity the cause of the metabolic syndrome? Ann Med. 2006;38(1):52-63.

31 Buchwald H, Avidor Y, Braunwald E, et al. Bariatric surgery: a systematic review and meta-analysis. JAMA. 2004 Oct 13;292(14):1724-37.

32 Flatt JP. Conversion of carbohydrate to fat in adipose tissue: an energy-yielding and, therefore, self-limiting process. J Lipid Res. 1970 Mar;11(2):131-43.

33 Wolinsky H. Disease mongering and drug marketing. EMBO Rep. Jul 2005;6(7):612-614.

34 Bergman EM, Verheijen IW, Scherpbier AJ, et al. Influences on anatomical knowledge: The complete arguments. Clin Anat. 2014 Apr;27(3):296-303.

35 Hegele RA, Pollex RL. Genetic and physiological insights into the metabolic syndrome. Am J Physiol Regul Integr Comp Physiol. 2005 Sep;289(3):R663-9.

36 Young J, Barton M, Richards-Dawson MA, et al. Knowledge, perception and practices of healthcare professionals at tertiary level hospitals in Kingston, Jamaica, regarding neonatal pain management. West Indian Med J. 2008 Jan;57(1):28-32.

37 Lenggenhager B, Pazzaglia M, Scivoletto G, et al. The sense of the body in individuals with spinal cord injury. PLoS One. 2012;7(11):e50757.

38 Crippen D. Brain failure in critical care medicine. Crit Care Nurs Q. 1994 Feb;16(4):80-95.

39 Chakraborty S, Zawieja S, Wang W, et al. Lymphatic system: a vital link between metabolic syndrome and inflammation. Ann N Y Acad Sci. 2010 Oct;1207Suppl 1:E94-102.

40 Uchino BN. Social support and health: a review of physiological processes potentially underlying links to disease outcomes. J Behav Med. 2006 Aug;29(4):377-87.

41 Marshall AM, Nommsen-Rivers LA, Hernandez LL, et al. Serotonin transport and metabolism in the mammary gland modulates secretory activation and involution. J Clin Endocrinol Metab. 2010 Feb;95(2):837-46.

42 Karasov WH, Martínez del Rio C, Caviedes-Vidal E. Ecological physiology of diet and digestive systems. Annu Rev Physiol. 2011;73:69-93.

43 Aronson D, Sella R, Sheikh-Ahmad M, et al. The association between cardiorespiratory fitness and C-reactive protein in subjects with the metabolic syndrome. J Am Coll Cardiol. 2004 Nov 16;44(10):2003-7.

44 Qiao Q, Gao W, Zhang L, et al, Metabolic syndrome and cardiovascular disease. Ann Clin Biochem. 2007 May;44(Pt 3):232-63.

45 Padhi T, Garima. Metabolic syndrome and skin: psoriasis and beyond. Indian J Dermatol. 2013 Jul;58(4):299-305.

46 Kupelian V, McVary KT, Kaplan SA, Association of lower urinary tract symptoms and the metabolic syndrome: results from the Boston area community health survey. J Urol. 2013 Jan;189(1 Suppl):S107-14; discussion S115-6.

47 Rostom S, Mengat M, Lahlou R, et al. Metabolic syndrome in rheumatoid arthritis: case control study. BMC Musculoskelet Disord. 2013 Apr 26;14:147.

48 Reaven G. Metabolic syndrome: pathophysiology and implications for management of cardiovascular disease. Circulation. 2002 Jul 16;106(3):286-8.

49 Nguyen QT, Thomas KT, Lyons KB, et al. Current therapies and emerging drugs in the pipeline for type 2 diabetes. Am Health Drug Benefits. 2011 Sep;4(5):303-11

50 Giovannucci E1, Harlan DM, and Archer MC. Diabetes and cancer: a consensus report. Diabetes Care. 2010 Jul;33(7):1674-85.

51 Fulgoni V III. High-fructose corn syrup: everything you wanted to know, but were afraid to ask. Am J Clin Nutr. 2008 Dec;88(6):1715S.

52 Fulgoni V III. High-fructose corn syrup: everything you wanted to know, but were afraid to ask. Am J Clin Nutr. 2008 Dec;88(6):1715S.

53 Miller A, Adeli K. Dietary fructose and the metabolic syndrome. Curr Opin Gastroenterol. 2008 Mar;24(2):204-9.

54 Lanaspa MA, Ishimoto T, Li N, et al. Endogenous fructose production and metabolism in the liver contributes to the development of metabolic syndrome. Nat Commun. 2013;4:2434.

55 Jensen J, Rustad PI, Kolnes AJ, et al. The role of skeletal muscle glycogen breakdown for regulation of insulin sensitivity by exercise. Front Physiol. 2011 Dec 30;2:112.

56 Goran MI. Energy metabolism and obesity. Med Clin North Am. 2000 Mar;84(2):347-62.

57 Wlodarczyk A, Strojek K. Glucose intolerance, insulin resistance and metabolic syndrome in patients with stable angina pectoris. Obesity predicts coronary atherosclerosis and dysglycemia. Pol Arch Med Wewn. 2008 Dec;118(12):719-26.

58 Bumgarner NR, Scheerens JC, Kleinhenz MD. Nutritional yield: a proposed index for fresh food improvement illustrated with leafy vegetable data. Plant Foods Hum Nutr. 2012 Sep;67(3):215-22.

59 Song S, Lee JE, Song WO. Carbohydrate intake and refined-grain consumption are associated with metabolic syndrome in the Korean adult population. J Acad Nutr Diet. 2014 Jan;114(1):54-62.

60 Marchiori D1, Waroquier L, Klein O. Smaller food item sizes of snack foods influence reduced portions and caloric intake in young adults. J Am Diet Assoc. 2011 May;111(5):727-31.

61 Pereira MA, Fulgoni VL III. Consumption of 100% fruit juice and risk of obesity and metabolic syndrome: findings from the national health and nutrition examination survey 1999-2004. J Am Coll Nutr. 2010 Dec;29(6):625-9.

62 Brown RJ, de Banate MA, Rother KI. Artificial sweeteners: a systematic review of metabolic effects in youth. Int J Pediatr Obes. 2010 Aug;5(4):305-12.

63 Stewart KJ, Bacher AC, Turner K. Exercise and risk factors associated with metabolic syndrome in older adults. Am J Prev Med. 2005 Jan;28(1):9-18.

64 Gillespie SJ, Kulkarni KD, Daly AE. Using carbohydrate counting in diabetes clinical practice. J Am Diet Assoc. 1998 Aug;98(8):897-905.

65 Hofmann SM, Tschöp MH. Dietary sugars: a fat difference. J Clin Invest. 2009 May;119(5):1089-92.

66 Reis JP, von Mühlen D, Kritz-Silverstein D, et al. Vitamin D, parathyroid hormone levels, and the prevalence of metabolic syndrome in community-dwelling older adults. Diabetes Care. 2007 Jun;30(6):1549-55.

67 Muller M, Grobbee DE, den Tonkelaar I, et al. Endogenous sex hormones and metabolic syndrome in aging men. J Clin Endocrinol Metab. 2005 May;90(5):2618-23.

68 Maggio M1, Lauretani F, Ceda GP, et al. Association between hormones and metabolic syndrome in older Italian men. J Am Geriatr Soc. 2006 Dec;54(12):1832-8.

69 Rahmanpour H1, Jamal L, Mousavinasab SN, et al. Association between polycystic ovarian syndrome, overweight, and metabolic syndrome in adolescents. J Pediatr Adolesc Gynecol. 2012 Jun;25(3):208-12.

70 Rustia M. Role of hormone imbalance in transplacental carcinogenesis induced in Syrian golden hamsters by sex hormones. Natl Cancer Inst Monogr. 1979 May;(51):77-87.

71 Goh VH1, Tong TY, Mok HP, et al. Interactions among age, adiposity, bodyweight, lifestyle factors and sex steroid hormones in healthy Singaporean Chinese men. Asian J Androl. 2007 Sep;9(5):611-21.

72 Dubuc PU. Effects of estrogen on food intake, body weight, and temperature of male and female obese mice. Proc Soc Exp Biol Med. 1985 Dec;180(3):468-73.

73 Bianchi GP, Zaccheroni V, Solaroli E, et al. Health-related quality of life in patients with thyroid disorders. Qual Life Res. 2004 Feb;13(1):45-54.

74 Johannessen AC1, Nilsen R, Matre R. In situ demonstration of Fc gamma-receptors in human chronic marginal and apical periodontitis. J Oral Pathol. 1987 Nov;16(10):492-8.

75 Shahar E, Redline S, Young T, et al. Hormone replacement therapy and sleep-disordered breathing. Am J Respir Crit Care Med. 2003 May 1;167(9):1186-92.

76 Dorgan JF, Hunsberger SA, McMahon RP, et al. Diet and sex hormones in girls: findings from a randomized controlled clinical trial. J Natl Cancer Inst. 2003 Jan 15;95(2):132-41.

77 Reimold M, Knobel A, Rapp MA, et al. Central serotonin transporter levels are associated with stress hormone response and anxiety. Psychopharmacology (Berlin). 2011 Feb;213(2-3):563-72.

78 Weinbroum AA1, Hochhauser E, Rudick V, et al. Multiple organ dysfunction after remote circulatory arrest: common pathway of radical oxygen species? J Trauma. 1999 Oct;47(4):691-8.

79 Van Griensven M, Calzia E, Jafarmadar M, et al. Circulatory kinetics of the cellular and humoral immune response in peritonitis. Shock. 2006;26(4):33.

80 Jericó C, Knobel H, Montero M, et al. Metabolic syndrome among HIV-infected patients: prevalence, characteristics, and related factors. Diabetes Care. 2005 Jan;28(1):132-7.

81 Vlassoff C. Gender differences in determinants and consequences of health and illness. J Health Popul Nutr. 2007 Mar;25(1):47-61.

82 Adibhatla RM, Hatcher JF. Altered lipid metabolism in brain injury and disorders. Subcell Biochem. 2008;49:241-68.

83 Kim HJ, Park JM, Kim JA, et al. Effect of herbal Ephedra sinica and Evodia rutaecarpa on body composition and resting metabolic rate: a randomized, double-blind clinical trial in Korean premenopausal women. J Acupunct Meridian Stud. 2008 Dec;1(2):128-38.

84 Haffor AS, Mohler JG, Harrison AC. Effects of water immersion on cardiac output of lean and fat male subjects at rest and during exercise. Aviat Space Environ Med. 1991 Feb;62(2):123-7.

85 Mukamal KJ. The effects of smoking and drinking on cardiovascular disease and risk factors. Alcohol Res Health. 2006;29(3):199-202.

86 Friedel N, Viazis P, Schiessler A, et al. Recovery of end-organ failure during mechanical circulatory support. Eur J Cardiothorac Surg. 1992;6(10):519-22.

87 Wagner EH, Austin BT, Von Korff M. Improving outcomes in chronic illness. Manag Care Q. 1996 Spring;4(2):12-25.

88 Khosh F, Khosh M. Natural approach to hypertension. Altern Med Rev. 2001 Dec;6(6):590-600.

89 Hamilton MT, Hamilton DG, Zderic TW. Role of low energy expenditure and sitting in obesity, metabolic syndrome, type 2 diabetes, and cardiovascular disease. Diabetes. 2007 Nov;56(11):2655-67.

90 Naura AS, Hans CP, Zerfaoui M, et al. High-fat diet induces lung remodeling in ApoE-deficient mice: an association with an increase in circulatory and lung inflammatory factors. Lab Invest. 2009 Nov;89(11):1243-51.

91 Rowland TW. The circulatory response to exercise: role of the peripheral pump. Int J Sports Med. 2001 Nov;22(8):558-65.

92 Sousa MM, Krokan HE, Slupphaug G. DNA-uracil and human pathology. Mol Aspects Med. 2007 Jun-Aug;28(3-4):276-306.

93 Kalra SP, Kalra PS. NPY and cohorts in regulating appetite, obesity and metabolic syndrome: beneficial effects of gene therapy. Neuropeptides. 2004 Aug;38(4):201-11.

94 Keller KB, Lemberg L. Obesity and the metabolic syndrome. Am J Crit Care. 2003 Mar;12(2):167-70.

95 Sun SS, Grave GD, Siervogel RM, et al. Systolic blood pressure in childhood predicts hypertension and metabolic syndrome later in life. Pediatrics. 2007 Feb;119(2):237-46.

96 Rutter MK1, Meigs JB, Sullivan LM, et al. Insulin resistance, the metabolic syndrome, and incident cardiovascular events in the Framingham Offspring Study. Diabetes. 2005 Nov;54(11):3252-7.

97 Vgontzas AN, Bixler EO, Chrousos GP. Sleep apnea is a manifestation of the metabolic syndrome. Sleep Med Rev. 2005 Jun;9(3):211-24.

98 Calvin AD, Albuquerque FN, Lopez-Jimenez F, et al. Obstructive sleep apnea, inflammation, and the metabolic syndrome. Metab Syndr Relat Disord. 2009 Aug;7(4):271-8.

99 Chopra R, Chander A, Jacob JJ. Ocular associations of metabolic syndrome. Indian J Endocrinol Metab. 2012 Mar;16 Suppl 1:S6-S11.

100 El Safoury OS, Ezzat M, Abdelhamid MF, et al. The Evaluation of the Impact of Age, Skin Tags, Metabolic Syndrome, Body Mass Index, and Smoking on Homocysteine, Endothelin-1, High-sensitive C-reactive Protein, and on the Heart. Indian J Dermatol. 2013 Jul;58(4):326.

101 Tulipani S, Llorach R, Jáuregui O, et al. Metabolomics unveils urinary changes in subjects with metabolic syndrome following 12-week nut consumption. J Proteome Res. 2011 Nov 4;10(11):5047-58.

102 Shin DW, Kwon HT, Kang JM, et al. Association between metabolic syndrome and Helicobacter pylori infection diagnosed by histologic status and serological status. J Clin Gastroenterol. 2012 Nov-Dec;46(10):840-5.

103 Yamanaka T1 Fukuda T, Sawai Y, et al. Clinical analysis of metabolic syndrome in vertiginous diseases [Article in Japanese]. Nihon Jibiinkoka Gakkai Kaiho. 2011 Jan;114(1):24-9.

104 James PT, Rigby N, Leach R, et al. The obesity epidemic, metabolic syndrome and future prevention strategies. Eur J Cardiovasc Prev Rehabil. 2004 Feb;11(1):3-8.

105 Gautam S, Meena PS. Drug-emergent metabolic syndrome in patients with schizophrenia receiving atypical (second-generation) antipsychotics. Indian J Psychiatry. 2011 Apr;53(2):128-33.

106 Song YM, Lee K, Sung J. Genetic and environmental relationships between change in weight and insulin resistance: the Healthy Twin Study. Twin Res Hum Genet. 2014 Jun;17(3):199-205.

107 Misra A, Khurana L. Obesity and the metabolic syndrome in developing countries. J Clin Endocrinol Metab. 2008 Nov;93(11 Suppl 1):S9-30.

108 Ferland A, Eckel RH. Does sustained weight loss reverse the metabolic syndrome? Curr Hypertens Rep. 2011 Dec;13(6):456-64.

109 Malmstrom R, Packard CJ, Caslake M, et al. Defective regulation of triglyceride metabolism by insulin in the liver in NIDDM. Diabetologia. 1997 Apr;40(4):454-62.

110 Oh K1, Hu FB, Cho E, et al. Carbohydrate intake, glycemic index, glycemic load, and dietary fiber in relation to risk of stroke in women. Am J Epidemiol. 2005 Jan 15;161(2):161-9.

111 Finley CE, Barlow CE, Halton TL, et al. Glycemic index, glycemic load, and prevalence of the metabolic syndrome in the cooper center longitudinal study. J Am Diet Assoc. 2010 Dec;110(12):1820-9.

112 Tamashiro KL, Sakai RR, Shively CA, et al. Chronic stress, metabolism, and metabolic syndrome. Stress. 2011 Sep;14(5):468-74.

113 Carlson JJ, Eisenmann JC, Norman GJ, et al. Dietary fiber and nutrient density are inversely associated with the metabolic syndrome in US adolescents. J Am Diet Assoc. 2011 Nov;111(11):1688-95.

114 Kochan Z, Karbowska J, Babicz-Zieliska E. Dietary trans-fatty acids

and metabolic syndrome [article in Polish]. Postepy Hig Med Dosw. 2010 Dec 27;64:650-8.

115 Soleimani M. Dietary fructose, salt absorption and hypertension in metabolic syndrome: towards a new paradigm. Acta Physiol (Oxf). 2011 Jan;201(1):55-62.

116 Motamed S, Ebrahimi M, Safarian M, et al. N Am J Med Sci. Micronutrient intake and the presence of the metabolic syndrome. 2013 Jun;5(6):377-85.

117 Yu M, Xu CX, Zhu HH, et al. Associations of cigarette smoking and alcohol consumption with metabolic syndrome in a male chinese population: a cross-sectional study. J Epidemiol. 2014 Sep 5;24(5):361-9.

118 Sisson SB, Camhi SM, Church TS, et al. Leisure time sedentary behavior, occupational/domestic physical activity, and metabolic syndrome in U.S. men and women. Metab Syndr Relat Disord. 2009 Dec;7(6):529-36.

119 Braunschweig CL, Gomez S, Liang H, et al. Obesity and risk factors for the metabolic syndrome among low-income, urban, African American schoolchildren: the rule rather than the exception? Am J Clin Nutr. 2005 May;81(5):970-5.

120 Grundy SM, Cleeman JI, Daniels SR, et al. Diagnosis and management of the metabolic syndrome. An American Heart Association/National Heart, Lung, and Blood Institute Scientific Statement. Executive summary. Cardiol Rev. 2005 Nov-Dec;13(6):322-7.

121 Goodman E, Daniels SR, Meigs JB, et al. Instability in the diagnosis of metabolic syndrome in adolescents. Circulation. 2007 May 1;115(17):2316-22.

122 Kumbasar B, Yenigun M, Ataoglu HE, et al. The prevalence of metabolic syndrome in different ethnic groups in Turkey. J Int Med Res. 2013 Feb;41(1):188-99.

123 Schneiderhan ME, Batscha CL, Rosen C. Assessment of a point-of-care metabolic risk screening program in outpatients receiving antipsychotic agents. Pharmacotherapy. 2009 Aug;29(8):975-87.

124 Grievink L, Alberts JF, O'Niel J, et al. Waist circumference as a measurement of obesity in the Netherlands Antilles; associations with hypertension and diabetes mellitus. Eur J Clin Nutr. 2004 Aug;58(8):1159-65.

125 Jaworski K, Sarkadi-Nagy E, Duncan RE, et al. Regulation of triglyceride metabolism. IV. Hormonal regulation of lipolysis in adipose tissue. Am J Physiol Gastrointest Liver Physiol. 2007 Jul;293(1):G1-4.

126 Isezuo SA. Is high density lipoprotein cholesterol useful in diagnosis of metabolic syndrome in native Africans with type 2 diabetes? Ethn Dis. 2005 Winter;15(1):6-10.

127 Ishizaka N, Ishizaka Y, Toda E, et al. Hypertension is the most common component of metabolic syndrome and the greatest contributor to carotid arteriosclerosis in apparently healthy Japanese individuals. Hypertens Res. 2005 Jan;28(1):27-34.

128 Wassink AM, Van Der Graaf Y, Soedamah-Muthu SS, et al. Metabolic syndrome and incidence of type 2 diabetes in patients with manifest vascular disease. Diab Vasc Dis Res. 2008 Jun;5(2):114-22.

129 Strazzullo P, Barbato A, Siani A, et al. Diagnostic criteria for metabolic syndrome: a comparative analysis in an unselected sample of adult male population. Metabolism. 2008 Mar;57(3):355-61.

130 Haffner SM. Risk constellations in patients with the metabolic syndrome: epidemiology, diagnosis, and treatment patterns. Am J Med. 2006 May;119 (5 Suppl 1):S3-9.

131 Yasein N, Masa'd D. Metabolic syndrome in family practice in Jordan: a study of high-risk groups. East Mediterr Health J. 2011 Dec;17(12):943-8.

132 Horvath B, Bodecs T, Boncz I, et al. Metabolic syndrome in normal and complicated pregnancies. MetabSyndrRelatDisord. 2013 Jun;11(3):185-8.

133 Bayard M, Peeples CR, Holt J, et al. An interactive approach to teaching practice management to family practice residents.Fam Med. 2003 Oct;35(9):622-4.

134 Reeves D, Campbell SM, Adams J, et al. Combining multiple indicators of clinical quality: an evaluation of different analytic approaches. Med Care. 2007 Jun;45(6):489-96.

135 Desplan M, Mercier J, Sabaté M, et al. The metabolic syndrome in patients with chronic obstructive pulmonary disease. Sleep Med. 2014 Aug;15(8):906-12.

136 Buscemi S, Re A, Batsis JA, et al. Glycaemic variability using continuous glucose monitoring and endothelial function in the metabolic syndrome and in Type 2 diabetes. Diabet Med. 2010 Aug;27(8):872-8.

137 Baruah MP, Kalra S, Unnikrishnan AG. Endocrine hypertension: Changing paradigm in the new millennium. Indian J EndocrinolMetab. 2011 Oct;15Suppl 4:S275-8.

138 Eyzaguirre F, Silva R, Román R, et al. Prevalence of metabolic syndrome in children and adolescents who consult with obesity [Article in Spanish]. Rev Med Chil. 2011 Jun;139(6):732-8.

139 Carek PJ1, Diaz V, Dickerson LM, et al. Preparation for practice in family medicine: before and after duty hours. Fam Med. 2012 Sep;44(8):539-44.

140 Green ML, Aagaard EM, Caverzagie KJ, et al. Charting the road to competence: developmental milestones for internal medicine residency training. J Grad Med Educ. 2009 Sep;1(1):5-20.

141 Qureishi R. Metabolic syndrome: a silent killer. Med Today. 2005 Mar;3(1):3.

142 Shea S, Basch CE, Zybert P. Correlates of internists' practices in caring for patients with elevated serum cholesterol. Am J Health Promot. 1990 Jul;4(6):421-8.

143 Rashed MS. Clinical applications of tandem mass spectrometry: ten years of diagnosis and screening for inherited metabolic diseases. J Chromatogr B Biomed Sci Appl. 2001 Jul 5;758(1):27-48.

144 Mattar SG1, Velcu LM, Rabinovitz M, et al. Surgically-induced weight loss significantly improves nonalcoholic fatty liver disease and the metabolic syndrome. Ann Surg. 2005 Oct;242(4):610-7.

145 Arslan AA, Helzlsouer KJ, Kooperberg C, et al. Anthropometric measures, body mass index, and pancreatic cancer: a pooled analysis from the Pancreatic Cancer Cohort Consortium (PanScan). Arch Intern Med. 2010 May 10;170(9):791-802.

146 Israili ZH, Lyoussi B, Hernández-Hernández R, Metabolic syndrome: treatment of hypertensive patients. Am J Ther. 2007 Jul-Aug;14(4):386-402.

147 Wagh A, Stone NJ. Treatment of metabolic syndrome. Expert Rev Cardiovasc Ther. 2004 Mar;2(2):213-28.

148 Hutley L, Prins JB. Fat as an endocrine organ: relationship to the metabolic syndrome. Am J Med Sci. 2005 Dec;330(6):280-9.

149 Duran A, Runkle I, Matía P, et al. Family physician and endocrinologist coordination as the basis for diabetes care in clinical practice. BMC Endocr Disord. 2008 Jul 31;8:9.

150 Iwen KA, Schröder E, Brabant G. Thyroid hormones and the metabolic syndrome. Eur Thyroid J. 2013 Jun;2(2):83-92.

151 O'Donnell M, de Siún A, O'Mullane M, et al. Differences in the structure of outpatient diabetes care between endocrinologist-led and general physician-led services. BMC Health Serv Res. 2013 Nov 25;13:493.

152 Johannsson G, Bengtsson BA. Growth hormone and the metabolic syndrome. J Endocrinol Invest. 1999;22(5 Suppl):41-6.

153 SchlaffWD. Responding to change in reproductive endocrinology fellowships. Fertil Steril. 2014 Jun;101(6):1510-1.

154 Zeller M, Steg PG, Ravisy J, et al. Prevalence and impact of metabolic syndrome on hospital outcomes in acute myocardial infarction. Arch Intern Med. 2005 May 23;165(10):1192-8.

155 Kondilis BK, AkrivosPD, Sardi TA, et al. Readability levels of health pamphlets distributed in hospitals and health centres in Athens, Greece. Public Health. 2010 Oct;124(10):547-52.

156 Leino-Kilpi H, Johansson K, Heikkinen K, et al. Patient education and health-related quality of life: surgical hospital patients as a case in point. J Nurs Care Qual. 2005 Oct-Dec;20(4):307-16.

157 OxenkrugGF. Metabolic syndrome, age-associated neuroendocrine disorders, and dysregulation of tryptophan-kynurenine metabolism. Ann NY Acad Sci. 2010 Jun;1199:1-14.

158 Scott JG, Sochalski J, Aiken L. Review of magnet hospital research: findings and implications for professional nursing practice. J Nurs Adm. 1999 Jan;29(1):9-19.

159 Mascia D, Di Vincenzo F, Cicchetti A. Dynamic analysis of interhospital collaboration and competition: empirical evidence from an Italian regional health system. Health Policy. 2012 May;105(2-3):273-81.

160 Duffin C. Raising awareness to support people with dementia in hospital.Nurs Older People. 2013 Jun;25(5):14-7.

161 Germain CP. Nursing the dying: implications of Kübler-Ross' staging theory. Ann Am Acad Pol Soc Sci. 1980 Jan;(447):46-58.

162 Jordan IB, Haworth A. The contribution of counseling in hospital and home-based care in a small town and surrounding rural area in Zambia. Trop Doct. 1995 Jan;25(1):21-4.

163 Marley KA, Collier DA, Goldstein SM. The role of clinical and process quality in achieving patient satisfaction in hospitals. Decision Sciences. 2004 Jul;35(3):349 - 369.

164 Zhou MS, Wang A, Yu H. Link between insulin resistance and hypertension: What is the evidence from evolutionary biology? DiabetolMetabSyndr. 2014 Jan 31;6(1):12.

165 Gorter PM, OlijhoekJK, van der GraafY, et al. Prevalence of the metabolic syndrome in patients with coronary heart disease, cerebrovascular disease, peripheral arterial disease or abdominal aortic aneurysm. Atherosclerosis. 2004 Apr;173(2):363-9.

166 Lopez-Jaramillo P, Lopez-Lopez J, Lopez-Lopez C. The goal of blood pressure in the hypertensive patient with diabetes is defined: now the challenge is go from recommendations to practice. DiabetolMetabSyndr. 2014 Mar 4;6(1):31.

167 SheuWH, Jeng CY, Shieh SM, et al. Insulin resistance and abnormal electrocardiograms in patients with high blood pressure. Am J Hypertens. 1992 Jul;5(7):444-8.

168 Sechi LA, Griffin CA, Giacchetti G, et al. Abnormalities of insulin receptors in spontaneously hypertensive rats. Hypertension. 1996 Apr;27(4):955-61.

169 Masuo K. Roles of beta2- and beta3-adrenoceptor polymorphisms in hypertension and metabolic syndrome.Int J Hypertens. 2010 Oct 21;2010:832821.

170 Pravenec M, Landa V, Zidek V, et al. Transgenic rescue of defective CD36 attenuates insulin resistance, dyslipidemia, and hypertension in spontaneously hypertensive rats. Hypertension. 2000;36:690.

171 Lembo G, Iaccarino G, Rendina V, et al. Insulin blunts sympathetic vasoconstriction through the alpha 2-adrenergic pathway in humans. Hypertension. 1994 Oct;24(4):429-38.

172 Kim YJ, Kim YJ, Cho BM, et al. Metabolic syndrome and arterial pulse wave velocity. ActaCardiol. 2010 Jun;65(3):315-21.

173 Sowers JR, Frohlich ED. Insulin and insulin resistance: impact on blood pressure and cardiovascular disease. Med Clin North Am. 2004 Jan;88(1):63-82.

174 Li C, Ford ES, McBride PE, et al. Non-high-density lipoprotein cholesterol concentration is associated with the metabolic syndrome among US youth aged 12-19 years. J Pediatr. 2011 Feb;158(2):201-7.

175 Risérus U, Berglund L, Vessby B. Conjugated linoleic acid (CLA) reduced abdominal adipose tissue in obese middle-aged men with signs

of the metabolic syndrome: a randomised controlled trial. Int J Obes-RelatMetabDisord. 2001 Aug;25(8):1129-35.

176 Taverne F, Richard C, Couture P, et al. Abdominal obesity, insulin resistance, metabolic syndrome and cholesterol homeostasis. PharmaNutrition. 2013 Oct;1(4):130-136.

177 Cahill LE, Chiuve SE, Mekary RA, et al. Prospective study of breakfast eating and incident coronary heart disease in a cohort of male US health professionals.Circulation. 2013 Jul 23;128(4):337-43.

178 Barrios V, Escobar C, CalderónA,et al. Prevalence of the metabolic syndrome in patients with hypertension treated in general practice in Spain: an assessment of blood pressure and low-density lipoprotein cholesterol control and accuracy of diagnosis. J CardiometabSyndr. 2007 Winter;2(1):9-15.

179 Barrios V, Escobar C, CalderónA,et al. Prevalence of the metabolic syndrome in patients with hypertension treated in general practice in Spain: an assessment of blood pressure and low-density lipoprotein cholesterol control and accuracy of diagnosis. J CardiometabSyndr. 2007 Winter;2(1):9-15.

180 Wang J. Consumption of added sugars and development of metabolic syndrome components among a sample of youth at risk of obesity. ApplPhysiolNutrMetab. 2014 Apr;39(4):512.

181 Kodama S, Tanaka S, Saito K, et al. Effect of aerobic exercise training on serum levels of high-density lipoprotein cholesterol: a meta-analysis. Arch Intern Med. 2007 May 28;167(10):999-1008.

182 Keller KB, Lemberg L. Obesity and the metabolic syndrome. Am J Crit Care. 2003 Mar;12(2):167-70.

183 Demerath EW, Reed D, Rogers N, et al. Visceral adiposity and its anatomical distribution as predictors of the metabolic syndrome and cardiometabolic risk factor levels. Am J Clin Nutr. 2008 Nov;88(5):1263-71.

184 Soyer MT, Ergin I, Gursoy ST. Effects of social determinants on food choice and skipping meals among Turkish adolescents. Asia Pac J Clin Nutr. 2008;17(2):208-15.

185 Hamilton MT, Hamilton DG, Zderic TW. Role of low energy expenditure and sitting in obesity, metabolic syndrome, type 2 diabetes, and cardiovascular disease. Diabetes. 2007 Nov;56(11):2655-67.

186 Sonko BJ, Prentice AM, Murgatroyd PR, Effect of alcohol on postmeal fat storage. Am J Clin Nutr. 1994 Mar;59(3):619-25.

187 Rice TM, Zhu M. Driver obesity and the risk of fatal injury during traffic collisions. Emerg Med J. 2014 Jan;31(1):9-12.

188 Hassan MO, Jaju D, Albarwani S, et al. Non-dipping blood pressure in the metabolic syndrome among Arabs of the Oman family study. Obesity (Silver Spring). 2007 Oct;15(10):2445-53.

189 Ryan AS, Nicklas BJ, Berman DM. Hormone replacement therapy, insulin sensitivity, and abdominal obesity in postmenopausal women. Diabetes Care. 2002 Jan;25(1):127-33.

190 Martyn-Nemeth P, Penckofer S, Gulanick M, et al. The relationships among self-esteem, stress, coping, eating behavior, and depressive mood in adolescents. Res Nurs Health. 2009 Feb;32(1):96-109.

191 Bose M, Oliván B, Laferrère B. Stress and obesity: the role of the hypothalamic-pituitary-adrenal axis in metabolic disease. Curr Opin Endocrinol Diabetes Obes. 2009 Oct;16(5):340-6.

192 Muennig P, Lubetkin E, Jia H, et al. Gender and the burden of disease attributable to obesity. Am J Public Health. 2006 Sep;96(9):1662-8.

193 Tong W, Lai H, Yang C, Ren S, Dai S, Lai S. Age, gender and metabolic syndrome-related coronary heart disease in U.S. adults. Int J Cardiol. 2005 Oct 10;104(3):288-91.

194 Poirier P, Eckel RH. Obesity and cardiovascular disease. Curr Atheroscler Rep. 2002 Nov;4(6):448-53.

195 Thomsen M, Nordestgaard BG. Myocardial infarction and ischemic heart disease in overweight and obesity with and without metabolic syndrome. JAMA Intern Med. 2014 Jan;174(1):15-22.

196 Filipovský J, Ducimetiére P, Eschwége E, et al. The relationship of blood pressure with glucose, insulin, heart rate, free fatty acids and plasma cortisol levels according to degree of obesity in middle-aged men. J Hypertens. 1996 Feb;14(2):229-35.

197 Bjorntorp P. Metabolic implications of body fat distribution. Diabetes Care. 1991 Dec;14(12):1132-43.

198 La Rovere MT, Bersano C, Gnemmi M, et al. Exercise-induced increase in baroreflex sensitivity predicts improved prognosis after myocardial infarction. Circulation. 2002 Aug 20;106(8):945-9.

199 SerembusJF. The healthy heart: health promotion and maintenance. Holist NursPract. 1998 Jan;12(2):44-51.

200 Lakka TA, Laaksonen DE. Physical activity in prevention and treatment of the metabolic syndrome.ApplPhysiolNutrMetab. 2007 Feb;32(1):76-88.

201 Tuso P. Prediabetes and lifestyle modification: time to prevent a preventable disease. Perm J. 2014 Summer;18(3):88-93.

202 Wu WC, Wang CY. Association between non-alcoholic fatty pancreatic disease (NAFPD) and the metabolic syndrome: case-control retrospective study. Cardiovasc Diabetol. 2013 May 20;12:77.

203 Esteghamati A1, Morteza A, Khalilzadeh O, et al. Association of serum cortisol levels with parameters of metabolic syndrome in men and women. Clin Invest Med. 2011 Jun 1;34(3):E131-7.

204 Rezzonico J, Rezzonico M, Pusiol E, et al. Introducing the thyroid gland as another victim of the insulin resistance syndrome. Thyroid. 2008 Apr;18(4):461-4.

205 Cherednichenko LK, Zaripova ZKh, Nogteva OV. Changes the lipids, blood sugar levels, glucose tolerance and energy metabolism of rats with different forms of obesity. Probl Endokrinol (Mosk). 1977 Jul-Aug;23(4):76-80.

206 Hofeldt FD. Reactive hypoglycemia. Endocrinol Metab Clin North Am. 1989 Mar;18(1):185-201.

207 Ohba K, Koibuchi H, Matsuura Y, Morning blood glucose determination in the monitoring of metabolic control in type 2 elderly diabetic cases treated by oral hypoglycemic agents [article in Japanese]. Nihon Ronen Igakkai Zasshi. 1999 Feb;36(2):122-7.

208 Woerle HJ, Szoke E, Gosmanov N, et al. Abnormal postprandial splanchnic and peripheral glucose disposal in type 2 diabetes. Diabetes. 2004;53(suppl 2):A374.

209 Given JE, O'Kane MJ, Coates VE, et al. Comparing patient generated blood glucose diary records with meter memory in type 2 diabetes. Diabetes Res Clin Pract. 2014 Jun;104(3):358-62.

210 Johnson RJ, Segal MS, Sautin Y, et al. Potential role of sugar (fructose) in the epidemic of hypertension, obesity and the metabolic syndrome, diabetes, kidney disease, and cardiovascular disease. Am J Clin Nutr. 2007 Oct;86(4):899-906.

211 Fraser R. Metabolic disorders in diabetes. Br Med J. 1972 Dec 9;4(5840):591-6.

212 Lipson KL, Fonseca SG, Ishigaki S, et al. Regulation of insulin biosynthesis in pancreatic beta cells by an endoplasmic reticulum-resident protein kinase IRE1. Cell Metab. 2006 Sep;4(3):245-54.

213 Gale EA. The rise of childhood type 1 diabetes in the 20th century. Diabetes. 2002 Dec;51(12):3353-61.

214 Temelkova-Kurktschiev T, Stefanov T. Lifestyle and genetics in obesity and type 2 diabetes. ExpClinEndocrinol Diabetes. 2012 Jan;120(1):1-6.

215 Catalano PM1, Kirwan JP, Haugel-de Mouzon S, et al. Gestational diabetes and insulin resistance: role in short- and long-term implications for mother and fetus. J Nutr. 2003 May;133(5 Suppl 2):1674S-1683S.

216 Leslie RD. Predicting adult-onset autoimmune diabetes: clarity from complexity. Diabetes. 2010 Feb;59(2):330-1.

217 White B. Making diabetes checkups more fruitful. FamPractManag. 2000 Sep;7(8):51-2.

218 Funnell MM1, Brown TL, Childs BP, et al. National Standards for diabetes self-management education. Diabetes Care. 2011 Jan;34Suppl 1:S89-96.

219 Foltz JL1, Cook SR, Szilagyi PG, et al. US adolescent nutrition, exercise, and screen time baseline levels prior to national recommendations. ClinPediatr (Phila). 2011 May;50(5):424-33.

220 Bennett WL, Maruthur NM, Singh S, et al. Comparative effectiveness and safety of medications for type 2 diabetes: an update including new drugs and 2-drug combinations. Ann Intern Med. 2011 May 3;154(9):602-13.

221 Mellbin LG1, Malmberg K, Rydén L, The relationship between glycaemic variability and cardiovascular complications in patients with acute myocardial infarction and type 2 diabetes: a report from the DIGAMI 2 trial. Eur Heart J. 2013 Feb;34(5):374-9.

222 Grundy SM. A constellation of complications: the metabolic syndrome. Clin Cornerstone. 2005;7(2-3):36-45.

223 Nguyen T, Chai J, Li A, Akahoshi T, Tanigawa T, Tarnawski AS. Novel roles of local insulin-like growth factor-1 activation in gastric ulcer healing: promotes actin polymerization, cell proliferation, re-epithelialization, and induces cyclooxygenase-2 in a phosphatidylinositol 3-kinase-dependent manner. Am J Pathol. 2007 Apr;170(4):1219-28.

224 Coerper S1, Wolf S, von Kiparski S, et al. Insulin-like growth factor I accelerates gastric ulcer healing by stimulating cell proliferation and by inhibiting gastric acid secretion. Scand J Gastroenterol. 2001 Sep;36(9):921-7.

225 Michalakis K, Mintziori G, Kaprara A, Tarlatzis BC, Goulis DG. The complex interaction between obesity, metabolic syndrome and reproductive axis: a narrative review. Metabolism. 2013 Apr;62(4): 457-78.

226 Leishangthem GD, Mabalirajan U, Singh VP, et al. Ultrastructural changes of airway in murine models of allergy and diet-induced metabolic syndrome. ISRN Allergy. 2013:1-11.

227 Maloney EM, Boneva RS, Lin JM, et al. Chronic fatigue syndrome is associated with metabolic syndrome: results from a case-control study in Georgia. Metabolism. 2010 Sep;59(9):1351-7.

228 Mikirova N, Casciari J, Hunninghake R. The assessment of the energy metabolism in patients with chronic fatigue syndrome by serum fluorescence emission. Altern Ther Health Med. 2012 Jan-Feb;18(1):36-40.

229 Chaudhuri A, Watson WS, Pearn J, et al. The symptoms of chronic fatigue syndrome are related to abnormal ion channel function. Med Hypotheses. 2000 Jan;54(1):59-63.

230 Innes KE, Selfe TK, Taylor AG. Menopause, the metabolic syndrome, and mind-body therapies. Menopause. 2008 Sep-Oct;15(5):1005-13.

231 Pandey S, Srinivas M, Agashe S, et al. Menopause and metabolic syndrome: A study of 498 urban women from western India. J Midlife Health. 2010 Jul;1(2):63-9.

232 Bassi N, Karagodin I1, Wang S1, et al. Lifestyle Modification for Metabolic Syndrome: A Systematic Review. Am J Med. 2014 Jul 5. part II:S0002-9343(14):00576-2.

233 Xia X, Weng J. Targeting metabolic syndrome: candidate natural agents. J Diabetes. 2010 Dec;2(4):243-9.

234 Katcher HI, Legro RS, Kunselman AR, et al. The effects of a whole grain-enriched hypocaloric diet on cardiovascular disease risk factors in men and women with metabolic syndrome. Am J ClinNutr. 2008 Jan;87(1):79-90.

235 Lumaga RB, Azzali D, Fogliano V, et al. Sugar and dietary fibre composition influence, by different hormonal response, the satiating capacity

of a fruit-based and a -glucan-enriched beverage. Food Funct. 2012 Jan;3(1):67-75.

236 Hardwick JP, Eckman K, Lee YK, Abdelmegeed MA, Esterle A, Chilian WM, Chiang JY, Song BJ. Eicosanoids in metabolic syndrome. Adv Pharmacol. 2013;66:157-266.

237 Lai YH, Petrone AB, Pankow JS, et al. Association of dietary omega-3 fatty acids with prevalence of metabolic syndrome: the National Heart, Lung, and Blood Institute Family Heart Study. ClinNutr. 2013 Dec;32(6):966-9.

238 Yuan GF, Sun B, Yuan J, et al. Effects of different cooking methods on health-promoting compounds of broccoli. J Zhejiang UnivSci B. 2009 Aug;10(8):580-8.

239 Akita S, Sacks FM, Svetkey LP, et al. Effects of the Dietary Approaches to Stop Hypertension (DASH) diet on the pressure-natriuresis relationship. Hypertension. 2003 Jul;42(1):8-13.

240 Jones PJ, Varady KA. Are functional foods redefining nutritional requirements? ApplPhysiolNutrMetab. 2008 Feb;33(1):118-23.

241 Panickar KS. Beneficial effects of herbs, spices and medicinal plants on the metabolic syndrome, brain and cognitive function. Cent NervSyst Agents Med Chem. 2013 Mar;13(1):13-29.

242 Hamdy O, Ledbury S, Mullooly C, et al. Lifestyle modification improves endothelial function in obese subjects with the insulin resistance syndrome. Diabetes Care. 2003 Jul;26(7):2119-25.

243 McGill AT, Stewart JM, Lithander FE, et al. Relationships of low serum vitamin D3 with anthropometry and markers of the metabolic syndrome and diabetes in overweight and obesity. Nutr J. 2008 Jan 28;7:4.

244 Watkins LL, Sherwood A, Feinglos M. Effects of exercise and weight loss on cardiac risk factors associated with syndrome X. Arch Intern Med. 2003 Sep 8;163(16):1889-95.

245 Stewart KJ, Bacher AC, Turner K, et al. Exercise and risk factors associated with metabolic syndrome in older adults. Am J Prev Med. 2005 Jan;28(1):9-18.

246 Pencek RR, Fueger PT, Camacho RC, et al. Mobilization of glucose from the liver during exercise and replenishment afterward. Can J Appl Physiol. 2005 Jun;30(3):292-303.

247 Pitsavos C, Panagiotakos D, Weinem M, et al. Diet, exercise and the metabolic syndrome. Rev Diabet Stud. 2006 Fall;3(3):118-26.

248 Larsen I, Welde B, Martins C, Tjønna AE. High- and moderate-intensity aerobic exercise and excess post-exercise oxygen consumption in men with metabolic syndrome. Scand J Med Sci Sports. 2014 Jun;24(3):e174-9.

249 Drigny J, Gremeaux V, Guiraud T, et al. Long-term high-intensity interval training associated with lifestyle modifications improves QT dispersion parameters in metabolic syndrome patients. Ann PhysRehabil Med. 2013 Jul;56(5):356-70.

250 Perry CG1, HeigenhauserGJ, Bonen A, et al. High-intensity aerobic interval training increases fat and carbohydrate metabolic capacities in human skeletal muscle. ApplPhysiolNutrMetab. 2008 Dec;33(6):1112-23.

251 Hunter SD, Dhindsa MS, Cunningham E, et al. The effect of Bikram yoga on arterial stiffness in young and older adults. J Altern Complement Med. 2013 Dec;19(12):930-4.

252 Sundell J. Resistance Training Is an Effective Tool against Metabolic and Frailty Syndromes. AdvPrev Med. 2011;2011:984683.

253 Ingham SA, van Someren KA, Howatson G. Effect of a concentric warm-up exercise on eccentrically induced soreness and loss of function of the elbow flexor muscles. J Sports Sci. 2010 Nov;28(13):1377-82.

254 Carpinelli R. Berger in retrospect: effect of varied weight training programmes on strength. Br J Sports Med. 2002 Oct;36(5):319-24.

255 Olsen O, Sjøhaug M, van Beekvelt M, et al. The effect of warm-up and cool-down exercise on delayed onset muscle soreness in the quadriceps muscle: a randomized controlled trial. J Hum Kinet. 2012 Dec;35:59-68.

256 Bennard P, Doucet E. Acute effects of exercise timing and breakfast meal glycemic index on exercise-induced fat oxidation. ApplPhysiolNutrMetab. 2006 Oct;31(5):502-11.

257 Bangsbo J, HellstenY.Muscle blood flow and oxygen uptake in recovery from exercise. ActaPhysiol Scand. 1998 Mar;162(3):305-12.

258 Ruxton CHS. Smoothies: one portion or two? Nutrition Bulletin. 2008;33(2):129-132.

259 Colberg SR, Sigal RJ, Fernhall B, et al. Exercise and type 2 diabetes: the American College of Sports Medicine and the American Diabetes Association: joint position statement executive summary. Diabetes Care. 2010 Dec;33(12):2692-6.

260 Kubota T1, Kubota N, Kumagai H, et al. Impaired insulin signaling in endothelial cells reduces insulin-induced glucose uptake by skeletal muscle. Cell Metab. 2011 Mar 2;13(3):294-307.

261 McAdam-Marx C, Yu J, Bouchard J, Aagren M,et al. Comparison of daily insulin dose and other antidiabetic medications usage for type 2 diabetes patients treated with an analog basal insulin. Curr Med Res Opin. 2010 Jan;26(1):191-201.

262 Aquilante CL. Sulfonylurea pharmacogenomics in Type 2 diabetes: the influence of drug target and diabetes risk polymorphisms. Expert Rev Cardiovasc Ther. 2010 Mar;8(3):359-72.

263 Musini VM, Nazer M, Bassett K, et al. Blood pressure-lowering efficacy of monotherapy with thiazide diuretics for primary hypertension. Cochrane Database Syst Rev. 2014 May 29;5:CD003824.

264 Taylor AA, Bakris GL. The role of vasodilating beta-blockers in patients with hypertension and the cardiometabolic syndrome. Am J Med. 2010 Jul;123(7 Suppl 1):S21-6.

265 Ryan PW. Beta blocker side-effects. Can Fam Physician. 1987 Apr;33:831.

266 Heran BS, Galm BP, Wright JM. Blood pressure lowering efficacy of alpha blockers for primary hypertension. Cochrane Database Syst Rev. 2012 Aug 15;8:CD004643.

267 Scheinfeld N. A comprehensive review and evaluation of the side effects of the tumor necrosis factor alpha blockers etanercept, infliximab and adalimumab. J Dermatolog Treat. 2004 Sep;15(5):280-94.

268 Montecucco F, Mach F. Statins, ACE inhibitors and ARBs in cardiovascular disease. Best Pract Res Clin Endocrinol Metab. 2009 Jun;23(3):389-400.

269 Hebert LA. Optimizing ACE-inhibitor therapy for chronic kidney disease. N Engl J Med. 2006 Jan 12;354(2):189-91.

270 Dieterich HA, Wendt C, Saborowski F. Cardioprotection by aldosterone receptor antagonism in heart failure. Part I. The role of aldosterone in heart failure. Fiziol Cheloveka. 2005 Nov-Dec;31(6):97-105.

271 Guichard JL, Clark D 3rd, Calhoun DA, et al. Aldosterone receptor antagonists: current perspectives and therapies. Vasc Health Risk Manag. 2013;9:321-31.

272 Martínez Martín FJ. Calcium channel-blockers for managing meta-

bolic syndrome-associated hypertension. Trials with manidipine [article in Spanish]. Nefrologia. 2007;27 Suppl 6:26-35.

273 Bray GA. Drug Insight: appetite suppressants. Nat Clin Pract Gastroenterol Hepatol. 2005 Feb;2(2):89-95.

274 Ryan DH. Use of sibutramine and other noradrenergic and serotonergic drugs in the management of obesity. Endocrine. 2000 Oct;13(2):193-9.

275 Yamada Y, Kato T, Ogino H, et al. Cetilistat (ATL-962), a novel pancreatic lipase inhibitor, ameliorates body weight gain and improves lipid profiles in rats. Horm Metab Res. 2008 Aug;40(8):539-43.

276 Harvey BH, Bouwer CD. Neuropharmacology of paradoxic weight gain with selective serotonin reuptake inhibitors. Clin Neuropharmacol. 2000 Mar-Apr;23(2):90-7.

277 Livingston EH. Procedure incidence and in-hospital complication rates of bariatric surgery in the United States. Am J Surg. 2004 Aug;188(2):105-10.

278 Sjöholm K, Anveden A, Peltonen M, et al. Evaluation of current eligibility criteria for bariatric surgery: diabetes prevention and risk factor changes in the Swedish obese subjects (SOS) study. Diabetes Care. 2013 May;36(5):1335-40.

279 PoriesWJ. Bariatric surgery: risks and rewards. J Clin Endocrinol Metab. 2008 Nov;93(11 Suppl 1):S89-96.

280 Carlin AM, Zeni TM, English WJ, et al. The comparative effectiveness of sleeve gastrectomy, gastric bypass, and adjustable gastric banding procedures for the treatment of morbid obesity. Ann Surg. 2013 May;257(5):791-7.

281 OchnerCN, Gibson C, Shanik M, et al. Changes in neurohormonal gut peptides following bariatric surgery. Int J Obes (Lond). 2011 Feb;35(2):153-66.

282 Guijarro A, Kirchner H, Meguid MM. Catabolic effects of gastric bypass in a diet-induced obese rat model.CurrOpinClinNutrMetab Care. 2006 Jul;9(4):423-35.

283 Kehagias I, KaramanakosSN, Argentou M, et al. Randomized clinical trial of laparoscopic Roux-en-Y gastric bypass versus laparoscopic sleeve gastrectomy for the management of patients with BMI < 50 kg/m2. Obes Surg. 2011 Nov;21(11):1650-6.

284 Ukleja A. Dumping syndrome: pathophysiology and treatment. NutrClinPract. 2005 Oct;20(5):517-25.

285 Gentileschi P. Laparoscopic sleeve gastrectomy as a primary operation for morbid obesity: experience with 200 patients. Gastroenterol Res Pract. 2012;2012:801325.

286 Dillard BE III, GorodnerV, Galvani C, et al. Initial experience with the adjustable gastric band in morbidly obese US adolescents and recommendations for further investigation.J PediatrGastroenterolNutr. 2007 Aug;45(2):240-6.

287 Marceau P, HouldFS, Simard S, et al. Biliopancreatic diversion with duodenal switch.World J Surg. 1998 Sep;22(9):947-54.

288 SugermanHJ, KellumJMJr, DeMariaEJ, et al. Conversion of failed or complicated vertical banded gastroplasty to gastric bypass in morbid obesity.Am J Surg. 1996 Feb;171(2):263-9.

289 Eldar S, Heneghan HM, Brethauer S, et al.A focus on surgical preoperative evaluation of the bariatric patient—the Cleveland Clinic protocol and review of the literature.Surgeon. 2011 Oct;9(5):273-7.

290 Inabnet WB III, Winegar DA, Sherif B, et al. Early outcomes of bariatric surgery in patients with metabolic syndrome: an analysis of the bariatric outcomes longitudinal database. J Am Coll Surg. 2012 Apr;214(4):550-6; discussion 556-7.

291 Adamo KB,Tesson F. Gene-environment interaction and the metabolic syndrome. Novartis Found Symp. 2008;293:103-19; discussion 119-27.

292 Speakman JR.Thrifty genes for obesity and the metabolic syndrome—time to call off the search? Diab Vasc Dis Res. 2006 May;3(1):7-11.

293 Carulli L, Rondinella S, Lombardini S, et al. Review article: diabetes, genetics and ethnicity. Aliment Pharmacol Ther. 2005 Nov;22 Suppl 2:16-9.

294 Schober E, Rami B, Grabert M, et al. Phenotypical aspects of maturity-onset diabetes of the young (MODY diabetes) in comparison with Type 2 diabetes mellitus (T2DM) in children and adolescents: experience from a large multicentre database. Diabet Med. 2009 May;26(5):466-73.

295 Butler MG. Genetics of hypertension. Current status. J Med Liban. 2010 Jul-Sep;58(3):175-8.

296 Soutar AK, Naoumova RP. Mechanisms of disease: genetic causes of familial hypercholesterolemia. Nat Clin Pract Cardiovasc Med. 2007 Apr;4(4):214-25.

297 Herrera BM, Lindgren CM. The genetics of obesity. Curr Diab Rep. 2010 Dec;10(6):498-505.

298 Yamada Y, Kato K, Hibino T, et al. Prediction of genetic risk for metabolic syndrome. Atherosclerosis. 2007 Apr;191(2):298-304.

299 Verhaak PF, HeijmansMJ, Peters L, Chronic disease and mental disorder. Soc Sci Med. 2005 Feb;60(4):789-97.

300 Newcomer JW. Metabolic syndrome and mental illness. Am J Manag Care. 2007 Nov;13(7 Suppl):S170-7.

301 Rintamaki R, Grimaldi S, Englund A, et al. Seasonal Changes in Mood and Behavior Are Linked to Metabolic Syndrome. PLoS ONE 2008 Jan;3(1):e1482.

302 Vancampfort D, Vansteelandt K, Correll CU, et al. Metabolic syndrome and metabolic abnormalities in bipolar disorder: a meta-analysis of prevalence rates and moderators. Am J Psychiatry. 2013 Mar 1;170(3):265-74.

303 Kemp DE, Gao K, Chan PK, et al. Medical comorbidity in bipolar disorder: relationship between illnesses of the endocrine/metabolic system and treatment outcome. Bipolar Disord. 2010 Jun;12(4):404-13.

304 Antonius D, Kline B, Sinclair SJ, et al. Deficits in implicit facial recognition of fear in aggressive patients with schizophrenia. Schizophr Res. 2013 Feb;143(2-3):401-2.

305 Burghardt KJ, Ellingrod VL. Detection of metabolic syndrome in schizophrenia and implications for antipsychotic therapy : is there a role for folate? Mol Diagn Ther. 2013 Feb;17(1):21-30.

306 Heiskanen TH, Niskanen LK, Hintikka JJ, et al. Metabolic syndrome and depression: a cross-sectional analysis. J Clin Psychiatry. 2006 Sep;67(9):1422-7.

307 Dunbar JA, Reddy P, Davis-Lameloise N, et al. Depression: an important comorbidity with metabolic syndrome in a general population. Diabetes Care. 2008 Dec;31(12):2368-73.

308 Butnoriene J, Bunevicius A, Norkus A, et al. Depression but not anxiety is associated with metabolic syndrome in primary care based community sample. Psychoneuroendocrinology. 2014 Feb;40:269-76.

309 Yoo S, Kim H, Cho HI. Improvements in the metabolic syndrome and stages of change for lifestyle behaviors in korean older adults. Osong Public Health Res Perspect. 2012 Jun;3(2):85-93.

310 Reilly S, Planner C, Gask L, et al. Collaborative care approaches for people with severe mental illness. Cochrane Database Syst Rev. 2013 Nov 4;11:CD009531.

311 WoudenbergYJ, Lucas C, Latour C, et al. Acceptance of insulin therapy: a long shot? Psychological insulin resistance in primary care. Diabet Med. 2012 Jun;29(6):796-802.

312 Loevinger BL, Muller D, Alonso C, et al. Metabolic syndrome in women with chronic pain. Metabolism. 2007 Jan;56(1):87-93.

313 Guldiken B, Guldiken S, Taskiran B, Koc G, Turgut N, Kabayel L, Tugrul A. Migraine in metabolic syndrome. Neurologist. 2009 Mar;15(2):55-8.

314 Winsvold BS, Sandven I, Hagen K, et al. Migraine, headache and development of metabolic syndrome: an 11-year follow-up in the Nord-Trondelag Health Study (HUNT). Pain. 2013 Aug;154(8):1305-11.

315 Dessein PH, ShiptonEA, Joffe BI, et al. High frequency of insulin resistance and hyperlipidemia in fibromyalgia. XIV European League Against Rheumatism Congress. Ann Rheum Dis. 1999;S553:137.

316 Roca MartínezFJ, Rubio RubioJM, Martín Gómez R, et al. Evaluation of immunoreactive serum levels of insulin, C peptide and glucagon in patients with acute pancreatitis and acute abdominal pain of non-pancreatic origin [article in Spanish]. Med Clin (Barc). 1982 Jan 10;78(1):13-6.

317 Husby S, Hoost A. Recurrent abdominal pain, food allergy and endoscopy. ActaPaediatr. 2001 Jan;90(1):3-4.

318 Locatelli F, Pozzoni P, Del Vecchio L. Renal manifestations in the metabolic syndrome. J Am Soc Nephrol. 2006 Apr;17(4 Suppl 2):S81-5.

319 Cojocaru M, Cojocaru IM, Silosi I, et al. Metabolic syndrome in rheumatoid arthritis. Maedica (Buchar). 2012 Jun;7(2):148-52.

320 Nakanishi-Minami T, Kishida K, Nakagawa Y, et al. Metabolic syndrome correlates intracoronary stenosis detected by multislice computed tomography in male subjects with sleep-disordered breathing. Diabetol Metab Syndr. 2012 Mar 1;4:6.

321 Ray L, Lipton RB, Zimmerman ME, et al. Mechanisms of association between obesity and chronic pain in the elderly.Pain. 2011 Jan;152(1):53-9.

322 Greisen J, Juhl CB, Grofte T, et al. Acute pain induces insulin resistance in humans. Anesthesiology. 2001 Sep;95(3):578-84.

323 Centers for Medicare & Medicaid Services (CMS), HHS. Basic health program: state administration of basic health programs; eligibility and enrollment in standard health plans; essential health benefits in standard health plans; performance standards for basic health programs; premium and cost sharing for basic health programs; federal funding process; trust fund and financial integrity. Final rule. Fed Regist. 2014 Mar 12;79(48):14111-51.

324 Sanders LM, Shaw JS, Guez G, et al. Health literacy and child health promotion: implications for research, clinical care, and public policy. Pediatrics. 2009 Nov;124 Suppl 3:S306-14.

325 Jafarov E, Gunnarsson V. Government spending on health care and education in croatia: efficiency and reform options. IMF Working Paper 2008 May;8:136.

326 Marks PA. Academic health centers and the federal government: a partnership in research, education, and patient care. Bull N Y Acad Med. 1981 Jul-Aug;57(6):470-5.

327 Roberts JN. Funding alternatives for corporate-sponsored health benefit plans. J Corp Acct Fin. 1991;2(3):345-51.

328 Lemmens C. Pharma Goes to the Laundry: Public Relations and the Business of Medical Education. Hastings Center Report. 2004 Sep-Oct;34(5):18-23.

329 Cegala DJ, Marinelli T, Post D. The effects of patient communication skills training on compliance. Arch Fam Med. 2000 Jan;9(1):57-64.

330 Frampton SB, Guastello S, Lepore M. Compassion as the foundation of patient-centered care: the importance of compassion in action. J Comp Eff Res. 2013 Sep;2(5):443-55.

331 Erskine PJ, Idris I, Daly H, Scott AR. Treatment satisfaction and metabolic outcome in patients with type 2 diabetes starting insulin: one-to-one vs group therapy. Pract Diab Int. 2003;20(7):243-46.

332 Kirk K. Confidence as a factor in chronic illness care. J Adv Nurs. 1992 Oct;17(10):1238-42.

333 Raleigh ED. Sources of hope in chronic illness. Oncol Nurs Forum. 1992 Apr;19(3):443-8.

334 Puhl RM, Heuer CA. Obesity stigma: important considerations for public health. Am J Public Health. 2010 Jun;100(6):1019-28.

335 Croker JE, Swancutt DR, Roberts MJ, et al. Factors affecting patients'

trust and confidence in GPs: evidence from the English national GP patient survey. BMJ Open. 2013 May 28;3(5). part II:e002762.

336 Vilhena E, Pais-Ribeiro J, Silva I, et al. Optimism on quality of life in Portuguese chronic patients: moderator/mediator? Rev Assoc Med Bras. 2014 Jul;60(4):373-80.

337 Frich JC, Malterud K, Fugelli P. Experiences of guilt and shame in patients with familial hypercholesterolemia: a qualitative interview study. Patient Educ Couns. 2007 Dec;69(1-3):108-13.

338 Trickett EJ. From "Water Boiling in a Peruvian Town" to "Letting them Die": culture, community intervention, and the metabolic balance between patience and zeal. Am J Community Psychol. 2011 Mar;47(1-2):58-68.

339 Zolnierek KB, Dimatteo MR. Physician communication and patient adherence to treatment: a meta-analysis. Med Care. 2009 Aug;47(8):826-34.

INDEX

Dear Reader,

I really can't express how flatte
grateful I am to Harlequin Boo
collection of my published works. It came as a great surprise. I never think of myself as writing books that are collectible. In fact, there are days when I forget that writing is work at all. What I do for a living is so much fun that it never seems like a job. And since I reside in a small community, and my daily life is confined to such mundane things as feeding the wild birds and looking after my herb patch in the backyard, I feel rather unconnected from what many would think of as a glamorous profession.

But when I read my email, or when I get letters from readers, or when I go on signing trips to bookstores to meet all of you, I feel truly blessed. Over the past thirty years, I have made lasting friendships with many of you. And quite frankly, most of you are like part of my family. You can't imagine how much you enrich my life. Thank you so much

I also need to extend than
husband, James, son
Christina, and
best friend, An
wonderful peo
editor of many y
talented people w
Thanks to all of yo
private life so worth living.

Thank you for this tribute, Harlequin, and for putting up with me for thirty long years! Love to all of you.

Diana Palmer

DIANA PALMER

The prolific author of more than one hundred books, Diana Palmer got her start as a newspaper reporter. A multi–*New York Times* bestselling author and one of the top ten romance writers in America, she has a gift for telling the most sensual tales with charm and humor. Diana lives with her family in Cornelia, Georgia.

Visit her website at www.DianaPalmer.com.

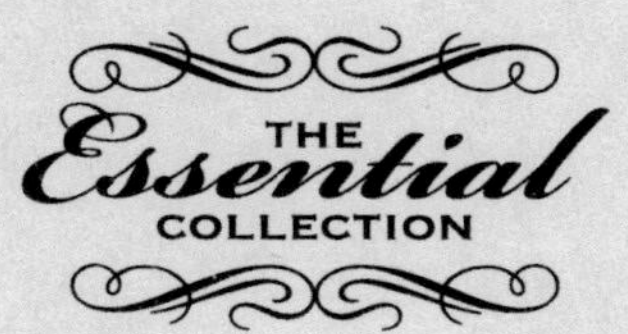

DIANA PALMER

New York Times and *USA TODAY* Bestselling Author

SEPTEMBER MORNING

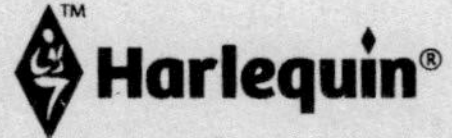

TORONTO NEW YORK LONDON
AMSTERDAM PARIS SYDNEY HAMBURG
STOCKHOLM ATHENS TOKYO MILAN MADRID
PRAGUE WARSAW BUDAPEST AUCKLAND

To Ann, Anne, "George," "Eddard," Dannis and Dad

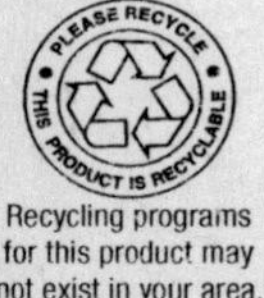

Recycling programs for this product may not exist in your area.

ISBN-13: 978-0-373-36411-4

SEPTEMBER MORNING

This edition published by arrangement with Harlequin Books S.A.

For questions and comments about the quality of this book please contact us at Customer_eCare@Harlequin.ca.

www.Harlequin.com

Printed in U.S.A.

New York Times* and *USA TODAY
Bestselling Author

Diana Palmer

The Essential Collection
Long, Tall Texans...and More!

AVAILABLE FEBRUARY 2011

Calhoun
Tyler
Ethan
Connal
Harden
Evan

AVAILABLE MARCH 2011

Donavan
Emmett
Regan's Pride
That Burke Man
Circle of Gold
Cattleman's Pride

AVAILABLE APRIL 2011

The Princess Bride
Coltrain's Proposal
A Man of Means
Lionhearted
Maggie's Dad
Rage of Passion

AVAILABLE MAY 2011

Lacy
Beloved
Love with a Long, Tall Texan
(containing "Guy," "Luke" and "Christopher")
Heart of Ice
Noelle
Fit for a King
The Rawhide Man

AVAILABLE JUNE 2011

A Long, Tall Texan Summer

(containing "Tom," "Drew" and "Jobe")

Nora

Dream's End

Champagne Girl

Friends and Lovers

The Wedding in White

AVAILABLE JULY 2011

Heather's Song

Snow Kisses

To Love and Cherish

Long, Tall and Tempted

(containing "Redbird," "Paper Husband" and "Christmas Cowboy")

The Australian

Darling Enemy

Trilby

AVAILABLE AUGUST 2011

Sweet Enemy

Soldier of Fortune

The Tender Stranger

Enamored

After the Music

The Patient Nurse

AVAILABLE SEPTEMBER 2011

The Case of the Mesmerizing Boss

The Case of the Confirmed Bachelor

The Case of the Missing Secretary

September Morning

Diamond Girl

Eye of the Tiger

Chapter One

The meadow was dew-misted, and the morning had the nip of a September breeze to give it life. Kathryn Mary Kilpatrick tossed her long black hair and laughed with the sheer joy of being alive. The sound startled the chestnut gelding she was riding, making it dance nervously over the damp ground.

"Easy, boy," she said soothingly, her gloved hand reaching out to touch his mane gently.

He calmed, reacting to the familiar caress. Sundance had been hers since he was a colt, a present from Blake on her sixteenth birthday. Sundance was a mature five-year-old now, but some of his coltish uncertainties lingered. He was easily startled and high-strung. Like Kathryn Mary.

Her dark green eyes shimmered with excitement as

she studied the long horizon under the pink and amber swirls of the dawn sky. It was so good to be home again. The exclusive girls' school had polished her manners and given her the poise of a model, but it had done nothing to cool her ardor for life or to dampen the passion she felt for Greyoaks. Despite the fact that the Hamiltons' South Carolina farm was her home by adoption, not by birth, she loved every green, rolling hill and pine forest of it, just as though she were a Hamilton herself.

A flash of color caught her attention, and she wheeled Sundance as Phillip Hamilton came tearing across the meadow toward her on a thoroughbred Arabian with a coat like polished black leather. She smiled, watching him. If Blake ever caught him riding one of his prize breeding stallions like that, it would mean disaster. What luck for Phillip that Blake was in Europe on business. Maude might indulge her youngest, but Blake indulged no one.

"Hi!" Phillip called breathlessly. He reined in just in front of her and caught his wind, tossing back his unruly brown hair with a restless hand. His brown eyes twinkled with mischief as they swept over her slender figure in the chic riding habit. But the mischief went out of them when he noticed her bare head.

"No helmet?" he chided.

She pouted at him with her full, soft lips. "Don't scold," she accused. "It was just a little ride, and I hate wearing a hard hat all the time."

"One fall and you'd be done for," he observed.

"You sound just like Blake!"

He smiled at her mutinous look. "Too bad he missed your homecoming. Oh, well, he'll be back at the end of the week—just in time for the Barringtons' party."

"Blake hates parties," she reminded him. Her eyes lowered to the rich leather of her Western saddle. "And he hates me too, most of the time."

"He doesn't," Phillip returned. "It's just that you set fire to his temper, you rebellious little witch. I can remember a time when you all but worshiped my big brother."

She grimaced, turning her eyes to the long horizon where thoroughbred Arabians grazed on lush pasture grass, their black coats shimmering like oil in the sunlight. "Did I?" She laughed shortly. "He was kind to me once, when my mother died."

"He cares about you. We all do," he said gently.

She smiled at him warmly and reached out an impulsive hand to touch his sleeve. "I'm ungrateful, and I don't mean to be. You and your mother have been wonderful to me. Taking me in, putting me through school—how could I be ungrateful?"

"Blake had a little to do with it," he reminded her wryly.

She tossed her hair back impatiently. "I suppose," she admitted grudgingly.

"Finishing school was his idea."

"And I hated it!" she flashed. "I wanted to go to the university and take political science courses."

"Blake likes to entertain buyers," he reminded her.

"Political science courses don't teach you how to be a hostess."

She shrugged. "Well, I'm not going to be here forever, despite the fact that you and Blake are my cousins," she said. "I'll get married someday. I know I owe your family a lot, but I'm not going to spend my whole life playing hostess for Blake! He can get married and let his wife do it. If he can find anyone brave enough," she added waspishly.

"You've got to be kidding, Cuz," he chuckled. "They follow him around like ants on a sugar trail. Blake could have his pick when it comes to women, and you know it."

"It must be his money, then," she said tightly, "because it sure isn't his cheerful personality that draws them!"

"You're just sore because he wouldn't let you go away with Jack Harris for the weekend," he teased.

She flushed right up to her hairline. "I didn't know Jack had planned for us to be alone at the cottage," she protested. "I thought his parents were going to be there, too."

"But you didn't think to check. Blake did." He laughed at her expression. "I'll never forget how he looked when Jack came to get you. Or how Jack looked when he left, alone."

She shivered at the memory. "I'd like to forget."

"I'll bet you would. You've been staring daggers at Blake ever since, but it just bounces right off. You don't dent him, do you?"

"Nothing dents Blake," she murmured. "He just stands there and lets me rant and rave until he's had enough, then he turns that cold voice on me and walks away. He'll be glad when I'm gone," she said in a quiet voice.

"You're not going anywhere yet, are you?" he asked suddenly.

She darted a mischievous glance at him. "I *had* thought about joining the French Foreign Legion," she admitted. "Do you think I could get my application accepted before the weekend?"

He laughed. "In time to escape Blake? You know you've missed him."

"I have?" she asked with mock innocence.

"Six months is a long time. He's calmed down."

"Blake never forgets," she sighed miserably. She stared past Phillip to the towering gray stone house in the distance with its graceful arches and the cluster of huge live oaks dripping Spanish moss that stood like sentries around it.

"Don't work yourself into a nervous breakdown," Phillip said comfortingly. "Come on, race me back to the house and we'll have breakfast."

She sighed wearily. "All right."

Maude's dark eyes lit up when the two of them walked into the elegant dining room and seated themselves at the polished oak table.

She had the same olive skin and sharp, dark eyes as her eldest son, the same forthright manner and quick temper. Maude was nothing like Phillip. She lacked his gentleness and easy manner, as well as his pale coloring. Those traits came from his late father, not from his maverick mother, who thought nothing of getting a congressman out of bed at two in the morning if she wanted a piece of pending legislation explained to her.

"It's good to have you home, baby," Maude told Kathryn, reaching out a slender, graceful hand to touch the younger woman's arm. "I'm simply surrounded by men these days."

"That's the truth," Phillip said wryly as he helped himself to scrambled eggs from the bone china platter. "Matt Davis and Jack Nelson nearly came to blows over her at a cocktail party last week."

Maude glared at him. "That isn't so," she protested.

"Oh?" Kathryn asked with an impish smile as she sipped her black coffee.

Maude shifted uncomfortably. "Anyway, I wish Blake were home. It was bad timing, that crisis at the London office. I had a special evening planned for Friday night. A homecoming party for you. It would have been perfect..."

"I don't need Blake to make a party perfect," Kathryn burst out without thinking.

Maude's pencil-thin gray brows went up. "Are you going to hold it against him forever?" she chided.

Kathryn's fingers tightened around her coffee cup. "He didn't have to be so rough on me!" she protested.

"He was right, Kathryn Mary, and you know it," Maude said levelly. She leaned forward, resting her forearms on the table. "Darling, you have to remember that you're just barely twenty. Blake's thirty-four now, and he knows a great deal more about life than you've had time to learn. We've all sheltered you," she added, frowning. "Sometimes I wonder if it was quite fair."

"Ask Blake," she returned bitterly. "He's kept me under glass for years."

"His protective instinct," Phillip said with an amused grin. "A misplaced mother hen complex."

"I wouldn't let him hear that, if I were you," Maude commented drily.

"I'm not afraid of big brother," he replied. "Just because he can outfight me is no reason…on second thought, you may have a point."

Maude laughed. "You're a delight. I wish Blake had a little of your ability to take things lightly. He's so intense."

"I can think of a better word," Kathryn said under her breath.

"Isn't it amazing," Phillip asked his mother, "how brave she is when Blake isn't here?"

"Amazing." Maude nodded. She smiled at Kathryn. "Cheer up, sweetheart. Let me tell you what Eve Barrington has planned for your homecoming party Saturday night…the one I was going to give you if Blake hadn't been called away…"

The arrangements for the party were faultless, Kathryn discovered. The florist had delivered urns of dried flowers in blazing fall colors, and tasteful arrangements of daisies and mums and baby's breath to decorate the buffet tables. The intimate little gathering at the nearby estate swelled to over fifty people, not all of them contemporaries of Kathryn's. Quite a number, she noticed with amusement, were politicians. Maude was lobbying fiercely for legislation to protect a nearby stretch of South Carolina's unspoiled river land from being zoned for business. No doubt she'd pleaded with Eve to add those politicians to the guest list, Kathryn thought wickedly.

Nan Barrington, Eve's daughter, and one of Kathryn's oldest friends, pulled her aside while the musicians launched into a frantic rock number.

"Mother hates hard rock," she confided as the band blared out. "I can't imagine why she hired that particular band, when it's all they play."

"The name," Kathryn guessed. "It's the Glen Miller ensemble, and Glen spells his name with just one 'n.' Your mother probably thought they played the same kind of music as the late Glenn Miller."

"That's Mother," Nan agreed with a laugh. She ran a finger over the rim of her glass, filled with sparkling rum punch. Her blond hair sparkled with the same amber color as she looked around the room. "I thought Blake was going to come by when he got home. It's after ten now."

Kathryn smiled at her indulgently. Nan had had a crush on Blake since their early teens. Blake pretended not to notice, treating both girls like the adolescents he thought them.

"You know Blake hates parties," she reminded the shorter girl.

"It can't be for lack of partners to take to them," Nan sighed.

Kathryn frowned at her. She cupped her own glass in her hands and wondered why that statement nagged her. She knew Blake dated, but it had been a long time since she'd spent more than a few days at Greyoaks. Not for years. There was too much to do. Relatives she could visit in faraway places like France and Greece and even Australia. Cruises with friends like Nan. School events and girlfriends to visit and parties to go to. There hadn't been much reason to stay at Greyoaks. Especially since that last bout with Blake over Jack Harris. She sighed, remembering how harsh he'd been about it. Jack Harris had turned every color in the rainbow before Blake got through telling him what he thought in that cold, precise voice that always accompanied his temper. When he'd turned it on Kathryn, it had been all she could manage not to run. She was honestly afraid of Blake. Not that he'd beat her or anything. It was a different kind of fear, strange and ever-present, growing as she matured.

"Why the frown?" Nan asked suddenly.

"Was I frowning?" She laughed. She shrugged, sipping her punch. Her eyes ran over her shorter friend's pale blue evening gown, held up by tiny spaghetti straps. "I love your dress."

"It isn't a patch on yours," Nan sighed, wistfully eyeing the Grecian off-the-shoulder style of Kathryn's delicate white gown. The wisps of chiffon foamed and floated with every movement. "It's a dream."

"I have a friend in Atlanta who's a budding designer," she explained with a smile. "This is from her first collection. She had a showing at that new department store on Peachtree Street."

"Everything looks good on you," Nan said genuinely. "You're so tall and willowy."

"Skinny, Blake says." She laughed and then suddenly froze as she looked across the room straight into a pair of narrow, dark eyes in a face as hard as granite.

He was as tall and big as she remembered, all hard-muscled grace and blatant masculinity. His head was bare, his dark hair gleaming in the light from the crystal chandelier overhead. His deeply tanned face had its own inborn arrogance, a legacy from his grandfather, who had forged a small empire from the ashes of the old confederacy. His eyes were cold, even at a distance, his mouth chiseled and firm and just a little cruel. Kathryn shivered involuntarily as his eyes trailed up and down the revealing dress she was wearing, clearly disapproving.

Nan followed her gaze, and her small face lit up. "It's Blake!" she exclaimed. "Kathryn, aren't you going to say hello to him?"

She swallowed. "Oh, yes, of course," she said, aware of Maude going forward to greet her eldest and Phillip waving to him carelessly from across the room.

"You don't look terribly enthusiastic about it," Nan remarked, studying the flush in her friend's cheeks and the slight tremor in the slender hands that held the crystal glass.

"He'll be furious because I haven't got a bow in my hair and a teddy bear under my arm," she said with a mirthless laugh.

"You're not a little girl anymore," Nan said, coming to her friend's defense despite her attraction to Blake.

"Tell Blake," she sighed. "See?" she murmured as he lifted his arrogant head and motioned for her to join him. "I'm being summoned."

"Could you manage to look a little less like Marie Antoinette on her way to the guillotine?" Nan whispered.

"I can't help it. My neck's tingling. See you," she muttered, moving toward Blake with a faint smile.

She moved forward, through the throng of guests, her heart throbbing as heavily as the rock rhythm that shook the walls around her. Six months hadn't erased the bitterness of their last quarrel, and judging by the look on Blake's rugged face, it was still fresh in his mind, too.

He drew deeply on his cigarette, looking down his straight nose at her, and she couldn't help noticing how dangerously attractive he was in his dark evening clothes. The white silk of his shirt was a perfect foil for his olive complexion, his arrogant good looks. The tang of his Oriental cologne drifted down into her nostrils, a fragrance that echoed his vibrant masculinity.

"Hello, Blake," she said nervously, glad Maude had vanished into the throng of politicians so she didn't have to pretend more enthusiasm.

His eyes sketched her slender figure, lingering at the plunging neckline that revealed tantalizing glimpses of the swell of her small, high breasts.

"Advertising, Kate?" he asked harshly. "I thought you'd learned your lesson with Harris."

"Don't call me Kate," she fired back. "And it's no more revealing than what everyone else is wearing."

"You haven't changed," he sighed indulgently. "All fire and lace and wobbly legs. I hoped that finishing school might give you a little maturity."

Her emerald eyes burned. "I'm twenty, Blake!"

One dark eyebrow went up. "What do you want me to do about it?"

She started to reply that she didn't want him to do a thing, but the anger faded away suddenly. "Oh, Blake," she moaned, "why do you have to spoil my party? It's been such fun..."

"For whom?" he asked, his eyes finding several of the politicians present. "You or Maude?"

"She's trying to save the wildlife along the Edisto River," she said absently. "They want to develop part of the riverfront."

"Yes, let's save the water moccasins and sandflies, at all costs!" he agreed lightly, although Kathryn knew he was as avid a conservationist as Maude.

She peeked up at him. "I seem to remember that you went on television to support that wilderness proposal on the national forest."

He raised his cigarette to his firm lips. "Guilty," he admitted with a faint, rare smile. He glanced toward the band and the smile faded. "Are they all playing the same song?" he asked irritably.

"I'm not sure. I thought you liked music," she teased.

He glowered down at her. "I do. But that," he added with a speaking glance in the band's direction, "isn't."

"My generation thinks it is," she replied with a challenge in her bright eyes. "And if you don't like contemporary music, then why did you bother to come to the party, you old stick-in-the-mud?"

He reached down and tapped her on the cheek with a long, stinging finger. "Don't be smart," he told her. "I came because I hadn't seen you for six months, if you want the truth."

"Why? So you could drive me home and bawl me out in privacy on the way?" she asked.

His heavy dark brows came together. "How much of that punch have you had?" he asked curtly.

"Not quite enough," she replied with an impudent grin and tossed off the rest of the punch in her glass.

"Feeling reckless, little girl?" he asked quietly.

"It's more like self-preservation, Blake," she admitted softly, peeking up at him over the empty glass as she held its coolness to her pink lips. "I was getting my nerves numb so that it wouldn't bother me when you started giving me hell."

He took a draw from his cigarette. "It was six months ago," he said tightly. "I've forgotten it."

"No you haven't," she sighed, reading the cold anger very near the surface in his taut face. "I really didn't know what Jack had in mind. I probably should have, but I'm not very worldly."

He sighed heavily. "No, that's for sure. I used to think it was a good thing. But the older you get, the more I wonder."

"That's just what Maude was saying," she murmured, wondering if he could read people's minds.

"And she could be right." His eyes narrowed to a glittering darkness as he studied her in the revealing little dress. "That dress is years too old for you."

"Does that mean it's all right with you if I grow up?" she asked sweetly.

One dark eyebrow rose laconically. "I wasn't aware that you needed my permission."

"I seem to, though," she persisted. "If I try to do anything about it, you'll be on my neck like a duck after a June bug."

"That depends on what sort of growing-up process you have in mind," he replied, reaching over to crush the cigarette into an ashtray. "Promiscuity is definitely out."

"Not in your case, it isn't!"

His head jerked up, his eyes blazing. "What the hell has my private life got to do with you?" he asked in a voice that cut like sheer ice.

She felt like backing away. "I...I was just teasing, Blake," she defended in a shaken whisper.

"I'm not laughing," he said curtly.

"You never do with me," she said in a voice like china breaking.

"Stop acting like a silly adolescent."

She bit her lower lip, trying to stem the welling tears in her soft, hurt eyes. "If you'll excuse me," she said unsteadily, "I'll go back and play with my dolls. Thank you for your warm welcome," she added in a tiny voice before she pushed her way through the crowd away from him. For the first time, she wished she'd never come to live with Blake's family.

Chapter Two

For the rest of the evening she avoided Blake, sticking to Nan and Phillip like a shadow while she nursed her emotional wounds. Not that Blake seemed to notice. He was standing with Maude and one of the younger congressmen in the group, deep in discussion.

"I wonder what they're talking about now?" Phillip asked as he danced Kathryn around the room to one of the band's few slow tunes.

"Saving water moccasins," she muttered, her full lips pouting, her eyes as dark as jade with hurt.

Phillip sighed heavily. "What's he done now?"

"What?" she asked, lifting her flushed face to Phillip's patiently amused eyes.

"Blake. He hasn't been in the same room with you

for ten minutes, and the two of you are already avoiding one another. Talk about repeat acts!"

Her rounded jaw clenched. "He hates me, I told you he did."

"What's he done?" he repeated.

She glared at his top shirt button. "He said…he said I couldn't be promiscuous."

"Good for Blake," Phillip said with annoying enthusiasm.

"You don't understand. That was just what started it," she explained. "And I was teasing him about not being a monk, and he jumped all over me about digging into his private life." She felt herself tense as she remembered the blazing heat of Blake's anger. "I didn't mean anything."

"You didn't know about Della?" he asked softly.

She gaped up at him. "Della who?"

"Della Ness. He just broke it off with her," he explained.

A pang of something shivered through her slender body, and she wondered why the thought of Blake with a woman should cause a sensation like that. "Were they engaged?"

He laughed softly. "No."

She blushed. "Oh."

"She's been bothering him ever since, calling up and crying and sending him letters…you know how that would affect him." He whirled her around in time to the music and brought her back against him loosely. "It hasn't helped his temper any. I think he was glad for the European trip. She hasn't called in over a week."

"Maybe he's missing her," she said.

"Blake? Miss a woman? Honey, you know better than that. Blake is the original self-sufficient male. He never gets emotionally involved with his women."

She toyed with the lapel of his evening jacket. "He doesn't have to take his irritation out on me," she protested sullenly. "And at my homecoming party, too."

"Jet lag," Phillip told her. He stopped as the music did and grimaced when the hard rock blared out again. "Let's sit this one out," he yelled above it. "My legs get tangled trying to dance to that."

He drew her off the floor and back to the open veranda, leading her onto the plant-studded balcony with a friendly hand clasping hers.

"Don't let Blake spoil this for you," he said gently as they stood leaning on the stone balustrade, looking out over the city lights of King's Fort that twinkled jewel-bright on the dark horizon. "He's had a hard week. That strike at the London mill wasn't easily settled."

She nodded, remembering that one of the corporation's biggest textile mills was located there, and that this was nowhere near the first strike that had halted production.

"It's been nothing but trouble," Phillip added with a hard sigh. "I don't see why Blake doesn't close it down. We've enough mills in New York and Alabama to more than take up the slack."

Her fingers toyed with the cool leaves of an elephant-ear plant near the balcony's edge as she listened to Phillip's pleasant voice. He was telling her how much more solvent the corporation would be if they bought two more yarn mills to add to the conglomerate, and how many spindles each one would need to operate, and how new equipment could increase production...and all she was hearing was Blake's deep, angry voice.

It wasn't her fault that his discarded mistresses couldn't take "no" for an answer, and it was hardly prying into his private life to state that he had women. Her face reddened, just thinking of Blake with a woman in his big arms, his massive torso bare and bronzed, a woman's soft body crushed against the hair-covered chest where muscles rippled and surged...

The blush got worse. She was shocked by her own thoughts. She'd only seen Blake stripped to the waist once or twice, but the sight had stayed with her. He was all muscle, and that wedge of black, curling hair that laced down to his belt buckle somehow emphasized his blatant maleness. It wasn't hard to understand the effect he had on women. Kathryn tried not to think about it. She'd always been able to separate the Blake who was like family from the arrogant, attractive Blake who drew women like flies everywhere he went. She'd kept her eyes on his dark face and reminded herself that he had watched her grow from adolescence to womanhood and he knew too much about her to find her attractive in any adult way. He knew that she threw things when she lost her temper, that she never refilled the water trays when she emptied the ice out of them. He knew that she took off her shoes in church, and climbed trees to hide from the minister when he came visiting on Sunday afternoon. He even knew that she sometimes threw her worn blouses behind the door instead of in the clothes hamper. She sighed heavily. He knew too much, all right.

"...Kathryn!"

She jumped. "Sorry, Phil," she said quickly, "I was drinking in the night. What did you say?"

He shook his head, laughing. "Never mind, darling, it wasn't important. Feeling better now?"

"I wasn't drunk," she said accusingly.

"Just a little tipsy, though," he grinned. "Three glasses of punch, wasn't it? And mother emptied the liquor cabinet into it with our hostess's smiling approval."

"I didn't realize how strong it was," Kathryn admitted.

"It has a cumulative effect. Want to go back in?"

"Must we?" she asked. "Couldn't we slip out the side door and go see that new sci-fi movie downtown?"

"Run out on your own party? Shame on you!"

"I'm ashamed," she agreed. "Can we?"

"Can we *what?*"

"Go see the movie. Oh, come on, Phil," she pleaded, "save me from him. I'll lie for you. I'll tell Maude I kidnapped you at gunpoint..."

"Will you, now?" Maude laughed, coming up behind them. "Why do you want to kidnap Phillip?"

"There's a new science fiction movie in town, and..." Kathryn began.

"...and it would keep you out of Blake's way until morning, is that how this song goes?" Phillip's mother guessed keenly.

Kathryn sighed, clasping her hands in front of her. "That's the chorus," she admitted.

"Never mind, he's gone."

She looked up quickly. "Blake?"

"Blake." Maude laughed softly. "Cursing the band, the punch, the politicians, jet lag, labor unions, smog and women with a noticeable lack of tact until Eve almost wept with relief when he announced that he was going home to bed."

"I hope the slats fall out under him," Kathryn said pleasantly.

"They're box springs," Maude commented absently. "I bought it for him last year for his birthday, remember, when he complained that he couldn't get any rest..."

"I hope the box springs collapse, then," Kathryn corrected.

"Malicious little thing, aren't you?" Phillip asked teasingly.

Maude slumped wearily. "Not again. Really, Kathryn Mary, this never-ending war between you and my eldest is going to give me ulcers! What's he done this time?"

"He told her she couldn't be promiscuous," Phillip obliged, "and got mad at her when she pointed out that he believed in the double standard."

"Kathryn! You didn't say that to Blake!"

Kathryn looked vaguely embarrassed. "I was just teasing."

"Oh, my darling, you're so lucky you weren't near any bodies of water that he could have pitched you into," Maude said. "He's been absolutely black-tempered ever since that Della toy of his started getting possessive and he sent her packing. You remember, Phil, it was about the time Kathryn wrote that she was going to Crete on that cruise with Missy Donavan and her brother Lawrence."

"Speaking of Lawrence," Phillip said, drawling out the name dramatically, "what happened?"

"He's coming to see me when he flies down for that writers' convention on the coast," she said with a smile. "He just sold another mystery novel and he's wild with enthusiasm."

"Is he planning to spend a few days?" Maude asked. "Blake has been suspicious of writers, you know, ever since that reporter did a story about his affair with the beauty contest girl…who was she again, Phil?"

"Larry isn't a reporter," Kathryn argued, "he only writes fiction…"

"That's exactly what that story about Blake and the beauty was," Phillip grinned. "Fiction."

"Will you listen?" Maude grumbled. "You simply can't invite Lawrence into the house while Blake's home. I've got the distinct impression he's already prejudiced against the man."

"Larry isn't a pushover," Kathryn replied, remembering her friend's hot temper and red hair.

Maude frowned, thinking. "Phillip, maybe you could call that Della person and give her Blake's unlisted number just before Kathryn Mary's friend comes, and I'll remind him of how lovely St. Martin is in the summer..."

"It will only be for two or three days," Kathryn protested. Her soft young features tightened. "I thought Greyoaks was my home, too..."

Maude's thin face cleared instantly and she drew Kathryn into her arms. "Oh, darling, of course it is, you know it is! It's just that it's Blake's home as well, and that's the problem."

"Just because Larry's a writer..."

"That isn't the only reason," Maude sighed, patting her back. "Blake's very possessive of you, Kathryn. He doesn't like you dating older men, especially men like Jack Harris."

"He has to let go someday," Kathryn said stubbornly, drawing away from Maude. "I'm a woman now, not the adolescent he used to buy bubble gum for. I have a right to my own friends."

"You're asking for trouble if you start a rebellion with Blake in his present mood," Maude cautioned.

Kathryn lifted a hand to touch her dark hair as the breeze blew a tiny wisp of it into the corner of her mouth. "Just don't tell him Larry's coming," she said, raising her face defiantly.

Phillip stared at Maude. "Is her insurance paid up?" he asked conversationally.

"Blake controls the checkbook for all of us," Maude reminded her. "You could find yourself without an allowance at all; even without your car."

"No revolution succeeds without sacrifice," Kathryn said proudly.

"Oh, good grief," Phillip said, turning away.

"Come back here," Kathryn called after him. "I'm not through!"

Maude burst out laughing. "I think he's going to light a candle for you. If you're planning to take Blake on, you may need a prayer or two."

"Or Blake may," Kathryn shot back.

Maude only laughed.

The house was quiet when they got home, and Maude let out a sigh of pure relief.

"So far, so good," she said smiling at Kathryn and Phillip. "Now, if we can just sneak up the stairs..."

"Why are you sneaking around at all?" came a deep, irritated voice from the general direction of the study.

Kathryn felt all her new resolutions deserting her as she whirled and found herself staring straight into Blake's dark, angry eyes.

She dropped her gaze, and her heart thumped wildly in her chest as she dimly heard Maude explaining why the three of them were being so quiet.

"We knew you'd be tired, dear," Maude told him gently.

"Tired, my foot," he returned, lifting a glass of amber liquid in a shot glass to his hard, chiseled mouth. He glared at Kathryn over its rim. "You knew I'd had it out with Kate."

"She's been gorging herself on the rum punch,

Blake," Phillip said with a grin. "Announcing her independence and preparing for holy revolution."

"Oh, please, shut up," Kathryn managed in a tortured whisper.

"But, darling, you were so brave at the Barringtons," Phillip chided. "Don't you want to martyr yourself to the cause of freedom?"

"No, I want to be sick," she corrected, swallowing hard. She glanced up at Blake's hard-set face. The harsh words all came back, and she wished fervently that she'd accepted Nan's invitation to spend the night.

Blake swirled the amber liquid in his glass absently. "Good night, Mother, Phil."

Maude threw Kathryn an apologetic glance as she headed for the staircase with Phillip right behind.

"You wouldn't rather discuss the merger with the Banes Corporation?" Phillip grinned at Blake. "It would be a lot quieter."

"Oh, don't desert me," Kathryn called after them.

"You declared war, darling," Phillip called back, "and I believe in a strict policy of non-interference."

She locked her hands behind her, shivering in her warm sable coat despite the warmth of the house and the hot darkness of Blake's eyes.

"Well, go ahead," she muttered, dropping her gaze to the open neck of his white silk shirt. "You've already taken one bite out of me, you might as well have an arm or two."

He chuckled softly and, surprised, she jerked her face up to find amusement in his eyes.

"Come in here and talk to me," he said, turning to lead the way back into his walnut-paneled study. His big Irish Setter, Hunter, rose and wagged his tail, and Blake ruffled his fur affectionately as he settled down in the wing armchair in front of the fireplace.

Kathryn took the chair across from his, absently darting a glance at the wood decoratively piled up in the hearth. "Daddy used to burn it," she remarked, using the affectionate name she gave Blake's father, even though he was barely a distant cousin. He was like the father she'd lost.

"So do I, when I need to take the chill off. But it isn't cool enough tonight," he replied.

She studied his big, husky body and wondered if he ever felt the cold. Warmth seemed to radiate from him at close range, as if fires burned under that darkly tanned skin.

He tossed off the rest of his drink and linked his hands behind his head. His dark eyes pinned Kathryn to her chair. "Why don't you get out of that coat and stop trying to look as if you're ten minutes late for an appointment somewhere?"

"I'm cold, Blake," she murmured.

"Turn up the thermostat, then."

"I won't be here that long, will I?" she asked hopefully.

His dark, quiet eyes traveled over the soft, pink skin revealed by her white dress, making her feel very young and uncomfortable.

"Must you stare at me like that?" she asked uneasily. She toyed with a wisp of chiffon.

He pulled his cigarette case from his pocket and took his time about lighting up. "What's this about a revolution?" he asked conversationally.

She blinked at him. "Oh, what Phil said?" she asked, belatedly comprehending. She swallowed hard. "Uh, I just..."

He laughed shortly. "Kathryn, I can't remember a conversation with you that didn't end in stammers."

Her full lips pouted. "I wouldn't stammer if you wouldn't jump on me every time you get the chance."

One heavy dark eyebrow went up. He looked completely relaxed, imperturbable. That composure rattled her, and she couldn't help wondering if anything ever made him lose it.

"Do I?" he asked.

"You know very well you do." She studied the hard lines of his face, noting the faint tautness of fatigue that only a stranger would miss. "You're very tired, aren't you?" she asked suddenly, warming to him.

He took a draw from the cigarette. "Dead," he admitted.

"Then why aren't you in bed?" she wanted to know.

He studied her quietly. "I didn't mean to ruin the party for you."

The old, familiar tenderness in his voice brought an annoying mist to her eyes and she averted them. "It's all right."

"No, it isn't." He flicked ashes into the receptacle

beside his chair, and a huge sigh lifted his chest. "Kate, I just broke off an affair. The silly woman's pestering me to death, and when you said what you did, I over-reacted." He shrugged. "My temper's a little on edge lately, or I'd have laughed it off."

She smiled at him faintly. "Did you…love her?" she asked gently.

He burst out laughing. "What a child you are," he chuckled. "Do I have to love a woman to take her into my bed?"

The flush went all the way down her throat. "I don't know," she admitted.

"No," he said, the smile fading, "I don't suppose you do. I believed in love, at your age."

"Cynic," she accused.

He crushed out the cigarette in his ashtray. "Guilty. I've learned that sex is better without emotional blinders."

She dropped her eyes in mortification, trying not to see the unholy amusement on his dark face.

"Embarrassed, Kate?" he chided. "I thought that experience with Harris had matured you."

Her green eyes flashed fire as they lifted to meet his. "Do we have to go through this again?" she asked.

"Not if you've learned something from it." His gaze dropped pointedly to her dress. "Although I have my doubts. Are you wearing anything under that damned nightgown?"

"Blake!" she burst out. "It's not a nightgown!"

"It looks like one."

"It's the style!"

He stared her down. "In Paris, I hear, the style is a vest with nothing under it, worn open."

She tossed her hair angrily. "And if I lived in Paris, I'd wear one," she threw back.

He only smiled. "Would you?" His eyes dropped again to her bodice, and the boldness of his gaze made her feel strange sensations. "I wonder."

She clasped her hands in her lap, feeling outwitted and outmatched. "What did you want to talk to me about, Blake?" she asked.

"I've invited some people over for a visit."

She remembered her own invitation to Lawrence Donavan, and she held her breath. "Uh, who?" she asked politely.

"Dick Leeds and his daughter Vivian," he told her. "They're going to be here for a week or so while Dick and I iron out that labor mess. He's the head of the local union that's giving us so much trouble."

"And his daughter?" she asked, hating herself for her own curiosity.

"Blond and sexy," he mused.

She glared at him. "Just your style," she shot at him. "With the emphasis on sexy."

He watched her with silent amusement. Blake, the adult, indulging his ward. She wanted to throw something at him.

"Well, I hope you don't expect me to help Maude keep them entertained," she said. "Because I'm expecting some company of my own!"

The danger signals were flashing out of his deep brown eyes. "What company?" he asked curtly.

She lifted her chin bravely. "Lawrence Donavan."

Something took fire and exploded under his jutting brow.

"Not in my house," he said in a tone that might have cut diamond.

"But, Blake, I've already invited him!" she wailed.

"You heard me. If you didn't want to be embarrassed, you should have consulted with me before inviting him," he added roughly. "What were you going to do, Kathryn, meet him at the airport and then tell me about it? A *fait accompli?*"

She couldn't meet his eyes. "Something like that."

"Cable him. Tell him something came up."

She lifted her eyes and glared at him, sitting there like a conqueror, ordering her life. If she buckled under one more time, she'd never be able to stand up to him. Never. She couldn't let him win this time.

Her jaw set stubbornly. "No."

He got to his feet slowly, gracefully for such a big man, and the set of his broad shoulders was intimidating even without the sudden, fierce narrowing of his eyes.

"What did you say?" he asked in a deceptively soft tone.

She laced her fingers together in front of her and clenched them. "I said no," she managed in a rasping voice. Her dark green eyes appealed to him. "Blake, it's my home, too. At least, you said it was the day you asked me to come live here," she reminded him.

"I didn't say you could use it as a rendezvous for romantic trysts!"

"You bring women here," she tossed back, remembering with a surge of anguish the night when she had accidentally come home too early from a date and found him with Jessica King on the very chairs where they were now sitting. Jessica had been stripped to the waist, and so had Blake. Kathryn had barely even noticed the blonde, her eyes were so staggered by the sight of Blake with his broad, muscled chest bared by the woman's exploring hands. She'd never been able to get the picture of him out of her mind, his mouth sensuous, his eyes almost black with desire…

"I used to," he corrected gently, reading the memory with disturbing accuracy. "How old were you then? Fifteen?"

She nodded, looking away from him. "Just."

"And I yelled at you, didn't I?" he recalled gently. "I hadn't expected you home. I was hungry and impatient, and frustrated. When I took Jessica home, she was in tears."

"I…I should have knocked," she admitted. "But we'd been to that fair, and I'd won a prize, and I couldn't wait to tell you about it…"

He smiled quietly. "You used to bring all your triumphs straight to me, like a puppy with its toys. Until that night." He studied her averted profile. "You've kept a wall between us ever since. The minute I start to come close, you find something else to put up in front of you. Last time it was Jack Harris. Now, it's that writer."

"I'm not trying to build any walls," she said defensively. Her dark eyes accused him. "You're the mason, Blake. You won't let me be independent."

"What do you want?" he asked.

She studied the delicate scrollwork of the fireplace with its beige and white color scheme. "I don't know," she murmured. "But I'll never find out if you keep smothering me. I want to be free, Blake."

"None of us are that," he said philosophically. His eyes were wistful, his tone bitter. He stared at her intently. "What is it that attracts you to Donavan?" he asked suddenly.

She shrugged and a wistful light came into her own eyes, echoing his expression the minute before. "He's fun to be with. He makes me laugh."

"That's all you need from a man—laughter?"

The way he said it made shivers run down her stiff spine, and when she looked at him, the expression on his hard face was puzzling. "What else is there?" she asked without thinking.

A slow, sensuous smile turned up the corners of his mouth. "The fires a man and woman can create when they make love."

She shifted restlessly in her chair. "They're overrated," she said with pretended sophistication.

He threw back his head and roared.

"Hush!" she said. "You'll wake the whole house!"

His white, even teeth were visible, whiter than ever against his swarthy complexion. "You're red as a summer beet," he observed. "What do you know about love, little girl? You'd pass out in a dead faint if a man started making love to you."

She stared at him with a sense of outrage. "How do you know? Maybe Lawrence..."

"...maybe not," he interrupted, his eyes confident, wise. "You're still very much a virgin, little Kate. If I'd had any fears on that account, I'd have jerked you off Crete so fast your head would have spun."

She grimaced. "Virginity isn't such a prize these days," she sighed, remembering Missy Donavan's faintly insulting remarks about it.

His silent appraisal lasted so long that her attention was caught by the faint ticking of the big grandfather clock in the hall. "Don't get any ideas about throwing yours away," he warned softly.

"Oh, Blake, don't be so old fashioned," she grumbled. "Anyway," she added with a faint, mischievous smile, "where would you be today if all the women in the world were pure?"

"Rather frustrated," he conceded. "But you're not one of my women, and I don't want you offering yourself to men like a nymphomaniac."

She sighed. "There's hardly any danger of that," she said dully. "I don't know how."

"That dress is a damned good start," he observed.

She glanced down at it. "But it covers me up," she protested. "It's a lot more modest than what Nan was wearing."

"I noticed," he said with a musing smile.

She peeked at him through her lashes. "Nan thinks

you're the sexiest man alive," she said lightly. "She knew you'd be at the party."

His face hardened. "Nan's a child," he growled, turning away with one hand rammed in his pocket. "And I'm too old to encourage hero worship."

Nan was Kathryn's age, exactly. Her heart seemed to plummet, and she wanted to hit out at him. He always made her feel so gauche and ignorant.

She studied his broad back. He was so good to look at. So big and vibrant, and full of life. A quiet man, a caring man. And a tyrant!

"If you won't let me invite Larry here," she murmured, "I suppose I could fly down to the coast and go to that writers' convention with him."

He turned, staring at her, hard and intimidating even at a distance. "Threatening me, Kate?" he asked.

"I wouldn't dare!" she replied fervently.

His dark face was as unreadable as a stone sculpture. "We'll talk about it again."

She scowled at him. "Tyrant," she grumbled.

"Is that your best shot?" he asked politely.

"Male chauvinist!" she said, trying again. "You do irritate me, Blake!"

He moved toward her lazily. "What do you think you do to me, little Kathryn?" he asked, his voice a low growl.

She looked up into his arrogant face as he came within striking distance. "I probably irritate you just as much," she admitted, sighing. "Pax?"

He smiled down at her indulgently. "Pax. Come here."

He tilted her chin up and bent his head down. She closed her eyes, expecting the familiar brief, rough touch of his mouth. But it didn't come.

Puzzled, she opened her eyes and looked straight into his at an unnerving distance. She was so close that she could see the flecks of gold in his dark brown irises, the tiny crinkled lines at the corner of his eyelids.

His fingers touched the side of her throat, warm and strangely caressing.

"Blake?" she whispered uncertainly.

His jaw tautened. She could see a muscle jerk beside his sensuous mouth.

"Welcome home, Kate," he said roughly, and started to move away.

"Aren't you going to kiss me?" she asked without thinking.

All the expression drained out of his face to leave his eyes smoldering as they looked down into hers. "It's late," he said abruptly, turning away, "and I'm tired. Good night, Kate."

He walked out the door and left her standing there, staring at the empty doorway.

Chapter Three

Blake was strangely reserved for the next few days, and Kathryn found herself watching him for no reason at all. He was just Blake, she kept telling herself. Just her guardian, as familiar as the towering old house and its ring of live oaks. But something was different. Something…and she couldn't quite grasp what.

"Blake, are you angry with me?" she asked him one evening as he started upstairs to dress for a date.

He scowled down at her. "What makes you think that, Kathryn?" he asked.

She shrugged, and forced a smile for him. "You seem… remote."

"I've got a lot on my mind, kitten," he said quietly.

"The strike?" she guessed.

"That, and a few other assorted headaches," he

agreed. "If you're through asking inane questions, I am on my way out."

"Sorry," she said flippantly. "Heaven forbid that I should keep you from the wheat fields."

"Wheat fields?"

"Where you sow your wild oats, of course," she said with what felt like devastating sophistication as she turned to go back in the living room where Phillip and Maude were talking.

He chuckled softly. "Your slip's showing."

She whirled, grasping her midi-length velveteen skirt and staring down at her shapely calf. "Where?"

He went on up the stairs with a low chuckle and she glared after him.

Later, she watched him come back downstairs, dressed in a pair of dark slacks with a white silk shirt open at the neck and a tweed jacket that gave him a rakish look. What woman was he taking out, she wondered, and would she know how to appreciate all that dark, vibrant masculinity? Just the sight of him was enough to make Kathryn's pulse race, and involuntarily she thought back to the night of her homecoming party and the strange look in Blake's eyes when he started to kiss her and didn't. That hesitation had puzzled her ever since, although she tried not to think about it too much. Blake would be frighteningly dangerous in any respect other than that of a cherished adopted brother.

Nan Barrington came over early the next morning to go riding with Kathryn. Petite and fragile-looking in her jodhpurs, she was wearing a blue sweater, very tight, that was the exact shade of her eyes.

She brushed by Kathryn with a tiny sigh, her eyes immediately on everything in sight as she searched the area for Blake.

"He's gone out," Kathryn said with an amused smile.

Nan looked wildly disappointed. "Oh," she said, her face falling. "I just thought he might be going with us."

Kathryn didn't bother to mention that Blake was doing everything short of joining a monastery to avoid her. That would have led to questions she didn't want to face, much less answer.

"Well, there she is, the golden girl," Phillip said from the staircase, gazing with exaggerated interest at the petite blonde. "You luscious creature, you."

Nan laughed delightedly. "Oh, Phil, you're such a tease," she said. "Come riding with us and let me prove that I can still beat the socks off you."

He made a mock pose. "No girl exposes my naked ankles," he scoffed. "You're on!"

Kathryn led them out the door, tugging her green velveteen blouse down over her trim hips as she went, delighting in its warmth in the chill morning air. "It's nippy out here," she murmured. Her slender hand went up to test the strength of the pins that held the coiled rope of hair in place on top of her head. The wind was brisk, invigorating.

"Nice and cool," Phillip agreed. "Strange how Blake's run out of time to ride," he mentioned with a curious glance at Kathryn. "He's literally worked every minute he's been home. And with the Leedses arriving Saturday, he's going to be lucky if he can manage time to pick them up at the airport."

"Fighting again?" Nan probed, shooting a glance at Kathryn.

Kathryn lifted her head and watched the path in front of her as they took the old shortcut to the big barn, with its white-fenced paddocks. The path led through a maze of high, clipped hedges, in the center of which was a white gazebo, carefully concealed, and ringed all the way around with comfortable cushions. Kathryn had always thought it a wildly romantic setting, and her imagination ran riot every time she saw it.

"Blake and I are getting along just fine," she said, denying her friend's teasing accusation.

"Nothing easier," Phillip agreed with a grin. "They never see each other."

"We do," Kathryn disagreed. "Remember the other night when Blake was going out on that date?"

Nan glanced up at Phillip. "Who's he after now?" She laughed.

Phillip shrugged fatalistically. "Who knows? I think it's the little blonde he's got in the office. His new secretary, if office gossip can be believed. But I hear she can't spell cat."

"Blake likes blondes, all right." Kathryn laughed with an amusement that she was far from feeling.

"Here's one he sure avoids," Nan groaned. "What's wrong with me?"

Phillip threw an avuncular arm across her shoulders.

"Your age, my dear," he informed her. "Blake likes his women mature, sophisticated and thoroughly immoral. That leaves you out of the running."

Nan sighed miserably. "I always have been."

"Blake used to pick us up after cheerleading practice, remember," Kathryn said, eyeing the gazebo longingly as they passed it. "He still thinks of us chewing bubble gum and giggling."

"I hate bubble gum," Nan pouted.

"So do I," Phillip agreed. "It leaves a bad…well, hello," he broke off, grinning at Blake.

The older man stopped in their path, dressed in a sophisticated gray business suit, with a spotless white silk shirt and a patterned tie. He looked every inch the business magnate, polished and dignified.

"Good morning," Blake said coolly. He smiled at Nan. "How's your mother?"

"Just fine, Blake," Nan sighed, going close to catch his arm in her slender fingers. "Don't you have time to go riding with us?"

"I wish I did, little one," he told her. "But I'm already late for a conference."

Kathryn turned away and started for the barn. "I'm going ahead," she called over her shoulder. "Last one in the saddle's a greenhorn!"

She almost ran the rest of the way to the barn, shocked at her own behavior. She felt strange. Sick. Hurt. Empty. The sight of Nan clinging to Blake's arm had set off a rage within her. She'd wanted to slap her friend of many years, just for touching him. She didn't understand herself at all.

Absently, she went into the tackroom and started getting together bits and bridles and a saddle. She barely noticed when the lithe chestnut gelding was saddled and ready to mount. He pranced nervously, as if he sensed her uneasy mood and was reacting to it.

Nan joined her as she was leading Sundance out into the bright morning.

"Where's Phil?" Kathryn asked, trying to keep the edge out of her voice.

Nan shrugged curiously. "Blake dragged him off to the office for some kind of council of war. At least, that's what it sounded like." She sighed. "Blake seemed very angry with him." Her face brightened. "Almost as if he didn't like the idea of Phillip going riding with me. Kate, do you suppose he's jealous?" she asked excitedly.

"It wouldn't surprise me a bit," Kathryn lied, remembering Blake's remarks about her friend. But, frowning, she couldn't help wondering if he'd meant it. Why in the world didn't he want Phillip to ride with the girls?

Kathryn knew that Blake felt Phillip's attitude toward the multi-company enterprise was a little slack sometimes. But why drag him off at this hour of the morning unless… She didn't want to think about it. If Nan was right, she didn't want to know.

"Get saddled and let's go!" Kathryn called. "I'm itching for a gallop!"

"Why did you run off back there?" Nan asked before she went into the stable to saddle her mount.

"Do hurry," Kathryn said, ignoring the question. "Maude wants me to help her plan some menus for the Leedses' visit."

Nan hurriedly saddled her mount, a little mare with the unlikely name of Whirlwind, and the disposition of a sunny summer day.

The two girls rode in a companionable silence, and Kathryn gazed lovingly at the rolling green hills in their autumn colors, trees in the distance just beginning to don the soft golds that later would become brilliant oranges and reds and burgundy. The air was clean and fresh, and fields beyond the meadows were already being turned over to wait for spring planting.

"Isn't it delicious?" Kathryn breathed. "South Carolina must be the most beautiful state in the country."

"You only say that because you're a native," Nan teased.

"It's true, though." She reined in and leaned forward, crossing her forearms on the pommel to stare at the silver ribbon of the Edisto River beyond.

"Do you know how many rice plantations there were in Charleston just before the Civil War?" she murmured, remembering books she'd read about those great plantations with their neat square fields and floodgates.

"I'm afraid I don't share your passion for history, Kate," Nan said apologetically. "Sometimes I even forget what year they fought the War of 1812."

Kathryn smiled at her friend, and all the resentment drained out of her. After all, Nan couldn't help the way she felt about Blake. It wasn't her fault he was so wickedly attractive…

"Let's ride down through the woods," she said abruptly, wheeling Sundance. "I love to smell the river, don't you?"

"Oh, yes," Nan agreed. "I'm with you!"

Blake was home for dinner that night, an occurrence rare enough to cause comment.

"Run out of girls?" Phillip teased as they sat around the table nibbling at Mrs. Johnson's chicken casserole.

"Phillip!" Maude chided, her dark eyes disapproving as she paused in the act of lifting a forkful of chicken to her mouth.

Blake raised an eyebrow at his brother. His blue-checked sports shirt was open at the neck, and he looked vibrant and rested and dangerously attractive to Kathryn, who was doing her best to keep her eyes away from him.

"You had more than your share this morning," Blake remarked dryly.

"Was that why you dragged me off to the office before I could enjoy being surrounded by them?" Phillip laughed.

"I needed your support, little brother."

"Sure. The way Samson needed a herd of horses to help him tug the pillars down."

"I would like to point out," Maude said gently, "that Mrs. Johnson spent an hour preparing this excellent chicken dish, which is turning to bile in my stomach."

Kathryn darted an amused glance at the older woman. "You should have had daughters," she suggested.

Maude stared at Blake, then at Phillip. "I'm not sure. It's very hard to picture Blake in spike heels and a petticoat."

Kathryn choked on her mashed potatoes, and Phillip had to lean over and thump her on the back.

"I'm glad Kathryn finds something amusing," Blake said in that cold, curt tone that she hated so much. "She wasn't in the best of humors this morning."

Kathryn swallowed a sip of coffee, and her dark green eyes glared at Blake across the table. "I don't remember saying anything to you at all, Blake," she murmured.

"No," he agreed. "You were too busy flouncing off to offer a civil greeting."

How could he be so blind? she wondered, but she only glared at him. "Excuse me," she said haughtily, "but I never flounce."

He lifted his coffee cup to his chiseled lips, but his eyes never left Kathryn's face. Something dark and hard in them unnerved her. "Push a little harder, honey," he challenged quietly.

Her small frame stiffened. "I'm not afraid of you," she said with a forced smile.

His eyes narrowed, and a corner of his mouth went up. "I could teach you to be," he said.

"Now, children," Maude began, her eyes plainly indicating which of the two she was referring to as they glared at Kathryn. "This is the meal hour, remember? Indigestion is bad for the soul."

Phillip sighed as he tasted his lemon mousse. "It's never stopped them before," he muttered.

Kathryn crumpled her napkin and laid it beside her plate before she got to her feet. "I think I'll play the piano for a while, if no one minds."

"Not for too long, dear, you'll keep Blake awake," Maude cautioned. "Remember, he has to get up at five in the morning to drive down to Charleston to pick up the Leedses at the airport."

Kathryn threw a gracious smile in Blake's direction. "Of course," she said with honey in her voice. "Our elders must have their beauty rest."

"By heaven, you're asking for it," Blake said in a voice that sent chills down her spine.

"Go, girl!" Phillip said, pushing her in the direction of the living room. He closed the door behind them with an exaggerated sigh and leaned against it. "Whew!" he breathed, and his dark eyes laughed at her when he opened them again. "Don't push your luck, sweet. He's been impossible to get along with for days now, and this morning he made a barracuda look tame."

"Doesn't he always?" she grumbled.

"Yes," he conceded. "But if you had his secretary, it might give you ulcers as well."

She glanced at him as she went to the piano and sat down, flexing her fingers. "If he wants secretaries who decorate instead of type, that's his business. Just hush, Phil, will you? I'm sick of hearing about Blake!"

She banged away at Rachmaninoff's Second Piano Concerto, while Phillip stared at her profile thoughtfully for a long time.

Chapter Four

Maude had the housekeeper, buxom Mrs. Johnson, and the two little daily maids running in circles by late afternoon. It was almost comical, and Kathryn had to force herself not to giggle.

"Don't put the urn of dried flowers *there,*" Maude wailed when one of the maids placed it in the entrance to the living room.

Kathryn decided she had better go outside and keep out of the way.

Phillip was just getting out of his small sports car as she emerged from the house. He hesitated for an instant when he saw Kathryn coming, then got the rest of the way out and closed the door.

"What's the matter with you?" he asked cheerfully.

"It's the dried flowers," she explained enigmatically.

Phillip blinked. "Have you been into Blake's whiskey, Kathryn?"

She shook her head. "You had to be there to understand," she told him. "Honestly, you'd think the head of state was coming. She's rearranged the furniture twice, and now she's going crazy over flowers. And just think, Phil," she added in a conspiratorial whisper, "Leeds can't even save the river!"

He chuckled. "Probably not. Blake should be back soon," he said, after a glance at his watch.

Kathryn looked out over the sculptured garden with its cobblestone path leading through hedges to the concealed white gazebo. "I wonder what Miss Leeds looks like?" she murmured thoughtfully.

"Vivian?" he asked, smiling. "The cover of a fashion magazine. She's an actress, you know, quite well-known already, too."

She felt ill. "Old?" she asked.

"Twenty-five isn't old, sweet." He laughed. "Blake can't be without a woman for long. He really can pick them."

She wanted to hit him. To scream. To do anything but stand there with a calm smile plastered to her face and pretend it didn't matter. Suddenly, terribly, it mattered. Blake was her… She stopped, frowning. Her *what?*

"Kathryn, you aren't listening," Phillip said patiently. "I said, would you like to go into King's Fort with me and buy a new dress or two?"

She looked up at him. "Whatever for?" she asked indignantly. "I don't dress in rags!"

"Of course not," he said, placating her. "But Maude suggested that you might like some new clothes since we're having guests."

She drew a deep, angry breath. "Put on my best feathers, you mean?" She thought about it, imagining an outfit daring enough to make even Blake take notice. A tiny smile touched her pink mouth. "All right. Take me someplace expensive. Saks, I think."

"Uh, Kathryn…" Phillip said.

"Blake won't get the bill until next month," she reminded him. "By then, I can be in St. Martin, or Tahiti, or Paris…"

He chuckled. "All right, incorrigible girl, come on. We've got to hurry or we won't be here when Blake's guests arrive."

Kathryn didn't tell him, but that was just what she had in mind. The idea of greeting Vivian Leeds made her want to spend several days in town. She disliked the woman already, and she hadn't even met her.

She left Phillip in a small, exotic coffee shop on the mall while she floated through the plush women's department in the exclusive shop, dreaming of Blake seeing her in one expensive dress after another. She'd show him! She'd be the most beautiful woman he'd ever seen, and she'd make him stand back and take notice!

But when she tried on one of the elegant dresses she'd picked out, all she saw in the mirror was a little girl trying to play dress-up. She looked about fifteen. All the excitement drained out of her face. Her whole body seemed to slump as she stared at her reflection.

"It doesn't suit you, does it?" the pleasant blond saleswoman asked her.

Kathryn shook her head sadly. "It looked so beautiful on the model..."

"Because it was designed for a taller, thinner figure than yours," the statuesque older woman explained. "If I may suggest some styles...?"

"Oh, please!" Kathryn said, wide-eyed.

"Wait here."

The three dresses the woman brought back looked far less dramatic than those Kathryn had picked out. They were simple garments with no frills at all, and the colors were pale pastels—mint, taupe and a silky beige. But on Kathryn, they came to life. Combined with her black hair and green eyes, the mint was devastating. The taupe emphasized her rounded figure and darkened her eyes. The beige brought out her soft complexion and its simple lines gave her an elegance far beyond her years.

"And this is for evening," the woman said at last, bringing out a burgundy velvet gown with a deep V-neck and slits down both sides. It's a dream of a dress, Kathryn thought, studying her reflection in the mirror, her face glowing as she imagined Blake's reaction to this seductive style—the light went out of her suddenly when she remembered the warning he'd given her, about provoking him. But surely she had the right to wear what she pleased...

"Kathryn, we've got to go," Phillip called to her.

One expressive eyebrow went up, and her eyes danced mischievously. What would this gorgeous gown do to Phillip?

She opened the curtains and walked out. He stared at her, with lips slightly parted, his brown eyes stunned.

"Kathryn?" he asked, as if he didn't trust his eyes anymore.

"Yes, it's me," she assured him. "Oh, Phil, isn't it a dream?"

He nodded dubiously. "A dream."

"What's the matter?" she asked, going close to look up at him, while the saleswoman smiled secretively from a distance.

"Are you sure it's legal to wear something like that in public?" he asked.

She smiled. "Why not? It's very fashionable. Do you really like it?"

He caught his breath. "Honey, I love it. But Blake…"

She glared at him. "I'm grown. I keep having to remind Blake…"

"You won't have to remind him anymore if you wear that dress," he said, staring down at the soft, exposed curves of her breasts in the plunging neckline. "He'll be able to see for himself."

She tossed her long, waving hair defiantly. "I'll bet that actress wears more revealing clothes than this."

"She does," he agreed, "but her lifestyle is different from yours, kitten."

"You mean she sleeps with men, don't you, Phillip?" she persisted.

"Hush, for heaven's sake!" he said quickly, looking around to see if anyone was listening. "Remember where we are."

"But she does, doesn't she?" she kept on, glaring.

"I know you've been at it with Blake about your writer friend coming," Phillip told her quietly. "But don't think you'll retaliate by insulting his latest female acquisition. He'll cut you into little pieces, Kate."

She felt the rage welling up in her like rain catching in a vat. "I'm tired of Blake telling me how to live my life. I want to move into an apartment."

"Don't tell him yet," Phillip pleaded.

"I already have," she replied, her eyes sparkling with temper.

"And what did he say?"

"He said no, of course. He always says no. But it won't work anymore. I'm going to get a job, and an apartment, and you're going to help me," she added, with a mischievous glance upward.

"Oh, like hell I am!" he replied. "I'm not taking on Blake for you."

She stamped her small foot. "That's what's wrong with men today!"

His eyebrows went up amusedly. "What is?"

"That no one's brave enough to take on Blake for me! I'll bet Larry will," she added stubbornly.

"If he does, he'll wish he hadn't," Phillip said. "And if you buy that dress, Kathryn, I'm going away for the weekend." He made a mock shudder. "I can't stand the sight of blood."

"Blake won't do anything," she said smugly. "Not in front of his guests."

"Blake will do anything, anytime, in front of anybody, and if you don't know that by now, you're even crazier than I thought you were." He shook his head. "Give it up, Kathy. Blake's only trying to do what's best for you."

"That's beside the point, Phillip," she replied, smoothing the velvet under her slender fingers. "I don't want to spend the rest of my life being told what to do. Blake's not my keeper."

"If you go out after dark in that dress, you'll need one," he murmured, staring at her.

She leaned up and kissed his cheek. "You're a nice man."

"Kathryn, are you sure…?"

"Don't be such a worrywart," she told him. She motioned to the saleswoman. "I'll take all of them," she said with a smile. "And that green velvet one, as well."

Phillip frowned. "What green velvet one?"

"It's ever so much more daring than this," she lied, remembering the high halter neckline and soft lines of the other dress she'd tried on. "It doesn't have a back at all," she added in a wicked whisper.

"Lord help us!" Phillip said, lifting his eyes upward.

"Don't bother Him," Kate said, "He has wars and floods to worry about."

"And I have you," he groaned.

"Lucky man," she said, patting his cheek before she

went to charge her purchases. "Come on. You have to sign the ticket."

"Whose name would you like me to sign on it?" he asked.

"Oh, silly!" she laughed.

She and Phillip had managed to sneak in the back way and dart upstairs to dress for dinner without being seen. Recklessly, Kathryn slid into the burgundy velvet dress after she had her bath, and tacked up her long hair in a seductively soft bun on top of her head with little curling wisps trailing down her blushing cheeks. She used only a little makeup—just enough to give her a mysterious look, a hint of sophistication. The woman looking back at her in the mirror bore no resemblance to the young girl who'd left that room the same day to go shopping.

Satisfied with what she saw, she added a touch of Givenchy perfume and sauntered downstairs. She heard voices coming from the living room, and Blake's was among them. She felt suddenly nervous, uneasy. That would never do. She lifted her head, baring the soft curve of her throat, and, gathering her courage, walked straight into the white-carpeted, blue-furnished room.

She noticed two things immediately: the possessive blonde clinging to Blake's sleeve like a parasite, and the sudden, blazing fury in Blake's eyes as he looked at Kathryn Mary.

"Oh, there you are, darl…ing," Maude said, her voice breaking on the word as she noticed the dress. "How…

different you look, Kathryn," she added with a disapproving glance.

"Where did you get that dress?" Blake asked in a harsh, low voice.

She started to speak, then darted a glance at Phillip, who was burying his face in his hand. "Phillip bought it for me," she said in a rush.

"Kathryn!" Phillip groaned.

Blake smiled, like a hungry barracuda, Kathryn thought shakily. "I'll discuss this with you later, Phil."

"Could we make it after Kathryn's funeral?" Phillip asked, with a meaningful glance at Kathryn.

"Aren't you going to introduce me to your guests?" Kathryn asked brightly.

"Dick Leeds and his daughter, Vivian," Blake said, indicating a tall, white-haired man with twinkling blue eyes and the equally blue-eyed blonde at Blake's side. "This is Kathryn Mary."

"Kilpatrick," she added proudly. "I'm the youngest, next to Phillip."

"How do you do?" Dick Leeds asked pleasantly, and extended a thin hand to be shaken. He smiled at her. "Not a Hamilton, then?" he asked.

"I'm a cousin," she explained. "Maude and the family took me in when my parents died, and brought me up."

"Apparently not too successfully," Blake said darkly, his eyes promising retribution as they seared a path down her body, lingering on the plunging neckline.

"If you don't stop picking on me, Blake," she said

sweetly, accepting a glass of sherry from Phillip, "I'll hit you with my teddy bear."

Vivian Leeds didn't look amused, although her lips managed a thin smile. "How old are you, Miss Kilpatrick?" she asked listlessly.

"Much younger than you, Miss Leeds, I'm sure," Kathryn replied with an equally false smile.

Phillip choked on his drink. "Uh, how was your trip, Viv?" he asked the blonde, quickly.

"Very nice, thanks," she replied, her eyes cutting a hole in Kathryn. "Lovely dress," she said. "What there is of it."

"This old rag?" Kathryn said haughtily, her eyes speaking volumes as they studied the rose silk gown the blonde was wearing. "It's warm, at least," she added. "I don't really care for these new fashions—some of them look more like nighties than dresses," she said pointedly.

Miss Leeds's face colored expressively, her blue eyes lighting like firecrackers.

"Let's eat," Maude said suddenly.

"Lead the way, Mother," Blake said. Amusement was vying with anger in his dark eyes, and just for an instant, amusement won. But then his dark gaze slid sideways to Kathryn, and the smile faded. His eyes curved over the creamy, exposed skin at her neckline, and she felt as if he had touched her. Her lips parted under a rush of breath, and he looked up suddenly and caught that expression on her young face. Something flared in his dark eyes, like a minor volcanic upheaval, and Kathryn knew that she was going to be in the middle of a war before the night was over. But she managed to return Blake's glare with bravado, and even smiled. If she was going to be the main course on his menu, she might as well enjoy the appetizer first.

Phillip dropped back beside her as they made their way into the dining room. "Feeling suicidal?" he asked under his breath. "He's blazing, and that sweet little smile didn't help."

"Revolutionaries can't afford to worry about tomorrow," she replied saucily. "Besides, Blake can't eat me."

"Can't he?" he asked, casting a wary glance toward his brother, who was glaring at them over Vivian's bright head.

"Phillip, you aren't really afraid of him, are you?" she teased. "After all, you're brothers."

"So," he reminded her, "were Cain and Abel."

"Don't worry, I'll protect you."

"Please don't," he asked mournfully. "Why did you have to tell him that I bought you that dress?"

"But, you did sign for it," she said innocently.

"I know, but buying it wasn't my idea."

"Be reasonable, Phil," she said soothingly. "If I'd told him it was my idea, he'd have gone straight for my throat."

He gave her a measuring look. "And having him go for mine was a better idea?"

She smiled. "From my point of view, it was," she laughed. "Oh, Phil, I am sorry, really I am. I'll tell him the truth."

"If you get the chance," he muttered under his breath, nodding toward his brother.

Blake seated Vivian and then turned to hold out a chair for Kathryn. She approached it with the same aplomb as a condemned terrorist headed for the gallows.

"Nice party," she murmured under her breath as she sat down.

"And it's only beginning," he said with a smile that didn't reach his eyes. "Make one more snide remark to Vivian, and I'll grind you into the carpet, Kathryn Mary."

She spared him a cool glance. "She started it," she said under her breath.

"Jealous?" he taunted softly.

Her eyes jerked up to his, blazing green fire. "Of her?" she asked haughtily. "I'm not fifteen anymore," she said.

"Before the night's over, you're going to wish you were," he said softly. "I promise you."

The deep anger in his voice sent chills running all over her. Why did she have to open her mouth and challenge him again? Hadn't she had enough warning? She felt a surge of fear at what lay ahead. It seemed that she couldn't stop fighting Blake lately, and she wondered at her own temerity. Was she going mad?

One glance at his set face down the table from her was enough to make her want to run upstairs and bar the door.

Dinner was an ordeal. Vivian monopolized Blake to such an extent that he was hardly able to carry on a conversation with anyone else, but her cold blue eyes made frequent pilgrimages to Kathryn's quiet face. The animosity in them was freezing.

"You're not doing much for international relations," Phillip remarked as they retired to the living room for after-dinner drinks.

"Blake's doing enough for both of us," she replied, darting a cool glance toward the blonde, who was clinging to Blake's big, muscular arm as if he were a life raft. "He has bad taste," she said without thinking.

"I wouldn't say that," Phillip disagreed. His brown eyes danced as they surveyed the blonde's graceful back. "She's pretty easy on the eyes."

"Is she?" she asked with magnificent disdain. "Frankly, she doesn't do a thing for me."

"Don't be sour," he said. "You forget why she's here, darling. Remember the strike?"

"Oh, I remember," she told him. "But does Blake? I thought her father was the focal point."

"Part of it, at least," he said.

She stared up at him. "What do you mean, Phil?" she asked curiously.

He avoided her sharp eyes. "You'll know soon enough. Look, Mother's motioning to you."

Maude was showing some of her antique frames to Dick Leeds, but she left him with a smile and drew Kathryn aside.

"You're doing it again, my darling," she moaned, darting a wary glance in Blake's direction. "He's ready to chew nails. Kathryn, can't you manage not to antagonize him for just one evening? The Leedses are our guests, remember."

"They're Blake's guests," came the sullen reply.

"Well, it is Blake's house," Maude said with a placating smile. "Johnny left it all to him. He felt Blake would keep me from frittering it away."

"You wouldn't have," Kathryn protested.

Maude sighed. "Perhaps," she said wistfully. "But it's a moot point. You aren't improving Blake's disposition, you know."

"All I did was buy a new dress," she said defensively.

"It's much too old for you, Kathryn," she said quietly. "Phillip hasn't taken his eyes off you all evening, and every time he looks at you, Blake scowls more."

"Phillip and I aren't related, after all," Kathryn pointed out.

Maude smiled. "And there's no one I'd rather see him marry, you know that. But Blake doesn't approve, and he could make things very difficult for you."

She scowled. "He doesn't approve of any man I date," she grumbled.

Maude started to say something, but obviously thought better of it. "It will work itself out. Meanwhile, please at least be civil to Miss Leeds. It's terribly important that we make a good impression on them both. I can't tell you any more than that, but do trust me."

Kathryn sighed. "I will."

Maude patted Kathryn's slender shoulder. "Now be a dear, and help me entertain Dick. Blake is going to drive Vivian into King's Fort and show her how the city looks at night. She was curious, for some reason that escapes me."

It didn't escape Kathryn, and it didn't improve her mood, either. Especially when she watched Vivian and Blake go out the door without a backward glance. She wanted to pick up the priceless Tang dynasty vase in the hall and heave it at Blake's dark head. In the end, she consoled herself with the fact that at least she didn't have to face Blake until the morning. That was a blessing in itself.

Dick Leeds was interesting to talk to. She liked the elderly man, who seemed to have the same kind of steel in his makeup that Blake did. All too soon, he went upstairs to his room, pleading fatigue from the long trip. Maude followed suit with a sigh.

"Like Dick," she told Phillip and Kathryn, "I'm beginning to feel my age a little. Good night, children."

Phillip challenged Kathryn to a game of gin rummy after Maude went out the door, but she protested.

"You'll just beat me again," she pouted.

"I'll give myself a ten-point handicap," he promised.

"Well…just a couple of hands," she agreed finally.

He held out a chair for her at the small table by the darkened window. "Sit down, pigeon…I mean, partner," he grinned.

She smiled across the table at him. "Why can't Blake be like you?" she wondered absently as he shuffled the cards. "Friendly, and easy to get along with, and fun to be around…"

"He used to be, when you were younger," he answered, and his warm brown eyes twinkled. "It's only since you've started growing up that you think he's changed."

She stuck out her tongue at him. "I don't think, I know! He growls at me all the time."

"You light the fires under him, my sweet. Like tonight."

Her face closed up, like a fragile flower in a sudden chill. "I don't like her."

"And the feeling seems to be mutual. I don't think attractive women ever really like each other." He studied her unobtrusively. "But I have an idea that her dislike stems from your own. You've hardly been friendly toward her."

She drew in a defeated sigh. "You're right, I haven't," she admitted.

"Trying to get back at Blake?" he persisted.

"My arsenal is limited when it comes to fighting your brother," she sighed.

He laid down three cards in sequence and discarded. "That goes for all of us."

She held the cool cards up to her lips absently while she drew a card, looked at it, grimaced, and laid it down on the discard pile. "I don't see why I can't have an apartment," she said. Her full lips pouted against the cards. "I can get a job and pay for it."

"A job doing what?" he asked politely.

She glared at him. "That's the problem. Finishing school didn't prepare me for much of anything. I know," she said, brightening. "I'll advertise to be a rich man's mistress! I'm eminently qualified for that!"

Phillip buried his face in his hands. "Don't you dare say that to Blake when I'm in the room! He'll think I suggested it!"

She laughed at the expression on his face. Phillip was such fun, and such a gentleman. She was fonder of him than she liked to say. He was truly like the brother she wished she'd had. But Blake...she turned her attention back to her cards.

She was so caught up in the game of gin rummy that she forgot the time. She was one card short of winning the game when all of a sudden she heard the front door open and she froze in her seat.

"Oops," she murmured weakly.

Phillip smothered a grin at the look on her soft features. "Sounds like they're home," he commented, as Vivian's high-pitched voice called good-night from the staircase.

Before she could reply, Blake, looking big, dark and formidable, came in the door. He glanced at the tableau they made as he slung his jacket onto a chair and tugged his tie loose, tossing it carelessly onto the jacket.

"Have a good time?" Phillip asked slyly, his sharp gaze not missing the smear of lipstick just visible on Blake's shirt collar.

Blake shrugged. He went to the bar and poured himself a jigger of whiskey, neat.

"Uh, I think I'd better get to bed," Phillip said, gauging Blake's mood with lightning precision. "Good night, all."

"I think I'll go up, too," Kathryn began hopefully, rising as Phillip made his hasty exit and disappeared into the hall.

Kathryn was only a step behind him when Blake's curt voice stopped her with her hand on the doorknob.

"Close the door," he said.

She started to go through it.

"From the inside," he added in a tone that was honeyed, yet vaguely threatening.

She drew a steadying breath and went back into the living room, closing the door reluctantly behind her. She leaned back against it, flashing a nervous glance at him.

"Did you have a nice drive?" she asked.

"Don't hedge," he growled. His angry eyes slid down her body in the velvet dress with its side slits and plunging neckline, and she felt as if his hands were touching her bare flesh.

"Dick's gone to bed. He's very nice," she murmured, trying to postpone the confrontation as long as possible. She'd seen Blake in plenty of bad tempers, but judging by the control she read in his face, this one was formidable. The courage she'd felt earlier, in company, dissolved now that she was alone with him.

"So is his daughter," he replied. "Not that you've taken the trouble to find out."

She shifted against the cold wood at her back. "She bites."

"So do you, honey," he replied, lifting his glass to his lips. "I want the truth, Kate. Did Phillip buy you that dress?"

She felt weary all of a sudden, defeated. Blake always seemed to win. "No," she admitted. "That is, he signed for it because I don't have a charge account, but Maude said herself that I needed some new clothes," she added defensively.

"I said the same thing. But I hadn't planned on your dressing like a Main Street prostitute."

"It's the style, Blake!" she shot at him.

"Almost exactly the same words you used after the Barringtons' party," he reminded her. "And I told you the same thing then that I'm telling you now. A dress like that raises a man's blood pressure by five points while it's still on the mannequin. On you..." He let his eyes speak for him, dark and sensuous as they caressed her.

"Vivian was wearing less," she replied weakly, feeling the heat in her cheeks. "I could almost see through *her* dress."

"Throwing stones?" he asked. "Your breasts are barely covered at all."

Her face went hot under the words, and she glared at him with outrage in her sparkling green eyes. "Oh, all right, I'll never wear the silly dress again, Blake! But I can't see what difference it makes to you what I wear!"

His eyes narrowed, and his hand tightened on the thick glass. "Can't you?"

She squared her small shoulders. "You're just being

a tyrant again," she accused. Her hands slid down the sensuous burgundy velvet over her hips as she lifted her face defiantly. "What's the matter, Blake, do I disturb you?" she challenged. "Would you rather I wore my gym suit from high school?"

He set the glass down on the bar and strode toward her deliberately, his eyes blazing, his face harder than granite. She saw the purpose in his eyes and turned with a feeling of panic, grabbing for the doorknob. But the action was too late. He caught her and whirled her around with rough, hurting hands to hold her, struggling against the door.

Chapter Five

She stared up into the face of a stranger, and her voice caught in her throat. "Blake, you wouldn't…!" she burst out finally, frightened by what she read in his dark eyes.

He moved, and his big, warm body crushed her against the door. She felt the pressure of his hard, powerful thighs against hers, the metal of his belt buckle sharp at her stomach. There was the rustle of cloth against cloth as his hands caught her bare arms and stilled her struggles.

"Oh, wouldn't I?" he growled, as his eyes dropped to her tremulous lips.

Stunned by the sight of his dark, leonine face at such a disturbing proximity, she looked up at him helplessly until he suddenly crushed her soft mouth under his, forcing her head back under the merciless pressure.

She kept her mouth tightly closed, her body trembling with sudden fear at what Blake was asking of her. She stiffened, struggling instinctively, and his mouth twisted against hers to hold it in bondage, his teeth nipping her lower lip painfully.

A sob broke from her tight throat as she yielded to the merciless ardor that was years beyond her few experiences with men. Nothing that had gone before prepared her for the adult passion she felt in Blake, and it sparked a response that was mingled fear and shock. This was no boyfriend assaulting her senses. This was Blake. Blake, who taught her to ride. Blake, who drove her to cheerleading practice and football games with her friend Nan. Blake, who was a confidant, a protector, and now…

He jerked his head up suddenly, surveying the damage in her swollen, bruised lips, her wounded eyes, her wildly flushed cheeks and disordered hair.

"You're…hurting me," she whispered brokenly. Her fingers went to her drooping coiffure, nervously, as tears washed her eyes.

His face seemed to harden as he looked down at her. His breath came hard and fast. His eyes glittered with unfathomable emotions.

"This is what happens when you throw that sweet young body at me," he said in a voice that cut. "I warned you before about flaunting it, and you wouldn't listen. Now, maybe I've managed to get through to you."

She drew in a sobbing breath, and the tiny sound

seemed to disturb him. His eyes softened, just a little, as they wandered over her face.

"Please let me go, Blake," she pleaded in a shaken whisper. "I swear, I'll wear sackcloth and ashes for the rest of my life!"

His heavy brows drew together and he let go of her arms to lean his hands on either side of her head against the door, pushing back a little to ease the crush of his powerful chest and thighs.

"Afraid?" he asked in a deep, lazy voice.

She swallowed hard, nodding, her eyes mesmerized by his.

He let his eyes move down to her swollen, cut lip as he bent toward her again. She felt his tongue brushing very softly against it, healing, tantalizing and she gasped again—but this time, not in pain.

He drew back and caught her eyes. The expression he found was one of curiosity, uncertainty. She met that searching gaze squarely and felt the breath sigh out of her body. Her heart went wild under the intensity of it. She wanted suddenly to reach up and bring his dark head back down again, to feel his mouth again. To open her lips and taste his. To kiss him hungrily, and hard, and feel his body against the length of hers as it had been, but not in anger this time.

His jaw went rigid. His eyes seemed to burst with light and darkness. Then, suddenly, she was free. He pushed away from her and turned to walk back to the bar. He poured himself another whiskey, and paused long enough to dash a jigger of brandy into a snifter for her before he moved back to the door where she stood frozen and handed it to her.

Wordlessly, he caught her free hand and drew her back to his desk with him. He perched against it, holding her in front of him while she nervously sipped the fiery amber liquid.

He threw down his own drink and put first his own glass, then hers, aside. He reached out to catch her by the waist, drawing her gently closer. He stared down at her flushed face for a long time before he spoke, in a silence heady with new emotions.

"Don't brood," he said, in a tone that carried echoes of her childhood. Blake's voice, gentle, soothing her when her world caved in. "The tactics may have been different, but it was only an argument. It's over."

She pretended a calm she didn't feel, and some of the tension went out of her shocked body. "That doesn't sound very much like an apology," she said, darting a shy glance up at him.

One eyebrow lifted. "I'm not going to apologize. You asked for that, Kathryn, and you know it."

She sighed shakily. "I know." Her eyes traced the powerful lines of his chest. "I didn't mean to say what I did."

"All you have to remember, little innocent one," he said indulgently, "is that verbal warfare brings a man's blood up. You can be provocative without even realizing it." He shook her gently. "Are you listening?"

"Yes." Her dark, curious eyes darted up to his for an

instant. "You...I didn't think that you..." she stopped, trying to find words.

"There's no blood between us to protect you from me, Kate," he said in a deep, quiet tone. "I'm not in my dotage, and I react like any normal man to the sight of a woman in a revealing dress. Phillip could have lost his head just as easily," he added gruffly.

She felt her heart pounding and caught her breath. "Perhaps," she whispered. "But he would have been... gentle, I think."

He didn't argue the point. His big, warm hand tilted her face up to his quiet eyes. "Another of the many differences between Phillip and me, young Kate," he said. "I'm not a gentle lover. I like my women...practiced."

The flush made bright banners in her cheeks. "Do they get combat pay?" she asked with a hint of impudence and a wry smile as she touched her forefinger gingerly to her cut lip.

His lips turned up, and his dark eyes sparkled. It was as if there had never been a harsh scene to alienate them. "It works both ways, honey," he replied musingly. "Some women would have returned the compliment, with interest."

Her eyes looked deep into his. This, she thought dazedly, is getting interesting. "Women...bite men?" she asked in a whisper, as if it was a subject not fit for decent ears to hear.

"Yes," he whispered back. "And claw, and scream like banshees."

"I...I don't mean *then,*" she said. "I mean when...oh,

never mind, you just want to make fun of me. I'll ask Phillip."

He chuckled softly. "Do you really think he's ever felt that kind of passion?" he asked.

She shrugged. "He's a man."

"Men are different," he reminded her. His eyes dropped to her mouth. "Poor little scrap, I did hurt you, didn't I?" he asked gently.

She drew away from him, and he relaxed his hold to free her. "It's all right," she murmured. "As you said, I did ask for it." Her eyes glanced off his. "You're…very sophisticated."

"And you're a delicious little innocent," he replied. "I didn't mean to be so brutal with you, but I do want to impress on you what you invite from a man with a dress like that." He smiled drily. "I've got a low boiling point, Kate, and I do recall warning you."

"I didn't think you were serious," she said with a sigh.

His dark eyes swept over her again. "Now you know better."

"And better," she agreed. She turned, almost knocking over Maude's priceless porcelain vase on its marble-topped table on the way out. "I'm taking back every dress I bought while there's still time."

"Kate, don't be ridiculous," he growled after her. "You know what I meant. I don't want you wearing dresses with necklines cut to the waist, that's all. You're still too much a child to realize what you could be letting yourself in for."

She turned at the door with great dignity, her carriage so perfect that Mademoiselle Devres would have cheered. "I'm not a child anymore, Blake," she told him. "Am I?"

He turned away, bending his head to light a cigarette with steady hands. "When does that writer get here?"

She swallowed nervously. "Tomorrow morning." She watched him walk to the darkened window and draw the curtain aside to look out. His broad back was toward her and unexpectedly, she remembered how warm and sensuous it had felt under the palms of her hands.

"Aren't you going to tell me to call it off again?" she asked, testing him, feeling a flick of danger run through her that was madly exciting.

He stared at her across the room for a long moment before he answered. "At least I won't have to worry about you sneaking off to go to that convention with him while he's under my roof," he remarked carelessly. "And he'd have his work cut out to seduce you, from what I've seen tonight."

Her eyes flashed at him. "That's what you think!" she shot back.

He only laughed, softly, sensuously. "Before you flounce off, hugging your boundless attractions to your bare bosom, you might remember that I wasn't trying to seduce you. You ought to know by now that my taste doesn't run to oversexed adolescents. Not that you fall in that classification," he added with a mocking smile. "You're green for a young woman just shy of her twenty-first birthday."

That hurt, even more than the devastating taste of him as a lover. "Larry doesn't think so," she told him.

He lifted the cigarette to his hard mouth, his eyes laughing at her. "If I had his limited experience, I might agree with him."

That nudged a suspicion in the back of her mind. "What do you know about his experience?" she asked.

He studied her for a long, static silence. "Did you really think I'd let you go to Crete with him and that harebrained sister of his without checking them out thoroughly?"

Her face flamed. "You don't trust me, do you?"

"On the contrary, I trust you implicitly. But I don't trust men," he said arrogantly.

"You don't own me," she cried, infuriated by his calm sureness.

"Oh, go to bed before you set fire to my temper again," he growled at her.

"Gladly," she returned. She went out the door without even a good night, and then lay awake half the night worrying about it.

Her dreams were full of Blake that night. And when she woke to the rumble of thunder and the sound of raindrops, she had a vivid picture of herself lying in his big arms while his mouth burned on her bare skin. It was embarrassing enough to make her late for breakfast. She didn't think she could have looked at Blake without giving herself away.

But her worries were groundless. Blake had already

left to go to the office when Kathryn came downstairs to find Vivian sitting by herself at the breakfast table.

"Good morning," Vivian said politely. Her delicate blond features were enhanced by her buttercup yellow blouse and skirt. She looked slim and ultra-chic. She eyed Kathryn's jeans and roll-neck white sweater with disgust. "You don't believe in fashion, do you?" she asked.

"In my own home, no," she replied, reaching for cream to add to her steaming cup of coffee as Mrs. Johnson hustled back and forth between the kitchen, adding to the already formidable breakfast dishes.

Vivian watched her add two teaspoons of sugar to her coffee. "Don't count calories either, do you?" She laughed.

"I don't need to," Kathryn said quietly, refusing to display her irritation. Where in the world were Maude and Phillip and Dick Leeds?

Vivian watched her raise the cup to her mouth, and her hawk eyes lit on the slightly raw lower lip, which was faintly throbbing this morning—a painful reminder of Blake's shocking intimacy.

The blonde's narrow eyes darted down to her plate as she nibbled at scrambled eggs. "You and Blake were downstairs together a long time last night," she said conversationally.

"We...had some things to discuss," Kathryn murmured, hating the memory of him that came back to haunt her with a vengeance. She was being forced to see Blake in a new, different way, and she wasn't at all sure that she wanted to. She was more afraid of him now than ever: a delicious, mushrooming fear that made her pulse race at just the thought of his mouth crushing hers. What would it have been like, she wondered reluctantly, if he hadn't been angry...

"You missed Blake this morning," Vivian remarked, her eyes strangely wary as she watched Kathryn spoon eggs and ham onto her plate. "He asked me particularly to come down straightaway when the alarm went off so that we could have breakfast together."

"How nice," came the stilted reply.

Kathryn's head was bent, and she missed the faintly malicious smile that curled Vivian's full lips.

"He was anxious to leave before you came down," the blonde went on in a low, very cool voice. "I think he was afraid you might have read something more than he intended into what happened last night."

Kathryn's fork fumbled through her fingers and hit the china plate with a loud ringing sound. Her startled eyes jerked up. "W-what?" she faltered. "He *told* you?" she asked incredulously.

Vivian looked the picture of sophistication. "Of course, darling," she replied. "He was bristling with regrets, and I just let him talk. It was the dress, of course. Blake is too much a man not to be swayed by a half-naked woman."

"I was not...!"

"He makes love very well, don't you think?" Vivian asked with a secretive smile. "He's such a vibrant lover, so considerate and exciting..."

Kathryn's face was the color of red cabbage. She sipped her coffee, ignoring the blistering touch of it.

"You do understand that it mustn't be allowed to happen again?" the older woman asked softly, smiling at Kathryn coolly over her china cup. "I quite realize why Blake hasn't told you the true reason I came over here with my father, but..." she let her voice trail away insinuatingly.

Kathryn stared at her, feeling her secure, safe little world dissolving around her. It was like being buried alive. She could hardly breathe for the sudden sense of suffocation. "You mean...?"

"If Blake hasn't told you, I can't," Vivian said confidingly. "He didn't want to make the announcement straight away, you know. Not until his family had a chance to get to know me."

Kathryn couldn't manage words. So that was how it was. Blake planned to marry at last, and this blond barracuda was going to swim off with him. And after last night, she'd actually thought... Her face shuttered. What did it matter, anyway? Blake had always been like a brother, despite his brutal ardor last night. And that had only been to warn her, he'd said so. He was afraid she'd read something into it, was he? She'd show him!

Vivian, seeing the look of despair that came into the young girl's face, hid a smile in her coffee cup as she drained it. "I see you understand," she remarked smugly. "You won't let Blake know that I said anything?" she asked with a worried look. "He'd be so unhappy with me..."

"No, of course not," Kathryn said quietly. "Congratulations."

Vivian smiled sweetly. "I hope we're going to become great friends. And you mustn't think anything about what happened with Blake. He only wants to forget it, as you must. It was just a moment out of time, after all, nothing to be concerned about."

Of course not, Kathryn thought, feeling suddenly empty. She managed a bright smile, but fortunately the rest of the family chose that moment to join the two women, and she was able to bury her grief in conversation.

Kathryn had always liked the airport; it excited her to see the travelers with their bags and bright smiles, and she liked to sit and watch and speculate about them. A long-legged young woman, tall and tanned and blond, ran into the arms of a big, dark man and burst into tears. Studying them as she waited for Lawrence Donavan's plane to get in, Kathryn wondered if they were patching up a lovers' quarrel. They must have been, because the man was kissing her as if he never expected to see her again, and tears were running unchecked down her pale cheeks. The emotion in that hungry kiss made her feel like a peeping Tom, and she looked away. The depth of passion she sensed in them was as alien to her as the Andes. She'd never felt that kind of hunger for a man. The closest to it that she could remember coming was when Blake had kissed her the second time—that sensuous, aching touch that kindled fledgling responses in her untried body. If he'd kissed her a third time…

A movement caught her eye and she rose from the chair to find Larry Donavan coming toward her. She ran into his outstretched arms and hugged him, lifting her face for a firm, affectionate kiss.

His blue eyes laughed down into hers under the shock of red hair that fell rakishly across his brow.

"Miss me?" he teased.

She nodded, and the admission was genuine. "Would I fight half my family to drive this distance to pick you up if I hadn't?" she asked.

"I know. It is a pretty long drive, isn't it? I could have caught a bus…"

"Don't be silly," she said, linking her hand with his as they walked toward the baggage conveyor. "How would you like a grand tour of Charleston before we head home? Blake's guests got it, and you're just as entitled…"

"Guests?" he echoed. "Have I come at an inopportune time?" he asked quickly.

"Blake's courting a labor union and a woman at the same time," she said with a trace of bitterness in her tone. "We'll simply keep out of the way. Phillip and Maude and I will take care of you, don't worry."

"Blake's the guardian, isn't he?" he asked, pausing to grab his bag from the conveyor as it moved past.

"That, and a distant cousin. The Hamiltons raised me," she murmured. "I'm afraid it isn't the best weather for a visit," she apologized, gesturing toward the rainy gray skies as they stepped outside and walked toward the parking lot. "It's been raining off and on all day and we're expecting some flooding before we're through. Hurricanes really get to us in the low country."

"How low is it?" he asked.

She leaned toward him, taking the cue. "It's so low that you have to look up to see the streets."

"Same old Kat," he teased, using his own nickname for her, and he hugged her close. "It's good to be down south again."

"You only say that because you're glad to get away from all that pollution," she told him.

He blinked at her. "Pollution? In Maine?" he asked incredulously.

She batted her eyelashes up at him. "Why, don't you all have smokestacks and chemical waste dumps and bodies floating in the river from gang wars?" she asked in her best drawl.

He laughed brightly. "Stereotypes?"

She grinned. "Didn't you believe that we wore white bedsheets to the grocery store and drank mint juleps for breakfast when you first met me?"

"I'd never known anyone from the south before," he defended himself as they walked toward her small foreign car. "In fact," he admitted, "this really is the first time I've spent any time here."

"You'll learn a lot," she told him. "For instance, that a lot of us believe in equality, that most of us can actually read and write, and that..."

The sky chose that particular moment to open up,

and rain started pouring down on them in sheets. She fumbled with her keys, barely getting them into the car in time to avoid a soaking.

Brushing her damp hair back from her face, Kathryn put the small white Porsche into reverse and backed carefully out of the parking space. It wasn't only due to her drivers' training course that she was careful at the wheel. When Blake had given her this car for her birthday last year, he'd been a constant passenger for the first week, watching every move she made. When he talked she listened, too, because in his younger days, Blake had raced in Grand Prix competitions all over Europe.

She swung into gear and headed out of the parking lot onto the busy street.

"It's raining cats!" She laughed, peering through the windshield wipers as the rain shattered against the metal roof with deafening force. It was hard to see the other cars, despite their lights.

"Don't blame me." Larry laughed. "I didn't bring it with me."

"I hope it lets up," she said uneasily, remembering the two bridges they had to cross to get back to King's Fort and on to Greyoaks. When flash floods came, the bridges sometimes were underwater and impossible to cross.

She saw an opening and pulled smoothly out into it.

"I see palm trees!" Larry exclaimed.

"Where did you think you were—Antarctica?" she teased, darting a glance at him. "They don't call us the

Palmetto State for nothing. We have beaches in the low country, too, just like Florida."

He looked confused. "Low country?"

"The coastal plain is called that because...well, because it's low," she said finally. "Then there's the up country—but you won't see any of it this trip. King's Fort, where the family lives, is low country, too, even though it's an hour and a half away." She smiled apologetically. "I'm sorry we couldn't fly down to pick you up, but the big Cessna's having some part or other replaced. That's why Blake had to drive down for his guests. There's a company executive jet, too, but one of the vice-presidents had to fly down to another of the mills in Georgia."

He studied her profile. "Your family must own a lot of industries."

She shrugged. "Just three or four yarn mills and about five clothing manufacturing companies."

He lifted his eyes skyward. "Just, she says."

"Well, lots of Blake's friends own more," she explained. She headed straight down I-26 until she could exit and get onto Rutledge Avenue. "We'll go the long way around to the Battery, and I'll show you some of the landmarks on Meeting Street—if you can see them through the rain," she said drily.

"You know the city pretty well?" he asked, all eyes as they drove down the busy highway.

"I used to have an aunt here, and I stayed with her in the summer. I still like to drive down on weekends, for the night life."

She didn't mention that she'd never done it alone before, or that she was making this trip without Blake's knowledge or permission. Maude and Phillip had protested but nobody had ever stopped Kathryn except Blake, and they couldn't find him before she left. She could still see Vivian Leeds's smug expression, and her pride felt wounded. If he was involved with the blonde, he should never have touched Kathryn...but, then, she'd provoked him. He'd accused her of it, and she couldn't deny it. All she didn't know was why.

"I'd like to use this as a location for a book," he said after they reached the turnoff onto the Battery, with its stone sea wall, and drove along it to Old Charleston.

She smiled at his excited interest as he looked first out at the bay and then across her at the rows of stately old houses.

They passed the Lenwood Boulevard intersection and he peered through the slackening rain. "Do you know any of the history of these old houses?" he asked.

"Some of them. Just a second." They drove on down South Battery Street and she pointed to a white two-story antebellum house on the right with long, elegant porches. "That one dates back to the 1820's. It was built on palmetto logs sunk in mud in an antiearthquake design later used by Frank Lloyd Wright. It was one of only a few homes to survive the 1886 Charleston earthquake that destroyed most of the city."

"How about that!" He laughed, gazing back toward the house enclosed by its neat white picket fence.

She gestured toward White Point Garden where a

small group of people were just disembarking from a horse-drawn carriage. "There are several carriage tours of the old part of town," she told him. "They're fun. I'm just sorry we don't have time today, but, then, it's not really the weather for it, either."

He sighed. "There wasn't a cloud in the sky when I left home."

"That's life," she told him. "Look on the left over there," she added when traffic let her turn onto Meeting Street. "That first house was once owned by one of the Middletons who owned Middleton Place Gardens. The second house is built in the Charleston 'double house' style—brick under cypress weather-boarding. It's late eighteenth century."

"Lady, you know your architecture," he said with grudging praise.

She laughed, relaxing in the plush leather seat. "Not like Aunt Hattie did. She taught me. A little farther down, there's a good example of the Adams-style construction—the Russell House. It's now the headquarters of the Historic Charleston Foundation."

He watched for it, and she caught a glimpse of smiling appreciation in his eyes as they studied the three-story building through its brick and wrought-iron wall.

"I wish we had time to go through Market Street," she said regretfully as she gave her attention to traffic. "There's a place where you can get every kind of food at individual stalls, and there are all kinds of shops and little art galleries..." She sighed. "But I guess we'd better stop at a restaurant a little closer to home. The wind's getting up, and I don't think the rain's any closer to quitting."

"Maybe on the trip back," he said with a smile, and winked at her.

She smiled back, flicking the radio on to a local station. The music blared for a few seconds, and then the weather report came on. She listened with a face that grew more solemn by the minute. Flash-flood warnings were being announced for the area around King's Fort as well as the rivers near Charleston.

"I hope you're not hungry," she murmured as she turned back into Rutledge Avenue. "We've got to get home, before that flooding covers the bridges."

"Sounds adventurous," he chuckled, watching her intense concentration as she merged into traffic.

"It is. Are you hungry?" she persisted gently.

"I was rather thinking along the lines of a chilled prawn cocktail," he admitted with a grin.

"I'll have Mrs. Johnson fix you one when we get home," she promised. "We keep it, fresh-frozen, because it's Blake's favorite dish."

He stared out the window at the gray, darkening skies, lit by shop lights and car lights. "Some of those trees are bending pretty low," he remarked.

"I've seen them bend almost to the ground during a hurricane," she recalled nervously. "That's what this is about to be, I'm afraid. If I thought I could spare the time, I'd stop and call home. But I'm not going to risk it."

"You're the driver, honey," he said.

She smiled wryly. If Blake had been with her, he'd be at the wheel now, whether or not it was his car, taking over. She shifted in the seat. Comparisons were unfair, and she had no right to even be thinking about Blake now that he was practically engaged. But she couldn't help wondering what was going to happen when she got home. As Phillip had once said, Blake didn't particularly care how many people happened to be around if he lost his temper.

The rain followed them all the way to King's Fort, and despite Larry's periodic reassurances, Kathryn couldn't help worrying. The little sports car, in spite of its brilliant engineering and design, was too light for some of the deep puddles of water they soared through. Once, Kathryn almost went into a mailbox as the car hydroplaned over the center line. She recovered it in time, but she was getting more nervous by the minute. There was no place to stop until they got to King's Fort, or she'd have given it up.

She gritted her teeth and drove on, refusing to let her passenger see how frightened she really was. If only Blake had been with her!

They were approaching the first river bridge now, and she leaned forward with anticipation, peering through the heavy rain as she tried to see if the bridge was still passable.

"How does it look?" he asked. "I think I can still see the road…I can!"

"Yes," she breathed, relieved. She geared down to get a better view of the rising water. It was already over the banks and only inches below the low bridge. A few more minutes...she concentrated on getting across and didn't think about it.

"Is it much farther to the next bridge?" he asked.

"About twenty miles or so," she said tightly. He didn't say anything, but she knew he was thinking the same thing she was—that those few minutes might mean the difference between getting across or not.

There was almost no traffic on the road now. They only met two vehicles, and one of them was the state police.

"I hate to mention this," Larry said quietly, "but what if we can't get across the second bridge?"

She licked her dry lips "We'll have to go back to King's Fort and spend the night in the hotel," she said, thinking ahead to Blake's fury when he caught up with her. "But the river shouldn't be that high yet," she said soothingly. "I think we can make it."

"Just in case," he asked with a speaking glance, "what kind of temper does your guardian have?"

She tightened her hands on the wheel without answering.

When they reached the long river bridge, her worst fears were confirmed. Two uniformed men were just putting up a roadblock.

She rolled down her window as one of them approached. He touched his hat respectfully. "Sorry, ma'am," he said quietly, "you'll have to detour back to King's Fort. The river's up over the bridge."

"But it's the only road into Greyoaks," she protested

weakly, knowing no argument was going to open up the road.

The uniformed man smiled apologetically. “The Hamilton estate? Yes, ma’am, I’m afraid it is. But there’s no way across until the water level drops. I’m sorry.”

She sighed. “Well, I’ll have to go into King’s Fort and call home…”

“You’re out of luck there, too,” the officer said with a rueful grin. “The telephone lines are down. One way or another, it’s been a rough day. I wish we could help.”

She smiled. “Thanks anyway.”

She rolled the window back up and hesitated just a minute before she put the small car into reverse, turned it neatly around, and started back toward King’s Fort.

“I feel bad about this,” Larry said gently.

“Oh, don’t be silly,” she replied with a smile, “it’s all right. We’ll just be…a little late getting home, that’s all.”

He studied her wan expression. “I’ll explain it to him,” he promised.

She nodded, but under her brave smile she felt like a naughty student on her way to the principal’s office. Blake wasn’t going to understand, and she sincerely hoped the river didn’t go down until he cooled off.

Chapter Six

Kathryn pulled up in front of the King's Fort Inn and cut off the engine. She sat there for a minute with her hands tight on the wheel.

"Well, we tried," she said wryly, meeting Larry's sympathetic blue gaze. "I hope my insurance is paid up."

"Will he really be that mad?" he asked.

She drew in a hard breath. "I didn't have permission to come after you," she admitted. "I think I'm old enough to do without it. But Blake doesn't."

He patted her slender hand where it rested on the steering wheel. "I'll protect you," he promised, smiling.

She couldn't return the smile. The thought of Larry protecting her from Blake was almost comical.

The rain was still coming down as they ran into the hotel, and Kathryn held up her raincoat, making a tent over her wild, loosened hair. She laughed with exhilaration as they stopped under the awning to catch their breath.

He grinned down at her, his red hair unruly and beaded with rain. "Fancy meeting you here!"

"Not very fancy, I'm afraid." She laughed, putting a tentative hand up to her disorderly hair. "I must look like a witch."

He shook his head. "Lovely, as always."

"Thank you, kind sir." She darted a quick look at the hotel entrance. "It's the only hotel in town," she sighed, "and I'm sure we're going to cause some comment, but just ignore the stares and go ahead. We'll pretend we don't see any familiar faces."

"This town isn't all that small, surely," he remarked.

She smiled uncomfortably. "It's not. But, you see, the headquarters of the textile conglomerate is located here, and the family is fairly well known."

"I should have realized. Sorry."

"No need. Let's go in, shall we? You can get your bag later."

He followed her into the carpeted lobby. "What will you do for a change of clothes?" he asked.

She shrugged. "Do without, I suppose. Maybe in the..." Her voice trailed off, and she paled visibly.

Larry looked at her with a puzzled frown. She was staring at a big, dark man who was sitting in an armchair by the window reading a paper. He seemed vaguely weary, as if he'd been in that particular chair a long time. Even at a distance he looked threatening. As

Larry watched, he deliberately put down the paper and got to his feet, to saunter over toward them.

Larry knew without being told who the man was. Kathryn's young face was stiff with apprehension. "Blake, I presume?" he murmured under his breath.

Kathryn's fingers dug into her slacks, making indentations in the soft beige fabric. She couldn't get the words out.

Blake rammed his big hands into his pockets, towering over her, his face expressionless. "Ready to go home?" he asked curtly.

"How…did you find me?" she whispered.

His dark eyes swept over her face. "I could find you in New York City at rush hour," he said quietly. Those fierce eyes shot across to Larry's face, and the younger man fought the urge to back away. He thought he'd met every kind of personality in the book, but this man was something beyond his experience. Authority clung to him like the brown slacks that hugged his muscular thighs, like the red knit shirt that emphasized the powerful muscles of his chest and arms.

"Donavan, isn't it?" Blake asked in a cutting tone.

"Y-yes, sir." Larry felt like a boy again. There was something intimidating about Blake Hamilton, and he knew without being told that he hadn't made the best of first impressions.

"The bridge is underwater," Kathryn said softly.

"I know." He started toward the exit, leaving them to follow.

"What about my poor car?" Kathryn persisted.

"Lock it and leave it," he threw over his shoulder. "We'll send back for it when the river goes down."

Kathryn looked at Larry helplessly. He nodded, and left them in front of the hotel under the awning. "I'll get my suitcase out, and lock the car for you," he told her.

She stood beside Blake, miserable and shivering from the chill of the rain.

"Why?" he asked, the single blunt word making her want to cry.

She sucked in a steadying breath. "It was only a short drive."

"With hurricane warnings out," he growled, looking down at her with barely contained fury behind his half-closed eyelids.

She drew her eyes away. "How are we going to get home?" she asked weakly.

"I ought to let you and your boyfriend walk," he replied coldly, staring out at the traffic in the wet street.

She looked down at her wet canvas shoes and then back up at him. He was only wearing a lightweight jacket with his shirt and trousers, and no raincoat.

"Don't you have an umbrella?" she asked gently.

He shifted his big shoulders, still not looking at her. "I didn't take time to look for it." His eyes glittered down at her, and his face hardened. "Have you any idea how long I've been sitting here wondering where you were?" he asked harshly.

She reached out and tentatively touched his sleeve. "I'm sorry, Blake, really I am. I wanted to call, but I was afraid to take the time..."

She suddenly noticed the new lines in his face, the bloodshot eyes. "Were you really worried?" she asked.

One big hand came out and ruffled her hair with rough affection. "What do you think?" he asked. Something in his face seemed to relax as he looked down into her soft eyes. "I've been out of my mind, Kate," he whispered, with such emotion in his voice that her heart seemed to lift up and fly.

"Blake…"

"Here I am!" Larry said merrily, joining them with his suitcase in his hand. "All locked up."

Kathryn folded her arms across her chest and tried to look calm. "How are we going to get across the river?" she asked Blake.

"I chartered a helicopter," he said with a wry smile.

She smiled. Leave it to Blake to make the most insurmountable problem simple.

Maude and Phillip had shared Blake's apprehension about the bad weather and Kathryn's absence, but they played it down. Vivian only shrugged when Kathryn told them about the rough trip home. She was much more interested in meeting another man to bat her false eyelashes at, Kathryn thought maliciously. The blonde was still glued to Blake and, remembering what was going on between them, Kathryn felt a twinge of pain. Blake had been worried about her, of course he had. But as his ward. Nothing more.

"You're very quiet tonight, darling," Phillip remarked when the rest of the family was gathered in the music room to hear Vivian play the grand piano. Kathryn had to admit that she was good. Larry, who played a little himself, sat and watched her with a rapt expression. It had all been a bit much for Kathryn, after the rough afternoon. She had slipped out into the hall and gone into the deserted kitchen to pour herself a cup of coffee. Phillip had followed her.

Sitting, her slender hands contracted around the cup, she crossed her legs, making her beige silk dress swish with the motion.

"I like that dress," Phillip remarked, perching himself on the edge of the table facing her. "One of the new ones, isn't it?"

She smiled and nodded. "Larry liked it, too."

"I like Larry," he grinned. "He makes me feel mature and venerable."

Her eyebrows flew up. "He what?"

"He's young, isn't he?" he asked drily, eyeing her over his cup.

"Ouch," she murmured impishly.

He laughed at her. "You know what I mean, don't you? Beside him, Blake looks even more formidable than usual." The grin faded. "Did he cut you up?"

"Blake?" She shook her head. "Surprisingly, no. I guess I should have told him I was going in the first place."

"Maude finally reached him in Atlanta." He emptied his cup and let it dangle in his hands. "He flew to Charleston, you know. It was a devil of a risk, but he took the chance. You were headed home by then. He had the state troopers after you."

Her face went pale. "I didn't realize…!"

"He'd been waiting three-quarters of an hour at the hotel when you got there," he added. "Sweating out every minute—along with the rest of us. Small cars are dangerous when it floods. I'm surprised he didn't really blow up. I imagine he felt like it."

She studied the coffee in her cup. "Yes, I imagine so," she whispered. Her eyes closed. She'd never have done it anyway if she hadn't been upset by what Vivian had told her at the breakfast table, but she couldn't tell Phillip about that. "It was a stupid thing to do."

"Just foolhardy," he corrected. "When are you going to stop fighting Blake?"

"When he lets go of me," she said curtly.

He only shook his head. "That could be a very long time…"

Greyoaks was imposing in the morning sunlight, and Kathryn reined up beside Larry to admire it.

She sighed. "You should see it in the spring when all the flowers are in bloom."

"I can imagine." His eyes swept over her slender body in her riding clothes. "You look completely at home on a horse."

She patted the Arabian mare's black mane. Sundance had been a little sluggish this morning, so she'd brought the mare instead. "I've been riding for a long time. Blake taught me," she added, laughing at the memories. "It was grueling, for both of us."

Larry sighed, studying the reins in his pale hands. "He doesn't like me."

"Blake?" She avoided his eyes. "He's hard to get close to," she said, knowing full well that wasn't completely true.

"If I planned to be here longer than three days," he admitted, "I think I'd buy a suit of armor. He makes me feel like an idiot."

"He's in the middle of labor disputes," she told him soothingly. "He and Dick Leeds are trying to work out some kind of agreement."

Larry smiled. "It looks like he's putting more effort into working on the daughter. A dish, isn't she? And talented, too."

Kathryn forced a smile onto her full lips. "Yes, she is."

"Are they engaged?" he asked with a sly glance. "I get a strong feeling that something's happening there."

"I think they are," she replied. "Let's head back, Larry. Mrs. Johnson hates to serve breakfast twice." She wheeled the mare and shot off ahead of him.

The question brought it all back. Of course they were engaged, and she couldn't understand why Blake was so concerned about keeping it a secret. The whole business made her angry. And Blake had told Vivian about... Her face flamed. She could never forgive him for that. And the conceit of the man, thinking that she was naive enough to read anything into that kiss. She'd put his treachery out of her mind yesterday, in the face of Blake's obvious concern for her safety. But now, with the danger over, it was burning holes in her temper. Damn Blake, anyway!

What you need, Kathryn Mary, she told herself as she leaned over the mare's black mane and gave her her head, is a place of your own!

She dismounted at the barn and waited for Larry to walk up to the house with her.

Blake and Vivian were the only ones at the breakfast table. Kathryn, smiling like a film star on display, clung to Larry's thin arm as they joined the others at the table.

"What a lovely ride," Kathryn sighed. She glanced at Vivian. "Do you like horses?" she asked.

"Can't stand them," Vivian said with a smile at Blake's taciturn face.

Kathryn's green eyes flashed, but she held on to her temper.

"The estate is very impressive," Larry remarked as he helped himself to bacon and eggs from the generous platters. "How many gardeners does it take to keep the grounds so neat?"

"Oh, Blake has three yard men, don't you, darling?" Vivian answered for him, leaning her muslin-clad shoulder briefly against his.

Kathryn wanted to sling scrambled eggs at her. She quickly lowered her eyes before any of her companions could read them.

"My parents have a garden about a fourth the size

of yours," Larry continued, "without the gazebo. Dad's hobby is roses."

Blake lit a cigarette and leaned back in his chair to study the younger man with an unnerving intensity. "Do you grow flowers too?" he asked cuttingly.

"Blake!" Kathryn protested.

He didn't even glance at her. His whole attention was concentrated on Larry, who reddened and looked as if he might explode any minute. Despite his easygoing nature, he did have a temper, and it looked as if Blake was trying his best to make him lose it.

"Do you?" Blake persisted.

Larry put his cup down carefully. "I write books, Mr. Hamilton," he said tightly.

"What about?" came the lightning reply.

"Pompous asses, mostly," Larry grated.

Blake's dark eyes glittered dangerously. "Are you insinuating something, Donavan?"

"If the shoe fits..." Larry returned, his blue eyes icy.

"Stop it!" Kathryn burst out. She stood up, throwing her napkin onto the table. Her lower lip trembled, her eyes flashed. "Stop it, Blake!" she whispered furiously. "You've done nothing but pick on Larry since he got here! Do you have to...!"

"Be quiet," he said coldly.

She closed her lips as if he'd slapped her. "You're horrible, Blake," she whispered shakily. "Larry's a guest..."

"Not mine," he replied, glaring at Larry, who was standing now, too.

"You're right there," Larry replied gruffly. He turned to Kathryn. "Come and talk to me while I pack."

He left the room and Kathryn turned back at the doorway to glare at Blake. "If he leaves, I'll go with him, Blake," she told him furiously.

"You may think you will," he said in a soft, dangerous tone.

"We'll see about that," she choked, whirling.

Kathryn's pleas didn't deter Larry. He packed in record time and had started to call a cab when Dick Leeds came out into the hall and stopped him.

"Vivian wants to do some shopping in Charleston," he said with a quiet smile, "and since the river's down, it's quite safe. Phillip's going to drive us, and you're welcome to ride along. We'd be happy to drop you at the airport."

"Thank you," Larry said. He reached down and pecked Kathryn lightly on the cheek. "Sorry, love. I'm very fond of you, but not fond enough to take on your guardian."

She stiffened. "I'm sorry it worked out like this. Give my best to Missy."

He nodded. "Goodbye."

She watched him walk away with a sense of loss. It had all happened so fast. Her head was still spinning with the suddenness of it. She tried to piece together Blake's unreasonable behavior. He'd done his best to break up her friendship with Larry from the beginning.

But why? He had Vivian. Why did he begrudge Kathryn a boyfriend? She hated him. Somehow, she had to get out from under his thumb….

She stayed out of sight until they left. Blake wasn't to be found, and she thought he'd gone with the rest. Maude had tried to persuade her to come along, to Vivian's obvious irritation, but she'd refused. She couldn't have borne being shut up in the same car with Larry and Blake both.

She walked through the damp hedges to the gazebo. The grass and shrubs were still wet from the previous day's heavy rains, but inside the quiet confines of the little white building with its delicate latticework and ring of cushions, it was dry and cozy.

She sat down on the plush cushions and looked out over the cobblestone walks that led around and through the well-kept gardens. Although the azaleas and dogwoods that bloomed gloriously in the spring were not in season now, the roses gave the gardens a dash of color. The fragrance of the white ones was delicious. She closed her eyes and drank it in, along with the warm breeze that made the September day more like summer.

"Sulking?"

She jumped at the sound of Blake's deep, curt voice. Her startled eyes found him in the entrance of the small building, a smoking cigarette in his hand. He was wearing the same beige slacks and yellow knit shirt he'd had on at the breakfast table, and the same forbidding scowl.

She scowled back, curling her jodhpur-clad leg under

her slender body, tugging her white sweater down. "Haven't you done enough for one morning?" she asked angrily.

One dark eyebrow went up. "What have I done? I didn't ask him to leave."

"No," she agreed hotly. "You just made it impossible for him to stay and hold on to his pride."

He shrugged indifferently. "In any case, it's no great loss."

"To you," she added. "Your girlfriend's still here."

He eyed her carefully. "Yes," he said. "She is."

"Naturally. She's *your* guest."

He shouldered away from the entrance and walked toward her, stopping just in front of her. "Would you really want a man who was afraid of me?"

Her eyes shot up to his. "No," she admitted sharply. "I'd like one who'd beat the devil out of you."

A slow, mischievous smile touched his mouth. "Had any luck yet?"

She tore her gaze away, remembering Jack Harris and a string of others. "Why didn't you go with them? Vivian seemed to have taken a shine to Larry last night."

"Vivian's tastes are not necessarily mine."

Kathryn stared down at the dark green cushions, tracing a pattern on the one where she was sitting with a nervous finger.

"Why wouldn't you let him stay, Blake?" she asked bitterly. "He wasn't bothering you."

"He wasn't?" He finished the cigarette and flung it out on the cobblestones, where it lay smouldering briefly until the dampness doused it. "The damned young fool, letting you drive in that downpour! I should have broken both his legs!"

She gaped at him. "It was my car, he couldn't very well tell me to let him get behind the wheel!"

"I could," he replied gruffly. "And I would have. If I'd been with you, you'd never have left Charleston."

She couldn't repress a tiny smile: It was exactly what she'd been thinking on the way home. "There was a moment or two there when I wish you had been," she said lightly.

He didn't reply, and when she looked up, it was to find his face strangely rigid.

"You shouldn't have worried," she added, aware of a new tension between them. "You taught me to drive, remember?"

"All I remembered was that you were in danger in the company of a fool, a boy who didn't know how to take care of you," he said tightly. "If anything had happened to you, I'd have killed him."

He didn't raise his voice. But the words had as much impact as if he'd shouted them.

"What a violent thing to say," she laughed nervously.

He didn't smile. His dark eyes narrowed, spearing her with an intensity that made flames kindle in her blood. "I've always been violent about you. Are you just now noticing it?"

She gazed up at him quietly, stunned by the words, by the emotion in them, her lips slightly parted, her eyes curious and soft.

Blake leaned one big hand on the back of the seat over her shoulder and his eyes dropped to her soft mouth. The action had brought him closer; so close that she could smell the clean, masculine fragrance of soap and cologne, feel the warmth of his big body.

"Blake," she whispered, yielding without words, without thought, longing for him.

He bent his dark head and brushed his mouth against hers, a whisper of delicious sensation that quickened her pulse, her breathing. He drew back, and she lifted a finger to trace, tremulously, the hard, sensuous curve of his mouth. Emotion trembled between them in the silence, broken only by the whispering breeze, and the distant sound of a songbird.

His lips moved, catching her exploring finger, and she felt the tip of his tongue moving softly against it. Her eyes looked straight into his, and she read the excitement in them.

He searched her flushed young face quietly. "Stand up, Kathryn," he said at last. "I want to feel you against me."

Like a sleepwalker, she obeyed him, letting him draw her so close that she could feel his powerful thighs pressing against hers, the muscles of his chest like a wall against her soft breasts.

His thumb brushed against her mouth and he studied it as if he needed to memorize it. "Are you afraid?" he asked in a strange, husky voice.

She shook her head, meeting his eyes with the hunger and need plain in her own. "Last time..."

"It's not going to be like last time," he breathed. "Kate…!" Her soft mouth parted eagerly as his lips met hers.

Her slender arms reached up around his neck, holding him, and she kissed him back feverishly, trying to show that she could be anything he wanted her to be.

His big hand tangled in the thick strands of hair at her nape, and his devouring mouth forced hers open even wider. He explored it with a deepening intimacy that made her tremble. With a sense of wonder she felt his hands at her back, sliding under the sweater and up to move caressingly against her silken skin.

"No bra?" he murmured against her mouth, and she could feel the amused smile that moved his lips.

She flushed at the intimacy of the question, and suddenly reached around to catch his wrists and hold them as he started to slide his exploring hands around under her arms.

"Blake…" she protested.

He chuckled softly and drew his hands away, to replace them at her waist over the thick fabric. "You said you weren't afraid," he reminded her.

She lowered her eyes to his broad chest. "Must you make fun of me?" she asked miserably. "You know I'm not sophisticated."

"It's quite obvious," he laughed softly. "If you were, you would know better than to plaster yourself against a man when he kisses you. Ten years ago, I'm not sure I'd have been able to draw back."

She looked up, startled. "But in the movies…"

"Plastic people, contrived situations; this is real, Kathryn." He took her hand and pressed it inside the opening of his shirt, against the hard, warm flesh and thick mat of hair. She felt the heavy rhythm of his heart. "Do you feel it?" he asked softly. "You make my blood run like a river in flood, Kate."

She was lost in his dark eyes, in the gentleness of his deep voice. Her fingers lingered inside his shirt, liking the feel of his muscular body, remembering suddenly and vividly the way he looked that night long ago with Jessica.

He seemed to read the thoughts in her mind. Abruptly he caught her hands and slid them under the shirt to lie against the broad, hard chest. Her fingers trembled on the hair-rough skin.

"I've never touched…anyone like this," she whispered, awed by the new longings surging through her body, making her tremble in his big arms. "I never wanted to, until now."

His lips brushed against her forehead, his breath warm and a little unsteady, while her curious fingers explored the powerful muscles.

She raised her eyes to Blake's. "I…Blake, I feel…"

His fingers pressed gently against her lips. "Kiss me," he whispered. "Don't think, don't talk. Just kiss me." His lips teased hers delicately, softly, causing a surge of hunger that dragged a moan from her tight throat.

She went on tiptoe to help him, to tempt him, her lips parting under the lazy pressure of his mouth as he began to deepen the kiss. She felt his hands caressing her back, moving surely around to her ribcage. But, this time, she didn't catch his wrists.

His thumbs edged out to trace the gentle slope of her high, firm breasts and she stiffened instinctively at the unfamiliar touch.

"It's all right," he whispered at her lips. "Don't pull away from me."

Her eyes opened, wide and curious and a little frightened. "It's…new," she whispered.

"Being touched?" he asked quietly. "Or being touched by me?"

"Both," she admitted.

His fingers moved higher, and he watched her face while they found the hard peaks and traced them tenderly, just before his hands swallowed the velvet softness and pressed against it with warm, sensuous motions.

"How does it feel, Kate?" he asked in a deep, honeyed tone. "Is it good?"

Her nails dug into his chest involuntarily as the magic worked on her, and she moaned softly.

"I shouldn't…let you," she whispered.

"No, you shouldn't," he agreed, moving closer. "Tell me to stop, Kate," he whispered. "Tell me you hate it."

"I…wish I could," she whispered. His mouth was on her closed eyelids, her nose, her high cheekbones, while his hands made wild shivers of sensation wash over her bare skin.

His mouth bit at hers tenderly in a succession of teasing kisses that made her want to cry out. "God, you're sweet," he whispered huskily. "As soft as a whisper where I touch you."

Her fingers tangled in the mat of hair over his strong chest. "I…dreamed about how it would be with you," she whispered shakily. "Ever since that night I saw you with Jessica, I've wondered…"

"I know," he whispered back, "I saw it in your eyes. That was what wrung me out so, Kate, because I wondered, too. But you were so damned young…"

She drew a deep, unsteady breath, lifting her body higher against his deft, sure hands. "Blake…?" she moaned.

"What do you want?" His dark eyes burned into hers. "There's nothing you can't ask me, don't you know that? What do you want, Kate?"

Her body ached with the newness of wanting and she didn't know how to put into words what she needed. It had never been like this, never!

"I don't know how to say it," she admitted in a breathless whisper. "Blake…please…"

He bent, lifting her in his big arms without a word, and carried her to the cushioned seat that ringed the gazebo. Then he came down beside her with something in his hard, dark face that was faintly shocking after all the years of banter and camaraderie and deep affection. She was just beginning to see Blake as a lover, and the effect it was having on her defied description. She looked up at him with all her confusion in her green eyes, and in her flushed, expectant face.

"I won't hurt you," he said softly.

"I know." She lifted her fingers to his hard, chiseled mouth and traced it gently. "I've never kissed a man lying down."

"Haven't you?" He smiled as he lifted himself to ease his formidable torso down onto her, so that they were thigh to thigh, hip to hip, breast to breast. She gasped at the intimate contact and her fingers dug into the rippling muscles of his shoulders.

His fingers cupped her face as he bent. "Am I too heavy, Kate?" he whispered against her soft mouth.

She flushed at the question, but she didn't look away. "No," she managed shakily.

He brushed his mouth across hers. "Pull your sweater up," he whispered.

"Blake..."

He kissed her closed eyelids. "You want it as much as I do," he breathed. "Pull it up, Kate...then help me pull up my shirt."

She looked into his eyes, trembling. She wanted him until she ached from head to toe, but he was suggesting an intimacy she'd never experienced before, and once it happened, there wouldn't be any going back.

"It's...I mean, I've never..." she stammered.

His thumbs brushed against the corners of her mouth while his tongue lightly traced the trembling line of her lips.

"Don't you want to feel me against you like that, Kate?" he whispered sensuously. "With nothing between us?"

She gasped against his invading mouth. Her eyes

closed tightly. "Yes," she ground out, and even her voice trembled. "Oh, Blake, yes, yes…!"

"Help me," he whispered huskily.

With trembling fingers, she lifted the hem of his yellow knit shirt and eased it up over the warm, hard muscles under their mat of crisp black hair, and her fingers savored the sensuous contact with him, while her heart pounded out a mad rhythm.

His mouth coaxed hers open, tasting it, gentling it, his fingers tenderly caressing her face.

"Now yours, love," he whispered softly. "There's nothing to be afraid of, nothing at all, I won't hurt you, I won't force you. Now, Kate…"

She looked into his darkening eyes while she slid the soft sweater up over her taut breasts and with a shuddering pleasure, she felt him ease down again until her taut nipples vanished into the dark pelt over his chest. She felt his body against hers in a contact that made magic in her mind and she gasped.

"My God, isn't it delicious?" he whispered tautly, shifting his powerful torso slowly, sensuously, across her breasts in the utter silence of the gazebo.

Her fingers hesitated on his hard collarbone, lightly touching him, feeling him. Her eyes widened as the intimacy sent her pulse racing, as her breath caught in her throat.

"You're…so warm," she whispered.

"A man being burned alive does feel warm," he replied half-humorously. He moved then, holding her eyes while his body eased completely onto hers.

"It's all right," he breathed, calming her as she stiffened involuntarily at the greater intimacy with his body. His hands stroked her hair lightly, his forearms taking the bulk of his weight. He studied her closely. "Now I can feel you completely," he whispered, "and you can feel me. We can't hide anything from each other when we touch like this, can we, Kate? You know without words how much I want you, don't you?"

She flushed wildly as the exact meaning of his words got through to her, and she noticed for the first time all the differences between his body and hers.

Pleasure surged up in her like spring sap in a young tree as she sensed her own awakening to emotions and sensations that had lain dormant inside her, waiting for a catalyst.

Her fingers touched his face, his mouth, his arrogant nose, his thick dark brows, and when she breathed, she was made even more aware of the warmth and weight of his hair-roughened chest against the sensitive warmth of her bareness.

The weight of him crushed her yielding body down into the soft cushions and her arms went up to hold him even closer as he bent to take her mouth under his.

She opened her lips, her fingers tangling in his thick, cool hair as the kiss went on and on. His tongue darted into her mouth, demanding, tormenting, while his hands slid under her thighs and lifted her body up against his with a bruising pressure, until she was achingly aware of how much he wanted her.

She shifted restlessly under the crush of his body, and

a hard groan tore out of his throat while he kissed her. A shudder ran the length of him.

"Don't do that," he whispered against her lips. "I may be past my first youth, but I can lose my head with you so easily it isn't even funny."

She watched him, fascinated. "I...I like the way it feels, to lie with you like this," she admitted in a whisper.

"My God, I like it, too," he groaned. "Kiss me, honey...!"

His hungry ardor flared like wildfire between them. She stopped trying to understand and melted into him. It was glorious, the hungry crush of his mouth, the feel of his arms, the long, hard contact with his powerful body, the warmth of him that seemed to burn her everywhere they touched. She never wanted this kiss to end. She wanted to spend the rest of her life in his arms like this, holding him, loving him. Loving him!

He caught her wrists abruptly and tore her clinging hands away from his back. He looked down at her as if he'd been temporarily out of his mind and had only just realized what he was doing. He shook his dark head as if to clear it. With a violent movement he got to his feet and pulled his shirt down, keeping his back to Kathryn while she fumbled, embarrassed, with her sweater. She stared at his broad back incredulously. She'd forgotten what had happened just an hour ago, forgotten the anger and frustration she'd felt. In the shadow of Blake's blazing ardor she'd even forgotten Vivian. How could she have let him...!

He turned, catching that expression of shock in her eyes, and something seemed to harden his face, take the soft light out of his eyes. He smiled mockingly.

"Now tell me you miss Donavan," he said in a voice that cut through her heart like a razor.

She licked at the inside of her swollen lips, tasting the lingering touch of his mouth there, her eyes vulnerable, hurt.

"Was that why?" she asked in a sore whisper getting to her feet.

He rammed his hands into his pockets. His face was harder than she could ever remember seeing it.

"Or was it…because you don't want another man to have me?" she asked painfully.

"I've got all the bodies I need, Kate," he said tightly "I didn't raise you to take you into my bed the minute you came of age."

"But, just now…" she began hesitantly.

"I want you, all right," he admitted, scowling down at her. "I have for a long time. But just because I lost my head with you a minute ago, that doesn't mean I plan to do anything about it."

Of course not, how could he, when he planned to marry Vivian? "Don't worry," she said bitterly, stepping away from him. "I'm not going to 'read anything' into it this time either."

"What?"

"That's what you told Vivian, isn't it?" she asked in a broken voice, slanting a glance back at him as she stepped down into the garden. "That you were afraid I might 'read something' into what happened the other night? I'm not a child, Blake, I quite realize that men can be attracted physically by women they don't even like, much less love."

"Just what are you talking about?" he demanded, his eyes blazing.

"Vivian told me yesterday how much you regretted your actions the other night!" she threw at him.

The expression on his hard face puzzled her, if a fleeting shadow could be called that. "She told you that?" he asked.

She whirled. "No, I just made it up for the fun of it!"

"Kate…!"

"Don't call me Kate!" She glared back at him through her tears, missing the sudden glint in his dark eyes. "I hate you. And I'm going to get a job and my own apartment, and you can drag Vivian off into gazebos and make love to her! I don't ever want you to touch me again, Blake!"

"You will," he said in a strange, deep tone.

She turned and ran back toward the house as if invisible phantoms were chasing after her. She locked her bedroom door behind her and threw herself down onto the bed, venting the stored-up tears. She loved Blake. Not as she always had, as a protector, but newly, differently, as a man. She could barely believe it had happened, and she didn't want to admit it even in the privacy of her own mind. She loved Blake. And he was going to marry Vivian. Her eyes closed in pain. Vivian, living here, loving Blake, too, touching him, kissing that hard, beautiful mouth…

She groaned out loud with anguish. She'd have to get a job. There was no way around it now. She sat up, drying her tears. She'd start looking first thing in the morning, Blake or no Blake, and find something that she could do to make a living for herself. There was no way she could go on living under the same roof with Blake and his wife!

Chapter Seven

She was purposely late for breakfast, and when she got downstairs she glanced around quickly, hoping to find that Blake had already eaten.

Maude was just finishing a piece of toast across from Phillip, who was sipping his coffee. Blake, Dick Leeds and Vivian were nowhere in sight.

"My, aren't you dressed up," Maude commented, her approving glance resting on Kathryn's pretty beige suit and crepe de chine eggshell blouse with its neat bow. Her hair was drawn into a soft chignon, with wisping curls around her face, her feet encased in spike-heel open-toed sandals in beige and brown. She looked the picture of working womanhood.

"Trendy-looking," Phillip added with a wink. "Where are you off to in your fine feathers, little bird?"

"I'm going to get a job," she said with a cool smile.

Maude choked on her toast and had to be thumped on the back by Phillip.

"A job?" she gasped. "Doing what, Kathryn?"

"It depends on what I can find," the younger woman said with a stubborn light in her green eyes. "Now, don't argue, Maude," she added, catching the quick disapproval in the pale, dark-eyed face.

"I wasn't going to, dear," Maude protested. "I was just going to ask how you planned to tell Blake."

"She already has," Blake told them, appearing in the doorway dressed in a becoming gray suit with a patterned tie that emphasized his darkness. "Let's go, Kate."

She sat there almost trembling with emotion, her wide green eyes pleading with him, even as she knew she wasn't going to fight. All her resolutions vanished when Blake confronted her. After yesterday, all the fight was gone, anyway. She didn't have the heart for it anymore.

"She hasn't had breakfast," Phillip observed.

"She'll learn to get downstairs in time, won't she?" Blake replied, and there was something vaguely menacing about the way he was looking at his younger brother.

Phillip grinned sheepishly. "Just an observation, big brother." He laughed.

Blake's dark eyes went to Kathryn, skimming over her possessively. "I said, let's go."

She got up, leaving a cup of fresh coffee and a plate

of scrambled eggs behind her as she followed him out into the hall apprehensively.

"Where are we going?" she asked.

Both heavy brows went up. He opened the front door for her. "To work, of course."

"But, I don't have a job yet."

"Yes, you do."

"What as?" she asked.

"My secretary."

She followed him out to his dark sedan in a daze, only speaking when they were going down the driveway at Blake's usual fast pace.

"Did I hear you right?" she asked, and stared at his profile with unconcealed disbelief.

"You did." He took out his cigarette case and extracted a cigarette from it as he drove, leaning over to push in the cigarette lighter.

"But, Blake, I can't work for you," she protested.

His dark eyes scanned her face briefly. "Why not?"

"I can't type fast enough," she said, grasping at straws. Having to be near him all day, every day, would be more agony than ecstasy.

"You're about average, little one. You'll do." He lit his cigarette and pushed the lighter back in place. "You said you wanted a job," he reminded her.

She watched cars in the other lane passing by them, not really seeing anything as she sat stiffly beside Blake.

"Where was Vivian this morning?" she asked quietly. "The two of you were out late last night."

"So we were," he said noncommitally.

"It's none of my business, of course," she said tightly, avoiding his eyes.

He only smiled, keeping his attention on the road.

The Hamilton Mills complex was located in a sprawling ground-level facility in the city's huge industrial park, modern and landscaped. Kathryn had been inside the building many times, but never as an employee.

She followed Blake into his attractive carpeted office, where the dark furniture was complemented by elegant furnishings done in chocolates and creams. Her eye was caught and held by a portrait that spanned the length of the big leather sofa under it. She stared at the sweeping seascape, the sunset colors mingling in the clouds, the palm-lined beach a swath of white and silver. In the foreground were the shadowy outlines of a man and a woman.

"Like it?" he asked as he checked the messages on his desk.

She nodded. "It's St. Martin, isn't it?" she asked quietly. "I recognize that spot."

"You ought to. We shared a bottle of champagne under that spread of trees on your eighteenth birthday. I nearly had to carry you back to the beach house."

She laughed, remembering her own bubbling pleasure that night, Blake's company and the sound of the surf. They'd talked a lot, she recalled, and waded in the foaming surf, and drunk champagne, while Phillip and Maude visited one of the casinos and lost money.

"It was the best birthday party I ever had," she murmured. "I don't think we had a cross word the whole trip."

"Would you like to do it again?" he asked suddenly.

She turned. He was standing in front of his desk, his legs slightly apart, his hands on his lean hips.

"Now?" she asked.

"Next week. I've got some business in Haiti," he explained mysteriously. "I thought we might stay in St. Martin for a few days and I could go on to Haiti from there."

"Why Haiti?" she asked, curious.

"You don't have to come on that leg of the trip," he said with a finality that permitted no further questioning.

She studied the painting again. "We?" she asked in a bare shadow of her normal voice.

"Vivian and Dick, too," he admitted. "A last-ditch effort to get his cooperation."

"And hers?" she asked with more bitterness than she knew.

There was a long pause. "I thought you knew by now why she came along."

She dropped her eyes to the huge wood frame of the painting, feeling dead inside. So he was finally admitting it. "Yes," she whispered. "I know."

"Do you? I wonder," he murmured, scowling at her downcast face.

"Is anyone else coming?" she asked. "Phillip?"

"Phillip?" he said harshly. His face hardened "What's going on between you two, Kathryn Mary?"

"Nothing," she said defensively. "We just enjoy each other's company, that's all."

Blake's dark eyes seemed to explode in flames. "By all means, we'll take Phillip. You'll have to have someone to play with!" His voice cut.

"I'm not a child, Blake," she said with quiet dignity.

"You're both children."

She squared her slender shoulders. "You didn't treat me like one yesterday!"

A slow, faint smile touched his hard mouth. "You didn't act like one." His bold, slow eyes sketched her body in the becoming suit.

She felt the color creeping into her cheeks at the words, remembering the feel of his warm chest, the hair-roughened texture of it against her breasts.

"Phillip," he scoffed, catching her eyes and holding them. "You'd burn him alive. You're too passionate for him. For Donavan, too."

"Blake!" she burst out, embarrassed.

"Well, it's true," he growled, his eyes narrowing on her face, darkening with memory. "I barely slept last night. I could feel your hands touching me… Your body like silk, twisting against mine. You may be green, little girl, but you've got good instincts. When you finally stop running from passion, you'll be one hell of a woman."

"I'm not running…" she whispered involuntarily before she realized what she was saying.

She stood there watching him, suddenly vulnerable, hungry as she remembered the touch of his hands against her bare skin and the violence of his emotion. She wanted to touch him. To hold him. To feel his mouth against hers… He read that surge of longing accurately. His eyes darkened violently as he rose and came around the desk toward her. There was no pretense between them now; only a thread of shared hunger that was intense and demanding.

"You'd damned well better mean what I read in your eyes," he growled as he reached her, his big hands shooting out to catch her roughly by the waist and pull her close.

She gloried in the feel of his big, muscular body against the length of hers. Her face lifted to his and her heart floundered as her eyes met his from a distance of scant inches. His head started to bend, and she trembled.

His mouth was hungry, and it hurt. She reached up, clinging to him, while his lips parted hers and burrowed into them ardently.

"Blake," she whispered achingly.

His big hand moved up from her waist to cover her breast, taking its slight weight as his tongue shot into the warmth of her mouth.

"You're in my blood like slow poison, Kate," he whispered roughly. His fingers contracted, and he watched the helpless reaction on her flushed face. "I look at you, and all I can think about is how you feel under my hands. Do you remember how it was between us yesterday?" he whispered against her mouth. "Your breasts crushed against me and not a stitch of fabric to stop us from feeling each other's skin…"

"Oh, don't," she moaned helplessly. "It isn't fair..."

"Why isn't it?" he demanded. He lifted her until her eyes were on a level with his. "Tell me you didn't want what I did to you in the gazebo. Tell me you weren't aching every bit as much as I was when I let you go."

She couldn't, because she had wanted him, and it was in every line of her flushed face, in the wide green eyes that searched his helplessly in the silence of the office.

"I'd like to take you to Martinique alone, do you know that?" he breathed huskily. "Just the two of us, Kate, and I'd lay you down in the sand in the darkness and taste every soft, sweet inch of your body with my lips."

Her breath caught at the passionate intensity in the words. "I...I wouldn't..."

"Like hell you wouldn't," he whispered. His mouth took hers hungrily, his hands slid down to grasp her hips and grind them sensuously into his until she cried out at the sensations it caused.

"Want me, Kate?" he taunted in a deep whisper. "God knows, I want you almost beyond bearing. It was a mistake for me to touch you the way I did. Now all I can think about is how much more of you I want. Kiss me, honey. Kiss me..."

She did, because at that moment it was all she wanted from life. The feel of him, the touch and taste and smell of him, Blake's big arms riveting her to every inch of his powerful body while his mouth took everything hers had to give. It seemed like a long time later when he finally raised his head to let his eyes blaze down into hers.

With a suddenness that was almost painful, the door swung open and Vivian's high-pitched voice shattered the crystal thread of emotion binding them.

"Well, hello," she said in her clear British accent. "I do hope I'm not interrupting anything?"

"Of course not," Blake said, turning to her with magnificent composure and a smile. "I promised you a tour, didn't I? Let's go. Kate," he said over his shoulder, "you come along, too."

She was still trembling, and she longed to refuse. But Vivian's eyes were already suspicious, and she didn't dare.

Blake escorted them through the huge manufacturing company, pointing out the main areas of interest—the training room where the new seamstresses were taught how to use the latest modern equipment; the pants line, where each sewing machine operator performed a different function in the manufacture of a pair of slacks; the cutting room, where huge bales of cloth were spread on long tables and cut by men with jigsaws through multiple layers of thickness. Kathryn remembered the terms peculiar to the garment industry from her childhood: "bundle boys" who carried the bundles of pattern pieces out to the sewers; "foreladies" who were the overseers for each group of seamstresses; "spreaders" who spread the cloth; "cutters" who cut it; and "inspectors" who were responsible for catching second- and third-quality garments before they could be shipped out as "firsts." Then there were the pressers and packers and the "lab lady" who washed test garments. Hundreds of sewing machines were running together in the room where the shirt line was located, and this section had button-holing machines as well as the other equipment found on the pants line. Kathryn's eye was caught by the brilliant colors.

"That shade of blue is lovely!" she exclaimed.

Blake chuckled. "I'll have to take you through the yarn mill sometime and show you how it's made. Bales of cotton go through a process that takes a rope of raw material and runs it through a volley of spindles in different rooms to produce a thread of yarn. We use cotton and rayon now. In the old days, the mill ran strictly on cotton."

"How interesting," Vivian said with little enthusiasm. "I've never actually been in a mill."

Kathryn gaped at her. This wasn't *her* first trip by a long shot. She was forever tagging along after Blake and Phillip in her younger days, because the whole process of making clothing had fascinated her. But she hadn't been in a yarn mill since her childhood, and she'd been too young to understand much of what she'd seen then.

"How many blouses come out of here in a week?" Kathryn asked, watching blouses in different states of readiness at each machine row as they walked past. She had to practically yell in Blake's ear to make him hear her above the noise.

"About ten thousand dozen," he told her, smiling at her shocked expression. "We've added a lot of new equipment here. We have over six hundred sewing machine operators in this plant, and it takes about a hundred and fifty thousand yards of material a week to keep these women busy."

Kathryn looked back the way they'd come. "The slacks…?"

"That's a separate plant, honey," he reminded her, glancing toward the door that linked the two divisions. "We only have about three hundred machines on the pants line. Our biggest business here is blouses."

"It's enormous!" she exclaimed.

Blake nodded. "We do a volume business. We have contracts with two of the biggest mail-order houses, and you'll remember that we have our own chain of outlet stores across the country. It's a hell of a big operation."

"It must make lots of money," Vivian commented, and Kathryn saw dollar signs in the older woman's eyes.

Blake's eyebrow jerked, but he didn't reply.

When they finished the tour, Vivian persuaded Blake to take her out for coffee, and he left Kate with a dictaphone full of letters to be typed. It rankled her that Vivian, who had gotten her breakfast at home, was being treated to coffee and doughnuts while Kathryn, who had been dragged away from her breakfast, got nothing. She was somewhat mollified a half hour later when Blake came back and set coffee in a styrofoam cup and a packaged pastry in front of her on the desk.

"Breakfast," he said. "I seem to recall making you miss yours."

She smiled up at him, surprised and pleased, and her face lit up.

"Thanks, Blake," she said gently.

He shrugged his powerful shoulders and strode over to the dividing door between her office and his. "Any problems with the dictaphone?" he asked over his shoulder.

"Only with your language," she remarked, tongue-in-cheek.

He lifted an amused eyebrow at her. "Don't expect to reform me, Kate."

"Oh, I don't know a woman brave enough to try, Blake," she said with angelic sweetness to his retreating back. Switching off the electric typewriter, she opened her steaming coffee.

It was almost quitting time when Phillip stopped by the office to see Blake. He leaned his hands on Kathryn's desk and grinned at her.

"Slaving away, I see," he teased lightly.

She sighed. "You don't know the half of it," she groaned. "I never realized how much correspondence it takes to keep a plant like this one going. Blake even writes to congressmen and state senators and the textile manufacturers association—by the way, I didn't realize he was president of it this year."

"See how much you're learning?" Phillip teased. He reached out a hand and tipped her chin up, bending close to whisper, "Has Blake flicked you with his whip yet?"

Her eyes opened wide and she smiled. "Does he have one?" she whispered back.

It was pure bad luck that Blake should choose that moment to open his office door. He glared at Phillip so blackly that the younger man backed away from the desk and actually reddened.

Blake jerked his office door shut. "Take Kathryn home with you," he told his brother curtly. "Vivian and I are going out to supper."

And he left the office without even a backward glance, while Kathryn sat there with her heart in her shoes, wondering how Blake could have been so loving earlier in the day and so hateful now. What had she done? Or was it just that Blake was already feeling regrets?

The days fell into a pattern. Kathryn rode to work with Blake every morning, and back with him in the evenings. Although he was business-as-usual in his dealings with her, Vivian seemed to purple when Kathryn and Blake left together. The blonde did everything except lobby for a job of her own to try to take up Blake's free time. And she succeeded very well.

By Saturday, Kathryn was ready for some relaxation, and since Vivian had talked Blake into taking her by plane for a shopping trip to Atlanta, Kathryn asked Phillip to go with her to one of the new malls in town. The request seemed to irritate Blake, but Kathryn ignored his evident displeasure. After all, what right did he have to interfere with her life? He was too wrapped up in Vivian to care what she did. Even the thought of going to the islands with him was frightening now—although she knew she'd never be strong enough to renege on her promise to accompany him. She loved him too much, wanted to be with him too much, to refuse. He might marry Vivian, but at least Kathryn would have a few memories to tuck away.

"You're walking me to death," Phillip groaned, hobbling with exaggeration to the nearest bench in the busy mall. He eased down with a stage sigh and smile.

"We've only been in five shops," she reminded him. "You can't possibly be tired."

"Five shops, where you tried on fifteen outfits each," he corrected.

She plopped down beside him, sighing wearily. "Well, I'm depressed," she said. "I had to do something to cheer me up."

"I'm not depressed," he said with a sigh. "Why did I have to come along?"

"To carry the packages," she said sensibly.

"But, Kathryn, love, you haven't bought anything."

"Yes, I have. In that little boutique we just came from."

His eyebrows lifted. "What?"

"This." She handed him a small sack containing a jeweler's box with a pair of dainty sapphire and diamond earrings inside. "Aren't they lovely? I charged them to Blake."

"Oh, no," he groaned, burying his face in his hands.

"Anyway, you can carry them," she said, "so you'll feel necessary."

"How will I ever survive all these honors you confer upon me?" he asked with mock humility.

"Don't be nasty," she chided, pushing against his shoulder with her own as they sat side by side. "I really am depressed, Phil."

He studied her dejected little face. "What's wrong, kitten? Want me to slay a dragon for you?"

"Would you?" she asked hopefully, her green eyes wide. "You could sneak up on her while she's sleeping, and…"

"Your eyes need checking," he remarked, lifting an eyebrow at her as he folded his arms and leaned back against the wooden bench. "Vivian isn't a dragon."

"That's what you think," she muttered. "Wait until she's your sister-in-law and see if you still like her."

"Vivian? Marry Blake?" He sat up abruptly, staggered. "Where did you come by that piece of utter nonsense?"

"It isn't nonsense," she told him, sulking. "She's just his style. Beautiful, sophisticated and blond."

"That's his taste, all right. But do you really think he's got marriage on his mind?" he asked with a wry grin. "That *isn't* his style."

"Maybe she's something special," she grumbled, hating everything about the woman. She glared into space, hurting in ways she never had before. "She told me that Blake wanted her over here to meet us."

"I know. She's the power behind her father. She controls everything he does, or haven't you noticed her ordering him around?"

She shifted on the bench and crossed her legs. "Blake spends all his time with her. Don't tell me it's just for business reasons," she replied, smoothing the close-fitting designer jeans over her thighs. Her eyes dropped to her cream-colored cowboy boots and she grimaced at a scuff on the toe.

"You and I spend a lot of time together, too," he reminded her. "But we're just friends."

She sighed. "That's true."

"And Blake hates it."

Her eyes jerked up. "What?"

He grinned. "He's jealous," he laughed.

She went cherry pink and averted her gaze. "You're nuts!"

"Am I? He's crazily possessive about you. He always has been, but in the past few days I'm almost afraid to sit beside you when he's at home."

She felt her heart racing at the words. She hoped against hope that they were true, even while she knew they weren't. "He's just the domineering type," she corrected nervously.

"Really? Is that why he deliberately picked a fight with your boyfriend to send him packing?" Phillip eyed her narrowly. "When we got home from Charleston, Blake was gone and you were hiding in your room with a headache. What happened between you two while we were gone?"

The blush went all the way to her toes. She couldn't answer him.

"You light up when he walks into a room," he continued, smiling. "And he watches you when he thinks no one's noticing. Like a big, hungry panther with its eyes on a tasty young gazelle."

She hadn't known that, and her heart went wild. "Oh, Phil, does he, really?" she asked involuntarily, and everything she felt was in the starved look in the soft eyes she lifted to his.

He nodded quietly, studying her. "That's just what I thought," he said gently. "Adding your heart to the string he drags behind him, kitten?"

"Is it so obvious?" she sighed miserably. She turned her attention to the passersby.

"To me, because we've always been close," he replied. "I knew why you bought that sexy dress even before you did. You wanted to see what effect it would have on Blake. Dynamite, wasn't it, girl?" he asked knowingly, with a teasing smile.

She flushed wildly. "Do you hide behind the curtains?" she whispered, embarrassed by his perception.

"I'm not in my adolescence, Kate," he reminded her. "You and Blake have always been passionate with each other. You push him hard—it isn't hard to guess at the reaction you get. Blake's not a gentle man."

How little he knew his brother, she thought, her mind going back longingly to that lazy morning in the gazebo…

"Or is he?" he whispered, reading her dreamy expression.

She glared at him. "Don't pry."

"I'm not trying to mind your business," he said gently. "But I don't want to see you end up the loser.

Blake's a very experienced man. He may be tempted by a bud about to blossom, but he's shy of nets. Don't try to cut your teeth on him. You might as well try to build a fence around the wind."

"What you really mean is that I can't compete with Her Ladyship," she threw at him.

"That's exactly what I mean," he said with gentle compassion. He patted her hand where it lay on the wood bench. "Kathryn, an experienced woman can attract a man in ways that an inexperienced one wouldn't even think of. I don't want to see you hurt. But you must know you're no competition for Vivian."

"Who said I was trying to be?" she asked. Her face shuttered. "You make Blake sound like a..."

"Blake is my brother," he reminded her. "And I'd do anything for him. But he's just noticed what a delicious little thing you've grown into, and he's lost his bearings. It won't take him long to find them, but that tiny space of time could be enough to destroy you." He squeezed her hand and grimaced. "Love him as a brother. But not as a man. I don't have to tell you how Blake feels about love."

She felt the life draining out of her. Her shoulders slumped, and she nodded weakly. "He doesn't believe in it," she whispered shakily.

"Blake wants one thing from a woman," he said. "And he can't have it from you."

She smiled wistfully. "He wouldn't take it even if I offered," she said quietly, darting a look at him.

"Not deliberately," he agreed. "But you could make

him forget every scruple he has, little one. Or didn't you know that men are particularly vulnerable to women they want?"

She sighed softly. "And Blake being Blake, he'd marry me, wouldn't he? Even though he hated the idea of it, and me, he'd do the honorable thing."

"That's exactly what I mean." He held her hand gently. "Nothing would make me happier than to see you happily married to my brother. But I know Blake too well, and so do you. He's too much a cynic to change overnight."

"You don't think he could…care for a woman?" she asked haltingly.

He shrugged. "Blake is a private man. I've lived with him all my life, but there are depths to him that I've never been allowed to explore. Perhaps he's capable of love. But I think in a way he's afraid of it. He's afraid of being vulnerable." He glanced at her with a dry smile. "He may marry eventually to provide Greyoaks with an heir. He may even fall in love. I don't know."

"You said he was possessive of me," she reminded him.

"Naturally, he's taken care of you half your life," he said. "But what he really feels, no one knows."

She bit her lower lip and nodded, turning away to stare at the pavement. "You're right, of course." She forced a smile to her frozen face. "Let's go get an ice-cream cone."

He caught her arm gently and kept her from getting up. "I'm sorry," he said suddenly. "I didn't mean to hurt you."

"What makes you think you have?" she asked with a smile that was too bright.

"You're in love with him."

She felt her face go white. She was only just beginning to admit that to herself. But, confronted with the accusation, she found she couldn't deny it. Her mouth tried to form words, but her tongue wouldn't cooperate.

He read the confusion in her face and stood up. "Ice cream. Right. What flavor would you like, Kathy... vanilla or strawberry?"

It was only two days until Blake planned to fly them to St. Martin. The pace at the office was hectic. Kathryn took dictation until her fingers felt numb, and Blake's temper, always formidable, seemed to be on a permanent hair trigger.

"You know damned well I don't use my middle initial in a signature," he growled at her, slamming the letters she'd just typed down on his desk violently. "Do them over!"

"If you don't like the way I do things," she complained tightly, "why don't you let Vivian come in and work for you?"

"She'd have been in tears by now," he admitted, with a faintly amused smile.

She straightened in the chair beside his desk, crossing her slender legs impatiently in the gray skirt that matched her silk blouse. "Afraid you might tarnish your shining armor?" she asked.

He studied her through a veil of smoke from his cigarette, his dark eyes thoughtful. "There isn't much danger of that happening with you, is there, Kate?" he asked quietly. "You know just about everything there is to know about me, my faults, my habits."

"Do I really know you at all, Blake?" she wondered absently. "Sometimes you seem very much a stranger."

He lifted his cigarette to his mouth. "Like that day in the gazebo, Kate?" he asked softly, watching the burst of color that shot into her face.

Her eyes darted back to her pad, and her heart ran away. "I don't know what you want from me anymore, Blake."

He got up and moved in front of her, leaning down to catch her chin in his big hand and lift her face up to his piercing gaze. "Maybe that works both ways," he said gruffly. "You're very young, Kathryn Mary."

"Oh, yes, compared to you, I'm a mere child," she returned.

"Little spitting kitten," he chided. Something wild and dangerous smoldered in his eyes. "Would you hiss and claw if I made love to you, Kathryn, or would you purr?"

She caught her breath sharply. "Neither!"

His eyes glittered down at her. "You don't think I could teach you to purr, Kate? Your mouth was wild under mine that day. I can still taste it, even now."

"I...didn't know what I was doing," she whispered weakly, embarrassed at the memory of her abandoned response.

"Neither did I, really," he murmured absently, watching her mouth with a disturbingly intense scrutiny. "I touched you and every sane thought went out of my head. All I wanted to do was make love to you until I stopped aching."

She caught her breath, meeting his eyes squarely. It was like the impact of lightning striking. It had been that way for her, too, but all he was admitting to was a purely physical attraction—just as Phillip had warned her. He'd lost his head out of desire, not love.

"Doesn't Vivian make you ache?" she asked in a tight voice, hurting with the certainty that what she felt for him was hopeless.

He searched her eyes quietly. "Not that way."

She dropped her gaze to her lap. "You can always find a woman, Blake," she choked.

He leaned down, placing his hands on either side of her against the chair arms, the curling smoke from his cigarette pungent in her nostrils.

"Not one like you, honey," he growled. "Or are you going to try to convince me that you've ever let another man touch you the way I did?"

She felt the heat creeping up from her throat, and her eyes riveted themselves to his tie, remembering the feel of his hands on her bare back, slightly rough, expertly caressing.

"You were afraid, because it was the first time. But if I'd insisted on making love to you, you wouldn't have stopped me. We both know that."

She felt the embarrassment, like a living thing, and she hated him for what he could do to her with words.

He made her vulnerable. She'd never been vulnerable to any man before, it was new and disconcerting, and to cover her fear she sought refuge in temper.

"You flatter yourself, don't you?" she asked crisply, raising her sparkling eyes to his. "Maybe I was experimenting, Blake, did you think about that?" She watched the darkness grow in his eyes. "What makes you think I don't feel exactly that way with other men?"

"What other men?" he shot at her. "Phillip?"

She tore her eyes away and stared down at her pad blankly. There was suppressed fury in his voice, and she knew better than to deliberately goad him. If he touched her, she'd go crazy. It was her basic reaction to that vibrant masculinity that rippled in every hard muscle of his body. She was too vulnerable now, and the only way to keep him from seeing it was to make sure she kept him at arm's length.

"We'd better get this work out of the way," he said coolly, and sat down behind his desk again, idly crushing out his cigarette. "How about that shipment of polycotton we never received from our Georgia mill?" he asked quietly. "Check with the office there and find out if it was shipped. The spreaders will need it for the next cut."

"Yes, sir," she replied in her best businesslike tone. "Anything else?"

"Yes," he said gruffly, watching her. "Send a dozen red roses to Vivian at the house."

That hit her like a ton of bricks, but she didn't even flinch. Methodically, she made a note on her pad and nodded. "One dozen. I'll call the florist right away. How would you like the card to read?"

He was still eyeing her. "Have them put, 'Thanks for last night' and sign it 'Blake.' Got that?"

"Got it," she replied. Her voice sounded vaguely strangled, but she kept the expression out of her face. "Anything else?"

He swiveled his chair around to stare out the window. "No."

She went out and closed the door quietly behind her. Tears were welling in her eyes by the time she got back to her own desk.

Chapter Eight

"Just imagine, a week in St. Martin," Maude sighed, studying the list of chores she'd outlined for Mrs. Johnson and the daily maids while the family was away. "How sweet of Blake to take us all with him, especially when he's getting along so well with Vivian!"

"Oh, it's delightful," Kathryn agreed dully.

"They've hardly been apart at all," she sighed. "And they do make such a striking pair, Blake so dark and Vivian so fair.... I think he's really serious this time." She clasped her slender hands together and beamed. "I'd love to plan a spring wedding. We could decorate the house with orchids..."

"Excuse me, Maude, but I really have to start getting my things together," Kathryn said brightly, rising from the sofa. "You don't mind?"

Maude was deep in her plans. "No, dear, go right ahead," she mumbled absently.

Kathryn went up the winding staircase, feeling dead inside. As she passed by Vivian's room, her eye was caught by the vase full of red roses sitting on the dresser in full view of the open door. Vivian had done that deliberately, no doubt, and Kathryn felt as if she'd been shot. At least Blake hadn't suspected how she felt about him. That would have been unbearable, especially since he was taking such a sudden and intense interest in the seductive blonde. They were going nightclubbing together, later that evening, and they'd been locked up in Blake's study ever since dinner. As had happened so many times since her return to Greyoaks, Kathryn sought out Phillip for companionship. And that seemed to catch Blake's attention in the most violent way.

The following morning he found Phillip sitting on her desk and he seemed to erupt.

"Don't you have anything to do, Phillip?" he growled at his younger brother.

"Why, yes, I do," Phillip replied.

"Then why the hell don't you go and do it?" came the terse, irritable question.

Phillip stood erect, his hands in his pockets, and studied the bigger, older man quietly, frowning. "I was asking Kate to take in a movie with me tonight," he said. "Any objections?"

Blake's jaw tautened. "Make your dates at home. Not on my time."

"I do have an interest in the corporation," Phillip reminded him. "Just like all the other stockholders."

"Try acting like it," Blake said coldly. His eyes darted to Kathryn. "Bring your pad. I've got some letters to dictate." He went back into his office and roughly closed the door.

Phillip stared after him, not taking offense at all. He knew Blake too well. A slow smile flared on his lips. "Now, in a lesser man, I'd swear that was jealousy," he teased, eyeing Kathryn.

She stood up with a sigh, clutching her steno pad to her chest. "But not in a man with someone like Vivian practically engaged to him," she reminded him. "We'd better get to work before he gives us a pink slip."

He shrugged. "With the temper he's been in lately, I'm not sure it wouldn't be a relief."

"Speaking of relief," she said, lowering her voice, "you promised to help me look for an apartment."

"Not until we get back from St. Martin," he said stubbornly. "And only then if Blake's temper improves. I don't have a suicidal bone in my body, Kate, and I'm not taking on Blake for you."

She sighed. "You won't have to," she said bitterly. "He'll be glad to see me go now, and you know it."

He studied her. "Will he, really?" he murmured.

"Kathryn!" Blake thundered over the intercom.

She flinched and hurried into his office.

He was sitting behind his desk, leaning back in his chair, and he glared at her when she walked in.

"From now on, don't encourage Phillip to waste time

talking to you during working hours," he said without preamble, his eyes blazing. "I don't pay either of you to socialize."

She stared at him belligerently. "Do I have to have your permission to say good morning to him now?" she wanted to know.

"In this building, yes," he replied curtly. His dark eyes held hers fiercely. "You practically live in each other's pockets already. I shouldn't think it would work a hardship for you to spend just eight hours away from him!"

He whipped his chair forward and grabbed up a letter, his leonine face as hard as the oak desk under his powerful hands. She remembered without wanting to the warmth and tenderness of those hard fingers on her bare skin…

"Are you ready?" he asked curtly.

She sat down quickly, positioning her pad on her lap. "Any time you are," she said in her most professional tone.

For the rest of the day, Kathryn and Blake maintained a cool politeness between them that raised eyebrows among the staff. There had been numerous arguments, ever since Kathryn's appointment as his secretary, but this was different. Now they were avoiding each other completely. They didn't argue, because there was no contact between them.

"I say, have you and Blake had a falling out?" Vivian asked Kathryn that evening as she waited for Blake to change for their dinner date. "You've hardly spoken to each other for the past couple of days."

Kathryn, curled up on the sofa in her ivory-colored jumpsuit with a book, glanced at the older woman coolly. The blue Qiana dress the actress was wearing left nothing to the imagination, and even Kathryn had to admit it flattered her figure, her lovely face, and her elegantly coiffured blond hair. Just Blake's style, she thought bitterly.

"Not at all," Kathryn replied finally. "Blake and I were never close," she lied, remembering happier times when there was never a cross word between them, and Blake's eyes were tender.

"Oh, really?" Vivian probed. She smiled a little haughtily, primping at a mirror on the wall between two elegant bronze sconces. "I do hope you and I will get on together. Living in the same house, you know..." She let her voice trail away insinuatingly.

"Have you set a date?" Kathryn asked with careful unconcern.

"Not quite," the blonde replied. "But it won't be long."

"I'm delighted for both of you," she murmured as she stared blankly at her book.

"Are you ready, darling?" Vivian gushed as Blake came into the room. "I'm simply famished!"

"Let's go, then," he replied with a sensuous note in his voice that Kathryn didn't miss. But she didn't raise her eyes from the book, didn't look at him or speak to him. She felt dead, frozen. It wasn't until the door slammed behind them that she was able to relax. How fortunate, she thought, that Dick Leeds and Maude had also gone out for the night, and that she'd convinced Phillip to go to the movies alone. There was no one to watch her cry. Now, for certain, she'd have to leave Greyoaks. There was no way she could live in it with Vivian.

The following day dawned bright and sunny, perfect for their flight to St. Martin. Kathryn and Phillip were bringing up the rear. Vivian, in a stunning white lace pantsuit, was clinging to Blake's arm like ivy while Dick Leeds and Maude followed along deep in conversation. Kathryn was wearing a simple peasant dress in green and brown patterns that brought out the deep green of her eyes and set off her long, waving dark hair. She was dressed for comfort, not for style, and she knew she was no competition for the blonde. She wasn't trying to be. She'd lost Blake, even though she'd never really had a chance to win him. There were too many years between them.

"You're tearing at my heart," Phillip said quietly, watching her as she watched Blake and Vivian.

She lifted her sad eyes to his. "Why?"

"I've never seen a woman love a man the way you love Blake," he replied quietly, with none of his usual gaiety.

She lifted her shoulders in a careless gesture. "I'll get over it," she murmured. "It…it's just going to take a little time, that's all. I'll land on my feet, Phil."

He caught her hand and held it gently as they walked toward the small jet owned by the corporation. "I honestly thought it was infatuation, at first," he admitted gently. "But I'm beginning to realize just how wrong I was. You'd do anything for him, wouldn't you? Even stand aside and watch him marry another woman, as long as he was happy."

Her long eyelashes curled down onto her cheeks. "Isn't that what love is all about?" she asked in a soft whisper. "I want him to be happy." Her eyes closed briefly. "I want everything for him."

He squeezed her hand. "Stiff upper lip, darling," he said under his breath. "Don't let him see you suffer."

She forced a laugh through her tight throat. "Oh, of course not," she said brightly. "We revolutionaries are very tough, you know."

"That's my girl. But why are you giving up the battle so soon?"

"Who said I was giving up?" she asked, glancing at him. "I've got the job I wanted, but not the apartment. Just wait until we come back!"

He chuckled. "That's my girl. I knew you could work it out."

"Of course we can," she said with a gleeful smile.

"We?" he asked, apprehensive.

"You know lots of people in real estate," she reminded him. "I'm sure you can find me something I can afford. In a good neighborhood."

"Now, just a minute, Kathy..."

But she was already boarding the plane.

* * *

The executive jet was roomy and comfortable, and as long as Kathryn didn't look out the window of the pressurized cabin, she was fine. She'd never gotten over the bouts with airsickness that were a carryover from her childhood, despite Blake's expert handling of the airplane.

Vivian was sitting in the co-pilot's seat, for which Kathryn was eternally grateful. She couldn't have borne her haughty company, her gloating smile.

"You look very pale, dear," Maude said sympathetically, reaching out to pat Kathryn's cold hand. "How about an airsick pill?"

"I've already had two," came the subdued reply. "All they do is make me dizzy."

"A spot of brandy might help," Dick Leeds suggested gently, as he appeared briefly beside her.

She shook her head, feeling even more nauseated. "I'll be all right," she assured them.

"Lie down for a while," Phillip said as the older passengers moved away. "Take off your shoes and just sleep," he coaxed, helping her stretch out in one of the plush, comfortable seats. "We'll be there before you know it."

They landed at Queen Juliana airport on Sint Maarten—the Dutch side of the divided island. As they stepped out onto the ground, the first thing Kathryn noticed was the hot, moist air that enveloped her. She stared at the blue skies and palm trees and the flags flying proudly at the terminal. She remembered the island with pleasure, as she had stayed many times at the family's villa.

A customs official took their immigration cards, and their passports, with a minimum of fuss. Blake obtained a rental car, and they were on their way.

"Where is your house?" Vivian asked, staring out at the red-roofed homes they passed as they drove along the paved road.

"On St. Martin," Blake replied as he drove. "The French side of the island, which is, by the way, very French. The Dutch side, which we're in now, tends to be more Americanized."

"It's confusing," Vivian laughed.

"Not really," Maude told her. "One gets used to it. The division is political as well as lingual, but the people are delightful on both sides of the island. And you'll love the shops in Marigot—that's very near our villa."

"And the restaurants," Phillip grinned. "You've never had better seafood."

"What do you like about it, darling?" Vivian asked Blake.

"The peace and quiet," he replied.

"Which you don't find much of during peak tourist season," Phillip laughed.

"Well, this is hurricane season, not tourist season," Maude said, shivering at the thought. "I do hope we don't run into any rough weather."

"Amen," Blake said with a faint smile. "I've got to fly over to Haiti on business while we're here."

"What for?" Vivian asked with blunt curiosity.

Blake gave her a lazy sidelong look. "I might have a woman stashed away there," he said.

It was the first time Kathryn had ever seen Vivian blush, and she made a good job of it. Her pale face turned a bright pink. "Oh, look, cattle!" she said quickly, gazing out the window toward a green meadow nestled between mountains.

Blake only chuckled, concentrating on the road as they passed from the Dutch side of the island to the French.

Maude jumped as they hit a pothole. "Oh, you can always tell when we pass into St. Martin," she moaned. "The roads over here are just terrible!"

"Just like home, isn't it?" Phillip asked, winking at Kathryn.

"I think we have very good roads at home, Phillip," Maude said, "an excellent county commission and a superb road department. Remember, darling, I helped Jeff Brown get appointed to the state highway board, and I think he's done a fine job."

"Forgive me for that unthinking comment," Phillip pleaded. "Heaven forbid that I should sully the name..."

"Oh, do be quiet," Maude moaned. "Vivian, here's Marigot," she said, pointing out the window toward the bay where fishing boats dotted the Baie de Marigot past the powdery beach. There were red-roofed houses stretching all the way down the beach, thick in places, mingling with hotels. Kathryn felt a shiver of girlish excitement as they stopped at one of them minutes later. It was Maison Baie—roughly, Bay House—and her eyes lovingly traced the white stone building with its graceful wrought-iron balconies and breezeways and long windows. It, too, had the classic red roof, and carved wood doors.

"Is this yours?" Vivian asked, her eyes also taking in the graceful lines of the house and its colorful setting with palm trees, bougainvillea, and sea-grape trees farther out on the powder-fine sand.

"Yes," Blake replied, cutting the engine. "Maison Baie. It's been in the family since my father was a boy, and the second generation of caretakers—a retired sea captain named Rouget and his wife—live here year round, looking after it."

"It's very pretty," Vivian said enthusiastically.

Kathryn stayed beside Phillip, feeling the coolness of the house wash over her as they walked inside. Rouget, a tall, thin man with white hair, came to meet them, welcoming them in his native French. Blake replied, his accent faultless, and Kathryn had to work to keep up with the translation. She'd forgotten just how French this side of the island really was. Her rusty attempts to speak the language had always amused Blake. Glancing at him, she wondered if anything she did would ever amuse him again.

The look on her young face was revealing, and Phillip drew her away before Blake could see it. She smiled at him gratefully as they left the spacious living room to settle into their respective rooms. Already she was hoping the visit would be a brief one.

* * *

That afternoon Vivian persuaded Blake to take her back to Marigot to look in the shops. Maude and Dick Leeds, deciding that the sun was a bit much, lounged on the balcony with chilled burgundy provided by Rouget. Kathryn spent the rest of the day lying quietly in bed, feeling out of sorts. The combination of the flight and the sultry, tropical climate had put her flat on her back. When night came, she was barely aware of Maude's fingers gently shaking her.

"Darling, we're going into Marigot to have seafood. Do you feel like coming with us?" she asked.

Kathryn sat up, surprised to find that the nausea and weariness were completely gone. "Of course," she said, smiling. "Just give me a minute to change..."

"What's wrong with what you have on?" Blake asked from the doorway, and she felt his dark eyes sliding up and down her slender body in the peasant dress that had ridden up above her knees while she rested. She pulled it down quickly and, smoothing it nervously, got to her feet.

"I...I suppose it would do, if we're not going anywhere fancy."

"The restaurant isn't formal, Kathryn," he said, moving inside the room. "Still queasy?" he added gently.

That soft note in his voice almost brought tears to her eyes. She turned away to pick up her brush. "No," she replied. "I'm all right. Just let me run a brush through my hair."

"Don't be long," Maude teased. "I feel as if I haven't eaten for days."

Kathryn nodded, expecting Blake to go, too. But he didn't. He closed the door quietly, an action that made Kathryn's heart go wild. She watched him in the mirror.

He moved up behind her, his dark eyes holding hers in the glass, so close that she could feel the blazing warmth of his big body. He was dressed in a red and white patterned tropical shirt, open at the throat, revealing a sensuous glimpse of curling dark hair and bronzed flesh. His slacks were white, hugging the powerful lines of his thighs. She could hardly drag her eyes away from him.

"Do you really feel up to this?" he asked quietly. "If you don't, I'll stay home with you."

The concern in his deep voice would have been heaven, if it had been meant differently. But it was the compassion of a man for a child, not of a man for his woman.

"I always get airsick," she reminded him dully. "I'm all right, Blake."

"Are you?" he asked tightly. "The light's gone out of you."

"It's been…a long week," she whispered unsteadily.

He nodded, dropping his narrow gaze to her long hair, her shoulders. His big hands went to her waist, testing the softness of her flesh through the thin dress, rough and vaguely caressing.

"I…I think we all needed a vacation," she laughed

nervously. The feel of his hands made her heart turn over in her chest.

"Yes." He drew her slowly back against his big, hard-muscled body, so that she could feel his breath against her hair. "You're trembling," he said in a deep, lazy tone.

Her eyes closed. Her hands went involuntarily to rest on top of his as he slid them closer around her waist. "I know," she managed weakly.

His fingers contracted painfully. "Kate..."

She couldn't help herself. Her head dropped back against his broad chest and her body openly yielded to him. In the mirror, she watched his dark, broad hands move slowly, seductively up her waist until they cupped her high breasts over the green and brown pattern of the low-cut peasant dress. She let him touch her, helpless in his embrace, the hardness of his thighs pressing into the back of her legs as he moved even closer.

His dark eyes held hers in the mirror, watching her reaction. His cheek brushed against the top of her head, ruffling the soft dark hair while his fingers brushed and stroked, the action even more erotic because she could watch it happening.

Her fingers came up to rest on top of his, pressing them closer to the soft curves, while her heart threatened to choke her with its furious thudding.

His face moved down and she felt the heat of his lips at the side of her neck brushing, teasing, his tongue lightly tracing the line of it down to her shoulder.

"You smell of flowers," he whispered. His hands

moved up and under the low neckline to surge down and capture her taut, bare breasts.

She moaned helplessly and bit her lip to stifle the sound that must surely have passed even through the thick stone walls of the house.

"I wish to God we were alone, Kate," he whispered huskily. "I'd lie down with you on that bed over there and before I was through, you'd be biting back more than one sweet moan. You'd be biting me," he whispered seductively, while his hands made magic on her arching body. "Clawing me, begging me to do more than touch your breasts."

"Blake..." she moaned, with a throb in her voice that broke the sound in the middle of his name.

She whirled in his arms, rising against his big body, her arms going around his neck, her lips parted and pleading.

"Kiss me," she whispered, trembling. "Blake, Blake, kiss me hard...!"

"How hard?" he whispered huskily as he bent. His mouth bit at hers sensuously, lightly bruising, open, taunting. "Like that?"

"No," she whispered. She went on tiptoe, her green eyes misty with mindless hunger, her lips parted as she caught his head and brought his open mouth down on hers. Her tongue darted into his mouth and she withdrew tauntingly just a half-breath away. "Like that..."

His mouth crushed hers, his tongue exploring the line of her lips, thrusting past them in to the warm darkness of her mouth, his arms contracting so strongly that they brought the length of her body close enough to feel every hardening line of his.

"Do you…want me?" she whispered achingly.

"God in heaven, can't you feel it?" he ground out. "Stop asking silly questions…closer, Kate," he whispered. "Move your body against mine. Stroke it against me…"

She eased up on tiptoe. "Like this, Blake?" she whispered shakily.

His mouth bit at hers. "Harder than that," he murmured. "I can't feel you."

Trembling, she repeated the arousing action and felt a small shudder go through his powerful body. "Do you like this?" she managed in a stranger's seductive voice.

"Let me show you how much I like it," he whispered. He bent and lifted her off the floor, looking down into her green eyes as he started toward the huge mahogany posted bed against the wall.

Her arms clung to him, her lips answering the suddenly tender kisses he was brushing against her lips, her eyelids, her eyebrows, her cheeks. The chaste touch of his mouth was at odds with the heavy, hard shudder of his heartbeat against her body, the harsh sigh of his breath that betrayed the emotions he was experiencing.

"Are you going to make love to me?" she whispered against his lips, knowing in her heart even as she asked the question that she was going to give him everything he wanted.

"Do you want me to, Kate?" he whispered back. "Are you afraid?"

"How could I be afraid of you?" she managed in a

tight voice. "When I..." Before she could get the confession out, before she could tell him how desperately she loved him, there was a sharp, harsh knock on the door, and he jerked involuntarily.

Vivian's abrasive voice called, "Blake, are you there? We're starving!"

"My God, so am I," he whispered, and the eyes that met Kathryn's as he set her back on her feet were blazing with unsatisfied desire.

She moved unsteadily away from him, her heart jerking wildly, her breath coming in uneven little gasps. She went back to the mirror and picked up a lipstick, applying it to her swollen mouth while Blake took a steadying breath and went to answer the door.

"I'm so hungry, darling," Vivian murmured with a smile, her hawklike eyes catching the slight swell of his lower lip, the unruly hair that Kathryn's fingers had tangled lightly. "Can't we go to dinner now that you're through talking to sweet little Kate?"

"I'm hungry myself," Kathryn said, avoiding Blake's eyes as she edged out the door past him, managed a tight smile in Vivian's direction, and almost ran from the room. What in heaven's name had possessed her to allow Blake such liberties? Now the fat was really going to be in the fire. She had let him know how desperately she wanted him, and she was afraid that he'd take advantage of it. What Phillip had said was true—Blake could lose his head. If he did, he'd be gentleman enough to marry her. But she didn't want Blake on those terms. She only wanted his love, not a forced marriage. What was she going to do?

* * *

The little French restaurant was as familiar to Kathryn as Maison Baie, and she remembered the owners well—a French couple from Martinique who served the most delicious lobster soufflé and crêpes flambées Kathryn had ever tasted. Her appetite came back the instant she saw the food, and Phillip's pleasant company at her elbow made it even more palatable.

She avoided Blake's piercing gaze all through the meal and when they got back to the house, she quickly excused herself and went to bed.

That night set the pattern for the next two days. Blake wore a perpetual scowl at Kathryn's nervous avoidance of him, and Phillip's efforts to play peacemaker met with violence on Blake's part. He stayed away during the day with Vivian, taking her on tours of nearby Saba and St. Eustatius—known to the locals as "Statia." But in the evenings he and the slinky blonde stayed close to home while he discussed the mill problem with Dick Leeds. It was at the end of one of these endless discussions that Kathryn accidentally came across him in the deserted hall upstairs.

His dark eyes narrowed angrily as she froze in front of him, on her way to change for supper in Marigot.

"Still running away from me?" he asked scathingly.

"I'm not running," she replied unsteadily.

"Like hell you're not," he returned gruffly. "You practically dive under things to keep out of my way lately. What's wrong, Kathryn, do you think you're so damned irresistible that I can't keep my hands off you?"

"Of course not!" she gasped.

"Then why go to so much trouble to avoid me?" he persisted.

She drew a slow, steady breath. "Phillip and I have been busy, that's all," she managed.

His face tightened. A cold, cruel smile touched his hard mouth. "Busy? So you finally decided to taste the wine, did you, honey?" His voice drew blood. "It's just as well. You're too much of a baby for me, Kathryn. I hate like hell to rob cradles!"

He turned on his heel and left her standing there.

She couldn't bear for Blake to think that about her, to look at her with eyes so full of contempt they made her shiver. But what could she do? The impact of his anger made her reckless and when the delicious white wine was passed around at the restaurant that night, she had more than her share of refills. Throwing caution to the wind, she sipped and swallowed until all her heartaches seemed to vanish. When Blake announced that he was flying to Haiti the next morning, she barely heard him. Her mind was far away, on pleasant thoughts.

"Honey, you're drunk," Phillip said with some concern when they got back to the villa. "Go to bed and sleep it off, huh?"

She smiled at him lazily. "I'm not sleepy."

"Pretend, before you give Vivian something else to laugh about," he asked softly. "And don't push Blake's temper any further tonight. I'm surprised he hasn't lectured you about the amount of wine you drank. He didn't like it, that's for sure."

"Be a pet and stop preaching," she murmured, fanning herself with one hand. "It's so hot!"

"Feels like storm weather," he agreed. "Go to bed. You'll cool off."

She shrugged and, to Phillip's quiet relief, went up to her room before the others came inside the house.

Chapter Nine

But once she got into bed, she was only hotter. It was too sultry, too quiet, and her thoughts began to haunt her. Blake's harsh words came back like a persistent mosquito—too much of a baby, he said. *Too much of a baby.*

She tossed and turned until it became unbearable. Finally she got up, put on her brief white bikini and grabbed up a beach towel. If she couldn't sleep, she might as well cool off in the bay. Just the thought of the cold water made her feel better.

She made her way downstairs in the dark house with the ease of long practice, and walked a little unsteadily out onto the beach. Her bare feet smarted on the grainy pebbles until she reached the softer sand where the foaming surf curled lazily. The air was static, the beach completely deserted. She stood and breathed in the delicious scent of blooming flowers that merged with the tangy sea smell.

"What are you doing out here?" came a harsh, deep voice from the shelter of a nearby palm.

She watched Blake move into view in the moonlight, wearing a pair of white shorts and the same red and white patterned silk shirt he'd been wearing the other night. Only tonight it was unbuttoned all the way down his massive chest.

"I asked you a question," he said, and even in the moonlight she could see the boldness in his dark eyes as they sketched her slender body in its brief white covering. The way he was looking at her made her pulses pound.

"I came out for a swim," she said, very carefully enunciating each word. "I'm hot."

"Are you?"

Her eyes traced the hard lines of his body, lingering on his massive chest with its wedge of dark, curling hair that disappeared below his waistline. Her lips parted as she felt a surge of longing so great, it moved her toward him without her even being aware of it until she was close enough to touch him.

"Don't be angry with me," she pleaded in a husky voice. Her fingers went to his broad chest, touching the bronzed skin nervously, feeling the sensuous masculinity in those muscles that clenched under her soft touch.

"Don't," he said harshly, catching her hands roughly.

"Why not, Blake?" she asked recklessly. "Don't you

like for me to touch you? I'm just a baby, remember," she taunted, moving her fingers under his deliberately. She could feel his heartbeat quicken until it was heavy and hard, hear the rough intake of his breath as she moved closer and let her body rest against him. The naked brush of her thighs against the hair-roughened muscles of his was intoxicating, and the feel of his hard chest against the softness of her body caused her to sigh.

"Blake," she whispered achingly. The alcohol she'd consumed made her uninhibited; she'd never been so dangerously relaxed with him before. But now she touched his shoulders and the muscles of his big arms in a desperate surge of longing, drowning in the nearness of him, the feel of his big, warm body under her exploring hands.

Her head moved forward, and she pressed her mouth against his chest, drinking in the tang of his cologne and the smell of some spicy soap on his bare skin.

He caught his breath sharply, and his hands suddenly gripped her bare waist. "Don't, Kate," he whispered roughly. "You'll make me do something we'll both regret. You don't know what you're doing to me!"

Her body moved sensuously against his, and she heard the hard groan that broke from his throat. "I know," she moaned, lifting her face to meet his blazing eyes. "Oh, Blake, love me!"

"On a public beach?" he growled huskily, before bending his head to take her mouth.

Her arms lifted around his neck, and his hands dropped to her thighs, lifting her body abruptly against his so that it was molded to every masculine line of him in a joining that tore a moan from her lips. His fingers contracted, and she felt the shudder rip through his body with the force of a blow, felt the arms holding her begin to tremble as his mouth invaded hers, devouring it in the silence of the night.

They swayed together like palm trees in a hurricane, tasting, touching, burning with a hunger that seemed incapable of satisfaction. Her fingers buried themselves in his thick, dark hair, ruffling it as she yielded to the violent passion she'd aroused.

She felt his fingers at the strings that held her bikini top in place, and she was too lost in him to notice what was happening until she felt with a sense of wonder the curling hair of his chest against the bare softness of her own, and she cried out with pleasure.

"This is how it felt that day in the gazebo, isn't it, Kate?" he breathed roughly at her ear as he pressed her breasts against the thickness of the dark hair that matted his muscular chest. "I want all of you against me like this, I want to lie down on the beach with you and let you feel every delicious difference between your body and mine."

Her thighs trembled where his broad fingers caressed them, drawing her hips to his. Her nails bit deeply into his hard back and she sobbed at the wave of emotion that trembled over her weak body.

"Kate, Kathy, sweet, sweet love," he whispered as his mouth touched her lips again and again, brief, hard kisses that aroused her almost beyond bearing so that she pressed even closer against his big, warm body and felt the shudder that went through it.

His mouth moved down her throat and her body arched as he found the thrust of her breasts and let his lips brush warmly, moistly, against flesh that had known no man's touch except his.

"Blake," she whispered achingly. I love you, she thought, I love you more than my own life, and if I have nothing else, I'll have this to remember when I'm old, and you and Vivian have children and I'm alone with my memories… Her fingers tangled in his hair and pressed his exploring mouth closer.

"God, you're soft," he breathed, lifting his head at last to move his mouth sensuously over hers. "Soft, like silk, like velvet against my body… Kathy, I want you. I want you like I want air to breathe, I want to make love to you…" His mouth took hers again, deeply possessive, his arms swallowing her, rocking her while the waves pounded rhythmically against the white sand, the sound just penetrating her mind while she got drunker on pleasure than she ever had on wine.

"We've got to stop this," he groaned, dragging his mouth away to look down at her in the darkness that wasn't darkness at all, his eyes black and tortured as they met hers. "I can't take you here!"

Her hands ran lovingly over his hair-matted chest, feeling the roughness of it, the strength of those well-developed muscles. She wanted to touch all of him, every sensuous inch of him.

"We could go inside," she suggested in a husky whisper.

"Yes, we could," he said roughly. "And you'd wake in my arms hating me. Not like this, Kate. Damn it, not like this!"

He pushed her away, and for just an instant, his eyes possessed the small high curve of her breasts like a thirsty man gulping water. Then he swooped and retrieved the bikini top. He dropped it into her shaking hands and turned his back.

"Put it on," he said harshly. His fingers dug into his shirt pocket for his crushed cigarette package and matches. "Let me cool off for a minute. My God, Kate, do you see what you do to me?" he growled, half-laughing as his fingers fumbled with the cigarette.

She tied the top back in place with trembling fingers, avoiding his direct gaze. Out of the corner of her eye, she saw the orange tip of his cigarette glow suddenly as he took a draw from it.

"I'm sorry, Blake," she said miserably. "I…I didn't mean to…to…"

"It's all right, Kate," he said gently. "You had too much to drink, that's all."

Her eyes closed and she folded her arms around her trembling body. "I'm so ashamed," she ground out.

He stiffened. "Ashamed?"

She turned away. "I can't think what got into me," she laughed harshly. "Maybe it's my age, maybe I'm going through my second childhood."

"Or maybe you're just plain damned frustrated," he

said, a whip in his deep voice. "Is that it, Kate? Can't Phillip give you what you need?"

Shocked, she turned, lifting her puzzled eyes to his across the distance. She'd never seen his face so hard. "What?"

He laughed shortly. "You make no secret of your preference for his company, honey," he reminded her. "But he isn't passionate. You're just finding that out, aren't you? Can't he satisfy those wild hungers in you, Kate? Can't he give you what I can?"

"I don't...I don't feel that way about Phil," she stammered.

"Don't expect me to stand in for him again," he shot back. "I draw the line at being used for a damned substitute."

"But I wasn't...!"

He turned away. "Go back inside and sober up," he said, stripping off his shirt.

She stared after him, watching as he walked forward, flicking the cigarette away, and abruptly dived into the moonlit water.

Kathryn wanted desperately to follow him, to make him understand how she felt. To tell him that she loved him, not Phillip, that she'd give anything to be to him what Vivian was. But she knew he'd never listen to her in his present mood. He might never listen to her again, regardless of his mood. She wanted to hit herself for putting away all that wine. She'd killed Blake's respect for her, and along with it, every chance she'd ever had of making him love her. With a sigh, she turned away and picked up her beach towel. She trailed it aimlessly behind her as she walked past the gnarled sea-grape trees back to the house, the flower-scented breeze making sultry whispers at her ear.

She overslept the next morning, and when she awoke it was with a bursting headache. She got to her feet to get an aspirin, glancing toward the rain-blasted window and the darkness of the clouds.

Phillip was the only one in the living room when she went downstairs.

"Where is everybody?" she asked, lifting a hand to her throbbing head as she sat down with the coffee she'd poured herself from the tray in front of the sofa.

"They drove Blake to the airport," he replied, watching her closely. "He was bent on flying to Haiti today, despite the storm warnings. He left before this started; I guess they stopped to do some shopping on the way back."

Her eyes stared blankly out the window at the pouring rain, whipped by the wind. "It looks bad out there," she remarked, her heart aching when she remembered what had happened last night and why Blake might have decided to take a risk like this. Had she made him reckless? Had her stupidity caused him to lose his temper so badly that he had to get away from the island, from her, at any cost?

"Yes, it does," he said. He raised his cup of coffee to his lips, watching her over the rim of it. He sipped some of the hot liquid and then abruptly put the cup down with a clatter. "What happened?"

The question was so unexpected that she stared at him for several seconds before she spoke. "What?"

"What happened last night?" he asked again. "Blake looked like a thunderhead when he came downstairs this morning, and he didn't say a word all through breakfast. He didn't ask where you were, but he kept watching the stairs, as if he expected you to come down them any second. He looked like a starving man with his eye on a five-course meal."

Tears formed in her own eyes, ran down her cheeks. She put her cup down and buried her face in her hands, crying brokenly.

He sat down beside her and patted her awkwardly on the shoulder. "What did you do to him, Kathy?"

"I'd had too much to drink," she whispered through her fingers, "and he'd said I was a child—"

"So you went out and proved to him that you weren't," he said softly, smiling at her.

A nagging suspicion formed in the back of her mind and she raised her tear-wet eyes to his with the question in them.

"It's a very public beach, Kathryn Mary," he said with a mischievous grin. "And the moon was out."

"Oh, no," she whispered, going red. She buried her face in her hands a second time. "You saw us."

"Not only me," he replied drily. "Vivian. Watch yourself, little one. I got a look at her face before she stormed off upstairs."

She swallowed. "Did anyone else...?"

He shook his head. "No. Mom and Dick were arguing politics. I'd taken Vivian for a stroll along the porch to see the view...and what a view we saw. Whew!"

The blush got hotter. "I could die," she moaned. "I could just die!"

"It's nothing to be embarrassed about," he said gently. "I'd give anything to have a woman care that much about me. And if you wondered how Blake really felt, I imagine you found out."

"I found out that he wants me," she replied miserably. "I knew that before. It's not enough, Phillip."

"How do you know that's all he feels?" he asked quietly. He leaned forward, studying the coffee table. "Blake's deep, Kathryn. He keeps everything to himself."

"I couldn't have faced him this morning," she said bitterly. "Not after what I did. Oh, Phillip, I'll never have another glass of wine as long as I live, I'll never touch another drop."

"Don't give up, girl," he said.

"Phillip, I don't have anything to give up," she reminded him.

"Don't you?" he asked, frowning. "I'm not so sure about that."

Vivian and Kathryn were left alone briefly while Maude supervised the evening meal and Dick and Phillip talked shop on the long porch. The rain had finally

vanished, but the wind had only let up a little, and Kathryn couldn't help wondering if Blake was all right. He wasn't due back until the next morning, but that didn't stop her from worrying.

"You really did get smashed last night, didn't you?" Vivian asked, shooting a quick glance at Kathryn's subdued expression as she poured herself a small sherry at the bar.

Kathryn stiffened. "I'm not used to alcohol," she said defensively, eyeing the coffee cup she was holding.

"What a pity you had to overdo it," the blonde said with a pitying glance. "Blake was utterly disgusted."

Her face flamed. "Was he?" she choked.

"I saw you, of course," she sighed. "Poor man, he didn't stand a chance when you absolutely threw yourself at him like that. Any man would be… stirred," she added. Her eyes sharpened. "For my part, I'm furious with you. Blake and I…well, I've told you how things are. And I should think you'd have enough pride not to offer yourself to an engaged man."

The coffee cup crashed to the floor. Kathryn got up and ran for the stairs. She couldn't bear to hear any more.

Blake was due by mid-morning, but when Phillip came back from the airport his face was grim.

"What's wrong? What happened?" Kathryn asked frantically.

"He left Haiti at daylight," Phillip said through tight

lips. "And filed a flight plan. But he hasn't been heard from since takeoff." He caught her hand and squeezed it warmly. "They think he's gone down in some rough winds off the coast of Puerto Rico."

Chapter Ten

She couldn't remember a time in her life when she'd been so afraid. She paced. She worried. She cried. When Phillip finally took pity on all of them and agreed to let them wait it out at the airport, she hugged him out of sheer relief. At least they'd be a little closer to the communications network.

The airport wasn't crowded, but it wasn't as comfortable as the restaurant in the adjoining motel, so the five of them waited there. Vivian was worried, but it didn't deter her from flirting with Phillip or casting a wandering eye around the restaurant for interested looks. There were several Europeans staying in the motel, and a good many of the customers were men.

Kathryn had eyes for no one. Her worried gaze was fixed on her lap while she tried not to wonder how she could go through life without Blake. She'd never thought about that before. Blake had always seemed invincible, immortal. He was so strong and commanding, it didn't occur to her that he was as vulnerable as any other man. Now, she had to consider that possibility and it froze her very blood.

"I can't stand it," she whispered to Phillip, rising. "I'm going out to the airfield."

"Kathryn, it may be hours," he protested, walking with her as far as the door, only to cast a concerned look back at Maude, who was deep in conversation with Dick Leeds, her thin face drawn and taut with fear.

"I know," she said. She managed a wan little smile. "But if he...*when* he comes back," she corrected quickly, "I think one of us should be there."

He clenched her shoulders hard. His face was older, harder. "Kate, it's not definite that he's coming back. You're got to face that. His plane went down, that's absolutely all I know. The rescue crews are searching, but heaven only knows what they'll find!"

She bit her lower lip, hard, and her eyes were misty when she raised them, but her jaw was set stubbornly. "He's alive," she said. "I know he's alive, Phillip."

"Honey..." he began piteously.

"Do you think I'd still be breathing if Blake were dead?" she asked in a wild, choked whisper. "Do you think my heart would be beating?"

He closed his eyes momentarily, as if searching for words.

"I'm going outside," she said gently. She turned and left him there.

* * *

The skies were still gray, and the sun hadn't come out. She paced the apron with an impatient restlessness, starting every time she heard a sound that might be a plane.

Minutes later, Maude came out to join her, her thin arms folded, her eyes pale and troubled. "I wish we knew something," she murmured. "Just whether or not they think he could be alive."

"He's alive," Kathryn said confidently.

Maude studied the brave little face, and a dawning light came into her eyes. "I've been very dense, haven't I, Kathryn?" she asked gently, studying the younger woman's face.

Kathryn watched the ground, reddening. "I..."

Maude put an arm around her shoulders comfortingly. "Come in and have another cup of coffee. It won't make that much difference."

"They found him!" Phillip yelled from the doorway of the terminal, his face bright, his voice full of sunlight. "The rescue plane's on its way in now!"

"Oh, thank God," Maude murmured prayerfully.

Kathryn let the tears run silently down her face unashamedly. Blake was safe. He was alive. Even if she had to give him up to Vivian, if she never saw him again, it was enough to know he'd be on the same planet with her, alive. Alive, praise God, alive!

Maude stayed outside with her, while Phillip went back inside with the others after they'd all been told the news. Kathryn couldn't be budged, and Maude stood quietly with her, waiting. Minutes passed quietly until there came the drone of a twin-engine plane. It circled the landing strip and dropped down gently, its wheels making a squealing sound briefly, lifting, then settling onto the runway.

Kathryn watched the plane with tears shimmering in her eyes, until it stopped, the engine cut off, the door opened.

A big, dark man in an open-necked shirt stepped out of it, and Kathryn was running toward him before his feet ever touched the ground.

"Blake!" she screamed, oblivious to the other members of the family coming out of the terminal behind her. She ran like a frightened child seeking refuge, her face tormented, her legs flying against the skirt of her white sundress.

He opened his arms and caught her up against him, holding her while she ground her cheek against his broad chest and wept like a wind-tossed orphan.

"Oh, Blake," she whimpered, "they said you'd gone down, and we didn't know...oh, I'd have died with you! Blake, Blake...I'd have died with you, Blake," she whispered, over and over, her voice muffled, almost incoherent, her nails stabbing into his back as she clung to him.

His big arms tightened around her, his cheek scrubbing roughly against her forehead. "I'm all right," he said. "I'm fine, Kate."

She drew away a breath and looked up at him with tears streaming down her pale face, lines of weariness and worry making her look suddenly older.

He looked older, too, his face heavily lined, his dark eyes bloodshot as if he hadn't slept in a long time. She searched his beloved face, everything she felt for him showing plainly in her green eyes.

"I love you so," she whispered brokenly. "Oh, Blake, I love you so!"

He stood there frozen, staring down at her with eyes so dark they seemed black.

Embarrassed at having been so stupidly blunt, she tugged weakly at his arms and stepped back. "I…I'm sorry," she choked. "I…didn't mean to…to throw myself at you a second time. Vivian told me…how disgusted you were yesterday," she added in a whipped tone.

"Vivian told you what?" he asked in a strange, husky whisper.

She stepped away from him, but she still clung helplessly to his big, warm hand, walking quietly beside him, the top of her head just coming to his chin, as they moved to join the others.

"It doesn't matter," she said with a painful smile. "It's all right."

"That's what you think!" he said in a voice she didn't recognize.

Vivian came running to meet him, shooting a poisonous glance at Kathryn. "Oh, Blake, darling! We were so worried!" she exclaimed, reaching up to kiss him full on the mouth. "How lovely that you're safe!"

Maude and Phillip echoed the greeting, Maude with tears misting her eyes.

"Close call?" Phillip asked with keen perception.

Blake nodded. "Too close. I wouldn't care to repeat it."

"What about the plane?" Maude asked gently.

"I'm glad it was insured," Blake replied with a faint smile. "I came down in the rain forest on Puerto Rico. The plane made it, barely, but I clipped off the wings."

Kathryn closed her eyes, seeing it in her mind.

"I'll buy you a drink," Phillip said. "You look like you could use one."

"A drink, a hot bath, and a bed," Blake agreed. He glanced at Kathryn as she moved away toward Phillip. She wouldn't meet his eyes.

"I…I'm going to pack," she murmured, turning away.

"Pack?" Blake asked gruffly. "Why?"

"I'm going home," she said proudly, letting her eyes meet his, only to glance off again. "I…I've had enough sun and sand. I don't like paradise…it's got too many serpents."

She turned toward the car. "Phillip, will you please drive me back to the house?" she asked with downcast eyes.

"Let Maude," he said, surprising her. "Would you mind, darling?" he asked his mother.

"No, not at all," Maude said, taking the younger girl's arm. "Come along, sweetheart. Vivian, Dick, are you coming?"

They declined, preferring to go with the men into the bar. Maude drove Kathryn home in a smothering silence.

"Don't go," Maude pleaded as Kathryn went upstairs to get her things together. "Not yet. Not today."

She turned at the head of the stairs with eyes so full of heartache they seemed to glow with it. "I can't stay here anymore," she replied softly. "I can't bear it. I…I want to look for an apartment before he…" She turned and went on upstairs. The tears choked her voice out.

She had packed everything in her bags and had changed into a neat pin-striped blue blouse and white skirt for traveling when the door opened suddenly and Blake walked in.

She stared wide-eyed at him across the bed. He looked more relaxed, but he still needed a shave and sleep.

"I…I'm almost ready," she murmured, brushing back a wild swath of long, waving dark hair from her flushed cheek. "If Phillip could drive me…"

He leaned back against the closed door and watched her. He was wearing a white shirt open halfway down the front, with dark blue trousers. His thick hair was ruffled, his face hard, his eyes narrow and dark and searching.

"The Leedses are leaving," he said quietly.

"Oh, are they?" she murmured, staring down at the white coverlet. "For how long?"

"For good. I went to Haiti to sign a contract. I'm switching the London mill to Port au Prince," he replied.

She stared at him. "But, Vivian…"

"Kathryn, I brought her over because I knew she was the power behind her father," he said wearily. "I knew if I could convince her to meet my terms, she'd convince him. But you misread the situation completely, and I suppose it was partially my fault. I wanted you to misread it."

She glanced at him and away. "It doesn't matter now."

"Doesn't it?" he asked softly.

"I'm going to look for an apartment when I get home, Blake," she told him, lifting her flushed young face proudly. "I want to be by myself."

He searched her eyes. "You told me you loved me, Kathryn," he said quietly, watching the color flush into her cheeks at the impact of the words.

She swallowed nervously, and traced an idle pattern on the coverlet with her finger. "I…was upset," she faltered.

"Don't play games. Don't hedge. You said you loved me. How? As a big brother—a guardian—or as a lover, Kate?"

"You're confusing me!" she protested feverishly.

"You've confused me for a solid year," he said flatly. His eyes smoldered with reined emotion. "All I do lately is slam my head against a wall trying to get through to you."

She gaped at him. "I don't understand."

He jammed his hands in his pockets and leaned back against the door, letting his eyes trace the line of her body with an intimate thoroughness.

"You never have," he replied roughly.

Her soft eyes touched the worn, weary lines in his face. "Blake, you look so tired," she said gently. "Why don't you go to bed for a while?"

"Only with you, Kate," he said shortly, watching the color go back and forth in her cheeks. "Because I'm not going to close my eyes only to open them again and find you gone.

"Donavan," he growled. "And then Phillip. My own brother, and I hated him because he could get close to you and I couldn't. And you thought that I just *wanted* you!"

Her face opened like a bud in blossom, and she stiffened, barely breathing as she listened to his deep, harsh voice.

"Wanted you!" he repeated, eyes blazing, jaw tightening. "My God, I've been out of my mind wondering whom I substituted for that night on the beach, and all along...!" He drew a short breath. "How long had you planned to keep it from me, Kathryn?" he demanded. "Were you going to go home and lock it away inside you?"

Tears were misting her eyes. She moved to the foot of the bed and held onto the bedpost, smoothing over the silky mahogany. "Blake?" she whispered.

"You told Phillip that I had to be alive, because your heart was still beating," he said in a strange, husky voice. "It was that way with me over a year ago. As long as I'm still breathing, I know you are, because there is no way on earth I could stay alive without you!"

She ran to him blindly, seeing only a big, husky blur as she reached up to be folded against him in an embrace that all but crushed the breath from her slender body.

"Kiss me," he whispered shakily, bending to take her

soft mouth under his. "Kathy, Kathy, I love you so…!" he ground out against her soft, eager lips.

They kissed wildly, hungrily, and she could feel the rhythm of steel drums in her bloodstream as the pressure of his mouth became deep and intimate, expertly demanding a response she gave without restraint.

He tore his mouth away finally and buried it against her soft throat. With a sense of wonder, she felt the big arms that were holding her tremble.

"I thought you hated me," she whispered, drowning in the unbelievable sensation of loving and being loved.

"For what?" he asked gruffly. "Trying to seduce me on the beach?"

"I wasn't," she protested weakly.

"It felt like it. You'll never know exactly how close to it you came."

"I loved you so," she whispered, "and I thought I'd lost you, and I wanted one perfect memory…"

"It was that," he said softly. His arms contracted lovingly. "I'll always see you the way you looked in the moonlight, with your skin like satin, glowing…"

"Blake!" she whispered, reddening.

"Don't be embarrassed," he said quietly. "Or ashamed. It was beautiful, Kate, every second of it was beautiful. It's going to be like that every time I touch you, for the rest of our lives."

She drew away and looked up at him. "That long?" she asked.

He searched her soft green eyes. "That long. Will you marry me?"

"Yes."

He reached down and brushed her mouth with his, very gently—a seal on the promise. "I hope you like children," he murmured against her soft lips.

She smiled lazily. "How many do you want?"

"Let's get married next week and talk about it."

"Next week!" Her mouth flew open. "Blake, I can't! The invitations, and I'll have to have a gown...!"

He stopped the flow of words with his mouth. Through a fog of sensation, she felt his hands moving slowly, expertly, on her soft body and she moaned.

He drew back a breath. "Next week," he whispered unsteadily.

"Next week," she agreed under her breath and reached up to draw his head back down.

Outside, the sunset was lending a rose glow to the bay, where fishing boats rocked gently at the shore. And in the orange and gold swirls of color on the horizon there was a promise of blue skies ahead.

* * * * *

ROBIN WILLIAMS

Andy Dougan

THUNDER'S MOUTH PRESS
NEW YORK

First THUNDER'S MOUTH PRESS edition 1998
Published by THUNDER'S MOUTH PRESS
841 Broadway, 4th Floor, New York, NY 10003

First published in 1998 by Orion Media
An imprint of Orion Books Ltd
Orion House, 5 Upper St Martin's Lane, London WC2H 9EA

Library of Congress Cataloging-in-Publication Data

Dougan, Andy.

Robin Williams: a biography / by Andy Dougan.

p. cm.

Filmography: p.

Includes bibliographical references and index.

ISBN 1-56025-196-4

1. Williams, Robin, 1952, July 21– 2. Comedians—United States—-Biography. 3. Actors—United States— Biography. I. Title.

PN2287.W473D68 1998

791.43'028'092—dc21

[B] 98–34078

CIP

Trade paperback ISBN 1-56025-213-8

Typeset in Minion by Selwood Systems, Midsomer Norton
Printed and bound in Great Britain by Butler & Tanner Ltd, Frome and London

Distributed by PUBLISHERS GROUP WEST
1700 Fourth Street
Berkeley, CA 94710
(800) 788–3123

CONTENTS

To Christine, Iain and Stuart

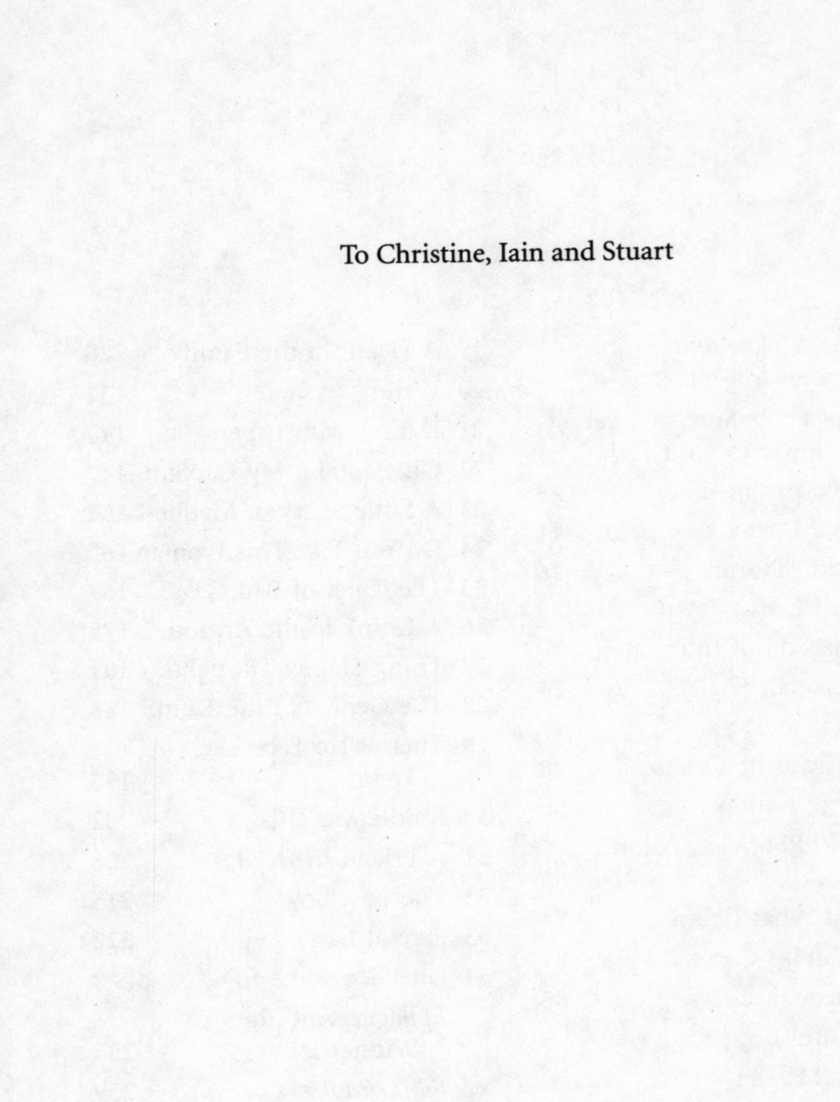

AUTHOR'S NOTE AND ACKNOWLEDGEMENTS

This is an unauthorised biography and does not pretend to be anything other than an unauthorised biography. This book has actually been in the pipeline for a number of years. As a film journalist one of the great joys of my professional life is to watch Robin Williams work a room. It is a pleasure and a privilege and it was as a result of this that I first started to think about this book. When I started to make contact with a number of his colleagues and co-workers I very quickly received a fax from his lawyers advising me that he would not 'authorize [sic] a biography of him to be written or encourage his close associates to cooperate in the writing of such a book'.

Since the purpose of the book was to try to explore some of the influences behind the creative process of 'the funniest man alive', this was discouraging but not altogether unexpected. However over the past few years I have interviewed a number of Robin Williams' co-stars and directors as well as, of course, interviewing him on his frequent publicity junkets for his films. This book draws from these interviews as well as subsequent conversations with friends and colleagues, some named, some not.

I would particularly like to thank those who took the time to talk to me, especially Adrian Cronauer, Barry Friedman and Dan Holzman. I am also grateful to those who were so helpful on my trips to New York and San Francisco, especially the staff at the Billy Rose Theater Collection in New York and Susan Krauss in California. My grateful thanks too to Kristine Krueger from the National Film Information Service at the Center for Motion Picture Study in Los Angeles, for once again guiding me through the maze.

A number of colleagues were also kind enough to help. I would like to thank Siobhan Synnot of BBC Radio Scotland for making available her interviews with Robin Williams for *Flubber* and *Good Will Hunting*, as well as Chris Columbus for *Mrs Doubtfire*, and Alison Maloney for access to her interview with Gus Van Sant as well as for asking questions on my behalf. My thanks too to Anwar Brett for having a better filing system than me and invaluably managing to retrieve the transcripts of press conferences for *Hook* and *Mrs Doubtfire* which I had misplaced.

For their help and encouragement along the way I would like to thank my agent Jane Judd, as well as Trevor Dolby and Pandora White at Orion.

And finally, once again, my thanks to my wife and children for putting up with the beast in the attic for another three months.

Andy Dougan

PROLOGUE

Be Sure to Wear a Flower in your Hair

America in 1969 was in the middle of tremendous civil unrest. At its heart was an unpopular war in Vietnam. American involvement in Vietnam reached a peak in 1969 with 541,000 US troops committed to serving in South East Asia. In addition to the notion of their boys being slaughtered in the jungle, Americans at home had also become sickened and horrified by revelations about the conduct of their troops in Vietnam. Only a year previously American soldiers had slaughtered Vietnamese villagers at My Lai. By the end of 1969 the mood on the home front had changed dramatically, with millions of Americans taking part in protest marches against the most unpopular war in the country's brief history.

The average age of the American combat soldier in Vietnam was only 19. By comparison the average age of a GI in the Second World War was 26. The youthful nature of the combatants was matched by the equally youthful nature of the protesters. This was very definitely a student revolution as millions of young people demonstrated and protested about their classmates and contemporaries being sent overseas to fight. The heart of this revolution could be found on the West Coast, specifically in the colleges and universities in and around San Francisco. The American protest movement has its origins in the so-called Summer of Love which was centred in San Francisco two years previously. That summer of 1967 was seen by the establishment as a symbol of the moral decline of American youth. Instead it would go on to define a whole generation as well as the ones which followed.

Since it was taken from Mexico in 1846, the whole of what became the state of California has had a frequently tenuous association with the rest of the country. Self-styled sophisticates in New York will refer disparagingly to California as America's 'left coast'. They do things differently out there to be sure, and this is largely because of the strong European influences on their culture and politics. Los Angeles, for example, had become the home of Stravinsky, Isherwood and Huxley. San Francisco similarly had been subject to strong European influences from the hundreds of thousands who came from all over the world, drawn by the discovery of gold in the Sierras in 1846, and later settled there because they had struck it rich or were too poor to go home. As a consequence of this melting-pot of cultures San Francisco has always taken a perverse pride in being *in* America without necessarily being *of* America.

In the Fifties, the city had become the home of the Beat Generation and its charismatic poets and writers such as Alan Ginsberg, Neal Cassidy and Jack Kerouac. They had turned the city's North Beach into the western annexe of New York's Greenwich Village. Their world revolved around the City Lights bookstore in Columbus Avenue and the bars and cafés which dotted the nearby streets. The word 'beatnik' was originally coined as a derogatory term by Herb Caen, one of San Francisco's best-known newspaper columnists. Within a few years the Beat Generation had grown up and moved on and left behind another movement which would shape America's future.

The hippies were an offshoot of the Beats. The word was originally a not altogether complimentary beat term to describe those well-intentioned young people who followed in their footsteps without always understanding what they were really about. Both groups believed in the rejection of materialism, but their rejection took different forms. While the Beats wrote novels and poems raging against the capitalist nine-to-five life and extolling the virtues of personal freedom, the hippies were more heavily influenced by drugs and music. They were more inclined to light up a joint than to write a poem. The hippie movement began in the coffee bars of the university campuses of the Bay Area but quickly found a home in the Haight-Ashbury district just to the west of downtown San Francisco. Here they established communal squats in formerly impressive but now run-down mansion houses and took the advice of their guru Timothy Leary by turning on, tuning in and dropping out.

The hippie movement was based on three things: music, love and drugs. And the greatest of these was drugs. The writer Hunter S. Thompson estimates that in 1965 almost everyone on the streets of Haight-Ashbury 'between twenty and thirty was a "head", a user of either marijuana, LSD, or both. To refuse the proffered joint is to risk being labelled a "nark" – a narcotics agent – a threat and a menace to almost everybody.'

The hippies had discovered LSD, a powerfully hallucinogenic, 'mind-expanding' drug. Not only that, many of them were bright enough to manufacture it safely and cheaply. A tab of good-quality acid would cost around $5 and leave you high as a kite for hours at a time. The money for the drugs could be quickly raised by begging on the streets. This so-called 'panhandling' was the principal source of income for many hippies, and the money was easily obtained from the tourists who were beginning to flock into the area. For their part it was a cheap price to pay for what was the best freak show in town.

Music was also an important part of hippie culture. Bands like Jefferson Airplane and The Grateful Dead were required listening for those who were not hearing the music of the spheres after dropping a tab or two. The defining moment of the hippie movement came in the summer of 1967 when their non-materialistic instincts led them to put on a free concert in San Francisco's Golden Gate Park. What was intended to be a tiny local event drew a crowd of 20,000 and took the media by storm. Suddenly world-wide attention was focused on this small Californian neighbourhood, and by the end of the year there were an estimated 100,000 hippies living in and around Haight-Ashbury.

The hippie lifestyle was a protest, however mild, against the American Way of Life. Elsewhere in San Francisco, at the universities of Oakland and Berkeley on the other side of the Bay Bridge, a more hard-line protest was taking shape from another group of disaffected young people. The Free Speech Movement was founded at Berkeley in 1964 as a means of evading a ban on student political activity. Within a few years this had hardened into a protest against America's involvement in Vietnam. In 1968 there had been pitched battles in San Francisco's Telegraph Hill area when rioting broke out after students attempting to show solidarity with their protesting contemporaries in Paris were met by a strong show of force from the police. The fighting and rioting went on for several days before order was eventually restored. Another protest at the so-called People's Park, a piece of university land which had been taken over by the students, ended when the police moved in to end the four-day occupation, firing tear gas into the crowd and wading in with night-sticks. One person died and more than 100 were injured.

The campus of the University of California at Berkeley became a symbol for America's rapidly increasing protest movement. It was the heart and soul of a new generation which was finding its own voice and fighting for a say in its own destiny. At first dismissed by the establishment as a bunch of rabble-rousing malcontents, the students from California rapidly began to define the mood of the country. Encouraged by the students' example, there were other protests in San Francisco in 1969. Under cover of darkness a group of American Indians took over the now abandoned former Federal penitentiary at Alcatraz in the middle of San Francisco. Their plan, among other things, was to convert the building into their own university. Their aims were idealistic and their methods were non-violent. Recognising that they were buoyed up by public opinion, the authorities decided to wait them out. It was a long wait, but eventually internal dissension on the part of the protesters and a rising tide of public indifference meant that Alcatraz was eventually reclaimed in 1971.

Even though the Indians finally surrendered these were heady times in 1969. The hippies were getting stoned, the students were getting tear-gassed, and the Indians were on The Rock.

Into the midst of all this came a shy, slightly overweight teenager from an exclusive private school in Detroit.

'That was the transitional year for me,' Robin Williams would later recall. 'San Francisco in 1969 changed everything.'

1

I Love You in Blue

The dawning of the American Century, that period when America began to dominate the world economically, politically and culturally, came with the end of the Second World War. After the restrictions of the war years America suddenly found itself in the years immediately after 1945 with one of the greatest consumer booms of modern times. Men who had fought and killed on the battlefields of Europe and the Pacific Theatre for four years returned home with new dreams and desires. Those dreams and desires boiled down to two things: their own car and their own home.

A new car was a convenient status symbol in the immediate postwar years. A plentiful domestic supply of petrol from the oilfields of Texas and Oklahoma meant that fuel was cheap and the automobile industry was set for its golden age. The mass production techniques originally pioneered by Henry Ford were honed and refined but they would not be used to churn out boxy, basic black Model Ts. This was the age of automotive opulence, where bigger was definitely better.

If one company came to symbolise American industrial might of that period it was General Motors, which dominated the automobile industry and with it America's manufacturing sector. This was the period when one of the company's senior executives, Charlie Wilson, was misquoted as saying that what was good for General Motors was good for America. What he actually said, when he left GM to become Secretary of Defence for President Eisenhower, was 'We at General Motors have always felt that what was good for the country was good for General Motors as well'.

Regardless of what he actually said, everyone knew what he meant and his point was well made. General Motors had a near monopoly on the car industry. Their main rivals Ford had deteriorated markedly from the company which Henry had founded. Indeed Ford's performance had fallen so badly that GM bosses genuinely feared that, such was their dominance, they might one day be liable to an anti-trust suit. In 1953, GM had 45 per cent of the American market, and by 1956 this had risen unchecked to a staggering 51 per cent.

The symbol of GM's power was the car which became America's dream machine, the Cadillac. This was the ultimate aspirational target for the American working man. Everyone dreamed that, in the land of opportunity, they would one day be driving their own Caddy, just like their boss. A Cadillac in the early Fifties would cost around $5000. Wages in the manufacturing sector ranged from $2400 to $3000 a year, with those in the motor industry not surprisingly at the top end of the scale. However, with an annual trade-in a Cadillac could be owned for a net cost of $700 per year. This meant that with hard work and a little initiative the dream car could become a reality.

It was hard for America's other automobile manufacturers to compete with the glamour, the price and the reliability of the Cadillac. Ford, even though it was second by a long way, was GM's chief rival and it attempted to lure motorists away from the Cadillac with its own luxury car, the Lincoln Continental. It was a hard row to hoe, but all they could do was try.

Robert Fitzgerald Williams was a senior executive at Ford in charge of the Midwest sales division of the Lincoln-Continental operation. He was a ramrod and a trouble-shooter. It was his job to go where the problems were and make sure that Ford could hold their own in the battle with General Motors at the top end of the market. Although he was a captain of industry, Robert Williams was cut from a different cloth from most of his fellow executives in the car industry. Williams had been born in Evansville, Indiana to a family which was a mixture of English, Welsh and Irish stock. The Williams family was seriously wealthy, having made its fortune in the lumber and mining industries. But like so many family fortunes, the businesses had fallen on hard times during the Depression. Eventually things had reached such a poor pass that Williams had to work in the family strip mines himself for a time. He was, by all accounts, possessed of talent and a fierce will, and through the combination of these and sheer hard work he was able to reach the upper echelons of industry once again. The experience had scarred him, however, and he would remain deeply cynical and mistrustful for the rest of his life.

Williams was a tall, imperious, patrician man who is said to have resembled the broadcaster Alastair Cooke. His wife Laurie was a former model and society beauty. Her family was French from New Orleans and she was blessed with the fine bone structure and gamine charm of Audrey Hepburn or Leslie Caron. They were the perfect couple who had found each other relatively late in life – each had been married before – and in the summer of 1952 they produced a son.

Robin McLaurim Williams first saw the light of day on 21 July 1952 in Chicago, Illinois. Robert Williams was a senior executive and was paid accordingly, so the family were not exactly short of a dollar. When his job required that he move to Detroit, the capital of the American auto industry, he took his wife and child to a 30-room mansion in 20 acres of grounds in the exclusive Bloomfield Hills district. This was the real deal for Robert Williams. It was the American dream writ large, with the big house, the good job, the servants and the high income. The problem was that he was frequently not around to share it with his family. Williams' work took him all over the Midwest and he spent days and weeks at a time away from the family home. Even when he was working in Detroit the hours would be long, requiring him to leave early in the morning and not return until late at night.

While he was away, young Robin had to grow up without him. And with his mother also busy modelling and organising charity benefits he spent a great deal of time without either parent. He had the whole third floor of this huge mansion to himself. Literally to himself. Bloomfield Hills was not exactly teeming with school-age children, and as Williams remembers there were no other children in the neighbourhood at all. There was just him, his dog Duke, and Carl his pet turtle. On a good day the son of the family's maid might come over and play. Duke was a constant companion but his value as a playmate was somewhat limited.

> We would play hide and seek [Williams recalled] and I would always find him. Duke thought that if he couldn't see me then I couldn't see him. Duke was dumb. I could always see – or at least hear – his big tail going whop! whop! whop! on the parquet floors. Pretty early on I banished myself to the attic where I had a huge army of toy soldiers. I had about 10,000 of them and I would have them all separated by periods in boxes. I would have time-machine battles with Confederate soldiers fighting GIs with automatic weapons and knights fighting Nazis.

As well as his toy soldiers – an army whose size appears to vary from 2000 to 10,000 depending on who he was speaking to – Robin Williams also had a full and rich fantasy life. When he tired of mock battles he would retreat into his imagination and fill his days with imaginary friends. But imaginary friends are no substitute for the real thing. Even when he was ten and discovered that he had in fact two half-brothers from his parents' previous marriages, the excitement was tempered by the fact that they were both much older than him. Lauren, his mother's son, was four years older, and Todd, the son of his father's first marriage, was 13 years older. Williams never saw them much when he was growing up, and his recollection of Todd in particular is of someone who would come into his room and 'borrow' from his piggy bank for beer money.

Although he was lonely, Robin Williams insists that he still felt loved. However, many years later, and with the benefit of therapy, he would look back and recall that his childhood was not necessarily as he had remembered it.

> I'm just beginning to realise that it wasn't always that happy [he told *Esquire* magazine in 1989]. My childhood was kind of lonely. Quiet. My father was away, my mother was working, doing benefits. I was basically raised by this maid and my mother would come in later, you know, and I knew her and she was wonderful and charming and witty. But I think maybe comedy was part of my way of connecting with my mother – 'I'll make mommy laugh and that will be okay' – and that's where it started.

Williams did, he realises now, grow up with an acute fear of abandonment. Such feelings are not uncommon in young children, but in his case, with his father coming and going so much, the fear must have been that little bit more real. Performing was a means of getting attention as well as providing a little bit of added value. He wasn't just their son, he could be entertaining too. If Williams' love of performing came from being eager to please his mother, he also acknowledges the debt he owes to both parents in contributing to his talent.

Laurie Williams was the perfect audience for her son's fledgling efforts as a performer. She is bubbly and effervescent, with a bizarre sense of humour which belies her Southern Belle upbringing. She once turned up at a society ball in an exclusive Illinois country club dressed to kill but with her two front teeth obscured by tape as a joke to make it appear that they were missing. Naturally all the women there were wondering, to her delight, why someone who could dress so well would not be able to afford to get her teeth fixed. Laurie Williams would regale young Robin with tales from a favourite book which was supposedly written by a nineteenth-century English society hostess which she insisted was called *Balls I Have*

Held. And among the inexhaustible supply of jokes and stories with which she would amuse her son, there was also her penchant for faintly *risqué* doggerel. One favourite rhyme was

> Spider crawling on the wall
> Ain't you got no sense at all
> Don't you know that wall's been plastered
> Get off that wall you little . . . spider.

Another of his mother's rhymes which amused the young Williams was

> I love you in blue
> Love you in red
> But most of all
> I love you in . . . blue.

Robert Williams on the other hand was stern without actually being strict. He was a great believer in children knowing their place and wasn't wild about the notion of youngsters acting up. Williams, however, cannot recall his father raising his voice to him, except on one occasion, when he made a rude gesture of defiance to his mother. That was the only time he remembers being smacked – but only once. According to Laurie Williams, Robert Williams was 'strict but fair' and his son absolutely adored him. She and Robin would affectionately refer to her husband as 'Lord Stokesbury, Viscount of India' for his elegance and patrician manner.

Williams himself recalls the advice his father gave him, a relic of the bitter cynicism which his own family's misfortunes had left in him. 'He was this wonderful elegant man who thought the world was going to hell in a hand basket. It was basically "You can't trust them. Watch out for them. They'll nail ya. Everybody's out to nail ya".'

There is no doubt that Robin Williams loved his father deeply and the feeling was reciprocated. It would be false to assume that Williams grew up feeling rejected by a cold and aloof paterfamilias. What there was between them was distance; sometimes geographical, sometimes emotional. There was also the problem of Robert Williams approaching middle age – he was 46 – when his son was born. It is often difficult for older parents to match their children's energy levels, and children of older parents frequently grow up feeling a little more distant from their families than they would like.

But between them Robert and Laurie Williams have passed on to their son the gifts which he has used to make him the man he is today. His mother gave him an extravagant sense of comedy, and the still, wry humour of his father gave him a sense of theatre. The combination of the two is what makes Williams a unique package.

'I got her energy and funkified sense of humour,' Williams concedes, 'and I got a grounding thing from Dad. I never met my grandmother on Mom's side, but Mom says she was a great character who just loved to watch men wrestle. There's probably a lot of happy madness which has been passed down in the family, with characters from *Arsenic and Old Lace* all over the place.'

2

School Daze

For someone who had effectively grown up in isolation, no matter how privileged that isolation may have been, school must have been a brave new world for Robin Williams. It was a whole exciting realm of adventure, stimulation and – most important – other children. Williams must have thought he had died and gone to Heaven on his first day of school.

Although he remembers his early days at Gorton Elementary School in Chicago as being unspectacular, his classmates have a slightly different recollection of the period. One former classmate remembers him as having a perpetual smile as early as the fourth grade when he was taught by Miss Granice, a teacher with a reputation for discipline. That was also, one assumes, the beginning of his talents for vocal mimicry. Friends recall that Williams would sit engrossed in his school work but at the same time emitting a variety of strange sounds – a forerunner of Mork from Ork – as he went about his business. Miss Granice would move his desk further and further away from the other children to minimise the distraction to them, but there was nothing to be done until eventually the desk ended up out in the corridor, where Williams would spend the rest of the lesson. Later on, by the time he reached the sixth grade at Gorton, Williams had found a favourite teacher. Miss Turner, who had a penchant for playing opera when the children were supposed to be studying maths, obviously appealed to the eccentric side of his nature.

If the story of Williams' noise-making is true, and there seems no reason why it shouldn't be, it is also perfectly understandable. Having spent hours occupying himself at home on his own, he was probably unaware of the habit. Whatever disruptive effect he might have had on the class can be put down to excitement and exuberance rather than mischief. Here was a whole new group to pay attention to him to overcompensate for the loneliness he frequently felt at home. It's also worth remembering that growing up without other children would also have left Williams' social and play skills considerably underdeveloped. That often meant that school could be a painful experience for the young Robin Williams, who was terminally shy. Class photographs of the period show Williams as a sturdy, pale, round-faced child with a rather severe crew cut. He sits with his back straight, his arms folded across his lap and his hands thrust between his thighs. And there is, as his classmates reported, just the hint of a sly smile; a suggestion that he knows something that no one else does. But for Williams, who was a quiet little boy, school could also be a trial.

'Kids can be quite cruel to one another, we all know that,' Williams concedes. 'And at one time I did get bullied at school, because I was little and I was fat, and I got called names.'

Occasionally the bullying manifested itself in more physical ways. Perhaps because they were aware that he had grown up without other kids, his parents had made a conscious effort to educate their son through the public school system rather than the more cocooned environment of a private school. For a short, fat kid with crippling shyness there were times when every day was sheer purgatory. There was, he realised, only one way to deal with it.

> I started telling jokes in the seventh grade as a way to stop getting the shit kicked out of me [he remembers]. Mom and Dad had put me in a public school and most of the kids there were bigger than me and wanted to prove they were bigger than me by throwing me into the walls. There were a lot of burly farm kids and sons of auto plant workers there. I'd come to school looking for new entrances and thinking, 'If only I could come in through the roof.' They'd nail me as soon as I got through the door.

It can't have been easy for Williams, the rich, well-spoken new boy, to be such an obvious fish out of water. Frequently, as Williams also recalls, the humour only worked up to a point. The school toughs thought he was funny but they decided they were going to pick on him anyway. Williams' physical torment was ended by a stroke of luck. For once the peripatetic nature of his father's job worked in his favour. The move to Bloomfield Hills in Detroit meant that Robin Williams ended up at the Detroit

Country Day School, a private school where he could at least mingle with boys of his own background and finish the seventh grade. To his horror he quickly found out that he had merely switched one form of abuse for another. The privileged pupils of his new school would never have soiled their hands with the physical battering Williams had suffered previously. But, in the casually callous manner of children all over the world, they found a new and possibly even more hurtful form of torture.

'I was picked on not only physically but intellectually too,' says Williams. 'People used to kick George Sand in my face,' he says trying to make light of it. 'It's a whole other thing when you get both.'

The irony is that Williams was by no means an intellectual lightweight. He was a studious and intelligent boy who was more than a match in terms of academic ability for any of his schoolmates. Where they had the advantage, however, was in terms of confidence. Williams was still hampered by his shyness, which meant he was less likely to say anything in his own defence, and more likely to say the wrong thing at the wrong time.

> All these hyperintellectuals would lay into me with lines like 'That was a very asinine thing to say, Williams' [he remembers]. I remember one kid was into heavy calculus in the seventh grade and everyone would go, 'Wow, cross sections of a cone. Gee, Chris, I wish I could do that.' That was one side. The other side was physical abuse. The real problem was that everyone was going through puberty or just about to, which produces a lot of tensions.

Perhaps as a defence against the bullying of his WASP classmates, Williams found himself gravitating towards the Jewish boys at the school. They were obvious targets for discrimination because of their background and that perhaps provided some common ground between them. Most of his school friends were Jewish and they proved to be much more accepting of Williams than the other classmates had been. Williams says, with some pride, that as an 'honorary Jew' he went to 14 bar mitzvahs in a single year. His new friends also provided him with a working knowledge of Yiddish which survives now in the words and phrases that sprinkle his conversations and his stage act.

It would be fair to say that Robin Williams endured rather than enjoyed his early years at school. But now with high school looming a number of important decisions would have to be made. One of the first was that he was going to have to do something with his life. Robin Williams had finally had enough of being bullied physically and intellectually. He had decided to take charge of his life and do something about it. At roughly the same time that he was due to go to high school he had started to get into shape. He took up running, which has remained a lifelong passion, he was doing calisthenics and had lost weight, and in addition he had begun playing sport.

One of the sports he had taken up was wrestling and he found that it brought him immediate and uncharacteristic popularity; the shy youngster who had been a target for everyone was now maturing into a successful and well-adjusted young man. Williams made the wrestling team and was undefeated in his freshman year. He was good enough to reach the state finals but there he met someone older, more experienced, and probably a bit heavier. Williams lost that bout and also picked up a shoulder injury which led to him having to give up the sport in his sophomore year. But wrestling had been good for him. He was naturally small and compact – by now he weighed just 103 pounds – which gave him an advantage, but he was also tenacious. More importantly, wrestling meant something to him. After years of being pushed around and picked on, he now had the chance to get his own back. It wasn't just about being big and tough, wrestling was also about guile and agility. This was a sport where quickness of the mind was as important as brute strength. Williams admits he got rid of a lot of pent-up aggression and frustration on the wrestling mat.

Although his shoulder injury meant he had to give up a promising career in wrestling, Robin Williams was by now well and truly hooked on sport. His running helped to keep his weight down and his mind focused. It was only a matter of time before he found another arena in which he could excel as he had at wrestling. Before that though there was the obligatory and disastrous try-out for the school football team. Williams was put in at safety with the job of stopping the other team from scoring. Given that he weighed just over 100 pounds and the average running back can weigh twice that, the experiment was not a success. By the end of the first game Williams was left with stud marks up one side and down the other. His football career lasted only a week. Such was the reputation of Detroit Country, however, that it attracted a lot of foreign-exchange students. This meant that as well as playing football they also played soccer. Again it is a sport where the small and nippy can excel against the large and slow, providing they are willing to take their lumps. Williams quickly made his mark in the burgeoning sport and became a team favourite.

His time at high school had changed Robin Williams completely. Gone was the shy, tubby boy who had been tormented in grade school. He was now a sturdy and compact youth who was not only scholastically bright but athletically successful and popular with it.

'By the end of my junior year I had my act together,' says Williams. 'I was a good student – a member of the Magna Cum Laude society, in fact – and I was going to be president of the senior class. I was looking forward to a very straight existence and was planning to attend either a small college in the Midwest or, if I was lucky, an Ivy League school.'

A bright and shining future beckoned Robin Williams. He could have gone on to study law, business, economics, whatever he chose. The world was pretty much his oyster. But while he was looking forward to his career, his father was becoming more and more disillusioned with his. The car industry in the late Sixties was not the industry that Robert Williams had joined. He was becoming increasingly frustrated with the declining standards and lack of concern for quality and value for money which he had once held so dear. As in almost every other industry, the grey men in suits were starting to take over and he wanted no part of it.

In 1968, at the age of 62, Robert Williams decided he had had enough and announced that he was retiring. Not only that, he was retiring to California. The family was on the move once again, and Robin Williams was about to find out that his way in the world would not be along the path he thought he had chosen.

3

In Old Tiburon

Tiburon is a quiet, residential town just 18 miles north of San Francisco on the other side of the Bay. It's a 40-minute rush-hour commute by car or bus to downtown San Francisco. The ferry sailing takes half the time and on a fine day it's an enjoyable trip. Tiburon is a pleasant retreat for the upwardly mobile, and during working hours the town empties as most of its population heads to either San Francisco or nearby Oakland.

The Spanish discovered Tiburon when they first explored San Francisco Bay in 1776. They named the peninsula Punta de Tiburon or Shark Point, *tiburon* being the Carib Indian word for shark. Some 220 years later Tiburon is a quiet residential community but it is one with an interesting past. Tiburon Town was created in 1884. It sprung up when the North-western Pacific railroad reached the north side of San Francisco Bay and completed a rail-ferry link with the city of San Francisco. Wealthy San Franciscans had been steadily migrating to the North Bay to buy property in nearby Belvedere, which had been subdivided as a 'residential park' and leisure retreat for those who could afford it. The rail-ferry link provided a fast, safe and convenient service across the Bay, and Tiburon grew steadily over the years. Sailing was another popular pastime and during Prohibition the town achieved a deal of notoriety because its safe harbour provided the ideal landing site for bootleggers smuggling booze.

Bootlegging was a lucrative but short-lived revenue source but it did attract the tourists, who continued to visit even after the Volstead Act was repealed in 1933. The heart of Tiburon remained the railroad yard and through the years the town grew around it. It was a thriving community. As well as the railroad there was good dairy farmland and herds of cattle grazed on the lush green hills surrounding the cove. It seemed that the railroad would be there for ever, but eventually it fell victim to the nationwide drift to private transport and the last train left the depot in 1967.

Tiburon has responded well to the challenge of change. A visitor to the town now would be hard pressed to recognise its railroad origins. The railyard is long gone. A clutch of chic shops and restaurants and a discreet row of condos now nestle where the trains once ran. The former pasture land has similarly been turned into high-priced housing. The old waterfront is now a shoreline park and the only trace of its heritage is in the historic Ark Row. In the old days the more Bohemian houseboat-dwellers of Tiburon would moor their boats here in the winter. A couple of the originals are still here, surrounded by shops and stores built in the same design. It's a quiet town, an upmarket Bedford Falls, and if it's not quite at the stage where everyone knows everyone else, it has a strong and well-developed sense of community. It's the sort of town where shops can close for maternity leave and the birth of the new baby is announced in the shop window to the delight of passing customers. It's the sort of town where a business can announce it's closing early because the entire staff are going on a skiing weekend. It's the sort of town, in fact, which guarantees a quiet and contented life.

It was to Tiburon that Robert Williams came when he retired from the rat race which the motor industry had become. Tiburon was in something of a period of transition then. The railyard had just closed and the redevelopment was about to begin. Tiburon and Belvedere have now reached maximum density, but in the late Sixties there was still plenty of space for a home befitting the Williams's status. In Tiburon Robin Williams very definitely was a rich kid. He has acknowledged as much in his act with gags to the effect that he wasn't really that rich – after all he had to wait until he was 16 for his first Mercedes.

Although he had been doing well at school, there was no resentment on Williams' part over being taken out of boarding school in the Midwest and shipped half-way across the country to California. For one thing, he wanted to go home to be with his family, and for another he would relish the chance to spend more time with his father. Williams completed his high-school education at Redwood High School in Larkspur, just a ten-minute drive from his new home. The drive was made not in a Mercedes, but in a Land Rover which his parents had bought for him. Williams admits that compared with the Midwest his new home in Marin County was something of a culture shock, but nothing was quite as shocking as his new school. At Detroit Country Day School he had worn the uniform – a fetching blue-and-gold blazer – and carried a briefcase. At Redwood the dress code was a little different.

> Well at first I still carried my briefcase [he remembers] and guys would either ask, 'Who's the geek?' or stare at me and say, 'Wow, a briefcase – how unmellow. You're really creating negative energy.' In the Midwest if your classmates thought you were creating negative energy, you'd hear 'Yo!', followed by a right cross to the jaw. It took me a few weeks before I showed up at Redwood without a tie on, and within a couple of months, I finally took the big step and went to school in jeans . . . Right after I started wearing jeans, somebody gave me my first Hawaiian shirt and I was gone; I got into a wild phase and I learned to totally let go.

The atmosphere inside the classrooms of Redwood High was every bit as different from Detroit Country as the dress code. The school had courses in film-making and psychology courses based on group encounters where the entire class would stop what they were doing for a group hug. Redwood also had a Black Studies department, although Williams insists there was only one black student at the school and he wanted nothing to do with it. The overall effect was an eye-opening and invigorating experience for the teenage Williams.

> I went from this all boys private school to a gestalt high school where some of the teachers were taking acid [he remembers]. It was great to go into a history class and find teachers saying 'I'm Lincoln'. It changed me, [going] from this private school which was very rigid to this full-out crazy school which was amazing. I thought, 'This is certainly different. I guess we won't be speaking Latin here.' This was in 1969 when there was rioting in certain places, when people were tripping their heads off. That was the transitional year for me. That was the year that changed everything.

Things were different in California in 1969 from almost anywhere else in the United States. The drug culture was almost *de rigueur* and it was at Redwood that Williams began to experiment with drugs for the first time. Before he came to California he claims he didn't even know what marijuana looked like; now he was smoking it. But at that stage he never got into it in a big way. Williams' hero at the time was the marathon runner and Olympic champion Frank Shorter – Williams even grew a moustache to look more like him – and he thought smoking grass might harm his endurance. He had just made the school cross-country team and didn't want to do anything which might damage his stamina. His only experience with serious drugs came just before he graduated when someone gave him some peyote without telling him. Watching his friend's face turn to rubber and melt before his eyes was apparently a salutary experience.

Redwood also did one more thing for Robin Williams. It made him realise that he was funny. Up till then he had been entertaining his mother with his routines at home. Obviously the strict regime at Detroit Country was not conducive to Williams' character 'schtick', but in the liberal surroundings of Redwood he blossomed.

'In the last year of high school it just sort of kicked out,' Williams explains. 'It wasn't like I had gone all through school being the class clown. It was like being a closet comedian – better latent than never – and then it finally happened in my first year at college and it was such fun.'

After his mother, his schoolmates at Redwood were Robin Williams' first serious audience and he left them rolling in the aisles. When he graduated he was voted 'Most Humorous Boy in School' and hand in hand with that he was also voted 'Least Likely to Succeed'.

In terms of his success after high school both Robin Williams and his parents had a fair idea what they wanted from life. When they sat down to choose a college his parents were keen that it should be one which would equip their son for a useful working life. His background thus far meant he would be studying liberal arts, but the idea of education in abstraction did not appeal to either Williams or his parents. They wanted their son to be able to take his obvious academic talent and wed that to some useful application in the working world. The syllabus and outlook of Claremont McKenna College seemed to fit the bill exactly. It was relatively new, having been founded in 1946, and was perfectly in tune with America's muscular take-charge view of the postwar world. The founder of the college, Donald McKenna, had envisaged an institution which would provide the basic grounding and preliminary training for business and the law. His 'Statement of Purpose' from 1946 explains his aims succinctly.

> Business administration and public administration are to be taught in combination so that their numerous interlocking aspects can be clearly studied from a bi-partisan viewpoint. The emphasis on training for leadership in public and private administration does not, however, imply a narrow vocational training. The new School will require its students to complete courses in the same broad fields of human knowledge as do

> the social science majors in the customary liberal arts college ... It is a fundamental part of the purpose of this institution that all who engage in the life and work of the college shall experience some of the great ethical and spiritual influences which are essential in building the character and effectiveness of individuals. For those who are to guide the corporate and public affairs in modern society, the importance of ethical foundations can hardly be overestimated.

At Claremont, Robin Williams would be groomed to take his place among America's élite. His parents were already looking to their son taking up a career in the diplomatic service where he could fully utilise his mother's grace and charm and his father's pragmatism. Claremont McKenna seemed to be the ideal place to equip him for that life. Williams had a sharp mind and was keen on politics and philosophy, and since Claremont specialised in political science it seemed like an ideal fit. In addition, the college also set great store by athletic achievement. Although it is a small school with around a thousand students, more than one in three of those students take part in team sports, so his new-found athletic skills would also be challenged.

The choice of this relatively staid college after a year at Redwood may seem surprising. According to Robin Williams his career choice was the last vestige of his Midwestern upbringing before becoming a fully-fledged Californian free spirit. He went to Claremont, which is some 35 miles north of Los Angeles, with the intention of studying politics and joining the foreign service. Williams took eight classes in his freshman year, mostly political theory and economics, but his choices also included one elective in theatre studies. After only an hour in class he was hooked. It was, as he remembers, 'a gas'.

'The school theatre seated about 80 people and we formed an improv group called The Synergy Trust and we filled the place every Friday night. I'd never had so much fun in my life, which was probably why I didn't show up for any of my other classes.'

Williams' work did suffer drastically and his absences from his other classes became so noticeable that at the end of the year some of the teachers who were supposed to be lecturing to him hadn't even met him. Williams maintains that his answer to the end-of-year essay in his macroeconomics course consisted of the five words 'I really don't know, sir'. It was obvious that Williams and Claremont would not remain in each other's company for long. Claremont was in the business of producing America's élite, not improvisational artists, and, having failed every course, Williams left at the end of the year. His sojourn at Claremont had been enough to convince Robin Williams that the life of a diplomat was not for him – he wanted to be an actor. When he broke the news to his parents his mother's reaction was entirely as you might expect. Laurie Williams, who believes that 'man was put on earth to know great joy', wished him good luck and told him his grandmother would have been very proud of him.

Under the circumstances his father's response was remarkably restrained. Robert Williams understood what it was like to have a dream; his had been beaten out of him by an industry obsessed with the bottom line. He was not therefore about to stand in the way of his son's dream. His only caveat, quite reasonably, was that there was no point in him paying Claremont's pricey tuition fees if Williams wasn't going into the foreign service.

'My father was wonderful,' remembers Williams. 'He said, "I'm not going to pay for you to go to that college, but if you want to come home and keep going with it [acting], that's okay. I also want you to study welding, just in case." '

Robert Williams was nothing if not a practical man. He knew that nothing could be achieved other than alienating his son by standing in his way. On the other hand he also knew that in a fickle business like acting his son would do well to have a second string to his bow – a career like welding would be perfect to fall back on. Both aims could be satisfied at Marin Junior College, a community college on Williams' side of the Golden Gate Bridge and within easy travelling distance of the family home. Robin Williams was delighted with his parents' reaction, and he was eager to fall into line with his father's wishes, but welding proved a little more than he was capable of.

'I went for one day to welding class and this man put on a mask and said, "Basically, you can be blinded if there's an accident." So I thought I would pass on that and keep on with the theatre.'

At Marin College, Williams threw himself whole-heartedly into learning more of the craft of acting. Improvisational theatre had appealed initially, he says, because there were no lines to learn. Now he was becoming more disciplined. Marin College had an excellent theatre department which would make demands on Williams' ambition. The school auditorium also had a replica of the Globe Theatre stage, and it was here that Robin Williams got his first taste of Shakespeare. He loved every minute of it.

'I was off and running,' he says about the adrenalin rush of his early days in improv. 'It was a chance to build on all the knowledge that you had acquired in school. When it works it's wonderful, but when it doesn't it's really a little scary.'

Williams' experience at Claremont had been a cathartic one. The whole world had opened up to him with the discovery that he could act and he could make people laugh. The shy little boy had been banished to the background, the grown-up Robin Williams had found a way to compensate and a way to ensure that he would never be picked on again.

4

It's a Helluva Town

The theatre course at Claremont McKenna College had opened up Robin Williams' eyes to a lot of things, and not just creative ones. In his short time in California Williams had discovered girls in a big way. Back in Michigan at the all-boys Detroit Country Day School, girls were like strange creatures from another planet. They were encountered once or twice a year when they were bused in for school dances. Having been placed in front of them they were then whisked away again, usually just as things were getting interesting, leaving behind a testosterone-drenched hall full of hormonally excited pubescent males.

But in California things were different. Williams jokes that the difference between a California girl and a Michigan girl is a handgun, but he certainly found that California girls were everything that the Beach Boys had led him to believe they might be. And they found him every bit as attractive as he found them. Williams was in good shape physically, the running and the wrestling and exercising having all contributed to a compact but athletic physique. More importantly, he could make them laugh, always a plus in any courtship ritual. The scales started to fall from Williams' eyes in the summer of 1969 when he took a holiday job before going to Claremont. Williams was working in the Trident restaurant in Sausalito, a place which would effectively be his finishing school in terms of California culture. Sausalito is now a glorified tourist trap and popular ferry destination about half-way round the coast between San Francisco and Tiburon. When Williams first knew it, the small coastal town was firmly in the vanguard of the counter-culture. It still retained much of the atmosphere of the Bohemian haven which had given the world such disparate talents as Jack London and William Randolph Hearst. Williams remembers the Trident – which is now long gone – as having the most beautiful waitresses in the world.

> It also had the strangest waitresses in the world [he recalls]. They wore spray-on two-piece macramé outfits that looked like a pair of socks. It was like 'Sonja, your nipple's hanging out'. And she'd say, 'I know, I'm trying to get tips'. Girls literally had to audition for their jobs. They'd come in and get their pictures taken and most of them were these lovely earth princesses. They'd go up to a table and say, 'Hello, I'm your waitress. How's your energy today?'

The effect of all of this on a boy from the Midwest who was dealing with the last remnants of his sexual repression must have been considerable. Not even a year at Redwood High had prepared him for this. And by the time he got to Claremont at the end of the summer his sexual hang-ups were well and truly behind him. The trip to Claremont wasn't just the beginning of college, it was a rite of passage.

> I really made the transition to manhood when I went away to college, moving away from home to where there was no one dictating what choices I had to make and I went berserk for one year. I just went 'Fuck this! There are girls to sleep with! And improvisational theatre classes where you don't have to learn any lines and people laugh.' I did all the shit that I ever wanted to do. Flunked out of all the political science classes but found what I'm doing now. It was this weird catharsis. Total freedom . . . Everything opened up. The whole world just changed in that one year.

By the time Robin Williams went to Marin Junior College he had more or less come to terms with his new identity. He was not as wild and he was much more focused on doing what he now knew he wanted to do with his life. He was, he believed, going to be an actor. Although he could make people laugh, he was convinced that his talents lay in the more legitimate theatre. And he wanted to learn and stretch himself. When they did *Romeo and Juliet* Williams chose to play Mercutio, Romeo's sidekick, rather than Romeo himself. The reason was simple: although Romeo is the one with his name in the title, Mercutio is the one with all the best lines. Robin Williams thrived on Shakespeare although his acting idols were people like Marlon Brando and Jason Robards. Privately he fancied himself following in the footsteps of someone like Robards, perhaps the quintessential American actor of his generation.

By day Williams was studying Shakespeare at Marin Junior College, but by night he was honing his improvisational skills. One of the country's leading improvisational groups, The Committee, was based in San Francisco. The first time he saw them Williams was completely knocked out. He had some experience of improvisational theatre from The Synergy Trust at Claremont, but by his own admission he was still a little naïve about the way things actually worked: 'I always thought, "Oh God, that's so brilliant." I didn't realise that some of it was scripted and they may have been doing that scene for the past three years.'

The Committee with its ground-breaking work was definitely the group to be with in the early Seventies, and Williams combined his time at Marin with studying with The Committee as well. It was an intense two-and-a-half-year period in which he did a lot of performing in almost every type of production it was possible to mount. He also came to realise that if he was serious about his ambitions as an actor then he would have to leave San Francisco. For all its European influences, San Francisco is something of a backwater theatrically. It could not compete with New York, Chicago, or even its deadly rival Los Angeles – the self-styled Athens of the West. If he stayed in San Francisco Williams faced the dubious prospect of becoming world famous in the Bay area. He could earn a living but he would not be stretched as an actor. There would be no way of maintaining the forward momentum which is vital to the growth of a performer.

The heart of the American theatrical establishment is New York, with the bright lights of Broadway as well as the chance to try out off-Broadway or, if you're really ambitious, off-off-Broadway. Either way Robin Williams knew that sooner or later he was going to have to leave San Francisco, and with his course at Marin Junior College coming to an end it was a decision that would need to be made sooner rather than later. The Juilliard School in New York is a world-wide centre of excellence as far as training in the arts is concerned. The school itself is a concrete oasis just beside the Lincoln Center in Columbus Circle at the north end of Broadway. As they make their way along its corridors and across its plazas, students can hear the roar of traffic coming from the Great White Way; they can see the glare of the neon and almost smell the greasepaint. Juilliard had primarily been concerned with teaching music, but in 1968 it had set up a drama department for those for whom the lure of Broadway was irresistible. Juilliard prides itself on its high standards and it will go to almost any lengths and travel any distance to find a promising student.

As a matter of course it regularly holds auditions in major cities throughout the United States.

Williams had heard that Juilliard had started a drama school. He had also heard that they were auditioning in San Francisco. If he could get an audition and if he was successful then he would qualify for a full scholarship which would take him to New York without being a drain on his family. Any audition is a daunting process, and even though Williams had got over his shyness it was still a fear-drenched experience, especially with so much riding on the outcome of those few minutes. The regional auditions usually attract hundreds of would-be students and on the day Williams was told to attend there were about fifty others trying out. Williams had prepared two contrasting pieces for his audition. The first piece was a speech by Malvolio from Shakespeare's *Twelfth Night*, the second a scene from John Knowles' novel *A Separate Peace.* Both were legit pieces – the Knowles book is an allegory about love and death in the Second World War which is a standard high-school text – and there was no improvisational comedy. In any event the audition was successful and Robin Williams was offered a three-year scholarship to the Juilliard School.

Going to Juilliard in September 1973 was the biggest step of Robin Williams' life. He was 21 years old, and despite his having reached the age of maturity, his family could not have been anything but concerned. He had lived a life of privilege, he had been born to money, and although he had been away from home before there was a world of difference between surviving at boarding school or college and surviving on his own in New York. There would be no support system, no schoolmates – even bullying classmates are better than none at all – and no friends. He would be completely alone. For all that, however, Williams was perversely keen to go. He knew it would be difficult and possibly emotionally painful, but he also knew that he was in danger of 'becoming terminally mellow' if he remained in San Francisco. New York held a sense of danger, a threat which Williams genuinely found appealing. He suspected the city would force him to toughen up mentally as well as physically, although he couldn't have expected it would have happened quite so quickly.

> On my first day in New York [he remembers] I went to school dressed like a typical California kid. I wore tie-up yoga pants and a Hawaiian shirt, and I kept stepping in dog shit with my thongs. My first week there I was in a bus going uptown to see an apartment when an old man two seats in front of me suddenly collapsed and died. He slumped over against a woman sitting next to him and she said 'Get off me!' and moved away. Somebody

> told the driver what had happened, so he stopped the bus and ordered everybody off, but I wanted to stay and help. The driver told me, 'He's dead, motherfucker, now get off! You can't do shit for him, so take your raggedy California ass and get outta my bus!' I knew that living in New York was certainly going to be different.

That's a story which sounds as though it may have been embellished somewhat over the years, but the point is still well made. Life in New York was different and, like Dorothy, Robin Williams knew he wasn't in Kansas any more. One thing helped; he found a friend very quickly. Because he was 21 when he went to Juilliard, Robin Williams was much older than most of the other students. He was being taken in as an advanced student which meant he would then have to work much harder to catch up with those who had already been at Juilliard for at least a year. Williams was one of two advanced students, the other being a young man called Christopher Reeve who had similarly been studying elsewhere.

Christopher Reeve was the ideal Juilliard student. He was dashing, handsome and prodigiously talented. Like Williams he was a privileged child; his mother was a journalist and his father a college professor. Unlike Williams he came from a broken home; his parents divorced when he was four although his mother was later married again, to a stockbroker. He had also started in the public school system but was so gifted that he switched to a private school so he might be more challenged academically. Something of a prodigy, Reeve studied music and voice and worked as an assistant orchestra conductor. When he was only nine years old he made his stage début in a professional production of a Gilbert and Sullivan operetta at the McCarter Theater in Princeton. By the time he was 16 he had an agent and immediately after graduating from high school he played Hollywood star Celeste Holm's leading man in a touring production of a play called *The Irregular Verb to Love.* He continued to combine professional acting with his studies at Cornell University thanks to an understanding agent who arranged auditions to suit his academic schedule.

Reeve had been at Cornell – where he majored in English and graduated with honours – while Williams had been at Marin. However, when they were thrown together in adverse circumstances they became fast friends. Reeve, who is a native New Yorker, is a few months younger than Williams but it seems reasonable to assume that Williams would have been somewhat in awe of a man who could be so effortlessly talented and still so likeable. Reeve for his part recalls being both amused and intrigued by 'this California kid who walked around in tie-dyed shirts and a track suit and knew about Eastern religions and Tai Chi'. Reeve was fitting in pretty well at Juilliard, but Williams was finding the work more difficult than he could have imagined and it was only his friendship with Reeve which made life bearable. They were near-neighbours, as it turned out, and after a day of being mauled by his teachers, Williams would walk the half-mile or so to Reeve's apartment building. The two young men would open a bottle of the cheapest wine they could stomach and talk about cabbages and kings long into the night.

If the first few months in New York were hard, there was worse to come for Robin Williams. Christmas rolled around and everyone, including Reeve, had gone home for the holidays. Williams couldn't afford to go back to Tiburon and was too proud to ask his parents for the cash they would doubtless have gladly given. Instead he chose to stay on his own in New York.

> It was the first cold winter I'd experienced in many years and New York seemed unbearably bleak and lonely. One day, I started sobbing and I couldn't stop. When I ran out of tears my body just kept on going; it was like having emotional dry heaves. I went through two days like that and finally hit rock bottom and realised I had a choice; I could either tube out or level off and relax. At that point, I became like a submarine on the bottom that blows out some ballast and gets back up again . . . Once in a while it's good to have a nervous breakdown. A little emotional house cleaning never hurt anybody. Once all my anxieties were behind me, the rest of the year was easy.

5

Damaged but Interesting

Robin Williams' breakdown in December of 1973 was simply an accident waiting to happen. He had gone to New York just three months earlier convinced that he was doing the right thing, determined that he was no longer going to be a big fish in a small pond. What he found was that he didn't know a fraction of what he thought he knew and if Juilliard was the pond in which he was now swimming, then he was barely at the level of plankton. Basically his teachers at Juilliard told him in pretty short order that almost everything he thought he had learned up to this point was completely and totally wrong.

'It's a little like the Army,' says Williams by way of comparison. 'They break you down and then they build you back up. In my first few days at school I learned that I didn't project out, that I talked too fast, and that I swallowed my words.'

Williams' confidence was shot to pieces. It also wasn't helped by the fact that, coming in as advanced students at an age where they should have been in their third year, he and Christopher Reeve were frequently in classes by themselves. Williams would almost certainly have suffered in comparison to Reeve at this stage, but now his shortcomings were being exposed almost on a one-to-one basis. The teaching methods at Juilliard contributed to this. At Marin Junior College and at The Committee, the method was to take scenes, break them down, and then discuss them. At Juilliard, however, the teaching focused on the individual skills and techniques that were required for an actor. Williams at this stage was an intuitive performer rather than a disciplined one, and he was quickly very aware of how much he needed to learn.

> One of the first things I tried in class was a religious monologue Dudley Moore had done in *Beyond the Fringe*. I thought I had done fine but my teacher, a man named Michael Kahn, hated it so much that he said to me, 'You have two choices. Come back and do it again or give up any thoughts you have about an acting career.' He really was furious with me and it was because I had only imitated what I had heard and hadn't tried to find new things that would make the piece mine.

Williams was shocked by Kahn's criticism but he also acknowledges that it had the desired effect. It was supposed to shake him up and make him think about what he wanted to do, rather than regurgitate other people's ideas.

> A lot of teachers were intense [Williams continues], including a New Yorker named Gene Loesser who would stop you in the middle of a reading and shout, 'What the fuck do you think you're doing?' What we were doing was working our asses off; between all the acting, speech, movement and even fencing classes, we'd be at Juilliard from eight in the morning until nine or ten o'clock at night.

Although Michael Kahn may have loathed Williams' monologue, there were others, including Christopher Reeve, who did not share that opinion. 'John Houseman had an idea of what the Juilliard actor should be, well spoken but a bit homogenised, so it's not surprising the teachers were thrown by Robin,' according to Reeve. 'That monologue from *Beyond the Fringe* made us laugh so hard we were in physical pain. They said it was a "comedy bit, not acting".'

John Houseman was the head of the Juilliard drama department. Houseman was one of America's most distinguished and respected actors and writers. With Orson Welles he had founded the Mercury Theater and helped write and produce some of their most famous work, including the notorious *War of the Worlds* broadcast in 1938. Houseman had also contributed significantly to *Citizen Kane* both as a writer and producer, but he and Welles parted company when Welles insisted on taking all the credit. Undeterred by the acrimonious split, Houseman went on to a successful career as a producer working with directors such as Vincente Minnelli, Max Ophuls and John Frankenheimer. In 1973, the year that Williams went to Juilliard, Houseman had made his film début at the age of 70 when he starred in *The Paper Chase.* The role of a sadistic law professor was originally intended for Edward G. Robinson, but terminal illness prevented Robinson from taking the part. When it was offered to James Mason he said he wasn't interested, so director James Bridges then went to Juilliard to find Houseman. The part made Houseman an international name and he won an Oscar for Best Supporting Actor, joining an élite band who have won Oscars for their film débuts. He would also reprise the role in a short-lived but highly-praised television series based on the film. By any standard Houseman was the jewel in Juilliard's drama crown.

It was undoubtedly at Houseman's suggestion that Williams was taken out of the third-year advanced class and made to start all over again at the first-year level. Christopher Reeve believes it was simply because they didn't know what to make of Williams. Reeve was always convinced of Williams' ability. The first time he saw his friend act it was in *The Night of the Iguana* in which Williams played Nonno, the old man. According to Reeve it was 'an amazingly full characterisation'. It seems certain that although he was a long way from the finished article, Houseman saw something in this young man whom he described as 'damaged but interesting'. By taking him back and grounding him in the basics he perhaps hoped that the talent he recognised would reach its potential. In many ways it was a real-life version of his screen persona as the tyrannical Professor Kingsfield.

Whatever the reason, Williams responded to Houseman, whom he took as a kind of role model. He admired Houseman's passion and saw the sense in Houseman's argument that if he was classically trained then he could go anywhere. During his early days at Juilliard Williams was having particular problems with an English Literature course which he looked liked failing. It was Houseman who took the time to sit him down for a very elegant pep talk in which he advised him that perhaps it was time to pull himself together. Williams quickly became one of John Houseman's biggest fans. He knew that he was having a hard time at the hands of his mentor, but at the same time he could see what Houseman – described by Williams as 'a card-carrying radical' – was trying to do.

'I don't think he wanted us just to crank out classical actors,' says Williams – at odds with Christopher Reeve for once – 'but people who would go out and change things.'

Houseman by this stage, with the Oscar and the television series, had become a man of some influence as well as something of a household name. Williams could not have been the only one who saw the irony in the situation.

'John Houseman gave a speech one day,' Williams recalls, 'in which he said, "The theatre needs you. Don't be tempted by television or the movies. The theatre needs new plasma, new blood." And then a week later, we saw him [on television] in a Volvo commercial.'

Although it was never completely easy, life at Juilliard became progressively easier after that first cathartic Christmas. Williams' comedy may not have gone down well with the teachers, but his fellow students loved it. Between classes and after school the locker-room became an impromptu improv comedy club as Williams and his friends tried constantly to outdo each other – the atmosphere was intensely competitive. Money worries had also eased quite considerably. Williams took his new-found skill in movement classes and began to perform at lunchtime as a mime on the steps of the Metropolitan Museum. Williams' skill and gift for physical comedy made him a very successful draw for the tourists and office workers. On a good week he could make up to $100, which helped to pay for his food, clothes and rent.

During his second year at Juilliard Robin Williams fell in love. He had been in love before, having had a spectacular crush on a young girl he had met at Marin Junior College, but this, he felt, was the real thing. The girl in question – Williams has never revealed her name – had come to New York from California and Williams was completely captivated by her. She was, he remembers, a free spirit, and when the two of them went back to Marin County at the end of his second year the relationship really deepened. His girlfriend was staying in California and Williams was so much in love that he did not want to go back to Juilliard.

As he saw it there wasn't a lot to go back for. Christopher Reeve had graduated from Juilliard the previous year and had gone first to England and then to France, where he worked at the Old Vic and the Comédie Française. When he came back to the United States he landed a leading role as Ben Harper on the long-running daytime soap opera *Love of Life.* Without his best friend Juilliard held little charm for Williams, and he was also concerned about the amount of actual training that he would now be getting. In their third year Juilliard students spent a lot of time out on the road performing shows in community theatre projects. They could go from playing the toughest neighbourhood in the Bronx one night to playing the rarefied social climes of Park Avenue on the next. Life was hard for Williams. Maintaining a long-distance romance was an incredible strain. He was racking up phone bills of around $400 a month just to keep in touch and by the time he paid these there was barely enough money left to pay the rent.

As Williams saw it there was only one thing left to do. He would leave

Juilliard and go back to California to be with the woman in his life. He was just over two years into his three-year course, but it was not as difficult a decision as he had thought it might be. Once again, as he had in San Francisco, Williams felt he had reached a point where he had gone as far as he could. It was time to move on. He wasn't sure where to in career terms, but he knew he had reached the end of the line at Juilliard. Geographically at least he was moving on to San Francisco. When he got back, however, things didn't work out anything like he had planned. He and his girlfriend set up home together, but after little more than a month of living with each other they parted company. The relationship ended and Williams went into a massive depression, which only got worse when he couldn't find any work.

Juilliard had been good for Robin Williams. He is not slow to acknowledge the debt he owes to the institution for providing him with the grounding which enabled him to make such a success of his career. But it undoubtedly also exacted its pound of flesh from the young man. He was a square peg whom they had resolutely but unsuccessfully tried to force into a round hole without much regard for the consequences.

'They were trying to mould Robin into a standardised Juilliard product,' says Christopher Reeve, citing Kevin Kline as the perfect example of what he believes they were looking for. 'But Robin was too special, too original, to be that. They kept breaking him down. It's amazing how he tried, how much he took.'

6

Fly Like an Eagle

Once again Robin Williams was in the middle of a deep depression. His early days back in San Francisco after dropping out of Juilliard were among the unhappiest of his life. His relationship with his girlfriend, which had seemed so full of promise back in New York, had now come to a sudden and abrupt end. It's interesting to speculate on the reasons, even though Williams himself seldom speaks publicly about it. In an interview in *Playboy* magazine some years later, the subject turned to the Bush administration's stance on abortion. Williams agonised about the plight of the poor who would be forced into a terrible dilemma of either having an unwanted child or consulting a potentially deadly backstreet abortionist. Williams offered that making the decision to have an abortion was not an easy one, which begged the obvious question from interviewer Lawrence Gróbel about whether he had ever found himself in that position.

'Long, long, long time ago,' Williams replied candidly, 'and it was because we were too young and it wasn't right.'

The time period between the 1992 *Playboy* interview and the break-up of his relationship in 1976 would certainly constitute a 'long, long, long time ago'. That being the case, did Williams and the love of his life split up because she had become pregnant?

Whatever the reason, Robin Williams' relationship had come to a dead end, but so too, it seemed, had his career. Williams had set aside the promise of a successful career three years earlier to go to New York. Surely, he reasoned, with almost three years of training at one of the world's finest schools behind him it would not be difficult to find work in his home town. As it turned out, however, when he tried to join some of the city's professional theatre companies, no one wanted to know. Williams couldn't get arrested in San Francisco in 1976. If he thought he had come to the end of the line in Juilliard, he must have begun to realise that in San Francisco he had well and truly hit the buffers.

Williams' only recourse was to go back to the only other thing he knew he could do. He put his legitimate acting career on hold and decided he would try his hand at making people laugh. San Francisco in 1976 was one of the breeding grounds for America's nascent generation of stand-up comedians.The city teemed with comedy clubs, and if Williams could be as successful with an audience as he had with his school fellows at Redwood and Marin and his classmates at Juilliard then he might have a chance.

> Comedy had always been an outlet for me [he explains], but I'd always treated it a bit like a guerrilla activity. It became primary for two reasons. It was a form of therapy which helped me get over the relationship and it also allowed me to support myself for the first time. I'd do $25 a night gigs and I'd actually make enough to pay my $100 a month rent. I was self-sustaining and I could say, 'No Pop, I don't need that cheque. But thanks.'

Williams' comment about his parents is interesting. Obviously they would not have been unconcerned about how their son was feeling, but they were caring enough to stay at arm's length to let him work out his problems for himself. The fact that his father was more than willing to subsidise him in order for his son to follow his dream also gives the lie to the notion of Robert Williams being aloof and uncaring.

Robin Williams quickly joined a comedy workshop which was run by a man called, appropriately, Frank Kidder. While the students worked in classes during the week, Kidder encouraged them to put what they had learned into practice by performing at the weekend. Williams quickly put a stand-up routine together and made his comedy début at a now defunct club called The Intersection on Union Street. The club was a former coffee-house in the basement of an old church. Since the comedians would generally come on after some avant-garde feminist poetry readings it wasn't necessarily the easiest room he would ever play. Another veteran of The Intersection, Lorenzo Matawaran, remembers it being a tough room. But he also remembers how Williams made it his own: 'Robin got up and blew everyone away, but he was meek the way he still is. He'd do a monster set and then come sit down and ask us in that little voice, "Did

I go over?" We used to have an Indian name for him – "Squirrel-Boy-Who-Turns-Into-Golden-Eagle-Onstage". When that grew too long we just shortened it to "Eagle".'

Williams quickly established himself and began to make the rounds of the clubs, touring the 'open mike' nights – generally in the quieter earlier part of the week – when just about anyone could get up and do their stuff. As he became more successful the bookings started to get better. The Boarding House was a San Francisco comedy club which prided itself on bringing in the best comedy talent from Los Angeles, New York and right across the country. Robin Williams became the first local comedian to play The Boarding House in what amounted to a major coup. His success there meant that he had opened the doors for other local comics to follow.

'Robin has a tremendously inquiring mind,' says David Allen, the owner of The Boarding House, who became a close friend of his new find. 'He was a street performer back in New York, so he knows how to look into people's lives, but he's got a number of other interests. He roller-skates, has a very serious concern about environmental issues, has a deep and abiding interest in the theatre, and he gets a kick out of sports cars. Everything he does for fun seems to end up in his act somehow because he is such a fantastic observer.'

Robin Williams was nonetheless still a fairly troubled young man at this stage. He admits himself that, had he not been doing stand-up, he shudders to think what the consequences might have been. The comedy was a release which enabled him to deal with the frustrations of the world. What he referred to as his 'duck and cover' technique allowed him to hide his real self away while dealing with his problems through a variety of different characters. The traditions of stand-up comedy are rooted in verbal violence. Old-time vaudevillians and the comedians who plied their trade in the early days of radio and television would talk of their work in the most aggressive terms. Audiences were 'killed' or 'slayed' or 'murdered'. It was almost an act of gladiatorial defiance as the lone comedian stepped into the spotlight in front of the baying mob.

But in the case of Robin Williams his stand-up comedy was a defence. Even when he went into his complete, frenetic, borderline psychotic routine – what he describes as 'full tilt bozo' mode – it was an act of self-defence. Williams was hiding from his problems, just as he had at school. His solution was to make people laugh while showing nothing of his real self for fear it might be used against him. His routines were a collection of fears, neuroses and repression – usually sexual repression.

'You're trying to keep the world out by being aggressively funny,' says

Williams, 'or by mocking it. Because somewhere along the line, when you let it in, it will hurt.'

Although the quickfire synaptic rhythms of his word-associative patter routines quickly became his trademark, the basis of Williams' comedy at this stage came in portraying different characters. The comedians he most admired were Peter Sellers and Jonathan Winters.

'Jonathan because of the pure madness,' he says of a man who used to do a routine in which he played King Quasi of Quasiland, a country which was five feet wide and eleven miles long. Its main exports were string and spaghetti. 'Jonathan transforms himself. He's like Buddha meets Gumby. He becomes it. With Sellers it's mostly the characters, that he could become so many different things. People who knew him said he just locked off and became the character.'

Those who knew Sellers would also point out that he was a man who would hide behind a number of comic personae, so that when the characters were stripped away there was almost nothing left of Sellers himself. Williams put together a rapidly expanding repertory company of weird and wonderful characters to hide behind. Over the years these would come to include Nicky Lenin, the Soviet Union's only entertainer, the Rev. Ernest Lee Sincere, a holy-rolling evangelist, Little Billy, a child who performed the Death of a Sperm ballet, a blind bluesman, and himself as an older man looking back on his life. These characters gave him a platform from which to free-associate and work the room while at the same time giving him something to hide behind. The characters also gave him a chance to develop a rapport with his audience; Williams' relationship with those who've paid money to see him is a good deal more gentle than that of some of his colleagues.

> I don't like to attack them [he explains]. There's a real fine line there, but if someone attacks me, like a heckler, then it's open season. I guess at the end you have to be prepared to take it yourself. If you're a character then you can get away with it, but if you're yourself then it's you who's doing the attacking and that's different. I used to do an evangelist who would heal people. I could do 'You with the bad wig, come forward. You could fly to Persia on that rug. Let's get a tight weave for Jesus.' You can do that when you're a character, you can play with those kinds of things.

Having left The Intersection behind and having cracked The Boarding House, Williams continued to ply his trade at a number of well-known clubs. One of the toughest was the Salamander in Berkeley, where he claims a bartender once shot a customer for having the temerity to ask for change. He was also becoming a regular at the Holy City Zoo, a club near Golden Gate Park where he had begun in the open mike nights on Mondays and Tuesdays. It was a small club which would hold no more than 60 people on a good night, but Williams liked the atmosphere. He built up something of a following and began to work in the club as a barman to supplement his comedy income. Also working in the same club was a cocktail waitress called Valerie Velardi. Like Williams she had her eye on bigger things while she was working at the Holy City Zoo. Her waitressing work was helping to put her through school. She was a dancer with ambitions to become a choreographer, and through a mixture of talent and determination she finally earned her Masters degree in Modern Dance.

The first night that Robin Williams and Valerie Velardi met he was coming on for 24 and she was 26. He pretended to be a Frenchman and she let him maintain the pretence even though she knew better. They quickly started a relationship and were soon inseparable.

'Was it love at first sight?' Williams wondered later. 'More like lust. She was this Italian woman, a Napoletana girl. She didn't dress sexy, she just looked . . . hot. Caliente. We hung out, we started living together.'

After the collapse of his last relationship Valerie Velardi was exactly what Robin Williams needed. Valerie was, by all accounts, a hard-headed and pragmatic young woman. The way her life had panned out up till now had given her little option to be anything else. She was the daughter of a building contractor, whose parents split up when she was 12 years old, leaving her to become a surrogate mother to three younger siblings. Valerie was used to providing a maternal influence; emotionally Robin Williams was still a mess and she provided a centre and a focus for his life. But it wasn't always easy.

'Since he didn't grow up with other children, he [Robin] is an only child as far as I'm concerned,' she said. 'The result is that he has a very rich private life, and it's hard to filter in. It's hard to get in deep with someone who's used to taking care of himself only. It's such a cliché but they make their own world.'

Within a month of meeting in the Holy City Zoo, Robin Williams and Valerie Velardi had moved in together. He thrived on the new-found stability in his life, and the work started to pour in. The money was getting better, the clubs were getting bigger, and the audiences were growing more and more enthusiastic. Once again Williams was faced with the prospect of being a big fish in a middling-sized pond. Both he and Velardi knew there was only one thing to do. They would have to make the leap of faith and try their luck in Los Angeles. It's debatable who actually had the idea of going to Los Angeles. In different interviews both Velardi and Williams have taken the credit. It seems more likely, however, that with so many other comedians from San Francisco heading for Los Angeles, Williams would naturally have wanted to prove himself in the bigger arena. The notion of heading south probably just grew organically out of the events of their daily lives. But no matter who made the decision, there was no doubt that it was Valerie Velardi who was making the sacrifice. She was mid-way through her studies and she would have to put her ambition on hold to further her boyfriend's career. In interviews of the period she never seems to have had less than 100 per cent faith in Williams' ability to succeed.

'I guess I always knew Robin was spectacularly talented,' she says, 'but I didn't trust the show business industry to pick up on it so quickly.'

Williams was well aware of what he was asking Valerie to give up. He knew that she would be passing up the chance of a career for herself because there wasn't a lot of call for choreographers in Los Angeles, a city not noted for its dance companies.

> Val supported me . . . kept me sane and most important she kept me happy. I always wanted to hit it big, but I thought it would be easier in San Francisco, where there was less competition. It was Val who made the sacrifice. She dropped her own career to help me with mine. She encouraged me, almost ordered me, to go to Hollywood. I trust Val completely. She's the best friend I have. Because she is on the outside looking in she sees things a lot clearer than I can ever possibly see them. Every so often she'll tell me to come and wash the dishes, and I like that because she knows it will keep my feet on the ground.

Of such mundane domesticity are show-business careers made. Six months after they met, Robin Williams and Valerie Velardi were on their way to Los Angeles and the Mecca for all stand-up comics, The Comedy Store on Sunset Boulevard. With its three showcase rooms The Comedy Store is effectively a multiplex for comedians. Agents, managers and other comics trawl the club like a comedy meat market looking for a hot comic or a routine they can lift. Robin Williams described his first viewing of it as 'a terrorising combination of the Roman arena and The Gong Show'. In the space of a week some 200 comedians will get up in front of the microphone and look for his or her fifteen minutes of fame; that magic moment which will propel them to sitting on the late-night couch swapping anecdotes with Dave or Jay or Conan. Robin Williams' audition was scheduled for only a few days after they had arrived in Los Angeles.

Typically he would have to show his mettle on open mike night on a Monday and prove his worth against anyone who wanted to pick up the microphone and tell a gag. The worst moments of Robin Williams' life have always been just before he goes on-stage. These are the moments when the fear has to be recognised, acknowledged and locked away before he goes out to face a crowd of complete strangers.

'My stomach was in my shoes, I was so scared,' he remembers of that first night in Los Angeles. 'But after less than a minute I felt comfortable. I knew I could make these people laugh.'

To borrow a phrase from the vernacular of Henny Youngman or Milton Berle, Williams slayed them. He had them laughing themselves sick and he was hired on the spot for a residency at a basic $200 a week. The Comedy Store was just one stop on the LA circuit. Williams worked the circuit vigorously, sometimes being billed as Robin McLaurim Williams. Among his early triumphs was an audition at the equally famous The Improv. This was typical Williams – a five-minute penis joke. The routine involved a man masturbating and watching his penis grow so large that he couldn't get out of the room. Once again they laughed until they were begging for mercy. Within weeks of leaving San Francisco to seek the big time Robin Williams was basking in the glow of being the hottest new talent in town. Williams hooked up with the late Harvey Lembeck who was running one of Los Angeles' best-known improvisational comedy ensembles. The Harvey Lembeck Comedy Workshop was the place to be if you wanted to be noticed. Lembeck was rigorous in his methods. He would simply stand there and yell out a subject and the comedians would then have to come up with a funny routine. One of his topics was a request that the class members improvise a phone call to explain that they were going to be late for an appointment. While the other comedians came up with the predictable responses, Williams improvised a routine about calling God. Lembeck knew that he had a rare talent on his hands.

Among his fellow comedians at the Lembeck company was John Ritter, who was still some years away from his TV fame on *Three's Company.*

> I saw the way this dude was dressed [remembers Ritter of their first meeting]. In baggy pants, suspenders, a beaten-up tux over high-topped sneakers, a straw hat with the brim falling off, and John Lennon glasses with no glass in the frames. I thought, 'Well, this guy is definitely going for the sight gag.' I was almost a big suspicious. So I watched carefully and he turned out to be the funniest guy I've ever seen.

Ritter and Williams became fast friends, behaving like poster boys for arrested development. They would run around like overgrown kids with water pistols or firing suction dart guns at each other. But at the same time they were capable of crafting the most brilliant improvisations. Ritter naturally settled into the classic role of the comic feed, providing Williams with the wind beneath his wings and allowing him to transform from Squirrel Boy to Golden Eagle. Ritter never once resented the arrangement. He says he saw right from the start how talented Williams was and how much potential he had. He hadn't a moment's hesitation in taking the part of the straight man. 'The first bit I ever saw him do,' remembers Ritter, 'was as a kiddie-show host. And it was the most demented thing you can imagine. He brought these puppets on-stage and did those weird voices and wound up doing an S&M routine with the puppets which is indescribable.'

Wherever he went Robin Williams was making a big impression. Nowhere more than at The Comedy Store, where his resident spots were among the biggest draws of the week. One of the people who had caught word of the buzz about the new kid in town was television producer George Schlatter. He came in one night and found that everything he had heard was true, and then some. 'I saw Robin doing a fragmented free-association act that was very, very funny,' says Schlatter. 'He was doing what I'd call dirty material. He had a full beard and hair down to his shoulders, he was barefoot and he wore overalls and a cowboy hat. But it was his originality that knocked me out.'

With the memory of that performance fresh in his mind, Schlatter approached Williams sometime later at The Comedy Store to pitch an idea to him. He was putting together a revival of *Rowan and Martin's Laugh-In* with an entirely new cast and he wanted Williams to be in it. Williams agreed almost immediately and found himself as the first cast member in what was supposed to be a pioneering new comedy show.

Williams was signed for six shows at the princely sum of $1500 a week. He was about to go from being a big fish in a small pool to being a household name. Or at least, that was the theory.

7

Sock it to Me

In 1968 radio announcer Gary Owens took American audiences for the first time to 'beautiful downtown Burbank' and brought possibly America's most revolutionary television show into their homes. Not since the great days of *Your Show of Shows* with Sid Caesar, which virtually defined television comedy in its earliest days, had a show had the impact of *Rowan and Martin's Laugh-In.*

Hosted by Dan Rowan and Dick Martin, a couple of actor-comedians in the classic pairing as suave straight man and dumb stooge, the show broke the mould as far as American television was concerned. Its formula of fast-moving, often pointless sketches with inanely repeated punchlines took America by storm. The humour, with its references to sex and drugs, was *risqué* by the standards of the period, and the whole psychedelic layout of the studio set was directly influenced by the West Coast drug culture. It made household names of Arte Johnson, Ruth Buzzi and Judy Carne, who became known as the 'Sock it to me' girl since her sole function seemed to be saying the line and then getting smacked in the head with a gag boxing glove. Other jokes were delivered by a body-painted go-go dancer, but those few moments of fame launched Goldie Hawn to stardom.

America loved it. It was a show which was directly in tune with the mood of the period. Sex and drugs were on the agenda and the establishment was there to be lampooned in the form of big-name guests who would turn up to get the treatment every week. One memorable show featured John Wayne no less in a giant pink bunny suit. *Rowan and*

Martin's Laugh-In was an instant success. Phrases like 'Sock it to me', 'You bet your bippy' and Dick Martin's lascivious 'Blow in her ear and she'll follow you anywhere' became part of the national vocabulary. The show was launched in the 1968–69 television season and stayed at number one in the Nielsen ratings for two years. But it was a programme which was very definitely of its time. After two years at the top the ratings bombed in the third season. What had once been fresh and pioneering now seemed stale and repetitive, and the show was cancelled. Even so, it left behind a rich legacy both in terms of the talent it produced and the influence it had. Rowan and Martin paved the way for shows like *Saturday Night Live* and comedians like Chevvy Chase, Eddie Murphy, John Belushi, Carrie Fisher, Dana Carvey and indeed Robin Williams himself.

Since he was away at boarding school in the great days when *Laugh-In* was in its pomp, it is debatable whether Robin Williams would have been able to see the show in first run. But he was certainly aware of its image and its reputation, which is why he was so enthusiastic when George Schlatter approached him that night at The Comedy Store. Williams was so keen that he even took Schlatter's advice and spruced himself up by shaving, getting his hair cut, and wearing something approximating to a conventional suit for his meeting with the television executives. Schlatter is a veteran television writer and producer with a number of shows such as *The Cher Show*, *Funny People*, and a Sinatra 80th birthday tribute to his credit before and since. He had a fair idea that with the growth of comic talent in the mid-Seventies there might be a possibility to recapture some of the magic of *Rowan and Martin's Laugh-In* with a whole new cast. After spotting him in The Comedy Store, Schlatter suspected that Williams would be the corner-stone of his new show, called simply *Laugh-In*.

Williams was as excited as he had ever been. When he knew he'd landed the part and realised that it paid $1500 a week, he thought he had made the big time. Mentally he was dreaming of the big house and the pool and everything else that comes with the trappings of a smash hit TV show. It didn't take long before his illusions were shattered.

'Unfortunately doing a remake of a show which had been one of the milestones of TV was a little like doing *Jaws VI*. How are you going to top the original? Are you going to have the shark come up on land and gum people to death? *Laugh-In* sure sobered my ass up. The show lasted 14 weeks and most of the time I played a redneck or a Russian.'

Schlatter had hired Williams and then put him in a show which stopped him doing what he did best. He simply wanted a clever mimic and a character comedian and there was nowhere in the show to use the more mercurial side of Williams' comic nature. *Laugh-In* became a personal if lucrative purgatory for Williams, but he never once gave anything less than his total effort. He was not happy but he wasn't about to stop working. Joan Rivers, who met Williams for the first time in the *Laugh-In* revival, says he seemed to be living off his nerves.

'You know how it is. You're struggling, you want to be noticed, and the only way to be noticed is to be the funny boy,' she recalls. 'We took a picture together and he never stopped mugging. You wanted to tie him down and say "Stop".'

George Schlatter quickly found that Dan Rowan and Dick Martin had caught lightning in a bottle with their show. It simply could not be repeated. The mood of the country had changed, and the mood of the television audience had changed along with it. Comedy in 1977 was bland and safe; it was *Welcome Back Kotter* and *Three's Company.* Within weeks it was obvious that the show was not going to work and Schlatter announced that he would be cancelling the run. It was something of a pre-emptive strike on his part: to cancel before they were cancelled, and also to try to attract the attention of the other two networks. There was no response, so *Laugh-In* ended, but its demise would have repercussions for Robin Williams further down the track.

Laugh-In had done nothing for Williams in career terms except to give him experience of working in television. It also provided him with what he now believes may be one of the single most embarrassing moments of his life. Like the original show the *Laugh-In* revival featured big-name guest stars coming on to act effectively as stooges for these young comics. Williams got to work with Hollywood legends like James Stewart, Frank Sinatra and Bette Davis, which was the up-side of the job. It also, unfortunately for him, provided a down-side which almost ended his fledgling career in ignominy.

'Frank Sinatra was on *Laugh-In* one week,' Williams recalled later. 'I went up to him and said, "Mr Sinatra, I'm so happy to meet you I could drop a log." I was afraid they would want to fire me and that I would have to explain that I never meant to upset Uncle Frank. Thank God he laughed,' said a relieved Williams.

Williams left *Laugh-In* after 14 weeks a little older, a whole lot wiser, and quite a bit better off financially. Whatever doubts he may have felt about appearing in a flop show were quickly quelled when he was hired almost straight away for another show. This time he would be working with one of his comedy idols, Richard Pryor.

For many Pryor is possibly the greatest stand-up comedian America has ever produced. He is certainly among the most influential, and his work has been an inspiration to a generation of black American comedians such as Eddie Murphy, the Wayans brothers, Martin Lawrence and Chris Rock. Given Pryor's background, it's astonishing he survived, far less became a comedian. He was born in Peoria, Illinois and raised by his grandmother in the brothel where his mother worked. He was abused physically and sexually as a child and abandoned completely by his mother when he was ten years old. The acorn plainly did not fall far from the tree in Pryor's case, and he dropped out of high school, became a teenage father himself, and spent many of his waking hours stoned on drink or drugs. Surprisingly, when he began stand-up comedy at the age of 17 his routines were safe and non-confrontational, in the mould of his role model Bill Cosby. Pryor was carving out a solid career for himself on stage and in cabaret until one night in 1969 when he had a breakdown on stage in Las Vegas.

When Pryor returned to performing he was a changed man. In 1969 he moved to the West Coast, became a black activist and was heavily involved in the counter-culture. His new stage act reflected his newly politicised status. His unashamedly excoriatingly confrontational routines about white versus black, especially in the twin areas of sex and drugs, were both shocking and rib-achingly funny. Before he ruined his health and his career with substance abuse – the lowest point came when he set himself on fire while free-basing – Pryor was as good as it got; he was the comedian to whom all others aspired. He took no risks and he took no prisoners. His 1979 concert movie *Richard Pryor – Live in Concert* is generally held to be the best stand-up routine ever committed to celluloid and one of the rare examples of Pryor's uncompromising genius caught on camera. Comedians idolised Pryor, and Robin Williams was no exception. There are comedians who make him laugh, such as George Carlin or the late Sam Kinison or Jay Leno. But Pryor was one of the few comedians that he actively envied, especially in his daring and courage in doing what Williams after all could not – talking about his own life on stage in the most frank and candid terms.

'When he kicks there is no one in the world better,' says Williams of Pryor. 'No one has ever done what he does. He is the king of that . . . And his stand-up, he sets the rules. Then he destroyed the boundaries.'

NBC, the network which had bombed with the *Laugh-In* revival, had signed Pryor to a weekly series, and Williams was also signed as a regular member of the supporting cast. Pryor had worked in television before. In his Cosby clone days he had starred in the *Kraft Summer Music Hall* for NBC in 1966. Even after his conversion Pryor had been successful as part of the Emmy-winning writing team for *The Lily Tomlin Show* and *Lily*.

Looking back, it is astonishing that anyone could have thought even for a moment that the scatology of Richard Pryor could fit on prime-time television in those pre-cable days. He had been on his best behaviour for a successful comedy showcase *The Richard Pryor Special?* Nevertheless both the network and Pryor felt that it could be made to work. NBC was obviously gambling on his new-found status as a wholesome film star in *Silver Streak*, the first of a successful series of films with Gene Wilder. It took only the first shot of the first episode of *The Richard Pryor Show* to prove both the comedian and the network catastrophically wrong. Pryor had planned to start the series by poking fun at the fact that he, possibly America's most threatening and seditious comedian, was now on prime-time television. The idea was to start with a tight shot on Pryor's face with him saying, 'I'm on TV – me, Richard Pryor – and I didn't have to give up a thing.' The camera would then simultaneously pull back and track down to reveal that Pryor was in fact naked. Not only was he naked but from the waist down, he had no genitalia, making him look like a Motown version of Barbie's boyfriend Ken. The point being, of course, that he hadn't given up a thing for prime-time television except that which every man holds dear.

The shot was instantly seized on when the show was previewed for the media, and it appeared in almost every newspaper in the country and on every television news show. But when the first episode of *The Richard Pryor Show* screened it wasn't there; the network had ordered that it be removed. This was the beginning of a long-running battle with the network which would bring Pryor close to breaking-point.

> Richard got nailed by the censors in the opening shot of the first show and that was the beginning of his frustration with TV [says Robin Williams]. It was sad, because he went into it with such hope ... After six or seven weeks he was so disillusioned that he would just do his old night club act as his monologue. They'd run film on him for 45 minutes and by the time the Broadcast Standards people got through with editing it, they could use maybe three minutes.
>
> In spite of all that, we had some great times on the show. In one sketch I played a liberal white Southern lawyer defending a black man charged with raping a girl who was a steaming hunk of white trash. I had a couple of ideas for lines but I wasn't sure if I should use them, but Richard said 'Just go for it', so I did. At one point in the trial I got up and told the jury, 'Negro – what a wonderful word. Say it with me: Negro, from the Latin word "negora" meaning "to tote".'

Williams would have given the Standards and Practices people as many headaches as Pryor with that particular sketch. It wouldn't be the last time he would be engaged in a battle of wits with the network censors over the next few years. Naturally, as Pryor became more and more disenchanted, the ratings slipped and the show was cancelled. Williams had now been on two shows which were cancelled in the space of a year, but it didn't matter. Richard Pryor had succeeded where *Laugh-In* had failed in allowing a little of Williams' natural humour to be transplanted from the stage to the tube. It was the first time Robin Williams had really had the opportunity to let himself go in comedic terms on television. It wouldn't happen again for a while, but at least he now knew that it could be done.

All the while that he was appearing on television, Williams had not neglected his stand-up work. Stand-up was where he felt most alive, and he continued to appear in Harvey Lembeck's troupe to keep the creative juices flowing and develop new material. Like The Comedy Store, Harvey Lembeck's Comedy Workshop was another required stop on the circuit for managers and agents. It was a tough gig for the comedians. They would effectively compete against each other in 'improv wars', trying to top their opponents before time-up was signalled by a buzzer or the lights going out. One night in the spring of 1978 Larry Brezner happened to stop by. Brezner was part of Joffe, Rollins, Morra & Brezner, one of the major management organisations which already looked after the interests of the likes of Woody Allen and Martin Mull. Brezner, who hadn't got where he was by not being able to spot talent, settled into his seat and quickly became absorbed in the proceedings.

> Harvey ... would throw out situations and the students would react [he recalls]. I watched this one kid get up and, no matter what situation was thrown at him, he never got lost. In an improv, right before the black-out, you've either won or lost; you either hit the big line or it lays there. I watched two hours of this kid never losing, reacting off the top of his head, working off nerve impulses – not intellect at all. Incredible.

The kid of course was Robin Williams, and Brezner was so impressed with what he had seen that night that he signed him as a client and became his first manager. 'He wasn't that different on-stage then; the attitudes were the same,' Brezner remembers. 'He's like Holden Caulfield, a guy walking around with all the nerve endings completely exposed.'

8

My Favourite Orkan

Despite two failed television shows Robin Williams was still a spectacularly talented comedian; possibly the most talented in America. But talent frequently is not enough on its own; sometimes talent needs a helping hand. Two men are responsible for making Robin Williams the success that he is today; one of them directly, the other indirectly. Williams may well be one of San Francisco's most famous citizens, but he owes a great deal to another near neighbour. George Lucas, who also lives across the Golden Gate Bridge in Marin County, is the man who is indirectly responsible for Robin Williams' meteoric rise. It is debatable whether we would ever have seen Mork, the alien from planet Ork, had it not been for two phenomenally successful films by George Lucas.

The influence of Garry Marshall on Robin Williams' career was felt much more directly. Marshall is the son of a classic showbiz mom who desperately wanted her son to be a dancer. Marshall had rhythm but not much aptitude for dance, and as a young man his ambition was to be drummer in a jazz band. He'd become a drummer when his mother finally despaired of him ever being a dancer and bought him a drum-kit so he could keep the beat for his sisters. Between gigs he supplemented his income by writing jokes and skits for the comics he met on the cabaret circuit. Marshall could turn a phrase and eventually he became a gag writer for the comedian Joey Bishop. On his own account Bishop was a good comedian without ever threatening to be a great comedian. But as one of Frank Sinatra's notorious Rat Pack, the men who defined masculinity for a generation of postwar Americans, Bishop was, by association, one of America's hottest funnymen. As his star rose, so too did Marshall's, and he eventually became a full-time writer supplying the gags on *The Dick Van Dyke Show*, the programme which became the prototype for American television comedy. From writing Marshall moved into production and became the producer of *The Odd Couple*, the television series based on the Neil Simon play which had also been a hugely successful film. By the early Seventies he was a recognised hyphenate, a writer-producer, a man of some weight who had done his duty in the trenches of television's ratings war. And it was with this kind of pedigree behind him that he made a reasonably confident pitch to the ABC network in 1971 for a new comedy.

Marshall's show was called *New Family in Town*, but no one at ABC seemed sufficiently interested to commission a series. The show eventually aired on the anthology comedy series *Love, American Style* on 25 February 1972 under the title *Love and the Happy Day*. In this case the happy day in question was the arrival of the first TV set into the lives of a Fifties' family played by Marion Ross, Harold Gould, Ron Howard and Susan Neher. Although it had not been commissioned as a series, *Love and the Happy Day* was not a total loss and would, bizarrely, play a key role in the development of American cinema. It had been seen by George Lucas and inspired a rites of passage movie he was developing about a group of teenagers in a small American town. Lucas was one of the new breed of American film-makers whose passionate love for cinema had led them to film school as a way of breaking into the business. Lucas, from Modesto in northern California, had been the *de facto* leader of an emerging group of diverse talents at the University of Southern California which also included John Carpenter, Robert Zemeckis and John Milius. From there he had gone on to be an assistant to Francis Ford Coppola, who in turn had now agreed to produce a movie which Lucas would direct from a script he had co-written with former college friends Willard Huyck and Gloria Katz. Lucas' film, *American Graffiti*, was set on a single night in an American small town in the summer of 1962 as the graduating class take their first tentative steps towards the adult world. Ron Howard, a popular TV star in his own right, had been cast in the film after appearing in the *Love, American Style* episode. *American Graffiti* also starred Richard Dreyfuss, Charlie Martin Smith, Candy Clark, Cindy Williams and, in a small role, Harrison Ford. With the exception of Howard, who had become something of an institution through his appearances on *The Andy Griffith Show*, all of them were unknown. That did not stop *American Graffiti* from being a runaway hit in the summer of 1973. It had cost just over $1 million and made more than $55 million at the US box-office. Suddenly it seemed that nostalgia was a hot property after all. Garry Marshall got the call from ABC; and happy days would soon be here again.

Marshall retooled his original proposal. For one thing the title was deemed to be a loser and the show would now be called *Happy Days* after the *Love, American Style* episode. It would now focus on the lives of one family – the Cunninghams – in small-town America in the Fifties. There were some changes from the pilot, but Marshall still put together a talented and likeable cast. Ron Howard is now at the top of Hollywood's directorial 'A' list as the man behind films such as *Splash*, *Cocoon*, *Apollo 13* and *Ransom*. In the Seventies this was all still in front of him but he was then one of American television's best-loved stars and he took the key role of Richie Cunningham. Marion Ross again played his mother, Tom Bosley was drafted in as his father, and his sister was played by Erin Moran. In the early shows Richie also had an older brother, played by Gavan O'Herlihy, but he was quickly written out. The series added two best friends – Potsie and Ralph Malph – who were played by Anson Williams and Donnie Most. But the one who would make most impression was Henry Winkler as Arthur Fonzarelli – The Fonz – who lived above the Cunninghams' garage. With a nod to Marlon Brando's biker-chic in *The Wild One*, Fonzie instantly became the coolest role model in America. A leather-clad stud muffin who was a cross between Elvis and James Dean with a heart of gold to boot, he became the idol of millions, male and female alike.

Happy Days débuted on 15 January 1974 and after a season and a half of solid ratings it eventually cracked the top ten and then remained one of America's most watched shows. It would stay in the top three in the Nielsen ratings for three years and spawn its own spin-off show *Laverne and Shirley*.

This spin-off, which starred Garry Marshall's sister Penny and Cindy Williams, came about when The Fonz and Richie Cunningham double-dated with Laverne Di Fazio and Shirley Feeney in an episode in series three of *Happy Days*. The girls ended up with their own series which was also a top-three show. If anything it was more popular than *Happy Days*, charting in the top three for four consecutive seasons. In the 1977–78 season *Laverne and Shirley* took over from *Happy Days* as America's top show, and it was about this time that Marshall started looking for fresh material. Like all sensible producers he did some market research and asked a sample of TV's biggest demographic group what should be on *Happy Days*. The sample actually consisted of Marshall's own son.

> My seven-year-old son, Scott, was reluctant to watch *Happy Days* or *Laverne and Shirley* or any show that I did [recalls Garry Marshall]. So I asked him, 'What do you like?' He said, 'I only like space.' I told him, 'I don't do space.' 'Well you could do it,' he said. So I asked him, 'How would you do space in *Happy Days*?' And he said, 'It could be a dream.'

Scott Marshall's choice was probably influenced by the massive legitimisation of science fiction in American popular culture which had been inspired by the huge success of another George Lucas film. The box-office clout of *American Graffiti* had allowed Lucas to make his long-cherished sci-fi saga *Star Wars*, until recently the most successful film ever released domestically in the United States. This had led to an explosion of science fiction-related films and television shows as space opera suddenly became the in thing.

Garry Marshall saw the potential for the idea. The show was now in its fourth year and they were running out of intriguing situations for Fonzie. An alien might be just what the show needed. America had been crazy about flying saucers in the Fifties after all, he reasoned, and he and his *Happy Days* writers came up with an episode called 'My Favourite Orkan', its title a reference to the popular Sixties' TV show *My Favourite Martian* which had starred Bill Bixby and Ray Walston. The basic plot was that an alien visitor from outer space would drop in on The Fonz while he was house-sitting for the Cunninghams. The visitor had come to take back a typical earthling for closer study. He had Richie Cunningham in mind but found The Fonz instead. The visitor would ask Fonzie's advice on terrestrial dating rituals, which would set up a slapstick sequence with the alien being fixed up with an Earth girl. The Earth girl in question was Laverne Di Fazio from *Laverne and Shirley*, alias Penny Marshall. All that remained was finding the right alien.

Garry Marshall's first choice for the role of the alien, who would be called Mork, was an established actor called John Byner. Byner was well known in the industry as an impressionist and a good ensemble player. He had done a number of sitcoms in the Sixties and Seventies, but none of them had gone on to be successful. His best-known role was probably as Detective Donahue in the cult comedy series *Soap*. Byner was perfect for what Marshall saw as basically a bit of fun. He was a seasoned pro, a recognisable face for the TV audience, and would do a good job on what was no more than a one-shot deal. Byner, for reasons best known to himself, turned the job down. Time was tight and the popular myth is that the casting dilemma was resolved by the tried and trusted formula of the cattle call, an open audition. From this audition, the story goes, a young man whom no one knew walked in off the street and announced himself as Robin Williams. He then, so the publicity material would have it, proceeded to slay them in the aisles and landed the part which would make him a household name.

In fact, Williams was nowhere near as unknown as the later *Mork and Mindy* publicity material would have had people believe. He did have a fair amount of television experience from *Laugh-In* and *The Richard Pryor Show*, and his new manager Larry Brezner had done a fair amount of shopping him around town. He would bring film and television executives to wherever Williams was playing in the hope that they would get a taste of his happy madness.

'Robin was doing stuff from Shakespeare, carrying on, dancing on tables,' says Brezner. 'I brought some United Artists executives to see him at The Comedy Store. They said "He's crazy" and walked out.'

Brezner in the meantime had found Williams more television work with guest spots in *Fernwood 2 Night*, *The Great American Laugh-Off* and *The Alan Hamel Show*. This was really just a question of trading on volume and getting experience in front of the cameras. With the exception of *Fernwood 2 Night*, none of the shows was especially distinguished. *Fernwood* is a neglected gem in America's television canon. Martin Mull, another Brezner client, starred in a parody of a small-town talk show. It was one of the first of the 'show within a show' genre which Garry Shandling has now made his own. As well as Mull and co-star Fred Willard, Williams also got to work with people such as Harry Shearer, Jim Varney and Kenneth Mars, who would all go on and establish themselves as major comedy names.

The real version of Robin Williams being cast as Mork is nowhere near as romantic as the press release would have it, although luck still played a part. Marshall is a man who in his work as a producer and director – he has gone on from television to direct movies such as *Pretty Woman*, *Soap Dish* and *Frankie and Johnny* – likes to surround himself with people he can trust. In many key positions these people turn out to be members of his family. He has cast his sister Penny many times and he uses another sister, Ronny Hallin, as his most trusted casting adviser. It was Ronny who suggested Robin Williams, whom she had found at Harvey Lembeck's Comedy Workshop in Los Angeles. Lembeck had pointed him out specifically when she had asked to see his top comedian. Because of her recommendation Williams found himself auditioning for Garry Marshall along with 20 other young comedians who were just as keen to land the part. Marshall was a little sceptical of his sister's choice, though he conceded that Williams did at least look as if he might be from another planet after the actor turned up wearing a pair of glasses made from two soupspoons with a white feather hanging from each of them. By good luck Williams had recently seen Steven Spielberg's *Close Encounters of the Third Kind* and had incorporated a character called 'The Alien Comedian' into the repertory company which was his stage act. Williams admits he was intimidated by the audition process, which is hardly surprising when you consider the shyness which had dogged him all his life. In addition he didn't think much of his chances and seems to have compensated for his lack of confidence by simply not taking things too seriously.

'When I auditioned for Mork I made every bizarre noise and gesture I could think of,' he recalls, 'and the director Jerry Paris hired me and pretty much let me play it the way I wanted to. The show got some positive feedback and for whatever reason ABC decided to use the Mork character in a spin-off series.'

Guest stars had come and gone on *Happy Days*, but Robin Williams made a big impression, especially with Henry Winkler. 'My job stopped being about remembering lines or moves, but to keep from laughing,' says Winkler of his guest star. 'And yet Robin was so shy, it was hard for him to speak. He did ask me, "After a day of this, how do you perform at The Comedy Store?" I told him, "After this, you really don't have the energy to perform at night".'

Garry Marshall jokingly insists Williams got the part because 'he was the only Martian who applied'. But only weeks after that episode had aired, he knew what he was going to do with his favourite Martian. 'We said, "No it's not a dream, it's real",' recalled Marshall in response to his son's original suggestion. 'It's another series.'

Marshall and ABC were simply giving the public what it wanted. Mork's lesson in love from The Fonz and his pursuit of Laverne around the Cunninghams' sitting-room had been a huge and entirely unexpected success. The network had received more letters about that one show than any other in the series and since almost all the letters wanted to see more of Mork, the next step seemed obvious. In the Seventies, American television followed the trends set by the movies, but where cinema had sequels, television had spin-offs. Ed Asner was one of the early successes when his Lou Grant character was successfully spun out of *The Mary Tyler Moore Show*; *Three's Company* would give rise to *The Ropers*; and *Happy Days* had already been responsible for *Laverne and Shirley*. No show had ever produced two spin-offs, until now.

While Marshall was negotiating with the network for his new spin-off show, he was also trying to put the show together. His first priority was to hire good writers, but the first two he approached – writer-producers

Dale McCraven and Bruce Johnson – were not keen. McCraven told him in no uncertain terms that he 'didn't do Martians'. Marshall had a trump card in the shape of the *Happy Days* episode which neither man had seen. Once they saw 'My Favourite Orkan' both McCraven and Johnson were so impressed with Robin Williams and his comic potential that they agreed to take on the writing responsibilities. McCraven and Johnson's first order of business was to work out a format for the show. Obviously three series set in the Fifties might strain credulity somewhat, so it was decided to place the show in a contemporary setting. Williams, who was brilliant at improvisational comedy, would also need someone to play against. What he needed was a straight man who didn't appear to be a straight man.

Pam Dawber was born in Detroit in October 1951. She grew up in the suburb of Farmington, which was only a half-hour drive from Bloomfield Hills, where Williams grew up. She had moved to California and begun a modelling career while she was at Oakland Community College. After becoming tired of what was essentially a small-town modelling scene, she headed for New York, where she joined an agency and became a busy and successful model. Dawber also had notions of a theatrical career and had started taking singing lessons. In 1977 she made her début in a production of *Sweet Adeline* in Connecticut and the following year she was cast by Robert Altman in *A Wedding*. In her movie début Dawber plays the jilted girlfriend of Desi Arnaz Jr, who has to ride a horse into the reception and announce that she may be pregnant. In between *Sweet Adeline* and *A Wedding*, Dawber had also auditioned for the title role in *Tabitha*, a proposed series based on the daughter of Elizabeth Montgomery's character in *Bewitched*. Dawber didn't get the part, which, given the short life of the series, was no bad thing. Instead she was given a one-year contract with ABC which led to another pilot. In *Sister Terri* Dawber would play a feisty nun whose mission was to bring God to the streets, but – perhaps not surprisingly – the show was not commissioned. Like all young actresses Dawber was anxious but reassured by the soothing promises of her agent who assured her that there was something much more satisfying in the offing. A few days later without ever, to her knowledge, having met or auditioned for Garry Marshall – or even having heard of Robin Williams – Pam Dawber read in the industry trade papers that she and Williams were being signed to do a show called *Mork and Mindy*.

McCraven and Johnson had come up with a comedy staple for the new show. It was a basic 'fish out of water' format, with Williams as Mork arriving from Ork on a scouting mission. He would then meet up with a sweet-natured Earth girl Mindy McConnell and eventually – in a prime-time friendly, sexually non-threatening way – move in with her the better to observe our quaint customs. Once the format had been decided on, Garry Marshall realised that he needed a female foil for Williams' free-wheeling humour. He was looking around for the right girl when he came across the *Sister Terri* pilot. With the help of a skilful editor, Marshall had Williams' scenes from the *Happy Days* episode cut together with Dawber's scenes from *Sister Terri.* The finished product looked as if the two characters were appearing in the same scene, and Marshall instinctively knew that the chemistry would work.

Garry Marshall now had his cast, his writers and his format. He was ready to launch his show but, even coming on the back of the huge response to 'My Favourite Orkan', they were still taking a big chance. Everyone knew that the show was risky, not least Williams and Dawber.

Williams is on record as voicing doubts about how the character of Mork could be developed satisfactorily for a series, while Dawber was reportedly worried that the show would turn out to be some 'real dumb thing'. Even ABC seemed a little uncertain about the show's ability to deliver an audience. They were initially going to schedule the programme in a notorious ratings graveyard. It was originally planned to run against *Monday Night Football*, a time slot which was effectively the kiss of death for any new show. With the bulk of the male television-watching, remote-controlling population watching the NFL's game of the week, there was next to no chance to build an audience. The show went into production in July 1978, still with that graveyard slot in mind. It was only when an ABC executive saw the finished versions of the first couple of episodes that the network realised they might have another hit on their hands. On the strength of these first few shows *Mork and Mindy* was switched to Thursday night at eight. This is historically the plum slot in American prime-time television, and Robin Williams was about to add another jewel to television's crown.

9

Nanoo, Nanoo

The summer of 1978 was an extremely important period for Robin Williams both personally and professionally. Being cast in *Mork and Mindy* – his first leading role – meant that his career was poised on the launch pad, but before it would finally take off there was something more important that he had to do. He and Valerie Velardi got married. Williams had spoken of Velardi in nothing but glowing terms, he was aware of all that she had sacrificed for him, and now he wanted to make a public declaration of how much she meant to him. He called her his 'stabilisation point', and perhaps their wedding near the family home in the hills above Tiburon in June 1978 was exactly what he needed. Velardi was much more pragmatic and hard-headed than Williams and, at a time when he was about to be exposed to all sorts of temptations, having at least one anchoring force in his life was no bad thing.

That same summer in San Francisco Williams performed the comedy gig of his life. He was part of a bill which also included Steve Martin and Joan Baez, but it was Williams who got the standing ovation from a crowd of more than 7000 people. This was a pre-*Mork and Mindy* appearance when Williams was very definitely a supporting act. The combination of television success and the audience reaction would mean that very soon he could play to crowds like this on his own.

Robin Williams had never actively sought television success. It had never been his ambition to star in his own TV show, far less a sitcom about a funny alien. But now that the opportunity was here he was not about to pass it up. However, even before he got the chance, the opportunity was almost snatched from him by a piece of legal red tape. When Williams had signed on to do the *Laugh-In* revival, his initial contract was for six shows, but he had also signed an option agreement. This agreement gave George Schlatter the right to renew his services annually for up to five years if the show was picked up as a series. NBC of course did commission a series, which meant that the option clause in Williams' contract could be activated. The consequences of this contract would not be felt for some time and in the process it would involve Williams in a serious political wrangle between producer Schlatter and the network. It was obvious within a few weeks that the new *Laugh-In* was not going to work, audience tastes had changed and the ensemble collected for this one, Williams notwithstanding, was nowhere near as talented as the original cast. George Schlatter announced that he was going to cancel the show. It seems, though, that this was simply a fishing expedition. He had got word that NBC was not going to renew the show, so he decided to go public in the hope that one of the other two networks would pick it up. The strategy came to nothing, and the show ended with Williams free of any obligation, or so he thought, and about $20,000 better off for the experience.

Once Williams had been confirmed as ABC's choice for *Mork and Mindy*, George Schlatter appeared on the scene again to announce that Williams was still tied to him under the terms of the *Laugh-In* contract. That being the case, then he would not be available for the series. It seems pretty certain that Schlatter was attempting to exert a little leverage on ABC, who could not, he reasoned, do the show without Williams since the whole concept was built around him. Whether he wanted some sort of financial settlement, or whether he wanted some kind of screen credit for what he would have perceived as a hit show, or whether he wanted a piece of Robin Williams is not clear. It is significant, however, that when Williams was cast in *The Richard Pryor Show* there wasn't a word from Schlatter. It seems reasonable to assume that the deciding factor was the huge buzz from the *Happy Days* appearance and the fact that Williams was now the star of the show. Robin Williams was undoubtedly stunned and surprised by the development. He insisted that he had, perhaps naïvely, believed Schlatter when he announced that *Laugh-In* was being cancelled and also believed that his contract was terminated. At the end of the day the issue was settled at a hearing held under the auspices of the American Arbitration Association. At the hearing Schlatter was very candid about his intentions with *Laugh-In.* He told the hearing that his announcement that he was scrapping the show was indeed merely a negotiating tactic to alert the other two networks in the hope that they might pick it up. Williams again argued that he believed he had no obligation to Schlatter whatsoever. The arbitrators agreed that Williams had acted in good faith and they dismissed Schlatter's claim. Williams was now free to star in *Mork and Mindy* without any legal encumbrances.

The first episode of *Mork and Mindy* was broadcast by ABC at 8.00 p.m. on Thursday, 14 September 1978. The show drew heavily on the *Happy Days* guest appearance which had played so well earlier that year. Initially Mork is given something of a back story in which it is revealed that life on Ork is rather dull. Orkans, according to Mork, are the white bread of the universe. Mork is something of a free spirit and his unconventional behaviour has brought him to the attention of the authorities more than once. The show opens with Mork awaiting another interview with Orson, supreme leader of Ork. Mork's sin this time is to have painted a moustache on The Solar Lander – whatever that is – and to have referred to Orson variously as 'Fatso', 'Rocketship Thighs' and 'Star-Twit'. As a punishment exercise Mork is sent to Earth – 'an insignificant planet on the far side of the galaxy' – where he will study our primitive ways and, conveniently, report back to Orson telepathically each week.

Mork arrives on Earth on the outskirts of what turns out to be Boulder, Colorado. It is late, and through a combination of darkness and cluelessness he manages to put on the one suit he has with him – his luggage was lost somewhere in the vastness of the universe – back to front. As he begins to walk into town he meets Mindy, who has been ditched by her date after being less than enthusiastic about his amorous advances. Seeing Mork and mistaking him for a priest because he has his collar back to front, Mindy is relieved to find some company out there on the road, and the two walk back into town together. Mindy invites him back to her apartment for a sociable drink, but when they get there she realises to her horror that he is not a priest, he simply has his suit on back to front. Once the rest of his luggage arrives at her front door, in an egg powered by some sort of anti-gravity device, Mork comes clean and reveals that he is in fact an alien. After the obligatory comic histrionics Mindy takes the news quite well, considering, and offers Mork a place to stay, temporarily, and realises that it will do her budding career as a writer the world of good if she studies him while he is studying us.

One of the first things Mindy has to do is make Mork more like a human by getting rid of his Orkan voice, which sounds a bit like Mickey Mouse on helium. This gives Williams the chance to engage in a wild improvisational riff in which he assumes the voices of variously Jackie Gleason, Shirley Temple and both Lucille Ball and Desi Arnaz. Later in the show he would settle on a modified Shakespearean accent which was modified still further to approximate to Williams' own soft-spoken tones. In the process of doing all of this Mork reveals that he has been to Earth before when he was sent by his biology class to collect a specimen. This is the cue for a flashback episode in which the bulk of 'My Favourite Orkan' with Henry Winkler and Penny Marshall is repeated. Once Mork's reminiscence is out of the way the story moves on to introduce the remainder of *Mork and Mindy*'s ensemble cast. Conrad Janis plays Mindy's father Fred, who runs a music store; Elizabeth Kerr plays her grandmother Cora; and young Jeffrey Jacquet plays Eugene, a kid from the neighbourhood who becomes one of Mork's first friends.

The formalities of introducing the dramatis personae completed, the plot, such as it is, for the rest of the show concerns Mork's ability to stay on Earth. Fred McConnell, grabbing the wrong end of the stick, is concerned about Mork and Mindy cohabiting. Not knowing that Mork is from Ork, he begins to suspect he might be at best mentally ill or at worst some kind of dope-head. His policeman friend Officer Tilwick – a guest appearance by Geoffrey Lewis – also has suspicions and eventually arrests Mork. Tilwick's excuse is that he thinks Mork is insane. A competency hearing has been arranged for the following day at which Mork's fate will be decided.

Mork conveniently spends the night before the hearing watching *Perry Mason* re-runs and the courtroom drama *Inherit the Wind*. He elects to conduct his own defence, which consists of another sparkling improvisation based on a Frederic March speech from *Inherit the Wind*. He is getting nowhere, however, and seems destined to be thrown into gaol. Eventually Mindy and Fred McConnell burst in to act as character witnesses for Mork, who is eventually found to be eccentric but sane. The episode concludes with Mork's first report to Orson – the heard but never seen Ralph James – in which he marvels at the human emotions which led Mindy to rush to his defence. Orson is similarly intrigued and modifies Mork's mission to study human emotions without getting involved with them.

One of the more prescient lines in this first episode of *Mork and Mindy* comes from Michael Prince, who plays the judge at the competency hearing. Mork, he concludes, 'adds a new dimension to the word eccentric'. Whether the line was written by Dale McCraven or Bruce Johnson, they were right on the money. Williams as Mork did take an audience to new realms of comic fantasy, much as his own hero Jonathan Winters had done for Williams as a boy. It was a question of looking at the world and seeing it exactly as it was, taking everything at its face value. One memorable moment from that first show remains a highlight of the programme's entire run. It comes when Mork encounters eggs for the first time. Having seen him and his luggage arrive in eggs, the audience already knows that on Ork eggs, like everything else, are different.

'Little hatchling brothers, you must revolt against your oppressors,' Williams tells a bowl of eggs which he finds on a kitchen worktop. 'You have nothing to lose but your shells. Fly, be free,' he encourages one egg, throwing it into the air where it demonstrates its natural aerodynamic properties and smashes on to the bench. Mork then offers it a quick burial at sea – in the sink – before sorrowfully telling the remaining eggs, 'Your brother bit the big one.' It's a piece of vintage Williams improvisation and was typical of the sort of humour which Williams brought to *Mork and Mindy*. It was humour born out of the freedom which he had been given by Garry Marshall.

> I wasn't restrained at all [Williams recalls], because they basically took what I did and put it into TV. They would take whole sections of my act and write episodes around them. They would come in and watch me perform and then write an episode of Mork doing this. There used to be a thing I did in my act about what it's like when a comedian bombs and I would talk about that, and they put that into an episode of *Mork and Mindy* where he split up into different personalities. The fact is I was very lucky to break through at a time when they [the network] didn't know what was happening. The fact that we had a live audience was the only thing that saved us – they saw it working. They didn't know what it was and they were scared but they said, 'People are laughing. Let's see what happens.' They gave me total freedom, carte blanche, and the first year was incredible because they didn't know what hit them.

People were indeed laughing. Within two weeks *Mork and Mindy*, the show destined for the graveyard opposite *Monday Night Football*, had broken into the top ten most watched programmes in the United States. By the end of its first season it would finish at number three in the charts with a weekly average audience of around 55 million viewers. In some weeks it reached as high as 70 million.

But Williams insists the men and women in suits at ABC were never quite certain what to make of the show. And were even less certain what to make of him.

> They really didn't know what I was [he remembers]. When we started the series the network guys would come in and sit together and, at first, they didn't laugh, but then they couldn't help laughing. Starting with the first

> taping in front of an audience it seemed like everyone was having a good time, and the more freedom I was given, the more I enjoyed it. It was the kind of playfulness I had experienced in night clubs, but never thought I would be able to get on television. I had guested on certain TV shows where they were very specific: 'Mr Williams, your line is "Lola, Jimmy's home".' There was no deviating from the script, but in *Mork and Mindy* I was allowed to work the way I do on-stage. In the middle of a monologue, I could suddenly go off into different accents and characters and nobody would blink.

Whether they understood him or not, the network certainly knew the series was a hit, and by the end of the first season Williams' salary had doubled from an initial $15,000 per show to $30,000 per show. As Williams has hinted, however, there was still some doubt about who was responsible for what on the show.

Certainly the physical characterisation of Mork was entirely the product of Williams' imagination and theatrical talent. The striped shirts and rainbow braces favoured by Mork were a direct reflection of Williams' own off-screen preferences for thrift-store attire. Williams also brought his own influences to bear on the way Mork moved. His strangely flat-footed childlike gait and the equally childlike manner in which he would cock his head quizzically at our Earth customs are a throwback to his days as a white-faced mime on the steps of the Metropolitan Museum in New York. Certainly it was a winning combination. The rainbow braces became fashion items, and Mork's everyday Orkisms – the greeting 'Nanoo, nanoo' and the all-purpose expletive 'Shazbot' – became Seventies' catchphrases.

As for the content of the programme, Williams continued to insist that much of the humour on the show was inspired either directly or indirectly by his improvisation. He maintains, probably with some accuracy, that the show would not have been as successful had it been completely scripted. Whether it would have been off the air in seven weeks, as he maintained, is debatable. In a 1982 interview with *Playboy* magazine Williams alleged that Garry Marshall and the other producers on the show had been aware of a chemistry between himself and Pam Dawber which they didn't want to interfere with. Williams would be encouraged to do his own thing while she was also encouraged to be completely natural in her reactions to it. According to Williams, it eventually reached the stage where the writers would simply offer notes in some scenes and he would then extemporise on the themes they had suggested. In another interview Williams claimed to improvise about a third of his dialogue and that he did so to prevent the TV writers from being forced into constant repetition.

Williams agreed that this was an unusual way to run a TV show.

> As far as I know it is [he conceded]. But you have to remember that Mork was basically an open book, a sieve who had picked up his knowledge of the planet from years of watching Earth television. He was a little like a comic-book character called Zippy the Pinhead, someone who absorbs everything that comes in but who puts it back out a little out of context, like a word processor with dyslexia. It helped that Mork was an alien, because in some ways there were no real boundaries as to what he could say or do.

This sounds like a perfect arrangement, but it's an argument which, whether Williams intended to or not, undervalues the contribution to the show made by McCraven and Johnson. Although Williams was the star, there was more to the show than just him. *Mork and Mindy* still had an ensemble of other characters who all had to be written for, and written for skilfully, so that they could provide springboards for Williams' humour while still remaining interesting to the audience.

> A half-hour TV show couldn't possibly be done that way [said Dale McCraven of Williams' explanation]. Robin contributes a great deal but we don't leave holes in the scripts. Robin can take lines which have been written and make them sound like ad-libs, which is great. He comes off as being spontaneous but he is a very studied man. He may try some ad-libs during rehearsals, but when we film the show on Thursday he knows exactly what he's doing.

The real truth is probably somewhere between the two. Williams has always been one to be fairly unrestrained during rehearsals and between takes, and there is no doubt that a lot of his own zaniness would have acted as inspiration for the scripts that Johnson and McCraven wrote. Those who know Robin Williams' stand-up work also suggest that one of his great strengths is the ability to take familiar lines and make them sound like ad-libs. But because of the logistics of camera set-ups and other actors' cues, the show cannot be improvised to the same extent as a stand-up set. What Williams was doing was improvisation, but only within some pretty well-defined parameters. And it was Williams' genuine improvisations which came closest to landing the show in trouble with the network.

> We were sneaking in with a lot of stuff [Williams remembers]. They had to get new censors every other week because they kept going 'What's he saying? What does he mean?' We would sneak in lines like 'Mindy, I just bought this book, the Catherine the Great story called *My Friend Flicka*.' They would get them a week later and realise, 'Damn, he got another one through.' It was a nice time because the network executives were just lost. Another part of the censorship is not the nudity or the words but the products you can't mention because you might upset a sponsor. Like you couldn't make jokes about McDonalds not serving red meat. I used to say things like 'Mindy, do you think McDonalds are using kangaroo meat, because I bought a hamburger and it had a pouch with another hamburger inside it.' And they went 'What?' and they cut out stuff like that. You couldn't do anything about religious groups either because they were such a powerful lobby. They would lobby against the products and then the sponsor would cut off the money, so that was it.
>
> But it was nice because parents could still watch it with their children. There were enough adult references and the children loved the innocence of it. I would have kids come up and throw an egg in the air and shout 'Fly' and you could hear their parents go, 'Our kitchen's all screwed up because of you.'

Mork from Ork was an instant success. Williams brought an innocence to what would be the first of a series of what might be termed 'man-child roles' that he would play both on television and in film over the next two decades. That mixture of naïveté and a literal interpretation of everything that was said to him struck a chord with audiences and critics alike. When the show first appeared there were some who compared it unfavourably with *My Favourite Martian*, but within a few episodes they were raving about the programme and hailing Robin Williams as a remarkable new talent.

One of the first to champion the show and Robin Williams in particular was *People* magazine, the ultimate arbiter of American popular taste. 'Even earthlings prepared to sneer,' it said, 'were won over by the elastic-faced, ineffably alien Robin Williams.' In a later article *People* would claim that Williams' 'brilliantly sophisticated mixture of wisecracks, double-talk and improvisations make *Mork and Mindy* sizzle'. *TV Guide* also heaped praise upon the show. 'What keeps it from bogging down is Williams' hundred inventions – his eerie vocal noises, babyish walk and crazy handshake, his virtuoso mangling of Earth language and his straight-faced ability to carry on a conversation with a talking space suit . . . The moments are a lot funnier than the plots but so far they are enough.'

Even the *New York Times*, America's newspaper of record, could not fail to notice the new kid on the television block. 'The season's biggest new face,' said the *Times*, 'undoubtedly belongs to Robin Williams of ABC's *Mork and Mindy*, another singularly unmemorable series except for the bizarre antics of its decidedly off-beat aggressively hilarious star. Mr Williams . . . not only exhibits a fine madness, but he also nurtures and protects it fiercely.'

While lavish in its praise for Robin Williams, the *Times* had noticed the show's fatal flaw. Robin Williams was bigger than *Mork and Mindy*. Without him there was no show. No single memorable moment was contributed by any other member of the cast. Every highlight of the series involved Williams and, more frequently than not, only Robin Williams. And the *New York Times* was not alone in noticing this. The suits in the ABC network offices, the ones Williams insisted didn't have a clue, were slowly wising up.

10

'Mork, Robin . . . Robin, Mork'

By any standard the first season of *Mork and Mindy* was a runaway success. Audiences loved it, critics were crazy about Robin Williams, and the show ended its first run in December 1979 as the number three show of the year. The success of *Mork and Mindy* helped give the ABC network an almost total ratings dominance. The top six shows on television were products of the so-called 'alphabet web', and with *Laverne and Shirley* in first position and *Happy Days* in fourth, three of the top four shows were Garry Marshall productions. Overall ABC had 12 of the top 20 shows, and the bulk of them were the half-hour sitcoms which were the network's speciality at that time.

Fast forward a year and the picture is entirely different. ABC finishes the 1979–80 season with only two shows in the top ten and a mere six in the top 20. The network had taken a big gamble and it had failed disastrously. Network television programming depends on holding an audience throughout the commercial breaks, especially those breaks between shows. The successful scheduler will carve out a whole slab of television time by carefully programming individual shows into what amounts to a whole evening of viewing. One of the most impressive examples in recent years is NBC's creation of 'Must See TV' on Thursday nights by packaging shows such as *Seinfeld*, *Friends* and *e.r.* together. This is standard practice now, but at the end of the Seventies it was less common. Most networks were happy to sweep certain nights, but ABC decided that with so many top-rated shows it could use these as a platform to sweep the ratings on consecutive nights, maybe even the whole week. So at the end of the

1978–79 season the schedulers started changing things around. Shows which had been popular in one time slot were suddenly switched to a different slot, sometimes even a different night, and often against stronger opposition in the hope that they could take their audience with them. *Mork and Mindy* was one of those shows which ABC hoped would be a hard-hitting weapon in the ratings arsenal. It was taken from its winning slot on Thursday night, where it had had barely three months to establish itself, and ended up on Sunday nights opposite *Archie Bunker's Place*, a hugely popular spin-off from the ground-breaking *All in the Family.* The redneck, politically incorrect Archie, played by the much-loved Carroll O'Connor, beat *Mork and Mindy* like a drum. For the rest of its run *Mork and Mindy* would never again feature in the ratings top 20. And, as it plunged in the ratings, the quality of the show suffered drastically.

> It was a simple case of greed and it didn't work out [says Robin Williams]. Then when the network realised things were going poorly for our show, it got panicky and started putting in all these sexually-oriented stories: 'Mork becomes a cheerleader for the Denver Broncos'. I think people who had always watched the series just looked at that stuff and said 'Jesus, what's this?' . . . It didn't piss me off so much as make me wonder why. Everyone was then doing T&A [tits and ass] shows, so I guess the network guys said 'Let's put Mork in drag – that's always funny.' But that was going far away from what we had originally had, a gentle soul who was suddenly becoming kind of kinky. The producers were torn between the network's saying 'We need stories we can promote' and their own feelings about supporting the characters. Well, because the network wanted a show it could promote, there I was with 32 cheerleaders.

The supporting cast was also changed to try and boost the flagging ratings in the second series. Conrad Janis was dropped as Fred McConnell, though the character was later restored in series three. Elizabeth Kerr had also been dropped as Mindy's trendy grandmother, as had Jeffrey Jacquet as Eugene, the kid who had proved an effective comic foil for Mork. Jay Thomas, Gina Hecht and Jim Staahl were added to give Mork and Mindy some friends of their own age, and Tom Poston joined the cast as grumpy downstairs neighbour Mr Bickley, who allowed Mork to examine less wholesome sides of the human condition. But the strangest addition was that of Robert Donner as Exidor, a man who believed that the Venusians were coming to reclaim him and a character who was even more bizarre than Mork. Donner is a fine comic actor with an excellent sense of timing, but the whole point of the show was how Mork interacted with normal people; to have someone behaving even more strangely than him seems odd to say the least. The network presumably felt that if one weird guy was funny, two would be even funnier. The real effect, however, was to make Mork look a little more normal by comparison, which was hardly the point of the show.

> I think the stories just got too complex and we got away from the simplicity of the character [explains Williams]. *Mork and Mindy* originally worked because it was about this cheerful man from outer space doing very simple things – 'Mork buys bread' or 'Mork deals with racism'. Mork and Mindy were both very strait-laced, and the charm of the show, I think, was in having Pam Dawber deal with me in normal, everyday situations to which I would react in bizarre ways. The show began with very human roots and Pam was responsible for a lot of that; she's a fine actress and a friend, and there was a wonderful exchange of humanity between us.

The second series of the show was also beset by rumours of professional jealousy between Williams and Dawber. She strenuously denied this, and his comments to *Playboy* magazine in 1982 also seem to give the lie to those suggestions.

> I think people really connected with the characters we played [Williams continued], and in our first year, the series was exactly what it was designed to be, a situation comedy. When you think of, say, *The Honeymooners*, you know who Ralph Kramden was and you know who Norton was; they were at their best in everyday situations and the simpler the better. If the stories ever became too complex – as they did on *Mork and Mindy* – there still would have been some funny things going on, but the show wouldn't have been nearly as effective. I didn't want to see *Mork and Mindy* bastardised in that way, but it was.

Shows in the second series did become increasingly off-beat. As well as having Mork almost join the Denver Broncos cheerleaders, another two-part episode had him fighting for his survival against the Necrotons, a race who had declared war on Ork. The fact that the Necrotons were led by Raquel Welch and included *Playboy* playmate Debra Jo Fondren among their number puts it fairly and squarely in the T&A category. In other shows Mork was shrunk and ended up in an alternative universe, brought home an abandoned chimpanzee, and even considered plastic surgery.

There's a certain irony here, because when they were developing the show McCraven and Johnson had consciously toned down Mork's abilities. Mork in the series has very few alien 'powers' compared with his appearances on *Happy Days.* They felt it was important dramatically that Mork be strange, but not too strange. Now the series was thrashing around, with its writers desperately searching for ideas and gimmicks of any kind that the networks could sell in a one-line teaser. According to Williams, by the time the show reached its third series it was all about getting a story which could be reduced to one line and then promoted to the audience. Williams himself was beginning to tire of the show by this stage. He still loved the character but was becoming increasingly frustrated at being used as a glorified network hustler to drum up audiences. He was also driving himself at an increasingly hectic pace. He would finish his day's shooting on *Mork and Mindy* at the Paramount lot and then spend his evenings doing gigs at local comedy clubs before making the one-hour journey back to his home in Topanga Canyon. It was not uncommon for him to work until two or three in the morning and then head for home – to be back on set a few hours later. In the autumn of 1978, not long after *Mork and Mindy* had become a ratings success, Williams collapsed from sheer exhaustion. His new wife Valerie Velardi, who had put her career on hold to support his, had to nurse him back to health. And, as Williams himself admitted, his sudden rise to fame so soon after getting married had caused some early tensions in their relationship. 'It was a little trying at first because Valerie felt like she was riding on my coat-tails,' he says. 'It has to cause tensions, but we came through that with flying colours.'

Velardi for her part seemed to realise that there was only so much you could do to control Robin Williams. He needed the free rein to exhaust himself if necessary; performing was for him like a drug which he could not do without. 'I love to see him work,' she says. 'I think it's a gift and so does he. If I knew what it was I'd package it. You have to take everything as it comes. You've got to live minute to minute.'

Although he was among the hottest names on television Williams was still, in many ways, an innocent abroad in showbusiness. The naïveté of Mork was not that much of a stretch from his own trusting nature. The incident with the *Laugh-In* contract had made that abundantly clear. 'He's still naïve about the business,' said screenwriter friend Bennett Tramer. 'He'll still talk to anyone who comes up to him.'

Valerie Velardi was equally aware of her husband's constant accessibility to fans, to agents, to bookers, to almost anyone who had a cause they needed to raise funds for. Williams was still a fit man who continued to run several miles a day, but she introduced him to health foods and mineral and vitamin supplements. She also put him in touch with a chiropractor to deal with chronic tension-induced back pain. But, more importantly, she was teaching her husband to say no.

There was one area where Williams was still not saying no. He had begun to take drugs. He admitted in the 1982 *Playboy* interview to smoking marijuana and taking cocaine but, in an eerily prophetic statement which echoes the views of addicts everywhere, he insisted he was in control. To be fair to him, at the time he probably thought he was. He told the magazine he had never got into hard drugs – and 'I never will', he insisted. 'Most times, anything I try, I have the opposite reaction to what I'm supposed to have,' he told interviewer Lawrence Linderman.

He was equally categorical about the effect cocaine had on him. 'I get passive and just hold back,' he said. 'Most people get talkative, I don't say anything to anybody. It's always weird, because I don't have regular reactions to any of these things. I don't like doing any of the heavies, because normally my energy is just up when I'm performing.'

There is nothing inherently contradictory in Williams' statement. In Hollywood in the late Seventies cocaine use was endemic in the film industry. It was almost a social grace and those who used it did not really consider themselves to be drug users. This is why on the one hand Williams can freely admit to doing coke, but on the other hand excuse himself because he isn't doing anything heavier like heroin, morphine or speedballs. It was a fine moral tightrope to walk and it would not be long before he would fall off.

Professionally, however, Williams was rapidly gaining the reputation as a man who just couldn't say no. Show him a crowd and he just had to perform. One close friend reckoned that if you had a kid and you had a way of getting to Williams, you could probably book him for a birthday party. For all that, Williams has always been an intelligent man with a fair amount of self-knowledge, and his own awareness of his problem led to what is probably the most remarkable *Mork and Mindy* show of the entire run.

'Mork Meets Robin Williams' was transmitted mid-way through series three. Although there may have been some doubt in the early days about who contributed what to the show, there seems little doubt that Williams was the guiding hand in this particular show. The set-up is simple. Mindy, who is now working for a local television station, has to get an interview with Robin Williams, who is doing a benefit concert in Boulder. Mork asks who Robin Williams is, and Mindy explains, pointing out that he and Williams look a lot alike. This is the cue for Mork/Williams to have a lot of fun at his own expense.

'You could pack a family in that nose, Mind,' says Mork of the cover of Williams' top-selling comedy album *Reality … What a Concept*. 'And look at that mouth! They had to airbrush this guy's entire face. I'm bright and cheery – this guy's got big problems.'

Mindy isn't the only one who notices the resemblance, and when Mork goes out into Boulder that afternoon he is spotted, mistaken for Williams, and mobbed. Mork barely manages to escape and, with his clothes in tatters through the efforts of souvenir hunters, it is a deeply traumatised alien who finally makes it back to their apartment. Mindy is having no luck arranging an interview, so she decides to go and doorstep Williams at the gig, and Mork tags along. The old mistaken identity bit works once again, this time in their favour. Mork, with Mindy in tow, is quickly ushered into Robin Williams' dressing-room by an eager security guard. A few moments later Williams himself walks in. The split-screen effect that was used to place Williams as Mork and Williams as himself in the same frame at the same time is crude and unsophisticated. Indeed its lack of subtlety is surpassed only by Mindy's interview technique which, through probing questions such as 'What's it like to be a celebrity?', finally elicits the fact that Williams is indeed the comedian who can't say no. Mindy thinks this may be a great line for her article and asks Williams why he thinks that might be.

> I don't know why I can't say no [says Williams as himself]. I guess I want people to like me. I hate myself for that. I used to be able to say no. Before all this craziness started my friends used to call me up and say 'Robin, come on, we're all going outside. There are some really gnarly waves. We can all hang out.' And I'd have to go, 'No, my momma says I have to stay inside and read Nietzsche tonight.' Later on I guess I felt really afraid to say no to them because then they'd all say, 'Oh, Robin Williams. Mr Smarty Pants. Big shot. You forgot your old friends. You can't lend me ten thousand dollars for a new car. You won't do the Save the Shrimp benefit.'

Seldom has a performer's sheer need to be liked and even loved by his audience been more nakedly exposed. And there was more to come, as Williams went on to describe how he had come to start out as a performer in the first place.

> Actually I became a performer by accident [he tells Mindy]. You see, my dad used to have this job where he had to move around a lot. And sometimes he'd leave a forwarding address. Just kidding [he said, presumably remem-

bering this is supposed to be a comedy show] – actually he'd pack me in the crates with the dishes.

I was always being the new kid in the neighbourhood. And since I was suffering from a case of the terminal shy I couldn't make friends that easily, and I always spent a lot of time in my room and I created my own little world full of all these little characters that had strange and unusual qualities. After a while, I realised that people found these characters funny and outrageous, and then it got to the point where I realised the characters could say and do things that I was afraid to do. And after a while, here I am.

It's interesting to consider the effect this scene would have had on the studio audience. By the time it was transmitted, in common with every other American comedy, a laugh track had been added to beef up the slow moments. To be honest 'Mork Meets Robin Williams' is self-indulgent, unsophisticated and not terribly funny to those who are unaware of his background. But, to those who are, it is an astonishing insight into what makes Robin Williams the performer that he is. The fear which had defined his stage act for years is articulated in one short speech. It was a catharsis via public confession to an audience of millions. It may also have been designed as something of a swan-song, because Williams had pretty well made up his mind that he wanted to leave the show. But the network had one powerful bargaining chip still to play. Williams would get the chance to appear regularly beside his comedy hero, Jonathan Winters.

The show had fallen to 49th in the ratings by the end of the second season, and not even a move back to its original Thursday time slot had been enough to halt the slide. Now Mork and Mindy were to be married in a move which smacked of sheer ratings desperation. Not only that, biological incompatibility aside, they were to have a baby only two shows later. The baby, Mearth, would be played by Winters, and Mork had to explain to Mindy that on Ork, unlike Earth, people are born old and grow younger over the years. So the audience was treated to the sight of the husky form of Jonathan Winters running around in romper suits and dungarees. Williams had nothing to do with getting Winters on the show, even though the older comedian had appeared as a different character in an earlier show and he and Williams had been terrific together. Given their particular comic chemistry it is surprising that Winters hadn't been introduced to the show sooner than this. But the network executives plainly felt that the presence of Winters would be enough now to get at least one more season out of Williams.

'Having him on the show was one of the main reasons I stayed with it,'

Williams agreed. 'For me, it was like the chance to play alongside Babe Ruth. I'd always wanted to just meet Winters. When I was a kid my parents would say, "All right, you can stay up a little longer to watch this wonderful man fly around the room and do all this crazy stuff".'

Winters appeared as Mearth in the final 18 episodes of *Mork and Mindy.* The chemistry between him and Williams is at times nothing short of magical. There is the occasional sense of the torch being passed between two of the great absurdist comedians of their respective generations. But even though Williams and Winters were inspired, the network was not, and it announced in the middle of the fourth series that *Mork and Mindy* was not being renewed. Winters, whose shows have attracted cult success rather than huge audiences, apparently blamed himself for the cancellation. But even though series three finished 60th in the ratings, Williams insists that the figures actually went up when Mearth was introduced to the show.

> But then [he adds] we got back to doing bizarre stories that had no semblance of reality, and the show's ratings went way down. For a little while I thought, 'God, maybe I'm not goosing up like I used to; maybe the old mad energy is gone.' But I decided it wasn't true, because people still liked my performances. I think the show just had a confused base. The combination of that and going up against *Magnum P.I.* was finally too strong.

Williams did at one point suggest that he thought ABC had deliberately manipulated things to get the show off the air, but that, he insists, was the initial rage against the coldness of the decision. No one had the decency to tell him in person. Everyone knew that the show was under threat, but Williams finally found out that it was cancelled from a newspaper.

> It was cancelled on 3 May [he remembers] . . . I think they tried to call me the day before; I just didn't return the call because I kind of knew what it was about. I knew it was coming. The ratings started off incredible with Pam and me going through the courting period. I guess the biggest was the honeymoon period – 'Mork is gonna get laid' – and then they stopped promoting it, and it went down the ratings list; the twenties, the thirties, the forties. It finally sort of bounced off the bottom. In the end it was like the last days in Berlin. We even shot one episode in 3-D.

When news of *Mork and Mindy*'s demise finally reached Williams he was filming a children's special, *The Frog Prince*, for his close friend the comedian Eric Idle. 'The end of that show wasn't unexpected,' says Idle, 'but you don't think you'll find out by having someone hand you a newspaper when you're on a set. Robin gathered the technicians around him and did a routine about TV executives. Everyone was on the floor and it was behind him. I thought that was the most useful example of comedy that I'd ever seen.'

Once his anger passed, Williams was at least grateful that *Mork and Mindy* was allowed to depart with some dignity, its 91-show run brought to an end with a three-part story in which Mork's existence is revealed to the world. The last show was broadcast on 12 August 1982. It had lasted four seasons; one more than *My Favourite Martian.*

'It was wonderful while it lasted, but I wouldn't want to bring the character back,' Williams said a few months later. 'The show was a crap shoot that worked out and the freedom I had on it was incredible.'

11

I Yam What I Yam

Robin Williams had always had his doubts about *Mork and Mindy.* He had never really believed that the character could be developed sufficiently well to last a single series, far less 91 shows. By the time ABC finally decided enough was enough, Williams was eventually branching out into other areas. With his success on the TV show it was inevitable that movies would be the next logical step. Already he and his now manager Larry Brezner were looking around trying to find the right vehicle to showcase his singular talents. By one of those happy Hollywood accidents it looked as though fate had steered them to the right project.

Popeye the Sailor Man was one of America's best-loved comic characters. He first made an appearance in 1929 in *Thimble Theatre*, a daily newspaper strip created by E. C. Segar. The previous star of the strip was the rake-thin Olive Oyl, but on 17 January 1929 Popeye made his début. Olive's brother Ham was looking for a sailor to take them on a trip when he spotted the unfeasibly muscled hero.

'Hey there,' he asked, 'are you a sailor?'

'Ja think I was a cowboy?' asked Popeye, before promptly telling Olive to get to the ship's galley. The first words she spoke to him – 'Shut up, you bilge rat' – were no indication of the decades-long romance which was to follow. After that first adventure Segar dropped Popeye from the strip, but reader demand was such that he was brought back at the expense of Ham. Popeye soon became the centre of a rich and varied repertory company of characters which included Olive Oyl, the villainous bully Bluto, the hamburger-mooching Wimpy, the evil Sea Hag and many others. *Thimble Theatre* was a weird and wonderful world where just about anything could and did happen, and only Segar's rules applied. The comic strip was a huge success and the spinach-guzzling seafarer became the star of a popular series of cartoons from Max Fleischer in the Thirties and Forties. The first of these appeared in 1933 and was called *I Yam What I Yam*, the phrase which would become his signature. In later years there would also be TV shows and hundreds of merchandising spin-offs from one of America's most enduringly appealing characters.

The huge box-office success of *Superman* in 1978 had made comic books and comic characters suddenly hot in Hollywood. Fantasy heroes were being optioned right, left and centre in the rush to jump on to a new bandwagon. One of the properties being actively pursued was *Popeye*, which producer Robert Evans wanted to turn into a live action movie. Evans was a mercurial New Yorker who had gone from being a child actor to a successful clothing manufacturer to a hot producer. With his lean, tanned good looks Evans looked more like a movie star than most movie stars, and his marriages to actresses Camilla Sparv and Ali McGraw, among others, merely cemented his Hollywood image. But beneath the tan and the dapper exterior, Evans possessed razor-sharp instincts. He had become head of production at Paramount Pictures in 1966 and over the next decade would turn out a stream of films which included *Rosemary's Baby*, *Love Story* and the first two *Godfather* films. In 1974 he started producing films for himself with a remarkable string of hits which began with *Chinatown*, and included *Marathon Man* and *Black Sunday*. *Popeye*, as far as he was concerned, was merely to be the next jewel in the crown.

The jewel, however, was proving a little too rich for Paramount Pictures' blood. *Popeye* was going to cost $20 million, a huge amount in 1979, and Paramount was unwilling to commit that much. Then Disney offered to share the load by taking on half the budget, so Paramount's exposure would only be $10 million. This was deemed more acceptable and the film got the go-ahead.

The production hit a snag early on when Evans' first choice for the role, Dustin Hoffman, decided that he didn't want to do it. Hoffman is an actor with impeccable instincts and he seems to have been right on the money here. It's hard to see him as the muscle-bound sailor man mixing it with Bluto. As they were looking around for a replacement, *Mork and Mindy* was going into its second series and Robin Williams was hotter than steam. You can see the attraction for Evans in having America's newest favourite comedian ready to make his screen début playing one of the country's most popular cartoon heroes. Everyone concerned felt that

Williams' physical comedy and his natural gifts as a mimic would be perfect for the role, and he was duly signed. Some of the other casting was not quite so smooth. Director Robert Altman wanted Shelley Duvall to play Olive Oyl. The slender Duvall could have passed as Olive's twin, but Paramount was holding out for *Saturday Night Live* star Gilda Radner. In the end, however, Altman got his way.

Although he was keen to make a film, Williams wasn't necessarily looking for a showy role that would net him hundreds of thousands of dollars; he simply thought it would be a good part. *Popeye* was not technically his screen début. He had recorded some skits for a lame sex revue called *Can I Do It . . . Till I Need Glasses.* The film was released in 1977 without Williams' contribution, but after the success of *Mork and Mindy* it was hastily re-edited to include Williams and re-released. *Popeye* was an entirely different proposition, and Charles Joffe from Joffe, Rollins, Morra and Brezner, who was an experienced negotiator, handled the deal with Paramount. Williams was so unconcerned with his actual pay-cheque that Joffe claimed it was three months before his client even asked him about the terms of his contract. So, having signed on, Williams spent his down time on the second series of *Mork and Mindy* punishing himself in the gym to learn the acrobatics which would be required for a very physical film. And when he wasn't in the gym he was taking dancing and singing lessons for this musical version of Segar's creation. Harry Nilsson was providing the music, and Williams as Popeye had one big number, *I Yam What I Yam*, based on the sailor man's oft-stated philosophy 'I yam what I yam and that's all that I yam'.

Popeye was to be directed by Robert Altman from a screenplay by writer-cartoonist Jules Feiffer. In retrospect you would have to question Altman's suitability for this particular job. Altman had gained rave notices and huge box-office returns for his first major movie, *M*A*S*H*, in 1970. Since then his work had been eclectic, ranging from the sublime *McCabe and Mrs Miller* to the frankly bizarre *Quintet.* Although he had established himself as a genuine American original, there was nothing to suggest that he was ideal to handle a musical comedy based on one of America's best-loved newspaper strips. Paramount executives were also less than thrilled by the choice of Altman, who was reported to have drink problems. Nonetheless Evans prevailed because of his fondness for hiring name directors after a flop, and there was no question that the bizarre *Quintet* had been a total disaster at the box-office.

Altman and Feiffer conceived *Popeye* as a morality tale about a young man searching for a lost father. Williams pitches up in the small seaside town of Sweethaven, impossibly muscled and with a permanent squint in one eye, looking for his pappy. He falls in love with the flighty Olive Oyl even though she is betrothed to Bluto, the man who rules Sweethaven with a fist of iron and a voice like thunder. Eventually Popeye and Bluto duke it out, Popeye wins and both gains the hand of his beloved Olive and is reunited with his pappy. Having been cast in the title role, Williams found himself surrounded by a quality selection of the Altman repertory theatre. Shelley Duvall played Olive, Paul Smith was Bluto, Paul Dooley played Wimpy, and respected Broadway star Ray Walston was Popeye's father, Poopdeck Pappy. Since Walston had starred in *My Favourite Martian* this was the first recorded meeting of a Martian and an Orkan.

Williams admits that he not only thought it was a good role, he also felt *Popeye* was the movie which could do for him what *Superman* had done for his good friend Christopher Reeve. His decision to wear the cape and tights and fly at the end of a Chapman crane in front of a blue screen had made him an international star. Williams took his research seriously, and he and Reeve had long talks about the difficulty of bringing a cartoon character to life and making him believable.

> When I was training for *Popeye* [says Williams], I thought this is it. This is my *Superman* and it's gonna go through the fuckin' roof. I also had the dream of getting up and thanking the Academy, but I got beyond the 'this-is-it' stage as soon as we started shooting. After the first day on *Popeye* I thought, 'Well, maybe this isn't it', and I finally wound up going, 'Oh God, when is this going to be over?'

Filming *Popeye* was a miserable experience for everyone concerned. Shooting took place in Malta, which has one of the world's largest marine tanks and is ideal for films with a nautical theme. A replica of Sweethaven was built on the coast, and the cast were more or less marooned for six months in a place which Williams describes as 'San Quentin on Valium'. Because Paramount were concerned with security, the cast and crew lived in a compound with wire fences and guards on the gates. This only added to the feeling of being held against their will and it was quickly dubbed 'Stalag Altman'. It was hardly surprising that drug-taking, especially cocaine use, was rife on the set.

> We were there for six months, working six days a week, and soon after we got to Malta it started raining and hardly ever stopped [recalls Williams]. That stretched out our shooting schedule, and we would just sit there for days, going bats and feeling trapped ... there are no great entertainment centres on Malta, and on weekends we used to drink. They had this very

strange wine available on the island; cabernet muck ... When the English had a naval base on Malta, they built a few pubs which are still there. We'd visit them on Saturday nights and get a little loaded and then sleep all day Sunday and go back to the grind on Monday.

It was a nightmare experience for anyone making their film début, especially someone who was obliged to carry the film by playing the title role. The pressure on Robin Williams must have been enormous, and it wasn't helped by the physical demands which the role made on him. Transforming him into Popeye took 90 minutes in the make-up chair every day, after which the trademark grotesquely inflated muscular forearms would be applied.

'They tied me off almost like a junkie,' he says. 'In some of the fight scenes I'd lose all the circulation in my arms and they'd lock up. I'd ask for a little blood and they'd untie me and say "Relax, Robin. Relax". Once the circulation got going they'd tie up my arms again so I could fight for another half-hour. It was very strange and very strenuous.'

Williams and the rest of the cast were not the only ones feeling the strain. As the shooting schedule wore on with no immediate end in sight, the executives at Paramount – who had never been keen on the project to begin with – started to become more and more anxious. Without warning they simply decided enough was enough, and Altman was told basically to finish up in Malta, come back with what footage they had and see if it could cut together into some kind of film. Williams in particular was devastated. He had felt the pressure throughout the film but hoped that, finally, as he had on *Mork and Mindy* and *The Richard Pryor Show* before that, he would get the chance to break free of the strait-jacket in a rousing finale. He had visions of a special-effects-laden final sequence in which he would perform impossible feats of spinach-fuelled derring-do and save the day. It wasn't to be. The final scenes, which involved Popeye rescuing Olive from a giant octopus, bordered on the farcical.

On the last day of shooting we were struggling desperately to come up with an ending [remembers Williams], and we all knew it would take great special effects to pull it off ... I know that I was supposed to punch an octopus out of the water and have it go whirling into space, but that didn't happen either ... when we were ready to shoot the ending the special effects guys had already left Malta. We were backed against a wall and we all knew it. Shelley Duvall, who was terrific as Olive Oyl, was supposed to be attacked by an octopus, but the one they built for the movie couldn't do anything. The Disney studios had half investment in *Popeye* and if anyone had let

> them know that the octopus couldn't even manipulate its arms, I think they would have sent over a couple of guys and we would have had an octopus that could blink, wink, blow bubbles and smoke underwater. Shelley had to do a scene with the octopus grabbing her, so she literally wrapped its tentacles around her like a wet rubber boa and had to sell the fucker as hand-to-hand combat. That's when I was supposed to show up and launch the octopus into outer space. We blew it up instead, but you couldn't tell what really happened.

Despite the Ed Wood-style finale there were more problems in store in post-production. Altman's obsession with the use of natural sound which he had pioneered in his earlier films meant that Williams had to re-dub his dialogue twice to get the right effect. He had spent a long time working on Popeye's voice, which he described as sounding like 'a frog farting under water'. But even with the benefit of two dubbing sessions much of his dialogue still sounds garbled and indistinct.

When the movie was released it was slaughtered by most of the American critics. Williams believes they went into the movie looking for the cartoon they had grown up on and were then instantly antagonistic to Altman's 'very gentle fable with music and a lot of heart', as Williams described the finished film. Given the circumstances under which the film was shot and the production was shut down, it's remarkable that there was anything to release at all. Williams for his part received generally non-committal reviews which praised his intuitive mimicry while pointing out that he had never really got into the character. It was a classic case of the prosthetics wearing the actor and not the other way round. Although some of the reviews wounded him deeply, Williams must have suspected that they were going to be like that. Especially after he had watched the film play in near total silence at its Hollywood première, an experience which he compared to a waking nightmare. But he also claims that he felt all along during shooting that something was missing.

> For instance [he explains], we needed a couple of slam-bang musical numbers that really tore the tits off the place. Same with the action. When the cartoon Popeye started dancing, walls would come down, windows would break, people would go flying out of the door, and Popeye would swinging Olive Oyl around with her body parallel to the floor. Instead of all that we shot in a real small space where you couldn't kick out the jams. A lot of the movie was filmed on a sunken steamer that was sitting on the end of the bay in Malta, and that kept things confined. So we wound up seeing the softer side of Popeye.

Williams dealt with the pain of the critical rejection of his efforts in *Popeye* by doing what he does best. He went on-stage and worked it out as a form of therapy. There were the inevitable heckles about the movie, and Williams would take them in his stride, zinging back with a one-liner. One of his favourites was to tell whoever asked 'What about *Popeye*?' that it was playing on a double bill in Hollywood with *Heaven's Gate*, the 1980 Michael Cimino folly which almost bankrupted United Artists. Williams felt aggrieved and hard done by about *Popeye*. His own feeling was that he had given a strong performance with some depth, but he had simply not been allowed to express himself. However, looking back on the film now you have to concede that the whole venture of a naturalistic *Popeye* was ill-conceived, with a clumsy script which was going to defeat even the most experienced of actors.

One thing that *Popeye* did teach Williams, however, was that he did not want to direct. He had done some directing on *Mork and Mindy* towards the end of the run and harboured genuine ambitions in that direction. Now, he cannot see any circumstance in which he would get behind a camera.

'People say to me, "Why don't you direct?"' he said recently. 'And I say, "It would be very difficult for me to say to someone, 'I'm sorry, you know that wasn't very good'" and then have them go "Well, what about *Popeye*?" ... I could never direct someone, I don't have the discipline.'

Since it was released in 1980, *Popeye* has become something of a Hollywood urban myth. The story is that the film was a complete disaster which lost millions of dollars for both studios. Some years after he had got over the trauma of the reaction to the film, Williams put the record straight: '... it wasn't that bad. There were some wonderful moments in *Popeye*,' he insists. 'Moments do not money make, but it did make some money because I got some cheques. And if I got money they must have made something. They must have made a lot of money, because before actors see any money, producers make a lot more.'

12

The Midas Curse

By the beginning of the Eighties Robin Williams was showing signs of running out of steam. He had been a sensation in the early days of *Mork and Mindy*, but he had been unable to translate that success into anything more meaningful. *Popeye*, while not a complete flop, had been nowhere near the career-making film everyone had expected. His next venture on to the big screen was more successful, but it was a qualified success.

Few movie débuts had been as anticipated as Robin Williams in *Popeye*. It seemed like the perfect combination, and the studios were bullish about his prospects. Once the box-office results were in, their enthusiasm waned somewhat and Williams found that the once plentiful supply of scripts was drying up. However, there was one among them which looked promising. John Irving's *The World According to Garp* was one of the most popular novels of the early Eighties. It was, as the title suggested, the story of a man's life and his view of the world.

T. S. Garp was raised by a formidable woman named Jenny Fields, who had wanted a child but not a husband. When she found herself nursing wounded soldiers the opportunity to solve her dilemma arrived in the form of Technical Sergeant Garp, a man with an unfortunate brain injury which had left him with a permanent erection. Jenny Fields took advantage of his condition and nine months later a son named T. S. Garp – after his 'father' – was born. Irving's rambling but fascinating novel is a story of life and love and loss as Garp grows up in a world full of women and becomes a successful writer himself.

It was a difficult novel to film, and once again the choice of director was not an obvious one. George Roy Hill was best known for films such as *Butch Cassidy and the Sundance Kid*, *The Sting* and *The Great Waldo Pepper*. These were all films which, in one way or another, celebrated maleness and male bonding. *Garp* on the other hand had a strongly feminist point of view. Williams was paid $300,000 to play the title role and found himself once again in the midst of an impressive cast. Glenn Close played his mother, John Lithgow was a transsexual former football star, Mary Beth Hurt played his wife, and Hume Cronyn and Jessica Tandy were his in-laws. Right from the start Williams was keen to play the role, sensing that it would provide him with the genuine dramatic challenge which Popeye had not presented. He also found that, unlike *Mork and Mindy*, this would require discipline, especially with a director who was not prone to giving Williams his head.

'I wasn't allowed to improvise,' says Williams. 'The first day I improvised George Roy Hill said, "Okay, that's a wrap." He made his point right away. Also he kind of forced me to stop. He'd say, "Okay, that's a joke. Let's go back to the next level and find out what's behind it." With comedy you can duck and dive out if it gets too serious. There you couldn't.'

The World According to Garp was a steep learning curve for Robin Williams, but he seems to have thrived on the challenge.

> Everything about *Popeye* and *Garp* is different [he says], starting with the directors. Altman and George Roy Hill represent two extremes. It was incredible to go from an Altman who gives you all that freedom to a Hill who says, 'You've got to do it this way.' They're like the yin and yang of the directing school. Hill knew exactly what he wanted . . . The roles themselves were opposites. *Garp* was like an oil drilling. I had to dig down and find things deep inside myself and bring them up. Heavy griefs and joys – births and deaths – *Garp* is an all-encompassing look at a man's life.

In the end Williams was pleased with his performance although, as he says now, he would play the role differently if he were playing it today with the benefit of being a parent himself. His performance as Garp is both funny and touching and, for audiences who only knew him from *Mork and Mindy*, a revelatory experience. It was the first time that audiences had seen a glimpse of the trained actor behind the manic performer. By and large they, and the critics, liked what they saw. Williams received a great deal of praise for a film which was generally admired by the critics but did only moderate box-office business. In the end, though, it was enough to re-establish Hollywood's faith in him and the scripts started to pick up again.

The World According to Garp was filmed during the final season of *Mork and Mindy* and released in July 1982, a month after the show had gone off the air. Williams filled in what was a fairly nervous period by going back on the road. A performance junkie, he sought solace in front of crowds, criss-crossing the country in a series of high-profile dates. For most of his life, whether as a lonely child in a huge mansion, or a shy bullied child at an intimidating boarding school, humour had been Robin Williams' sword and shield. It was his armour against the world, a way of being liked, and a way of dealing with his fear of being left on his own. Now he was finding that it was a double-edged sword.

'Humour is a dreadful curse,' says Eric Idle, 'and Robin was like Midas, being funny endlessly. Getting blasted was the only way he could stop.'

With the notable exception of those decent reviews he received for *The World According to Garp*, his film career had not panned out. His marriage was now in disarray, and he was becoming more and more reliant on vodka and cocaine.

His problems were largely self-inflicted and can be traced back to that very first series of *Mork and Mindy*. Williams has already alluded to the problems in the early days of his marriage, suggesting that Valerie Velardi was having some difficulty in riding the coat-tails of his success. In truth, if Velardi was having problems with anything it was with the way that Williams was handling his success. *Mork and Mindy* had made him a household name overnight, but it also made him a sex symbol. His little-boy-lost television persona, coupled with his athlete's physique and his devastating wit, made him something of a babe magnet. For someone to whom popularity had come relatively late in his life, the temptation must have been overpowering. One of his earliest magazine profiles, in *Playgirl* in March 1979, was already noting Williams' fondness for the perks of celebrity.

'He always grapples with Valerie when she shows up on the set,' wrote Richard J. Pietschmann, before noting, 'but he also continually grabs asses and squeezes tits and generally hugs and cuddles the best-looking women within range.'

Pietschmann also pointed out the relish with which Williams was responding to his new role as an 'alien sex symbol'. It wasn't long before others started to notice too. Williams had become a celebrity, which meant that, in their eyes, he was fair game for the gossip columnists and the supermarket tabloids. Less than a year after his marriage to Valerie Velardi the *New York Post* was suggesting that a divorce was in the pipeline.

The *National Enquirer*, which would become the bane of Williams' life, also suggested that he and Valerie and another woman were going out on triple dates. Williams was upset by the reports, according to *Mork and Mindy* co-star Pam Dawber quoted in the *New York Daily News*. On the other hand, she was also quoted as saying that he was not very secretive, suggesting that she too believed that he was the architect of his own misfortune.

One reason for Williams' behaviour may have been that he had deserted the one thing which had kept him reasonably sane up till now. He was no longer performing. Getting up on stage for Robin Williams was his entire *raison d'être*, and even when he had become famous with *Mork and Mindy* he continued to go back and perform at open mike nights at comedy hole-in-the-wall joints like the Holy City Zoo.

> It only sits 60 people, usually the same people [he explains]. I liked going in there late at night, after 12.30 when there's only about 12 people in there. Then it's really funny. There's something about it which strips away the pretensions. People still yell things at you and heckle you. They give you about five minutes grace. Then if you get them it's great, but after that five minutes you better have something. It's good, it really forces you to find stuff and tap into it.

Now Williams, who by the end of 1979 not only had a hit TV series but a hit album as well with his Grammy-winning *Reality . . . What a Concept*, appeared to be believing his own publicity. Far from finding something which would strip away the pretensions, he was now actively wallowing in them. He denies Pam Dawber's suggestion that he was making his behaviour too public, but he does admit that things got out of hand.

> Hollywood is so full of horseshit temptations. During the second year of the series, I kind of lost track of all kinds of stuff. I stopped performing. I mean, I did an album but when that was over, it was a kind of blaaah for a while. I lost track of everything, kind of ... When things started really peaking you had friends you didn't know you had before. You'd be spending time at clubs all night long and then going to work the next day expecting people wouldn't notice and they did. You'd come in the next day and people would say, 'Oh, pardon me. Refried shit?'
>
> There was always someone somewhere to keep partying with. Hollywood is designed that way. And the temptations are so many and varied. There is everything . . . The deadly sins of Hollywood. They wait for everyone.

While Williams was out partying the nights away, his wife would eventually make her way back home to the heights of Topanga Canyon. Valerie Velardi is a hard-headed woman. She was not the sort to sit back and accept this kind of behaviour from her husband, but at the same time she was aware that she was dealing with precious cargo. Williams was bright, very intelligent and supremely talented. Yet in spite of being all those things, he was still not terribly mature emotionally. He was behaving like a kid locked in a toy store. Velardi said once that she knew that if she had simply drawn a line in the sand and told Williams that it would all have to stop and stop now, he would simply have walked out. She knew that if she was going to stand by her man then it would require something a little different. Living in Hollywood had already required several adjustments on Valerie Velardi's part. In the first place she had had to become used to being, as far as the Hollywood movers and shakers were concerned, a Hollywood wife.

> Robin and I would go to a party and separate, wander around, looking for a good time, and I would take up with somebody, maybe a woman or maybe a group who wouldn't be giving me the time of day. And all of a sudden they'd see a photographer taking a picture of Robin and me and it was 'What a wonderful dress', or 'What you said before was simply fascinating'.
>
> Now in the past, the way I would deal with that would be to say, 'I wasn't good enough for you then; why am I good enough for you now? Just because I'm screwing Robin Williams I'm hot to you now? I don't need this shit.' But instead of reacting like a shit, or someone who is hurt or rejected, I'd say, 'Okay, this is the life we're living – enjoy it, have a ball, but don't take it too seriously.'

But Williams was taking it seriously. He was a born-again party animal and the effects began to show, not least in the fact that his weight began to balloon up. There were also anxiety attacks on the set of *Mork and Mindy*, which suggests a Catch-22 scenario. Was he taking drugs because he was anxious, or was he suffering from cocaine-induced paranoia? Williams goes for the former.

> Do you think that drug abuse isn't old? [he asked a journalist recently]. If you look back at old newspaper headlines, it's old. People from the Twenties did all these things. Cocaine has been in Hollywood since the beginning of Hollywood. I think it's the pressure – some people snap. I used it to try and kind of numb out and forget, it was a reaction to sometimes try and escape from it all. I had a reverse metabolic reaction to cocaine, I would do it and

> go catatonic. People think I must have been really wild; no, it was the exact opposite. It comes and goes because Hollywood is a high-pressure place. It isn't just the salaries, it's the nature of worrying about how you're doing. 'Am I still being creative?' It's also sometimes flirting with the dark side or whatever, chasing the dragon.

By his own admission Robin Williams was seriously messed up during this time of his life. Valerie Velardi, the woman he had often referred to as the stabilising influence on his life, did the best she could. She tried tough love by simply walking out and leaving him. There were a number of separations for about a month at a time when she had simply had enough. But she always came back, he was always pleased to see her, and before too long things were always back the way they had been. Another approach was called for. 'You can guide people,' Velardi says, 'you can make yourself interesting enough and important enough in your lover's life so that he'll always come back to you if you just keep growing along with it. If you just be part of their rhythm and give them a lot of freedom and be part of their growth instead of pulling them back from what is titillating and exciting. Let's face it, Robin is a stimulus junkie.'

Velardi's approach then was to accept Williams' womanising for what it was. She insists that he had a lot of female friends at the time but the relationships were nowhere as intense as people were speculating. Williams, according to his wife, loves women and loves their company. And, she says, that's mostly what it was about, simply spending time with friends who happened to be female. She never tried to stop him seeing female friends as long as he abided by one firm ground rule; no one would take her place.

> It doesn't sit right [she said at the time], but under extraordinary circumstances, which we are under, if you don't make the necessary adjustments, then you can lose precious things. That's not to say that it gives us the licence to go off and screw everything that's around. It's just the freedom to at least feel like we're free individuals as opposed to being married and locked in and 'You can't go out tonight because I know so-and-so is there, and she's hot and pretty and I'm afraid you're gonna get involved with her'. He's never going to get involved with anyone without me knowing about it. And the other way doesn't work. You can't hold somebody in. They resent you, hate you, and you become unattractive to them.
>
> If I had jumped the gun and divorced him I would have lost the most precious thing in my life and it would have curtailed our experience together, which is a lot richer than anything he can get off the streets.

There were also times when Velardi would take matters into her own hands. The guiding and giving space would simply give way to a pre-emptive strike.

'She would march right up to some girl sitting at [Robin's] table and say, "Hello, I'm Valerie Williams, Robin's wife" ', claims Pam Dawber. 'Or call up a girl. Or have lunch with a girlfriend. And say, "You think he's gonna leave me for you? You're crazy".'

While Valerie was able to take matters into her own hands when it came to her husband's flirting and womanising, his substance abuse was an entirely different matter. There was no reasonable threat she could make to a line of cocaine or a pitcher of kamikazes – vodka and lime – which had become his drink of choice.

> I was 26 or 27 then [says Williams, trying to put it all into some kind of perspective], and then bang, there's all this money, and there are magazine covers. Between the drugs and the women and all that stuff, it's all coming at you and you're swallowed whole . . . Even Gandhi would have been kind of hard pressed to handle it well . . . the reason I did cocaine was so that I wouldn't have to talk to anybody . . . For me, it was like a sedative, a way of pulling back from a world that I was afraid of.

The defining step for most addicts is the point where they accept the fact that they need help, the moment when they can realise for themselves that they have a problem. Williams, who could be so intuitive and aware in so many other areas, simply didn't see what was going on. Part of that was the drug culture which was pervasive in Hollywood at the time. Snorting cocaine was regarded in some quarters as almost a social skill and an outward symbol of your ability to compete in the hard world, play even harder, 24/7 lifestyle of contemporary Hollywood. Looking back, Williams recognises that what he needed was intervention.

'I think I was crying out for someone to say "Enough",' he admitted. 'In the end I had to make my own line. Anybody who finally kicks himself in the ass and wants to clean up makes his own line. You realise the final line is the edge.'

Williams' desire to get himself straight arose in the end from two disparate sources. A birth and a death.

13

Consequences

There was a nervous atmosphere on the set of *Mork and Mindy* on the afternoon of 5 March 1982. It wasn't just that the show was not doing well in the ratings and was only a matter of weeks away from being cancelled. There was something else, a sense of foreboding and deep concern about the star of the show. This time the concern was not about the harm he was doing himself; instead it was about the damage he might do himself. The comedian John Belushi had been found dead of a heroin and cocaine overdose at the Chateau Marmont hotel off Sunset Strip. He and Robin Williams were friends, and were related through their comedy and their fondness for recreational pharmaceuticals. Now that Belushi was dead, someone was going to have to break the news to Robin Williams.

> Somebody told me to tell him [says Pam Dawber], because they were afraid he would fall apart. You never knew how he was going to take something because he was so emotional. He was affected in the way, at first, that made it look as though he wasn't affected at all. He said, 'Wow, I was with him last night.' Then, as it absorbed, he became more and more devastated by it, because suddenly I think he began to see the parallels – just what fast living can do. And also, somebody the same age, somebody you just saw that night, to then suddenly be dead.

John Belushi was 33 years old when he died. He had risen to fame as one of the stars of the TV show *Saturday Night Live* and hit films such as

National Lampoon's Animal House. However, his prodigious talent was becoming increasingly overshadowed by his even more prodigious appetite for drugs. Belushi was capable of ingesting phenomenal amounts in his ever more desperate search for a high. On the night of his death he was contemplating what might be the ultimate creative achievement from his point of view: he was planning to inject himself on-screen with heroin for a part in a proposed movie. One of the reasons he was at Chateau Marmont that night was to seek the support of his friend and fellow Marmont resident Robert De Niro. Belushi felt De Niro was the greatest method actor who had ever lived and would undoubtedly have backed him up. Robin Williams was with Belushi briefly on the night he died. He spent no more than ten minutes in his friend's company – only long enough to do some drugs – and then left.

Even now Williams believes there was an element of conspiracy in his being there that night. It seems more likely that, in the absence of any obvious motive for involving him, he was there simply as a result of a misunderstanding.

> I was only there for five or ten minutes [he says]. I saw him and split. He didn't want me there, really. He obviously had other things he was doing. I do think I was set up in some way to go over there. A guy at the Roxy said that John wanted me to stop by his bungalow. But when I went he wasn't looking for me. He wasn't even there. When he arrived he said 'What are you doing here?' and offered me a line of cocaine. I took it and then I drove home. If I had known what was going on, I would have stayed and tried to help. It wasn't like he was shooting up in front of me. The next day on the set of *Mork and Mindy*, Pam Dawber came up to me and said 'Your friend is dead.'

Williams and Belushi had first met about three years previously. They were not close, but in the three or four months before Belushi's death they had begun to see more of each other and were becoming closer. Given that they were both *habitués* of the celebrity drug scene, it was inevitable that their paths would cross in exclusive clubs or private lounges where the stars hung out at night.

'I admired the shit out of him,' says Williams, who probably secretly envied Belushi's uncompromising wild-man behaviour. 'I'd had a wonderful time with him. One time he took me to a heavy hard-core punk club, and I was scared shitless. People were slam dancing, which I had never seen before. It was like being on tour with Dante, if Dante was James Brown . . . I was like Beaver Cleaver in the Underworld.'

One of the things Williams most admired about Belushi was the fact that he had a constitution like an ox. He could put his body through the most terrible punishment and still emerge virtually unscathed. The idea that someone of Belushi's iron-clad constitution could succumb to an overdose must have given Williams pause for thought. In the end he dealt with Belushi's death in the only way he knew how: he went on-stage and performed.

The day after John Belushi died Robin Williams spent the afternoon speaking to a *Playboy* reporter as part of his first major interview with the magazine. This, incidentally, was also the interview in which he claimed that he had not got into hard drugs and never would, which implies a great deal of self-delusion either on the part of the interviewer or the interviewee. That night Williams went on-stage at The Comedy Store as a surprise guest and did an impromptu 45-minute set. 'It was good,' Williams recalled later to interviewer Lawrence Linderman, 'but there was a strange mood in the air. It was just kind of up and down.'

Williams never mentioned Belushi once during his set. Neither did any of the other comics at The Comedy Store that night. Williams believes it was partially out of respect for a dead colleague, but also no one particularly wanted to open a can of worms by talking about drug use, especially with so many reporters in the audience. Williams says he felt no guilt over John Belushi's death. He could not possibly have known how the evening was going to turn out and, even if he had, he did not know Belushi well enough to make any kind of satisfactory intervention.

But it still gnawed away at the back of his mind. If this could happen to Belushi, a man who was as strong as a bull and only a couple of years older than himself, then what did the future hold for Robin Williams? Not long after Belushi's death, Pam Dawber came across Williams standing quietly on the *Mork and Mindy* set. He was on his own and lost in thought. 'Don't you worry, Dawbs,' he told her quietly. 'It'll never happen to me.'

He was as good as his word. Within a year he was clean, sober, and a father. But there was still a lot of fall-out from his friendship with John Belushi to deal with before then. The police had been investigating the death of Belushi since the afternoon his body was found in the back bedroom of bungalow number three at the Chateau Marmont. The officers who were investigating the case, Detectives Russell Kuster and Addison Arce, guided by a coroner's verdict that Belushi had died of a drugs overdose, were inclined to believe that it was just another accidental death. They were going through the protocol of following all the required leads and wrapping up all the loose ends when the case was blown wide open by comments from an unlikely source. Cathy Smith, a friend of Belushi's who had infiltrated his inner circle because of her easy access to drugs, told the *National Enquirer* that she had been with Belushi on the night he died. She also told the newspaper that she had mixed the speedball – a mixture of cocaine and heroin – which had killed Belushi. Then, to cap it off, she named Robin Williams and Robert De Niro as having been with Belushi on the night he died.

The police were caught on the horns of a dilemma. No one really believed Smith's story, and the fact that she had received $15,000 for it didn't help her credibility much. But with Smith having gone public, her claims had to be investigated. Smith made her comments in a recorded interview with the *Enquirer*, and Addison Arce is one of the few people who have heard this tape. He is in no doubt that Smith was being set up.

> By the time I got through listening to that tape it was obvious to me that they were getting her to say almost anything they wanted [he says]. It was almost like a controlled conversation where the interviewer would be providing 85 per cent or even 95 per cent of the information and she would just be sitting there saying 'That's right'. By the end of the conversation her voice was very slurred and her demeanour very casual. From that and the sucking noise during the interview it was obvious to me from working narcotics and being a policeman for so long that she was smoking a joint and enjoying a drink at the same time. It was a very relaxed atmosphere and they were having a conversation, but it was very definitely a controlled environment.

The *National Enquirer* had been the bane of Robin Williams' life for some time. They first crossed paths when Williams claims the paper tricked his mother into giving them an interview and supplying precious family photographs. These, according to Williams, were then used in a piece which suggested that he had grown up under the thumb of a bullying and tyrannical father. Now they had gone a step further and landed him in the middle of a homicide investigation. Perhaps this is what Williams suspected when he suggested that his presence at Belushi's bungalow had been a set-up? But is he suggesting that it was the *Enquirer* that set him up? Or that someone else set him up in the hope of selling the story to the *Enquirer*? We will never know.

Although the police did not necessarily believe the whole of Cathy Smith's story, there were parts which struck them as being plausible. According to Addison Arce, Smith described De Niro and Williams as attacking a bag of cocaine with straws 'like a Hoover vacuum cleaner'.

Williams' version was that he had called De Niro when he got to the Chateau, but the actor had company and obviously did not want to be disturbed. He never saw De Niro that night, but he did admit to doing some cocaine in Belushi's room. The police were duty bound to investigate now, if only to sort out what had happened leading up to the death of John Belushi. Los Angeles Deputy District Attorney Mike Genelin announced that the police were going to have to speak to both Williams and De Niro. It is technically possible that, had they been with Belushi that night, the two actors could have been charged under California's felony murder laws. Since Belushi had died as a result of a felony being committed, i.e. injecting drugs, then the person who had injected him with those drugs could be guilty of second-degree murder. However, in announcing that they wanted to speak to De Niro and Williams, Deputy District Attorney Genelin made it plain that neither man was a suspect. On her own admission, Smith had injected Belushi, who had something of a phobia about needles. The police were chiefly concerned with obtaining corroborative statements to piece together Belushi's final hours.

The investigation into Belushi's death brought on by Cathy Smith's interview flared up in the summer of 1982. Neither De Niro nor Williams was instantly available for questioning. De Niro had gone to Italy to make a film, and his publicists made it perfectly plain that he would not be returning to the United States for questioning. The LAPD, for its part, would not authorise the expenditure for detectives to go to Italy to speak to him. De Niro never spoke to the police and never gave any evidence about Belushi's death other than to a Grand Jury, which he spoke to by telephone some months later. Williams on the other hand did agree to cooperate, but only up to a point. The investigation could not have come at a worse time for him. He was in the midst of doing advance publicity for *The World According to Garp*, the film which might establish him as a serious actor, when he had to face up to being part of a police inquiry. Indeed, when the story broke that the police were now treating Belushi's death as homicide, Williams was in the middle of an interview for what would be a cover story for *Rolling Stone*. One of his managers, David Steinberg, went so far as to call the reporter later, asking for the tapes of the interview to check for references to Belushi.

David Steinberg and the rest of Williams' management team eventually struck a deal with the Police Department. Williams would be interviewed, but only with his lawyers present and with the questions vetted in advance. Detective Arce was not really expecting to find out anything significant from the session, but once it had been effectively neutered the interview became meaningless. 'I have no problems with attorneys being in an interview,' he said later, 'but when they have me write the questions out beforehand then that's no interview.'

In the end, as expected, no charges were brought against Williams, nor were they ever likely to have been. The only one who needed to fear indictment was Cathy Smith, and on 15 March 1983 – just over a year after Belushi died – she was charged with murder in the second degree as well as other drugs offences. She was extradited from Canada and after being found guilty, served a short jail sentence.

The death of John Belushi was a salutary lesson not just for Robin Williams but for the whole of Hollywood. A great many stars began to see that cocaine and heroin were no longer high-priced fashion accessories, and large numbers began to clean up their act. Robin Williams was among them. It was David Steinberg and others close to him who finally gave him the intervention he desperately needed and persuaded him to seek treatment. But the response that he initially received when he tried to quit is an indication of the prevailing social climate in the film industry at the time.

> The weird thing about the drug period is that I didn't have to pay for it very often [he recalled several years later]. Most people give you cocaine when you're famous. It gives them a certain control over you; you are at least socially indebted to them. And it's also the old thing of perfect advertising. They can claim, 'I got Robin Williams fucked up.' 'You did. Lemme buy a gram then.' The more fucked up you get, the more they can work you around. You're being led around by your nostril. I went to one doctor and asked, 'Do I have a cocaine problem?' He said, 'How much do you do?' I said, 'Two grams a day.' He said, 'No, you don't have a problem.' I said 'Okay.'

Williams kicked drugs on his own. He didn't check into the Betty Ford Clinic or any other celebrity enclave. He was encouraged by his mother's belief in the Christian Scientist doctrine of self-healing and he was determined to end his drug addiction on his own. He dealt with his alcoholism likewise by handling it on his own.

> With alcohol it was decompression [he explains]. The same way I started drinking I stopped. You work your way down the ladder from Jack Daniels to mixed drinks to wine to wine coolers and finally to Perrier. With cocaine there is no way to decompress yourself. It took a few months . . . People come up to you with twitching Howdy Doody jaws and you think, 'Hmmmm, I looked like that.' You realise that if you saw by daylight the people that you

> had been hanging out with at night, they'd scare the shit out of you. There are bugs that look better than that.

Along with kicking his drink and drugs addiction, Williams was especially keen to make a genuine attempt at rebuilding his relationship with Valerie. When that *Rolling Stone* article appeared in September 1982, Williams was already celebrating taking the first steps to getting himself clean and sober. He spoke of the strains on both of them of his becoming famous overnight; of going from being poor and newly married to being hugely successful and the centre of a huge national craze. He also spoke of his gratitude that they had survived.

'You go through this kind of phase … and then you're through it,' he said, trying to be serious and articulate his feelings. 'It's like you go through one of those blizzards and you lose each other's hands for a while, and then you come through on the other side.'

Very soon he had another reason for staying straight. Williams and his wife admitted in the interview that they had been trying for a child. Not long afterwards Valerie discovered she was pregnant. This gave Williams added resolve.

'Zach was about to be born,' he said later, 'and I didn't want to miss it because I was coked up or drinking. It was hideous enough feeling hung over without a baby screaming. I mean there are times when you think God made babies cute so you don't eat them – imagine if you're loaded.'

14

Beautiful Boy

Possibly the single defining moment in a man's life is when he becomes a father. Suddenly, from being really accountable only for and to himself, he becomes responsible for the life and well-being of someone else. It is a challenging vocation to which all men react with varying degrees of success. Robin Williams was determined that the birth of Zachary Tim Williams was going to be the moment when his life turned around.

He had already kicked alcohol and cocaine, and he was now seriously getting back into shape. He had taken up running again, and a strenuous and dedicated fitness regime saw him back at something close to his fighting weight when his son was born. Williams had grown up more or less on his own, although he was never in any doubt that his parents loved him. He was determined that he would be around for Zachary more than his own father had been for him. However, it was also a good deal easier for Williams to take charge of his own life that it had been for his father.

He was also taking time to be a new dad, and in the process becoming much closer to his own father. All men ultimately become their fathers, but the process speeds up considerably when you have a child. Suddenly fatherhood is the one thing you have in common. You realise that the problems you are now facing with your child are no different from the ones your father faced with you. The birth of his grandchild brought Robert and Robin Williams much closer together. Williams had a new respect for his father; he began to realise just how difficult a job it is. There had never been any serious strain between father and son, but there were undoubtedly times of great distance, brought on by the gap in their ages if nothing else. Robert Williams could not have failed to notice his son's binges on booze and drugs, but neither he nor his wife would have been inclined to intervene. If Robin wanted help then he would need first to realise that he needed help. And when he finally took matters into his own hands and cleaned up his act, his parents would have been overjoyed.

The birth of Zachary was the beginning of a new era in Robin Williams' life. Almost from the moment when Zach was born, he and his father each saw the other in a different light. They were no longer father and son; they were simply fathers. Zach's birth sparked a *rapprochement* and an understanding between the two men which grew and deepened over the remaining years of Robert Williams' life. It was a source of great comfort and enjoyment for both men.

In career terms, Williams was still considering his options. *Mork and Mindy* was now vanished into the mists of time, and neither *Popeye* nor *The World According to Garp* had done what he had hoped. There was still live performing, and Williams continued to jump on and off 'Das Bus', as he called his tour coach, and entertain crowds large and small across the country. He was keen to continue his movie career, and the warm critical response for his performance in *The World According to Garp* allowed him to do that. The scripts which had tailed off after *Popeye* had started to pick up again and he was being offered some interesting roles. But he appeared determined to do things a little differently next time out.

'I'm just interested in learning what I can about movies,' he said at the time, 'because there are two possibilities. I can act in other people's films or I can eventually write and act in my own. I hope I can play a supporting actor in the next film I do, so that I can sit back and watch people work rather than take the burden of being a major character, as in *Popeye* and *Garp*.'

In the end Williams did sign up for another film not long after that, but things didn't turn out quite the way he planned. He would be part of an ensemble cast but not in a supporting role. He and Walter Matthau would be joint male leads in *The Survivors*, a black comedy from Michael Ritchie. Again this was an atypical role for Williams in the sense that there was nothing in the script which suggested that it could be the vehicle for his particular talents. Williams plays a middle-management executive who lives the ideal suburban life while harbouring dreams of being on the corporate fast track to the executive washroom. Summoned to a meeting one morning, Williams rushes in expecting promotion at the very least, only to find he is being fired. In a final indignity he is fired by his boss's parrot which has been trained to deliver the downsizing eulogy. As he leaves his former office, Williams stops for petrol at a nearby filling station which is owned by Matthau and inadvertently triggers an explosion which destroys the whole place and puts Matthau out of business. Williams and Matthau cross paths again at the unemployment office and ultimately, in a barely credible plot twist, they get mixed up with Jerry Reed as a hit man and find themselves doing battle with a crowd of angry survivalists.

Certainly the black humour of the early part of *The Survivors* would have appealed to Williams. Politically he would have been in tune with a timely script which focused on the consequences of nothing actually trickling down from Ronald Reagan's trickle-down Reaganomics. However, the second half of the film is totally wrong-headed and Williams' particular brand of humour seems ill-suited to a dark comedy which descends into broad farce. He tried his best, but at the end of the day his performance was rather like throwing a match into a box of fireworks; spectacular, entertaining and ultimately too volatile to be kept in such a restricting container. None of Robin Williams' first three films had come close to stretching him comedically or dramatically. That was partly the result of his inexperience in picking the right projects; it was also the fault of directors who did not appreciate his talents or know how to use them; but mostly it was the fault of a studio system which was resolutely trying to hammer a square peg into a round hole. What Robin Williams really needed was someone who understood what he could do and how best he could do it.

In Hollywood terms Paul Mazursky is almost a Renaissance man. He is best known as a director, but he is also an actor, a comedian, a scriptwriter and a producer. He began as a night-club comedian in his native New York before graduating to television as a writer for artists such as Danny Kaye and for television shows like *The Monkees.* By the end of the Sixties he had made his directing débút with the then-controversial *Bob and Carol and Ted and Alice.* This was followed by a series of increasingly barbed studies of American society. Films such as *Blume in Love*, *Harry and Tonto* and *An Unmarried Woman* took a slightly skewed look at the American Dream. In the process they allowed Mazursky to build a reputation as one of the industry's most intelligent and literate directors, a genuine American *auteur.*

One of Mazursky's most perceptive looks at life in America came in 1984 when he made *Moscow on the Hudson.* It is the story of a Russian musician who defects on a visit to the United States; the actual defection takes place in Bloomingdale's – 'between Estée Lauder and Pierre Cardin'.

After being smuggled home by a security guard he marvels at life in the United States compared with the life he has left behind him. Then, after being mugged, he sees the other side of America – Mazursky shows the underbelly of the American Dream with crime, violence and poverty. Finally, however, the defector realises that, for all its faults, he is much better off in his new home. Although the film tends towards the sentimental too often for comfort, the central role of Vladimir the saxophonist could have been written for Robin Williams. For the first time in his film career, the actor also found a kindred spirit behind the camera. Paul Mazursky had been a stand-up comedian, he was one of Williams' gladiatorial fraternity, and he understood that Williams needed to be handled with care.

'At the time I knew Robin he was very manic,' recalled Mazursky some years later, suggesting that the toxin-free Williams hadn't quite found the calm that he was looking for. 'We went to several comedy clubs together and I once actually agreed to go on stage with him, but he was so funny I ran. On the set I always felt that what I had to work at was getting the tensions out, and I think we did it even though we had a couple of shouting matches at the beginning where I'd say "It's too much!" and he'd say "It's not anything!" I like the man very much. He's very sweet and he obviously wants to keep growing. He has a desperate need to be wonderful.'

If Williams did indeed have such a need, then he can thank Mazursky for allowing him to satiate his need on this film. Where Robert Altman had given him his head, and George Roy Hill had reined him in, Mazursky realised that Williams' artistic temperament had to be harnessed, not crushed. He needed direction, but he also needed to feel that he had an input into the creative process. The results are quite remarkable and, although it was not a huge commercial success, the film showed for the first time a glimpse of a maturing talent. As Vladimir the saxophonist, Williams submerged himself in a character for the first time. The accent, the mannerisms, the bewilderment of this stranger in a strange land were seamless. You could not tell where Williams stopped and Vladimir started and vice versa. Williams was not pretending to be someone else; he was playing a role. The strange alchemy between his Juilliard training and his mercurial comic gifts was showing signs of taking effect.

'I loved doing it,' said Williams of *Moscow on the Hudson*. 'Immersing yourself into another language and culture is wonderful. Oddly it was a little bit like Mork in that I was looking at American culture from the outside.'

Once again the reviews for *Moscow on the Hudson* were very good, maybe the best he had ever had, but once again the film failed to strike a chord with the people. It was at best a modest commercial success, meaning that he had now effectively struck out four times as a movie star. His career was not going as well as he or his managers had hoped. In addition his home life was rapidly declining into disarray. He and Valerie had come back together and Zach was the result of that. His birth, however, also threw into sharp focus the problems that still remained in the Williams marriage. Robin and Valerie were both devoted to Zach, they just weren't so sure they were still devoted to each other. Williams may have stopped drinking and doing coke, but he had not stopped his womanising. By the end of 1984 he had begun what would be a lengthy relationship with another woman. In addition he was spending more and more time performing. His comedy had always been his defence against the world; now it provided a hiding place. On the nights when he was performing on his concert tours he would finish his scheduled set and then the performance junkie would get into his car and prowl around looking for a fix. Eventually he would find another club, the smaller the better, and slip in quietly and do a late-night set. He got off on the buzz from the crowd when he stepped out of the shadows and into the limelight and they realised who it was. Some comedy fans effectively staked out certain of his favourite clubs in the seldom disappointed hope that he might turn up.

'As wonderful as he was, he was no prize package at that point,' recalled manager David Steinberg some ten years later. 'He was in a little trouble – there were four or five personalities trying to get out. The stage was the only place in his life where no one could fool with him.'

15

Enter Marsha

The strain on Robin and Valerie Williams' marriage was beginning to tell. Williams had begun a relationship with Michelle 'Tish' Carter, a women he had met while she was working as a waitress at a night-club. He was deeply involved in this relationship and spending less and less time at home. The times he spent with Valerie could not have been happy ones. Even though she was unwilling to draw that line in the sand for her husband, it was becoming more and more unbearable.

'Neither of us was prepared for the sudden life shift,' she said later. 'He never stops performing or partying. And the women! Very attractive women throw themselves at men in his position. You'd have to be a saint to resist. But I have to admit, the other women were harder to take after I'd had a child.'

In the cold light of sobriety, both sides of the Williams marriage would have to admit that it was little more than a sham. They could rub along as best they could for the time being, but their marriage was holed below the waterline and sinking fast. And it appeared to be having an effect on Zachary. Both Robin and Valerie loved the boy dearly, but friends began to notice changes in his behaviour. When he was about 18 months old he started to have serious temper tantrums, and his nanny was unable to do anything about it. Privately friends felt that the nanny was not as sympathetic as she might have been to the little boy's needs.

While all this was going on, Marsha Garces was working as a waitress in San Francisco. Working at night helped put her through San Francisco State College by day, where she was studying fabrics and textiles as well as Mandarin Chinese. She had met Robin Williams at a party some 12 years previously but, given his lifestyle at that stage, that hardly put her in an exclusive club. It's debatable whether she made any impression on him at all in that first meeting, and even if she did it would be nothing like the effect she was about to have on him. Marsha Garces was the daughter of Leon Garces, a chef born in Cebu in the Philippines who had moved to the States, and his wife Ina, who was the daughter of Finnish immigrants who had settled in Owen, Wisconsin. When Leon and Ina got married they settled in Milwaukee where Marsha was born. She was the youngest of four children – one boy and three girls – and as the youngest she tended to spend a lot of time on her own. Going to school and mixing with other children did not help much.

'I grew up in a German community, where all the other kids were blond and we were dark, so I know what it feels like to be considered different,' she explains. 'I was different even from my brothers and sisters. They were very social, I was always by myself.'

As she was growing up she discovered a passion for art and design. She subsidised her art studies at the University of Wisconsin in Milwaukee by working as a waitress in several places throughout the city. The waitressing seemed to come naturally to her as she learned that she had the knack of putting people at their ease. In addition it didn't take up any of her daylight hours, which allowed her to continue with her studies. Eventually she grew tired of the Midwest and decided to move to California to continue her studies in San Francisco.

Marsha Garces is an attractive, dark-haired woman with deep, dark eyes. She has a ready smile and, as she found out, the ability to make people feel comfortable. She would not, however, have considered herself maternal. She had been married twice and had not felt the need or the urge to have any children. That would account for her surprise when she met a mutual friend in 1984, who told her about the Williams' problems with Zachary and their current nanny, and the friend suggested that Marsha would be an ideal replacement.

When she had been working in those restaurants Marsha had often joked, 'If I'm thirty and still slinging hash, drag me out of here.' She had not yet reached her landmark age, but it was looming on the horizon and maybe a change of vocation might not be a bad idea. She was duly interviewed and got the job, and made preparations to move out to the Williams ranch which sat in 600 acres of its own land in the Napa Valley. Williams had bought the original spread in Sonoma some years previously and had added to it over the years to guarantee almost total seclusion. It was bought in 1982 as a refuge from the madness of the film industry and his overnight fame. His friend Eric Idle had encouraged him by pointing out that he didn't need to talk into a microphone when he could smell a flower instead. The Sonoma estate – which Williams occasionally referred to as 'The Fuckin' Ranch' – was, literally, an attempt to stop and smell the roses. That aspect of the purchase hadn't worked out, but it was still ideal for Marsha Garces. There was enough room there to allow her to look after her new young charge, and she also had enough time and space to continue with the hand-dyed fabrics in which she was starting to specialise.

To begin with, Marsha had all the time and space in the world. She seldom saw Robin and Valerie as they went about their business wrapped up in their own lives. Zachary became the centre of her universe, and the woman who had not previously shown any maternal urges quickly discovered that this little boy hung the moon. The feeling was mutual. Zach stopped the tantrums and he and his new nanny formed a deep and abiding bond.

For Robin Williams things were going from bad to worse. His marriage was a disaster and his career seemed to be heading in the same direction. He had made another two feature films which were near total disasters. *The Best of Times* featured Williams opposite Kurt Russell as two former high-school football team-mates whose lives had been scarred by one defining game. Russell was the quarterback who had thrown the ball for what should have been the winning touchdown; Williams was the running back who had dropped the ball. Their team had lost the game, and both men, their ambition stunted by this catastrophic blow to their self-esteem, seemed destined to live out their lives in a small-town hell without ever reaching their full potential. Eventually Williams, who is by now a manager in the local bank, gets the idea that they should replay the game. If the result is different, then perhaps their lives might be different. *The Best of Times* was written by Ron Shelton, who has gone on to corner the market in sports movies such as *Bull Durham* and *White Men Can't Jump*, and directed by Roger Spottiswoode, who also went on to success, most notably with *Tomorrow Never Dies.* As well as Williams and Russell the cast also boasted Pamela Reed, Donald Moffat and M. Emmet Walsh. A lot of talent, to be sure, but none of it adequately harnessed in a film which, like Russell and Williams, never reached its full potential. *The Best of Times* barely got a cinema release and made its way quickly to the video shelves without causing much of a blip on the box-office radar.

The same fate befell Williams' next film, *Club Paradise.* Later, as he became more experienced, he would confess to not being an especially good judge of a script. The fact that he agreed to star in this film simply confirms that. On paper it should have been a box-office smash. The cast was virtually a Who's Who of American comedy in the Eighties. As well as Williams and *Saturday Night Live* alumni Rick Moranis – who had just starred in the smash *Ghostbusters* – and Brian Doyle-Murray, the comic talent also included Eugene Levy, Andrea Martin and Mary Gross. British model-turned-actress Twiggy provided the glamour, Jimmy Cliff provided the music, and Peter O'Toole provided a touch of class. The film was being directed by Harold Ramis, another *Ghostbusters* star who was also one of the hottest comedy directors around after the success of *Caddyshack* and *National Lampoon's Animal House*. Ramis had co-written the script with Brian Doyle-Murray, and the Hollywood insiders felt that the whole package was simply a licence to print money.

Williams played a Chicago fireman who was being invalided out of the job after a work-related accident. He decides to use his sizeable severance payment to live in the Caribbean and spend his days lying in the sun listening to the surf. But when he discovers that his chosen resort, Club Paradise, is under threat from ruthless developers, he gets involved in a scheme to attract tourists to the island to raise enough money to keep the resort going. In the end, however, *Club Paradise* the movie turned out to be as big a disaster as Club Paradise the resort. In subsequent interviews Williams has insisted that he did the film purely and simply for the money. He knew that there were problems with the script but he believed they could be fixed. It's worth remembering that this would be his sixth film and he had yet to have a box-office hit. His television and stand-up popularity had yet to translate on to the big screen and, given the talent attached to this one, this must have seemed like a golden opportunity for a much-needed hit. It's hardly surprising that he put aside his misgivings and decided to sign on.

'They said it would be a box-office smash – "a great combination of people", "we'll kick ass",' he recalled later. 'And then it was my ass that got kicked. That's when you get screwed. Jump in with your passion. Not as a whore.'

Williams and his loyal managers could not have been anything other than deeply concerned about where his career was going. But just at this low point, Williams came up with something which remains one of the hidden gems of his career. Abandoning films for the time being, he went back to television. His experience with ABC on *Mork and Mindy* had left him justifiably leery of the big networks, but this time he would be working for PBS, America's public broadcasting network. Williams was taking the lead in a TV version of Saul Bellow's *Seize the Day* – a phrase which would have echoes later in one of his most successful roles – as part of the PBS Learning in Focus series. Williams played the central role of Tommy Wilhelm who, to all intents and purposes, is a Jewish Willy Loman. Tommy had wanted to be an entertainer, but his stern father, played by Joseph Wiseman, wanted him to follow in his footsteps as a doctor. Tommy had neither the ambition nor the aptitude for medicine and in the end he became a salesman. Now, as he approaches forty, his life is in complete disarray. Half of his territory – the better half – has been taken away and given to the boss's son-in-law; he is juggling both an ex-wife and a girlfriend and being crippled by alimony and support payments; and the nest egg he had been saving has all been eaten away in a series of bad investments. In desperation he approaches his father and asks for help, only to have his own father turn his back on him and refuse to bail him out. The film ends bleakly with Tommy sitting in the back of a synagogue raving to himself on the verge of a complete mental collapse.

It is very easy to look at *Seize the Day* and read into it a correlation between Tommy Wilhelm and his father and Robin Williams and his own father. Unfortunately the comparisons don't really stand up. Robert Williams may have been distant but he never once hardened his heart against his son, even when he decided – as Tommy does – to go against the family's chosen career path. Robert Williams had frequently been there and ready to support his son whenever it was needed; it was merely a point of pride on Robin Williams' part that he chose to make it on his own. If the film relates to any aspect of Robin Williams' life then it is to the state of his life at the time he was making it. This was a period where Williams would later refer to himself as walking through his personal life with all the certainty of a haemophiliac in a razor factory. Compared to Williams' life at that point, Tommy Wilhelm didn't really have too much to worry about. Nonetheless it is an extraordinary performance. Williams, frankly, is too young to play Tommy, but although he had logged a lower mileage, the panic in his eyes in this performance testifies to the fact that they had all been hard miles. Williams was struggling to find a role which showed off his comic skills but, almost as a by-product, he had found a role which marked him as a serious actor of considerable promise. If he was succeeding as an actor, however, he was failing miserably as a husband. The time had come to do something about it.

Looking back on the events leading up to the end of his marriage, Robin Williams is not especially proud of any of it. All things considered his behaviour may be, in his own eyes, the most shameful thing he has ever done. He continued to be completely self-absorbed. He continued in his relationship with Tish Carter, and as far as he and Valerie were concerned there was only one thing left to do.

> In the beginning when I started doing stand-up in coffee-houses, I wasn't looking to be famous to be recognised [he says]. I just wanted to have a good time performing. Valerie helped in a lot of ways. We were working hard together and then this thing took off. Fame came, and that was strange to me ... and Valerie. It's a type of life that tends to tear people asunder. Hollywood is a weird place. The industry affected our relationship – strained it horribly. Finally it just became impossible for us to stay together.

Williams admits that he and Valerie had always had a tumultuous relationship. There was Latin blood in her, she was fiery and she would fight for her man when she had to. But with all the separations and the constant womanising they both realised it was a losing battle, especially when Valerie also started seeing another man.

> There were things that were done that two people should never do to one another [says Williams]. I'd go off and run around because I didn't know what the fuck I wanted. I'd be a schmuck and she would respond in kind. And then we'd try to stop and deal with it and it wouldn't work. Finally I had to say, 'I can't do this to myself any more ... I'm tired of living this passive-aggressive shit.'

At the end of the day Robin and Valerie Williams had to consider the most important thing in each of their lives, Zach. 'Things ultimately went astray between me and Valerie,' says Williams. 'It was terribly painful but our marriage just was not functioning. The separation from her was difficult but it was also gentle. It was better to do that than to go at each other's throats.'

16

Growing Up

When Robin and Valerie Williams agreed to separate they were doing so as much in the best interests of their child as themselves. Williams moved out of the family home at Sonoma and into a beach house where he tried to get himself back together again. One of the important aspects of the separation was to make it as painless as possible for Zach. They arrived at a situation where, if Williams was on tour or on location, then the boy would stay with his mother. If Williams was in San Francisco, then he would have unhindered access to his son.

The split also had an effect on Marsha Garces. She had been feeling for some time that it was about time to move on anyway; she had held 15 jobs in as many years and was not really about making long-term career commitments to nannying. But she did love Zach and the boy was extremely fond of her. At the same time Williams was doing what he always did when he had a problem: he was exorcising them in public by going on tour. His working life was every bit as chaotic as his personal life, and what he really needed was someone to put things in order for him. He was looking around for an assistant at the same time as Marsha was looking to move on. As far as she was concerned, this would be an ideal way to take up a new challenge while keeping Zach in her life and she in his. So she became Robin Williams' secretary and personal assistant.

In the fullness of time and, as events unfolded, that simple action of changing careers would make Marsha Garces one of the most vilified women in show business. She was, according to the tabloids, 'the nanny who broke up Robin Williams' marriage'. It's a convenient label and, in newspaper terms, it's a sexy one too. But it doesn't bear closer scrutiny. For one thing, when she went to work for Robin Williams on his own, Marsha Garces was involved in her own long-term relationship and remained so for some time. Williams for his part was still involved with Tish Carter and, as David Steinberg had already hinted, given the shape he was in at that stage Williams was no catch for any woman. When Marsha Garces went to work for Robin Williams it was strictly business, nothing else. 'He was too screwed up and I wasn't interested in being sucked dry,' says Marsha of the early days of their professional relationship.

However, Marsha Garces quickly brought a sense of order to Williams' life. One of the first things he did when he started to get himself together was to go into therapy. Williams was still a fairly fragile individual. If he was to stay clean and sober then he would have to get through this crisis period in his life. One way of doing that was through a process of therapy which helped him discover more about his life.

'Therapy made me re-examine everything,' he admitted later. 'My life, how I related to people, how far I could push the "please like me" desire before there was nothing left of me to like. Therapy has helped me face my limitations, what I can and cannot do. And it's made me a much calmer and saner person.'

One of the people who undoubtedly forced Williams into therapy was Marsha Garces. From his earliest days as a little boy alone in a great big house Robin Williams has needed to be liked and feared being left alone. As a consequence of that he has required people to take charge of his life, to show him what needs to be done as opposed to what he wants to do. Someone needed to provide some no-nonsense assessment of where he was going with his life, and in this case it seems to have been Marsha.

'You've got two great careers,' she would tell him. 'You're really intelligent, you're healthy, you're strong, you're handsome, you have a great son – and you're totally depressed. You're an adult. Pull it together.'

And, slowly but surely, he did. Through the therapy he faced his anxieties and his fears. He was able to talk to someone seriously about the sort of things he used to hide from in his comedy.

> For me, going through therapy and stuff [he admitted in a revealing interview with *Esquire* magazine], I'm just beginning to realise that it [childhood] wasn't always that happy. My childhood was kind of lonely. Quiet. My father was away, my mother was working, doing benefits. I was basically raised by this maid, and my mother would come in later, you know, and I knew her and she was wonderful and charming and witty. But I think maybe comedy was my way of connecting with my mother – 'I'll make Mommy laugh and

> that will be okay' . . . Maybe it started off that I wanted the attention from my mother, but it was also that I could do something here. Comedy is something I was meant to do, whether it's that kind of divine purpose or not. I was meant to do this. I was not meant to sell insurance.

Williams then went on to talk candidly about his other greatest nightmare, being left by his parents:

> The fear of abandonment – the oldest, the deepest, fear of all: 'I'm ditched. I'm history'. But . . . you begin to know you'll survive. They [your parents] haven't been with you for a long time. You're okay. I can't deny the child inside me because obviously it's done kind of nice for me. And I love that. But to know what it comes from and let the genuine warmth grow . . . that's what I see changing. Knowing that fame is obviously like a drug and recognising that, yeah, I kicked other drugs. And once you recognise that, you can get up and do what you want to do.

Williams is an intelligent man with a knowledge that verges on the intuitive rather than the learned. But for all of his remarkable intellect and prodigious mental acuity there was always a gap. There was a blind spot in terms of self-knowledge and it is this which therapy helped him address. He doubts he will ever attain inner peace, whatever that might be, and although he became a better person he is sensible enough to realise that even cleaned up he is not easy to live with.

'I'm no great shakes,' he says. 'It's the "love me" syndrome coupled with the "fuck you" syndrome. Like the great joke about the woman who comes up to the comic after the show and says, "God I really love what you do. I want to fuck your brains out!" And the comic says, "Did you see the first show or the second show?"'

Williams remains riddled with enough insecurities to stay as a great comedian while at the same time becoming a better person. There will always be an element of one hand reaching out to someone while the other hand pushes them away. But there is no doubt that the therapy changed his life. For one thing it helped him deal with the end of his relationship with Valerie without renewing his acquaintance with vodka and lime or cocaine.

> It's not disappointing [he said of the failure of his marriage]. That's why therapy helps a lot. It forces you to look at your life and figure out what's functioning and what's not. You don't have to beat your brains against a wall if it's not working. That's why you choose to be separated rather than

call each other an asshole every day. Ultimately things went astray. We changed, and then with me wandering off again a little bit, then coming back and saying, 'Wait, I need help' – it just got terribly painful.

Therapy also enabled Robin Williams to deal with his constant need to perform. He had always been there with a quip or a routine or a benefit show at the drop of a hat. As he parodied himself in the 'Mork Meets Robin Williams' episode of *Mork and Mindy* he was the comedian who couldn't say no. Now he was learning.

> The hardest word of all to say is 'no' [he admitted]. Bette Davis, back when we were doing the revival of *Laugh-In*, told me, 'The one word you'll need is "no".' The secret is to be able to turn things down, to not take on projects like *Club Paradise* or *The Best of Times* just because they say they want you to. If they can't get you, they'll get anybody, so wise up.

This desire to take just about anything for fear that he might not be offered anything else is at the heart of some miserable film choices at the start of Robin Williams' film career. Of the seven films he had done, two – *The World According to Garp* and *Moscow on the Hudson* – had been worth his while; Williams claimed at the time that these were the two films of which he felt most proud. One film, *Seize the Day*, was overly ambitious in that he was just too young for Tommy Wilhelm. But the other four were unmitigated disasters in almost every way.

Williams was also learning to say no in his personal life, and not just to drugs and drink. Ironically it was Valerie who first spotted this character flaw when they were first married and had tried to straighten it out. Now, with a combination of harsh experience, Marsha Garces and a good therapist, he was finally getting the message.

> People expect you to be constantly 'on' but you can't [Williams said]. You'd be drained like a car battery. You'd have to have two guys pull up with a truck and jump leads at your house every morning. You can't do it all the time. It's fun to perform, but if you have to do it all the time it's a drain. If you do it when you're ready for it then it's wonderful, but not all the time. It used to be in the old days I thought you could, but you can't. You have to take time, you have to recharge. I thought I had to be on all the time because I thought I had to keep performing, but you'll flame out. There's only so many times you can do that. It's like dry heaving. You're real drunk and you're leaning over the porcelain altar going 'There's nothing left', and your

> body is going 'But there is'. At a certain point you run out of stuff. You have to recharge or find another stimulus.

For Robin Williams the answer really came in finding another stimulus, and in his case the stimulus was Marsha Garces. After about a year of their professional relationship they began to realise that this was more than an employer-employee thing. One of the turning-points came before Williams' landmark 1986 concert at the Metropolitan Opera House in New York; he was the first comedian to perform there.

'Robin was complaining, in a joking way, about the bimbettes who knocked on his door at the hotel,' Marsha recalled. 'I asked him, "Why are you so surprised? If I wasn't working with you and I didn't know how screwed up you are, I'd be interested in you." '

One thing that therapy had not changed that much in Robin Williams was the fear which still gripped him before he went on-stage. That night at the Metropolitan Opera it would have been worse than usual. This was a big gig. This was history in the making – and it was being filmed for television and video. The potential to die a horrible comic death was greater here than at any other time in his career. One of the little rituals that Williams had fallen into over the past year was that just before he would go on-stage Marsha, who was there for any last-minute panics, would give him a hug. That hug would probably have been more welcome at the Met than at any other time over the past year.

Marsha recalls: 'I told him, "You can do it. You're okay. I love you" – which is what I say to my friends all the time.'

On the stage that night Williams gave one of the greatest stand-up comedy performances of all time. It was lightning in a bottle and, fortunately, it was captured on film. But at the moment of his triumph he remembered what Marsha had told him as they waited in the wings.

'Marsha used to tell me I was a good person, and finally I believed it,' he says.

This is what he needed. All his life he had wanted other people to like him, but Marsha Garces convinced him that he had to like himself. By doing that he no longer felt the need to be loved. Marsha Garces saved Robin Williams' life, perhaps literally as well as figuratively.

> She would just talk me down [says Williams of Garces' role when his marriage was breaking up]. I was not suicidal but I was fucked up. My wife was living with another man. I was just out of my fucking mind. I was very indignant and very self-righteous and Marsha said, 'Listen, asshole, there's no reason to be indignant, you were no prince and she was no saint' …

> I was living in a house on the beach and started to get my life together and I fell in love with Marsha. And that's why my life was saved by her and not ruined by her.

Friends of Williams very quickly noticed the difference that Marsha Garces had made in his life. 'Marsha is Robin's anchor,' claims Pam Dawber. 'She's reality. Ground zero. She's very sane and that's what he needs. She's incredibly loving too. She knows who is bad for him and who is good, and she helps keep the good relationships going.'

In the early days of their relationship there may have been an element of the Stockholm Syndrome, a psychological oddity where people in extreme conditions tend to fixate on others in the same situation – as when bonds form between hostages and their captors. Williams was certainly in a mess, and the fact that Garces was not prepared to indulge him could have helped create that circumstance. But there is no doubt that once they had acknowledged their feelings for each other, this quickly established itself as a deep, meaningful and sustaining love.

> I moved out of the house and I was like goo. I was a babbling idiot [says Williams]. And then I became involved with Marsha. All of a sudden I started to calm down. I stopped running around with all this madness. I started to go, 'Wait, I can live a life. I don't have to live and die in my own sweat.' I slowly pulled myself up. I started to create and to work – kind of like the phoenix that rises out of its own ashes. Marsha is not someone who dragged somebody away. She's somebody who offered something, who said 'This is a way to live', and I went for it.
>
> Am I going to run around now? [he continues rhetorically]. No. I'm at peace with myself. It's not something like 'I – am – very – happy', like I've got a dart in the back of my neck. But it's something like 'God, I don't want to blow this. This is wonderful stuff.'

17

'Goood Mooorning, Heraklion!'

In 1965, Robin Williams was 13 years old and enjoying life as much as any bright and studious pupil would at a private school in Detroit. Half a world away the 25-year-old Adrian Cronauer was coming to the end of his stint in the Air Force in Greece.

Cronauer was the son of a Pittsburgh machinist and a schoolteacher. He had always loved radio. As a small boy he would sit in his darkened bedroom long after lights out listening to his favourites on a jerry-rigged set of headphones when he was supposed to be asleep. At the age of 12 he auditioned for a gig as the piano player on a radio variety show called *Happy's Party.* He got the job and thus began a lifelong love affair with the communications business. By the time he was in high school he had graduated to working for the educational TV station in Pittsburgh where he was involved in the backroom staff of a show hosted by Fred Rogers. This was Rogers' first foray into television but Mr Rogers, as he would become known, and his fictional television neighbourhood went on to shape the minds of millions of young Americans over the next four decades as one of television's best-loved presenters.

It was inevitable that Cronauer would go on to try to make a living in broadcasting, which is why he spent four years as a broadcasting major at the American University in Washington. Cronauer started school in 1960 but it would be 25 years before he finally completed his degree. Cronauer was combining his classes with some real broadcasting work and as such he was officially only a part-time student. Someone from the college administration informed the draft board and, since he was not actually exempt from the draft on education grounds, Cronauer was contracted by the draft board and given a hard choice. It was actually more of a dilemma than a choice; he had thirty days to decide whether to enlist or be drafted. Since enlistment gave him some say in his future in the military, Cronauer signed on with the US Air Force.

Cronauer had been passed 1-A by the draft board and had put in his application for flight training to be a pilot. But, to his horror, when he went to Texas for basic training he found that instead of releasing them at the end of three years, they were holding on to pilots. Figuring he could be in the Air Force until he was 30, Cronauer quickly cancelled his application and looked around for something else instead.

'They said, "What can we do with you?" I told them, "Here are my credentials. I majored in broadcasting, I've been a disc jockey, I've worked in television." And they said, "Oh, all right, we'll make you a radio and television production specialist".'

As a television and radio specialist, Cronauer's first job was to supervise the making of instructional films on how to prepare aircraft engines and launch missiles. Eventually he was sent to Crete in the Greek islands, where he ended up as the presenter of an early morning radio show at the US Air Force base on Heraklion. It was there, in the autumn of 1963, that he coined what would become his trademark phrase when he first uttered the deathless words 'Goood mooorning, Heraklion'.

'As a catchphrase it has more of a clang than a ring to it,' he admits.

Cronauer served at Heraklion for about a year and a half which was bringing him ever closer to the end of his three-year hitch. He would have to make a decision about his future and make it quickly.

> When my enlistment was coming to an end in Crete [he explains], the normal procedure would be to rotate back to the United States, and that would mean going back to another educational television facility and I didn't want to do that. I wanted to see a little bit more of the world. I had only a year left of my enlistment and there were only two places I could go that were one-year tours, Korea or Vietnam. I chose Vietnam. There was not that much fighting going on over there. We were still an advisory mission and at that time the American contingent was still very small. They were living in hotels in downtown Saigon. All the fighting was being done by Vietnamese out in rice paddies and the boondocks, and the Americans were sitting back in their hotels in a cheerleading position. I could see no problems in going to Vietnam. About four weeks after I had turned in my paperwork, by which time it was too late to retract it, we got word that the Viet Cong had blown up the radio station in Saigon.

So Cronauer was now going into a war zone, and one with an ever-increasing American presence. The Gulf of Tonkin incident at the end of 1964, in which the Americans accused North Vietnamese gunboats of attacking American ships on the Gulf, allowed President Lyndon Johnson to step up America's involvement in the war. In the space of a single year, 1965, American troop numbers almost doubled from just over 55,000 men to 100,000. Adrian Cronauer arrived in Vietnam just as the escalation was beginning and quickly found himself wrapped up in the siege mentality. He would present his morning *Dawn Buster* show with a loaded ·45 on the studio desk, and he was expected to use it if the situation arose.

> The first week I was there, I walked down the street and saw a little old lady with a basket over her arm [says Cronauer]. I said to myself, 'She's the one. She's got the grenade that's going to get me.' I immediately crossed the street only to find there was another little old lady with another basket on that side too. You quickly develop a fatalistic attitude. If the grenade or the bullet is going to get me then it has my name on it. It's not until about a month before you are due to rotate out that you start looking for the little old ladies with the baskets again.

Adrian Cronauer was something of a jack of all trades at the Armed Forces Radio station in Saigon. He presented the early morning show, where of course his signature call sign had now become 'Goood mooorning, Vietnam'. He was also, in the early days, the station's news director and latterly the production manager for the station.

> I grew up in Pittsburgh, and there was a morning man there by the name of Reeves Cordick and he sort of owned morning drive-time radio. My conception of what a good morning show should sound like was pretty much what Cordick did, so I deliberately fashioned and modelled my show on that. But since I was also the production manager I tried to make the station sound very much like Stateside radio. I expanded the range of top 40 music, we had Number One Hits and Golden Oldies and all these sorts of features. We also had on-air promotions and mock contests just to try to make it sound as much as possible like a Stateside station.

With thousands of raw recruits arriving every week, Cronauer's efforts at bringing a little slice of Americana to the Far East were much appreciated by the troops. Though, he concedes, they occasionally had a strange way of showing their appreciation.

> I was told that after a while, especially when they were out in the field, the troops had their own particular way of responding [he recalls]. When I would start my show by shouting 'Goood mooorning, Vietnam', they would usually respond by shouting in unison 'Get fucked, Cronauer'. I'm told that on at least one occasion when I yelled it, a guy picked up his M-16 and blew his radio away. I guess he was having a particularly bad day.

Cronauer served his 12-month tour of duty without major incident. He was never wounded but he insists, quite properly, that there is no one who served in Vietnam who doesn't bear some sort of scar. When he was finished with Vietnam he was finished with the Air Force, and after his discharge he went back to his first love, broadcasting. His first job was as a television anchor man in Lima, Ohio. Eighteen months later he went on to be programme director of a small TV station in Roanoke in Virginia. He liked Virginia and based himself there for almost eight years, including a stint working as a management consultant in San Francisco, and then going back to run a radio station in Virginia. Nothing apparently seemed to satisfy him during an increasingly peripatetic existence which also included starting up and then selling a successful advertising agency, and spending seven years in New York making commercials, teaching and working part-time at WQXR, a station for which he had always dreamed of working.

There is no doubt, though, that while he was criss-crossing the country in a number of well-paid and successful jobs, a large part of Adrian Cronauer was still in Vietnam. He was increasingly upset at the way the troops in South East Asia were being portrayed at home. He was particularly incensed at the ease with which people in the United States were able to believe the troops in Vietnam were little more than a bunch of drug-taking, baby-killing rapists. He was also angry, like so many veterans, that they had been forced to slink home with their tails between their legs and made to feel ashamed for doing nothing more than serving their country.

One of Cronauer's closest friends in Saigon was Ben Moses. Moses had a position in military intelligence but he was also a disc jockey who would later go on to be an Emmy-award-winning television producer. He and Cronauer had kept in touch over the intervening years and together in the late Seventies they hit on the idea of turning their Vietnam experiences into something more meaningful to a wider audience. It was Cronauer's idea to try to come up with an allegorical story about the effect of Vietnam on one man, reflecting the effect of the war on the United States as a whole.

> I served in Vietnam through 1965 and that was the year in which America became involved in the war in a major way [explains Cronauer]. I watched Saigon go in a single year from being this sleepy little French colonial town – the Paris of the Orient – to a nightmare because of this massive influx of troops and equipment and money. By the time I left, the black market was flourishing, the economy was in ruins, the traffic was unmanageable and the whole place was totally different from when I arrived there.

Cronauer and Moses originally tried to get their idea off the ground in 1979 as a television sitcom, hoping it might combine the popularity of two other hit shows, *M*A*S*H* and *WKRP in Cincinnati.* Not surprisingly, television executives were less than thrilled with the concept. They had difficulty in visualising any scenario in which the words 'comedy' and 'Vietnam' could reasonably coexist. To the average American, comedy in Vietnam meant Bob Hope entertaining the troops on a USO tour. Doors were politely but firmly shut in their faces, but Moses and Cronauer kept plugging away. Eventually they decided to try for a television movie rather than a weekly sitcom, and Moses wrote a script about an essentially fictional character who just happened to be called Adrian Cronauer. On the basis that no one had seemed to find Vietnam remotely funny, there was more drama in this version and fewer laughs. The TV movie brought largely the same response as the TV sitcom and it rattled around various companies and numerous executives for four years. It eventually made its way to the desk of Larry Brezner in the hope that it might be suitable for one of his clients. Unlike many others Brezner could see the potential in the script. He optioned it almost immediately and then passed it on to writer Mitch Markowitz in order to punch it up and make it funnier. Markowitz had written for *M*A*S*H*, as well as the ground-breaking cult comedy *Mary Hartman, Mary Hartman.* He was completely in tune with the ideas that Moses and Cronauer were trying to get across and had exactly the right sensibility to bring out the laughs without sacrificing the drama.

Larry Brezner was Robin Williams' personal manager. It is by no means certain that when he came across the script he saw it as the perfect vehicle for his client, but both men must have known that after seven films without a substantial hit – and including the disastrous *Club Paradise* – there were not going to be many more opportunities for stardom. Williams happened by Brezner's office one day and, looking through a pile of material, he came across Markowitz's script. Williams often describes himself as a poor judge of material, but after reading this one he decided it was for him.

For once, his instincts were spot on. Whether they knew it or not at the time, Brezner and Williams had just found the perfect role.

18

From the Delta to the DMZ

Larry Brezner was convinced that *Good Morning Vietnam*, as Moses and Cronauer's project was now known, would be a hit. There were others, however, who did not share his feeling. Paramount Pictures, for example, were interested but only if they were prepared to turn the movie into a broad, farcical, low comedy – a cross between *National Lampoon's Animal House* and *Stripes.* Brezner was adamant that the script should retain Cronauer's original allegorical notion of a man changed by the circumstances he faces in Vietnam, reflecting the changes faced by America in the same period. Eventually Paramount and Brezner disagreed so comprehensively that the studio put the script into turnaround. This is a fairly common occurrence in Hollywood and basically means that the producer has a certain amount of time to find someone else who will make the project and be prepared to reimburse the original studio for the money they had invested in developing it.

If Brezner was worried about the script languishing in Development Hell for any length of time he need not have been. Barely 24 hours after being put into turnaround *Good Morning Vietnam* was picked up by Jeffrey Katzenberg, the chairman of Walt Disney Studios. Katzenberg was known in the industry as 'the Golden Retriever' for his ability to sniff out commercial prospects, and his instincts once again had not let him down. He saw *Good Morning Vietnam* as a perfect project for Disney's Touchstone Pictures, the division which had been set up some three years earlier to allow Disney to escape from the strait-jacket of its family image and make slightly more adult pictures.

With the script having found a secure home, Brezner and Markowitz went to work on making sure that it would fit Robin Williams like a glove. None of his previous seven pictures had been so immaculately or carefully hand-tooled to suit the actor's needs. Whether they said it or not, everyone connected with the picture knew that this time they were going for all the marbles; this was the movie which would either make Robin Williams a star, or send him back to television. 'If this isn't a breakthrough,' joked Williams, 'then we've made a very expensive travel film.'

Good Morning Vietnam was still essentially a film about Adrian Cronauer, but the more it progressed the more it became about someone who was Cronauer in name only. In the film Cronauer arrives in Saigon from Greece in 1965 and quickly becomes a forces favourite with his madcap comedy and his unconventional methods. Before Cronauer, Armed Forces Radio consisted of Ray Connif music and bland announcements about avoiding foot rot and razor burns. Cronauer, in the movie at least, turned it into the bastard child of Howard Stern and Wolfman Jack with James Brown music and *risqué* stand-up routines. The Armed Forces Radio authorities in the shape of Bruno Kirby and the late J. T. Walsh don't take kindly to Cronauer's flouting of their regulations and his, in their eyes, mockery of their conventions. Cronauer is also pursuing an unrequited love affair with Trinh, a Vietnamese girl, in the process becoming very friendly with her brother, Tuan. It is Tuan who urges Cronauer to leave a favourite GI bar only seconds before it is blown up, and it is he who goes into the jungle to rescue Cronauer when he has fallen victim to a Viet Cong ambush. When his superiors discover that Tuan is in fact a wanted Viet Cong terrorist, they finally have the means to get rid of Cronauer. Five months into his tour Cronauer is manoeuvred into an honourable discharge and sent back to the United States.

'Larry Brezner played a very active role in developing the script,' recalls the real Adrian Cronauer. 'His first idea was that every good film has to be a love story and it doesn't have to be a traditional boy-girl love story.'

The example that Brezner quoted to Cronauer was the hit comedy *Arthur*, in which Dudley Moore played a drunken millionaire playboy who falls in love with shopgirl Liza Minnelli. But, as Brezner pointed out, the real love story in *Arthur* is not between Moore and Minnelli. Instead it is between Moore and his faithful butler played by John Gielgud, who has looked after Arthur all of his life and has become something of a surrogate father.

> In *Good Morning Vietnam* [Cronauer explains], Brezner felt that although the sex interest was between Robin Williams and the girl, the real love story

> was between Williams and her brother. That was one of his foundations. The script went through about five different versions – in one version they had me captured by the Viet Cong and put in a bamboo cage, in another I got married to the Vietnamese girl – and I was able to get hold of a copy of each version. Each time I got one I would sit down and write page after page of suggestions for additions and deletions. Some of them they accepted and some of them they ignored.

In the main Larry Brezner was generally very receptive to his notes, but Cronauer maintains that he found a real problem with Barry Levinson, who had been signed on to direct the film. With so much attention being lavished on the script, it was equally important that just as much care be taken in the choice of the director. Everyone agreed that Levinson was the right man for the job. Levinson, as it happened, had been a broadcaster in his youth and he had also been a successful comedy writer. He had a reputation as an actor's director. In films like the classic *Diner* and *Tin Men* he had taken a cast of quality actors and encouraged them to improvise and given them the freedom to find their roles within the confines of the script. Levinson would be perfect for handling someone like Robin Williams, who thrived on freedom but also needed to be told when he had gone too far.

> He puts up road cones [Williams says, describing Levinson's technique]. It's a bit like going to driving school. It's not like hitting a wall, you know when you run over it that you've gone too far, but there's no real harm done. So you know what the limits are and that's nice. The good part for me was the stuff that was done when I was out of the radio studio, Barry took all the pressure off me. He told me there were times when I didn't have to be funny. He told me, 'Just play off people. If you're quiet, then that's good.' That was very freeing, because the tendency is 'I have to find a joke here', but then you realise you don't have to. It's all right. That gives it another side completely, which helps.

While Robin Williams' fictional Adrian Cronauer was finding Levinson a joy to work with, the real Adrian Cronauer was less impressed:

> Barry Levinson was a strange person to deal with. I don't know what his problem was, but he became very much afraid of me. I had a deal where I would play a small cameo role in the movie, from the very beginning that had been my arrangement with Larry Brezner, but Levinson would have none of it. I don't know what his feelings were about it, I can't even speculate.

> It got to the point where I couldn't find out what was going on. I could get no feedback whatsoever once they had started shooting. It got to the point where I had almost to threaten to go public with my dissatisfaction.

From Cronauer's point of view you can understand his frustration, especially at being denied the opportunity to appear in the movie in however small a role. It would have been a nice gesture to have him in the movie, especially with Ben Moses getting a screen credit as co-producer. His frustration was made all the more acute because he considered himself a fan of Levinson's previous work. But, from Levinson's point of view, you can also appreciate that from the moment the cameras start turning it is his picture. Film-making is a collaborative process, to be sure, but there can be only one vision and that has to belong to the director. Levinson has made no public comments about Cronauer other than to say that he didn't find him funny either in person or on the tapes of shows. That being the case, he presumably felt that Cronauer had little to contribute, which makes Levinson guilty of gracelessness rather than actual malice.

Cronauer himself admits that there is a school of thought articulated by John Grisham, another lawyer who has done well out of Hollywood, which says that if you have a property which is being turned into a film then you should take the money and – not walk – run away without looking back. Instead of perhaps wisely following the Grisham dictum, Cronauer became so concerned about the lack of information coming from the set that he eventually insisted on a moral turpitude clause being introduced into his contract to control the way he would be portrayed in the film. He was anxious that he did not turn out to be a murderer, or a drug addict, or a baby-killer. This appears to be something of an over-reaction. Even though the film was being made for Disney's adult arm Touchstone Pictures, Robin Williams' film career was not yet in such dire straits that it would require such a radical change of image.

Williams and Cronauer never met at any stage during shooting or in the pre-production process. The official version is that Williams is such a gifted and intuitive mimic that the film-makers wanted the two men kept apart so that Williams did not end up imitating Cronauer on-screen.

> That's the story I usually see [says Cronauer], but I don't believe that was true. Something else was going on there and I have yet to figure out what it was. At one point my wife and I went to Hollywood to see a rough cut of the film and we had dinner with Barry Levinson and his wife. I could say charitably that the man is very shy, but there was no rapport, no attempt to

> talk to me about the film in any way, shape or form. My wife and I talked about this. I cannot understand what he was afraid of, or what he was worried that I could do to hurt him or his film.

Regardless of what Barry Levinson might have felt about Adrian Cronauer, there was another fear behind the scenes at *Good Morning Vietnam*, and it was a very genuine one. Was Robin Williams still funny? His previous seven films had been box-office disasters. Two of them – *Garp* and *Moscow on the Hudson* – had brought warm reviews for Williams, but there were no queues stretching round the block. Williams was 35 when he made *Good Morning Vietnam* – ten years older than Cronauer had been when he was in Saigon – and his off-screen life was in tatters. He had kicked his cocaine habit but his marriage had broken down. As well as being emotionally torn by the end of his relationship with Valerie Velardi, he was also distraught about his relationship with his son, Zach. The boy was four years old now and Williams was desperately beating himself up about what kind of father he would be to his son. Was Zach destined to grow up the same way he did, with a loving father who was unable to communicate that affection? Williams was in the process of turning his life around. He was in therapy for the first time in his life, but still there was a genuine concern that he might have lost his gift for mayhem and anarchy.

'When he said "That's it, enough",' according to his friend and manager Larry Brezner, 'there was a fear he'd lose his edge, but he's as free as ever he was.'

A lot of that freedom was brought about by the direct influence of Marsha Garces. When they were on location in Thailand she seldom left Williams' side. She was there for whatever he needed. She went over lines with him, she provided massages to ease his tensions, she found books about 1965 and went over them with him, they even wrote some of his dialogue together. 'She was the hardest working person on the set,' says producer Mark Johnson. 'She was there for him 24 hours a day. She truly loves him.'

Undoubtedly Levinson's careful direction also played a great part in making sure that Williams not only had not lost his edge, but was able to take his craft up another level. There is in fact a lot less comedy than people remember in *Good Morning Vietnam*. The first half of the film deals with Williams' microphone mania, with the audio meters pinning themselves into the red zone as he bawls out Cronauer's trademark greeting. But the second half of the film, in the aftermath of the restaurant bombing, concentrates more on the human drama of Cronauer's relation-

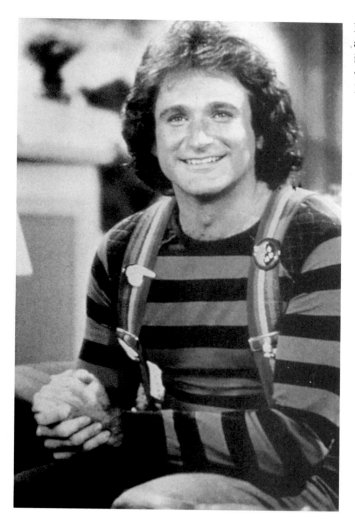

Robin Williams as Mork (1979) in what he assumed was traditional Earth garb.

Williams in his Orkan space suit in the early days of *Mork & Mindy.* He started out with a guest appearance on *Happy Days* in 1978 and ended up with a show which ran for 91 episodes from 1979 to 1983.

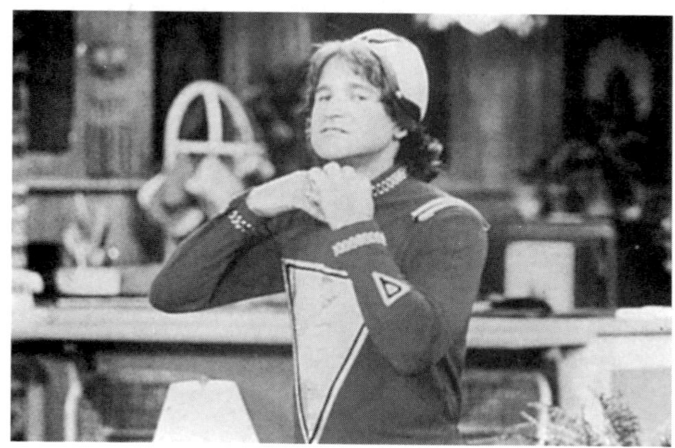

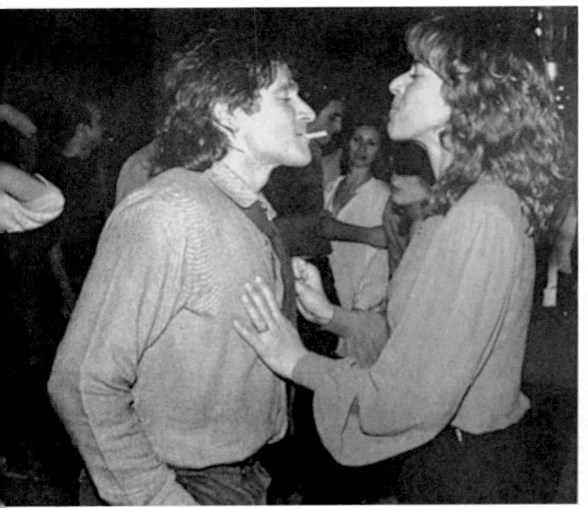

Party animal. Robin Williams and first wife Valerie were among the favoured who were allowed past the velvet rope and given free rein at New York's chic Studio 54 (1979).

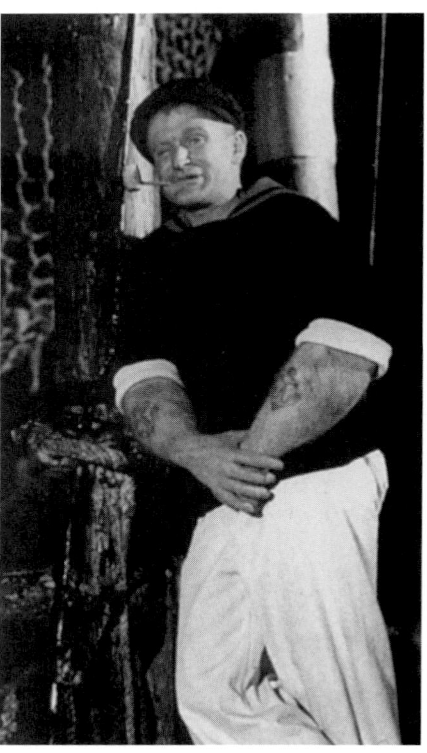

Williams underwent daily torture in his full Popeye make-up in 1980. The latex forearms were so tight they frequently cut off the circulation.

Old friends. Robin Williams and Christopher Reeve after a performance of Reeve's *The Fifth of July* in 1981. The friendship would be tested by adversity over the years but never broken. When Reeve met with his tragic accident Williams was at his bed-side making him laugh.

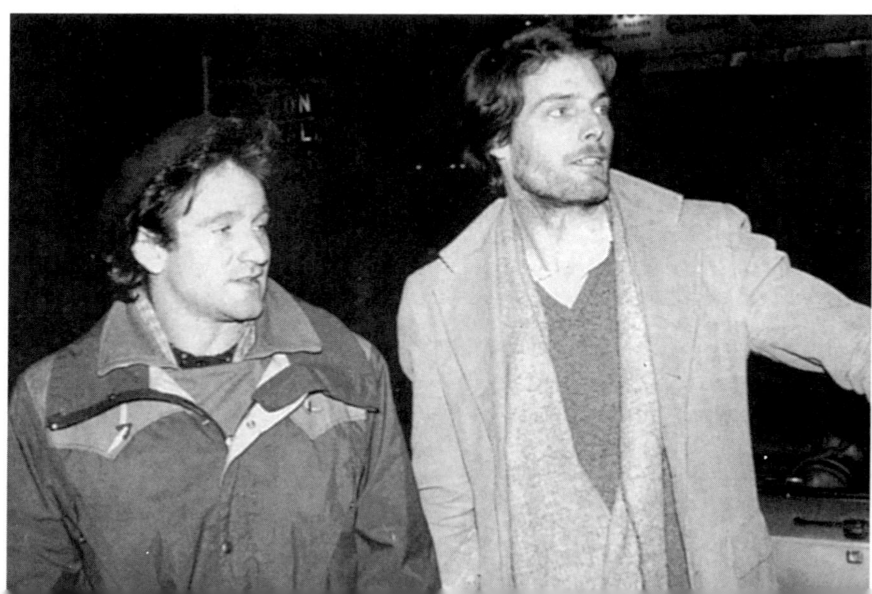

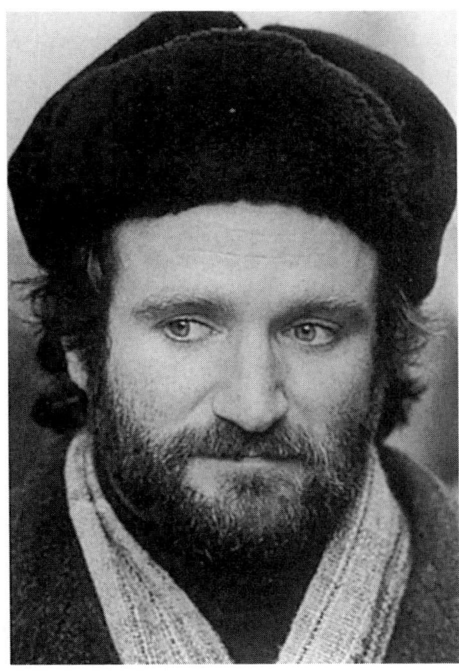

As asylum seeker Vladimir Ivanoff in *Moscow on the Hudson* (1984). Williams gave some hint of his potential as an actor. The fact that the film was directed by former comedian Paul Mazursky helped.

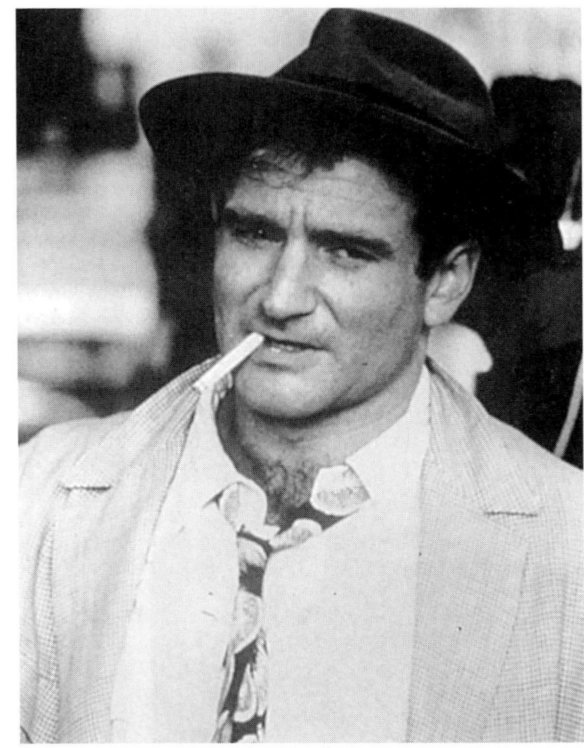

By deciding in 1986 to play Tommy Wilhelm in a PBS adaptation of *Seize the Day* Robin Williams went back to his dramatic roots. Despite being a shade young for the role it remains an impressive performance as a man at the end of his tether.

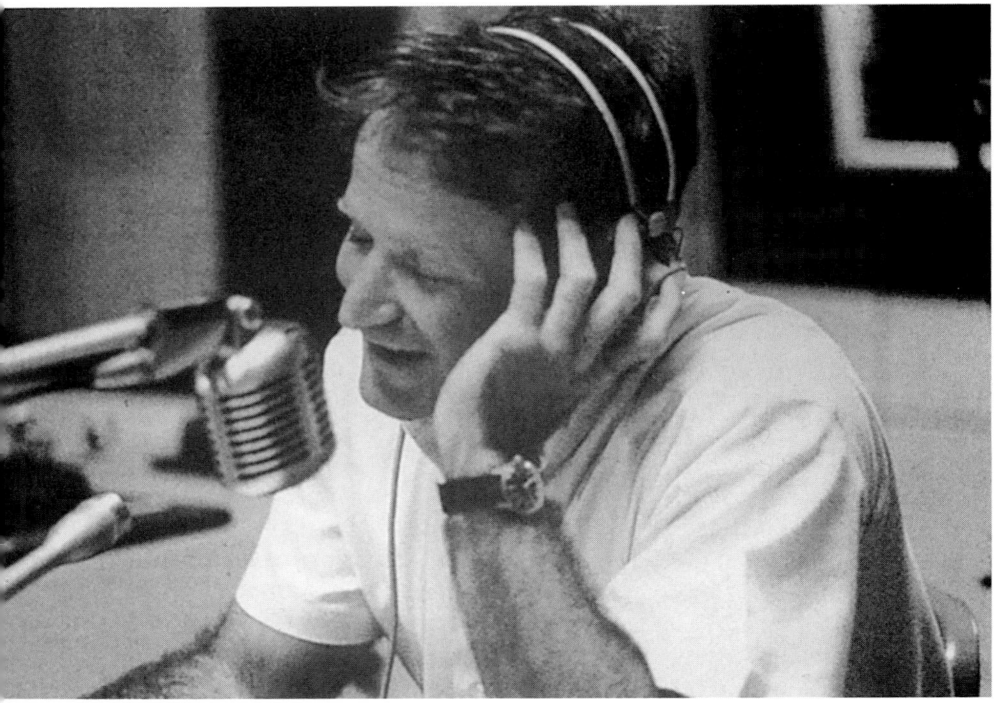

A star is born. After a string of cinematic failures Williams scored a smash hit and his first Best Actor nomination as DJ Adrian Cronauer in *Good Morning Vietnam* (1987).

Despite the personal problems which still beset him in 1987, everything was forgotten when Williams took the stage for his stand-up routine that December.

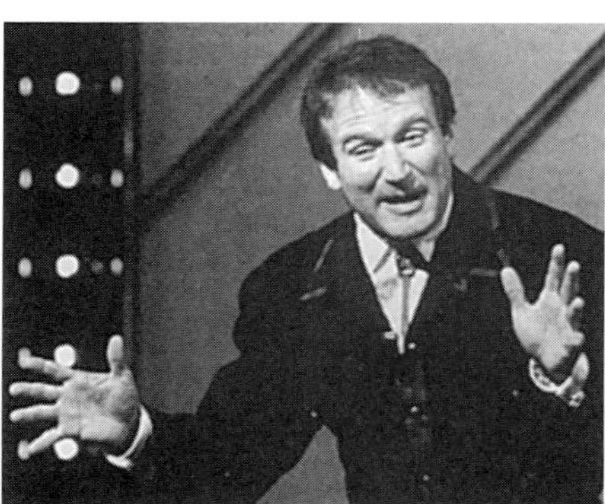

Robin Williams and Steve Martin as Estragon and Vladimir in the controversial Lincoln Center production of *Waiting for Godot* in 1988.

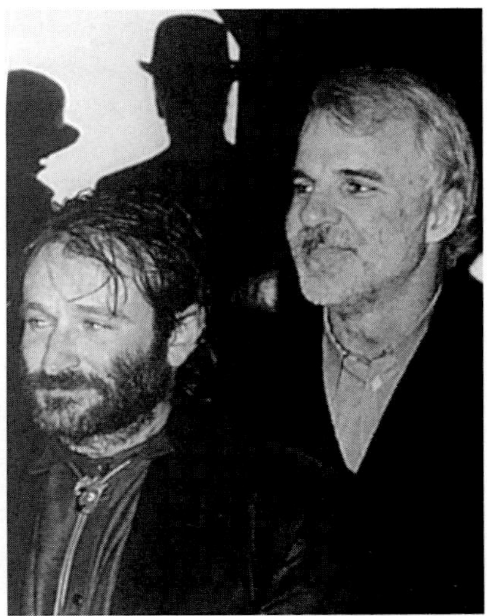

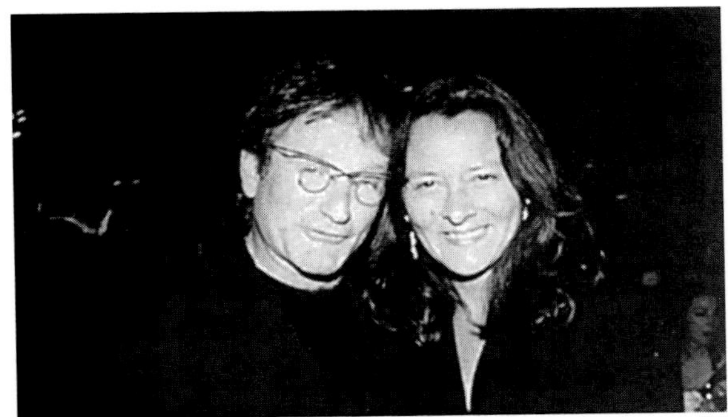

As well as turning his life around (in 1988), Marsha Garces Williams became Robin Williams' good right arm in terms of his career choices. It was she who found and produced *Mrs Doubtfire.*

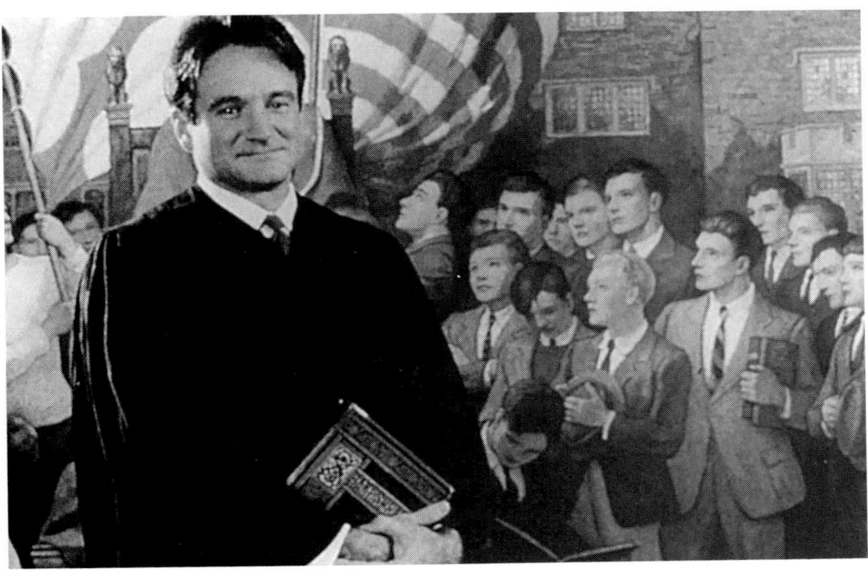

Carpe diem. Robin Williams as teacher John Keating and some of his young charges in *Dead Poets' Society* (1989). The script originally called for Williams to die at the end but this idea was junked by director Peter Weir.

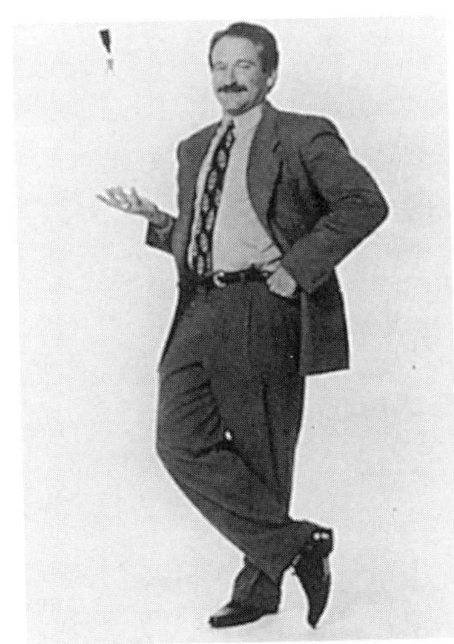

Would you buy a used car from this man? Robin Williams as Joey O'Brien in *Cadillac Man,* (1989) a film which – much like Joey's cars – never quite lived up to its promise.

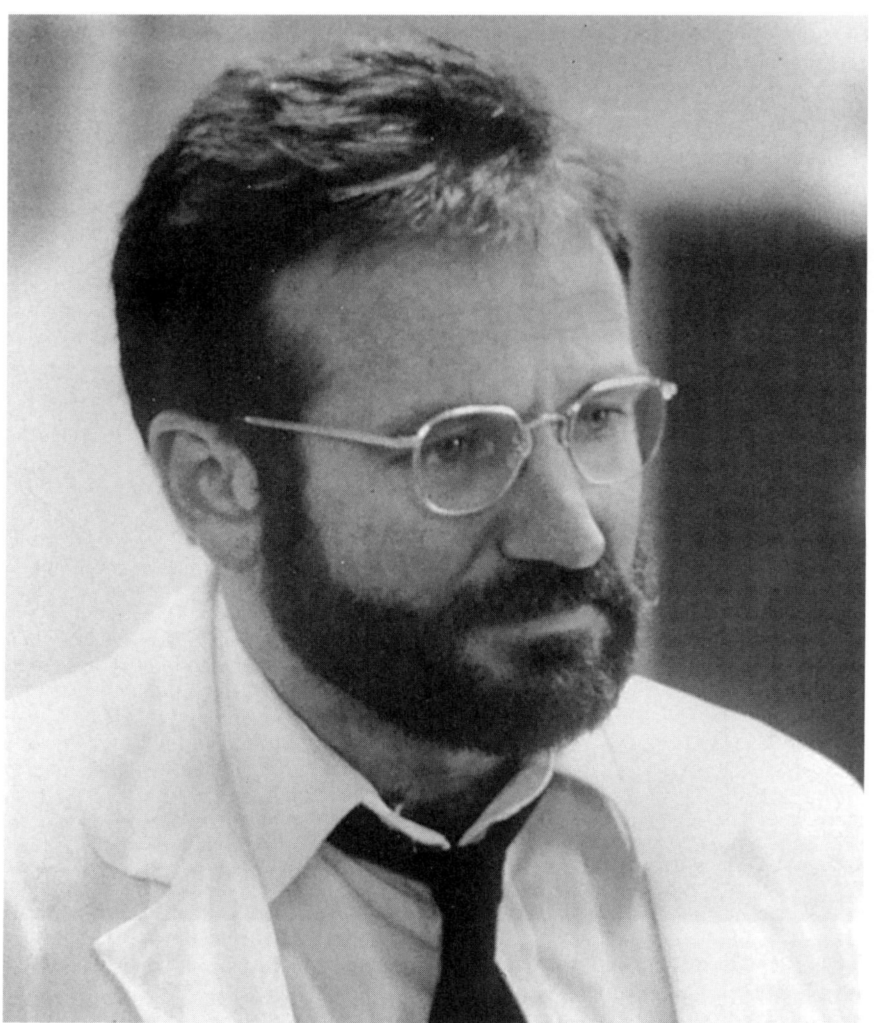

Williams was so moved when he read the script for *Awakenings* (1990) on a plane that he burst into tears. Playing Dr Malcolm Sayer, the fictional Oliver Sacks, lead to a long-lasting friendship and mutual admiration between Williams and Sacks.

Always the bridesmaid, never the bride. His performance as Parry in *The Fisher King* (1991) brought Williams a third Best Actor nomination but once again he came away empty-handed on Oscar night.

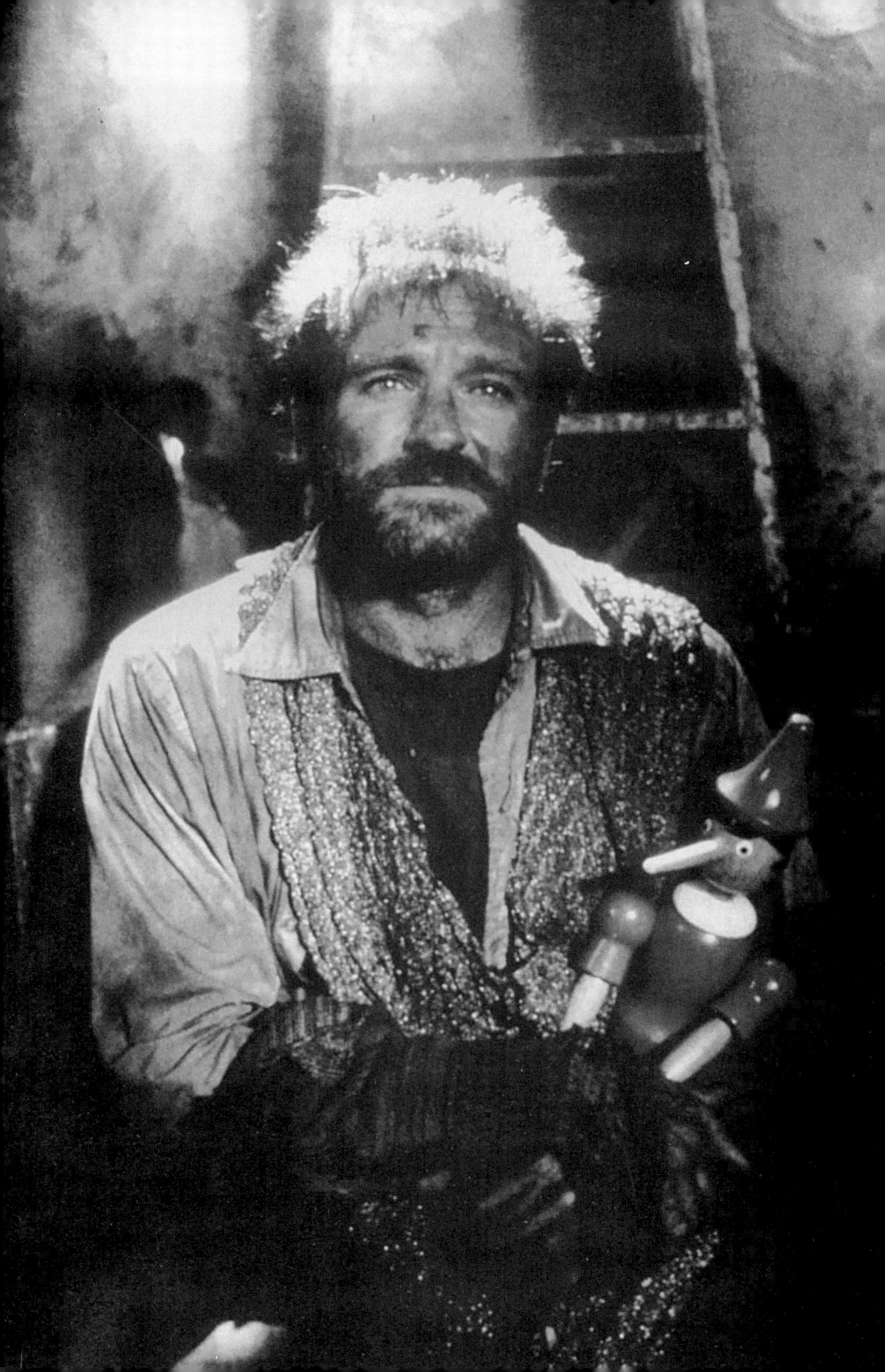

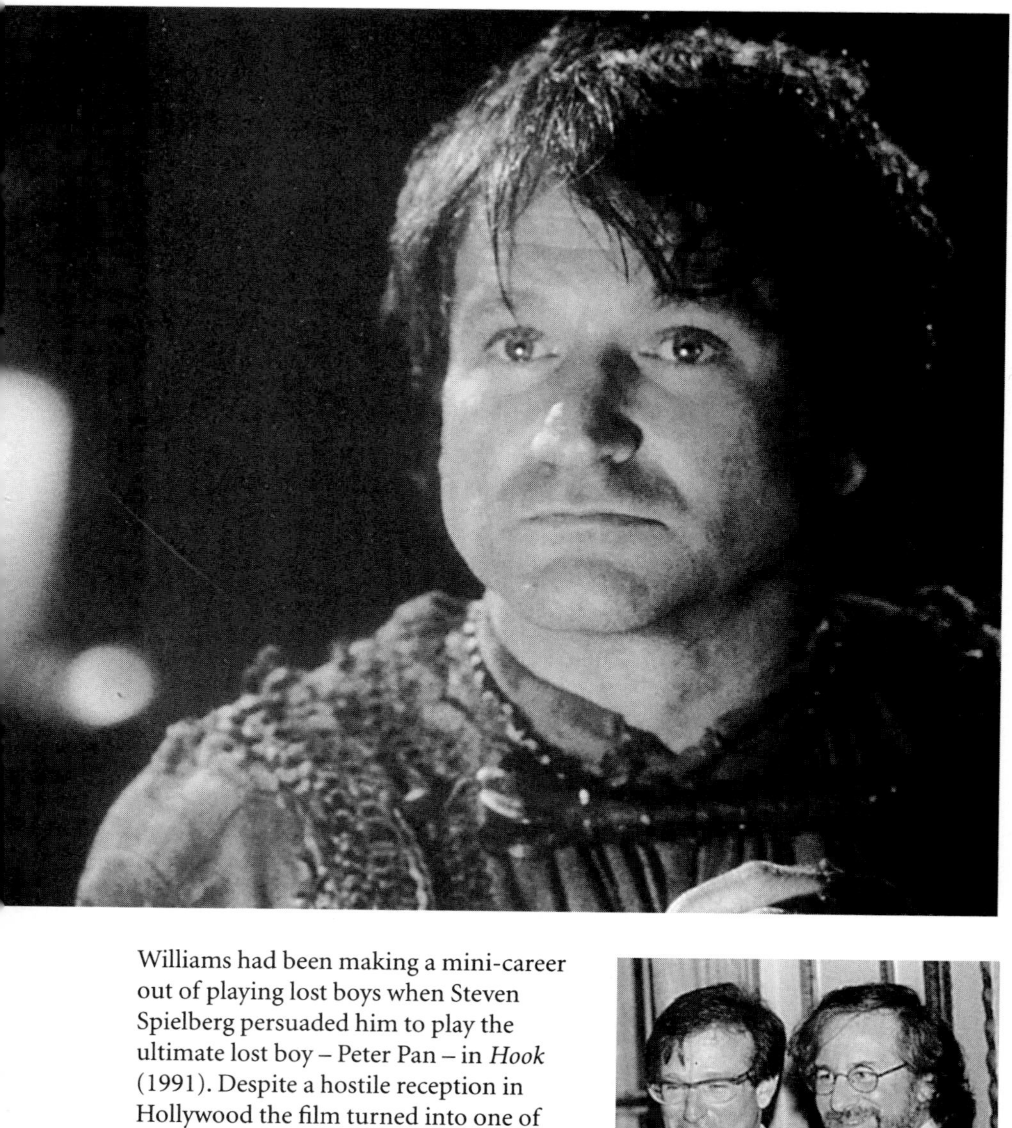

Williams had been making a mini-career out of playing lost boys when Steven Spielberg persuaded him to play the ultimate lost boy – Peter Pan – in *Hook* (1991). Despite a hostile reception in Hollywood the film turned into one of Williams biggest hits.

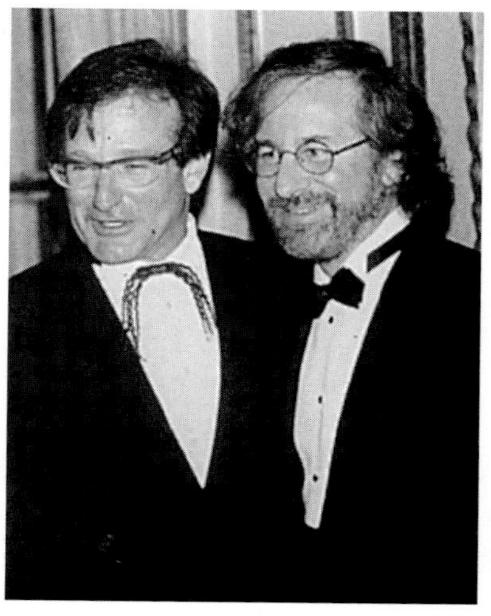

Williams and Steven Spielberg have been close friends for years. When Spielberg was feeling depressed during the shooting of *Schindler's List* he would spend hours on the phone being cheered up by Williams.

ship with Tuan and Trinh. There is very little comedy in this section of the film, and Williams is required to give a real performance as Cronauer changes and loses his innocence. Levinson's assurance that it was all right to be quiet removed from Williams the fear of silence which had been a weakness of some of his earlier work, on the stage as well as in films. Levinson gave Williams a safe place to express emotion. Undoubtedly Williams was able to draw on the turmoil of his personal life to portray some sense of Cronauer's loss and betrayal and disillusionment. But he was also, perhaps for the first time, able to do what he had originally been trained to do. Williams was an actor who became a comedian and this was the perfect vehicle.

> This combined two worlds that I'd kept separate [he explains]. One was stand-up comedy, the other was acting. Maybe there was a little bit left over from my Juilliard training – 'I'll be an actor, but I'm weak so I'll talk about my genitals'. So I combined the two and became an actor talking about my genitals. I was putting the two together because I had played characters like that in *Moscow on the Hudson* and *Garp*, or in *Seize the Day* where I played a guy having a nervous breakdown. In this one I thought I would try to put them together. The character is basically 98 per cent me. There is a slight veneer of a character but I can't say I studied immensely. It's me.

Williams' injection of himself into the Adrian Cronauer character extended to rewriting most of Cronauer's monologues. These captured for the first time on-screen the freewheeling word-associative adrenalin rush of Williams' stand-up performances. For the first time in the cinema, there was the realisation of the promise that had been shown in *Mork and Mindy*. The notion of eavesdropping on a performance was accentuated by Levinson's decision frequently not to tell Williams when the cameras were rolling. The results are some scenes of glorious spontaneity.

> They had it all written out but it wasn't very good [Williams admits], it was mostly a lot of jokes about food. So we said 'Okay, thank you' and threw it out. We came in with different character ideas like the military intelligence man who's not too tightly wrapped – this guy's coming in on one engine to begin with. We did them all. We would try things and Barry was so good because he would just tell us to try something else. Or he would throw in an idea because he's a comic himself. It's great, he really understands.

Levinson took an active part in the rewrites – by his estimate they discarded or changed about 40 per cent of the script – and his own comedy background made it very easy for him to understand his star. Like Paul Mazursky in *Moscow on the Hudson*, there was no one better equipped at that point to direct Robin Williams.

> Working with Robin on his routines was a little like playing football when we were kids [explains Levinson]. We used to say, 'Why don't you get over here? You there. Okay, let's go.' Robin would do a take and I would say, 'I like that thing about so-and-so. I don't think that bit works, but this bit is quite good. What about that thing you talked about the other day about the nudist monk? Let's give that a try.' Then he'd go and do another take, we'd go over it again and say, 'This is good, save this. Drop that. Add this. I think we're in fine shape. Let's see if you've got other ideas.' Then another idea would emerge that wasn't really developed; we'd talk about it and explore it a little more, and then start shooting again. We shot very fast, a lot of footage, and basically hammered out that whole section of the movie.

The use of the comic characters on air is one of the few similarities between Williams' interpretation and the real Adrian Cronauer. Cronauer's *Dawn Buster* show featured large helpings of comedy, but he's the first to admit that it was very different from Robin Williams' madcap monologues.

> What Robin Williams was doing wasn't really accurate – it was more 1988 radio than 1965 – but it was good [says Cronauer]. He was essentially doing Robin Williams with music. I did comedy but it was more situational comedy with pre-recorded material. We had characters like Sergeant Bassett who was a kind of Gyro Gearloose guy who was always coming up with weird inventions, and Boris the keeper of the Vault of Dusty Discs. He spoke like Boris Karloff and he always wanted me to play *Monster Mash.* And then there was a woman with a sultry voice who became the AFRS Friendly Thermometer. She was essentially just a seductive voice who came in to tell everybody how hot she was that day. The troops loved it, it was the theatre of the mind, which is a lot of fun.

Cronauer concedes that in terms of the resemblance to what actually happened to him in Saigon, *Good Morning Vietnam* is about 45 per cent accurate. For one thing he served his full 12-month tour of duty and wasn't bounced out of the country after five months. He did teach an English class to the Vietnamese but he had, for example, no Viet Cong friends, nor did he have a romantic relationship, unrequited or otherwise, with any Vietnamese girls. He did try to push the envelope in terms of breaking down the restrictions of military censorship of the news but again his confrontations were nowhere near as intense as Williams' battles. 'If I had done everything Robin Williams does in this film I'd have been court-martialled on the spot. I'd probably still be in Leavenworth,' says Cronauer.

The one dramatic incident in the film which is drawn from Cronauer's real-life experience is the bombing of Jimmy Wah's, the fictional GI bar in Saigon. The death of two soldiers in the blast is the catalyst, in the film at least, for an escalation in the conflict and a hardening of attitudes on both sides. It is also the beginning of the movie Cronauer's disillusionment with the military. In the film Williams escapes death by seconds when Tuan, who planted the bomb, warns him to get out. The sequence is based on the real-life bombing of the Mekong Floating restaurant, a popular haunt for American servicemen. Cronauer had left the restaurant only moments before it was blown apart by the Viet Cong using claymore mines. At that stage he was the news director on the station and he argued the case for broadcasting the news of the bombing. But in real life at least he lost.

Robin Williams finally met the man he had been playing in the movie when *Good Morning Vietnam* premièred in New York in December 1987. 'As I recall,' says Cronauer, 'when we were introduced we shook hands and he said "It's nice to meet you" and I said "It's nice to meet me too" and we both laughed at that. We never developed a real relationship. We still exchange Christmas cards but it's not like we're bowling buddies.'

The real Adrian Cronauer is now a successful media lawyer in Washington DC. There is perhaps a certain irony in the fact that he is and always has been a card-carrying Republican. He is still keenly involved in Veterans politics and was co-chairman of the Veterans for Dole group in the last US election. He also recorded a national TV commercial for the George Bush campaign in 1992 which effectively accused Bill Clinton of lying about his military service record. Quite a contrast to Williams himself, whose political leanings lie in the opposite direction, and who portrayed Cronauer as a man who gave the impression that he would be quite happy to leave the studio and join an anti-war demonstration.

The real Adrian Cronauer doesn't really have a problem with his screen characterisation. 'I have always been something of an iconoclast,' he explains. 'A lot of people have seen the movie and said to me, "Well you must be anti-military." That's not the case. What I am is anti-stupidity, and Lord knows in the military you encounter a whole lot of stupidity.'

> *Good Morning Vietnam* has certainly been a positive factor for me in my life [says Cronauer, looking back on the experience]. The film came along at

the right time because I was in the process of going to law school. I was going to the University of Pennsylvania, which is a fairly expensive school, and I planned to come out of three years in law school with a personal debt the size of a small South American country. Instead I came out in the black, which for a new lawyer is about the best feeling you can get with your clothes on. I have also become kind of an icon to many veterans. When the film came out my wife and I discussed this and she said, 'Adrian, you have to realise that you are now Adrian Cronauer Vietnam disc jockey' – and she was right. Of all the names that people remember from Vietnam there is probably General Westmoreland, William Calley of My Lai, Ron Kovic from *Born on the Fourth of July* – and me! And of those names I probably have the most positive image. So I have had a chance to get out and talk to a lot of the veterans.

I have also been told by many veterans that they think it's the first film that has shown Vietnam veterans as they really are, rather than as murderers and rapists and baby-killers, or dope addicts and psychotics. It has happened maybe a couple of dozen times or more that a man will come up to me and shake my hand and say quietly, 'Thank you for helping me get through that.' I never realised at the time how great an impact Armed Forces Radio had.

The impact that the film really had on the men and women who fought in Vietnam was forcibly brought home to Adrian Cronauer a few years after the film came out when he went along as a guest speaker at a veterans' reunion.

A lady came over and said her husband really wanted to meet me. The man was crippled and couldn't make it over, so I had to go and see him. I went over and he had arm braces on, and he was wearing his black beret and some of the military regalia. He started telling me how he was a lieutenant in charge of a platoon which was being shipped out into the field and they were in their truck when I came along in a jeep. I stopped and talked to the troops and entertained them for a while. And he wanted me to know how much that meant to his troops, and he was crying while he was telling me this. The problem is, that never happened. That was only in the film.

I talked with a friend who was a military psychologist who wasn't surprised to hear that. This man was suffering from Post Traumatic Stress Syndrome and had undergone some experiences that were so traumatic that he picked up the story of the film and substituted that for something that he couldn't deal with. Too often the media portrayed Americans in Vietnam as monsters and I really wanted this film to redress the balance.

For once, even if it is after the event, Adrian Cronauer and Barry Levinson are in complete agreement. 'What little political reaction there was to the film was very good,' says the director. 'I spoke to a number of veterans who felt it said a lot without actually showing the fighting. I think that because there was humour in the film and no graphic violence, the political implications were probably overlooked by some who simply saw it as a diversion.'

19

A Death in the Family

On the morning of Sunday, 18 October 1987 Robert F. Williams died. He was 81 years old and had been suffering from cancer for some time. He died peacefully in his sleep at the family home in Tiburon, where he and his wife had settled after their nomadic but comfortable existence throughout the Midwest with the Ford Company. Robin Williams was not with him when he died, but he was nearby at his own home in San Francisco. The death of his father was a devastating blow for Williams. It came in a year when his marriage was ending, his career was on the line, and his relationship with his own son was in some doubt. The death of Robert Williams was all the more affecting because it came at a point when father and son had finally begun to get to know one another.

It would be a misconception to see Robert Williams as a cold and distant father, perhaps not unlike the father figure Jonathan Hyde would play some years later in *Jumanji.* Robert Williams was a man of his time and a product of the work ethic of the Twenties and Thirties. The prime motivation in his life was providing for both his families. He was a hard worker and by all accounts good at his job. If his job took him away from home a lot, then it was not through desire but necessity. Similarly, if the family had to move from time to time, it was not always because they wanted to.

Robert Williams was a senior executive in the motor industry. He was by any consideration a captain of industry and thus a powerful man of influence and standing. Had he been alive in the Nineties, there is little doubt that he would have been one of Tom Wolfe's 'Masters of the Universe'.

There is also little doubt that Robert Williams loved his son, he just wasn't always there to show it. Robin Williams had frequently described his father as an elegant and sophisticated man with a very dry sense of humour. It is from his father, he claims, that he gets his love of theatre. Williams and his mother used to affectionately refer to Williams Senior as 'Lord Posh' as well as 'Lord Stokesbury', so urbane and sophisticated was his manner. Again as a product of his times, and through having been in his late forties when his youngest son was born, Robert Williams may have had difficulty in displaying his emotions, but all the evidence suggests he loved his son and was proud of him.

When his son announced that he was turning his back on his father's chosen career in the diplomatic corps for what amounted to a life as a vagabond player, Robert Williams did not behave like a dictatorial autocrat. He was pragmatic, as you would expect from a man in his position. His response was not to put any barriers in his son's way, but simply to cut his losses and bring him to a less expensive school closer to home. Likewise, when Williams then announced that he was going to New York to try to make a go of life as a performer, his father's only response was a perfectly sensible one. He merely suggested that his son acquire a back-up trade for when times would inevitably get tough. These are not the actions of a man who does not love his son.

Once Robin Williams became a father himself, he found that he could appreciate and understand the difficulties that his own father had gone through. By all accounts Robert Williams was the perfect grandfather for Zachary, and the support of both grandparents would have been invaluable to the boy during a difficult period. The little boy spent many weekends with his grandparents in Tiburon.

'It's a wonderful feeling when your father becomes not a god but a man to you,' says Williams. 'When he comes down from the mountain and you see he's this man with weaknesses, and you love him as this whole being, not this figurehead.' And father and son were now beginning to reach the stage where they were finally able to display their feelings for one another.

> My father loved boats [Williams recalled recently], and once for Fathers' Day I gave him a beautiful hand-made model of a whaling boat. He was just totally stunned by that because it was something that he really loved and it really touched him. And that was at the point also where I was getting to know him as a person. I had probably just started to make it and have a

career, and when I gave him that gift it was something very special for both of us.

The news of his father's death was broken to Robin Williams in a telephone call from his mother. She simply called him and told him without fuss or histrionics that his father was dead. Some months later, after *Good Morning Vietnam* had been a certified hit, Williams spoke frankly and movingly to *Rolling Stone* magazine about his father.

> I got to know another side [of him] in the last few years [he told writer Bill Zehme]. I saw that he was funkier, that he had a dark side that made the other side work. He was much older than me; he died at 81. Up until four or five years ago I kept distance out of respect. Then we made a connection ... He'd had operations and chemotherapy. It's weird. Everyone thinks of their dad as invincible, and in the end here's this little tiny creature almost all bone. You have to say goodbye to him as this very frail being.
>
> At least he was at home and died very peacefully in his sleep. My mother thought he was still asleep. She came downstairs and kept trying to shake him. She called me that morning and said, 'Robin, your father's dead.' She was a little in shock but she sounded happy in a certain way, if only because he went without pain.

You could argue that Robin Williams' life has been dominated by women. Whether it was Valerie Velardi, Marsha Garces, Tish Carter or his own mother, women have been the dominant and defining force in his life. But the relationship between a man and his father transcends those definitions.

'When I started to talk to my father,' he recalled, 'it was like *The Wizard of Oz* where you look behind the curtain and see the man for what he is. There was this little man behind the curtain going, "Take care of your mother and I love you and I've been worried about certain things. And I'm afraid but I'm not afraid." It's an amazing combination of exhilaration and sadness at the same time because the god turns into a man.'

Williams was speaking here as a father himself and, more importantly, a father who was facing the possibility of losing his son. With his marriage to Valerie on the rocks, the question of custody of Zach, who was now five, would loom large in his future. When he spoke of his hopes and fears for his son, there is an obvious echo of what he felt he had learned from his childhood relationship with his own father.

'I've learned to have the security not to worry that he will love me,' said Williams, 'as long as I keep the connection strong enough. I've learned not to try and force the love. You can't. All you can do is try and set up a world for him that's safe and stable enough to make him happy.'

Williams was very concerned that the separation from his wife should have as little effect on his son as possible. He was adamant that, wherever possible, Zachary would be kept out of the public eye, so he could grow up and have a life of his own.

'He's more comfortable with it now,' he says of Zach's attitude to the estrangement. 'He understands it . . . we have a good custody arrangement, so he comes and goes freely. He knows exactly how many days he's here and how many days he's there. Children at his age don't want to deal with the anger and volatility or whatever would develop. As long as things are peaceable, he's fine switching back and forth.'

Robin Williams had one final act to perform for his father. Robert Williams was a lifelong lover of water and boats, so, not long after the services, there was one last remembrance. Robin Williams and his two half-brothers – Todd, who was now a wine distributor, and Lauren, a high-school physics teacher – met to scatter their father's ashes in San Francisco Bay.

> It was sad but also cathartic and wonderful in the sense that it brought my two half-brothers and me closer together [Williams told Bill Zehme]. It kind of melded us closer as a family than we've ever been before. We've always been very separate.
>
> That day we gathered right on the sea in front of where my parents live. It was funny. At one point I had poured the ashes out, and they're floating off into the mist, seagulls flying overhead. A truly serene moment. Then I looked into the urn and said to my brother, 'There's still some ashes left, Todd. What do I do?' He said, 'It's Dad – he's holding on!' I thought, 'Yeah, you're right. He's hanging on.' He was an amazing man who had the courage not to impose limitations on his sons, to literally say, 'I see you have something you want to do – do it.'

20

Waitin'

Good Morning Vietnam opened in December 1987 just over two months after Robert Williams' death. Almost immediately the film proved that everyone from Adrian Cronauer through Jeffrey Katzenberg through Larry Brezner and ultimately through to Robin Williams himself had been absolutely right. The film was a huge commercial success and Robin Williams received some of the best reviews of his career. The critics believed that he had found the right role at last and the public seemed to agree. In three weeks of limited release – where it was playing on only four screens in the whole country – it was making $1 million a week. On its first weekend on wide release it grossed $12 million which is an impressive sum now, but in 1988 was a huge opening. By the end of its run the film had grossed $123.9 million in the United States alone – a figure roughly equivalent to the combined grosses of his first seven films. But later, when he was promoting the film in Europe, Williams revealed that he had had some misgivings about whether or not the audience would take to it. He had been genuinely concerned that young audiences in the latter part of 1987 and the early part of 1988 would not get references to 1965.

'That's why a lot of the jokes and references are about television like Gomer Pyle and Elvis,' said Williams, explaining the gamble. 'You tried to find some kind of broad reference. I worried that too many people would see it and wonder, "What the hell is he talking about?" But it worked. I've seen the film with all sorts of audiences and it does work. Maybe it just sounds funny.'

The timing of the release of *Good Morning Vietnam* was crucial. Putting out a movie about the trauma of Vietnam at Christmas may not have seemed on the surface to be the ideal marketing move. Other films like the James Brooks television satire *Broadcast News* or the Steven Spielberg-produced comedy adventure **batteries not included* may have seemed like surer commercial bets. But Disney felt that they had a potential Oscar candidate on their hands with *Good Morning Vietnam*, and the limited pre-Christmas release was designed to ensure that it would qualify for the following year's Academy Awards.

The closing date for qualification for the Oscars is the end of the calendar year, midnight on 31 December to be precise. To be eligible for an Academy Award a film has to have played at least one full week on at least one screen in Los Angeles, so the four-screen limited release in December was enough to fulfil the criteria. The ballot papers and a list of eligible films are sent to the 5000-odd members of the Academy of Motion Picture Arts and Sciences in January. After the usual intensive lobbying and advertising campaigns the nominations are announced in mid-February, and the awards themselves are handed out on or about the last Monday in March. Buoyed up by a groundswell of critical acclaim and box-office receipts, Robin Williams found himself nominated for an Academy Award for the first time. The other nominees were Michael Douglas – also a first-time nominee – for *Wall Street*, William Hurt for *Broadcast News*, Marcello Mastroianni for *Dark Eyes* and Oscar veteran Jack Nicholson for *Ironweed*. The competition was tough. Hurt, for example, was enjoying a run of three successive Best Actor nominations. Nicholson, on the other hand, was the nominations kingpin, his nod for *Ironweed* being his ninth Oscar nomination. Douglas, who had previously picked up an Oscar as a producer for *One Flew Over the Cuckoo's Nest*, was making his début as a nominee and also had in his favour the phenomenal success of *Fatal Attraction* which had been released in the same year.

Three-time nominee Mastrioanni was the obvious outsider of the quintet. His nomination was as much in recognition of his long and distinguished career as for his performance in *Dark Eyes*, a charming period comedy in which he played an Italian aristocrat. Leaving him out of the equation, Williams then became the longest-odds candidate for a number of reasons. First there was the fact that *Good Morning Vietnam* had not received nominations for either Best Picture or Best Director, which are generally seen as prerequisites for success. But most importantly, as Barry Levinson pointed out, a lot of people read the film the wrong way. Despite its considerable dramatic content it was marketed as a comedy and was perceived as a comedy. By extension Williams, although he had shown considerable subtlety as an actor in his performance, was still seen as a comedian. Oscar has not been kind to comedy over the years. Only horror movies have fared more poorly in terms of the statuettes they've been awarded. In the 70-year history of the Academy Awards only four men have won Best Actor Oscars for what might be termed comic performances: James Stewart in *The Philadelphia Story*, Lee Marvin for *Cat Ballou*, Richard Dreyfuss for *The Goodbye Girl* and Jack Nicholson for *As Good As It Gets*. All four of these wins were by straight actors in comic roles. No established comedian has ever won a Best Actor Oscar and that includes the comedy greats like Chaplin and Keaton. What's worse in the case of Robin Williams was that he was seen as a television comedian and therefore in the eyes of the Academy something of an *arriviste*. The Academy had been happy to turn to Williams a couple of years earlier when he replaced long-time Oscar night compère Johnny Carson in a bid to boost flagging TV ratings, but it was not yet ready to give him the coveted statuette.

In the end the Best Actor contest came down to a straight fight between Douglas and Hurt. It was Douglas who took away the prize for his performance as *über*-speculator Gordon Gekko, whose 'greed is good' mantra symbolised the mood of the post-Reagan Eighties. Douglas, incidentally, like Williams, was in a film with no nominations for Best Picture or Best Director, proving if nothing else that occasionally nothing is certain when it comes to the Oscars. What probably tipped the scales for him and against Hurt was the full trophy cabinet syndrome. Hurt already had one Best Actor Oscar for *Kiss of the Spider Woman*, and two statuettes in three years would have been just too much.

Williams however at least had the consolation of winning a Golden Globe from the Hollywood Foreign Press Association as Best Actor in a Musical or Comedy. It was his second Golden Globe; he had won for *Mork and Mindy* some years earlier. All told it wasn't a bad spell for Robin Williams in terms of awards. He also picked up an Emmy for Best Individual Performance in a Variety or Music Programme. The show in question was *ABC Presents a Royal Gala*, a benefit concert which had been staged in England in front of Prince Charles and Princess Diana. Although Williams was delighted to receive the honour, the Emmy brought back memories of one of the worst nights of his life.

'I was getting ready for The Prince's Trust concert and I went to a club in Windsor and I just blanked,' he recalls. 'It was like one of those old movies from the Fifties where they show the comic on-stage, and the lights are in your face, and I just opened my mouth and nothing came out.'

For someone like Williams, whose act is based on fear of so many different types, being confronted with any comedian's greatest fear must have been a terrifying moment. His act used to include a routine in which he pretended to be a comedian dying on-stage in a puddle of flop sweat. It was certainly a defining moment for Williams to go through it for real at such a stage in his career. Even ten years later he can recall the experience almost unbidden as one of the most salutary nights of his career.

> It really scared me and the next night I did the show and it was better. It's good to have one of those nights once in a while because it just scares you and it sobers you up real quick. I kept looking up to see if Prince Charles was laughing and they said he was so I thought 'Good, I can come back.' It was one of those nights where I could see the first ten rows of attitude going 'Who are you?'

There's no doubt that the sight of Williams in what he describes as 'full-tilt bozo' mode must have been curious to say the least to a typical British charity audience who had paid large amounts of money to be entertained by a man who appeared to be having a psychotic episode on-stage. For his part the culture shock for Williams must have been just as great. He wasn't in the Holy City Zoo now, and not even a little pre-show encouragement from Princess Diana could make him any more relaxed.

> Meeting the Princess was amazing [he admitted some years later]. She's exquisite. I knew he would have a certain presence, but with her you go 'Wow'. She's obviously been trained to do certain things, one of which is the look. She'll look at you, then turn away, then look at you again. It's beyond coquette. Before the show she asked me, 'Do you know what you're going to do tonight?' I said, 'I really don't know, but after you see it, I don't think you'll want me back.' She said, 'Oh, don't tell me that.' And she gave me one of those looks.
>
> At one point [says Williams recalling the performance itself], I came off the stage and into the audience. I said to one lady, 'Look at those jewels. You could wear them or feed Thailand.' And she looked at me and said, 'Yes. Yes, I could.' So I thought, 'Right, I'm going back up on to the stage.'

It was certainly safer on-stage for Williams, and with the security of the footlights between him and the audience he went on to give a devastating performance which was justly recognised with the Emmy award.

Although he had made his name as a comedian, first in stand-up and then in *Mork and Mindy*, it is important to remember that comedy was not Robin Williams' chosen field. He was a comedian by inclination but originally set out to be an actor as an avocation. Juilliard does not produce stand-up comedians as a matter of course. Williams had been classically trained and now in the early part of 1988 he was inclined to put his training to the test.

When he had finished *Good Morning Vietnam*, Williams had no other film projects in mind. Both he and his manager Larry Brezner were waiting for the reaction to the Vietnam movie before deciding on their next move. Brezner was keen to develop Williams into a fully-fledged movie star, the sort of bankable actor whose name was enough to raise finance for a picture and guarantee a good opening weekend. Williams on the other hand was keen to find projects which interested him in their own right and was less concerned with their overall effect on his career. However, both men were of the same mind when Williams decided he would make his stage début in a production of *Waiting for Godot* at the Lincoln Center in New York. The production was being put together by director Mike Nichols. With cinema hits such as *The Graduate* to his credit, as well as some landmark satirical performances with Elaine May, Nichols is one of America's most intelligent, literate and respected directors. He had held a number of readings of Beckett's play in the autumn of 1997 with a hand-picked group of actors. By the end of this unconventional auditioning process he had narrowed his choices for the four principals down to Robin Williams, Steve Martin, F. Murray Abraham and Bill Irwin. Rehearsals were to be held in May 1988, and the play would open for an eight-week run starting in mid-June. Having settled on their proposed cast, Nichols and Gregory Mosher, the artistic director of Lincoln Center, flew to Paris for discussions with Beckett himself, who approved their choice of cast.

'We're going to do a musical version called *Waitin*',' Williams joked, trying to make light of his first foray into legitimate theatre. But even though he joked in public, he was well aware of the size of the challenge which faced him and the risks he was preparing to take. 'It's wonderful stuff,' he continued. 'Beckett is like Pinter on valium. You do it, because the experience itself will change you.'

Williams was at a stage in his life where he not only needed change, he actively sought it out and embraced it. Having the courage to go on-stage as an actor was only part of it. His relationship with Marsha Garces was getting stronger and closer. He and Valerie had made public the news of their split. He was now living with Marsha and the stability he was beginning to find in his domestic life was being reflected in a greater willingness to stretch himself in his creative life. Scheduling problems meant that *Waiting for Godot*, which was not being done as any kind of musical, would not now be able to go ahead until the autumn of 1988. Williams and Garces moved from San Francisco to the Upper West Side of New York for most of the year, with Zach making frequent visits.

The production was formally announced in the Lincoln Center's newsletter to its members in September. The play would be staged at the Mitzi E. Newhouse Theater from 11 October until 27 November. The seven-week run was predicated on the availability of the five cast members – Nichols had added young Lukas Haas to his original quartet – and the small 299-seat auditorium instantly made this the hottest ticket in town. The Lincoln Center correctly anticipated that demand would be huge. There were not even enough tickets to satisfy their own members who would have the chance to buy them before the general public. To ensure as much fair play as possible an independent accounting firm was brought in to supervise a ballot of members to make sure that the tickets were distributed as fairly as possible. In a bid to play down accusations of élitism Mosher and Bernard Gersten, executive producer of Lincoln Center Theater, let it be known that they planned to make a TV film version of the production so that as many people as possible could see this stellar production. That never materialised, but there is at least a record of it on video in the New York Public Library for the Performing Arts.

Waiting for Godot was first performed in Paris on 5 January 1953. Beckett described it as a 'tragicomedy in two acts'. Its central characters are two tramps – Vladimir and Estragon – who wait on a deserted country road for a mysterious character called Godot. Their wait is long and to pass the time they hold rambling discussions on their own lives and the nature of life in general. In each of the two acts they meet an overbearing man named Pozzo, and Lucky, his improbably named slave. Each of the two acts ends with a young boy coming on-stage to tell them that Godot will not be here tonight but will certainly meet them if only they will come again tomorrow.

Waiting for Godot had enjoyed a chequered reputation in its 35 years; at one point it had been censored in England. But it had endured to become a classic and this Lincoln Center production was the first major New York revival of the play in more than ten years.

Nichols had chosen his cast with care. Steve Martin would be Vladimir, Robin Williams was Estragon, F. Murray Abraham played Pozzo, with Bill Irwin as Lucky. The young Haas appeared at the end of each act to announce the unfortunate delay of the eponymous Godot. In terms of billing the cast was listed in alphabetical order which put Abraham first and made Robin Williams last on the bill. Few theatrical events had been more keenly anticipated and, not surprisingly, there was not a seat to be had for the entire run.

The play begins with a darkened stage. Then with a drum roll and a clash of cymbals the lights come up to reveal a tramp struggling with an ill-fitting boot. This is Estragon, played by Williams. His costume looks like an explosion in a charity shop. A battered bowler hat lends a forlorn dignity to a blue-grey ruffled shirt with a huge wing collar, a hooded sweat top with cut-off sleeves, flared trousers which fit where they touch and are held up tentatively with an old piece of string. A swarthy growth of unshaven stubble gives him the look of an Emmett Kelly clown. After much struggling with the boot he is joined by Steve Martin as Vladimir, who cuts a slightly more presentable figure but not by much. Together they debate, bicker and squabble about their miserable lives as they wait for Godot. They are joined periodically by Pozzo, a man of self-styled wealth and taste who lives to abuse his mute slave Lucky. After a while Pozzo and Lucky go on their way and eventually the boy arrives to announce that Godot will not be coming. The second act more or less mirrors the first, except for some great tragedy having befallen Pozzo, who has been blinded between the two acts.

Williams' great genital dilemma quickly manifests itself in the performance. Should he be a straight actor like they told him in Juilliard, or should he talk about his genitals? There is very little actual discussion of his genitals in the play but, in the first half in particular, there is much fumbling and manipulation of them by Williams. He seems to lack the will, if not the desire, to make this final leap into straight acting. There is always something going on to remind the audience that they're watching Robin Williams and not Estragon. Whether it's pantomimed foot odour, inappropriate motor car noises, comic business with carrots, or a variety of accents including John Wayne and Gabby Hayes, Williams seems reluctant to subsume himself to the text. To be fair, he is not alone in this. Steve Martin similarly brings too much of his screen baggage to his role as Estragon, who might as well be playing in *The Jerk* or *The Man with Two Brains.* Only fitfully do they appear as anything other than Robin Williams and Steve Martin, and they are aided and abetted by an audience which seems to see its function as a sitcom laugh track, chiming in at every bit of business.

Neither Williams nor Steve Martin seems terribly concerned about serving Beckett's text, and director Mike Nichols must also bear some degree of responsibility. One of the *coups de théâtre* in Godot comes when Lucky finally speaks. Having been mute throughout, he has one magnificent stream-of-consciousness soliloquy which is a test of any actor's ability. It's not just a question of remembering the words, which spew out like a burst water main, it's capturing the sense of Lucky's frustration as an intelligent man trapped in this lumbering body and used for brute labour. It is a pivotal moment in the play and in most productions the speech is generally accompanied by a respectful silence from whoever is playing Vladimir and Estragon. Beckett's stage directions are normally quite explicit and they do not leave a lot of room for interpretation. In this production, however, the opening of Bill Irwin's soliloquy as Lucky is the cue for Martin and Williams to mime, caper and play shamelessly to the audience throughout his speech. Whether it is funny is neither here nor there, the effect is to distance the audience from the world of Beckett and make them aware they are doing nothing more than watching the Steve and Robin show.

Waiting for Godot was a sell-out, as expected, but its critical reception was less than rapturous. And criticism came from an unexpected quarter in a scathing letter from the playwright himself. The letter was the result of correspondence between Beckett and producer-director Jack Garfein, described by the *New York Post* as a long-time friend of Beckett. Garfein had sent Beckett copies of the reviews and also, apparently, a copy of the programme for the production. Beckett was in a nursing home in Paris receiving physiotherapy for his arthritis. This, coupled with the fact that he was now 82, meant it would have been almost impossible for him to travel to New York. Had he done so he might not have liked what he saw. In his letter to Garfein, reprinted in the *Post*, Beckett was scathing about the production. 'I deplore the liberties taken in N.Y. *Godot*, with text and on stage,' he wrote.

Beckett's reaction meant that any proposed television version of this particular production was dead in the water. He was unlikely to give his permission if he felt so strongly about this version. A Lincoln Center spokesman later admitted that they did not have the television rights, nor did they ever have them. Another spokesman, however, suggested that Gregory Mosher's original comments regarding a TV version had been made in good faith, although they were also aware that it would soften the criticism about no one being able to see the play. Garfein insisted that he was about to stage his own version of the play and that he also had Beckett's permission to film it, but as yet there is no sign of the film.

Williams did not react well to the criticism of the production and his performance. In the first place he criticised the exclusivity of the event by blaming the Lincoln Center subscription audience. 'They came because it was an event, the thing to do,' he said with uncharacteristic bitterness.

'We put our ass out and got kicked for it,' he would reflect some years later. 'Some nights I would improvise a bit and the hard-core Beckett fans got pissed off. We played it as a comedy team; it wasn't existential. Like these two guys from vaudeville who would go into routines that would fall apart into angst. Basically it's Laurel and Hardy, which is how Beckett had staged it in Germany.'

Beckett's own reaction to the Lincoln Center production suggests that he and Williams differ more in their interpretation of the piece than Williams thinks. Critics generally shared Beckett's view about the changes which had been made to the text. Williams lambasted them, accusing them of double standards in their treatment of the play. These were the ones, according to Williams, who 'used to despise Beckett and now hold him godlike'.

But he insisted that, even if he had been bloodied by the criticism, he would remain unbowed. He said that he would love to do another play in New York, possibly doing *Godot* again. He also pointed out that as you get older you learn how to play what he calls the 'frightening silences'.

> I thought, 'Wouldn't it be great to do *Godot* again?' [he said recently]. Except this time I would be Lucky, the one who has the big long speech, the five-minute monologue. *Godot* is one of the great pieces of writing of the twentieth century. It has great comic and tragic moments. It has everything you could ever want in a play. I would love to do that again.

Williams would mature as an actor over the years. He would learn to use the stillness of the silences instead of being intimidated by them. He would no longer feel it necessary to leap in and fill the void with noise. But he has never acted again on the stage from that day to this.

21

Dances with Lepers

It was Andy Warhol who said that one day everyone would be famous for 15 minutes. As far as a great many people were concerned, Robin Williams had pretty well used up his quarter of an hour almost ten years ago when *Mork and Mindy* became a hit. Now *Good Morning Vietnam* had made him a household name all over again and removed him from the province of the terminally hip and addicts of retro-television. Williams is in no doubt about what might have happened had *Good Morning Vietnam* gone the way of most of his other movies. On one occasion just before the film was released he was doing another night at the Holy City Zoo when he started being heckled by someone about his performance in *Popeye.*

'No ... no more *Popeye*,' Williams told him. 'But I have a new movie that just might work. If not I'll be off somewhere shouting "Show me a vowel". There's a scary thought.'

The prospect of a career as a perennial game-show celebrity guest might have been genuinely terrifying to Williams. But he had given some serious thought to what might have happened if, instead of being hailed by *Time* magazine as 'the best military comedy since *M*A*S*H*, *Good Morning Vietnam* had joined his other films in going down the box-office drain.

'You're not hosed totally,' he recalled. 'You simply slip down the comedy food chain of that list of people who get scripts ... It all kind of works that way. If this film had failed I'd go down another couple of notches. So you have to work your way back up again or do character parts – or you fall back and punt,' he said, reverting to an analogy from his brief and spectacularly unsuccessful football career. 'Now with this I knew I had the open fields to run through. The radio broadcasts obviously afforded me the freedom to improvise, yet the story had dramatic elements which provided some interesting turns.'

He had, he said – joining the consensus – found the right role at last. But he also conceded that not finding the right role up till now had been as much his fault as anyone else's.

> It was part ego, part stubbornness in trying to do something unexpected. Then there were other times when I took on slight projects thinking 'I can fix this'. I got suckered into a couple of films like that – *The Best of Times*, *Club Paradise* – I thought, 'Well, they'll give me the freedom to do my thing', but it turned out they didn't. Also for the first time I didn't have any fear or tension. Barry Levinson kind of took away the onus of being 'on' . . . I would ease into a scene and it helped me a lot. I started to relax.

In becoming famous all over again, Robin Williams once again came to the attention of the American media. Up until *Good Morning Vietnam* his marital situation was not really of interest to anyone. With the exception of the odd burst of notoriety such as the Belushi investigation, Robin Williams did not tend to register in the celebrity radar. However, once he had a $100-million-grossing movie, a Golden Globe award and an Oscar nomination, he became fair game for America's growing celebrity media circus. Williams' relationship with the media had been somewhat ambivalent. He was, in the main, accessible to the mainstream media and he plainly had his favourites, opening his heart to *Rolling Stone* on a number of occasions. As for the *National Enquirer* he had been having a running feud with the paper since the days of *Mork and Mindy.*

> My mother is so naïve about certain things [he explained, outlining the origins of his antipathy]. The *National Enquirer* called her and said, 'We're doing a story and we'd like to have some photos.' She gave them some photos of my father and me and some school photos. They used these pictures to imply that my father was this tyrant and I came from this horrible existence and that's why I was funny . . . She [his mother] felt used, and she was.

People magazine, however, sat somewhere between the *Enquirer* and *Rolling Stone.* It dealt in celebrity tittle-tattle but in such a way that it had become the defining force of American popular culture in the late

Seventies and Eighties. You knew you had arrived when you made the cover of *People* magazine. Indeed it was *People* that was among the first to recognise Williams' potential back in 1978 on that first series of *Mork and Mindy*, referring to his 'brilliantly sophisticated mixture of wise-cracks, double-talk and improvisations' which it said made the show 'sizzle'. Now that Williams had finally fulfilled the potential they had highlighted a decade earlier they were planning another cover story for their 22 February 1988 issue.

Celebrity profiling in the Nineties has become something of a domesticated animal. Contemporary stars frequently insist on choosing the journalist, vetting the questions, controlling the access and often getting approval on the finished article before they will consent to a few moments of their time. Ten years ago this practice was in its infancy and Williams was certainly not powerful enough to put too many preconditions on his interview. Indeed it was quite the opposite. He was intelligent enough to know that the events of his recent past were potentially the stuff that tabloid dreams were made of. So, he reasoned, rather than try to hide it, he would be honest about it. When he spoke to journalist Brad Darrach, Williams tried to explain that there were certain things that he did not want to talk about. But, as he later explained to *Playboy* magazine, it all went horribly wrong.

> I was trying to tidy up the last ends of my first marriage and get on with my life with Marsha [he told *Playboy* Contributing Editor Lawrence Grobel]. I didn't want to talk about that, because I was trying to be respectful of my first marriage and end it decently. And then it just exploded. But I was so angry and horrified that the interview turned this way, it was like being mugged. At the end they said, 'We have to ask you certain questions or you don't get the cover.' Fuck it, I don't need a cover that badly. I sat down and talked to the reporter very personally and said, 'This is what's up. This is the truth.' And they didn't put any of it in. They made it seem exactly what they wanted to do from the very beginning: Marsha broke up the marriage. Which is total horseshit.

Once again the last remnants of Williams' naïveté had been his undoing. He chose what he felt was the intelligent approach to the *People* journalists. Unfortunately it wasn't the smart approach. The smart approach would have been to volunteer nothing, indeed to turn down the interview in the first place. Instead Williams was, in journalistic parlance, 'stitched up' with a front page which has now become notorious. The headline read: 'Robin Williams. Public triumph, private anguish'.

If that wasn't enough, the rest of the cover – which contained only one small posed shot of Williams plus another, not terribly flattering shot of Williams and Garces – went on to say: '*Good Morning Vietnam* has made the comic genius into a movie star at last, but his life is a minefield. Having beaten alcohol and drugs, he's now entangled in a love affair with his son's nanny that has left his wife embittered – and Zachary, 4, in the middle. It's the emotional challenge of his life. "I'll do anything," he says, "to keep my son from harm".'

It was a remarkable piece of journalism which attempted to sensationalise a situation that had all but been resolved. Two years previously it might have been a story, now it was simply rehashing old events. However, as far as the majority of the *People* readership and, by extension, most of America were concerned it was news to them. Williams suddenly became some kind of coke-snorting booze-hound all over again, while Marsha – described as 'sloe-eyed, elegantly slender' – was one step removed from a man-eating home-wrecker. *People* made great play out of her refusal to be interviewed and quoted 'friends' in filling in her background details as sketchily as possible. Similar 'friends' and 'close observers' were used to put Valerie Velardi's side of the story. Unfortunately a great deal of the innuendo thrown around by the story did not quite square with the quotes from Valerie herself in the same article.

'Robin has been conducting himself very well,' she offered generously. 'We're acting together in Zach's interest. We separated to re-examine our lives. It's a time for personal growth for both of us. I see another man but I live alone, and I like it that way.'

Given that the paragraph which follows those quotes begins 'Who's kidding who?' in the voice of the journalist, this certainly seems to have been one of those articles where the angle has been decided before the interview and nothing anyone says subsequently will change that. Like Valerie Velardi, Robin Williams admitted that his prime concern in this unfortunate saga was his son.

> He's just wonderful [he enthused]. The most sobering and wonderful thing in my life. Blond. Valerie's blue eyes. My chin. Full lips. He looks like an Aryan poster child ... He's amazingly adaptive and we all try very hard to make the new arrangement work. We all love Zachary and Zachary loves us all. Also we're all in therapy, and that's helped a lot – Jesus, I should get a discount. Valerie and I have a good understanding too. The separation was difficult, but it was also gentle. Better to do that than to go at each other's throats ... I'll do anything to keep my son from harm. What I'm trying to do now is to work with Valerie to transform our marriage into a relationship

> in which we share Zachary and do all we can to make him happy. I expect my involvement with Valerie will go on until I die.

Although Valerie Velardi would talk about the state of their relationship now and the fact that she was seeing another man, she would offer no comment about Marsha Garces. 'You're not gonna get that out of me in 100 years,' she 'blurted', according to *People.* But on the other hand what did they really expect her to say? She is hardly going to be silly enough to humiliate publicly the woman who still meant so much to her son. That's not to say that Williams was unaware of how his wife – they were only separated and not yet divorced – felt about the new love of his life.

> The problem is intensified because Zachary loves Marsha and Marsha loves the child [he said]. So for Valerie, along with the feeling that Marsha took *me* away, there's the threat that Marsha might replace *her* in Zach's affections. That won't happen. Valerie is a very good mother. Nothing could shake his love for her. And I won't give her unnecessary pain. A relationship as long and close as ours can't be brushed aside. Besides we've got to work together for Zach. He's fine except when things get tense. He doesn't want tension . . . To live in this grey area is hard for everyone concerned. People have to get on with their lives.

Through all of the quotes from Robin Williams which appear in the article you can plainly see his sub-text. He is trying to do the decent thing by Valerie, by Marsha, by Zach, and even by *People* itself in attempting to lay all his cards on the table. Unfortunately his candour came back to bite him. The villain of this piece was very definitely Marsha Garces as far as *People* was concerned. Williams did not immediately condemn the article at the time. He felt it was better to allow things hopefully to blow over. That, he admitted later, was a mistake. He should have offered a more immediate and more robust defence, because without it what he came to call 'the nanny thing' would haunt them both for years.

People magazine also suffered as a consequence. Williams was and is a popular man in Hollywood, with lots of friends. His experience encouraged them to be a lot more careful in future, and ironically it was pieces like this article which helped usher in the more restrictive climate for entertainment journalists in the years to come.

'They went from being a magazine people wanted to do to a magazine people were wary of,' claims Williams. 'It was really a hatchet job, a set-up, an ambush. A very low blow. And it cost them. Celebrities got very worried. It was like "Why should I do a story with you?".'

The incident with *People* magazine and his frequent battles with the *National Enquirer* have inevitably coloured Robin Williams' relations with the press. These days he generally only does interviews when he has something to promote, and even then he is selective. On a recent visit to Britain, for example, his people insisted that he would not talk to any tabloid newspapers and only broadsheets were given access.

'It is a dance,' he admitted of the relationship between the famous and the press. 'It's like two lepers doing a tango – "Uh-oh, you walked away with an arm". It's difficult with journalists because they come in thinking, "Well I've got to find something", and we know. It's like a Bergman film where you are playing Parcheesi with Death.'

22

Oh Captain, My Captain

The cover story on the February 1988 issue of *People* magazine may not have done Robin Williams' public image many favours. On the other hand, even while he was railing at being set up by *People*, privately Williams and his handlers must have been breathing a sigh of relief. They would have been relieved because of the story that *People* missed, a scandal which was potentially more damaging to Williams than the tawdry claims that he had ditched his wife in favour of his child's nanny.

On Tuesday, 26 April 1988 a lawsuit was filed against Robin Williams in the San Francisco Superior Court. The suit was filed by Tish Carter and sought $6 million in damages after claiming that Robin Williams had infected her with herpes. Although the suit was filed in the San Francisco Superior Court some two months after the *People* story, it had been active for almost two years. It was originally filed in another court in 1986, and if *People* had found out about that, all the box-office magic in the world would have made it difficult for Williams to recover from the double whammy.

According to Carter's lawyer, Adolph B. Canelo, she met the comedian in December 1984 while she was working as a cocktail waitress at the Improv comedy club in Los Angeles. This would have been right in the middle of Williams' period of serious womanising. Williams has never denied having a relationship with Carter and, although a gagging order forbids him from talking about it directly, he has strongly indicated that it was this relationship which ultimately led to the breakdown of his marriage to Valerie Velardi. It's alleged that Williams and Carter had their affair from December 1984 until November 1985. According to her lawsuit she discovered on 20 November 1985 that she had been infected with the incurable, sexually transmitted disease herpes. She claimed that she told Williams, and that he told her on the same day that he had been infected since high school. Through Canelo, Carter then brought an action against Williams. It was originally filed in a small court in Stanislaus County, in California, with the express purpose of avoiding publicity while negotiations went on with Williams and his legal team. However, when those negotiations came to nothing, Canelo transferred the action from Stanislaus County to the San Francisco Superior Court, where it could not help but attract publicity.

As filed in the Superior Court, the suit charged Williams with being negligent and also responsible for the negligent infliction of mental suffering, and with fraud because he failed to tell Carter that he had herpes. The suit went on to say that Williams ought to have known that since herpes is a sexually transmitted disease it would be 'most likely' that Carter would be infected. As a consequence of that the suit alleged she would 'suffer a great deal of pain, worry and embarrassment not only after she first learned of the disease but for the rest of her life'.

According to Canelo, apart from denying that he had herpes, there had been little response from Williams' legal team. That appeared to be the general tactic of the Williams camp about the whole Carter business. They had made no comment to the media and were obviously taking the view that this was just one of the many nuisance suits that a man in Williams' position would get in the course of his career. However, the fact that this was originally filed in 1986, when Williams' career was in a trough, should perhaps have alerted them to the possibility that this was not necessarily a fame-inspired get-rich-quick scheme. Once the case was filed in the Superior Court it was only a matter of time before it came to the attention of the media. And so it did, although some treated it differently from others. The *San Francisco Chronicle* contained a relatively sober and straightforward account of the action on an inside page; the *National Enquirer*, renewing their battle with their old foe, splashed it across the front page with what appeared to be undisguised glee. Now that it was out in the open, Williams could no longer afford to play a waiting game. He had tried that before over the break-up of his marriage and found himself and his new love pilloried. This time he would have to take the offensive.

Robin Williams' legal affairs have been handled for many years by Gerald Margolis who, at the time of the action, was a partner in the Los

Angeles firm of Margolis, Ryan, Burrill, Besser. This was an extremely high-profile law firm which specialised in entertainment law and, as well as Williams, also represented big names such as Eric Clapton, Mick Jagger, Keith Richards and Paul Simon. In San Francisco, the showbiz responsibilities of Margolis, Ryan, Burrill, Besser, were generally looked after by Phil Ryan, another partner in the firm. As a consequence it was Ryan who looked after the Carter case for Williams. Ironically, as well as looking after Williams, Ryan was also Valerie Velardi's personal attorney, although he would not be involved in their divorce proceedings.

Ryan had built up a reputation for himself in the Bay Area for being almost as flamboyant as some of the people he represents. His standard fee for a civil action then was $250 an hour, and he generally indulged in what might safely be described as a rock-and-roll lifestyle. A self-described 'loudmouth trial attorney', he was the sort of flamboyant character who used rock videos as evidence, did not shrink from holding full-scale press conferences, and on one occasion, when defending a client accused of murder, handed out carnations to supporters going into court. But his extravagance could not disguise a shrewd legal mind and an uncompromising approach on behalf of those who engaged his services. The break-up of the cult Seventies band Jefferson Starship is a perfect example of how effective Ryan can be. When Paul Kantner, one of the founders of Jefferson Airplane – as the band was originally called – wanted to leave in 1984, it was Ryan who handled an increasingly acrimonious split. But when co-founder Grace Slick decided she too wanted to leave the band in 1988, the first person she turned to was Ryan, even though he had 'screwed her over' in the original action.

'Entertainers are strange beasts,' Robin Williams told the *San Francisco Chronicle* over lunch with a reporter, Phil Ryan and Marsha Garces. 'Most of the world looks at you like "Eeeech". But he [Ryan] understands. You need someone like that to kind of wade through the diverse things that happen.'

In acting for Williams, Ryan quickly found himself not so much wading as wallowing hip-deep in the Carter case. Rather than take the approach favoured by many celebrities and simply offer some cash to make it go away, Ryan was favouring a full-frontal approach in Williams' defence. That lunch was only the first step in a high-profile campaign to protect his client's interests. The first thing he did was to tell Williams not to utter a word about the case and, to this day, he has followed his lawyer's instructions. Any comment about Tish Carter would come from Phil Ryan; and come they did.

'We have examined Miss Carter's medical records,' he informed the

Chronicle, 'and they indicate she does not have herpes. She does have warts, however,' he added archly, 'and Mr Williams has no pet frogs ... Miss Carter seems to think there is public interest in her genital history. We don't think there is, just as there's no interest in Robin's. Or mine for that matter.'

But there was more to Phil Ryan than a few arch dismissals of Carter's claims. He was immediately going for the jugular by announcing that he would be filing a cross-complaint against Carter. Ryan gave only a few hints of what he might be claiming, but the details were finally revealed on Thursday, 6 October 1988, when he filed a complaint on behalf of Robin Williams in the San Francisco Superior Court. Basically Ryan was claiming that Carter had lied in an attempted extortion scam against his client to get money and a car.

Williams, according to the lawsuit, was claiming that Carter had used 'duress, coercion and fraud' to coax money from him since 1985. The *San Francisco Chronicle* went on to publish more details of Williams' complaint. 'Carter,' it alleged, 'intentionally and with extraordinary malice, made these representations to Williams, threatening damage to his public persona and damage to his family life in order to extort money and property from him.'

The suit also alleged that Carter began plotting against Williams after he had told her at the start of their relationship that he had herpes. She claimed to have contracted the disease in 1985, although Williams' suit said two herpes tests in 1986 proved negative. When Williams tried to break off the relationship, he claimed, Carter then told him she was pregnant and demanded $20,000 and a new car. She also threatened to go public with her allegations. Williams' lawsuit charged her with extortion, conspiracy and international infliction of emotional distress. It was also asking for an unspecified amount in damages.

Plainly this was a case which was going to run and run, and it would be several years yet before it would be finally resolved. In the meantime, while the drama was being played out by various teams of lawyers in San Francisco court rooms, Williams was on-stage in New York completing his run in *Waiting for Godot*. And immediately afterwards he was due to start work on another film.

Williams and Brezner had thought long and hard about the follow-up to *Good Morning Vietnam* and there were a number of possibilities in the pipeline. Far and away the most intriguing was the chance to play The Joker in *Batman*. Bob Kane's comic-book creation was finally being given the treatment he deserved with a big-budget screen version directed by Tim Burton, whose dark vision was closer to the comic book's sensibilities than anything before or since. *Batman* was being produced by Jon Peters and Peter Guber, and Burton ran into some problems with his casting choices. It seems that while Burton was keen on Williams for a role which probably more than any other would have given free rein to his manic abilities, Guber and Peters were more concerned with the star power of Jack Nicholson. In the end the producers prevailed and Nicholson got the role which eventually netted him a pay-day reported to be around $50 million once his cut of the box-office and merchandising revenues were taken into account.

Looking back on the *Batman* experience, Williams feels that perhaps he was a little naïve. He felt that his name had been used to get Nicholson interested and then he had been dumped once Nicholson bit.

> What they do a lot of times, they bait people [he explained]. They'll say, 'Robin might do this, are you in or out?' A lot of things are word of mouth and a lot of people are offered something and then immediately it's taken away and given to somebody else ... He [Nicholson] had been offered it six months before and then it was given to me. I replied, but they said I was too late. They said they'd gone to Jack over the weekend because I didn't reply soon enough. I said, 'You gave me till Monday, I replied before the deadline.' But it was just to get Jack off the pot.

His relationship with Marsha Garces had changed Williams' attitude to his profession; although he was angry about the *Batman* episode he could be sanguine at the same time. He had also learned a deal of humility and was now pursuing parts that he wanted and was not above auditioning to get them.

'I'm not going to play that game of "What do you mean audition? I'm Robin Williams",' he says. 'Fuck it. I'll go read. It's worth it to try. And it felt better to read with somebody than to get hired and not have the chemistry work out. It's sobering, too, because some of the parts have fallen through.'

One of the parts which did fall through was in *Midnight Run* in which Robert De Niro was to play a bounty hunter trying to bring back a Mob book-keeper. This would be the part which would spark something of a box-office renaissance for De Niro, but to begin with the studios were concerned about his pulling power. Ned Tanen, who was head of Paramount at the time, was looking for some box-office insurance. At one point they considered rewriting the book-keeper's role for Cher, who had just won an Oscar for *Moonstruck*. And one of those who actively campaigned for the role was Williams, who was keen to work alongside his friend De Niro.

> I met with them [De Niro and director Martin Brest] three or four times and it got real close [says Williams]. It was almost there and then they went with somebody else. The character was supposed to be an accountant for the Mafia. Charles Grodin got the part. I was craving it. I thought 'I can be as funny', but they wanted someone obviously more in type. And in the end he was better for it. But it was rough for me. I had to remind myself: 'Okay, come on, you've got other things.'

One of those other things turned out to be a man who was quickly turning into a fertile source for Robin Williams' films. Dustin Hoffman had passed on *Popeye* and *The World According to Garp*, and now he was about to pass on another film. Like the first two, *Dead Poets Society* ended up starring Robin Williams.

'I should be just hanging out by his house,' Williams jokes. ' "What did you pass on? Yeah? OK, that sounds good. What else?". '

Dead Poets Society was an original screenplay by Tom Schulman which was being directed by the Australian Peter Weir, who had carved out a Hollywood reputation with his success with the Harrison Ford film *Witness.* It is the story of John Keating, an English teacher at a select private school who believes that poetry is a living, breathing thing. His unusual methods earn the displeasure of the teaching establishment and some of the parents, but they touch the hearts of some of his young charges. In the end, when he leaves the school, he has changed their lives for ever. While *Good Morning Vietnam* had given him the opportunity to combine comedy and drama, this was an out-and-out dramatic role. Once he saw the screenplay Williams knew that he had to do *Dead Poets Society.*

'It talks about something of the heart and pursuing that which is a dream – and in some cases to a tragic end,' he explains. 'Originally my character was supposed to have leukaemia, which would have been *Dead Poets Love Story.* Then Peter Weir said, "Let's lose that. Focus on the boys." Lose the melodrama and it becomes much simpler and much better.'

Williams responds to good direction. Whether it was from John Houseman back in Juilliard or Barry Levinson on *Good Morning Vietnam*, Williams can see and recognise someone who is trying to help his performance. One of his greatest strengths is his intelligence, and he was smart enough here to see that Peter Weir was stretching him dramatically like no one else before. To find the character of John Keating, Williams drew from two sources. The first was one of his own teachers at Detroit Country Day School, John Campbell, whom he describes as a 'radical of the highest order, a crusader of conscience'.

'John Campbell is an abrasive man,' says Williams. 'He was my wrestling coach, a history teacher who basically said history would make a great farce, and that most wars would be hilarious except that massive numbers of people die from the madness.'

You can see why Campbell would appeal to Williams in the process of building John Keating's character. But the other guiding influence on Robin Williams' performance was much more profound. It came from his own father.

> They were yin and yang, my parents [Williams explains]. My mother is this outrageous character who is so sweet and basically believes in the goodness of people. And Dad had seen the nasty side of people. He had been in combat. She told me, 'There are no boundaries.' And he gave me this depth that helps with acting and even with comedy, saying, 'Fuck it. Do you believe in this? Do you really want to talk about it? Do it. Don't be frightened off.' Somewhere in his early life he had to give up certain things, certain dreams. And when I found mine he was deeply pleased.

Williams acknowledges that his father had worked hard in an industry which could be as thankless and heedless as the film industry. He also suggests it was his father who recognised those parallels. But Robert Williams had also seen that although his son's life was in transition, he was slowly becoming the master of his own fate.

> He was this wonderful elegant man who thought the world was going to hell in a hand basket [says Robin Williams]. It was basically 'You can't trust them. Watch out for them. They'll nail ya. Everybody's out to nail ya' ... I realise that what he gave me is what's been working now in some of these dramatic movies. He had a great stillness and power to him, a great kind of ... I can only use the word depth. He knew exactly what and where he'd been, who he was and why he did certain things. He was never pushed along. If things weren't done the way he felt was right, he left. That's coming into play now when I do movies like *Dead Poets Society*. I find myself thinking, 'That's for you, Pop.'

23

A Little Spark of Madness

Robin Williams felt Marsha Garces' influence most keenly in his private life. There was no more drinking, no more drugs, and no more womanising. What there was, was peace and quiet and time to take a breath. Even for his fans, however, the influence of Marsha Garces on Robin Williams could be keenly felt in his performance. Williams' comedy before and after Marsha came into his life was like chalk and cheese.

Most of America knew Williams as Mork from Ork, but it was not long after the initial impact of the success of that series that millions got to see the other side of Williams. The comedy special *Robin Williams: Off the Wall* was recorded at the Roxy in Los Angeles to be screened by the cable station HBO in 1978. This was a period when, by his own admission, Williams was drinking and using drugs, and the resulting performance is at times astonishing, and at other points simply painful. *Off the Wall* is a picture of a man on the edge; a man who cannot control his boundless energy.

Williams begins by surveying the celebrity-studded audience. Those out front included friends and colleagues such as Henry Winkler, John Ritter, Tony Danza and JoAnne Worley. 'Everyone I know is here,' quips an incredulous Williams. 'Some people I've slept with twice.'

He then proceeds to launch into an increasingly frenetic routine. Early in the show he takes leave of the stage and clambers hand over hand into the balcony where he does a *faux* Charles Laughton schtick from *The Hunchback of Notre Dame.* Back down on the stage much of the humour is drug-laced and drug-influenced. Describing himself as 'George Jessel on acid', Williams unveils the eclectic range of comic characters which vie for attention in his magpie mind as he prowls the stage sucking in stimuli from an eager crowd. He moves in the blink of an eye from an old blind bluesman to televangelist the Reverend Ernest Lee Sincere. In between we have the six-year-old Little Billy performing the by now famous 'Death of a Sperm' ballet and Williams as children's TV host Mr Rogers microwaving a hamster to teach children about the horrors of radiation. This is Williams using his famous duck and cover technique of comedy. It is brilliant, manic and entirely illusory.

Unlike most comedians his routine is not a revelatory process; we learn nothing about Robin Williams in the course of the show. In fact the opposite holds true, in that we are so bombarded by images that we leave the show even more confused about who Williams is than we were when we sat down.

There are, however, one or two moments of clarity in the obfuscatory hilarity. Williams starts into one of his other stock routines, the one about the comedian dying on-stage. This time it looks uncomfortably real. After about half an hour of his act Williams' wheels are spinning to the point where he comes close to being too hip for the room. By the time he gets to the dying comic, the audience are not quite sure what to make of it. There is the strong sense that as Williams makes comments about 'a gentle rose, dying here like me', he's getting uncomfortably close to the real thing. There is just a momentary glimpse of fear in his eyes, and the audience are just at the point where they are beginning to laugh because of who he is rather than what he's saying. At the last minute, like a pitcher at the bottom of the eighth inning, Williams makes a brilliant save and regains the day and with it the audience.

There are moments, too, when Williams goes into what he describes as 'Zen-lock', a period of total comedic freedom, a point where he is almost not in charge of what is going on around him. One such moment comes near the end when Williams leaves the stage and wanders among the audience in a spoof-Shakespearean soliloquy. In the middle of the monologue he wonders aloud whether it is 'nobler to suffer the slings and arrows or do some crazy shit on TV at eight o'clock'. Bearing in mind that the HBO show was recorded at the end of the first series of *Mork and Mindy*, it's pretty obvious that the disillusionment had set in at a fairly early stage. Then towards the last few minutes of the show Williams gets back on stage and adopts a variation of his Grandpa Funk persona; the old man who feeds heroin to pigeons because it keeps them coming back. This time Grandpa Funk is Williams himself looking back from the future to his own career. It's a painful little routine which shows signs of an extremely bleak worldview.

'We're only given a little spark of madness,' says Williams/Grandpa Funk. 'If you lose that you're nothing.'

After introducing Nicky Lenin, the Soviet Union's only entertainer, for an encore, Williams leaves the stage to tumultuous applause. The cameras follow him backstage where he collapses into a chair in a kind of post-orgasmic state, exhausted but satisfied and a little dislocated from the real world.

Off the Wall is rather like a distillation of everything that Robin Williams had been up to that point. The routines are brilliant but entirely fuelled by fear, a fear of rejection which had dogged him since childhood. This is the performance of a man who desperately needs and wants to be liked. This is Robin Williams, performance junkie par excellence.

Four years later Williams committed another stand-up routine for posterity with the release of *An Evening with Robin Williams.* This concert was recorded in the Great American Music Hall in his adoptive home town San Francisco, with Lovin' Spoonful founder John Sebastian providing a musical warm-up. If *Off the Wall* was a portrait of a man on the edge, *An Evening with Robin Williams* was an uncomfortable look at a man clawing his way back from the abyss. This was Williams after John Belushi had died and, more importantly, after Zachary had been born. There was much less drug humour here now; experience had taught him that it was no longer that funny. Williams appears on-stage like a man with every nerve-ending laid bare and twitching. Some of the routines – grabbing a camera from an audience member and taking a picture of his own penis, or heckling a woman who has the misfortune to require a bathroom break – are uncharacteristically cruel for a man who has never turned on his audience like some of his fellow Kalashnikov comedians. Williams here is nowhere near as innovative as he falls back on tried and trusted material. The penis jokes which are a staple of his act come thick and fast. A police siren sounds outside and he quips 'Here comes my ride', a line he has been using for 15 years now. It's like watching a drowning man swimming for shore: you don't necessarily enjoy the spectacle, but you can't help hoping that he reaches dry land.

An Evening with Robin Williams is a performance for a man in transition both in terms of his life and in terms of his material. The comedians Williams envies, such as Richard Pryor and Sam Kinnison, are those who are able to take their lives and turn them into comedy. Those for whom comedy is a catharsis. For the first time in his career Williams was starting to do that. *An Evening with Robin Williams* contains an early routine about childbirth and Zachary which he would hone and develop over the years. He acknowledged that it was a major change in direction.

> I need to work more on that [he said of incorporating personal material into his act], and if you do that it makes your work richer. That's one part that I think that I'll grow into. That'll give it a depth. If I look at the other stuff there is an energy and a mind, but it's still kind of flying all over the place. To have that thing that Richard Pryor has always had, it's so real that it's scary, that type of thing where you are not just opening a vein, you're basically pulling veins out of your arms. Scary stuff.

But Williams was able to deal with it and to incorporate it into his act. The quintessential Robin Williams stand-up performances came on the weekend of 9 and 10 August 1986, when Williams became the first solo comedian to perform at the Metropolitan Opera House in New York. The concerts were preserved and edited into a TV special which was later released on video. *Robin Williams: An Evening at the Met* is a remarkable piece of work – both on video and on live CD – which finally presents the sharpest comic mind of his generation functioning at the peak of its ability. This was Williams clean and sober and, thanks to Marsha Garces who was a vitally important part of his life at this stage, able to confront his life through his art. The man who had been not waving but possibly drowning in *An Evening with Robin Williams* had finally made it back to shore.

Taken as individual routines, *An Evening at the Met* is a very funny series of musings on drink, drugs, law enforcement, Ronald Reagan, penis jokes (again!), lust, sexual prowess and just about anything else that comes to mind. Taken as a whole, however, this is a very different Robin Williams performance. For one thing it is very tightly structured. There is still room for him to suck up all the creative energy in the room, but nothing is going to deflect him from where he is going. Hecklers are dealt with crisply and effectively as he heads for his pre-determined goal. Instead of the Williams who prowled the stage at the Roxy like a caged animal or who went through a fair approximation of a psychotic episode at the Great American Music Hall, this is a man in command of the medium. He strides around the stage at the Met with confidence and poise and delivers a routine which is almost a meditation on his life thus far.

We begin with alcohol and his confessional account of the fact that he is a recovering alcoholic – 'I'm the same asshole, I just have fewer dents in my car'. He knew he had an alcohol problem when he was found 'nude on the hood of my car with my keys in my ass'. After acknowledging that alcohol is designed to 'bring out the asshole in everybody' he heads off for more of his personal purgatory. From alcohol he moves on to cocaine – 'anything that makes you paranoid and impotent, gimme more of that' – and acknowledges how drugs almost destroyed him.

'Freebasing,' he says derisively. 'It's not free, it costs you your home. It should be called homebasing.'

Nothing is spared. After the drink and the drugs come the women, as he moves on to the period when he was 'driven to find Miss Right, or at least Miss Right-Now'. None of this is delivered in a remotely mawkish or maudlin manner. This is great material and he is in devastating form, so much so that anyone who didn't know Williams' background would simply see it as a trenchant commentary on contemporary mores. It is painful, but only if you know where he's been. Williams' comedic Stations of the Cross eventually take him through his Good Friday and into his Easter Sunday in the form of his son Zachary. Time and again he rails at the problems of parenthood, but each time he stops himself short with the phrase 'They handed me my son', and his voice softens and his eyes widen with wonder each time he says it. Eventually Williams uses his incredible mimetic skills to 'become' his son as he and Zach wander off the stage together.

The concert at the Met was and remains a high point in Robin Williams' career. This was still before *Good Morning Vietnam* and all of the success which would follow that, but it is a landmark in Williams' career in that it marks the first time that he was able to put it all together. For the first time, with Marsha's help, the fear had gone. He would still be scared before a performance but that was only stage-fright, not the paralysing primal fear he had felt before. That concert at the Met heralded a genuine purple patch in Robin Williams' comedy career. This was a period in which he could take the time to go on the road and play to thousands of people at a single venue. This was the last period in his life in which he could do that before he was swallowed up completely by his film career.

The men who had the dubious task of opening for Robin Williams on that tour were an incredibly gifted comedy juggling act called the Raspyni Brothers. Choosing an opening act for a comic is a very difficult decision. Williams had tended to use musicians before. John Sebastian had opened for him, and his opener of choice at that stage was San Francisco jazzman and vocalist extraordinaire Bobby McFerrin. However, the idea of going on the road did not appeal to McFerrin, so Williams needed a new opener. Billy Crystal suggested a comedy juggling act he had seen on *The Tonight Show*, and so the Raspyni Brothers – alias Barry Friedman and Dan Holzman – were hired on his recommendation. All things considered, they were perfect; funny enough to get the crowd laughing, but with an act that was sufficiently different from Williams' not to steal any of his thunder.

'Robin is definitely the best stand-up I have ever seen, out of all of them,' says Holzman. 'Billy Crystal is very good because he could do all these character pieces, very structured, a bit like watching a play. But Robin is the only one who I could stay and watch every night because he was always different.'

Holzman and Friedman are in a perfect position to judge Williams at this stage of his career. They have opened for a Who's Who of contemporary American comedians including Billy Crystal, Dana Carvey, Dennis Miller, Garry Shandling and David Brenner. Friedman shares his partner's endorsement of Williams as the best of the best.

> He has a huge library of material, so that when something did come up he had a good line or a good quip ready for it [says Friedman]. 'Like other comedians he has his standard things, but probably from his training at Juilliard, he has the ability to make it sound like he had never said it before. In comedy the beginning and the end are the most important parts of the act. They're bookmarks and the bit in the middle kind of takes care of itself. But Robin would close with something one night and the next night you'd see him open with it. We've worked with a lot of styles and some you can set your watch by. Dennis Miller, for example, is very scripted. But Robin can just go off at a tangent.
>
> Robin also has the ability to move you. That stuff about his kid at The Met moves you to tears. With other comedians, such as Howie Mandel, you get a lot of bathroom jokes but you don't expect them to touch you emotionally. Robin and Billy were the two who could do that.

Williams also honed his talent for improvisation on that tour, which took in a lot of college and university campuses. One of the few things he insisted on was that there should be a box of toys on stage every night. He also insisted that the choice of toys or props be entirely up to the concert organisers.

> That would be his encore [recalls Holzman]. He would just go over to the box and take something out and riff on it. Some comedians do that with their own boxes of props – Carrot Top for example always knows what's in there, that's the point of his act – but Robin never knew until he got there. It was just great to watch. I don't know anyone else who would take that kind of risk. He was also one of the few comedians you could interact with.

The relationship between a comic and his warm-up is a kind of strange one, it is basically employer-employee. A lot of them don't watch your show, they don't want anything to do with you. But every night we could hear Robin laughing backstage. It was great to hear that laugh. It was louder than anyone else.

He also liked to do our opening announcement for us, he would use a different comedy voice each time. Garry Shandling used to do that too. A lot of other guys take their role of being a celebrity a bit too seriously, but Robin was a lot of fun.

On one occasion, Williams took his status as the star of the show so lightly that he held up proceedings until the Raspynis could get there.

We were flying on Eastern Airlines into Miami for a show on Superbowl Weekend [remembers Barry Friedman]. The show was at eight but the plane was delayed and we didn't touch down until eight. We were changing into our stage clothes in the limo at the same time that we were on the phone to Robin, and he was just so cool about the whole thing. We could hear the stage manager in the background saying, 'Can we start, can we start?' and Robin was saying, 'Let's just talk a little while and calm these guys down.' Then he went out and did a whole routine about how bad Eastern Airlines were.

He was also very relaxed with his fans [remembers Dan Holzman]. One time in Oregon this girl came up to him and she was so excited to meet him that she was in tears, she was freaking out. His reaction was so genuine. He couldn't understand why she would respond like that, as far as he was concerned he was just a guy. He was so gentle with her when he could just have blown her off completely – I've seen some guys do that. Another time we were driving between gigs and we stopped at a fast food joint. Robin went in and everyone kind of freaked out. The manager came over and apologised but Robin said, 'Let me eat my meal, and then we can play around.' After he had finished his meal he stood up and did about 15 or 20 minutes, he fooled around with the drive-in speaker, he did all this stuff just for the benefit of the folk in the restaurant. It was very cool.

I think some people have a persona and they are not the people you think they are, but I think one of the reasons Robin is so popular is that people sense he has a good heart.

The most obvious public demonstration of Robin Williams' good-heartedness also came in the middle of this incredibly fertile comedic spell. In 1986, along with his good friends Billy Crystal and Whoopi Goldberg, Williams founded the American version of Comic Relief. This triumvirate of talent acts as the backbone for a series of live concerts and television specials which are designed to raise funds for the homeless in America. The first of those benefits – a live three-hour show screened on HBO on 29 March 1986 – raised $2.5 million. It's hardly surprising that Williams, who was raised in a spirit of radicalism by his father, who had found out at first hand what an unfair place the world could be, should have become involved in something like Comic Relief. That initial spirit was further fostered by his Juilliard mentor John Houseman, who felt that activism and drama went hand in hand. Now Williams felt confident enough to play a leading role in helping people who were being dealt seconds by the system.

> What's changed for me [he says] is that rather than just sit and criticise, you say OK, what can you actually do to start wading into it and make it work, instead of just saying 'You're wrong. That sucks. They're ripping us off'. Now we have to fight from our local community up and work on schools and for the homeless. All that's left now in a lot of our schools is reading, writing and arithmetic, everything else is considered ketchup ... We're raising a nation of overweight, unintelligent people. The cities have broken down, the educational systems suffer cutbacks. The reality is we're broke.

In the dozen or so years since that first Comic Relief event Williams has done his bit to address himself to the issues rather than just shouting about them. In the first ten years of its operating Comic Relief raised more than $35 million for charitable works.

24

Do You Take This Woman

On 30 April 1989 Robin Williams and Marsha Garces were married. The divorce settlement had taken three years to finalise and had come through at the start of the month. A few weeks later, at a quiet ceremony in Lake Tahoe, Williams married the woman who had been his redemption.

It was a small gathering with a wedding party of barely 30 guests. Those present on that day were among the most important people in Robin Williams' life. Apart from his immediate family the guests included fellow comedians Billy Crystal and Bobcat Goldthwait and their wives, Barry Levinson and his wife, as well as *Good Morning Vietnam* producer Mark Johnson and his wife. The wedding was the culmination of what had been a hectic and turbulent period in Robin Williams' life. There were still some outstanding issues – not least the Tish Carter lawsuit – but he could now move on.

Williams had been working fairly constantly for the past 18 months. After shooting *Good Morning Vietnam*, there had been a series of concert dates, there had been meetings over other roles, and finally there was the filming of *Dead Poets Society.* The shooting of Peter Weir's movie overlapped with the end of the run of *Waiting for Godot.* This meant that Williams was filming a movie in Delaware while he was also on-stage every night in New York, some 150 miles to the south. It was tough, but with some creative scheduling he was able to emerge relatively unscathed. By the time filming ended in January 1989, however, Williams and Marsha Garces had been away from home for a total of five months. They were both keen to get back to San Francisco. They wanted to spend some quality time with Zach for one thing, and Williams wanted to stay in touch with his recently widowed mother. But there was another pressing reason for their return to California.

Marsha Garces was pregnant. By the time *Dead Poets Society* was finished she was three months gone. That, however, did not prevent her from performing her usual tasks in supporting Williams in whatever he needed. By the time the couple were finally married, Marsha was almost six months pregnant. This was the ultimate declaration of Williams' commitment to this woman. He had put his old ways behind him and was now ready to start family life all over again. Valerie Velardi for her part was also building a new life for herself; she had had a baby early the previous year. For Williams it was a case of having his mid-life crisis a little early; whereas most men wait until their forties, he had his in his thirties.

'I guess I've been going through a mid-life crisis for about five or six years,' he admitted. 'When's it supposed to hit, forty? I think I got laid enough. Sport-fucking I explored. That's done, thank you. That was nuts. That was totally the opposite of intimacy.'

With Marsha it seemed he had found everything he never knew he was looking for: strength, stability, intimacy, and the space to get to know himself. This seemed to be the real thing. But perhaps he had already had the real thing in his marriage to Valerie Velardi and just wasn't aware of it.

'I don't know,' he told *Esquire* magazine in June 1989, just a few weeks after he had remarried. 'Part of me says no and part of me says maybe. Obviously it's like asking an amnesiac what happened. I don't know. That's something that'll take years to work out in therapy. Now, I know I have the real thing.'

Three months after they were married Marsha Williams gave birth to a baby girl. They decided to call her Zelda, but not for what might appear to be the obvious reasons. 'Most people think we named her after Zelda Fitzgerald,' Williams explains, 'But my son named her – after a character in a Nintendo game. He has a very fertile imagination.'

However, Williams did promise Marsha that if there were any more children there would be 'no more Z's'. While *Dead Poets Society* was in post-production and being readied for an end-of-year release to qualify for hoped-for Oscar nominations, Williams retreated to the Bay Area to spend time with his new family. They divided their time between a spacious apartment in San Francisco and the ranch in Sonoma. Both Williams and his wife decided that they no longer wanted to live in Los

Angeles, which had too many unpleasant associations with Williams' past.

'LA is like Disneyland staged by Dante,' says Williams. 'I lived there when I was doing *Mork and Mindy* and I was so paranoid about my career. In San Francisco, variety is a spice of life, it's not a magazine.'

When he went on retreat in San Francisco, Williams could indulge in two of his favourite pastimes: reading science fiction and playing with his children. The houses boast a room full of computers and electronic games, and Williams and Zachary fight for equal time on the consoles. When they're not playing computer games, they prefer to watch television together.

'Our favourites are *Sesame Street* and those old Warner Brothers cartoons,' Williams revealed. 'Sometimes while Zach and I are watching them, I do wacky voices, the same way I do in my act. And Zach will say, "Daddy, don't use that voice. Just be Daddy." And that's just what I want to do. Just be Daddy.'

While Williams was dividing his time being Daddy between San Francisco and Sonoma, the buzz was gathering in Hollywood about *Dead Poets Society*. The film in which his John Keating would exhort his young charges with the words 'Carpe diem' ('Seize the day') was gathering all sorts of praise. Williams had established himself as what he had always intended to be, a dramatic actor. The box-office results were quite remarkable. In the United States the film took a fraction under $96 million, not as much as *Good Morning Vietnam* but, bearing in mind that this was aimed at an older, more discerning audience, still a remarkable figure. Audiences were riveted, and moved to tears by the ending of the film, in which Keating leaves the school as the boys stand on their desks in tribute to the man who has changed their lives. The response overseas was even better than in the domestic market. Commercially the film took $140 million internationally, and overseas audiences were similarly moved by the story. In Japan, for example, the house lights remained down for five minutes after the film ended, to allow the emotional patrons time to compose themselves and regain face before leaving the cinema.

With this kind of response another Oscar nomination seemed a decent prospect. And indeed when the nominations were announced Williams found himself nominated in the Best Actor category for his second film in succession. This time Williams was nominated with a clutch of Best Actor débutants. His fellow nominees were Kenneth Branagh for *Henry V*, Tom Cruise for *Born on the Fourth of July*, Daniel Day-Lewis for *My Left Foot* and Morgan Freeman for *Driving Miss Daisy*. The tipsters seemed to be fairly evenly split about who might win the award. A case could be made for each of them, it seemed, although there was intense lobbying for Cruise as a disabled Vietnam veteran. Unfortunately for Williams, the one thing that all the pundits did seem to agree on was that he was once again the outsider of the bunch. Despite the quality of his performance, his background in television and especially comedy was once again working against him. It is, it seems, easier for the proverbial camel to pass through the eye of a needle than for a comic to win a Best Actor award. There was much talk before the event of split votes and candidates emerging through the gap. *Driving Miss Daisy* had most nominations and it was felt that Freeman might win on the momentum of what many thought might be a clean sweep for the movie. On the other hand Spike Lee's *Do the Right Thing*, which presented a much more uncompromising view of black life in America, had been completely overlooked by the Academy. As a consequence there was something of a backlash building against *Driving Miss Daisy* with its somewhat more sentimental view of race relations in the South.

Williams remained remarkably calm throughout. While other nominees fretted nervously in their rooms, Williams enjoyed a relaxed eve-of-awards dinner at the Bel Air hotel in Los Angeles with his best friend Billy Crystal, who would be hosting the event. In the end the Oscar went to Daniel Day-Lewis for his portrayal of disabled writer Christy Brown in *My Left Foot*. It was a remarkable performance and it once again confirmed the Academy's fondness for honouring actors playing characters who overcome devastating adversity. In the end *Dead Poets Society* won only one Oscar, for Tom Schulman's script. Williams had been passed over again, but this time he could be more sanguine about events. He had discovered there were more important things in life than Academy Awards.

The final postscript to the *Dead Poets Society* saga came more than a year later when John Campbell, the man on whom Williams had based his performance, was fired from Detroit Country Day School. The circumstances of his dismissal were uncannily similar to those of John Keating's in the film. Campbell, who was then 55 and had been at the school for almost 30 years, had been on probation for several years. After he had been dismissed the school headmaster Gerald Hansen claimed that Campbell 'had not satisfactorily demonstrated a willingness to adhere to all the academic and professional standards of the school'.

Campbell, it seemed, was keen that his students simply teach themselves. On one notable occasion he insisted that anyone could teach history. To prove his point he went out into the street, stopped the first car he found, and asked the driver to come in and take the class. When asked later how the class had gone, Campbell said he didn't know, he had left. The fact that he made such an indelible mark on obviously bright students, such as Robin Williams, testified to Campbell's ability. He also had the support of the PTA, who claimed he was 'one of the few who doesn't bore parents at Faculty Night'. But in the end it was all too much for the school administration and they got rid of him.

John Campbell saw *Dead Poets Society* and enjoyed it. Like Adrian Cronauer before him, he didn't think that Robin Williams' portrayal was terribly accurate. Unlike Cronauer, however, Campbell felt his former pupil had erred on the side of caution.

'Actually Robin Williams wasn't as radical a teacher as I am,' Campbell insists. 'He tells the students to rip out the pages in their books. I tell them to throw the whole thing in the garbage.'

25

The Thief of Bad Gags?

The folklorist and philosopher Joseph Campbell suggests that there are only seven basic stories. No matter what they are, everything else is simply a permutation of one or more of these seven elements. By extension there are probably no more than seven different jokes in the sense that whatever the gag is and whoever is telling it, it can be boiled down to easily classifiable basic components. One of the things which makes Robin Williams such a great comedian is his ability to recognise this. His steel-trap mind can take almost any scenario and instantly turn it into a joke by almost intuitively adapting it to the basic format.

But in the summer of 1989 there were suggestions that perhaps there was a little less to Williams than met the eye. It seemed to begin in an issue of *GQ* magazine which more or less accused Williams of stealing material. According to *GQ*, 'his [Williams'] reputation for taking jokes and quickly making them his own is unequalled'. These were serious charges, and Williams' friends sprang quickly to his defence. Whoopi Goldberg, for example, claimed that Williams was not doing anything different from any other comedian: 'They made it sound as if Robin were taking their [other comics'] livelihoods away,' she said. 'Comics do this all the time. Someone says a great line and it stays with you and you use it. We had "Make my day". Everybody was using it. Is that theft?'

Daniel Holzman of the Raspyni Brothers agrees with Goldberg, but suggests that it is Williams' own skill which is at the heart of the criticism: 'The bigger your library, the more chance there is of some comics thinking that your library and their library are kind of intersecting,' he explains.

'It's hard because you have to have so much material in your head that you're not sure whether you said it first or whether someone else said it first.'

The allegations eventually became a joke in themselves. Comics would point out that Lindy's famous diner in Times Square in New York, which has sandwiches named after famous comedians, has introduced a 'Robin Williams'. It's just two slices of bread – you have to steal the meat. Joking or not, Williams certainly took the allegations seriously and they began to affect him. He began to wonder whether he had in fact stolen material, and endured long bouts of self-doubt about just how original he was. Was this really all him, or was his undoubted mimetic ability simply soaking up other people's material and reprocessing it as his own? For a while Williams admits he even believed it. On his own admission, when you spend up to eight hours a day listening to comedy, some of it is bound to rub off. In Williams' case it was the nature of his celebrity which got him into difficulty.

'I hung out in clubs eight hours a night, improvising with people, playing with them, doing routines,' he explains. 'And I heard some lines once in a while and I used some lines on talk shows accidentally. That's what got me this reputation.'

Williams was simply doing what every other observational comedian was doing. His life and his surroundings, and that includes lines from other comedians, were informing his art. However, where another comic could use material he had heard elsewhere in front of an audience of a few hundred and no one would be the wiser, when Williams appeared on Johnny Carson or David Letterman he was repeating lines in front of audiences numbering millions. As a mark of common decency, Williams was genuinely and sincerely apologetic whenever he discovered he had used someone else's material inadvertently. So apologetic, in fact, that he would willingly pay them for the line. But even this had to stop.

'I started getting tired of just paying, of being the chump,' he says. 'I said, "Hey, wait a minute. It's not true." People were accusing me of stealing stuff that was basically from my own life. And then I went, "Wait, this is nuts. I didn't take that. That's about my mother." '

Williams admits that one of his most famously quoted lines, about cocaine, is not original. 'A drunken guy came up to me on the street years ago,' he recalls, 'and he said, "Robin, here's something for you. Cocaine is God's way of saying you're making too much fucking money." A lot of times people come up and tell you this stuff. And you have to be careful. Did they hear this somewhere else?'

The most absurd point in the whole situation came at a time when

Williams was accused of stealing material from a comedian he hadn't seen perform in two years. At the time Williams said this would be genuinely worth *National Enquirer*'s interest in him as the world's first psychic thief. Eventually Williams realised that he was as much sinned against as sinning. People were shamelessly lifting his material and he was supposed to be flattered, but if he used a line from someone else then it was comic larceny. After a time he came to terms with it, but it has left him more cautious. Those late-night sets which he so much used to enjoy performing would now be done a little differently. He would build precautions into his approach.

> I don't want to take anyone else's time [he explains]. I got tired of other comics giving me looks like, 'What the fuck are you doing here?' ... It's just hard to find the clubs right now because they are so jammed. You don't want to bump anybody. If I go on any place it's usually in the middle of the week, late at night, unannounced. When no one else is there, so no one can say 'You took my line'.

While this comic storm in a teacup was raging around him, Robin Williams was getting on with his film career. After taking some much-needed time off to get married and get adjusted to his new family, he was eager to get back into the fray. He had shown in *Good Morning Vietnam* that he could do screen comedy and in *Dead Poets Society* that he could do straight drama. For his next project he was going to mix them in a drama which bordered on black farce. In *Cadillac Man*, Williams was once again teamed up with an Australian director, as he had been in *Dead Poets*. The film was directed by Roger Donaldson, who was rapidly acquiring a solid commercial reputation after his successes with *No Way Out* and *Cocktail*. *Cadillac Man* must have been an appealing project on paper for Williams, who could reasonably have expected to provide another showcase for his full dramatic and comedic range.

Williams plays Joey O'Brien, a used-car salesman who is almost at the end of his rope. Life in Queens is one long hustle for Joey as he desperately attempts to keep his life together. He is under pressure from his ex-wife for more money, his teenage daughter is running wild, he has two mistresses whose names he can't remember, and he owes $20,000 to a local gangster. On top of all that, his boss is finally on to him and if he doesn't meet his quota of selling twenty cars in a single day then he is going to lose his job. This however is the least of his worries because gun-toting Tim Robbins has just ridden his motorcycle through the window of the car showroom. His wife, the showroom receptionist, is having an affair with one of the salesmen and he is going to hold everyone hostage until he finds out who it is. Ironically, in this instance, Joey is not the philanderer. But he pretends to be, in order to use his negotiating skills to the utmost to try to get everyone out alive.

Cadillac Man never quite lives up to the promise of its sales pitch, which was basically *Good Morning Vietnam* in a car showroom. Williams has one or two good moments. There is a gloriously sleazy opening in which he tries to peddle used cars to a stalled funeral cortège – the funeral director could certainly use a new hearse, and while he's at it perhaps the widow might like a luxury car as a tribute to the dear departed? Williams also excels in another delightfully frantic moment when he tries to juggle four customers at once as his time runs out to hit his quota. But for all Williams' skill, the material was just too thin to stretch him. Tim Robbins, however, who underplays gloriously while Williams tries to spin metaphorical plates, steals the film from under him.

Cadillac Man failed to strike a chord with the movie-going public. It's debatable whether it was a summer movie, and certainly in the summer of 1990 it got lost in the shuffle and was swamped by predictable hits such as *Die Hard 2, Total Recall* and *Dick Tracy.* Hopes that it might emerge as the sleeper hit of the summer were dashed when the previously unheralded *Ghost* proved to be a runaway success, breaking the $100 million barrier and leaving *Cadillac Man* to gather an unspectacular $27 million. But whatever disappointments Williams had over *Cadillac Man*, they would be short-lived. He was now about to embark on one of the most spectacularly successful periods of his career.

Dr Oliver Sacks is a neurological genius and acclaimed author of best-selling books such as *The Man Who Mistook His Wife for a Hat.* In the late Sixties he was responsible for ground-breaking work on a group of patients at the Beth Abraham Hospital in the Bronx in New York. These patients were survivors of the epidemic of sleeping sickness, encaphilitis lethargica, which had swept America after the First World War. Between 1916 and 1927 the disease struck down 5 million people. More than 1.5 million people died; others were attacked by a form of Parkinsonism which left them frozen, often in grotesque positions. It was some of these patients, who had effectively been locked away from public view, that inspired Dr Sacks to try to revive them after he had arrived at the hospital in 1966. By using trial and error with doses of a new wonder drug L-DOPA, Sacks was able to restore them to useful and constructive life. The drug, however, was not always successful and one of Sacks' greatest triumphs and disasters was Leonard L, a young man who awoke from his vegetative state to enjoy the world around him, only to lapse back after a relatively short time. The story of Sacks and his patients had already been told before in a British television documentary, as well as a Harold Pinter play called *A Kind of Alaska*. There had been some interest from Hollywood in a film, but Sacks had always resisted.

> I got approached by Hollywood in 1979 and the two would-be producers Walter Parkes and Larry Lasker came to the hospital in 1980 [explains Sacks]. Leonard L was alive then, a lot of the patients were alive. We talked about things and I was surprised by their interest. I was excited. I was intrigued. I was piqued. I was challenged. I was frightened. I was conflicted. I think one has to be. I didn't know how things would come out. I was very frightened of some exploitative film, but they seemed very good people who had an essential feeling of respect for the patients and the phenomena. I think that feeling of respect seemed to me a guarantee that if a film were made it would be a decent one. Then years passed and I didn't think a film would ever be made, not much happened until 1987 when a script suddenly arrived.

Despite the best efforts of Parkes and Lasker the script was gathering no interest whatsoever at Fox until it was found by director Penny Marshall. After her phenomenal success with *Big*, Marshall could have her pick of projects. Once she found the Oliver Sacks script she took it to Columbia who acquired it on her behalf and started to develop it. *Awakenings*, as the script was now called, concentrated on the relationship between Oliver Sacks and Leonard L. Marshall was hugely enthusiastic about the project and she very quickly brought it to the attention of Robert De Niro. The two had almost worked together in *Big* and, although she was keen for him to play the doctor, De Niro was equally keen to play the role of Leonard L. While she was casting around, Marshall went to see *Dead Poets Society* and was hugely impressed with Robin Williams' performance. She recommended it to De Niro, who agreed with her, and Williams was duly sent a script.

> I happened to read it on a plane [Williams recalls], and I was quite moved – to the point where a stewardess thought there was something wrong with me. It decimated me . . . It's weird because when you first read it you think, 'How will this play?' Because it's basically internal; a man going through all these realisations and putting together a medical puzzle. And then after that to read Oliver's book and go, 'My God, it's all true.' It reads like Greek drama. It's something like Sisyphus. To rise and then fall, the human struggle of it all.

Williams immersed himself in the study of Oliver Sacks. He spent time with him, he spent time with his patients, he absorbed everything there was to know about him. This concerned Penny Marshall, who was worried that Williams was actually impersonating Oliver Sacks rather than playing a character. This was solved by a small but significant change; the character's name was altered to Dr Malcolm Sayer.

'It freed both him and me simultaneously, it relaxed a certain stand-off,' says Williams of the change. 'Oliver had been coming to the set all the time to help us, and for him it was like walking into a three-dimensional mirror.'

Sacks, for his part, found the whole experience of becoming a character in a film about his own life as amusing as it was bemusing.

> The portrayer portrayed, the discloser disclosed [he smiles ironically]. I had it coming to me. I objected violently when I saw that I was a character in the script. 'I'm not a character,' I said. 'I'm the author, get me out of here.' They said, 'No, you have to be a character.'
>
> I was very closely involved in the patients' lives and they were part of my life, I still feel very strongly for them. I still have their charts out, I never put their charts away. On the other hand I didn't entirely like the idea of 'the doctor's story', which they wanted to do and to have a sort of symmetry. But I suppose there was something in it and I do recognise some resemblance between the shy, bumbling, awkward, diffident, but sort of quite tenacious and tough-minded young Dr Sayer and myself of thirty years ago.
>
> The phrase I used to describe Robin was 'a younger identical twin'. That was very uncanny. I didn't really feel as though I was being observed by him. We did things together and went around together, but he not only picked up my gestures and mannerisms such as they are – one isn't conscious of them, only other people have gestures and mannerisms. I've had to give most of them up because people feel I'm imitating Robin. But, more, he would sort of pick up opinions, interests, aspirations, really a whole identity. It was really extraordinary, I've never had an experience like this – a sort of mimesis, a sort of genius. Then there was more distance and he developed the character differently.

Sacks, a great bear of a man, was also amused by Williams' description of him as 'part Schweitzer – part Schwarzenegger'. But the two men formed a close and abiding friendship during that four-month shoot in often difficult conditions in New York. They remain friends still and frequently correspond or get together when their schedules allow. Science is one of Williams' great enthusiasms and he admits to being in awe of men like

Oliver Sacks. He has a passion for Einstein in particular, and one of his proudest possessions is Einstein's autograph. For Williams there are clear parallels between great science and great comedy.

> I love the idea that most of them will admit their major discoveries are accidents [says Williams of the scientists he admires]. They find out that something will trigger that one random association that allows the rest of the discovery. That, to me, is astonishing. It's the ultimate improvisation. When they find that thing, you see, the majority of them will say it was an accident or they had a dream. If you think of Einstein they would say it's his wife, there is a theory that it was actually his first wife who came up with the theory of relativity. And they have that child-like quality. When you see these interviews their eyes light up and they look like kids because they are talking about that which they find the joy in and it's incredible. My favourite scientist to see and see lecture is Richard Feynman. Here's this brilliant man, but he makes science so accessible, it's wonderful.

For Williams the experience of working with long-time friend Robert De Niro was as exhilarating as working with Oliver Sacks. The two had almost worked together before in *Midnight Run*, but this time it had come off and Williams suspected he would have to be on the top of his game.

> It's like hang-gliding nude over the grand canyon [says Williams of working with De Niro]. It can be kind of frightening sometimes. That kind of thing when you go 'Oh my God, it's him' ... But after a couple of weeks I finally went 'Oh stop – don't carry that whole thing'. You've got to work with the man, not the myth ... There's a wonderful thing in this movie that I don't think I've seen him do before – a kind of innocence. A shyness that people don't expect, and then he smiles and he's got this wonderful warmth, because normally he's playing very scary guys.

Warmth or not, there were still persistent reports from the set of *Awakenings* that Williams had lost his temper and broken De Niro's nose. Both actors, and director Penny Marshall, were keen to play down any talk of ill-feeling. The official version is that the two men were rehearsing a scene and Williams' elbow flew up and hit De Niro on the nose. The blow was such that the noise of De Niro's nose breaking was apparently picked up by the sound recordist on the soundtrack. De Niro, ever the trouper, did nine more takes with an increasingly stunned Williams before he decided to let wiser counsel prevail and went to a nearby hospital to have it checked. Ironically, De Niro says Williams actually did him a favour.

He had broken his nose some years ago, and he claims Williams' blow straightened it out again.

There's no doubt that, given his bulk and his weight and his athletic prowess, Williams probably could break a man's nose should he so desire. But it seems much too far out of character to have been deliberate. In fact, according to Penny Marshall, De Niro laughed so long and hard at Williams' pre-take routines that she was worried that he would look far too healthy for his scenes as the pallid Leonard.

'It was in various press accounts that I got angry and broke his nose,' Williams acknowledges. 'If that was true I don't think I'd be here saying "Let's talk". At least not with my own teeth.'

26

A Chink in the Armour

Awakenings was a solid commercial success for Robin Williams. It took just over $52 million domestically and more than made up for the box-office disappointment of *Cadillac Man.* Having won back-to-back Oscar nominations with *Good Morning Vietnam* and *Dead Poets Society* he could count himself unlucky not to have made it three out of four nominations with *Awakenings.* But for a quirk of billing he might yet have been wondering whether he should be preparing an acceptance speech for Oscar night. Although Williams has the larger role as Dr Sayer, there is no doubt that De Niro's supporting role as Leonard is the showier. Perhaps also thanks to De Niro's greater clout, he was the one who was first-billed and he was the one who ended up with the Academy Award nomination. In the end he would lose out to Jeremy Irons in *Reversal of Fortune,* and *Awakenings* itself would lose out to *Dances With Wolves* in the Best Picture race.

In any event by the time the 1991 Academy Awards were being played out in Los Angeles, Williams was hard at work on another film. He had worked for director Terry Gilliam some years before in Gilliam's magnificent folly *The Adventures of Baron Munchausen.* Although he is American born, Gilliam had spent a large part of his working life in Britain as a ground-breaking animator and founder-member of the Monty Python team. *Munchausen* was a distillation of all of his comic fantasies, but it proved so ruinously expensive that hardly anyone saw his delirious vision of the classic folk tales. Williams was roped in for an unbilled cameo in the 1988 movie as the disembodied head of the King of the Moon. Three years later Gilliam was back behind the camera for the first time since *Munchausen* with *The Fisher King*. There was no doubt in his mind that, once again, he wanted to work with Williams.

'The thing with Robin is, he has the ability to go from manic to mad to tender and vulnerable,' says Gilliam. 'He's the most unique mind on the planet. There's nobody like him out there.'

Gilliam's assessment of Williams may be exaggerated, but in terms of *The Fisher King* it is entirely accurate. It is debatable whether any other actor could have tackled the incredibly difficult role of Parry. The film is essentially a story of redemption. Jeff Bridges is a New York shock jock whose cavalier on-air manner is the fuse which ignites a gunman's murderous rampage in a quiet restaurant. The ensuing controversy ruins Bridges' career, and we find him all but down and out on the streets of New York. He is about to be set on fire by a street gang when he is rescued by a rag-tag man dressed in what approximates to a junkyard's version of a suit of armour. This is Parry, a former professor of medieval history. His wife was killed in the restaurant shooting and he has subsequently become unhinged by the tragedy. Feeling grateful and at the same time responsible, Bridges buys into Parry's quest for the Holy Grail in a final resolution which leaves both men changed and renewed by their adventure together.

For Williams it would be one of the most challenging roles of his career to date as well as one which he admitted he was only just beginning to feel sufficiently confident to tackle. In one location interview he conceded that ten years previously he would never have even come close to nailing Parry's character. Whatever characterisation he might have attempted then would have been largely comedic and taken the film in an entirely different direction. But for Williams *The Fisher King* was an important film to do; it was a film which spoke to him as an actor but also as an activist.

'*Fisher King* I did,' he recalls, 'because it's about bottom-line compassion, about redemption, about not taking people on initial value but looking deeper. It's about dependency and strange relationships that come and go.'

Williams was also enthusiastic about the film because the tragic circumstances in which Parry finds himself through no fault of his own are exactly the conditions which encouraged Williams to help set up Comic Relief.

'Laughing is better than a diatribe,' he explains. 'With comedy you can pull people in and say "Look at some of the things in the fun house mirror, but (really) look at them." That's what *The Fisher King* does –

starts out oh-wow funny and strange, but behind all that is a horrible vision Parry cannot deal with.'

The demands placed on him by Gilliam were considerable. As well as reacting to Bridges and other members of the cast such as Mercedes Ruehl and Amanda Plummer, Williams also had to convey Parry's own private madness. This was the vision he referred to as Parry is pursued by a knight in blood-red armour mounted upon a fearsome charger which is more monster than horse. 'Terry shoots stuff that has a half-life,' says Williams. 'You walk out and then it hits you ... Red knights. Sixty-foot samurais. Icarus. Simple things. He creates images that are shot into your skull.'

Although Gilliam and Williams had formed something of a mutual admiration society, there were some people connected with *The Fisher King* who were less certain. Jeff Bridges, for example, was not sure that Williams would be able to do anything other than go for the laugh. In the end he was delighted to find that Williams could not only handle the serious side of playing Parry but also keep the company in stitches during the lengthy down time in a long and tedious shoot. Screenwriter Richard LaGravenese was similarly surprised by the depth of emotion which Williams put into his pain-wracked performance.

Williams, however, had been working hard at his craft and was working hard at letting his defences down and simply being himself in front of the camera. It was a process, he claimed, which had been going on since *The World According to Garp*. 'For the first time I actually got comfortable even to be – and this sounds like a strange thing to say – to be myself. To be able to stop, relate, listen. To be interesting without doing all kinds of business ... It was [hard]. I'd built a whole thing and then I was asked to give it up, to work without the armour.'

For Terry Gilliam, *The Fisher King* was a difficult film. He was going into the movie with the reputation of an extravagant spendthrift, and if he wasn't exactly drinking in the last chance saloon he could certainly hear the tinkling of the victrola behind the bat-wing doors. It was also a hard movie to shoot, many of the sequences involved long night shoots and there was always the potential to go over-budget on a film where every dollar he spent would be scrutinised. But, in these difficult circumstances, Gilliam found Williams to be head and shoulders above almost any other actor he had worked with.

Robin sensed the weariness,' says Gilliam, recalling one particular night-time sequence, 'and suddenly went into a breathtaking 20-minute show. It was so specific. He knew every member of the crew. He knew their peculiarities, he had details and it was one of the great shows of our time. Afterwards everyone was just flying. We got back to work and zapped right through the evening. It was exactly what we needed.'

When *The Fisher King* was finished, Williams maintained what was becoming a prodigious work rate. He agreed to take one of two small cameo roles – the other was played by Andy Garcia – in *Dead Again*, a thriller from actor-director Kenneth Branagh. This, for the first time, gave him the chance to play a less than savoury character – a doctor who had been struck off for misconduct.

> It was a great experience [he said]. Sometimes when you come in and do a role where you are unbilled, or barely billed, you're not under the same pressure ... I just want to keep playing different characters to change the perception of just being 'the manic'. In *Dead Again* I played a slightly evil character. I think the job for me is to keep pushing the boundaries so I don't get labelled as one particular thing, that 'manic' thing. I'll save that for the performance, for the stand-up, when I'm in public.

While Williams was forging ahead in his professional life, matters were coming to a head in his private life. Tish Carter's lawsuit had been rumbling on for the better part of five years now and had recently been joined by his own countersuit. Williams' lawyer Phil Ryan had also filed a motion to dismiss Carter's suit, and it was this motion which was to be considered by the San Francisco Superior Court in September 1991. But Ryan was not finding things going quite the way he wanted. Instead of the summary dismissal he would doubtless have been expecting, Judge William Cahill further delayed his ruling. At a hearing on 10 September he decided that it could not be as simple as deciding which of the parties was in the wrong. Judge Cahill decided that first of all he would have to make up his mind on whether Williams actually had any legal duty to warn Carter that he was suffering from a sexually transmitted disease. Both sides were given a further five days to present their opinions on this issue and Judge Cahill tentatively set a trial date of 13 January 1992.

Judge Cahill's apparently simple ruling had now raised the stakes immeasurably in the Williams case. Instead of being a glorified ex-lovers' spat – albeit a high-profile one – the case was now beginning to take on a seriously precedential aspect.

It was now felt in some quarters that this had all the makings of a landmark case. If Judge Cahill ruled that Williams did indeed have a legal duty to inform Carter of any sexual diseases he may or may not have had, then the consequences could be awesome. In theory such a ruling would mean that anyone who failed to tell a partner of a potentially sexually transmitted disease could then be held liable if the partner then contracted an illness. Carter did eventually concede in pre-trial motions that she had never asked Williams whether he had any sexually transmitted disease, but with the wheels of justice grinding inexorably on, this was of little consequence.

The Williams legal team redoubled their efforts to have the case thrown out but there was more bad news when Judge Cahill finally delivered his ruling on 8 November 1991. The judge had decided that there were no grounds on which to dismiss the case. In a four-page written judgement he argued that only a trial would be able to ascertain whether Carter had asked Williams whether he had herpes, and whether Williams was obliged to warn her of any disease he might have had. The trial date remained set for 13 January, but Ryan was now promising to take Judge Cahill's ruling to the Court of Appeal.

Both sets of lawyers were adamant now that there would be no compromise. A settlement conference had been pencilled in for early December but no one was even remotely optimistic of any settlement being reached. Adolph Canelo, who was acting for Carter, said they had gone through settlement negotiations before which had amounted to nothing, and he saw no reason why this should be any different. Ryan for his part continued to insist that there would be no settlement because his client was not going to be extorted.

By going to the Court of Appeal, Phil Ryan succeeded only in dragging out the litigation further. The original trial date of 13 January 1992 came and went, and a few weeks later – on 21 February – the state Supreme Court finally handed down its ruling in which it refused to block the trial. Only one of the Supreme Court judges felt that Judge Cahill's ruling required to be reviewed. This meant that, the original ruling standing, a trial could now go ahead in late summer.

The trial in fact was due to take place in San Francisco Superior Court in the first week of August 1992. But, just six days before the case was due to go before the judge and jury, there was a surprising resolution. Williams quietly, and without fuss, settled out of court. In addition to the settlement, Williams and Carter also reached a confidential agreement in his countersuit that she had tried to extort money and a car from him. Williams, who is subject to a gagging order, has made no direct comment on the case since. Whether he settled because her case had merit or because he simply had become tired of it and wanted to make it go away, no one but he, and his legal team, will know.

Even after the settlement his lawyers were still referring to the suit as 'nothing but extortion'. And one of Williams' legal team gave the *New*

York Daily News a blunt but succinct explanation for why the case had been settled. 'At the last minute he got cold feet,' said the unnamed lawyer. 'He didn't want his reputation sullied by a money-grabbing attention seeker.'

27

Think Happy Thoughts

Los Angeles is one of the world's greatest tourist destinations for movie fans. Every year millions of them flock to Hollywood to visit theme parks such as Disneyland, or Universal Studios, or to stroll down the Walk of Fame on Hollywood Boulevard or simply to fit their own hands and feet into the cement imprints enshrined in the forecourt of the Chinese Theater. But in the summer of 1991, the biggest movie attraction in Hollywood was also the most exclusive. Nine stages at Columbia Studios at Culver City had been taken over by Steven Spielberg for his new film *Hook.* The film was a modernistic retelling of J. M. Barrie's *Peter Pan*, and Spielberg had spent $8 million on recreating Neverland here on what was once the old MGM back lot. Stage 30 – once the domain of Esther Williams – and stage 27 – where *The Bounty* once sailed – had been taken over by the giant tangle of tree houses which was home to the Lost Boys. Stage 15 was taken over by Pirate Town, complete with saloons and bawdy houses. But dominating all of this was *The Jolly Roger*, the 70-foot pirate galleon which was the flagship of Captain Hook.

Although it was in theory the most exclusive attraction in town, it may not have seemed so in practice. Day in and day out there was a constant stream of VIP visitors, often with their children, to look at the marvels Spielberg was creating. The list included Demi Moore, Tom Cruise, Whoopi Goldberg, Warren Beatty – who was filming *Bugsy* next door – Michelle Pfeiffer, Bruce Willis, Mel Gibson, Prince – before he became The Artist Formerly Known As Prince – and real royalty in the shape of Queen Noor of Jordan. As budgets spiralled and schedules lengthened,

Spielberg continued to receive his visitors with good grace, but no one was really surprised when he decided that his next film, *Jurassic Park*, would be shot on a closed set.

Hook is the story of Peter Pan as an adult. He has grown up and left Neverland and the Lost Boys and become a corporate lawyer going by the name of Peter Banning. Meanwhile his old nemesis Captain Hook has grown bored and tired of having no one to fight, so he comes to London to steal Peter Pan's children. Peter has become materialistic and inattentive, especially to his son. Hook attempts to seduce the boy away by becoming the father he has never had. Peter follows Hook to Neverland, but it is only by embracing his true heritage that he can hope to win the day and save his children.

The original idea came from the son of screenwriter Jim Hart who, while out in the family car one day, asked what if Peter Pan had grown up. Hart was intrigued by the idea and began to develop it, and in August 1990 TriStar Pictures announced plans for *Hook*, as Hart's script became known. Steven Spielberg, who had long wanted to make a live-action Peter Pan film, possibly with Michael Jackson, would direct. Dustin Hoffman would take the title role and Robin Williams would play Peter. *Hook*, which was due to start shooting in January 1991, was one of two projects that Williams had agreed to do as he was completing filming on *The Fisher King*; the other was *Toys*, with Barry Levinson, which he would begin once he had fulfilled his commitment to Spielberg.

Within weeks of the original announcement, TriStar revealed that it was putting not one, but two, Peter Pan movies into production. Hollywood had already seen the duelling Robin Hood movies of the previous summer, but they at least were from separate studios. It was unheard of for the same studio to set up rival projects. The idea was hatched by TriStar's mercurial boss Peter Guber. Although they had green-lit *Hook*, TriStar had also been developing a new version of *Peter Pan* itself. The rights to the Barrie classic were owned by Dodi Fayed, who was a near neighbour of Guber's in Malibu. One morning Guber turned up at Fayed's house and announced that he had acquired 'the sequel to *Peter Pan*'. From there it was a short step to an article which appeared in *Variety* on 6 September to the effect that *Peter Pan* and *Hook* would film back to back, a technique which had brought success with the second and third instalments of the *Back to the Future* trilogy. While *Hook* would have Williams and Hoffman and be directed by Spielberg and written by Jim Hart, *Peter Pan* would star two unknowns as Peter and Wendy, with Joe Dante directing from a Lasse Halstrom script. Fayed would produce *Peter Pan* and executive produce *Hook*. Although the idea of filming back to back seemed attractive it was wildly impractical given the relative stages of pre-production on both pictures. While Fayed continued to prepare *Peter Pan*, Spielberg got ready to start shooting *Hook*.

Spielberg was delighted when Williams accepted the role of Peter Banning. He felt that the actor embodied all of the hidden, and not so hidden, child-like qualities which were necessary to be convincing. Williams was keen to do the film and to work with Spielberg, but he was less certain of being able to get a handle on the character.

> I really had to convince myself that I could play this [he remembers] . . . It took a lot of hard work to get this really anal tone, to find one that is kind of lost but still believable as a man-boy – as a guy who suffers from a Peter Pan complex because he is, in reality, Peter Pan . . . And finding that tone to make it boyish, lost, yet still a guy who makes a living basically screwing people as quickly as he can . . . Steven has been amazing. At first you think here's a guy who basically deals in visuals. But no, he knows every movie that's ever been made. He's seen every movie twice. So he knows if someone did something before. And from that, he can give you an idea that goes beyond that.

Not long after filming started the pressure began to build. Playwright Tom Stoppard was brought on to do rewrites. Massive toy deals were done with Mattel, which increased pressure for the film to be in the cinemas for Christmas. More importantly, the film began to get more and more expensive. It was originally budgeted at $40 million, but as the real nature of the special effects needed to make Peter fly and the physical effects for the rest of the scenes became apparent, it was obvious that this figure would have to be taken with a liberal sprinkling of fairy dust. The budget quickly climbed to $50 million, then $60 million. Some sources put the final cost at $80 million, but the generally accepted figure seems to be closer to $60 million. Even so it was still one of the most expensive pictures ever made, despite the fact that Spielberg and his three principals – Julia Roberts had come on board as Tinkerbell – had deferred their salaries. They hadn't received a penny in wages for the film, choosing instead to take their fee in profit participation. But since this was 'first dollar' participation, it meant that TriStar could be committing up to 40 per cent of the film's gross receipts, making it harder still for the studio to turn a profit.

These problems may have confirmed some of the initial misgivings which Marsha Williams had about her husband taking part in *Hook*. Robin Williams and Marsha are very much a team, and although the final decision is his, the decision will not be taken without considerable input from her. In this case she had misgivings, both about the sheer scale and cost of the film, and the fact that they were essentially tampering with an icon. The fact that her husband stood to pick up the biggest pay-cheque of his life was neither here nor there.

'Money's never been the reason for me to recommend anything,' says Marsha Williams. 'Unless the entire country collapses we have as much as we'll ever need. I'm more interested in looking at what Robin hasn't done and seeing what's next. I'm prejudiced, but I've never seen anyone with his range.'

Hook ran into more production problems when Julia Roberts jilted her fiancé Kiefer Sutherland almost at the altar the week before she was due to start filming on *Hook*. At the same time she was beginning a relationship with the actor Jason Patric, and the two of them sought solace in Ireland as a respite from the packs of reporters and photographers who were following them. All of this put her participation in *Hook* in doubt, especially when she took off for Ireland. Although Spielberg now insists that there was never any real difficulty, there were growing suggestions at the time that he had threatened to replace her unless she turned up by an appointed date.

In the midst of all of this Williams and Hoffman were doing their best to keep things light on an increasingly difficult shoot. Having built a career on three films on which Hoffman had passed, Williams was delighted to finally be working with him. The two men enjoyed a fairly relaxed working relationship. Williams' prodigious mimetic skills meant he could do a spot-on impression of one of the parrots which was used to decorate Hook's galleon. Generally he would wait till things got slow and Hoffman was in the middle of a long speech before emitting a dead-on 'parrot' screech which brought proceedings to a halt. Hoffman would retaliate by teasing Williams about merely being a television actor. But together they conspired to keep the mood light. Williams, who had lost 20 pounds since *The Fisher King*, was often the target of his own humour as he pranced around in his green tights. And, just as he did in *The Fisher King*, he would entertain the cast and crew, especially the large numbers of child actors, with impromptu comedy spots between takes.

Still the film continued to run beyond its schedule. Studio bosses at TriStar were beginning to get nervous. The film was due to stop shooting at the end of July, but Spielberg told them he would need to shoot until at least the middle of August. This caused more pressure, because Hoffman was required to do re-shoots for Disney on his gangster movie *Billy Bathgate*. If filming on *Hook* went much past the end of August, then

Hoffman might not be available. The TriStar executives' anxiety was compounded by the fact that they still had not seen much evidence of what they were getting for their money. Spielberg had a clause in his contract which said they could not see daily rushes or assembled footage until he was ready. He did, however, reassure them that he was no stranger to this kind of pressure since he became used to tight deadlines on all three *Indiana Jones* pictures.

Williams' reaction to the pressure was similar to that of the rest of the cast. He chose to ignore it. 'I don't even ask,' he said in reply to a question about the rising cost of the film. 'I don't want to know. I just don't want that pressure. You can't go around worrying about the cost of the movie. No one took any money up front. We said, "Okay, we'll take it in the back end. We don't want to add any more to this".'

Williams clearly felt that he and Spielberg, Hoffman and Roberts had done their bit for the budget. Their only other responsibility was to make the best film they could. There are obvious parallels to be drawn between Williams' own childhood, in which he enjoyed a full and rich fantasy life, and Peter Pan himself. Peter Banning was the first of a number of man-child roles in which Williams would find himself locked over the next few years. But the notion of a lost childhood was reinforced not long before the film opened. On 25 November in San Francisco, Marsha Williams gave birth to their second child, a boy named Cody. As the film opened, it was inevitable that Williams' thoughts would turn to childhood and family.

> I believe childhood is a very precious time [he said], and I don't want to miss it with my children because I did miss it with my father. He was out working all the time and was always off round the country. So I didn't get a chance to see him very much and I miss that. I'm trying not to do the same thing with my children, and you have to balance it because it's a very precious thing. The line that sums it up in the movie is when Peter's wife says 'Don't miss it, because it's gone'. They only want to be with you up to a certain point, and they're basically looking at you going 'You're an asshole'. You have that time, maybe five or six years, when they want to know you and play with you and share with you. Then they start to grow away from you through biological necessity. I don't want to miss that with my children, but I did miss it as a child. My father loved me dearly, but I didn't spend time with him.

But Williams also conceded that, given what he does for a living, the magic of childhood may not last quite as long as in some other families.

> My son [Zach] is eight now [he said at the time], and he saw *Hook*. The first time I fly he turned to me and said, 'That's blue-screen. Right, Dad?' And I said 'Yeah'. So his sense of wonder is tempered by this heavy knowledge of all the technical stuff. But when my daughter saw it she just went 'Wow'. You get to experience that again, you get to see the world again through her, which is just wonderful.

TriStar chose an unconventional date to open *Hook*. It was released on Wednesday, 11 December, with special previews the previous evening. On the Tuesday night and the Wednesday the film took just over $2 million and the studios pronounced themselves thrilled. However, there were others who decided to reserve judgement until the opening weekend figures were in. By the following Monday, *Hook* had taken $14.2 million from its opening weekend and $17.7 million in its first six days. Although it was the clear box-office number one – taking almost twice as much as *Star Trek VI: The Undiscovered Country* in second place – the figures were still disappointing. There were some industry sources who called the film '*Hudson Hook*', a reference to the financially disastrous Bruce Willis film *Hudson Hawk*. That was overstating the case, but there is no doubt that the figures were not as high as TriStar had been expecting. One factor working against the film was its length – it ran for 144 minutes – which reduced the number of screenings cinemas could have in a day. Nonetheless the film was by no means a flop; the figures were solid if unspectacular. Ultimately TriStar had the last laugh after all. *Hook* turned out to have unexpected legs, and audiences defied the indifferent reviews to come out and see it. By the end of its run in the United States it had taken a respectable $119.7 million. It did even better in overseas markets, and when foreign grosses were taken into account the film took almost $300 million world-wide. It then went on to be a huge hit on video, selling millions of units and earning even more money.

By the time he had finished his chores on *Hook* both in terms of filming and his round of publicity interviews, Robin Williams simply wanted to go home to San Francisco. He had a new house and he wanted to spend time with his new family.

> This place is strange for me [he said of Los Angeles]. It's a fantasy life, just very surreal ... When you're in LA for more than a month, you bump into your career too much. You start reading the trades, looking for your name. You get paranoid about how you're doing. We're living in this rented house in Bel Air ... There's a gate, a little beeper, a guy that comes if you press the beeper. What is that? Is that the way it's supposed to be? No. But it's the

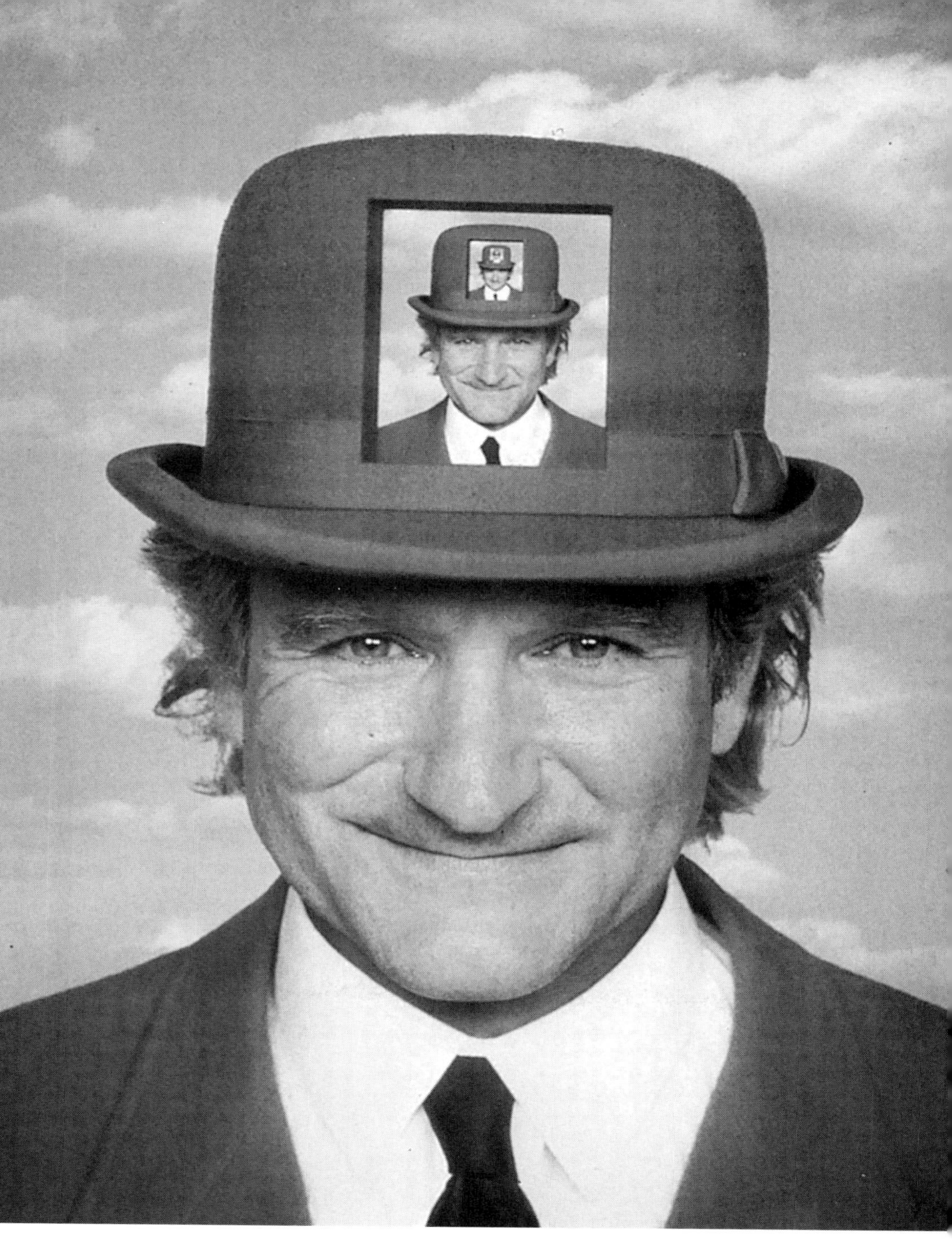

The surreal poster image for *Toys* (1992) evoked the work of surrealist artist René Magritte, but in the end the film was too much of an indulgence on behalf of Barry Levinson for a talented cast including Williams, Joan Cusack and Michael Gambon to save.

A family moment. Robin and Marsha with Zachary and Zelda in 1992. After Zelda was born, Williams promised if they had more children there would be 'no more Zs'. Their next child was Cody.

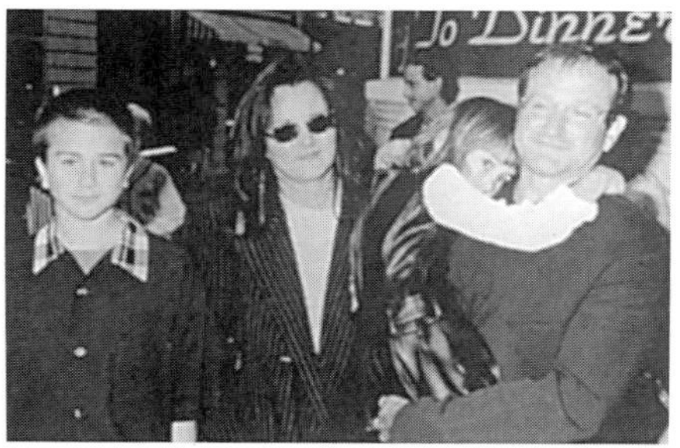

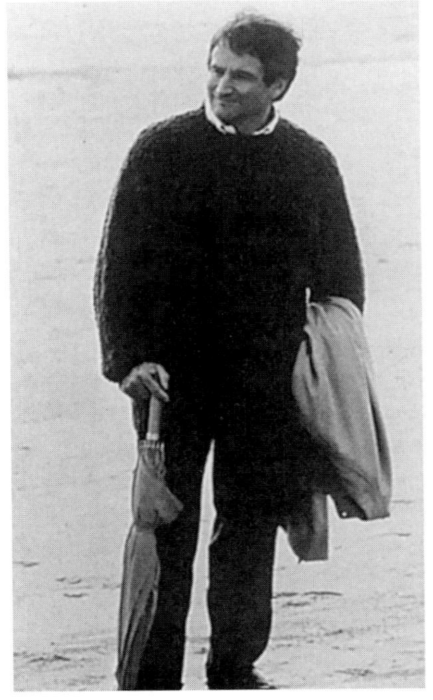

Robin Williams as the modern Hector, one of five characters he played in Bill Forsyth's rarely-seen *Being Human* (released 1994). Forsyth's Scottish accent gave Williams the inspiration for the voice of his next screen incarnation Iphagenia Doubtfire.

Robin Williams takes a breather on the front stoop of the Hillard household in *Mrs Doubtfire* (1993). Williams frequently went out into the street dressed in character just to see how people would react.

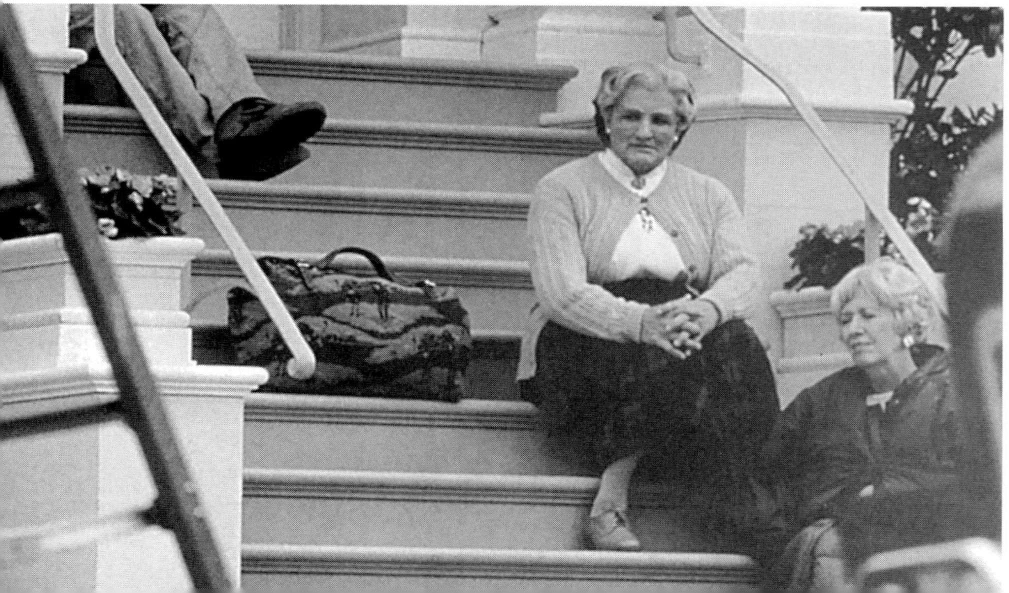

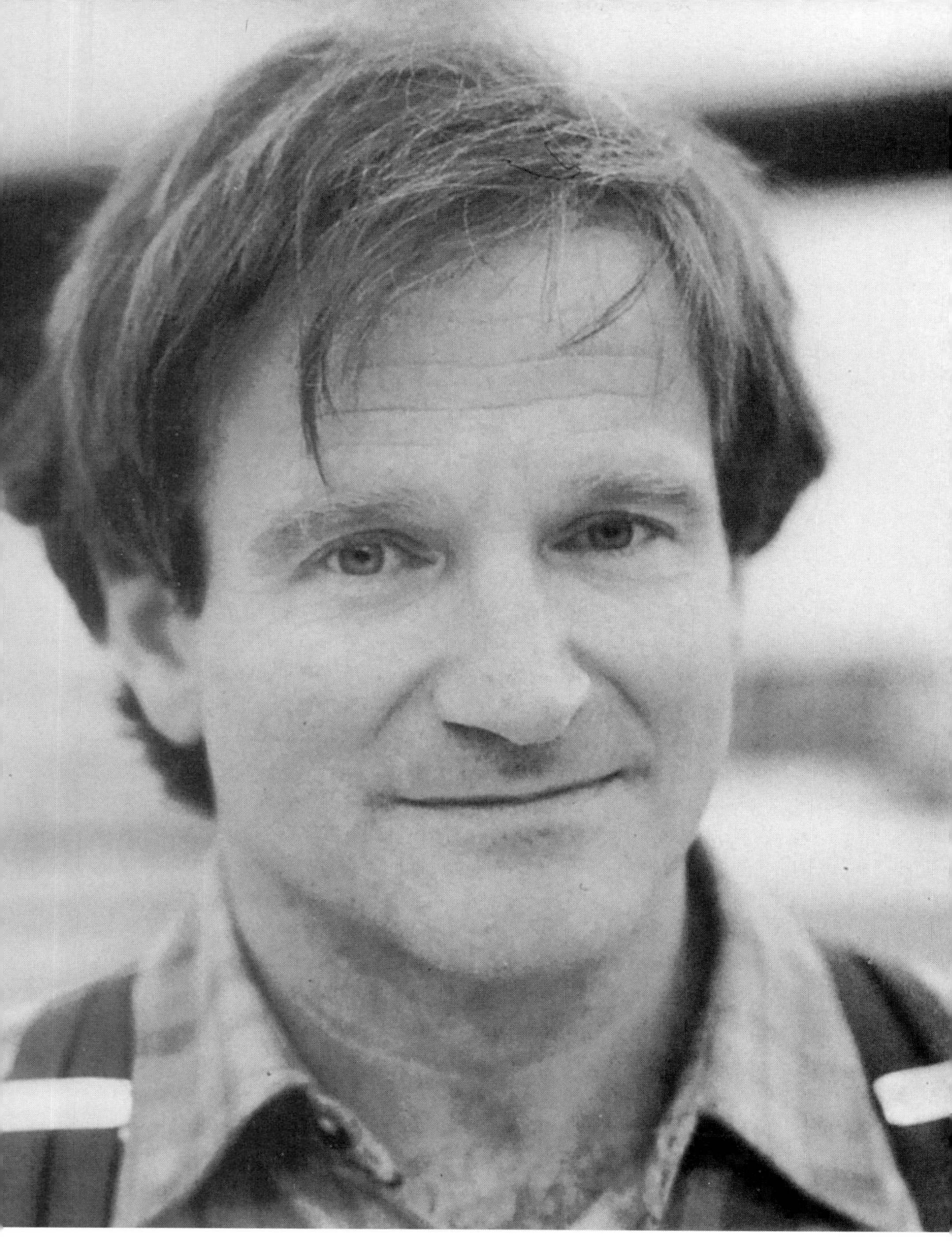

The last of his lost boy roles – or so he claimed. Robin Williams as the grown up Allan Parrish in *Jumanji* (1995).

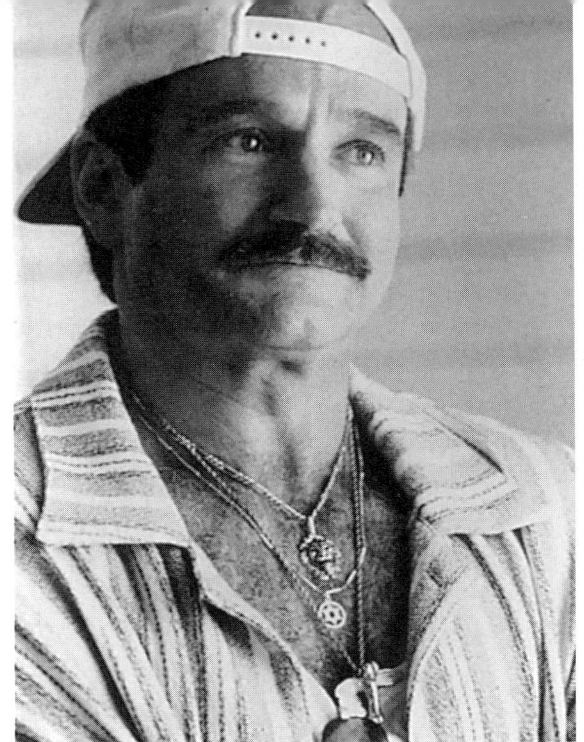

Robin Williams chose to play the straight role of Armand in the gay comedy *The Birdcage* (1996). He felt he had already done the drag stuff in *Mrs Doubtfire* and there were more possibilities with Armand. He was right.

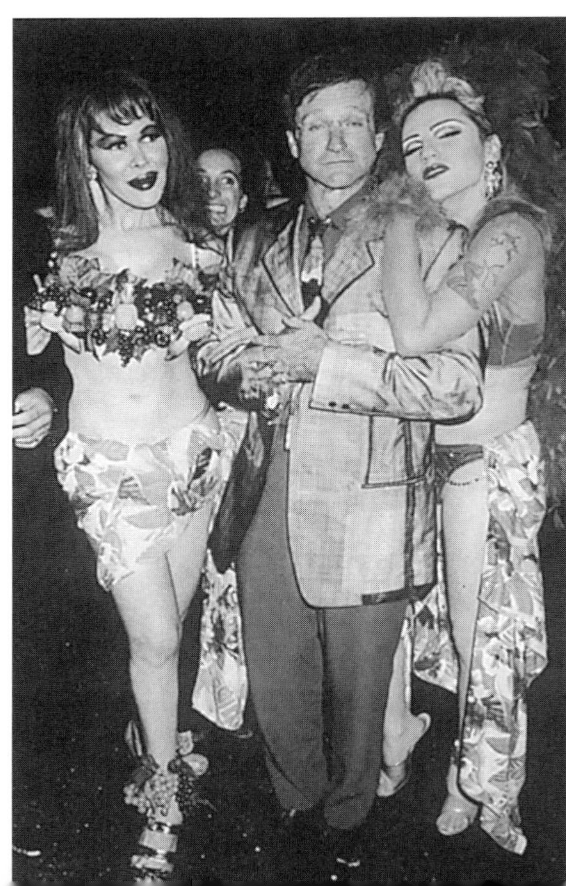

Robin Williams and two drag queens at the post-première party for *The Birdcage* (1996). Although he has often been criticized for his camp caricatures Williams has been a strong and vocal advocate on behalf of gay rights.

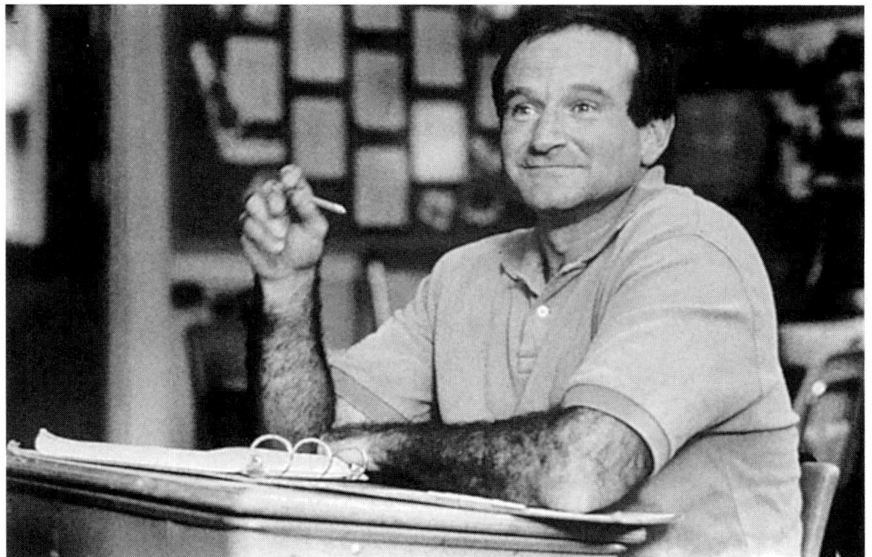

No really, this is the last of the man-child roles. Williams allowed his friend Francis Ford Coppola to talk him into doing *Jack* (1996) but the lukewarm response suggested that Williams' instincts were right. It was time to move on.

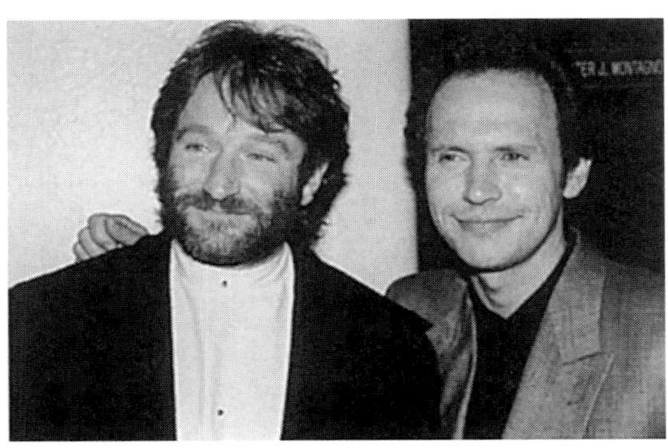

Robin Williams with his best friend Billy Crystal. Having not worked together on film before, they ended up doing three movies together – *Hamlet, Father's Day* and *Deconstructing Harry* – inside a year (1997).

Robin Williams, man of the people. Williams is mobbed at the video launch of *Aladdin and the King of Thieves* (July, 1996). He agreed to voice the genie again after settling his differences with Disney.

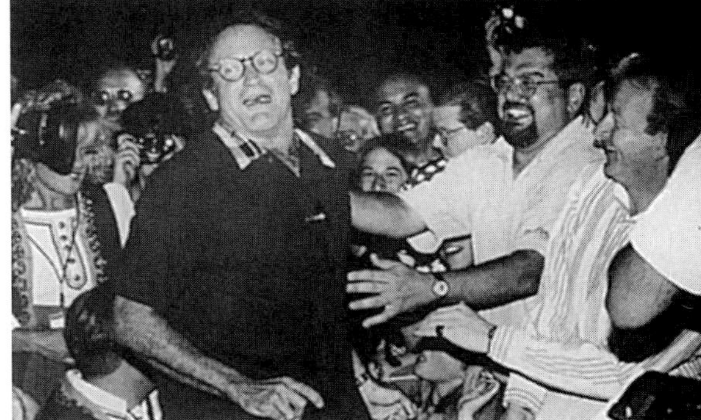

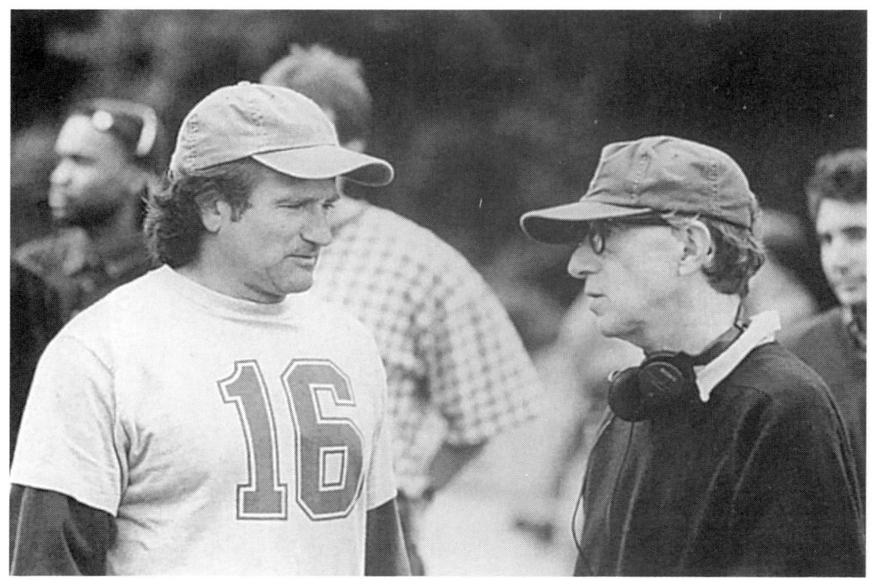

Two masters of their craft. Williams took a small role in *Deconstructing Harry* just so he could watch Woody Allen work.

Williams and Matt Damon on Boston Common in *Good Will Hunting* (1997). This emotional speech is one of the key scenes in the movie and went a long way to landing the Best Supporting Actor Oscar for Williams.

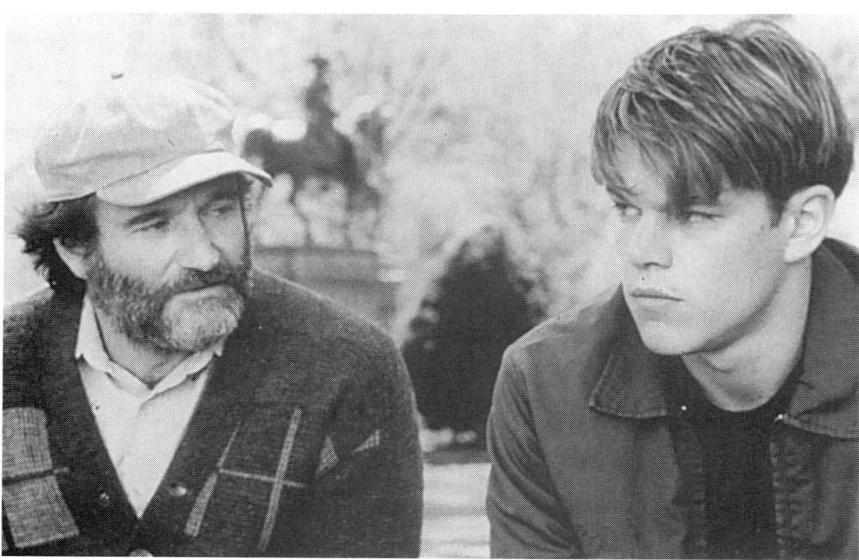

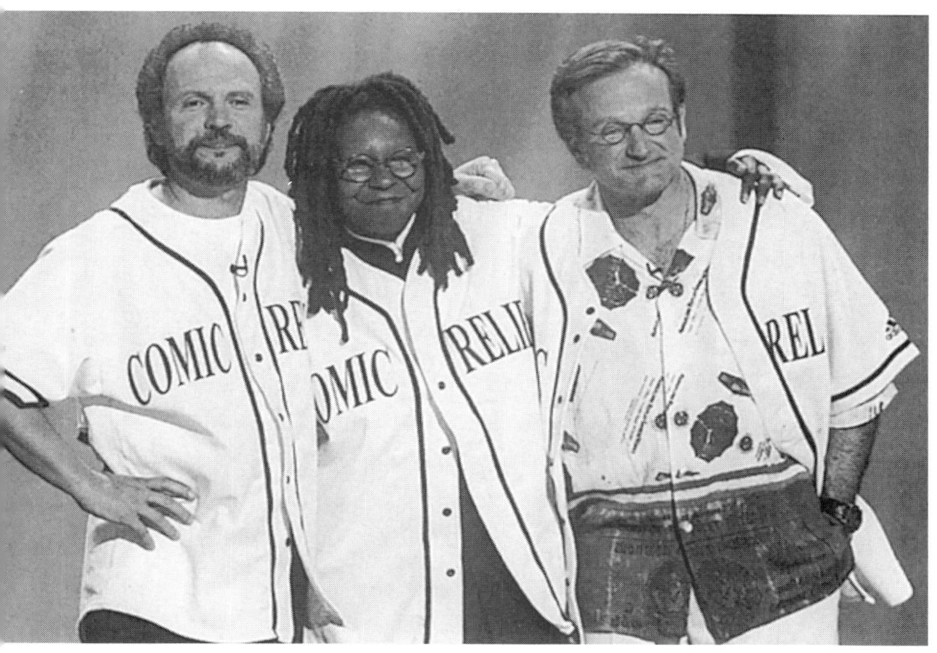

One for all and all for a good cause. Billy Crystal, Whoopi Goldberg and Robin Williams at *Comic Relief 1998.*

A nervous Robin Williams brought his wife Marsha and his mother Laurie to the 1998 Academy Award ceremony for some moral support.

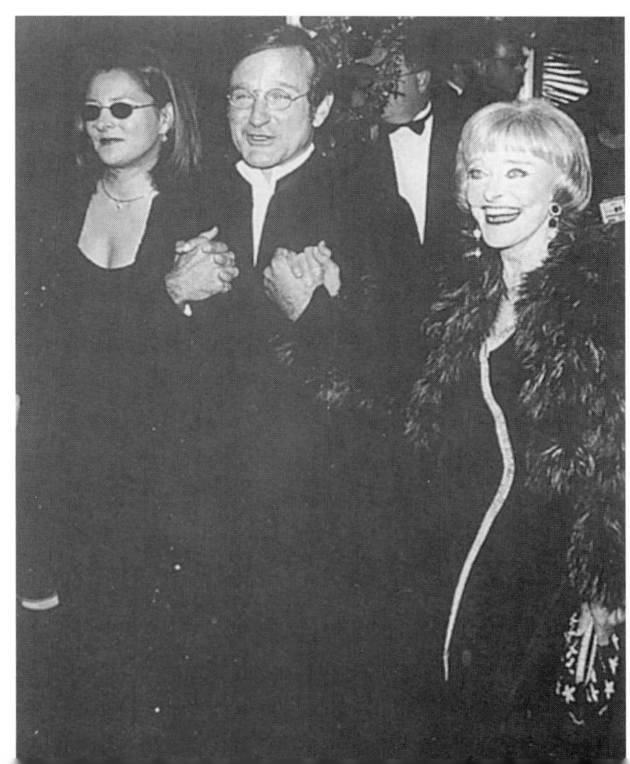

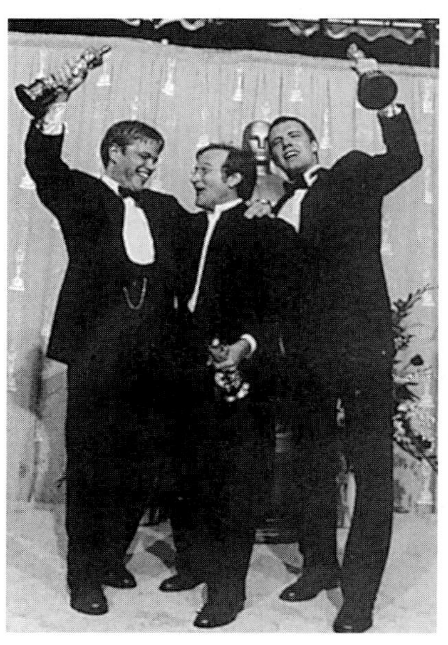

Williams and his fellow *Good Will Hunting* Oscar winners Matt Damon (left) and Ben Affleck celebrate backstage. Williams probably still wants to see some ID.

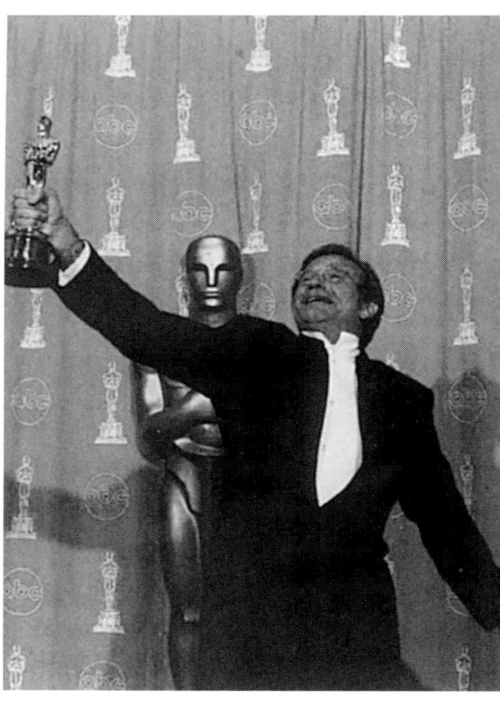

This one's for you Dad. Williams backstage at the Academy Awards when he dedicated his win for *Good Will Hunting* to his late father, Robert.

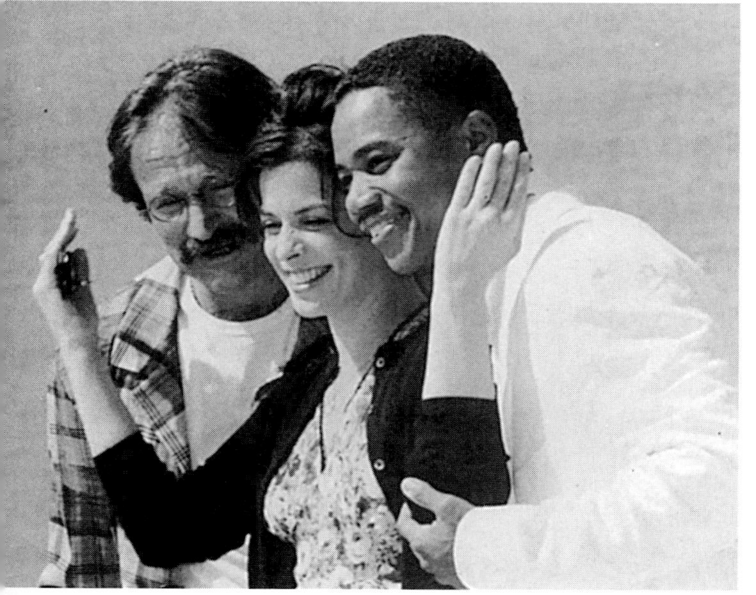

Williams with co-stars Cuba Gooding Jnr and Anabella Sciorra pose for the waiting photographers as they promote *What Dreams May Come* (1998) at Cannes.

reality of the place and that's why I don't live there. People do pretty horrible business things to each other and still try and hang socially there. I don't come down and hang out there. The house we just bought in San Francisco is at the mouth of the Bay, and you go from there through this beautiful park and up along the western beaches. It's incredible. It's nice to have distance between you and the world.

28

The Genius of the Lamp

When a man turns 40 it's time to take stock of his life. Robin Williams celebrated this particular landmark on 21 July 1991, while he was still filming *Hook*. As she had done with almost everything else in his life recently, Marsha took charge and arranged a surprise party for her husband at the ranch in Sonoma. She also organised a special birthday book. As early as March she had contacted all of the people who were important in Robin Williams' life and asked them to contribute to a book of memories. The book was duly presented to him at the party in front of a gathering which included major showbusiness names such as Steven Spielberg, Bette Midler, Billy Crystal, John Travolta, Bobcat Goldthwait, Kirstie Alley and Joan Baez, as well as people such as Adrian Cronauer, Dan Holzman and Barry Friedman who had also played their part in Williams' career.

As he looked back over his life at the age of 40, Williams must have been pleased with what he had accomplished. In personal terms the demons of drink and drugs had been defeated, he had a stable and happy relationship with a new wife, and, as he was heading into 1992, he had three children in whom he delighted. In career terms he was one of the top ten box-office draws in the country – his films had collectively grossed almost $600 million at the box-office – and he was able to command up to $8 million a picture; more importantly, he was able to move freely between serious roles and dramatic roles with relative ease and take his audience with him. He had also had two Best Actor nominations and was just about to pick up a third.

Of all the performances he had given since his renaissance in *Good Morning Vietnam*, the best was undoubtedly *The Fisher King*. Williams brought to Parry a touching pathos which made his madness all the more poignant and believable to the audience, without becoming maudlin. It is a performance which contains a large amount of sentiment without ever being sentimental. There was no real surprise when Williams was again nominated in the Best Actor category – his third in five years – when the Academy Award nominations were announced in February 1992. His fellow nominees were Warren Beatty for *Bugsy*, Robert De Niro for *Cape Fear*, Anthony Hopkins for *The Silence of the Lambs*, and Nick Nolte for *The Prince of Tides*.

This time round there was no clear favourite in what was generally regarded as one of the most even Oscar races for some years. The pre-Oscar tips were Nolte and Beatty. Nolte had surprised everyone with the sensitivity of his performance in *The Prince of Tides*, and he had also turned in an exceptionally strong performance in *Cape Fear*. Beatty on the other hand seemed to have gone out of his way to court the Academy. His film was the nominations kingpin with ten nominations, and he himself had gathered 13 nominations over the years as actor, director, producer and writer but had won only once, as Best Director for *Reds* in 1981. Beatty had even ended his status as Hollywood's most eligible bachelor by marrying his *Bugsy* co-star Annette Bening, and becoming a father. Surely, it was argued, such a track record could not easily be ignored. Williams and De Niro were both in with a shout, but the fact that neither *The Fisher King* nor *Cape Fear* had a Best Picture nomination might count against them. The only thing that was certain, according to Hollywood gossip, was that Anthony Hopkins had no chance. For one thing *The Silence of the Lambs* was perceived as a horror film – a category consistently ignored by the Academy – and for another it had been released in February of the previous year, six weeks before the last Oscars. In any event, after wins for Daniel Day-Lewis and Jeremy Irons in the two previous years it seemed unlikely that Oscar would leave the States three times in a row.

On the night, however, it was Hopkins, the rank outsider, who triumphed in what turned out to be a clean sweep for *The Silence of the Lambs*, which became the first film to take the five big awards – picture, director, actor, actress and screenplay – since *One Flew Over the Cuckoo's Nest* in 1975. Hopkins was as astonished as anyone. He was convinced that Nolte would win, but he admitted to having worn his lucky shoes just in case. For Robin Williams there was yet more disappointment. It was obviously easier for a camel to pass through the eye of a needle than for a former TV star and a comic to be recognised by the Academy.

By the time the Oscars had come around, Williams had almost completed another film. As he had said he would when he announced he was doing *Hook*, Williams had gone on from there to be reunited with his *Good Morning Vietnam* director Barry Levinson in *Toys*. Levinson had originally intended *Toys*, which he co-wrote with Jane Curtin, to be his début picture. It had been bought by Fox in 1978 on the understanding that he would direct it. But there was the inevitable change of studio regime and the new management didn't think the script was funny enough.

'Studio executives didn't know how to respond to it,' says Levinson, 'because they can't think of any other that it's like.'

Instead of making *Toys*, Levinson then went ahead and wrote and directed the seminal *Diner*, while *Toys* languished in Development Hell. It came close to being produced at Columbia, who wanted to make it with Levinson and Williams immediately after *Good Morning Vietnam*. But by the time the Vietnam comedy was finished, Columbia boss David Puttnam had left. The film would turn up from time to time in articles about Hollywood's best unproduced scripts, and that seemed to be where it would remain. Now, however, with the considerable combined clout of both Williams and Levinson the film was finally going into production. For Williams it was the chance to go back and do comedy after a lengthy absence.

> *The Fisher King* had some comedy, there was none in *Awakenings*, *Hook* has a few funny lines [he says]. It's nice to change the parameters and go against what people expect sometimes. It was nice to do *Dead Poets* because it suddenly allowed me much greater room to move. *Dead Poets Society* allowed me to do something like *Awakenings* because De Niro saw it and suggested I star with him. It gives me a much broader range, so that I can then go back and do the *Good Morning Vietnam* kind of thing, which is what I'm doing with *Toys*.

During pre-production for *Toys* Williams managed to squeeze in another memorable TV performance. Johnny Carson was retiring in May 1992 after 30 years as America's best-loved chat-show host on *The Tonight Show*. Carson, no mean comedian himself, was the king of late-night TV and Williams was one of his most favoured guests. In his final week on air Carson asked back some of his favourites. He had no studio guests for his farewell show, therefore the most important show of the week would be his second last. The show was broadcast on 21 May 1992 and Carson's guests were Robin Williams and Bette Midler. The programme aired not long after the Rodney King riots in Los Angeles, and Williams was on devastating form. He and Carson played off each other and each frequently reduced the other to tears of laughter. It was one of Carson's best interviews and it seemed appropriate that the best had been kept till last.

In *Toys*, Williams plays Lesley Zevo, son of a great toymaker – played by Donald O'Connor – who has to fight for the factory's future after his father dies. His uncle, a former military man played by Michael Gambon, takes over the company. All he wants to make are war toys until he then gets the idea of manufacturing war toys that shoot real bullets. Williams then has to enlist the aid of his sister, played by Joan Cusack, and some of the more peaceable toys to regain control of the family firm and his legacy.

Williams describes Gambon's character as 'F.A.O. Schwartzkopf', but behind the quick-witted pun on the world's most famous toy store, it's obvious that the strong anti-war message would have appealed to him. He was also delighted to be working with Hollywood legend Donald O'Connor, who plays his screen father before dying early in the film. Williams was so delighted to be working with O'Connor that he sent him a note when shooting was finished, thanking him for being 'such a great stiff'.

When Levinson originally conceived *Toys* almost 15 years previously, it had included ground-breaking ideas such as virtual reality and other concepts which were barely thought of at the time. Even if the finished film did not incorporate virtual reality itself, Levinson's wildly surreal vision was breathtaking to look at, but at the same time almost swallowed the actors whole. Williams was not alone in struggling to make an impact in a film which was a triumph of design over content. Bizarrely, given that it was Levinson who had finally provided an outlet for his comic potential in *Good Morning Vietnam*, Williams remains firmly shackled here by a very sentimental and cloying screenplay. Only once, in the scene where he delivers a pep talk to a series of nursery toys before the final battle for control of the company, is he allowed to cut loose. Williams' verbal gymnastics in that scene alone make you pine for what might have been had he been encouraged to do more.

Toys was aimed at the lucrative Christmas market. It was released in December 1992 to poor reviews and even worse box-office. The film ended up taking only $23.3 million at American cinemas, Williams' poorest return since he had originally teamed with Levinson for *Good Morning Vietnam*. But, bizarrely, even as *Toys* was flopping, Williams was already at the top of the box-office charts with another film.

Towards the end of shooting on *Hook*, Williams got a call from Jeffrey Katzenberg's office at Disney. Would he, wondered the Disney chairman, make some time to come over and have a look at some footage which they were putting together? Williams, a long-time animation fan, was intrigued and readily agreed. So, on a day off from *Hook*, he went across to Disney to meet animation directors Ron Clements and John Musker and animator Eric Goldberg. What they had to show him resulted in the most successful and popular role of Williams' career to date, as well as one which would plunge him into a bitter wrangle with the studio which had resurrected his career.

In April 1991, the Disney animation department was in the depths of despair. They had just screened an eight-minute black-and-white assembly of their new animated film. *Aladdin* was supposed to complete the 'fairy tale trilogy' of *The Little Mermaid* and *Beauty and the Beast.* But the consensus was that this version just didn't work. After a final viewing from Katzenberg the order came down to scrap it and start all over again.

Part of the problem was that the film simply didn't look right. The solution came from British animator Eric Goldberg, who was working on the genie. He had been searching every reference source he could find to come up with a look which would work on the genie. Almost by accident he came across the work of Al Hirschfeld, the brilliant caricaturist who can take an elongated curve and turn it into the most devastatingly accurate caricature. Goldberg started to work on the genie à la Hirschfeld and quickly realised that he had found the key. Using Hirschfeld as his starting-point, Goldberg came up with an elongated S shape which took the genie from being a puff of smoke coming out of the spout of Aladdin's lamp into a big-headed, lantern-jawed, sharp-witted comedy slave. This elongated S became the template for the rest of the design, and *Aladdin* was very quickly back in business.

As far as Clements and Musker, who had been responsible for *The Little Mermaid*, were concerned, there was only one person who could voice the genie. They had written the character with Robin Williams in mind, hoping that his quicksilver wit could be transformed into equally mercurial animation. Goldberg, who was in charge of animating the genie, agreed with Clements and Musker, but there were others who were less enthusiastic. Goldberg then went away and quietly assembled what amounted to a virtual screen test by taking samples of Williams' comedy and animating the genie to them. When Williams came over to Disney that late spring day in 1991, what he saw was the genie performing magic with his voice.

> There was one bit [recalls Goldberg], where he said 'Tonight I'd like to talk to you about schizophrenia'. Then another voice would say 'No he doesn't. Shut up'. To illustrate that I had the genie grow a second head to argue with himself, so we could see how far we could take that approach to the character . . . He [Williams] laughed his guts out. It was clear to him that we weren't going to take his comedy and make a mess of it.

Williams was convinced and, with the studio bosses, who had already seen the footage, equally certain, he became an enthusiastic conspirator in the comic mayhem of *Aladdin.* Williams already had some experience of animation. He had provided the voice for Batty Koda, a spaced-out, not too tightly wrapped bat in *FernGully . . . The Last Rain Forest.* But that was nothing like this. This was Disney. At this stage the genie was still not much more than a minor supporting character, but the more Williams did, the more the character grew. In the end he recorded about 30 hours of material, which encouraged Disney to change the entire focus of the film and turn the genie into a major character. One of the improvisational techniques during their recording sessions echoed Williams' own days on the road. He would come into a studio and find a lot of props covered in sheets. Williams never knew what they were until the sheets were taken away and, just as he used to do with his box of toys on-stage, he would improvise at length once the sheets were taken away. Every utterance was transcribed and passed on to the animators, who would then use it to craft sequences such as Williams' show-stopping song *A Friend Like Me.* In that one song alone he becomes Arnold Schwarzenegger, Jack Nicholson, a kilted Scotsman, a Scottie dog, Ed Sullivan, a sheep, and – in a nod to the classic comedy show *Let's Make a Deal* – Groucho Marx and his prop duck.

'We weren't sure whether Robin was going to bring out his whole bag of tricks,' says Goldberg, 'but he did. So for the funny stuff I had to go as visually nuts as possible.'

Williams had become more excited about *Aladdin* than any project in recent memory. Part of the reason was that he was now the father of young children, and he saw in this movie the chance to leave a permanent legacy for them and for future generations. It was a way of giving something back to them for the joy they had brought him and he went more than the extra yard for Disney. For one thing there was no question of him charging anything like his normal seven-figure fee. He said he would do the job for the union rate – around $75,000 – the only proviso he made being that Disney should not exploit his name or his voice in their advertising. Disney were more than happy to agree. But the agreement didn't seem to last very long and one day when Williams was watching television he saw a TV commercial using his voice as the genie to sell Disney merchandise. Williams had consistently turned down offers to endorse products. The hamburger chain McDonald's were apparently keen for him simply to name his price but he has always said no. His father's experience with the car industry has left him very cagey about his dealings with corporate America.

> It wasn't as if we hadn't set it out [recalls Williams of his deal with Disney]. I don't want to sell stuff. It's the one thing I won't do. In *Mork and Mindy* they made Mork dolls – I didn't mind the dolls; the image is theirs. But the voice is me. I gave them [Disney] my self. When it happened I said to them 'You know I don't do that'. And they apologised; they said it was done by other people.

Williams was not satisfied with the explanation. He felt that a deal was a deal and that Disney had broken their end of the agreement. The ill feeling deepened when *Aladdin* was released in November 1992 – a month before *Toys* – and went on to become the most successful film in Disney's history. There was no doubt in the minds of many people that the film's success was entirely down to Williams' extraordinary vocal performance. *Aladdin* took $217.4 million in the United States alone. It then went on to sell 15 million copies in its first month in video release. Analysts estimate that by the time revenues from international exhibition and ancillary sales are added in, the film could have made around $750 million for Disney. Most of this was clear profit for Disney, because once the production and advertising costs have been taken into account the rest is a massive windfall for the company, with no profit participation for the artists involved.

Williams was still smarting from the breach of the agreement not to use his voice, which he felt was a betrayal, but his fellow actors were aggrieved on his behalf at Disney's refusal to pay a bonus. There was, it was pointed out, a clear precedent. After *Pretty Woman* had been a huge success, Julia Roberts – who like Williams had no profit participation agreement – was given an *ex gratia* bonus of $750,000. *Pretty Woman* made $300 million for Disney, less than half what *Aladdin* was coining in for them. Various industry sources put different figures on the amount they felt was morally due to Williams. These ranged from $10 million to $25 million, and none of them seemed excessive. But Williams' old friend and *Awakenings* director Penny Marshall summed it up. 'I'd give him whatever he wants,' she said, 'because he doesn't want that much.'

Marshall was quite correct. The money was not important to Williams who is not, by all accounts, materially obsessed. There was a principle at stake here and he had learned from his father that principles are more important than almost anything. It may have been that, whereas Disney had felt an obligation to Julia Roberts, they felt no such duty to Williams because in producing *Good Morning Vietnam* when no one else wanted it they had effectively given him his career. However, the longer the row went on the more damage was being done. When Williams was awarded a special Golden Globe award, for example, Disney, unbelievably in the light of the row, included it in a new wave of advertising for *Aladdin*.

'The mouse only has four fingers,' said Williams in one stinging rejoinder. 'It can't write a cheque.'

Disney eventually sent Williams a Picasso which is reportedly valued at more than $1 million as a peace offering. Williams accepted the painting – one in which Picasso imagines himself as Van Gogh – and it hangs in the living-room of his San Francisco home. But the damage had been done. He swore he would never make another film for Disney. He remained true to his word even when Joe Roth took over Disney's films division. Roth had come from Fox and was not involved in the *Aladdin* débâcle. Nonetheless, when he sent Williams a script, Williams returned it with a note saying that he knew that Roth was a very nice man but he still had a problem with the studio.

It was Roth who finally ended the feud almost four years after *Aladdin*. The movie had spawned a straight-to-video sequel, *The Return of Jafar*, in which Dan Castellaneta, the voice of Homer in *The Simpsons*, provided the voice of the genie. When Roth took over at Disney he was looking over the books and was astonished to find that, even without Robin Williams, *The Return of Jafar* had generated more profit for Disney than *Pretty Woman*. Almost immediately Roth called Williams to apologise in person for the way in which his original agreement had been breached. Disney then put out a press release to that effect. The *rapprochement* was sealed when Williams agreed to reprise his role as the genie in 1996 in another straight-to-video movie, *Aladdin and The King of Thieves*. Not surprisingly it was a huge international success.

'We made up,' said Williams succinctly some time afterwards. 'They apologised and that was all I wanted. They basically said, "We screwed him. Yes, we put out negative press and we're sorry." I said, "Thank you, you're a mensch, welcome back."

'That's all I wanted and they did it, and they did it publicly.'

29

There's No Face like Foam

Even though they had been married for more than three years, Robin and Marsha Williams were still the subjects of a whispering campaign. If he had ever doubted it before, Williams was very definitely being made aware of the fact that mud sticks. The mud which had been thrown by that *People* magazine cover story was sticking like glue. In almost every major interview, in almost every magazine profile, there was the mention of Marsha having been Zachary's nanny and – by implication, however veiled – the woman who wrecked Robin Williams' life. It would be fair to say that, in some quarters at least, Marsha Williams was still regarded with caution if not downright suspicion.

The whispering campaign intensified after an article in *The New Yorker* magazine in September 1993. The article was a profile piece on Marsha as she made her début as a producer. The tone, however, was unfortunate to say the least. Journalist Lillian Ross depicted Marsha as some kind of *über*-producer and supermom; a cross between Martha Stewart and D. W. Griffith. This was heady stuff for a woman without a single production credit to her name, and when it emerged that Ross's son Steven was a production secretary on the film the rumours flew thick and fast.

Marsha Williams had become used to defending herself in public and this was no exception.

> First of all, it was something I really didn't solicit or want [she insisted]. I'm really pretty uncomfortable being interviewed and try to stay away from it . . . Personally I was a bit offended for Lillian that one would reduce her

> writing to thinking that she would come out of retirement because her son answered phones on the production for a couple of weeks and that she could write a flattering piece as a result. I'm going to get a lot more trash and, frankly, I'm not thrilled about it. The first set of press that came out when Robin and I were together was horrible for my parents. It's like a feeding frenzy; they're looking for dirt.

The project which had put Marsha Williams back in the firing line was the film which would be the most successful of her husband's career, *Mrs Doubtfire.* Marsha Williams had read the original children's novel, *Alias Madame Doubtfire* by Anne Fine, some years previously and saw it as the perfect vehicle for Robin Williams. The book tells the story of a struggling actor who is divorced by his wife and loses custody of his children. He may be a lousy husband, but he is still a devoted father and will do anything to stay in touch with his children, even if it means impersonating an elderly woman so he can get a job baby-sitting his own kids. The book had been optioned by Fox but, with no producer attached, it was offered to Marsha to develop. The first thing she did was to form a production company, something they had both been talking about for some time. So, Blue Wolf was set up – Marsha Williams says the name is inspired by her husband, 'the blue-eyed wolf' – with *Mrs Doubtfire* as its first production.

It doesn't take much of a stretch of the imagination to see some parallels between the Williams's own life and the story in the film. Marsha Williams is adamant that it simply never occurred to her.

> I never thought about it [she said at the time]. I can't think about what connections people are going to make. But there was a piece in a small movie magazine I saw recently. It talked about *Mrs Doubtfire* and then said, 'Are we the only movie magazine in America that noticed the parallel between Robin Williams' role and Marsha Garces Williams' role as nanny to the Williams clan?' But I was nanny to Zachary before we were involved, so what's the parallel? ... The thing for me that is sort of curious is that, had Robin picked me up in a bar, would that have made me a better choice? I have had 15 jobs in my life, and being a nanny was one.

Now being a producer was another, with both Robin and Marsha Williams receiving screen credits on *Mrs Doubtfire.* Although this was her first official job as a producer, Marsha Williams had been doing a similar job on a *de facto* basis for a long time.

'Actually, what I'm doing is to a great extent what I've been doing with Robin for several years,' she explained. 'I've been reading scripts for him, looking into possible projects, and giving him my opinions about all of it when he asks me. He doesn't always agree with me, and there have been movies he has embarked on without paying any attention to what I thought, but I've supported him in whatever decisions he's made.'

Marsha Williams had been around movie sets since *Good Morning Vietnam* and had been able to watch some highly effective producers at work. She had also worked closely with Robin on writing, rewriting and researching.

'She waded right into it,' says Williams of his wife's new job. 'She likes the challenge of producing. My name is on *Mrs Doubtfire* as producer, and we talk to each other about everything, but she does most of the work, and all that talking with other people. She has the patience to discuss a problem for hours and hours. I have to be busy preparing for my part. I tend to be more direct. I'll just say "That sucks".'

In making *Mrs Doubtfire*, Williams teamed up with another San Francisco resident, Chris Columbus. Columbus was a hugely successful director who had made his name with *Home Alone*, the most successful comedy in film history. He and Williams hit it off immediately when they met and they both had similar reasons for making the film. Columbus felt the film stressed the importance of family and he believes that they both made the film as a way of atoning for the amount of time they had each spent away from their children pursuing their careers. Both men agreed that the look of the character was vital to the success of the film. 'In the film,' says Columbus, 'if Robin's character doesn't fool the woman he'd been married to for 14 years, she won't hire him – and there's no movie.'

The key to Mrs Doubtfire herself came in the make-up and the costume. Williams had to draw once again on his experience at Juilliard, where he had taken a mask class in which they would put on masks and become a character.

> It was like the costume of dreams [he joked about his Mrs Doubtfire make-up]. If you wear it she will come. Once I put the mask on – it wasn't really a mask, it was twelve separate pieces that took four hours to fit. Once that was on, plus the body suit, plus the orthopaedic socks and everything else, plus the frock and the sweaters, she started to emerge. The first thing was learning to relax your body a little bit in the walk, and to walk in those heels. To get the gravity of all that helped. The first make-up test we did was with a make-up which was very real, but she had so many liver spots she looked like a Jack Daniels poster child. We had to tone her down and give her that look you see in old Scottish ladies from Inverness who look like they're lit from within – especially after a couple of Glenfiddichs. We just

tried to give her that softness, just as people see her, and they started to relate to her as an aunt or a relative.

Perhaps more than any of his other films, *Mrs Doubtfire* gave Williams the chance to combine comedy and drama very effectively. Mrs Doubtfire herself doesn't come into the film for more than half an hour, leaving Williams plenty of screen time to make an impression as the doting but feckless Daniel Hillard. Once she appears, however, it allows Williams to cut loose with both vocal and physical improvisation which makes the most of the man inside the woman. Finding the right voice for his *alter ego* had been somewhat problematic. Williams had experimented with a number of accents but nothing seemed quite right. Eventually the Scottish accent emerged as a result of Williams having spent months working with Glasgow film-maker Bill Forsyth on *Being Human*, a film which would be released after *Mrs Doubtfire.*

'The accent was in the back of my mind from working with Bill for four and a half months,' Williams recalls. 'Also, I had these teeth, kind of Julia Childs teeth, the kind that take you over. The first couple of tries sounded like Margaret Thatcher on steroids, then we pulled it back and softened it up a little bit.'

Although Mrs Doubtfire was supposed to be English rather than Scottish, Williams points out that most American audiences can't tell the difference. However, the choice of accent is appropriate since for years there had been a persistent rumour that Williams had been born in Edinburgh rather than Chicago.

'I think the story about me being from Edinburgh came about from an interview I did way before *Mork and Mindy*,' he explains. 'I was kidding with someone, a local paper reporter who was interviewing me, and I think he assumed because of the way I spoke I was from Edinburgh. I thought that was great. Sure, I performed once at the Festival, but he must have been on a lot of medication or something because he wrote that I was born there.'

The effect of transforming the chunky hirsute actor into a woman with whom you would cheerfully leave your children was quite remarkable. Chris Columbus compares the experience to a kind of multiple personality disorder: 'For me it was like working with two different actors. There were days when I worked with Robin and days when I worked with Mrs Doubtfire. It wasn't until the end of the shoot that I really started to treat her like Robin. Before that, whenever she came on to the set, everyone was a little more gentle with her, and I could almost feel myself wanting to help her across the street.'

Williams too noticed the change in the way people related to him and related to his character.

> It's a weird thing [he says], the cast and crew treated her with a sort of genteelness, even though the big air-conditioner I had to blow cool air up my skirt was a bit of a give-away. But they would literally walk me in and make sure everything was all right for me. The reality came when I would wander off the set in full make-up and saw how other people treat older women in America. It's different. There are people who are very nice, but also there's a strange kind of neglect that you pick up once in a while. You'd be standing there and feel that no one would ever come and help you if you needed it. That only happened once in a while. We shot in a place called North Beach in San Francisco which was the closest thing they had to a red light district. I walked into a sex shop one day as Mrs Doubtfire and actually tried to buy a vibrator. The guy went with me for a few minutes until he made the connection with my eyes or something. It was great wandering off as her, the make-up was so good that it held up that way.

Mrs Doubtfire was released on 24 November 1993 to catch the Thanksgiving weekend which is the start of a highly lucrative six-week box-office window going through to the Christmas holidays. The film was a huge success with both public and critics and ended up grossing $219.2 million in the United States – a shade more than *Aladdin*, although the Disney movie grossed more in the long run once ancillary sales were taken into account. But not everyone was happy with the film. The then Vice-President Dan Quayle, who had previously taken Murphy Brown to task for becoming an unmarried mother, was unhappy with the film. The fact that Murphy Brown was a fictitious TV anchorwoman played by Candice Bergen seemed to have slipped past Quayle. However, he felt that *Mrs Doubtfire* was sending a negative message about family values.

> Happy Dan has that Norman Rockwell painting view of American values [said a dismissive Williams]. The reality is that there are a lot of families that aren't necessarily first families, or families like Dan's ... the idea was that a family doesn't end with divorce. The reality in America – sad but true – is that it [divorce] is up to about 60 per cent, maybe higher, so second families move on from there. To have shown it as otherwise would have been a negative fantasy. It is a negative fantasy for a lot of therapists who work with children of divorced couples, because a child immediately thinks that the parents are going to get back together. Once they've established

> that they don't love each other but they love him, then it's something to work towards. That's the reality in America.

As a divorced father himself Williams knows whereof he speaks. Although his own split from Valerie Velardi was civilised, with no custody battles, there are moments when Daniel Hillard, the character he plays in the film, mirrors his own relationship with Zachary. And he admits that on occasion he did draw from life in his characterisation.

'What I wanted to do was just to try to put across something that my therapist was saying to me after my divorce,' he explains. 'Just focus on your child. Try and make things better for him. That's the only thing I bring to it.'

One of the things which so exercised Dan Quayle was the way the film ended. Daniel has forged a new relationship with his children as Mrs Doubtfire, and that relationship is strengthened when they discover his secret and realise how much he loves them. However, this is not the cue for a conventional happy ending. The film has an epilogue of sorts which shows that Daniel and his wife, played by Sally Field, do not get back together again. Instead their children have two parents who love them but simply choose to live apart. This epilogue was not in the original script from Randi Mayem Singer and Leslie Dixon. It was added in a director's rewrite by Chris Columbus with the full support of Robin Williams.

> I think it's important that when kids see this picture they realise we aren't giving them a dishonest ending [says Columbus]. The parents don't get back together again, but we wanted kids to know that their family, if they come from a divorced family, was just as valid as the family next door with two parents. Also it was important that kids seeing this picture knew it wasn't their fault just because their parents got divorced . . . In the original script Daniel and Miranda went off and got pizza together and reconciled. Robin, Marsha and I weren't interested in doing that kind of movie. We wanted a film which would be emotional where we could get a bit of a message across to kids.

30

Riddle Me This

From the moment he made his television début on *Mork and Mindy*, Robin Williams has been one of the entertainment industry's most endearing personalities. Audiences love him and this love is reflected in the roles he plays. Whether it's Adrian Cronauer, Peter Pan, Malcolm Sayer or Mrs Doubtfire, Williams does not play unsympathetic characters. For all that he talks about seeking variety in his work, it is only variety up to a point. He seems to want varied roles so long as they are varied likeable roles. Whether the audience would accept him as a villain is another matter entirely. Some actors, such as Morgan Freeman, have regrettably come to accept that their choice of roles is so inextricably linked with their screen persona that they simply cannot play a villain and take an audience with them. Robin Williams was perhaps reaching the same conclusion although, especially in the light of the success of *Mrs Doubtfire*, he did seem to be actively considering playing a villain.

> Anthony Hopkins said there is something very amazing when you play those characters [said Williams of villainous roles]. He said that even when he played Hitler there was an unexpected side that he found was very effeminate, and looking for those things was very interesting. That could be good for me, because I have been playing all these warm, giving characters. That's why in *Dead Again* it was nice to play this defrocked psychiatrist, who basically had his wires slightly crossed.

While no one seriously expected Williams to play Hitler, there was a hot role in Hollywood which seemed to have his name written all over it – and as an added bonus, it was a villain. The *Batman* franchise had become a huge money-maker for Warner Brothers since Tim Burton brought the character to the screen in 1989. *Batman*, in which Williams lost the role of The Joker to Jack Nicholson, made $250 million in the United States alone that summer. The sequel, *Batman Returns*, came along three years later and took in $163 million. Warner, however, were unhappy with the dark tone of the second film and wanted a lighter movie for the Caped Crusader's third outing. Tim Burton was reluctant to go in that direction, so he and Warner parted company over their creative differences and Joel Schumacher was drafted in for the third film. With *Batman* star Michael Keaton also leaving, the third film – *Batman Forever* – was the chance to reboot the whole franchise. Val Kilmer took over as Batman, and this time he would be battling evil in the form of The Riddler and Two-Face. Tommy Lee Jones, fresh from his Oscar success on *The Fugitive*, was pencilled in for Two-Face, and Robin Williams seemed tailor made for the part of The Riddler. In terms of *Batman*'s rogues' gallery, The Riddler was something of an oddity; he was not necessarily as dark as The Joker, but his compulsion to leave clues in the form of riddles made him a much quirkier character. Audiences knew him from Frank Gorshin's manic characterisation on the *Batman* television series, and with that in mind it seemed that this was the ideal role for Williams.

In public Williams was making all the right noises. 'I haven't read the script but if it's one that I think I can play then I'd love to do it,' he said when he was on the road promoting *Mrs Doubtfire*. 'I think I've played enough nice characters so it's time to play a villain. The Riddler was always a fascinating character in the comic books I've read. He's not as menacing as some of the others, but he's more interesting. I'd love to play it. If it was the right script, I'd do it in a second.'

While Williams was making positive noises, so too was Joel Schumacher, who conceded that in all probability Williams would play The Riddler in *Batman Forever*. However, he insisted that nothing was definite and even as he was saying so, Williams' management were denying that anyone had been in touch about the role. Having been bitten once before, Williams' agent was understandably reluctant to get drawn into any kind of mating dance to allow his name to attract another actor to the movie. Other actors had been mentioned – John Malkovich was considered for a time – but it seemed that the role was Williams' if he wanted it.

While negotiations were going on – there was some dispute over Williams' $7 million fee, and the actor also wanted rewrites before he would commit – another variable entered the equation in the shape of Jim

Carrey. Three smash-hit movies in a row with *Ace Ventura: Pet Detective*, *Dumb and Dumber* and *The Mask* had turned the rubber-limbed Carrey into Hollywood's hottest property. There wasn't a producer in town who didn't want Carrey's name on a contract and Warner Brothers was no different. On 2 June 1994 the shock announcement came that Robin Williams was out of *Batman Forever* and Jim Carrey was in. Carrey would be paid $5 million and apparently agreed to the role after only 30 minutes' negotiation.

Williams made no direct comment at the time, but let it be known that he had been unhappy with the script. He felt that the character in *Batman Forever* was too intellectual and not as comedic as the character Gorshin originated on television. He was also apparently concerned that The Riddler would end up playing second banana to Tommy Lee Jones' Two-Face. A few days later, however, Williams insisted that he had been ready to play the part, only to discover that it was no longer on offer. Schumacher for his part insisted that they simply became tired of waiting for Williams to make up his mind and moved on accordingly.

Losing a role like this to Jim Carrey must have been a salutary experience for Williams. Carrey was the only actor in years who could rival Williams for his verbal dexterity, and had the added bonus of incredible physical comedy. Carrey was hotter than steam. His success put him on the cover of *Newsweek* – the last comedian who had been there was Williams himself almost ten years previously. Ironically, Carrey also lists Williams as one of his biggest influences. But, even with the new kid in town, Williams insisted there was more than enough room for both of them.

> I think we do different things [he explained]. I think he does something quite unique and wonderful and I do something different. I'm still working, so as long as they don't say, 'I'm sorry, Robin, there's no more work for you. Jim has done everything and he's doing everything too. There are no more scripts for you, all comedy is Jim from now on. There'll be no more work for small hairy boys unless you want to do a musical of *Gorillas in the Mist*.' As long as they don't say that and I can do what I just did, then I'll be okay for a while. I appreciate what Jim does, it's great, and he does something so physical that it is wonderful. But I think there is room for different kinds of comedy.

While Robin Williams was losing the role of The Riddler to Jim Carrey, audiences were seeing another side of him in American cinemas. Or rather, a select few audiences were seeing another side of him. Williams had spent a large part of the late summer of 1993 in Scotland filming *Being Human* with director Bill Forsyth. The film is a meditation on the nature of humanity and follows five men, all of whom are called Hector and all played by Robin Williams, through various periods of history. In the 6000-year span of the film Hector is variously a caveman, a Roman slave, a medieval Crusader, a sixteenth-century Portuguese nobleman, and finally a contemporary divorced New Yorker trying to be reconciled with his children.

Williams enjoyed the experience immensely. 'It's an unusual film,' he conceded. 'But it was a great thing to work on, especially with Bill. He makes wonderful strange movies. He just tries to get it exactly right.'

Marsha Williams was equally enthusiastic about the film. 'I see it as basically the realisation that after 6000 years we all still have the same needs,' she says. 'How have we evolved? The reality is we're still just human beings.'

Despite Robin Williams' enthusiasm, Warner Brothers, who had funded *Being Human*, were nowhere near as enthusiastic. The film that had been delivered by Forsyth was not what they had expected, although given Forsyth's track record of beautifully judged whimsical observation, how could they have expected anything different? They had spent $30 million on the film and despite extensive re-editing they were about to wash their hands of it. *Being Human* was eventually given a minimal release in the United States and Europe and not surprisingly sank without trace at the box-office. Those critics who did see it didn't think much of it, and audiences were simply not given the opportunity to make up their own minds.

The failure of *Being Human* did not matter a jot when it came to Robin Williams' pulling power in Hollywood. In box-office terms he was still anointed. He had starred in four films which had passed the magic $100 million mark – including two that broke the $200 million barrier – as well as starring in another which fell just short of the $100 million mark. Audiences loved him and, with a gap in his schedule after *Batman Forever* fell through, so did studios. Williams had been making noises about going back on-stage for a concert tour, especially after the gruelling business of filming *Mrs Doubtfire.* Live performance was becoming more and more appealing, especially after his recent hectic filming schedule. For Williams, performing on-stage was still the wellspring of his creativity.

> Improvisation is total freedom [he says]. There's no dictating where or what you have to do. And it's a chance to use everything you know in one place. To do a Shakespearean play on George Bush – 'Neither a borrower nor a

> Savings and Loan defaulter be' – you see, you have that freedom. No one has to tell you. You can play with all that stuff. You can be anything you can be.

But nothing was set in stone yet as far as a concert tour was concerned, and if the right movie offer came along Williams could probably still be tempted.

One likely offer which looked like succeeding was a film called *Crazy*, which would have been produced by Ron Howard's Image company. The film would also have reunited Williams with Mike Nichols, with whom he had done *Waiting for Godot* at the Lincoln Center. Disney were also making overtures, now that Jeffrey Katzenberg had left, to be replaced by Joe Roth. Disney felt that Roth, who had given the go-ahead for *Mrs Doubtfire*, might be the man to settle their increasingly embarrassing row with Williams after *Aladdin*. Roth after all was the man who had been responsible for Williams now being established in the $15 million a picture bracket after the success of *Mrs Doubtfire*. Roth did indeed turn out to be the peacemaker, but not just yet. In any event it's debatable whether any amount of kissing and making up would have got Williams interested in the project which Disney most wanted. They were keen for a sequel to *Good Morning Vietnam* which would have put Adrian Cronauer at the turbulent Democratic convention in Chicago in 1968. The idea for the sequel came from Williams' manager Larry Brezner. Even though he wasn't at the convention, Adrian Cronauer himself was keen on doing another picture, which was tentatively titled *Good Morning Chicago*.

The fly in the ointment was Williams himself, who was simply not keen on the idea. 'They've written a couple of versions and they're getting better,' he said, 'but why do a sequel unless you can do something quite wonderful? You can't push it. The best sequels take the movie further. It's also a hard call because the real man never went there, so now you're fictionalising it.

In the end Williams decided that his next film would be another family comedy adventure. *Jumanji* is the story of Alan Parrish, a young boy who is having a difficult relationship with his father. One evening he discovers Jumanji, a strange board game with supernatural powers. The boy is drawn into the game where he survives for more than 30 years until two other children find the game and continue to play. Immediately the game starts to manifest its bizarre powers and strange creatures begin to appear. Amid all the weirdness the adult Alan Parrish, played by Williams, comes back after being trapped inside the strange world of Jumanji for all that time. Together the grown-up Alan and his new young friends have to play the game to its conclusion to save their town from being destroyed.

Jumanji is a special-effects romp directed by Joe Johnson, who had previously directed *Honey, I Shrunk the Kids.* For Williams there were once again parallels with his own life. How much of himself did he see in Alan Parrish, a little boy living alone in a big house with a stern and authoritarian father?

> I think maybe I was just possibly working out something from my own childhood [he admits]. Maybe I'm drawn to it because I sympathise with it. The character in *Jumanji* is an only child who gets picked on. I was that child who was picked on not only physically but intellectually too and it's like a whole other thing when you get both. But also there is a stage where you have to say 'Don't need to talk about that any more' and you can go on and play other characters.

Essentially *Jumanji* was a children's film. Williams abhors violence in real life, and as he grows older he admits to being drawn, just as he was with *Aladdin*, to films that he can take his own children to see. Unlike his earlier days Williams was now creating out of happiness rather than fear, and that was one of the overriding reasons for doing *Jumanji.*

> I love the fact that a film like *Mrs Doubtfire* can work for adults and children, [he says]. In *Aladdin* especially I used to get people coming up to me and going 'I was with my kid and I was laughing so much that my kid told me to shut up'. If the movie can be that funny, and there is stuff for children and there's stuff for you if you're there with your child, then that's great. It truly is a family film without being about talking down to children. You have to find something that works for both audiences, and that's why I do them. I do them because of my own children and for other people's children.

31

A Friend in Deed

In the life of actor Christopher Reeve, 15 September 1973 was an important date. At that stage Reeve was a prodigiously talented but still promising actor. International fame as Superman and with the Merchant-Ivory film-making partnership was still some years away. But on that autumn day when he turned up as an advanced student at the Juilliard school he met his fellow student – there were only two of them in the advanced group. Reeve remembers him as 'a short, stocky, long-haired fellow from Marin County, California, who wore tie-dyed shirts with track-suit bottoms and talked a mile a minute'. His classmate of course was Robin Williams. The two of them hit it off straight away and have remained close friends ever since. It was to Reeve that Williams would turn for advice for the lovelorn or just a kind word when he was feeling particularly miserable. It was also to Reeve that Williams turned when he thought he was about to make it big as Popeye, a role he hoped would do for him what Superman had done for his friend. There were no hidden agendas, no career points to be scored; Robin Williams and Christopher Reeve were simply as close as two friends could be.

More than 20 years after that first meeting, on 27 May 1995 the two friends had gone their separate ways in career terms. Williams was a household name with three Oscar nominations and a string of box-office hits to his name. Reeve was also a household name, but he had found the Superman tag a little difficult to shake off. The first three Superman films had been major successes, but the fourth one had done poorly at the box-office. Reeve was now carving out a new career on the stage and in character roles. On that day in May – Memorial Day weekend, the official start of summer in the United States – Reeve was indulging in another of his favourite pastimes. He had become passionate about horse-riding since he had had to learn it for a movie role some ten years earlier. Well and truly bitten by the bug, he had quickly become a passionate and accomplished equestrian. He was competing in a three-day event in Culpeper, Virginia on his favourite horse Eastern Express, which he had nicknamed Buck.

After the dressage round Reeve was handily placed and was looking forward to the cross-country event which was coming up next. Everything seemed to be going well and Buck took the first two fences with little difficulty. At the third fence, however, the horse simply stopped dead. Some reports said he had been startled by a rabbit, others that he had been spooked by some shadows. We will never be certain. What is certain is that the inevitability of Newtonian physics was demonstrated with sickening accuracy. Buck stopped and put his head down; Reeve, with nothing to stop him, went sailing over the horse's head. That would be bad enough, but normally a rider could try to do something to break his fall. Tragically and freakishly Reeve's hands were entangled in the bridle and he went crashing to the ground, taking the riding tack with him. Reeve landed on his head, breaking the first and second vertebrae in his neck. He was heard to say, 'I can't breathe.' Those were the last words he spoke until he woke up five days later in the University of Virginia hospital. Reeve had been flown there by helicopter when doctors at Culpeper realised that his injuries were so extensive they were well beyond the scope of their small hospital. He was paralysed, he could not breathe unaided, but all things considered he was lucky to be alive at all. The bones he had broken are the ones which are intended to be broken by a hangman's noose, causing almost instantaneous death.

The world was stunned by the news of Reeve's tragic accident. News bulletins the world over followed his progress during those first five days until he regained consciousness. His wife Dana never moved from his bedside, keeping vigil with his three children as he fought for his life. The news was also a devastating blow for Reeve's friends. Here was a man who was fit and vital and, at 43, in the prime of his life. This was a man who had made his name playing the most powerful man in the universe. But still he had been struck down suddenly and without warning. It was a powerful reminder if any were needed that celebrity does not automatically confer invulnerability.

When Robin Williams was told of his friend's accident he was shocked and stunned. When he finally discovered the extent of Reeve's injuries he was devastated almost beyond belief. The news was almost enough to tip him over into the sort of severe bout of depression he had not had for many years. 'When I heard about Chris that beat me up pretty bad,' he admits. 'Then I realised I couldn't be there for him like that. I had to be the friend that I had been before.'

Reeve, meanwhile, was still in hospital and still gravely ill. Doctors were waiting for him to recover his strength to the point where he would be strong enough to withstand a vital operation to reconnect his skull to his spine.

As he flitted in and out of consciousness he became aware of a new doctor in the room, one who appeared to be speaking with a strong Russian accent and a poor command of English. The new doctor was wearing a scrub hat and a surgical gown and he announced to the increasingly befuddled Reeve that he was his proctologist and that he had to conduct an immediate rectal examination.

'Five days after my accident I had a 50–50 chance to live,' Reeve would recall later. 'I was hanging upside down in a hospital bed and I looked and saw a blue scrub hat and a yellow gown and heard this Russian accent. There was Robin Williams being some insane Russian doctor.'

Robin Williams and Marsha had flown immediately from San Francisco to Virginia and quickly proved the old saw about laughter being the best medicine. 'I laughed,' Reeve recalls. 'And I knew for the first time I was going to be all right.'

There is no more passionate supporter of Reeve in his fight to regain the use of his legs than Robin Williams. If he was slightly in awe of Reeve's natural gifts when they were students together, he now yields to no one in his admiration of his friend's raw courage.

'How did he get through it?' Williams asks rhetorically. 'He has this amazing sense of purpose which drives him, and he gets through it with a sense of humour. His wife says he is the one who still uses phrases like "walk into the room". He's very focused on raising funds and raising consciousness.'

Nonetheless even the most optimistic scenario puts Reeve's recovery process at many years and at a cost of many millions of dollars. Williams' immediate aim was to get his friend off the respirator which had been helping him breathe. He was horrified to learn that a power cut near Reeve's home in Connecticut could have killed him had they not been able to hook up the respirator to a back-up generator. Williams has undoubtedly made some kind of direct financial contribution to Reeve's medical expenses as well as contributing his skills to the fund-raising efforts, but he is at pains to play down the extent of his involvement.

> They [the media] put out this myth that we had made a blood oath in college to help one another [says Williams]. We didn't have that. I've done some things for him and I'll do others if he needs it. But the wonderful thing is that he is going to take care of himself. If he needs help I'll be there, but that's not to say that I have taken care of all of his medical expenses until the year 2010 or something. I haven't.

The story of the Reeve/Williams pact, which appears to have originated in the *Washington Post*, claimed that Williams had promised to pay his friend's medical expenses when his medical insurance ran out towards the end of 1995. It was the *Post* which pointed out that Reeve's annual medical bill was somewhere around the $400,000 mark, and claimed that 'if either made it in showbiz they would help the other in time of crisis'. Whether the story is true or not, and we must take Williams at his word, it nonetheless led to Robin Williams being praised in the US Senate.

Paul Simon, the senator for Williams' home state of Illinois, used his native son's example, however erroneously, as a stick to beat the Clinton administration's health policy. Taking the *Post* story at face value, Senator Simon praised Williams for his loyalty and generosity.

'I applaud what Robin Williams is doing,' he told the House. 'But something is wrong with our system when Robin Williams has to do that. And what about the millions of Americans who have no Robin Williams to help them? ... Three cheers for Robin Williams! But three Bronx cheers [boos] for our short-sightedness in not protecting all of our citizens.'

Williams' reaction to Senator Simon's speech is not recorded, but it is likely to have been one of acute embarrassment. Williams was merely doing what he had been raised to do. He was helping a friend. He would do the same for Steven Spielberg when the director was shooting his Holocaust epic *Schindler's List*. At the end of a day spent recreating one of the most horrific and inglorious episodes in human history Spielberg would call Williams from the set in Poland and ask him to make him laugh. Williams would stay on the line no matter what the hour, telling jokes and doing 'schtick' until his friend had recovered his spirits sufficiently to tackle the next day's shooting.

Although Robin Williams and Christopher Reeve are not what you would call conventionally political animals, they are both driven by a strong sense of moral and social justice. It was this sense of decency and fairness which prompted Reeve to found The Creative Coalition in 1989. He set up TCC with two actor friends, Ron Silver and Susan Sarandon, as a lobby group to influence government policy on a number of issues including the environment, homelessness, funding of the arts and campaign funding reform. Every year TCC honours two people for their work in these fields. In January 1995, Reeve had told Williams that TCC wanted to honour him at its annual dinner in October for his work with Comic Relief, which was about to celebrate its tenth anniversary. Williams had agreed to accept the award, but it appeared that Reeve's accident a few months later had put paid to that plan. What only a handful of people, including Robin Williams, were privy to was that Christopher Reeve was planning on using that TCC annual dinner to re-enter public life.

Christopher Reeve was cheered to the echo as he was wheeled on-stage at the function room of the Hotel Pierre in Washington that October night. He was now in the process of coming off the ventilator and could speak haltingly through a 'sip-and-puff' process which involved taking in a small gulp of air and then speaking as he exhaled. Although he had forgotten to prepare anything, he managed to charm and entertain the audience of invited guests with a short but witty speech. He then introduced the main guest of the evening, Robin Williams.

In his inspiring and moving autobiography, *Still Me*, Reeve recalls that moment when Williams came on-stage and how effective his friend proved to be in normalising the situation.

> For the next twenty minutes he and I bounced off each other [recalls Reeve]. He took the curse off the wheelchair, going around behind it and pretending to adjust all the controls, referring to my breathing tube as a stylish new necktie and suggesting that I use the chair for a tractor pull. He told the audience that I had to be careful with the sip-and-puff control; if I blew too hard into the tube, I might pop a wheelie and blast off into the audience. The evening was transformed into a celebration of friendship and endurance.

His performance at that TCC gala may not have been the funniest in Robin Williams' career, but it was certainly one of the most meaningful. It re-established his friend as a man and not a cripple, and it was a typically warm and humane gesture by the comic. Williams remains uncompromising in his attitude towards Christopher Reeve. When people ask Williams how Reeve is doing, he will generally reply 'He's on a roll', just to watch the shock value. But Williams remains unstinting in his efforts. He and Reeve went to Puerto Rico together on a fund-raising trip for the American Paralysis Association in 1996, and in February 1998 Williams was one of the star guests at A Celebration of Hope, a gala evening in Los Angeles which raised more than a quarter of a million dollars for the Christopher Reeve Foundation.

'Tonight,' Williams told the glittering assemblage, 'we are here to help my friend and 250,000 other people get back on their feet again.'

It was a moving moment for a man who can frequently be moved to tears by the plight of others. When he spoke of Reeve in the early days after his accident it was not uncommon for Williams' eyes to fill with sadness. They are still prone to fill with tears, but these days they are prompted more by pride than anything else. To paraphrase the copy line from the first *Superman* film, he believes a man can walk.

Williams is an emotional man by nature, but especially where children are concerned. Steven Haft, who produced *Dead Poets Society*, recalls that his wife had a baby not long after Zelda Williams was born. As they were telling Robin and Marsha Williams the story of their own child's birth, Haft happened to mention that at one point in the delivery the nurse had to run out to deal with another mother whose baby was tragically stillborn.

'Robin and Marsha's first child had been born that year,' recalls Haft, 'and the story affected Robin so much he had to leave the room. A few minutes later I found him sitting by the crib, his hand on our son's back and tears streaming down his face.'

On the set of *Hook*, Williams was always available for child visitors. He was determined not to shatter the illusion of Peter Pan and would make time for the young tourists. He was also concerned that some of his co-stars, especially Julia Roberts who was going through a stressful period of her own, might not be able to give the youngsters the time he felt they deserved. Williams is also active in the StarBright Foundation, a charity which does its best to make wishes come true for terminally ill children.

Children respond to Williams' generosity of spirit. Their response is also very different and a good deal less hypocritical than the response he gets from some adults.

> They're very interesting and they're critical [says Williams]. They really let you know and it's wonderful when kids come up to you. I don't mind being Robert De Niro [from *Aladdin*] for a ten-year-old. It's really great that they respond. Before I went out to dinner with Chris one night I went to this thing at one of the hospitals for the StarBright Foundation. It's like a virtual world where these kids communicate with each other in different wards if they're in isolation. And all those kids came out about *Mrs Doubtfire* and the movies that affected them. One kid said he had seen *The Fisher King* when he was seven and it's wonderful when kids are affected like that. One child said he'd been in chemo for a while and he had watched *Aladdin* every day, twice a day and it had really helped him.
>
> They really want to hear the voice [he says of Mrs Doubtfire, who is

invariably the star of these private shows]. This little girl was at the hospital and they said 'He did *Jumanji*' and she went 'So'. And then they mentioned *Mrs Doubtfire* and I started to talk to her as Mrs D and she just started to laugh because the voice triggered something in her.

It's weird because sometimes kids will come up and do Jack Nicholson's voice from *Aladdin* and not even be aware of who they're doing.

32

The Lost Boy

Working in the film industry is a little like being in a different time zone on a semi-permanent basis. It can be particularly difficult for actors, who are the most conspicuous of the hired help in the film industry. A director can typically spend 18 months on a film from conception to final cut, and when he goes on the road to promote it, that is all he has to talk about. For some actors 18 months can encompass an entire career; Matt Damon, for example, went from being an unknown to a major player in less time. In the period that it takes a director to make one film an actor can make two or even three. Then, when the first of them is released and they have to do the publicity, they find themselves having to step back into a kind of time warp to try to remember what they were thinking about more than a year earlier in some cases.

That was exactly the situation in which Robin Williams found himself at the end of 1995 and beginning of 1996, when he was touring the world promoting *Jumanji*. Williams was well aware of the most frequently levelled criticism against him; namely that he was beginning to get stuck in a rut in his career choices. He had not been varying his roles of late, and after *Hook* and then *Jumanji*, and with the emotionally stunted Daniel Hillard in *Mrs Doubtfire* thrown in, he was becoming something of a poster boy for arrested development. *Jumanji* might possibly be the last time the audience would accept Williams as the man-child, no matter how well he did it.

'I think I have reached the limit,' he said. 'I think I have reached the end of the man-boy characters ... I think it was possibly just working something out from my childhood, but you reach a stage where you can play other characters.'

Quite why Williams wanted to work out these things from his childhood remains a mystery. He had been in therapy for a long time, since the break-up of his first marriage, and he must surely have addressed these issues many times in the privacy of the therapy sessions. Nonetheless he had been working it out and had realised that enough was enough. Williams claimed to be actively seeking other types of role. Indeed he was privately very pleased that he had just completed his first truly villainous performance. He had taken a small unbilled role – he was credited as 'George Spelvin' – in a film version of Joseph Conrad's novel *The Secret Agent.* Christopher Hampton was directing his own adaptation of the novel, and Williams had agreed to take a tiny role in a cast which included Bob Hoskins and Gérard Dépardieu. He was pleased with the end result and hoped it might help break the casting mould in which he was being set.

'I play the professor, the man who makes the bombs. It scared me quite deeply,' he said the morning after he had seen Conrad's political thriller for the first time. 'It was quite frightening and not warm in any way. I think it's time for me to play adults, no more cuddly folks.'

As it happened, no matter how convincing Williams is in *The Secret Agent* – and it is by no means a bad performance – it did him little good in career terms. The film, which was made by Twentieth Century Fox, was barely released in the United States and hardly anyone saw his first screen villain. Publicly Williams made no comment, but privately he must have been angry that a role which had been chosen with such care to enhance his dramatic range had been thrown into the cinematic dustbin. Ironically, however, when Williams was singing the praises of *The Secret Agent* while he was out promoting *Jumanji*, and when he was pledging to play more grown-up roles, he was just about to start work on his most obvious man-child role to date.

Francis Ford Coppola is one of the few genuine *auteurs* of American cinema. The first two parts of his *Godfather* trilogy are among the greatest American films ever made, and his Vietnam epic *Apocalypse Now* is an astonishingly surreal yet visceral look at the American involvement in Vietnam. But even icons have to eat. Coppola's films had not done especially well at the box-office recently and he had effectively become a director for hire. His version of *Dracula* was a success but it was scarcely his personal vision. Now he found himself working on a film which could only touch on his cinematic world view in the most tangential manner.

Coppola had signed on to direct *Jack*, a fantasy about a little boy with a rare but fictitious disease. This ailment means that he ages four years in biological terms for every calendar year. Hence by the time Jack is ten and in the fifth grade, he has the looks and physique of a 40-year-old man while still possessing the understanding and emotional maturity of a ten-year-old.

It's hardly surprising, given his recent track record, that Robin Williams was the first person the script went to. To his credit Williams did try to be true to his pledge about doing no more man-child roles. His initial response was a flat refusal. 'My first reaction was to say "No thanks, I've done this",' he recalls. 'But it was like they kept coming and then I kept saying "Please, I've done *Hook*, I've done *Jumanji*".'

Jack was being produced by Disney, but this had no effect on Williams' decision. As we have seen, Joe Roth's diplomatic courtship had paid off, and after Disney made a public apology Williams had willingly buried the hatchet. He bore no grudges and he wasn't deliberately holding out for more money or to make Disney squirm. He genuinely felt that there was nothing new that he could bring to the role. Disney, who were equally keen to have Williams back in their corporate fold, had one card left to play. They relied on Coppola's personal intercession. Williams and Coppola are neighbours in the Napa Valley, their properties backing on to each other. They are also partners in a San Francisco restaurant, The Rubicon, and they had been friends for 15 years. Williams had always wanted to work with Coppola and the feeling was mutual. The director went to work on his reluctant putative star and eventually wore him down.

> He started talking about it in a way that was very human [explains Williams]. I must say that I'm really glad that I went along for the ride. People might think that this movie is very bland, but it isn't. It talks about certain delicate things and there is a sadness to it. But it's what love is all about . . . It's about reaching out and making connections, about relationships between adults and between kids . . . It's a very human film and I'm very proud of it.

Filming *Jack* brought back memories of Williams' childhood both good and bad. In the early part of the film Jack is raised in virtual isolation from any other children, which must have recalled his own lonely early days in that big house. Inevitably too there were memories of the short, fat boy being bullied. But the film also rekindled memories of happier times from his childhood in Chicago. Times he had almost forgotten.

> I remember once we moved to a new neighbourhood near Chicago and there were lots of kids on bikes [he recalls]. I remember moving from backyard to backyard, doing kid things and riding my bike everywhere. I remember we had a tree fort just like Jack and his friends do in the film. In the movie they get Jack to go and buy a copy of *Playboy*, and he can of course because he looks like an adult. Well, with us it wasn't *Playboy*, it was *National Geographic*.

Coppola had signed on Diane Lane and Brian Kerwin to play Jack's anxious parents, trying to make the most of what will inevitably be the short time they have with their son. But the bulk of the film deals with Jack's relationships with other kids. To get Williams into the right mood for the part, Coppola sent him on a camping trip with his half-dozen young co-stars.

> I hung out with them at Francis's place for about three weeks [he says]. It was great because you assimilate behaviour without even knowing that you are picking it up. All of a sudden you have this weird combination shuffle and jump that a ten-year-old has and you don't bother about your shoes any more. It was really useful . . . The kids were like seven technical advisers and they would let you know when you went wrong. But you had to be in with them first, you had to know the dynamics of the group and how it worked. They form bonds and I had to be part of that.

As well as three weeks at Camp Coppola, as he came to call it, Williams also relied on his son Zach who was now 13. He remembered how difficult an age it can be for a boy and also how difficult it can be for a parent trying to deal with that. But for all of his efforts *Jack* was not a success. The film opened well enough on the strength of Williams' name, but reviews and word of mouth were against it. It seemed that Williams' instincts had been right; it had simply been a role too far. The public appeared to be tiring of watching Williams the man-child; they wanted the comedy of *Good Morning Vietnam* or *Mrs Doubtfire*, or the pathos of *The Fisher King* or *Dead Poets Society*. In the end *Jack* took $58.6 million at the American box-office, which was respectable but not what Williams was becoming used to.

By the time *Jack* was released in the autumn of 1996, Williams had had four films in a row which had broken $100 million at the American box-office. Ironically the most recent of these was *The Birdcage*, a film which he had completed before *Jack* and which gave him another shot at breaking out of those man-child shoes. *The Birdcage* was an Americanised version of the classic French comedy *La Cage aux Folles*, which had already been a huge international hit in its own right as well as spawning a successful stage musical. In the original two gay Frenchmen are thrown into a panic when the straight son of one of them announces that he is about to be married. The meeting of the prospective and very strait-laced in-laws is a potential nightmare. If they discover his father is gay and living with another man, then the whole thing will be off. In desperation his father's partner pretends to be the boy's mother and the whole things descends into hilarious farce.

The Birdcage, which was written by Elaine May and directed by Mike Nichols, the combination which effectively defined American satire in the Sixties, relocates the action from France to Miami's gay enclave on South Beach. Williams plays Armand, who has lived for 20 years with his flamboyant lover Albert, a career-making performance from Nathan Lane. Then Armand's straight son, played by Dan Futterman, turns up unannounced to reveal that he is to be married to his college sweetheart, played by Calista Flockhart. She is the daughter of Gene Hackman's right-wing senator, whose family values platform is being seriously undermined by a sex scandal. He decides that the wedding might be just the thing to take the political heat off, so he and his wife, Dianne Wiest, head for Miami to meet the new in-laws. The last thing they expect is a gay couple, so Lane drags up with hilarious consequences.

Williams' initial reaction when he was offered the movie was to turn it down. He felt it was a mistake to remake a classic, but once he read the few pages of the script that he had been sent he was laughing so loud that he knew it could work on its own terms. Williams had only one further reservation. He had been offered the part of Albert the drag queen, but he wanted the role of Armand.

'First of all I've done that,' he said to explain his choice. 'I wanted to try something different. I wanted to play off of him. I still get to go nuts many times, but it was like learning a whole different job.'

Subconsciously Williams' choice of Armand over Albert may also have been a reaction to another criticism. Over the years Williams had been criticised by gay groups for the extravagant way in which he had portrayed them in his stand-up performances. It was an issue that he had addressed at some length in his 1992 *Playboy* interview.

> I understand what they're talking about and I have tried to cut back a little [he conceded]. I can see their point because they have always been portrayed as being that way. But don't tell me, if you walk down a street in San Francisco, you won't see a lot of people like that . . . How do you not offend

> anyone? Finally you just say, 'Fuck it. I have to do what I do. If it pisses you off, I still do other things that piss other people off.' I've got the born-again Christians after my ass because I defend gays, and gays are mad at me because I do effeminate characters. You can't keep modifying or you're like a chameleon in front of a mirror.

Once he had got the choice of role squared away, the other major attraction for Williams was the chance to work on film with Mike Nichols, who had directed him on the stage in *Waiting for Godot*. Throughout his career Williams has made impeccable choices of the directors he works with. From Robert Altman through George Roy Hill through Peter Weir through Francis Ford Coppola he has worked with the best. He has also consciously chosen directors who will challenge him and stretch him and bring out the best in him.

> Working with Mike Nichols was amazing [he says]. In terms of comedy he is the best. He was amazing to work with. That's why in *The Birdcage* I took the more masculine of the two. I didn't want to do the drag part, not only because I had already done the drag thing in *Mrs Doubtfire*, but also because I had faith that if I worked with Mike I could find a different level of comedy, and I did. It was great. He really helped me find that other level. We would try wonderful outrageous things, but I knew he would pick the best. I wasn't afraid.

The lack of fear had come to typify Williams' whole life in the Marsha era. It had taken hold first of all in his private life, and now it was spilling over into his professional life as he began to create things out of happiness rather than stark terror. Williams' performance as Armand is a little gem. It is remarkably restrained for a man who was once described as 'the Tasmanian devil of comedy'. There is a touching and loving core about Armand which Williams manages to bring out while still being able to throw hissy fits with the best of them when the script demands.

The Birdcage, like *Mrs Doubtfire*, also allowed Williams to sermonise, however discreetly, about the importance of real family values as opposed to the false values of Gene Hackman's character.

> Lots of Americans look at San Francisco and say 'That place is crazy' [he explains]. But I used to live at 19th and Castro, and it's a neighbourhood. Yeah, there are a lot of gay men and gay women, but it has the same values as your neighbourhood. They want peace and quiet. They want to live their lives, and they do have children from previous marriages, artificial

insemination, a hundred different ways. It's family oriented. People don't acknowledge it, but that's the reality.

Whether audiences took Williams' subliminal message on board or not, they flocked to *The Birdcage* in droves. The film grossed $124.1 million in the States and in the process helped to kick-start the ailing MGM studio which was slowly getting back on its feet after years of financial limbo. It was strong and compelling evidence to back up what Williams already knew – that there would be no more man-child parts.

By the time *The Birdcage* came out he was already committed to *Jack* and indeed had begun filming. But he was adamant that *Jack* would mark the end of this particular phase of his career. The epiphany apparently came one day during shooting as he was sitting on a playground swing. 'This is the last one,' he said to himself. 'This is the ultimate one. This is the metaphor gone beyond hyperbole and into simile. I can't do it any more after this. I'm 45. This is way beyond the Peter Pan syndrome.'

So far, he has remained true to his word.

33

Free at Last

Robin Williams never set out to be a comedian. He wanted to be an actor; the comedy was a defence mechanism he happened to be good at. It was something he had started because he couldn't get work in legit theatre, and after a while it became too difficult for him to give up. Now in his mid-forties he was starting to have some second thoughts. There was only so long that he could continue doing comedy without become passé. Very few comedians have long shelf lives and Williams' had been longer than most. Perhaps it was time to stretch the acting muscles more rigorously than he had been doing of late.

Williams began to seek out projects which would challenge him as an actor. One was a film about the assassination of San Francisco's gay leader Harvey Milk. *The Mayor of Castro Street*, as the project was known, had been in development with Williams' good friend and fellow San Franciscan Gus Van Sant. The two men had wanted to work together for some time and the script was gelling slowly but surely, even if it wasn't quite there yet. Another project he was keen on was *Damien of Molokai*, the inspiring story of a priest who founded a leper colony on the island of Molokai. Father Damien eventually contracted the disease and died himself, but was later canonised by the Catholic Church. There was also the possibility of doing a new version of *Don Quixote*, with John Cleese as Cervantes' deluded hero and Williams as his faithful Sancho Panza. This looked like being his next project until the financing fell through inexplicably at the last minute.

Then, with his wife Marsha under the auspices of their Blue Wolf company, Williams was also developing the story of cartoonist and humorist John Callahan. Callahan is a quadriplegic and a recovering alcoholic, and Williams had been talking about doing this one since the time of *Mrs Doubtfire.*

> He's really been through it [says Williams], but he also has a great, totally uncompromising way of looking at his life. Here's someone who is very unsentimental about everything he does. His cartoons are deadly. One shows two people, a blind guy and a blind woman sitting in the daylight, with the sun just streaming in, and the blind man is courting her, saying 'The night is made for lovers'. He's not afraid to talk about it.

Most of these projects would remain in the pipeline for several years. In the meantime Williams was trying to concentrate on some character work and staying out of the limelight. As well as the sinister professor in *The Secret Agent*, he had also played Osric in Kenneth Branagh's version of *Hamlet*, and before that he had played a crazed Russian doctor – a rehearsal for his performance with Christopher Reeve – in *Nine Months* for Chris Columbus. He had also been obliging his friends. He did a brief cameo as a mime teacher for Bobcat Goldthwait in his directing début *Shakes the Clown.* Then he obliged Steven Spielberg with a single-scene cameo as a night-club owner in the drag comedy *To Wong Foo, Thanks for Everything, Julie Newmar*, which Spielberg was producing.

'I just want to work with characters, with great ensembles of people,' he insists. 'You kind of have to say [to the fans], "If you're disappointed I'm sorry, but I have to keep trying new things for the sake of my own sanity".'

Williams also did another film with Disney. He had agreed to reprise his role as the genie in a third *Aladdin* movie, *Aladdin and the King of Thieves.* The straight-to-video movie had actually started shooting, with Dan Castellaneta once again providing the voice of the genie. Then, with about a third of the film already animated, Joe Roth reached his *rapprochement* with Williams. When Williams signed on, Castellaneta was out and Williams was in.

'I went into a room and started improvising and these guys kept throwing things at me,' says Williams, describing an experience similar to that first turn on *Aladdin.* 'It just got wild. They let me play. That's why I loved it – it was like *carte blanche* to go nuts.'

Williams' fee for this one was more than the union scale of $75,000 that he got for *Aladdin*, but there was still no profit participation on a video which was expected to sell around 10 million units. Disney for their part were still forbidden to use his name or his voice to sell anything connected with the film.

'When your name's above the title, there's a lot of pressure on you,' says Williams, explaining his recent choices. 'When you're a supporting actor, you're just free to do the character.'

That's all very well, but nobody earns more than $20 million a year – Williams earned a reported $23 million in 1996 and $27 million in 1997 – by doing character roles. He still had to be on the look-out for those big starry vehicles which would enable him to pull down the $15 million pay-cheques. One such vehicle seemed to be *Father's Day*, like *The Birdcage* – and *Nine Months* for that matter – a Hollywood version of a successful French film. The French version was called *Les Compères* and starred Michel Richard and Gérard Dépardieu. The plot concerns a woman looking for her missing son. Unable to find him, she calls two old flames and enlists their aid by telling each of them that he is the father of the missing boy. Neither of them is aware of the other and in the course of the film they team up, discover their mutual secret, and at the same time find out by proxy about the joys of parenthood.

Although Robin Williams and Billy Crystal had been close friends since their early days on the comedy circuit, they had never made a film together. Their screen appearances had been limited to their Comic Relief specials with Whoopi Goldberg. Bizarrely, by the time they started shooting together in *Father's Day*, it was their third screen team-up in a year. Billy Crystal had also appeared in *Hamlet*, and Williams had taken a small but telling role in Woody Allen's *Deconstructing Harry*, in which Crystal was second lead. Williams' cameo about a man whose life is so unfocused he is literally out of focus in the film is one of the best jokes in Allen's movie. Williams has barely a handful of scenes, but he took the part just to be on a Woody Allen set and watch him work.

In *Father's Day*, Crystal is the sharper, more successful of the pair. Williams plays a struggling poet who is prone to lachrymose anxiety attacks at the drop of a hat. Appearing with such a close friend in such high-pressure circumstances could have been stressful, but Williams insists the experience was nothing but positive.

> For me it was great getting to know him as a friend over the years [he explains], and someone might think that doing a movie together would tax the marriage, but we still love each other. Actually I got to know him better because you spend so much time together doing a movie. I got to really know him and talk about things and in the process I learned a lot about his past. He was telling me about his father and that was great. These talks were

> actually in the movie at one point. He has a wonderful thing where he talked about a real dream he had about his father and I said, 'You have to use that. It's such an amazingly powerful thing.' It's something that may seem very specific, but I think anybody who has lost their father would relate to what it was. Then the movie ended up going more with the comedy stuff, but that is one of the things that was very powerful.

Father's Day was the sort of movie which everyone thought would be a huge hit in the summer of 1997. It had two popular stars, a proven formula, and the expectations were very high. They had even arranged a rare television appearance for Crystal and Williams on *Friends* in the week of the film's release. It was also opening in mid-May, just before the all-important Memorial Day weekend. The idea was that it would hit the box-office with a bang and then clean up before the perceived summer heavyweights, *The Lost World: Jurassic Park*, *Men in Black* and *Batman and Robin*, came along. It all went horribly wrong, however, and *Father's Day* finished a poor second on its opening weekend to the sci-fi epic *The Fifth Element*. It was a poor summer all round for Warner Brothers, who were hitting a box-office slump not only with *Father's Day* and the *Batman* movie but also their other summer entry *The Conspiracy Theory*. This one also underperformed despite the presence of Mel Gibson and Julia Roberts.

The fact that Warners were in such a slump meant that very little of the blame for the failure of *Father's Day* attached itself to any of the stars. Industry pundits blamed Warner's slightly old-fashioned way of packaging high-priced star vehicles when the rest of the industry had moved on from that. This set the bar so high in terms of movie costs that it would be difficult to make money in what Williams referred to as a 'Darwinian summer' at the box-office. Natural selection did come into play and *Father's Day* was a major loser.

Williams, however, was a prodigious and apparently tireless worker and he was able to turn this work ethic to his advantage. If he had missed out on the summer box-office there was always the Christmas holidays. Williams was already hard at work on a new film for Disney which was tipped to be one of the big holiday hits of 1997.

Disney was remaking *The Absent-Minded Professor*. The original starred Fred MacMurray as a scientist who invented a remarkable elastic compound which he called 'flying rubber' – or Flubber – which allowed anything it came into contact with to effectively defy gravity. *The Absent-Minded Professor* had been the highest-grossing film of 1961 and had spawned a sequel, *Son of Flubber*. Now Williams was taking on the

MacMurray role in a remake called simply *Flubber.* He was playing Professor Philip Brainard, a man so preoccupied with his work that he forgets everything else – even his wedding day. When he invents the miraculous Flubber it seems all his troubles are over, but before that can happen he has to prevent some unscrupulous rivals from getting their hands on it.

Williams claims to be not very astute when it comes to judging a script. He points out that he wanted to turn down *The Birdcage*, for example. On the other hand his instincts also told him not to go with *Jack* or *Father's Day* in their initial form, so his judgement may not be that bad. For *Flubber*, however, he did some market research. He held a private screening of *The Absent-Minded Professor* for five-year-old Cody and asked if he thought he should do his own version. When Cody said he should, Williams signed on.

'This film was made for kids, make no mistake about that,' says Williams. 'You can't say, "I was trying to achieve scientific reality." That's bullshit. It's a children's movie, and when I took mine to the première of *Flubber* they were laughing like crazy, which is a good sign. And the audience was full of kids and they were laughing too.

'My kids don't analyse what I do,' he continues. 'They don't say, "Hey Dad, your acting has less depth than Fred MacMurray." They just have a natural reaction to a film and they laugh if they think it's funny. And that's the way it should be.'

In *Flubber*, as in *Hook* and *Jumanji*, Williams was extensively involved in optical effects. He has a number of scenes in which his car flies, courtesy of a tank full of Flubber, and others where he bounces ceiling-high because of the effects of the stuff. And when he's not flying around himself, he has to share almost every scene either with Flubber, a green computer-generated goo with a personality of its own, or Professor Brainard's flying robot Weebo.

> There are other people in the room so I still had someone to talk to [he says of the lonely experience of acting to nothing for computer-generated imaging]. I was a mime so I had a running start on that stuff, so you start from there and you just play and improvise. The animators pick what they like, so it wasn't as hard as it seems . . . Once they have explosions and things breaking, then it becomes a little more precise. But in the scenes when you first see it [Flubber] when I discover it, they let me try a lot of different things.

Flubber also meant Robin Williams had to log more flight time in his flying harness for the aerial scenes.

> I've got more flying time than Mary Martin [he jokes]. They put you in the same kind of pants and they have this thing called a nitrogen ram which pulls you up in the air. They can go 50 or 60 feet up if you want to go that high, and they can bring you down to within an inch of the floor – or through the floor if you choose – and then back up again 15 or 20 times.
>
> It's a ride [he says enthusiastically]. They would go 'We've got it' and I would want to try again and again. It's fun. It's not a stunt in the sense that there is no real danger, or if there was they didn't tell me. On *Hook* they used to have eight guys on a pulley, but with this it's like a system of nitrogen ratchets. It's very precise and they test it with sandbags. It's a bit like watching a hanging.

Flubber was Disney's major family movie release for the Thanksgiving season in November 1997. It was opening on Thanksgiving weekend against what was perceived to be stiff competition in the shape of the keenly anticipated but twice-delayed *Alien Resurrection*. Not only that, but *Flubber* was also following on from Fox's high-priced animated version of *Anastasia* which had opened strongly over the previous weekend. The reviews for *Flubber* had not been overly enthusiastic. Director Les Mayfield seemed to be at a loss to know what to do with Williams' character. There are so many effects and so much mayhem in some scenes that Williams has nothing to do, and for much of the film he plays second fiddle to a lump of computer-generated green jelly. But, as Williams pointed out, *Flubber* was made for kids not critics. It finished the five-day Thanksgiving weekend in top spot at the box-office with a shade under $36 million. *Alien Resurrection* trailed well behind in second place with just under $26 million.

Although it started with a bang, *Flubber* didn't demonstrate the staying power for which Disney might have hoped. One of the box-office trends of the Nineties was that films tended to have shorter shelf lives – the total box-office take is now roughly three times the opening weekend, compared with five times around ten years ago. *Flubber* was a shining example of this theory, finishing up with just over $96 million at the American box-office.

Flubber had just fallen short of the $100 million mark, which was becoming a trademark of Robin Williams films in the Nineties. If Williams was concerned about his appeal slipping, however, he need not have been. The best was only a matter of weeks away.

34

Let's See Some I.D.

By the end of its second weekend *Flubber* was already running out of steam. The box-office charts showed that it had dropped off 58 per cent from its opening. That still meant a healthy $60 million in the first twelve days, but that would also turn out to be around two-thirds of its entire box-office take. Further down the charts on *Flubber*'s second weekend came an entry which made interesting reading. *Good Will Hunting* had entered the charts in 19th position. It was only playing on seven screens but it had taken more than quarter of a million dollars. Significantly its per screen average – often a better indicator of how a film is performing than the box-office total – was the highest in the chart at a thumping $38,897. This effectively meant that the film was playing to sell-out crowds. Robin Williams was also in *Good Will Hunting*, and this box-office chart provided a snapshot of the two sides of his career. *Flubber* was a popcorn movie he had made for his kids; *Good Will Hunting* was the movie he had made for himself. It was a serious movie which gave him his best role since *The Fisher King*.

Good Will Hunting stars Matt Damon, in the title role of Will Hunting, and Ben Affleck. They are lifelong friends from the South Side, the toughest part of Boston. Affleck is a demolition worker and Damon is a janitor at MIT (Massachusetts Institute of Technology). Damon is also a mathematical genius who has serious personality disorders as a consequence of his abusive childhood. When MIT professor Stellan Skarsgaard discovers him solving one of the complicated problems he has left on the blackboard for his students, he becomes intrigued by Damon. By this time Damon's temper has landed him in trouble with the law, again. Skarsgaard persuades the judge not to jail him on two conditions; the first that he is released into his custody, the second that he undergoes therapy. After trying a series of doctors without success, Skarsgaard finally turns in desperation to his old friend Robin Williams. At one time Williams was a brilliant psychiatrist doing ground-breaking work with traumatised Vietnam veterans, but the death of his wife has left him alone, bitter and brooding. He eventually agrees to see Damon, and after an inauspicious start they begin to build a relationship. Williams, like Damon, comes from the South Side and, like Damon, he too was abused as a child. In the course of their sessions together both find a way to deal with their own problems and get on with their lives.

Before *Good Will Hunting* was released, its co-writers Damon and Affleck, who are 28 and 26 respectively, were regarded as two of Hollywood's most promising young actors. Affleck was tipped for great things after his performance in Kevin Smith's *Chasing Amy.* Damon, however, was thought to be the brighter prospect after starring in *The Rainmaker*, which had just opened, and being cast by Steven Spielberg in the title role in his war epic *Saving Private Ryan.* Like the characters they play in *Good Will Hunting*, Damon and Affleck have been friends since they were ten years old. *Good Will Hunting* has its origins in a one-act play Damon wrote at Harvard before he dropped out. Over the years the two friends expanded it, honed it, and in the end transformed it into a movie script for which they both took equal credit. Although Damon has the lead role in this one, they have an understanding that Affleck will take the lead in their next script. Eventually they managed to interest Castle Rock Pictures in making the film, which was gathering a lot of interest in young Hollywood. Castle Rock however wanted to cast two actors who were the same age as Affleck and Damon, but better known. This proved to be a deal-breaker. Castle Rock gave them two months to come up with a buyer who would reimburse them for the money they had spent developing the script, otherwise it would stay with them and they would go with the big names. Happily Miramax was willing to step in, and also willing for Damon and Affleck to take the roles they had written for themselves. Gus Van Sant was then attached as director, and by one of those fortunate coincidences he and Robin Williams finally got the chance to work together. Damon and Affleck had written the role of Sean Maguire with Williams, or something they described as a Robin Williams type, in mind. When he saw the script he had no doubt in his mind that he was going to do this film.

'When I met the boys [Ben and Matt] for the first time I said "Let's see some I.D.",' says Williams, who could not believe that a script which dealt in such a mature way with so many life experiences could have been written by such young men. He also recognised that this was a long way from the man-child rut in which he had recently become mired.

> When I do a movie like *Good Will Hunting* I do it because the story works [he explains]. I read it and thought I would be insane to pass this up. A movie like *Awakenings* is a serious movie, a movie like *Deconstructing Harry* which is really dark comedy I did because I really just wanted to be in the same room with Woody Allen and see what it's like to work with him. It's not a duel (with lighter roles), it's a conscious choice. I do a children's movie because I have children and I want something for them to see, and then I do these serious movies and I like to have access to both. To do all these different movies is important to me, and to do a stand-up comedy routine like I still do in clubs is just as valuable.
>
> The writing is better for the serious roles [he continues]. So far in the serious films the scripts ... have a certain quality of writing about them. You've seen the quality of the writing that these two guys wrote, and then I met them and went 'Now who wrote this really?' Because you see the depth of perception in the things that they talk about and you go 'This is something that I want to be part of'. It's a supporting part, but it's a great ensemble. It's just like being in *The Birdcage*, it's a great ensemble, I like being in a supporting part more than I like being a star ... For me it's just as meaningful and in some ways more relaxing to do that and to work with someone like Gus Van Sant, who's very relaxed. I enjoy doing the effects movies. I love computers, I love being on-line and I love playing computer games, so for me an effects movie like *Flubber* or *Jumanji* is just another live-action computer game with myself as part of the game. To do a serious movie is really good exploration and it pushes the envelope of people's perceptions of what I can do. I was training to be an actor. John Houseman said, 'Mr Williams, you are damaged but interesting.' It's part of what I hope to do eventually is to be acting once again.

Although he still loves comedy, especially stand-up, and he still sneaks into comedy clubs late at night to do impromptu sets to keep his creative juices flowing, Williams appears to be coming round more and more to the fact that he really wants to be an actor. By this time he had reached the stage where the combination of commercial success and creative security meant that he was really enjoying film-making for the first time in his career.

Two of the most difficult scenes of Williams' career come in *Good Will*

Hunting. The first is after Sean and Will have had their first disastrous session together. The next time they meet Sean takes him out on to Boston Common and tells him about life, and how little Will really knows about life. It is a remarkable scene. Damon and Williams are sitting side by side on a bench, not looking at each other but staring straight ahead. Williams then pours out his soul to Damon and by extension to the audience. We hear of his Vietnam experiences, the death of his wife, his complete loss of faith, in a remarkable four-minute speech. The camera is on Williams almost continually; the only cut comes when Van Sant moves from right profile to left profile about half-way through. It is a searing and deeply affecting scene without a trace of mawkishness or sentiment. Similarly, towards the end of the film when Sean finally gets through to Will in his consulting room, Williams is faced with another tough challenge. Will has finally opened up and revealed his abusive childhood, and Sean has revealed that he had a similar experience with his own father. Sean then tells Will that it's not his fault, none of it is his fault. This is perhaps the first time in Will Hunting's life that anyone has understood the burden of guilt he has been carrying and attempted to lift part of it from his shoulders. The line is repeated nine times until Will finally breaks down and sobs in Sean's arms. As the camera pulls back, they are both weeping – as the script says, 'two lonely souls being father and son together'.

Each of these scenes is technically extremely difficult. In the Boston Common scene Williams has to be completely submerged in the character, there can't be so much as a gesture or a facial tic to distract the audience. Similarly, as he tells Will nine times that it's not his fault, there cannot be a variation of tone or inflection. Both scenes require Williams to totally serve the script, something he has not always been able to do in the past. There cannot be a trace of the sentiment which he allowed to creep in to *Dead Poets Society* to colour the audience's perception of the scenes. Williams nails both scenes so well that it's hard to imagine anyone else playing them. The combination of commercial success and creative security had given Williams a new confidence in his performance. According to Gus Van Sant, he now knew exactly what was required of him and how he was going to go about it.

> I didn't have to do a lot of directing [says Van Sant]. I was possibly doing things intuitively. When we discovered the role, he [Williams] said he was going to do something that he hadn't done before. I pretty much tried to stay out of his way and didn't give him specific pointers during the shoot. Generally, whatever I did say, he would disagree with. A number of times I would say 'You could do it this way' and he'd say 'No, no, no' and then do

> it a completely different way, the way he wanted to. So my direction was more as an observer, making sure everything was going right and staying out of the way. I once saw this Jack Lemmon interview on TV and the only criticism of directors he had was that if things are going really well, they didn't need to get involved because it only confused matters. If the actor was on a run it was better if the director stood back. That's what I did.

Williams continued in serious vein after *Good Will Hunting* by going into *What Dreams May Come.* This is a fantasy directed by New Zealand film-maker Vincent Ward about a man's journey through the Afterlife. This modern-day Orpheus tale combines both effects and drama, since the Afterlife is being created on a virtual set, with Williams and co-stars Cuba Gooding Jnr and Annabella Sciorra completing some location shooting in Montana.

> It's Vincent's sense of the visual that made me agree to this [explains Williams]. Have you ever seen his film *The Navigator*? If it had been anyone else I don't know if I would have done it. The guy I play is married to an artist who does all these landscapes, and when I die it's like I'm in one of her paintings. It's basically Orpheus and Eurydice. There's something quite wonderful and at the same time quite scary about this film.

After *What Dreams May Come*, which was due for release in the autumn of 1998, Williams went straight on to location filming in Poland and Hungary for another challenging role in *Jakob the Liar.*

> It's based on a novel by a survivor of the Lodz ghetto [he says]. It's a fictional account of a Polish Jew in 1944 who hears a radio in a German commandant's office and he figures out that it's about a battle being fought on the Polish border. From that he realises that the Russians aren't that far away. He's in the ghetto and they have no other news or access to other news, and it's about what he does when he tells people this news, the effect it has on them, the hope it brings them, and how it changes people's lives. He only hears one broadcast so he has to keep making things up – hence the title Jakob the Liar – so he keeps bringing more news and tries to keep people going with it, and it's that effect. It's basically a character-driven story. It has Armin Mueller Stahl, Alan Alda, Bob Balaban and I think it's quite unique. I made the film because the story is so powerful and so interesting, and that's what I want to do from now on.

His next interesting story is *Patch Adams*, in which he plays the real-life doctor who founded The Gesundheit Institute, a holistic health-care system which is based on the healing power of laughter. After *Patch Adams*, he moves on to *First Person Plural*, the true story of a man with multiple personality disorder, which Disney acquired for Blue Wolf for more than $1 million.

It's safe to say that Robin Williams is a much-changed man, not only personally but also as a performer. It is inconceivable to think of the man who struggled beneath the latex in *Popeye* being the same man who could star in *Good Will Hunting*. Williams has learned not to fear the silences any more. He has learned to cherish the down time and be grateful for his second chance. There was a time when he was defined by what he did on-stage; now he is defined by what he does off-stage, in his own home. His family has become the most important thing in his life. He no longer has fits of depression, instead he has constructively turned them to moments of quiet contemplation.

'People expect a certain level from you,' he says. 'I have learned to be quiet now, but if I am quiet, or just out walking along or watching something, they think something's wrong. It's that thing of people always wanting you to be on, but there are times when I am just very quiet.'

These quiet moments come most frequently at home with his family, where he retreats to find some sanity and decency in the world. He has acknowledged that it was his family who helped him combat and defeat his depression.

'I have great friends, and my wife and family are extraordinary,' he says. 'It's people who get me through all of that, but especially my children, who are stunning. We were sitting at breakfast one morning and my little girl said "Isn't it wonderful, Cody's not talking". My wife said "That's because he's eating". And Zelda said "I can dream can't I?" Stuff like that keeps me going, that simple human contact.'

His family have also helped him adjust to his fame. He is no longer driven by it and no longer a hostage to it. His celebrity has become a tool to help make his life easier, not a rod for his own back.

> You can't take it seriously [he says simply]. You can't worry if you make movies that don't make $100 million. It's a roulette wheel. You can only look at a script and say, 'Does the story appeal to me? Is it something that I should be doing? Is it something that only I can do?' The truth is with *Flubber* there are about 25 guys who could have played this part, honestly. It's an effects movie that I can bring a certain kind of fun to. A movie like *Good Will Hunting* on the other hand, while there are others who can play that part, I think I can bring something quite unique to it. When I get a

script now I try to find those things that you can do, that you can really kick the shit out of and yet explore and have a good time doing and push the envelope a little.

Will it make hundreds of millions? I don't know and I don't care [he continues]. If *Good Will Hunting* makes hundreds of millions of dollars that would be wonderful for the people who invested in it, but for me I got a chance to be in a good movie, to be in a story that has some depth, and that's worth it. I did *Flubber* for children and that's worth it too. I don't want to demean children's movies, they have a right to be entertained, just like adults have a right – if they want to go and see *Air Force One* with things blowing up and a guy hanging on the wing of a plane, they have a right to, that's entertainment. But in the process of doing that, if you can find other things good, that's the drill.

Fame for me has come and gone about 15 times [he says philosophically, considering the 'power lists' of *Premiere* magazine and *Entertainment Weekly*]. Been there, number 1, number 5, number 8, number 12, number 30. It's a very surreal thing. That's why I live in San Francisco – when you pass a nun dressed in leather that gives you a different perspective. I live there because you really don't want to have to worry about your career constantly. I mean parking lot attendants give you scripts in Los Angeles. In San Francisco people accept me as me, they know I've done movies, but that's just part of it. I can go to a bike shop and buy some weird bike and hang out and talk to bike messengers and then I can get on my bike and ride 40 miles across the Golden Gate to some other place, to woods, and be totally alone, and that's wonderful.

The other thing is surreal, it's like a Mardi Gras float. I'm not having to say it isn't fun and there aren't perks with being famous, but the other part is having a life and having a life as an adult. I'm a father, I'm 46 years old, I have three kids and I love them madly, and I have to be an adult.

EPILOGUE

And the Winner Is...

Despite what they say in public about acting not being a competitive sport, and awards not really meaning anything, all actors have entertained the notion at least once in their lives of standing on the stage on Oscar night thanking their parents, their agent, their guru, and everyone else they can think of. But for all that, an Academy Award remains a quixotic honour. Great actors such as Richard Burton and Peter O'Toole have never won. Martin Scorsese, possibly the most influential director of his generation, has also continually been overlooked by the Academy. At the same time less notable talents have picked up almost inexplicable Oscars.

Some bear the snub better than others. Martin Scorsese has now become philosophical about the fact that he may never win. However, he has made no secret of the fact that he genuinely wanted to win an Oscar. So too did Robin Williams. He had been nominated three times as Best Actor – for *Good Morning Vietnam*, *Dead Poets Society* and *The Fisher King* – and each time he came away with his acceptance speech unheard.

> It's so much fun to go along and go, 'Grrrr. Oh somebody else won? Oh good for you. La de da' [he says with some candour]. I'd like to win one so that I could pick it up and say, 'Look, Oscar hasn't got any balls.' I've had friends win and some day it would be nice. I don't want to win one of those awards for being 100.
>
> For a while I was trying to look for movies. It was like 'This is your Academy Award-winning movie'. But if you do that, it's like trying to kiss

> your own ass – you can't do it. I'm not that flexible. Now I just try and find movies that I just enjoy making, because if you are going to spend four, five, or six months of your life doing something, it had better be something that you enjoy doing. You have to be willing to put your heart and soul into it rather than trying to achieve some award that may not happen.

Good Will Hunting was a project that Williams had put his heart and soul into and had given him huge creative satisfaction. He also gained a great deal of financial satisfaction, since he waived his fee in return for a 15 per cent profit participation in a film which stayed in the US box-office charts for six months and earned almost $140 million. But his performance attracted a lot of attention during the annual end-of-year round of award ceremonies. Although his name was above the credits, Williams was playing a supporting role and it could be argued that going for Best Supporting Actor might give him a better shot at winning. However, the films competing for the 1997 Academy Award featured some of the best supporting performances of recent years. The candidates included Robert Forster and Robert De Niro from *Jackie Brown*, De Niro again from *Wag the Dog*, Anthony Hopkins and Morgan Freeman from *Amistad*, Guy Pearce, Russell Crowe, Kevin Spacey and James Cromwell from *L.A. Confidential*, Burt Reynolds from *Boogie Nights*, Billy Zane from *Titanic*, Greg Kinnear from *As Good As It Gets*, Billy Connolly from *Mrs Brown*, Al Pacino from *Donnie Brasco*, Tom Wilkinson and Mark Haddy from *The Full Monty*, and Williams and Ben Affleck from *Good Will Hunting*. This was bound to be one of the most competitive Best Supporting Actor categories in years, especially since most of the other Oscar categories seemed cut and dried.

In the end there were some shocks and some glaring omissions when the Academy Award nominees were announced in February 1998. The Academy voters had indeed nominated Williams, and his fellow nominees were Burt Reynolds, Greg Kinnear, Anthony Hopkins and Robert Forster. Pundits quickly decided it was a two-horse race. Hopkins could be eliminated for being a previous winner and for starring in a film which the Academy seemed to have overlooked; likewise Forster had appeared in a film which also seemed to have found little favour with the Academy, while Kinnear suffered from something which Williams knew all about in that he was a TV star and perceived as a comedian.

Two other award ceremonies have been deemed to be significant in deciding the final fate of the Academy Award. The first is the Golden Globe awards, which are voted on by Hollywood's Foreign Press Association. Some of their choices have been odd to say the least, but with national television coverage and support from the major studios, these awards have gained bell-wether status. Perhaps a more reliable indicator might be the relatively new Screen Actors Guild awards. These are seen as a better guide because the same people vote for them, i.e. SAG members, as vote for the Academy Awards.

Burt Reynolds drew first blood by winning the Golden Globe for his role as a porn-movie mogul in *Boogie Nights.* Reynolds' sly and ironic performance was seen by some as a self-deprecating nod to his old screen image, as well as capping a comeback which had been simmering for some years. However, by March the momentum seemed to be running away from Reynolds, especially when stories began to circulate that he hadn't been too enamoured of *Boogie Nights* in the first place.

Williams evened the score by taking Best Supporting Actor at the SAG awards. 'I was sitting over there sweating like Marlon Brando after Thai food,' he joked on accepting his award. 'I'm stunned.'

With the Oscars only three weeks after the SAG awards, Williams was deemed to have the edge in what was still being seen as a close race. On the night Williams went along with his wife and his mother. He and Marsha sat in the orchestra section of the Dorothy Chandler Pavilion, where the major names are seated, with the rest of the *Good Will Hunting* contingent. The film had nine nominations overall, including one for Affleck and Damon who would win for Best Original Screenplay.

In the end, when the envelope was opened and the winner's name was finally announced, it was Robin Williams. Burt Reynolds had to be as good as his pre-show quote when he had suggested that if he lost we would see the best piece of acting he had ever done. As a plainly stunned Williams hugged his wife before bounding up the steps to a standing ovation from the orchestra section, a tight-lipped Reynolds applauded but did not get to his feet. Williams embraced his best friend Billy Crystal, who was the Oscar night master of ceremonies, before admitting to a new phenomenon.

'Ah man!' he said. 'This might be the one time I'm speechless.'

A speechless Robin Williams is as likely as a politician declining a sound-bite. He did make a speech, in which he thanked Marsha eloquently, and then pointed to his *Good Will Hunting* co-star and said, 'Matt, I still want to see some I.D.'

In the midst of his greatest triumph he still found time to think of his parents. He thanked his mother, but especially his father. 'I want to thank my father up there,' he said, gesturing to the ceiling of the auditorium, and praised his father for not standing in his way when he made the decision to be an actor. Then the old performance junkie kicked in again as Williams recovered his composure sufficiently to impersonate Groucho Marx and duck-walk off the stage carrying his Oscar.

Afterwards Williams admitted to being genuinely stunned. He said he had not expected to win on any of his previous nominations and this was no exception. 'I didn't think I had a chance, and when they said it, I was shocked,' he said. 'This is a wild night. It's just insane. I'm very proud. This is an extraordinary piece and the first time I read it I wanted to do it.'

But Williams also said he hoped that his win might end the stigma against comedians. 'I was trained as an actor,' he pointed out. 'it's not like they had to medicate me. People think a comedian is a slightly damaged person. It's like "You're a comedian, go over there. Stay. Good".'

The irony of the evening would not have been lost on Robin Williams. He, as an alleged comic actor, had finally won an Oscar playing a straight role, while Jack Nicholson as a straight actor had won Best Actor for a comic role in *As Good As It Gets*.

Irony aside, it mattered not a jot. The camel had finally passed through the eye of the needle.

FILMOGRAPHY

Can I Do It . . . Till I Need Glasses? (1977)

Director I. Robert Levy; script supervisor Sandy King. Running time 72 mins.

Cast: Victor Dunlap, Moose Carlson, Walter Olkewicz, Joey Camen, Amy Kellog, **Robin Williams**

Williams filmed some sequences for this insipid sex revue after his success in *Mork and Mindy.* The film premièred without his contribution, which was added later.

Popeye (1980)

Director Robert Altman; producer Robert Evans; screenwriter Jules Pfeiffer. Running time 114 mins.

Cast: **Robin Williams (Popeye)**, Shelley Duvall, Ray Walston, Paul Dooley, Paul Smith, Linda Hunt

Robin Williams plays a latex-enhanced version of L. C. Segar's famous comic-strip sailor.

The World According to Garp (1982)

Director George Roy Hill; producers George Roy Hill, Robert L. Crawford; screenwriter Steve Tesich. Running time 136 mins.

Cast: **Robin Williams (T. S. Garp)**, Mary Beth Hurt, Glenn Close, John Lithgow, Hume Cronym, Jessica Tandy

Williams is the eponymous hero in John Irving's account of an unconventional young man and his remarkable mother.

The Survivors (1983)

Director Michael Ritchie; producer William Sackheim; screenwriter Michael Leeson. Running time 102 mins.

Cast: Walter Matthau, **Robin Williams (Donald Quinelle)**, Jerry Reed, James Wainwright, Kristen Vigard, John Goodman

Williams plays an insecure man who takes survivalist training to absurd levels after identifying a criminal.

Moscow on the Hudson (1984)

Director Paul Mazursky; producer Paul Mazursky; screenwriters Paul Mazursky, Leon Capetanos. Running time 115 mins.

Cast: **Robin Williams (Vladimir Ivanoff)**, Maria Conchita Alonso, Cleavant Derricks, Alejandro Rey, Savely Kramarov, Elya Baskin

Williams is a Russian musician who has to try to adapt to life in the United States after defecting in Bloomingdales.

The Best of Times (1986)

Director Roger Spottiswoode; producer Gordon Carroll; screenwriter Ron Shelton. Running time 104 mins.

Cast: **Robin Williams (Jack Dundee),** Kurt Russell, Pamela Reed, Holly Palance, Donald Moffat, Margaret Whitton, M. Emmet Walsh.

Williams is a mild-mannered bank manager whose life is frustrated by the memory of missing a big play in a football game 20 years previously.

Club Paradise (1986)

Director Harold Ramis; producer Michael Shamberg; screenplay by Brian Doyle-Murray, based on a story by Tom Leopold, Chris Miller III, Harold Ramis and Ed Roboto. Running time 104 mins.

Cast: **Robin Williams**, Peter O'Toole, Rick Moranis, Jimmy Cliff, Twiggy

Williams is a Chicago fireman who is persuaded to sink half his severance pay into a run-down Caribbean resort.

Seize the Day (1986)

Director Fielder Cook; producer Robert Geller; screenplay by Saul Bellow and Ronald Ribman, based on a story by Saul Bellow. Running time 93 mins.

Cast: **Robin Williams (Tommy Wilhelm)**, Joseph Wiseman, Jerry Stiller, Glenne Headley, Richard B. Shull, Tony Roberts

Williams' first genuinely dramatic performance as a salesman who seeks nothing more than the approval of his flint-hearted father.

Dear America: Letters Home from Vietnam (1987)

Director Bill Couturie; producers Bill Couturie, Thomas Bird; screenplay by Richard Dewhurst and Bill Couturie, based on the book *Dear America, Letters Home from Vietnam.* Running time 87 mins.

Voice cast includes narration from **Robin Williams**, Robert De Niro, Ellen Burstyn, Kathleen Turner, Michael J. Fox, Willem Dafoe and many others

Williams is one of many star names who contributed their voices to this intensely moving collection of letters from American soldiers in Vietnam to their loved ones at home.

Good Morning Vietnam (1987)

Director Barry Levinson; producers Mark Johnson, Larry Brezner, Ben Moses, Harry Benn; screenwriter Mitch Markowitz. Running time 120 mins.

Cast: **Robin Williams (Adrian Cronauer)**, Forest Whitaker, Tung Thanh Tran, Chintara Sukapatana, Bruno Kirby, Robert Wuhl, J. T. Walsh

Williams' breakthrough role as an Army radio disc jockey whose irreverent rantings make him a folk hero among the troops and a thorn in the side of his superiors.

The Adventures of Baron Munchausen (1989)

Director Terry Gilliam; producers Thomas Schuhly, Ray Cooper; screenplay by Charles McKeown and Terry Gilliam, based on the stories of Rudolph Erich Raspe. Running time 126 mins.

Cast: John Neville, Eric Idle, Oliver Reed, Charles McKeown, Bill Paterson, Uma Thurman, **Robin Williams (King of the Moon)**

Williams contributes a very funny but unbilled cameo in Gilliam's lavish interpretations of Raspe's flights of fantasy.

Dead Poets Society (1989)

Director Peter Weir; producers Steven M. Haft, Paul Junger Witt, Tony Thomas; screenwriter Tom Schulman. Running time 128 mins.

Cast: **Robin Williams (John Keating)**, Robert Sean Leonard, Ethan Hawke, Josh Charles, Kurtwood Smith

Williams plays an inspirational English teacher who encourages his impressionable young charges to 'carpe diem' – seize the day.

Awakenings (1990)

Director Penny Marshall; producers Walter Parkes, Larry Lasker; screenplay by Steve Zaillian, based on the novel by Oliver Sacks. Running time 121 mins.

Cast: **Robin Williams (Dr Malcolm Sayer)**, Robert De Niro, Julie Kavner, John Heard, Ruth Nelson, Penelope Ann Miller

Williams is a brilliant neurologist whose work with patients in a post-vegetative state enables them to have some semblance of a life.

Cadillac Man (1990)

Director Roger Donaldson; producers Charles Roven, Roger Donaldson; screenwriter Ken Friedman. Running time 97 mins.

Cast: **Robin Williams (Joey O'Brien)**, Tim Robbins, Pamela Reed, Fran Drescher, Zack Norman, Annabella Sciorra

Williams is a hustling car salesman who ends up negotiating for his life when a crazed gunman bursts into his showroom.

Dead Again (1991)

Director Kenneth Branagh; producers Lindsay Doran, Charles H. Maguire; screenwriter Scott Frank. Running time 107 mins.

Cast: Kenneth Branagh, Emma Thompson, Andy Garcia, **Robin Williams (Doctor Cozy Carlisle)**, Campbell Scott, Wayne Knight

Williams plays a cameo as a disbarred psychologist in Branagh's Hitchcockian mystery.

The Fisher King (1991)

Director Terry Gilliam; producers Debra Hill, Lynda Obst; screenwriter Richard La Gravenese. Running time 137 mins.

Cast: **Robin Williams (Parry)**, Jeff Bridges, Mercedes Ruehl, Amanda Plummer

Williams is a man driven to madness by the senseless killing of his wife.

Hook (1991)

Director Steven Spielberg; producers Kathleen Kennedy, Frank Marshall, Gerald R. Molen; screenplay by Jim V. Hart and Malia Scotch Marmo, based on the story by Hart and Nick Castle, adapted from the original stage play and books by Sir James M. Barrie. Running time 144 mins.

Cast: Dustin Hoffman, **Robin Williams (Peter Banning/Peter Pan)**, Julia Roberts, Bob Hoskins, Maggie Smith, Caroline Goodall

Williams is Peter Pan as a grown man who has lost his identity.

Shakes the Clown (1991)

Director Bobcat Goldthwait; producers Paul Colichman, Ann Luly-Goldthwait; screenwriter Bobcat Goldthwait. Running time 83 mins.

Cast: Bobcat Goldthwait, Julie Brown, Bruce Baum, Steve Bean, **Robin Williams (Mime Jerry)**

Williams makes an unbilled cameo as a mime teacher.

Aladdin (1992)

Directors John Musker, Ron Clements; producers John Musker, Ron Clements; screenwriters Ron Clements, John Musker, Ted Elliott, Terry Rossio. Running time 90 mins.

Cast (voices): Scott Weinger, **Robin Williams (Genie)**, Linda Larkin, Jonathan Freeman, Gilbert Gottfried

Williams is the voice of the genie in this animated adventure.

FernGully . . . The Last Rain Forest (1992)

Director Bill Kroyer; producers Wayne Young, Peter Faiman; screenplay by Jim Cox, based on the FernGully stories by Diana Young. Running time 76 mins.

Cast (voices): Tim Curry, Samantha Mathis, Christian Slater, Jonathan Ward, **Robin Williams (Batty Koda)**, Grace Zabriskie

Williams provides comic relief as a spaced-out bat in this ecological animated feature.

Toys (1992)

Director Barry Levinson; producers Barry Levinson, Mark Johnson; screenwriters Barry Levinson, Jane Curtin. Running time 121 mins.

Cast: **Robin Williams (Lesley Zevo)**, Michael Gambon, Joan Cusack, Robin Wright, LL Cool J, Donald O'Connor

Peaceable Williams tries to regain control of the family toy firm from his militaristic uncle.

Mrs Doubtfire (1993)

Director Chris Columbus; producers Marsha Garces Williams, Robin Williams, Mark Radcliffe; screenplay by Randi Mayem Singer and Lesley Dixon, based on the novel *Alias Madame Doubtfire* by Anne Fine. Running time 125 mins.

Cast: **Robin Williams (Daniel Hillard/Mrs Iphigenia Doubtfire)**, Sally Field, Pierce Brosnan, Harvey Fierstein, Polly Holliday

Williams is a struggling divorced actor who impersonates an elderly babysitter to see his kids.

Being Human (1993)

Director Bill Forsyth; producers David Puttnam, Robert F. Colesberry; screenwriter Bill Forsyth. Running time 122 mins.

Cast: **Robin Williams (Hector)**, Kelly Hunter, John Turturro, Anna Galiena, Vincent D'Onofrio

Williams plays five men named Hector in a story spanning 6000 years.

Jumanji (1995)

Director Joe Johnston; producers William Tietler, Scott Kroopf; screenwriters Jim Strain, Greg Taylor, Jonathan Hensleigh. Running time 104 mins.

Cast: **Robin Williams (Alan Parrish)**, Jonathan Hyde, Kirsten Dunst, Bradley Pierce, Bonnie Hunt

Williams is a small boy trapped in a board game who emerges as an adult 26 years later.

Nine Months (1995)

Director Chris Columbus; producers Ann Francois, Michael Barnathan, Mark Radcliffe; screenwriter Chris Columbus. Running time 103 mins.

Cast: Hugh Grant, Julianne Moore, Tom Arnold, Joan Cusack, Jeff Goldblum, **Robin Williams (Dr Kosevich)**

Williams contributes a short cameo as a Russian gynaecologist.

To Wong Foo, Thanks for Everything, Julie Newmar (1995)

Director Beeban Kidron; producer G. Mac Brown; screenwriter Douglas Carter Beane. Running time 109 mins.

Cast: Wesley Snipes, Patrick Swayze, John Leguizamo, Stockard Channing

Williams has a one-scene cameo as the owner of a gay night-club.

The Birdcage (1996)

Director Mike Nichols; producer Mike Nichols; screenwriter Elaine May. Running time 119 mins.

Cast: **Robin Williams (Armand Goldman)**, Gene Hackman, Nathan Lane, Dianne Wiest, Dan Futterman, Calista Flockhart, Hank Azaria

Williams is a gay but subdued night-club owner whose straight son is bringing his reactionary prospective in-laws to dinner.

Hamlet (1996)

Director Kenneth Branagh; producer David Barron; adapted screenplay by Kenneth Branagh, based on the play by William Shakespeare. Running time 238 mins.

Cast: Kenneth Branagh, Julie Christie, Derek Jacobi, Kate Winslet, Billy Crystal, **Robin Williams (Osric)**

Williams plays a courtier in this full-length adaptation of Shakespeare.

Jack (1996)

Director Francis Ford Coppola; producers Ricardo Mestres, Fred Fuchs, Francis Ford Coppola; screenwriters James De Monaco, Gary Nadeau. Running time 113 mins.

Cast: **Robin Williams (Jack Powell)**, Diane Lane, Brian Kerwin, Jennifer Lopez, Bill Cosby, Fran Drescher

Williams plays a boy who ages four times as fast as normal children.

Joseph Conrad's The Secret Agent (1996)

Director Christopher Hampton; producer Norma Heyman; screenplay by Christopher Hampton, based on Joseph Conrad's novel. Running time 95 mins.

Cast: Bob Hoskins, Patricia Arquette, Gérard Dépardieu, **Robin Williams (The Professor)**

Williams is billed as George Spelvin in his role as a sinister bomb-maker.

Father's Day (1997)

Director Ivan Reitman; producers Joel Silver, Ivan Reitman; screenplay by Lowell Ganz and Babaloo Mandel, based on the film *Les Compères* by Francis Veber. Running time 102 mins.

Cast: **Robin Williams (Dale Putney)**, Billy Crystal, Julia-Louis Dreyfuss, Nastassja Kinski, Bruce Greenwood

Williams plays one of two men searching for a missing boy each believes is his son.

Flubber (1997)

Director Les Mayfield; producers John Hughes, Ricardo Mestres; screenwriters John Hughes, Bill Hall. Running time 95 mins.

Cast: **Robin Williams (Professor Philip Brainard)**, Marcia Gay Harden, Christopher McDonald, Raymond J. Barry, Clancy Brown, Ted Levine, Wil Wheaton

Williams is an absent-minded scientist who invents a substance which defies gravity.

Good Will Hunting (1997)

Director Gus Van Sant; producer Lawrence Bender; screenwriters Matt Damon, Ben Affleck. Running time 126 mins.

Cast: **Robin Williams (Sean Maguire)**, Matt Damon, Ben Affleck, Stellan Skarsgaard, Minnie Driver, Casey Affleck

Williams is a therapist trying to help a troubled mathematical genius.

What Dreams May Come (1998)

Director Vincent Ward; producers Barnet Bain, Ronald Bass, Alan C. Blomquist, Stephen Simon, Ted Field, Erica Huggins, Scott Kroopf; screenwriter Ron Bass. Running time 113 mins.

Cast: **Robin Williams (Chris Nielsen)**, Annabella Sciorra, Cuba Gooding, Jr., Max von Sydow, Josh Paddock, Jessica Brooks Grant, Rosalind Chao

Williams is a man who has died and journeys from heaven to hell in search of his wife, who has committed suicide.

Patch Adams (1998)

Director Tom Shadyac; producers Allegra Clegg, Alan B. Curtis, Mike Farrell, Barry Kemp, Marvin Minoff, Devorah Moos-Hankin, Charles Newirth, Steve Oedekerk, Tom Shadyac, Marsha Garces Williams; screenwriters Patch Adams, Maureen Mylander, Steve Oedekerk. Running time 115 mins.

Cast: **Robin Williams (Patch Adams)**, Monica Potter, Daniel London, Philip Seymour Hoffman, Bob Gunton, Peter Coyote, Michael Jeter

Williams plays a medical student in the 70s who treats patients illegally, using humor.

Get Bruce (1999)

Director Andrew J. Kuehn; producers Joan Hyler, Andrew J. Kuehn, Susan B. Landau, Gregory McClatchy, Irwin M. Rappaport, Don Scotti. Running time 82 mins.

Cast: **Robin Williams (Himself)**, Bruce Vilanch, Bette Midler, Billy Crystal, Whoopi Goldberg, Lily Tomlin, Nathan Lane, Roseanne, Carol Burnett, Florence Henderson, Rosie O'Donnell

Williams plays himself in this documentary of comedian Bruce Vilanch.

Bicentennial Man (1999)

Director Chris Columbus; screenwriter Nicholas Kazan, based on a story by Isaac Asimov.

Cast: **Robin Williams (Andrew Martin)**, Embeth Davidtz, Sam Neill, Oliver Platt

Williams is an android with human emotions who tries to stop his creators from destroying him.

Jakob the Liar (1999)

Director Peter Kassovitz; producer Nick Gillott; screenwriter Peter Kassovitz.

Cast: **Robin Williams (Jakob Heym)**, Alan Arkin, Armin Mueller-Stahl, Liev Shreiber, Michael Jeter

Williams plays a Jewish café owner in World War II Poland who spreads false news in order to keep hope alive among the people.

BOX OFFICE

Robin Williams' films have grossed more than $1 billion at the American box-office. These are his top ten earners in the domestic market.

1. *Mrs Doubtfire*	1993	$219.2 million
2. *Aladdin*	1992	$217.4 million
3. *Good Will Hunting*	1997	$138.3 million*
4. *The Birdcage*	1996	$124.1 million
5. *Good Morning Vietnam*	1987	$123.9 million
6. *Hook*	1991	$119.7 million
7. *Jumanji*	1995	$100.4 million
8. *Dead Poets Society*	1989	$95.9 million
9. *Flubber*	1997	$92.9 million
10. *Nine Months*	1995	$69.7 million

**Good Will Hunting* was still on domestic release in the United States as at 1 August 1998.

AWARDS

Robin Williams has won awards in almost every sphere of entertainment. The only one to elude him so far is a Tony for a Broadway performance. Here are his other major honours.

1979
Golden Globe: Best Actor in a Comedy Series, *Mork and Mindy*
Grammy: Best Comedy Recording, *Reality . . . What a Concept*

1987
Emmy: Best Individual Performance in a Variety or Music Programme, *A Carol Burnett Special*
Golden Globe: Best Actor in a Comedy, *Good Morning Vietnam*
Grammy: Best Comedy Recording, *A Night at the Met*

1988
Emmy: Best Individual Performance in a Variety or Music Programme, *ABC Presents A Royal Gala*
Grammy: Best Comedy Recording, *Good Morning Vietnam*
Grammy: Best Recording for Children, *Pecos Bill*

1991
Golden Globe: Best Actor in a Comedy, *The Fisher King*

1992
Golden Globe: Special Achievement, *Aladdin*

1993
Golden Globe: Best Actor in a Comedy, *Mrs Doubtfire*

1998
Academy Award: Best Supporting Actor, *Good Will Hunting*
Screen Actors Guild: Best Supporting Actor, *Good Will Hunting*

SOURCES

I Love You in Blue

Playboy October 1982; *San Francisco Chronicle* 19 October 1987; *Esquire* June 1989; *New York Times* 11 November 1990; *Playboy* January 1992; *New York* 22 November 1993

David Halberstam: *The Fifties* Fawcett Columbine 1998

School Daze

Author's interviews with Robin Williams, January 1988 and February 1996; US press junket for *Jack* 1996

Playboy October 1982; *San Francisco Chronicle* 19 October 1987; *New York* 22 November 1993

In Old Tiburon

Author's interview with Robin Williams, January 1988

Playboy October 1982; *New York Times* 11 November 1990; *Playboy* January 1992; *New York* 11 November 1993

It's a Helluva Town

Author's interview with Robin Williams, January 1988

Harpers magazine February 1979; *Playboy* October 1982; *Premiere* January 1988; *New York Times* 11 November 1990; *Playboy* January 1992

Damaged but Interesting

Siobhan Synnot interview with Robin Williams, February 1998

Playboy October 1982; *Premiere* January 1988; *New York Times* 11 November 1990; *Los Angeles Times* 8 December 1991

Christopher Reeve: *Still Me* Random House 1998

Fly Like an Eagle

Author's interview with Robin Williams, January 1998

Rolling Stone August 1979; *Playboy* October 1982; *Premiere* January 1988; *New York Times* 11 November 1990; *New York Newsday* 24 September 1991; *Playboy* January 1992; *Esquire* November 1993

Mary Ellen Moore: *The Robin Williams Scrapbook* Tempo 1979

Sock it to Me
Rolling Stone August 1979; *Playboy* October 1982; *New York* 11 November 1993
People Entertainment Almanac 1988
Alex McNeil: *Total Television* Penguin 1996

My Favourite Orkan
Author's interview with Robin Williams, January 1988
Playboy October 1982; *Premiere* January 1988; *New York* 22 November 1993
Mary Ellen Moore: *The Robin Williams Scrapbook* Tempo 1979
People Entertainment Almanac 1988
Alex McNeil: *Total Television* Penguin 1996

Nanoo, Nanoo
Author's interview with Robin Williams, January 1988
Playboy October 1982
Mary Ellen Moore: *The Robin Williams Scrapbook* Tempo 1979
Alex McNeil: *Total Television* Penguin 1996
Mork and Mindy pilot episode viewed at the Museum of Television and Radio, New York

'Mork, Robin . . . Robin, Mork'
Author's interview with Robin Williams, January 1988
Playgirl March 1979; *Rolling Stone* September 1982; *Playboy* October 1982; *New York* 22 November 1993
People Entertainment Almanac 1988
'Mork Meets Robin Williams': *Mork and Mindy, Vol. 4* Paramount Video

I Yam What I Yam
Author's interview with Robin Williams, January 1988; Siobhan Synnot interview with Robin Williams, February 1998
Rolling Stone August 1979; *Rolling Stone* September 1982; *Playboy* October 1982; *Rolling Stone* February 1988; *New York Times* 11 November 1990
Peter Biskind: *Easy Riders, Raging Bulls* Simon & Schuster 1998

The Midas Curse
Author's interview with Robin Williams, January 1988
Playgirl March 1979; *Rolling Stone* September 1982; *Playboy* October 1982; *Rolling Stone* February 1988; *Los Angeles Times* 8 December 1991; *New York* 22 November 1993

Consequences

Author's interview with Addison Arce, July 1995
Rolling Stone September 1982; *Playboy* October 1982; *Rolling Stone* February 1988; *New York* 22 November 1993

Beautiful Boy

Playboy October 1982; *Rolling Stone* February 1988; *New York Times* 11 November 1990; *Playboy* January 1992; *New Yorker* September 1993; *New York* 22 November 1993

Enter Marsha

Rolling Stone February 1988; *People* 22 February 1988; *Redbook* January 1991; *Rolling Stone* February 1991; *Playboy* January 1992; *New Yorker* September 1993; *New York* 22 November 1993; *Cosmopolitan* April 1994

Growing Up

Author's interview with Robin Williams, January 1988
Rolling Stone February 1988; *People* 22 February 1988; *Esquire* June 1989; *Redbook* January 1991; *Rolling Stone* February 1991; *Playboy* January 1992; *New Yorker* September 1993; *New York* 22 November 1993

'Goood Mooorning Heraklion!'

Author's interview with Adrian Cronauer, February 1998
Premiere January 1988

From the Delta to the DMZ

Author's interview with Robin Williams, January 1988; author's interview with Adrian Cronauer, February 1998
Premiere January 1988; *People* 22 February 1988; *New York* 22 November 1993
Levinson on Levinson Faber & Faber 1992

A Death in the Family

San Francisco Chronicle 19 October 1987; *Rolling Stone* February 1988; *Playboy* January 1992

Waitin'

Author's interview with Robin Williams, January 1988; Siobhan Synnot interview with Robin Williams, February 1998
New York Post 12 December 1988; *New York Newsday* 24 September 1991; *Playboy* January 1992
Anthony Holden: *The Oscars* Little, Brown 1993
John Harkness: *The Academy Awards Handbook* Pinnacle 1997

Waiting for Godot, viewed at the Museum for the Performing Arts, New York

Dances with Lepers
Rolling Stone February 1988; *People* 22 February 1988; *Esquire* June 1989; *Playboy* January 1992

Oh Captain, My Captain
San Francisco Chronicle 27 April, 8 June, 10 October (all 1988); *Rolling Stone* February 1988; *New York Times* 11 November 1990; *Playboy* January 1992
Nancy Griffin and Kim Masters: *Hit and Run* Touchstone 1986

A Little Spark of Madness
Author's interview with Dan Holzman, March 1998; author's interview with Barry Friedman, March 1998
Esquire June 1989; *Playboy* January 1992; *Premiere* January 1990
Robin Williams: Off the Wall, viewed on Comedy Central 24 March 1998
An Evening with Robin Williams CIC Video
An Evening at the Met Vestron Video

Do You Take This Woman
Life 10 April 1989; *Esquire* June 1989; *People* 12 August 1991; *New York Newsday* 24 September 1991; *Redbook* January 1991; *Los Angeles Times* 8 December 1991; *New Yorker* September 1993
Anthony Holden: *The Oscars* Little, Brown 1993
John Harkness: *The Academy Awards Handbook* Pinnacle 1997

The Thief of Bad Gags?
Author's interview with Oliver Sacks, February 1991; Siobhan Synnot interview with Robin Williams, February 1998
Premiere January 1988; *Time* 21 May 1990; *New York Times* 11 November 1990; *Premiere* January 1991; *Rolling Stone* February 1991; *Playboy* January 1992

A Chink in the Armour
Author's interview with Robin Williams, February 1996
New York Times 11 November 1990; *New York Newsday* 24 September 1991; *San Francisco Chronicle* 10 September 1991; *San Francisco Chronicle* 8 November 1991; *Playboy* January 1992; *San Francisco Chronicle* 22 February 1992; *San Francisco Chronicle* 30 July 1992; *New York Daily News* 31 July 1992

Think Happy Thoughts

Author's interview with Robin Williams, February 1992; author's interview with Dustin Hoffman, February 1992

Daily Variety 7 August 1990; *Variety* 15 August 1990; *Daily Variety* 2 February 1991; *Variety* 18 February 1991; *Daily Variety* 9 June 1991; *Daily Variety* 16 June 1991; *Variety* 29 July 1991; *Daily Variety* 13 December 1991; *Daily Variety* 16 December 1991; *Variety* 23 December 1991; *Los Angeles Times* 8 December 1991; *People* 23 December 1991; *Playboy* January 1992; *Daily Variety* 1 December 1992; *New York* 22 November 1993

The Genius of the Lamp

Author's interview with Robin Williams, February 1992; author's interview with Robin Williams, February 1996; Siobhan Synnot interview with Robin Williams, February 1998

Premiere December 1988; *Premiere* December 1992; *New York* 22 November 1993; *Variety* 12 September 1994; *TV Guide* 16 December 1996; *Screen International* 12 December 1997

Anthony Holden: *The Oscars* Little, Brown 1993

John Harkness: *The Academy Awards Handbook* Pinnacle 1997

Levinson on Levinson Faber & Faber 1992

There's No Face like Foam

Author's interview with Robin Williams, January 1994; author's interview with Chris Columbus, January 1994; Siobhan Synnot interview with Chris Columbus, January 1994

New Yorker September 1993; *New York Newsday* 21 November 1993; *Los Angeles Times* 22 November 1993; *New York* 22 November 1993; *St Louis Post-Dispatch* 8 December 1993; *Screen International* 12 December 1997

Riddle Me This

Author's interview with Robin Williams, January 1994 and February 1996

Entertainment Weekly 1 October 1993; *Los Angeles Times* 21 November 1993; *Entertainment Weekly* 3 June 1994; *People* 23 May 1994; *USA Today* 8 June 1994

David Frost Interview (May 1991), viewed at the Museum of Television and Radio, New York

A Friend in Deed

Author's interview with Robin Williams, February 1996 and May 1997

New York 22 November 1993; *People* 30 October 1995; *USA Today* 3 February 1998

Christopher Reeve: *Still Me* Random House 1998

The Lost Boy

Author's interview with Robin Williams, February 1996; US junket for *Jack* 1996

Playboy January 1992; *USA Weekend* 3 March 1996; *TV Guide* 16 December 1996

Free at Last

US junket for *Father's Day* May 1997; US junket for *Flubber* November 1997; Siobhan Synnot interview with Robin Williams, February 1998

TV Guide 16 December 1996; *Forbes* 22 September 1997; *Los Angeles Times* 21 November 1993; AP news wire, 3 December 1997

Let's See Some I.D.

Author's interview with Robin Williams, February 1996 and May 1997; Siobhan Synnot interview with Robin Williams, February 1998; Alison Maloney interview with Gus Van Sant, March 1998

Matt Damon & Ben Affleck: *Good Will Hunting* Miramax Books 1997

And the Winner Is . . .

Siobhan Synnot interview with Robin Williams, February 1998

AP news wire, 9 March 1998; AP, Reuters news wires, 24 March 1998

Oscar telecast, 24 March 1998

INDEX

TEACHING TECHNICAL COMMUNICATION

TEACHING TECHNICAL COMMUNICATION

Critical Issues for the Classroom

EDITED BY

James M. Dubinsky
Virginia Tech

BEDFORD / ST. MARTIN'S Boston • New York

For Bedford / St. Martin's

Executive Editor: Leasa Burton
Executive Assistant: Brita Mess
Associate Editor, Publishing Services: Maria Teresa Burwell
Senior Production Supervisor: Joe Ford
Production Associate: Christie Gross
Project Management: DeMasi Design and Publishing Services
Text Design: Anna George
Cover Design: Donna Dennison
Composition: Macmillan India Limited
Printing and Binding: Haddon Craftsmen, an RR Donnelley & Sons Company

President: Joan E. Feinberg
Editorial Director: Denise B. Wydra
Editor in Chief: Karen S. Henry
Director of Marketing: Karen Melton Soeltz
Director of Editing, Design, and Production: Marcia Cohen
Manager, Publishing Services: Emily Berleth

Library of Congress Control Number: 2003115622

Manufactured in the United States of America.

9 8 7 6 5 4
f e d c b a

For information, write: Bedford / St. Martin's, 75 Arlington Street, Boston, MA 02116 (617-399-4000)

ISBN: 0-312-41204-5

The author extends special thanks to the reviewers who contributed valuable advice during the development of this project: Robert R. Johnson, Carolyn Plumb, Gerald J. Savage, Charlotte Thralls, and Thomas Warren.

Acknowledgments
Acknowledgments and copyrights appear at the back of the book on pages 627–628 which constitute an extension of the copyright page. It is a violation of the law to reproduce these selections by any means whatsoever without the written permission of the copyright holder.

PREFACE

The field of technical communication is growing. For evidence, one need only look at the number of undergraduate and graduate programs or the number of journals in the field that exist today in comparison with the number of programs or journals in existence twenty years ago. The field is also changing. What once was a field rooted almost exclusively in engineering education is rapidly becoming a field linked to such diverse areas as human-computer interaction, business information systems, and management.

Teaching students about a field this broad is no easy task because it requires a breadth of knowledge that is truly interdisciplinary. *Teaching Technical Communication: Critical Issues for the Classroom* has two goals: to introduce prospective teachers to the diverse, interdisciplinary field of technical communication and to give these teachers an overview of the art of teaching in this field. To accomplish those goals, this book collects and organizes articles about some of the critical issues that are shaping the field, issues as diverse as history, gender and intercultural communication, ethics, and working in online environments. Some of these issues result from the interdisciplinary nature of our field, and some are deeply embedded in the history of teaching language use. Each chapter focuses on an issue that has emerged over the past several decades as technical communication has grown as a discipline.

The book begins with an essay that offers an introduction to and a rationale for the concept of reflective practice. As reflective practitioners, teachers can adapt to our rapidly changing field and meet a diverse student body's needs. Following the introduction are eight chapters and an annotated bibliography. In chapter 1, "Introducing Theoretical Approaches," the focus is on a debate about humanism, rhetoric, and technical communication that has been ongoing for nearly twenty-five years, ever since the publication of Carolyn Miller's seminal article "A Humanistic Rationale for Technical Writing." This debate about finding a balance between pragmatic and humanistic concerns informs much of the work in our field as we seek to define ourselves and resist being pushed into binaries (e.g., theory and practice). Chapter 2, "Constructing a History of the Field," attempts to define and contextualize our field. We have a rich history, one that has roots in both classical rhetoric and in the very pragmatic concern of teaching engineers how to communicate their disciplinary knowledge effectively. Knowing about our history helps us to recognize the character of our discipline and its roots. Understanding, for instance, what happened in technical writing classrooms in the past and why can enable us to make informed pedagogical decisions about the present and future. Chapter 3, "Laying a Foundation for Ethical Praxis," expands upon some of the issues emerging from the debate in chapter 1, such as the social responsibilities associated with technical communication, issues linked to historical and philosophical concerns that have become embedded in the kinds of work we do as rhetoricians. In this chapter, questions about *what should be* in terms of human relations and such specific issues as communicating in networked environments are highlighted.

The next two chapters shift the emphasis from foundational and historical material to issues relating to the actual practice of technical communication. Chapter 4, "Following User-Centered Design Practices" and chapter 5, "Learning on the Job," offer an overview of the importance not only of understanding the writing process, which includes consideration of readers/users of the material, but also of understanding the importance of the situational contexts in which writing is produced. Chapter 4 addresses a variety of essential issues involving design practices, from the microscopic (looking at page design) to the macroscopic (thinking about the nature of involving readers in the design/writing process from concept to final production). The emphasis is on developing a mindset that highlights people and problem solving. In chapter 5, the focus is on recognizing the fact that there are few universals, that much of what we do in our field is contextual and situated. Thinking about genre, for instance, as a means to learn social dynamics (e.g., writers' roles and community values), will enable students to create more usable products. As teachers of technical communication, we need to understand the differences between our field and others in academe. Our students need to know that their audiences will use the materials they produce, and as a result, as writers, they need to be much more aware of the specific backgrounds and needs of their readers/users. In addition, because each organizational situation may be different, they will need to realize the constraints of style and genre. Simply put, our students need to learn *how to learn* and how to adapt what they learn to meet the many, diverse communication challenges they'll face.

These communication challenges include the ability to adapt to a changing workplace, one that is becoming more diverse in terms of both gender and nationality, and to changing technologies that influence the ways and places in which work is done. Chapter 6, "Working within and across Cultures," focuses on both gender and international/intercultural issues. Several of the articles provide an overview of the value of a feminist research perspective for both teachers and practitioners, and the others open up the discussion of how varying perspectives resulting from different cultural or national backgrounds can affect the ways in which material is learned and used. In chapter 7, "Writing and Working in Digital Environments," the articles offer various perspectives on learning, working, and teaching in online environments. Issues addressed include why, given the emphasis on technology in the workplace, teachers need to understand and think critically about technology, as well as its role in shaping values (individual and societal), and then apply that understanding to course and program design. As teachers of technical communication, we need to consider the ways that working in these environments affects the ways in which our students will collaborate, organize and present information, and (re)define their job responsibilities. Laying a foundation for working and collaborating in these environments will truly prepare our students for their future tasks.

Finally, the last section helps to orient teachers toward the future, while also grounding them in the specific issues they will face in their classrooms. Chapter 8, "Looking to the Future," offers insights from some of the field's influential scholars and teachers into the new directions we may be heading, while simultaneously offering some very practical advice for teachers who have to deal with those changes. The annotated bibliography is a list of pedagogical resources that emphasize classroom practices more explicitly. These references may be useful as teachers look for guidance in order to design and teach specific genres or assignments such as the résumé or the proposal, gain insight into topics common to writing classes (e.g., peer review, collaborative assignments), and reflect upon one of the most difficult tasks a writing teacher faces: evaluation.

Each section has a short introduction that outlines the key issues addressed, several articles that represent an overview of the issues, and a list of additional resources for further study. Among the articles, in order to demonstrate the Möbius loop of theory and practice, there is an article (and in one case two) that falls under what many in the field call applied theory. These articles, often taken from *Technical Communication*, one of the field's main journals, which is published by the Society for Technical Communication, are often written by and for practitioners. In addition, because ours is a pedagogical field, many of the articles in each section will have a pedagogical approach or at least offer some pedagogical strategies, highlighting the recursive nature of our field.

My hope is that this collection of essays, introductions, and suggested readings will give new teachers a lay of the land, so to speak. In addition, I hope that it will offer experienced teachers a way of organizing the various issues in the field, or, at a minimum, give them a framework that they can use to reshape their sense of the field's geography. The field of technical communication is rich and exciting, and teaching in it is both challenging and rewarding. This collection is not meant to be didactic or limiting in any way; rather, my goal is to open up avenues for exploration into the critical issues of our field so that, as teachers, you may prepare the students you teach to meet the many tasks they'll face now and in the future.

James M. Dubinsky

CONTENTS

INTRODUCTION

Becoming User-Centered, Reflective Practitioners

JAMES M. DUBINSKY

The morning of August 21, 1986 promised to be very hot. I was up early, at 0530, to jog and get ready for the drive over Storm King Mountain to teach my first college class. My destination was a classroom in Thayer Hall, a magnificent old stone building that had once been the largest riding hall in the world, containing the stables for cavalry soldiers stationed at this prestigious fort along the Hudson River known as West Point. I wanted to get in the classroom early, knowing the students would show up promptly at 0730.

Since completing my first graduate degree and moving with my family from California to New York, I had spent two months preparing for the first-year composition class, reading all of the essays I would teach as models, studying the syllabus, which asked the students to write nine assignments resulting in five completed essays, and talking to new and experienced faculty. But even with that preparation, I was nervous; I didn't know what to expect, having never taught writing before. The only classrooms I had worked in during the previous nine years were located in tracked vehicles, as soldiers working for me prepared to fire ninety-seven pounds of steel at targets six to twelve miles away; in staging areas or headquarters' buildings and tents, as we prepared to deploy to our next position; or in motor pools, as we stood in front of (or more often crawled under) vehicles that weren't working properly. In these "classrooms," I had worked with many men and women from varied backgrounds and socioeconomic situations; I knew they liked to talk given a chance, and I had discovered that if they felt they had a say in the matter at hand, they were more likely to respond and learn. I also learned that they had a lot to teach me, if I would listen.

As I stood in the front of the room, with Annie Dillard's words on the board behind me ("Seeing is of course very much a matter of verbalization. Unless I call my attention to what passes before my eyes, I simply won't see it" [30]), I watched as young men and women in crisp gray uniforms marched in quickly and silently and performed something known in the vernacular of West Point as "taking seats." Thus, we began. To their and my relief, the formalities, although never absent, faded quickly as I asked them to talk to me about what they had learned during the past ten weeks of their introductory military training and initiation, affectionately known at West Point as "Beast Barracks." And talk they did. That first day of class, even though we didn't actually discuss the material, proved to be important in establishing a context for future discussions as well as for building a classroom community. Much happened in class, and I tried to be attentive to it. After class, and after sharing some "opening day" stories with other new instructors, I thought about what had happened, and realized that something valuable had occurred in my class that I might want to remember, something about learning from students, about studying not only the material but also the context of teaching, seemed to be important to a class devoted to writing about ways of seeing and of knowing. I made some notes in the journal I kept.

Two days later, the department chair, Colonel Capps, came in to observe my 0730 class, unannounced. We were discussing Annie Dillard's essay "Seeing." The cadets were struggling with the essay. But realizing that the Colonel was in the room, they perked up and seemed to try even harder. Even with that extra effort, the discussion seemed rather lackluster, particularly when I compared it with their efforts the class before. Most of the students found Dillard fascinating, but they had a hard time finding connections to their own life or to their writing. Watching them struggle reminded me of the stories Dillard tells in the essay of the newly sighted, patients who had cataract operations that restored their sight. These patients often found the "tremendous size of the world" overwhelming (27).

I tried several strategies, including making connections between events in my life, such as watching my young children grow, learn to see, and articulate what they saw. I tried introducing a few poems, including Robert Frost's "Design," into the discussion. I asked the students to talk about walks in the woods or staring up at stars at night, activities Dillard discussed. Nothing worked well.

Afterward, when speaking with Colonel Capps in his office, I had a chance to talk about the class. He was positive about the class and my efforts, and I shared with him my concerns. We talked about ways to help students use the essays we were reading and wondered whether or not such professional models were the most effective means of teaching writing. We didn't reach any conclusive answers, but just talking about these issues seemed to help me as I struggled to make sense of what was going on inside my classrooms, as I wrestled with questions familiar to many writing teachers: Should you use models from professional writers? How explicit should you be when faced with confusion or what seems to be a lack of understanding? Should you resort to lecture when the dialogic, Socratic method seems to be stagnating?

I didn't know it at the time, but I was very lucky. As I talked with Colonel Capps, I was learning about teaching in ways that continue to serve me well today. In that classroom and afterward in Colonel Capps's office, I learned the importance of valuing my students' experiences, of creating a dialogic and democratic classroom, and of teacher talk, of trusting a person who due to "his long acquaintance with [his] subject [has] a right to judge" (Newman, qtd. in Dunne 35). Donald Schön calls what I was beginning to do "reflective practice": the practice of teachers proposing and investigating problems themselves (1983, *Reflective Practioner*).

Colonel Capps, a veteran teacher, obviously believed that teachers could learn about teaching and become more effective in the classroom. Not everyone shares his belief. In *The Vocation of a Teacher*, Wayne Booth describes an encounter with a recent winner of the Quantrell Prize for Undergraduate Teaching at the University of Chicago. The teacher, roused by a poster that advertised a presentation about "The Student as Text," said to Booth, "You know and I know that all that stuff is crap. Nothing is really known about how to teach well; the most that could be known would be how to make students like the class and the professor and thus believe, probably erroneously, that they have been taught something worth learning." As Booth, a teacher who believes in the value of reflective practice, continues the story, he adds that he asked another colleague to explain "what is really *known* about teaching," and the colleague said, "'Not much! . . . There's really not a lot of hard knowledge to report'" (209).

There may not be much "hard knowledge to report," and perhaps little or nothing is known, but it's odd and even a bit unsettling to hear college teachers, especially those who win teaching awards, make such assertions or hesitate to make pronouncements about teaching. My guess is the reason lies within: although they may know their content area well, few have ever taken a formal seminar on teaching or reflected upon their teaching (Eble; Allen et al.; Grossman). As Gilbert Highet said, "most people are clumsy at learning and teaching, not because they are stupid, but because they have not thought about it" (5).

The Möbius Loop, Reflective Practice, and Technical Communication

Assertions such as the one Booth's colleague made are anathema to those of us who teach technical communication. Ours, much like the field of composition studies, is a pedagogical discipline. We focus on ways language can be used to create meaning and effect change. To understand the complexity of our task, which involves an understanding of both language and strategies of use, I propose that the teaching of writing be refigured as an "art," a *technê* in which the form/content dichotomy becomes a Möbius loop. In such a loop, which is continuous and turning constantly on itself, theory becomes practice, and teaching becomes research. Refigured in this way, teachers shift from an instrumental approach to teaching, focusing on forms and genres, toward a rhetorical approach that explores how these forms and genres are adapted and appropriated by specific discourse communities to fit specific situations. By so doing, we can recognize not only the complexity of our discipline but also the knowledge-generating element of teaching and the fact that because what we do is so intimately tied up with how we do it, we benefit from studying and reflecting on our teaching. This work will help us become graceful teachers who reflect on and think about our work.

Few of us, even those very qualified ones who may even have been technical writers, come to the field with prior teacher training. Although some of us may be born teachers, most of us aren't. Those who aren't can, however, become more effective and learn our art by working with other teachers, those whom Aristotle calls master-craftsmen. As Kenneth Eble says, "teaching skill is not so much taught as it is nurtured into existence" (154). By working with others, what I've called *researching with teachers* (Dubinsky), and working collaboratively with our students, we can learn more than "how to" teach. Through dialogue, observation, and practice with those who have gathered an implicit knowledge over time, we can begin to acquire "know-how." This work would augment a course in methods or theories of teaching writing that you may be taking.

As we are nurtured and learn to think about our teaching, we begin to understand the methods by which we can become *user-centered, reflective practitioners*, a term I use to describe competent, knowledgeable practitioners (Dubinsky). Linking teaching and reflection is not something new, but it is critical to success in the classroom. Reflection, in terms of judgment and forethought, has long been associated with the concept of pedagogy, which, etymologically, is linked to the study or practice of guiding or rearing children (van Manen). Dewey, building on the notion of forethought, explained that reflective teaching "enables us to know what we are about when we act. . . . convert[ing] action that is merely appetitive, blind, and impulsive into intelligent action" (211, *Selected Writings*). He recognized, however, that reflective thought does not occur naturally; it involves an attitude and a method consisting of steps, which usually begin with "perplexity, confusion, or doubt," move through "conjectural anticipation" into "examination . . . exploration, [and] analysis," and, after clarifying the problem and tentative suggestions, concludes with "a plan of action" (1973, 494–506).

Embedded in this attitude is the importance of being aware of the theories behind your practice and taking the time to observe and reflect upon the practice of those theories. Through study and practice, we learn that teaching is more than a "technology that can be mastered; it is an art, and the artist is the researcher *par excellence*" (Rudduck and Hopkins 60). At that point, we occupy the Möbius loop of theory and praxis, and become graceful, reflective craftspersons who are mastering the *technê* of teaching.

Technê and Praxis

Teaching is both a making (*technê*) and a doing (*praxis*), concepts with roots in classical rhetoric. For many teachers and scholars in our field, classical rhetoric, which once was at the center of pedagogy in our country (Halloran), has again become central to our work because of its emphasis on the connection between the effective use of language and the public good. Because technical communicators work in the public forum in areas such as business, industry, and government, the work they do has a hand in shaping the affairs of human society. Thus, to prepare our students for the responsibilities they will face, we need to teach them not only to create good arguments and well-thought-through discourse, but also to consider the difference between "what is" and "what ought to be" (Whitburn). Our work involves more than teaching our students strategies or forms; it also involves asking them to consider the impact of those strategies and forms on public policy. We teach them to become user-centered practitioners, to take their audience and its needs into consideration always.

Aristotle was one of the first scholars and teachers to attempt to create a logical framework to explain rhetoric and its uses. For him, *technê* was an intellectual or rational state that was concerned with making, and to be an artist, he believed you must reflect upon your work by studying (*theorein*) how something is made. The interesting distinction he makes is that the end (*telos*) of productive knowledge (*technê*) is not in the product itself, but in the use of that product by the user (Johnson; Atwill). Therefore, the best judges of the *making* are not the makers but the users. As Aristotle said in his *Politics*, "There are some arts whose products are not judged of solely, or best, by the artists themselves . . . for example, the knowledge of the house is not limited to the builder only; the user, in other words, the master, of the house will actually be a better judge than the builder, just as the pilot will judge better of a rudder than the carpenter, and the guest will judge better of a feast than the cook" (*Politics* iii, 11, 1282a, 18–24).

This idea presents two difficulties for teachers. The first is that what we *make* isn't something tangible. What we *make* is an environment rich with possibility and ideas that we hope will lead to an awakening, a change, or some growth in the students themselves. The students may be the best judges of that awakening, change, or growth because they are the ones who will *use* what we have *made*. Unfortunately, we can't always *see* the change; we can't easily gauge the quality of our work. There is no way to *test* it consistently or effectively (although many have and continue to try). We, therefore, need to rely upon the users.

The second problem is that much of what we, as teachers, do is often directed toward some social goal relating to the function of education or the students' role(s) in society, which puts our work in a permeable zone that combines both *technê* and *phronesis* (the virtue of moral life that allows and enhances the prospects for ethical character). Joseph Dunne argues that for the kinds of fields that involve a "shifting field of forces" (315), where the material is not stable (as is woodcraft) but human, then what the artist must deploy is a "'phronetic' technê, i.e., one whose responsiveness to the situation is not fully specifiable in advance and which is experiential, charged with perceptiveness, and rooted in the sensory and emotional life" (355).

If we accept these conditions, then our art, the teaching work we do on a daily basis, becomes a matter of conduct. The questions or dilemmas we face concern *whose good* and *for what end*, and the teacher's ethos or character is always in the forefront (whether explicitly or implicitly).

These dilemmas or problems are quite real and often profound. There is a difference between the end a student may desire and one the teacher may seek. Because we are limited and our material and context are constantly changing and indeterminate, we can't *know* for certain what is best. Therefore, to achieve an end that can be evaluated by the user, we need to depend upon a clear knowledge of our students, which is usually achieved over time via reflection and dialogue with others (both other teachers and the users who will use that which we produce) to achieve an end that is good for them.

Learning from Stories

Maxine Greene has said, "The sounds of storytelling are everywhere" (ix). One reason is that storytelling helps human actions become intelligible by providing a means for people to negotiate their personal experiences. Such negotiations are important because experience is "the process by which, for all social beings, subjectivity is constructed" (de Laurentis), and this construction happens, whether we like it or not, in our own classes. We could ignore it, but by not doing so, by making it public, we can begin to deal with the vicissitudes of human intentions (Bruner, qtd. in Witherell and Noddings 3)—and, by dealing with those intentions, we can begin to come to terms with consequences resulting from those intentions. Dealing with the concepts of intentions and consequences is especially important in a narrative in which the author wants to acknowledge his goals openly.

To examine this notion of intentions and consequences, illustrate what it means to learn from and with someone, and emphasize how important it is for teachers to be aware of their students' needs, I would like to examine a story about learning and teaching from *Taran Wanderer*, a book in a series by Lloyd Alexander that I read to my children when I returned again to graduate school, after teaching at West Point, to learn to become a teacher in our field. Near the end of the book, Taran, who has been raised by a foster father, goes off in search of his identity, hoping to find knowledge of his parents and birthright. As he does, he apprentices at a series of different professions: blacksmith, weaver, and potter. What he learns is essential both to how he sees himself and to my discussion of *technê*, teaching, and learning.

Taran's first encounter is with the blacksmith, Hevydd. He greets him by calling out, "Master Smith . . . I am called Taran the Wanderer and journey seeking a craft to help me earn my bread. I know a little of your art and ask you to teach me more" (221). The smith is reluctant to help at first, but Taran persists and is given a chance. After an initial trial, the smith claims, "of the art, indeed, you know little. And yet . . . you have the sense of it" (223). He takes Taran on as an apprentice due to his possessing that "sense."

What happens next is important. Taran isn't put to work making a sword (his goal) immediately; instead he must learn the materials of the craft: the forge, with its roaring fire, the bars of metal, the hammer, and the anvil. The two work side by side, and after many ill-fated tries, Taran ultimately produces "a blade worth bearing" (226). However, he is not happy, claiming that he has learned that he is not a swordsmith (a master craftsperson). Hevydd's response illustrates a key point about the idea of teachability. He says: "How then! . . . You've the makings of an honest swordsmith, as good as any in Prydain" (227). What he tells Taran is that the art of swordsmithing *can be taught and learned*. It may be true that Taran may not be a natural artist, born to the craft. But, he can be "as good as any" *if* he continues to work at it.

In this example, Taran is able to achieve a relative mastery by learning the materials, practicing his skills, and testing them, while in a dialogic relationship with the master craftspeople. He achieves a measure of success because he studied, reflected, and dialogued with the masters of the individual crafts. At the same time, he also learns that what he was working toward couldn't be mastered and set into stone, so that if one followed a set of prescriptions, the result would always be the same. One must be flexible, willing to learn as the situations change.

Taran's teacher also demonstrates his skill of teaching. In each instance, the master takes time to talk with and listen to the young apprentice. Hevydd gives Taran a chance *because* he took the time to learn enough about him to recognize that he had "the sense of it." He studies his student, reflects on his abilities, and sets up a program of study to develop that "sense" into an art. That study involved another important step in the process: reflection. Joseph Dunne argues that "in being initiated into the practice of teaching, student-teachers need not only experience in the classroom but also the right conditions for reflecting on this experience—so that reflectiveness (which we have all the time been clarifying under the name 'phronesis') can become more and more an abiding attitude or disposition. . . . The main aim of 'educational studies' should be to contribute to the development of this disposition" (369).

Integrating Theory and Practice

Isocrates, speaking about teaching rhetoric, says, "For ability, whether in speech or in any other activity, is found in those who are well endowed by nature and have been schooled by practical experience. Formal training makes men more skillful and more resourceful in discovering the possibilities of a subject; for it teaches them to take from a readier source the topics which they otherwise hit upon in haphazard fashion" (48). Isocrates recognized that there are those who are naturally talented and who will succeed without much help, but he argued that "formal training makes men more skillful," *even if* they are naturally talented. This training is what leads to knowledge of the skill, for it helps one to think about it, which for Aristotle was a critical component of *technê*.

To become reflective practitioners who create knowledge, we have to learn about the art of teaching, which means understanding the concept of *know-how* and becoming aware of the theories we subscribe to and embed in our practice. Then by instituting changes that reflect the classical roots of rhetoric we draw from, we can become *technitai* and create a discipline devoted to dialogic practice.

Teachers Must Also Learn

I use the title of an article by Charles Gragg as the section heading to emphasize that just as there is a theory/practice binary we need to overcome, there is also a teaching/learning binary. Teachers who believe they have mastered a subject thoroughly will often become complacent about opening doors to new ideas or theories. This complacency is detrimental to developing a *technê of teaching*. Because, as Gragg says, "teaching is a social act," (15) it necessarily involves fostering relationships among people, and to successfully create such relationships, one must adopt an attitude of openness, of collaboration with our students and with other teachers (Comeaux; Dubinsky). We saw such an attitude in both Taran and Hevydd, and we need to develop it in ourselves and our students.

This book is designed to help you learn about the discipline by gaining an understanding of the critical issues those in the field face. My hope is that it will help you become more informed, more receptive to change, and more inclined toward reflection. One needs to understand that most situations are uncertain, unique, and require space for what Donald Schön calls "reflection-in-action." While the connection between "reflection" and "self-critical enquiry" may seem evident and while the two terms are often used interchangeably, there is an important distinction highlighted by Robert Tremmel. Citing Schön, Tremmel argues for a broader approach to "reflection," an approach with roots in the Zen Buddhist tradition of "mindfulness" (435). He calls it "the art of paying attention," and argues that such an art, akin to "thinking on your feet" (Schön, qtd. on 436), has roots as far back as Plato's belief that "'learning' is really 'recollection of what the soul has encountered in other worlds'" (435). "Paying attention" or "mindfulness" prods the teacher to formulate her implicit knowledge into explicit knowledge, which can provide her with the skills she needs to solve problems she encounters. It is this capacity for "mindfulness" or reflection that enables one to discover "know-how."

Thinking about this responsibility for "mindfulness" brings to mind lines from "Incantation," a poem by Czeslaw Milosz:

> Human Reason is beautiful and invincible
> No bars, no barbed wire, no pulping of books,
> No sentence of banishment can prevail against it.
> It establishes the universal ideas in language,
> And guides our hand so we write Truth and Justice
> With capital letters, lie and oppression with small.
> It puts what should be above things as they are.

As teachers, we always are working with things as they are but pushing toward things as they should be. We work in and with language, and regardless of our feelings toward the enlightenment or the "universal," most of us believe we're working on issues of justice. To accomplish our goals, we must recognize that the knowledge of the classroom is valuable because it is theoretical. We recognize the tension between "is" and "ought," between "theory" and "practice," all the while knowing that the our ability to understand those tensions, as well as the contradictions caused by these tensions that result in the classroom, can lead to a more productive knowledge. There is nothing certain about teaching, but there is a knowledge that is generated as a result of it. Recognizing that teaching is an art that generates knowledge for use by people will take you a long way toward becoming a reflective practitioner.

WORKS CITED

Alexander, Lloyd. *Taran Wanderer*. New York: Henry Holt, 1989.

Allen, Harold B., et al. "The Doctoral Program for the Teacher of College English." In *The Education of Teachers of English (NCTE Curriculum Series),* edited by Alfred H. Grommon, 539–63. New York: Appleton-Century-Crofts. 1963.

Aristotle. *Politics. The Basic Works of Aristotle*. Translated by Benjamin Jowett. Edited by Richard McKeon, 1113–324. New York: Random House, 1941.

Atwill, Janet. *Rhetoric Reclaimed*. Ithaca, NY: Cornell UP, 1998.

Booth, Wayne C. *The Vocation of a Teacher*. Chicago: U of Chicago P, 1988.

Comeaux, Michelle. "But Is It Teaching? The Use of Collaborative Learning in Teaching Education." In *Issues and Practices in Inquiry-Oriented Education,* edited by Robert B. Tabachnick and Kenneth M. Zeichner, 151–65. London: Falmer, 1991.

de Lauretis, Teresa. "The Essence of the Triangle or, Taking the Risk of Essentialism Seriously: Feminist Theory in Italy, the U.S., and Britain." *Differences: A Journal of Feminist Cultural Studies* 1 (1989): 3–37.

Dewey, John. *John Dewey: Selected Writings*. New York: Modern Library, 1964.

———. *The Philosophy of John Dewey*. Edited by John McDermott. Vols. 1 & 2. New York: G. P. Putnam's Sons, 1973.

Dillard, Annie. *Pilgrim at Tinker Creek*. New York: Harper Magazine P, 1974.

Dubinsky, James M. "More than a Knack: Techne and Teaching Technical Writing." *Technical Communication Quarterly* 11, no. 2 (2002): 131–47.

Dunne, Joseph. *Back to the Rough Ground: Phronesis and Techne in Modern Philosophy and in Aristotle*. Notre Dame, IN: U of Notre Dame P, 1993.

Eble, Kenneth. *The Craft of Teaching: A Guide to Mastering the Professor's Art*. San Francisco: Jossey-Bass, 1988.

Gragg, Charles I. "Teachers Must Also Learn." In *Teaching and the Case Method: Text, Cases, and Readings*, 3rd ed., edited by Louis B. Barnes, C. Roland Christensen, and Abby J. Hansen. 15–22. Boston: Harvard Business School P, 1994.

Greene, Maxine. Foreword to *Stories Lives Tell: Narrative and Dialogue in Education*. Edited by Carol Witherell and Nell Noddings, ix–xi. New York: Teachers College P, 1991.

Grossman, Pamela. *The Making of a Teacher: Teacher Knowledge and Teacher Education*. New York: Teachers College Press, 1990.

Halloran, Michael. "Rhetoric in the American College Curriculum: The Decline of Public Discourse." *Pre/Text* 3 (1982): 245–69.

Highet, Gilbert. *The Art of Teaching*. New York: Vintage, 1954.

Isocrates. "Against the Sophists." In *The Rhetorical Tradition: Readings from Classical Times to the Present,* edited by Patricia Bizzell and Bruce Herzberg, 46–49. Boston: Bedford, 1990.

Johnson, Robert R. *User-Centered: A Rhetorical Theory of Technology for Technical Communicators*. Albany, NY: SUNY P, 1998.

Milosz, Czeslaw. "Incantation." In *Four Poems*, edited by Robert Pinsky. *Slate*, September 21, 2001. http://slate.msn.com/id/115850.

Rudduck, Jean, and David Hopkins, eds. *Research as a Basis for Teaching: Readings from the Work of Lawrence Stenhouse*. London: Heinemann Educational Books, 1985. 60 .

Schön, Donald A. *Educating the Reflective Practitioner*. San Francisco: Jossey-Bass, 1987.

———. *The Reflective Practitioner*. San Francisco: Jossey-Bass, 1983.

Tremmel, Robert. "Zen and the Art of Reflective Practice in Teacher Education." *Harvard Educational Review* 63 (1993): 434–58.

van Manen, Max. "Pedagogy, Virtue, and Narrative Identity in Teaching." *Curriculum Inquiry* 24, no. 2 (1994): 135–70.

Whitburn, Merrill D. "The Ideal Orator and Literary Critic as Technical Communicators: An Emerging Revolution in English Departments." In *Essays on Classical Rhetoric and Modern Discourse*, edited by Robert J. Connors, Lisa S. Ede, and Andrea A. Lunsford, 226–47. Carbondale and Edwardsville, IL: Southern Illinois UP, 1984.

Witherell, Carol, and Nel Noddings, eds. Prologue to *Stories Lives Tell: Narrative and Dialogue in Education*. New York: Teachers College P, 1991.

CHAPTER ONE

Introducing Theoretical Approaches

Chapter One: Introduction

In 1956, C. P. Snow documented a split between humanists and scientists: "non-scientists have a rooted impression that scientists are shallowly optimistic, unaware of man's condition . . . [and] the scientists believe that the literary intellectuals are totally lacking in foresight, peculiarly unconcerned with their brother men." Snow argued that these impressions are, for the most part, "baseless," and rest upon "misinterpretations" of each side (5–6).

In the intervening years, some have argued that the split has begun to close at the theoretical level, particularly due to the work of theorists and philosophers of science (e.g., Michael Polanyi, Stephen Toulmin, Paul Feyerabend). In addition, both the broad acceptance of influential arguments such as Thomas Kuhn's *Structure of Scientific Revolutions* and the growing acknowledgment of the social construction of knowledge have had an impact. However, most scholars still see a split present at the institutional level, and many believe the chasm has widened.

The kind of split that Snow outlines is not new: Plato believed there was a clear, hierarchical division between science and poetry (literature), and he had grave doubts about the Sophists, some of the first teachers of rhetoric. Nor is it confined to the scientists and literary intellectuals Snow references. Indeed, such a split exists among many groups, and often within groups. In the field of English studies, scholars have documented the split between literature and composition (Horner), literature and technical communication (Smith; Miller in this volume), and even within technical communication (Dobrin). Within technical communication, this split often revolves around pedagogical decisions related to preparing students to handle the various skills and software they'll need to know to succeed in the workplace (often labeled as an instrumental approach) and preparing them to be reflective, responsible practitioners who have obligations to their discipline and society (often labeled as a rhetorical approach).

This chapter documents one of the many pedagogical debates in our field between an instrumental approach (Moore) and a rhetorical one (Johnson). Both Moore's and Johnson's articles rely on assumptions about language that are outlined in the first essay, "A Humanistic Rationale for Technical Writing." Miller's piece delineates a divide she sees between two views of science and knowledge that impact the way our discipline is perceived.

This chapter should help you begin to develop a sense of the range of possible pedagogical stances you may adopt. Before you begin teaching, you might find it useful to consider questions that arise from this debate, such as 1) whether or not you subscribe to a position that technical communication is clear, objective, and neutral; 2) whether or not "technical communication is constituted in and by the social, political, and economic interests it serves" (Savage 311); and 3) whether you think technical communicators transmit, translate, or mediate language (Slack, Miller, and Doak). These questions will lead you to beliefs about the field, about whether it is *just* technical communication or "our species' primary survival trait" (Smith 578). Prior to teaching your technical communication class, you will form ideas and beliefs about the subject, its importance, and its place in the curriculum. How you define technical communication and what you think its role is in society will affect how you teach.

WORKS CITED

Dobrin, David N. "What's the Purpose of Teaching Technical Communication?" *Technical Writing Teacher* 7 (1985): 146–60.

Horner, Winifred B., ed. *Composition and Literature: Bridging the Gap*. Chicago: U of Chicago P, 1983.

Savage, Gerald. "Redefining the Responsibilities of Teachers and the Social Position of the Technical Communicator." *Technical Communication Quarterly* 5, no. 3 (1996): 309–27.

Slack, Jennifer Daryl, David James Miller, and Jeffrey Doak. "The Technical Communicator as Author: Meaning, Power, Authority." *Journal of Business and Technical Communication* 7, no. 1 (1993): 12–36.

Smith, D. B. "Axioms for English in a Technical Age." *College English* 48, no. 6 (1986): 567–79.

Snow, C. P. "The Two Cultures." In *The Two Cultures and the Scientific Revolution*. New York: Cambridge UP, 1959. 1–22.

1 A Humanistic Rationale for Technical Writing

CAROLYN R. MILLER

In this seminal article, Miller works to expose what she considers to be unreflective and inaccurate perceptions of the role language plays in knowledge creation in order to demonstrate the validity of the work done by those in the field of technical communication. Her critique of the positivist or "windowpane theory of language," in which language "accurately and directly transmits reality" (p. 16 in this volume), has been influential and often cited. In the positivist or instrumental model, which she sees as "skills-based," language becomes "utilitarian" and rhetoric becomes "irrelevant" (p. 18). Those who teach writing from this perspective become more akin to trainers than teachers and are usually seen by others in the academy as working in a vocational field. Miller argues instead for a "rhetorical," postpositivist perspective (p. 18) that would grant technical communication "disciplinary respectability" (p. 18) because in such a perspective knowledge is not seen as a set of facts to be discovered but rather as a communally based enculturation. As a result, technical communication would not be merely a tool for transmitting knowledge from one mind to another, but rather a way of participating effectively in a community. Her article is included as essential background reading; it informs not only the debate between Johnson and Moore but also virtually every key issue in our field involving definition, ethics, and social responsibility.*

A question arose, during a committee discussion in our English department last year, whether students in our large technological university should be permitted to take a technical writing course to satisfy humanities requirements of their own schools and departments.[1] There were two opinions among those in my department with whom I talked. Those who teach literature believed that students should not satisfy a humanities, or "English," requirement with a technical writing course. And our department should prevent them from doing so by instituting a literature prerequisite for the

From *College English* 40, no. 6 (1979): 610–17.

*See Elizabeth Smith, "Intertextual Connections to 'A Humanistic Rationale for Technical Writing.'" *Journal of Business and Technical Communication* 11, no. 2 (1997): 192–222, for a discussion of how often Miller has been cited.

technical writing course. Those of us who teach technical writing responded differently. Mostly, we were baffled. Obviously we did not welcome what we considered an irrelevant prerequisite for our course, and we did not like the idea of our course being held hostage for the overstaffed literature courses. But were we willing to argue, indeed, *could* we argue that technical writing has humanistic value?

I believe that the argument can be made, and on firm and respectable grounds. But the way to it is not clear. The reasoning is obscured by a tradition of thought in both the sciences and the humanities, a tradition which has become a tacit understanding, a form of common sense. Making the argument requires articulating some new notions of what science is and does and some corresponding new notions of what technical and scientific rhetoric can be and do. I wish to argue that the common opinion that the undergraduate technical writing course is a "skills" course with little or no humanistic value is the result of a lingering but pervasive positivist view of science. In this view, human knowledge, of which we may take science to be a model, is a matter of getting closer to the material things of reality and farther away from the confusing and untrustworthy imperfections of words and minds. Technical and scientific rhetoric becomes the skill of subduing language so that it most accurately and directly transmits reality. It aims at being an efficient way of coercing minds to submit to reality.

Because the positivist view has supported both the rhetoric we call scientific and that we call technical and provides no systematic way to distinguish the two, in this essay I begin by treating them together. I shall first summarize the main features of positivist science and illustrate how this view of science pervades the way we define and evaluate technical writing. I shall attribute some of our pedagogical problems to the positivist legacy. Then I shall sketch the new thinking in the philosophy of science and suggest its particular relevance for technical writing. Finally, I shall be able to suggest how this altered view of science, and of the relationship between science and rhetoric, can provide a basis for seeing technical writing as a more humanistic and less coercive endeavor.

Let me illustrate some common notions about technical and scientific rhetoric with a passage from an article entitled, "How Rhetoric Confuses Scientific Issues":

> Rhetoric is defined as language designed to persuade or impress; the word may be considered a euphemism for loaded language. . . . Anyone who is convinced that only facts should persuade must, logically, condemn such rhetoric in the scientific literature. Realistically, of course, rhetoric cannot be eliminated entirely. But its use can be constricted significantly, and both readers and writers should be on guard against this violation of scientific principles. . . . Since scientists agree that their observations and conclusions should be presented as objectively as possible, rhetoric should be avoided assiduously in scientific writing.[2]

Obviously, in this view, science and rhetoric are mutually exclusive. Science has to do with observation and logic, the only ways we have of approaching external, absolute reality. Rhetoric has to do with symbols and emotions, the stuff of uncertain, incomplete appearances.

The technical writing textbooks are suffused with this view of both science and rhetoric. Some typical examples: "Technical writing is expected to be objective, scientifically impartial, utterly clear, and unemotional. . . . Technical writing is concerned with facts and the careful, honest interpretation of these facts."[3] Another: "Since technical writing is by definition a method of communicating facts it is absolutely imperative to be clear. . . . The point of view should be scientific: objective, impartial, and unemotional."[4] And again: "Technical communication has one certain clear purpose: to convey information and ideas accurately and efficiently."[5] And finally: "Because the focus is on an object or a process, the language is utilitarian, emphasizing exactness rather than elegance. . . . Technical writing is direct and to the point."[6] These characterizations have in common a conviction that content (that is, ideas, information, facts) is wholly separable from words. They all presuppose what has been called the "windowpane theory of language": the notion that language provides a view out onto the real world, a view which may be clear or obfuscated.[7] If language is clear, then we see reality accurately; if language is highly decorative or opaque, then we see what is not really there or we see it with difficulty.

This way of talking about technical writing is the legacy of what I am going to call for convenience the positivist view of science.[8] This is a complex and varied tradition, extending in some forms back to the ancient Greek philosophers, but reaching its most extreme expression in the logical positivism of the early twentieth century. Put simply, positivism is the conviction that sensory data are the only permissible basis for knowledge; consequently, the only meaningful statements are those which can be empirically verified. Sense data are correlated and systematized by logical (mathematical) means and culminate in lawlike generalizations. Scientific laws are thus nothing more than shorthand summaries of sensory observations. Theoretical terms, or mathematical symbols, must be explicitly defined in terms of sense data and are, in effect, abbreviations for phenomenal descriptions.

Since sense impressions must initially be described in some language, much effort has been expended in the attempt to devise a pure "observation language," free of the emotion and metaphysics which pollute ordinary language. Ideally, scientific discourse would consist of "observation sentences" using only logical terms and observation terms, or of assertions using theoretical terms explicitly defined by reference to the observation terms.[9] The culmination of this view of science and language was the attempt by Whitehead and Russell in *Principia Mathematica* to express the empirical content of science in the formulas of classical mathematics, to do away with ordinary language altogether and rely on the rock of logic.[10] Korzybski's *Science and Sanity* and the General Semantics movement subscribe to a similar conviction.

Such a view of science presupposes a mechanistic and materialistic reality. The goal of human knowledge is direct apprehension of that reality. Facts are self-evident entities existing out there in the real world—we have only to learn how to see them accurately or derive them logically. Objectivity on the part of the observer minimizes personal and social interference, reducing observation to the accurate recording of the self-evident; formal logic represents the underlying structure of mechanistic reality. Truth, then, is the correspondence of ideas to reality, and proof is the logical demonstration of that correspondence.[11] Science, which arrives at proven knowledge, is that process of demonstration, proceeding in Cartesian fashion by logical deduction from the self-evident.

In this epistemology, language, based as it is in personal psychology, is largely a distraction for science; and rhetoric is just irrelevant, because conclusions follow necessarily from the data of observation and the procedure of logic. Aristotle would have agreed: rhetoric, he said, has to do with "things about which we commonly deliberate—things for which we have no special art or science . . . things as appear to admit of two possibilities."[12] Rhetoric relies upon "artistic proofs," those which are created by the art of the speaker or writer. Science has to do with what Aristotle called "inartistic proofs," facts or artifacts which exist independently of human intentions and emotions and about which deliberation is unnecessary. Inartistic proofs are those which have only to be found; they are just *there*—self-evident and real and objective.

The most uncomfortable aspect of this non-rhetorical view of science is that it is a form of intellectual coercion: it invites us to prostrate ourselves at the windowpane of language and accept what Science has demonstrated. After all, if we do not see the self-evident, there must be something very wrong with us. I believe that this mystique of absolute scientific truth is as much responsible as our technical achievements for the power of science and technology in our culture today.

If rhetoric is irrelevant to science, technical and scientific writing become just a series of maneuvers for staying out of the way. A rhetorical discipline built on positivist theory must founder on this self-deprecation at its center. But because there has been no alternative basis for the discipline, technical writing as it is commonly taught is shot through with positivist assumptions, which destroy its aspirations toward disciplinary respectability and relegate it to its status as a skills course. I want to discuss four features of technical writing pedagogy which seem to me to illustrate problems due to this positivist legacy: unsystematic definitions of technical writing, emphasis on style and organization, insistence on certain characteristics of tone, and analysis of audience in terms of "level."

Definition of the subject has been a continuing problem in the teaching of technical writing. The textbooks and pedagogical literature are rife with attempts, all very similar and none very satisfactory.[13] Definition based on content seems at first obvious and then unworkable—no one is prepared to say which subjects are "technical." Engineering, certainly; science, of course; but linguistics? political theory? seventeenth-century music? urban planning? Reality doesn't come in packages clearly marked "technical" or "nontechnical."

But perhaps any aspect of reality might be treated in a technical or nontechnical manner. To return to the windowpane analogy, definition in terms of the window itself may be more promising than definition in terms of what is outside. Such definitions often take the form of an appeal to absolute clarity,[14] but clarity is a more elusive and less useful criterion than we have believed. It provides no way to distinguish poorly executed technical writing from writing that is not technical writing. For instance, the prose that many people find least clear, and which is the subject of much popular complaint these days, is writing that few would hesitate to call "technical"—government reports, sociological studies, insurance policies. Clarity is not a useful criterion especially if technical writing fails the test more often than other types of writing. Our definitions of technical writing leak badly. How can we teach a course, let alone develop a field of study, when we have no way to tell anyone what our subject matter is?

The second feature of our teaching that creates a problem is the emphasis on form and style at the expense of invention.[15] The collapse of invention as a rhetorical canon is complementary to the rise of empirical science. If the subject matter of science (bits of reality, inartistic proofs) exists independently, the scientist's duty is but to observe clearly and transmit faithfully. The whole idea of invention is heresy to positivist science—science does not invent, it discovers. Form and style become techniques for increasingly accurate transmission of logical processes or of sensory observations; consequently, we teach recipes for the description of mechanism, the description of process, classification, the interpretation of data. And, as one text indicates, stylistic problems are understood to result from the complexity of technical subject matter: the intricacy of that reality out there makes it difficult for me to transmit it accurately, to make my windowpane sufficiently transparent that you may see the details clearly. If we take this approach to form and style very seriously, there is not very much to teach in a technical writing class. Form and style become, in theory, as self-evident as content.[16] No wonder that technical writing is a course that anyone can teach and no one wants to teach. But why is it that students have difficulty writing effective prose if all they are doing is transmitting a reality about which they know more than the technical writing teacher?

A third problematic feature of our teaching is the insistence on certain characteristics of tone: be objective, be unemotional, be impersonal. These injunctions directly implement the positivist epistemology. But technical writing teachers are consequently always grappling with the dilemma that English syntax does not handle impersonality very gracefully. Under the sway of positivism, scientists adopted as conventions the obvious stylistic means for staying out of the way of the subject matter—third person constructions, personifications, passive voice.[17] Does it make sense to place a double burden on students by urging them to be impersonal on the one hand, but denying them, in the name of stylistic grace, these obvious syntactic tools on the other?

The fourth feature which our teaching owes to positivism is the tendency to analyze audiences in terms of "levels," as though we are concerned with how tall they have to be to look out of our window. Some audiences are capable of seeing some aspects of reality; others are more capable and can see more. Technical writing is sometimes characterized by its particular concern for audience analysis, but the positivist legacy encourages us to analyze only the relationship between the reader and the reality (and whether the reader is mentally adequate to the reality). As a result, audience adaptation too often becomes an exercise in vocabulary. If audience adaptation is to be central to technical writing, we need broader and more flexible methods which will permit analysis of the relationship between the writer and the reader. For we have not said anything very useful about the writer-reader relationship when we say that the purpose in technical writing is to be clear. Why has it been so difficult in a technical writing class to talk about the relationship between writer and readers and the reasons for saying anything about a subject in the first place?

Scientists, engineers, teachers of technical writing, and their students tacitly share the positivist theory about the role of rhetoric in science. Consequently, students look upon writing as a superfluous, bothersome, and usually irrelevant aspect of their technical work. I submit that our teaching reinforces that attitude. We encourage students to see writing as a necessary evil, necessary primarily because it is an amenity occasioned by the conditions of employment in business or industry. We teach writing as the ex post facto expression of a scientific idea or a technical effort, not as part of that idea or that effort.

My real point here is that although our thinking about technical writing seems to be heavily indebted to the positivist view of science (and of rhetoric), this view is no longer held by most philosophers of science or by most thoughtful scientists. Among the major objections to the theory are the complete failure of attempts to devise an observation language, the inability of theoretical terms defined as summaries of known effect to account for new effects observed later, the failure to account for the growth and change of scientific knowledge, and the serious limitations of logical systems.[18] In addition, a new epistemology, based on modern developments in cultural anthropology, cognitive psychology, and sociology, has challenged the positivist conception of knowledge. This new epistemology makes human knowledge thoroughly relative and science fundamentally rhetorical.

This epistemology has been developed at length in the journals of rhetoric and philosophy, and I will not attempt a full discussion here.[19] Briefly summarized, it holds that whatever we know of reality is created by individual action and by communal assent. Reality cannot be separated from our knowledge of it; knowledge cannot be separated from the knower; the knower cannot be separated from a community. Facts do not exist independently, waiting to be found and collected and systematized; facts are human constructions which presuppose theories. We bring to the world a set of innate and learned concepts which help us select, organize, and understand what we encounter.

Science, then, is not concerned directly with material things, but with these human constructions, with symbols and arguments. Scientific observation relies on tacit conceptual theories, which may be said to "argue for" a way of seeing the world. Scientific verification requires the persuasion of an audience that what has been "observed" is replicable and relevant. And logical procedure, as Thomas Kuhn has shown, is inadequate to account for scientific growth and change.[20] Science is, above all, a communal enterprise; it is, according to John Ziman, unique among the "faculties" in insisting on consensus.[21] Truth, or the knowledge for which science seeks, is thus the correspondence of ideas, not to the material world, but to other people's ideas. Certainty is found not in isolated observation of nature or in logical procedure but in the widest agreement with other people. Science is, through and through, a rhetorical endeavor.

It is the contention of this essay that we can improve the teaching and study of technical writing by trading our covert acceptance of positivism for an overt consensualist perspective. For one thing, as I have tried to show, our pedagogy is weakened by submerged inconsistencies and contradictions, which I attribute to an unthinking acceptance of positivist science. For another, we can stop engaging in and submitting to the intellectual tyranny to which our tacit epistemology has led us. Science understood as apodictic demonstration demands acknowledgement, an act of submission by the audience. Science understood as argument asks for assent, for an act of will on the part of the audience. Good technical writing becomes, rather than the revelation of absolute reality, a persuasive version of experience. To continue to teach as we have, to acquiesce in passing off a version as an absolute, is coercive and tyrannical; it is to wrench ideology from belief. Much of what we call technical writing occurs in the context of government and industry and embodies tacit commitments to bureaucratic hierarchies, corporate capitalism, and high technology. If we pretend for a minute that technical writing is objective, we have passed off a particular political ideology as privileged truth.[22]

Finally, if we revise the understanding of science that underlies our teaching, we may be able to reconceptualize our entire discipline in a more systematic way. I am not prepared to offer a complete reconceptualization here and now. There are many promising trends in the texts and the teaching literature, and growing awareness of the problems will help to change the way we teach and talk about technical and scientific writing.[23] But I would like to suggest a general approach to rethinking our discipline along the lines of the new rhetoric. This approach will also provide a way of distinguishing scientific from technical rhetoric, an issue which this essay has avoided until now. We can begin with a sociological and rhetorical truism: communication occurs in communities. Scientists form an epistemic community, consisting of smaller and overlapping disciplinary subcommunities. We can define scientific writing as written communication based within a certain community and undertaken for certain communal reasons. Technical writing occurs within a somewhat different community for somewhat different reasons.

The scientific community's objectives, methods, and values have been widely discussed. Bronowski, Kuhn, and Ziman, for example, have much to contribute to an understanding of the reasons and conditions for communication in science. Very little has been accomplished, however, to provide a similar characterization of the technological community and its rhetoric. My own hunch is that we should look in the direction of organizational and management theory, the sociology of technology, and the cultural history of industry and bureaucracy. These areas may provide a basis for distinguishing the reasons and values which underlie the rhetoric of technical writing.

Under this communalist perspective, the teaching of technical or scientific writing becomes more than the inculcation of a set of skills; it becomes a kind of enculturation. We can teach technical or scientific writing, not as a set of techniques for accommodating slippery words to intractable things, but as an understanding of how to belong to a community. To write, to engage in any communication, is to participate in a community; to write well is to understand the conditions of one's own participation—the concepts, values, traditions, and style which permit identification with that community and determine the success or failure of communication. Our teaching of writing should present mechanical rules and skills against a broader understanding of why and how to adjust or violate the rules, of the social implications of the roles a writer casts for himself or herself and for the reader, and of the ethical repercussions of one's words. We can thus ground our teaching and our discipline in a communal rationality rather than in contextless logic. Under this flagrantly rhetorical approach, the subject matter, syllabi, and assignments in a technical writing course may not change very much. But our attitudes might, and so might those of our students and colleagues.

Finally, let me return to my original problem, the humanities requirement. If we do begin to talk about understanding, rather than only about skills, I believe we have a basis for considering technical writing a humanistic study. The examination and understanding of one's own activity and consciousness, the "return of consciousness to its own center," is, as Walter Ong has suggested, the central impulse of the humanities.[24] I maintain that a course in scientific or technical writing can profitably be based upon this kind of self-examination and self-consciousness, and that, in fact, the rhetorical approach demands such a basis. It might, in addition, contribute to a more fruitful appreciation and critical understanding of two central forces in our culture, science and technology themselves.

NOTES

1. The question proved moot, for the university curriculum committee had previously decided that technical writing could not be allowed to serve as a humanities course.

2. Barbara G. Cox and Charles G. Roland, *IEEE Transactions on Professional Communication*, PC-16 (Sept. 1973), 140.

3. Thomas E. Pearsall, *Teaching Technical Writing: Methods for College English Teachers* (Washington, D.C.: Society for Technical Communication, 1975), p. 1.

4. Gordon H. Mills and John A. Walter, *Technical Writing*, 4th ed. (New York: Holt, Rinehart, and Winston, 1978), p. 7.

5. Joseph N. Ulman, Jr., and Jay R. Gould, *Technical Reporting*, 3rd ed. (New York: Holt, Rinehart, and Winston, 1972), p. 5.

6. Charles T. Brusaw, Gerald J. Oliu, and Walter E. Alred, *Handbook of Technical Writing* (New York: St. Martin's Press, 1976), p. 475.

7. See James L. Kinneavy, *A Theory of Discourse* (Englewood Cliffs, N.J.: Prentice-Hall, 1971), p. 39; also Joseph Gusfield, "The Literary Rhetoric of Science: Comedy and Pathos in Drinking Driver Research," *American Sociological Review*, 41 (February 1976), 16–34.

8. More technically known as the Received View; for a full discussion see Frederick Suppe, *The Structure of Scientific Theories*, 2nd ed. (Urbana: University of Illinois Press, 1977), chs. 1–3.

9. Suppe, p. 15.

10. J. Bronowski, "Humanism and the Growth of Knowledge," in *A Sense of the Future* (Cambridge, Mass.: MIT Press, 1977), p. 74.

11. Two relevant discussions of the philosophies involved here are: Barry Brummett, "Some Implications of 'Process' or 'Intersubjectivity': Postmodern Rhetoric," *Philosophy and Rhetoric*, 9 (1976), 21–51; and C. Perelman and L. Olbrechts-Tyteca, *The New Rhetoric* (Notre Dame, Ind.: University of Notre Dame Press, 1969), esp. pp. 1–10, 509–14.

12. *Rhetoric*, 1, 2; see *The Rhetoric of Aristotle*, ed. Lane Cooper (Englewood Cliffs, N.J.: Prentice-Hall, 1932), p. 11.

13. For attempts at systematic definition, see Mills and Walter, cited above, note 4, and W. Earl Britton, "What Is Technical Writing?: A Redefinition," in *The Teaching of Technical Writing*, ed. Donald H. Cunningham and Herman A. Estrin (Urbana, Ill.: National Council of Teachers of English, 1975), pp. 9–14.

14. An influential definition of this sort is Britton's: "The primary . . . characteristic of technical and scientific writing lies in the effort of the author to convey one meaning and only one meaning in what he says. That one meaning must be sharp, clear, precise. And the reader must be given no choice of meanings" (p. 11). The textbook definitions cited earlier are other examples.

15. This lack of interest in invention is, of course, consistent with the tradition of teaching composition; it may be traced to Renaissance rhetorical theory (Ramism), which is the complement of Cartesian and Baconian science.

16. The notion that form is self-evident may be related to the tendency for technical writing to be a listing of facts whose significance is supposed to go without saying; George Douglas has called this "cobblestone writing" in his recent article in *The Technical Writing Teacher*, 5 (Fall 1977), 18–21.

17. It is interesting that the social sciences, which still place a great deal of stock in positivism, adhere more strictly to impersonal stylistic forms than do the biological and physical sciences; compare, for example, the preferences on the use of the first person pronoun in the style manuals of the American Psychological Association and the Council of Biology Editors.

18. See Suppe, ch. 4.

19. See especially Michael C. Leff, "In Search of Ariadne's Thread: A Review of the Recent Literature on Rhetorical Theory," *Central States Speech Journal*, 29 (Summer 1978), 73-91, for a survey of this epistemic view of rhetoric.

20. *The Structure of Scientific Revolutions*, 2nd ed. (Chicago: University of Chicago Press, 1970).

21. *Public Knowledge: The Social Dimension of Science* (Cambridge: Cambridge University Press, 1968), p. 13.

22. For a critique of this problem in the area of technology assessment, see B. Wynne, "The Rhetoric of Consensus Politics: A Critical Review of Technology Assessment," *Research Policy*, 4 (March 1975), 108–58.

23. Recent discussions that explicitly recognize the rhetorical character of scientific and technical writing are: Dennis R. Hall, "The Role of Invention in Technical Writing," *The Technical Writing Teacher*, 4 (Fall 1976), 13–24; Dwight W. Stevenson, "Toward a Rhetoric of Scientific and Technical Discourse," *The Technical Writing Teacher*, 5 (Fall 1977), 4–10; S. Michael Halloran, "Eloquence in a Technological Society," *Central States Speech Journal* (forthcoming); and S. Michael Halloran, "Technical Writing and the Rhetoric of Science," *Journal of Technical Writing and Communications*, 8 (1978), 77–88.

24. *Rhetoric, Romance, and Technology* (Ithaca, N.Y.: Cornell University Press, 1971), p. 304.

2 *Complicating Technology: Interdisciplinary Method, the Burden of Comprehension, and the Ethical Space of the Technical Communicator*

ROBERT R. JOHNSON

Robert Johnson's article asks technical communicators to become concerned "with a broader band of activity than just the explanation of, and eventual dissemination of, technology" (pp. 24–25 in this volume). His goals include opening up the interdisciplinary nature of our field and demonstrating that, as a result of that interdisciplinarity, members of the discipline have obligations and ethical responsibilities that reach beyond the task of simply communicating. Johnson frames the dilemmas and binaries in other disciplines (history of technology, philosophy of technology) in ways that illuminate binaries in our own. He also offers reasons for adopting a complicated, critical stance by focusing on the users of technology. His emphasis on our "central role in instructing people how to use" and being "purveyors of how-to" (p. 26) is critical to understanding ways in which we can both see ourselves in more complex ways and help our students see their own value as they enter workplaces where they may encounter prejudice and resistance. Other issues to consider include Johnson's focus on our research methods, the importance of and ways to consider history, and his discussion of our use of "artifacts."

Technology. The word has become so commonplace in our culture that we take it for granted, unless, of course, technology doesn't do what we expect it to do (like when the soda machine takes our last quarter or the electricity in our house goes off). In traditionally practice-oriented professions like technical communication, we are frequently guilty of taking technology at its face value. We see technology for what it is—a tool that must be explained or documented in some fashion. When we do see it as something other than a tool, we often characterize it as a controlling phenomenon: an autonomous monster that has a life of its own.

Such an either/or attitude toward technology is problematic for technical communicators because it potentially limits our practice and, ultimately, our sphere of influence in the greater scheme of technology. Technical communication, as much as any technology-related profession, should be concerned with a

From *Technical Communication Quarterly* 7, no. 1 (1998): 75–98.

broader band of activity than just the explanation of, and eventual dissemination of, technology. However, recent proclamations within technical communication concerning "instrumental discourse" tell an opposite story. Instead of expanding the scope of the technical communicator, these arguments for an instrumental approach to technical communication illuminate vividly the profession's entrapment within, and comfort with, the role of the technical communicator as mere scribe (Moore; Hagge). To define narrowly the theoretical disposition of the profession as "instrumental" is to become defensively monodisciplinary. In so doing, we, unwittingly or not, pigeonhole ourselves as "nonrhetorical," "antihumanistic," or "pro-instrumental," and thus risk becoming subservient to disciplines that occupy the other side, usually the power-side, of the binaries: disciplines that are unlikely to relinquish even the smallest vestige of influence. To become comfortable with such a narrow-gauge view of our profession is to become too comfortable—a complacency in part due to unproblematic attitudes toward the defining influence of our profession: Technology.

An uncomplicated, reductive stance makes it far too simple to just perceive technology as an *is*: as something that predetermines our very thinking about who we are, what we do, and why we do what we do. We have a responsibility to more than just the technologies that we write about, and to the developers who so generously give them to us at the end of the design-development-packaging cycle. To be blunt, if technical communicators could expand their scope of influence beyond the instrumental how-to of ready-to-go technologies, then there might be fewer disasters like Bhopal, Chernobyl, or *Challenger* that need after-the-fact communication to assess the damage and, at best, cut the losses. (Two comments are in order here. First, my mentioning of these three technology disasters/accidents is a direct reference to Patrick Moore [115]. Second, as I write about "after-the-fact" assessment of technological damage, I am reminded of Langdon Winner's statement in his chapter "Technologies as Forms of Life," where he critiques the role of technology assessment. Winner explains the intent of such research is to determine that "[A]fter the bulldozer has rolled over us, we can pick ourselves up and carefully measure the treadmarks" [*Whale* 10].) To study the complexity of technology through its design, development, and dissemination stages—an activity that forces an examination of the human elements of technologies—is one possible way for technical communicators to begin the long process of becoming more influential in technological planning and decision-making.

More to the point, technical communicators are intimately connected with many of the actual users of technology—whether they are users of concrete artifacts like lawnmowers, sewing machines, and computers, or users of more complex technologies, such as medical institutions, legal systems, and educational systems—and thus we have an ethical responsibility to be cognizant of the larger (and sometimes more ominous) effects of technology on those who use and live with the technologies we "write." (See Christina Haas' *Writing Technology* for an elaboration of this concept.) If for no other reason, it is this ethical responsibility to our audiences that should drive our interest in complicating the essential binary of good technology/bad technology. All technologies (even the technology of language itself) have elements of "the good and the bad," but these cultural values are only apparent when technologies are put into *use* (Johnson).

That is, until humans activate technologies, they are for most intents and purposes inert objects. A knife on the table, an automobile in a showroom, a vacuum cleaner on the department store shelf: these all can be "read" and deconstructed, but they have little if any ethical value until they are used. As I have already noted, technical communicators play a central role in instructing people how to use; we are the purveyors of how-to. The ethical dimension of technology is squarely in our laps, and to complicate technology in a given situation of use may feel uncomfortable. Reactionaries may say that, in so doing, we are biting the hand that feeds us. Nevertheless, we must accept this ethical responsibility, along with any discomfort, by virtue of our relationship with technological artifacts and their eventual users. Our purpose should be to ensure that we (and our audiences) are not, so to speak, force-fed.

Approaching technology from a more complicated perspective, however, is not problem-free. It entails, among other things, journeys into other arenas of knowledge, into other disciplines. To stroll willy-nilly into another area of expertise is dangerous. You need look no further than the *Social Text* "event" of last summer, for instance, to consider the implications of discussing technology studies in an interdisciplinary arena. In the Spring/Summer volume of the journal *Social Text*, a special issue appeared that centered on discussions of technology from what might be called an "outsider's" perspective. The editor of this special collection, Andrew Ross, devoted an entire issue to discussions of science and technology by those who, for the most part, are outsiders of the academic disciplines of science and technology. In the introduction to the special issue, Ross clearly lays out the purpose of his collection as a response to conservative critics who have characterized those who study science and technology from the "outside" as "science bashers" (7). Ross, much to his credit, put together a collection of articles by scholars well suited to lead the counter charge (A side comment: It is interesting to note the propensity for scholars in STS [science/technology studies] to engage in battle and war metaphors to describe this arena of scholarship. In addition, this *Social Text* issue also displayed several articles that used the all too common marriage/divorce analogy to discuss the disciplinary debates surrounding STS—metaphorical ground that has been well plowed in rhetoric and composition studies [see Reichert]), a stellar array of some of the best STS scholars, including Sandra Harding, Winner, Dorothy Nelkin, Stanley Aronowitz, to name only a few. Unfortunately, there was a fly in the ointment.

The last article in the *Social Text* collection was written by a physicist, Alan Sokal, who was not readily known in STS. This "novice" to STS, however, wrote quite a piece. Complete with fifty-five explanatory footnotes and references to over two hundred works spanning the disciplines of philosophy, cultural studies, history, physics, biology, feminist studies, and literary criticism, Sokal gave to the collection, "Transgressing the Boundaries: Toward a Transformative Hermeneutics of Quantum Gravity." In a nutshell, Sokal focused on the study of quantum gravity, a new area of physics research that he described as

> the emerging branch of physics in which Heisenberg's quantum mechanics and Einstein's general relativity are at once synthesized and superseded. In quantum gravity, as we shall see, the space-time manifold ceases to exist as an objective reality; geometry becomes relational and contextual; and the foundational conceptual categories of prior science—among them existence itself—become problematized and relativized. This conceptual revolution, I will argue, has profound implications for the content of a future postmodern and liberatory science. ("Transgressing" 218)

Profound implications indeed, except for one problem—the entire article was a ruse. Shortly after it was published, Sokal proclaimed his scam in *Lingua Franca* ("Physicist"). The whole article was meant to discredit the advocates of social studies of science and technology and have them appear as intellectual frauds. Sokal's underhanded purpose was to have profound implications, but in an opposite direction from that which the editors of *Social Text* had envisioned for the special collection.

I suppose we could just look at this embarrassing moment and learn from it a simple lesson, like "walk softly and always carry a few good external reviewers." But I'm afraid the lessons are deeper and more far-ranging than to just call it a mere cautionary tale. One significant implication is the illumination of the difficulties we face as we cross disciplinary boundaries. In the case of Sokal's article ("Transgressing"), there are also blatant ethical issues regarding collegiality and professional respect when one crosses the "knowledge borders."

More subtle, though, are problems that result from an impatience to find the "right" answer: an answer we seek in the greener pastures of another discipline. Julie Thompson Klein describes such impatience as "evidence of a 'quick-fix mentality' rather than a long-term, integrated solution" (88), and she describes six problems common to the practice of interdisciplinary borrowing:

1. distortion and misunderstanding of borrowed material;
2. use of data, methods, concepts, and theories out of context;
3. use of borrowings out of favor in the original context (including an overreliance on "old chestnuts");
4. "illusion of certainty" about phenomena treated with a caution or skepticism in their original disciplines;
5. overreliance on one particular theory or perspective; and
6. a tendency to dismiss contradictory tests, evidence, or explanations. (88)

Klein goes on to explain that these problems are far from insurmountable, but that in order to overcome them it is the borrower's responsibility to accept the "*burden of comprehension* . . . that borrowers acquire at least a basic understanding of how something is used in its original context" (88). (Klein, in turn, borrowed the phrase "burden of comprehension" from Jancie Lauer's 1983 address to the Rhetoric Society of America at the Conference on College Composition and Communication in Detroit. See Lauer for a published rendition of this speech. For an example of how the burden of comprehension can be activated in a substantial project, see Lauer and Asher's *Composition Research*.)

It is the burden of comprehension—the responsibility we have to understand the contexts, values, and methods of those from whom we borrow—that I will address. The purpose of my discussion is four-fold. First, I want to come to some understanding of how technology has been approached—historically, methodologically, and ideologically—by scholars in disciplines that have for some time interrogated technological artifacts, systems, and the people who use them. Second, I bring this research to technical communication for the purpose of situating the arguments of other-disciplinary technology scholars into our own disciplinary framework. Third, I hope to experience some of the promise of interdisciplinary research that in the best of circumstances leads to what Klein calls "an inductive openendedness" (93): that interesting space in the world of research where we end up with more—and even more interesting—questions. Finally, I turn to some of these questions back toward the profession of technical communication for the purpose of rethinking our roles and responsibilities.

I will limit my discussion to the methodologies of several disciplines that have for some time been involved with the study of technology from historical, sociological, and philosophical perspectives. I have chosen disciplines that not only have some precedent in the field, but which also cover a fair stretch of methodological ground appropriate for technical communicators. For instance, I have chosen the history of technology because of its comparative longevity in technology studies; sociology because of its innovative techniques, specifically ethnography and case study, and its interest in feminist studies; philosophy due to its concerns with fundamental issues of human action, most importantly ethics and public decision-making. In line with Klein's suggestions for approaching interdisciplinary study, the following sections on these three disciplines are structured to 1) provide a historical and ideological context for each discipline, 2) discuss some of the methodological approaches of each discipline, and 3) pose questions that expose spaces relevant to technical communication. The final section discusses the implications for translating these three disciplines for use by technical communicators.

Telling Technology's Stories: The Historian's Approach

Historians of technology got off to an uncertain start when they formalized their profession through the founding of a society and accompanying journal in 1959. The problems they encountered in this formative period were steeped in disciplinary politics, and can be summed up in one succinct phrase: technology is *not* science. Consider the following anecdote told by Melvin Kranzberg concerning the beginnings of the Society of the History of Technology (SHOT) in 1957:

> We [John Rae, Carl Condit, Tom Hughes, and Mel Kranzberg] thought that an appropriate strategy would be to approach the History of Science Society and see if historians of science might widen their purview to include the history of technology. It so happened that Henry Guerlac, a leader in HSS, taught at Cornell. So a deputation went to see him. The meeting proved to be a disaster. . . . We were crestfallen as we walked down the hill from Guerlac's home in Ithaca. "Well," I said, "if the History of Science Society is not going to 'condescend' to include the history of technology and if *Isis* is not going to publish any articles dealing with it, then maybe we ought to form a society of our own. . . ." (qtd. in Staudenmaier 1)

So began the Society for the History of Technology and its journal, *Technology and Culture,* and here we also get a graphic description of a highly contentious issue in the study of technology. Namely, there is a problem if we conflate science and technology as though they are of the same cloth. Certainly the case can be made that they are related, maybe as a wall-mounted tapestry is akin to a rug on a floor. That they are the same in the eyes of academe (or even in the public sphere), however, is a misconception. Indeed, there have been subsequent improvements in the relationship between these two disciplinary schools (the historians of science and the historians of technology)—most evident in that the two societies held their first joint meeting in 1991 at the University of Wisconsin, Madison.

Nevertheless, the turn to technology has been slow for almost all disciplines that have turned to it as a focus of research. Sociologists, for instance, have begun to focus on technology only in the last fifteen years or so, a good decade after science had become an arena of research among sociologists (see Woolgar). Winner has claimed that researchers in the history and sociology of technology have revered the study of science to the point that they regard technology studies "as a kind of intellectual slumming" ("Opening" 62). Several researchers in our own field started with investigations of science long before there appeared to be any concerted interest in technical communication to focus on technology (Bazerman; Myers).

The important point here is that there are connections between the study of science and the study of technology, but within the disciplinary complex of intellectual life it can be debilitating to technology studies to pretend that it is one and the same locus of study with science studies because, like it or not, the study of science has the upper hand when it comes to academic respectability. As newcomers to the field of technology studies, it is important that technical communicators understand these differences, just as we would expect someone coming to English studies to understand that composition is not the same as literature. (A compelling example of how composition studies has been inappropriately applied to another discipline, see Frances Ranney's "Reading, Writing, and Rhetoric: An Inquiry into the Art of Legal

Language." Ranney explains how teachers of legal writing have appropriated composition pedagogy and theory with little knowledge of composition's context or history.)

To return more directly to the methods of historians of technology, I should make clear that the founding of SHOT was not the genesis of historical technology studies. There had been significant research conducted through several research methodologies for quite some time before SHOT appeared on the scene. For over three decades preceding the founding of SHOT, historians interested in the study of technology had used various methods to explore the nature of technology. These pre-SHOT methods (all of which have continued in varying degrees to be used after the formation of SHOT) consisted of three types: internalist history, nonhistorical analyses, and contextual history (Staudenmaier 8–9).

Internalist history derives its name from scholarship that focuses on technological artifacts themselves, especially their design characteristics and functions. This research is most likely the oldest form of technology history. John Staudenmaier, for instance, places its origins in the fifteeth century work of Giovanni Tortelli, who primarily viewed technology as a series of inventions. In the twentieth century, internalist history continued its quest to understand the nature of inventors and inventions, although other approaches finally began to compete with this artifact-centered view after 1950.

Just at the time other methods began to compete with the internalist paradigm, the internal methodologists witnessed the appearance of one of their most impressive publications—*The History of Technology*, edited by Charles Singer, E. J. Holmyard, and A. R. Hall. This five-volume encyclopedia-like collection stands as a hallmark of the internalist approach. Internalist history began to fade to some degree after the publication of *The History of Technology*, however, as this approach lacked much critical or contextual interest beyond the artifacts themselves. The time was ripe for a less mechanical-centered, complete-coverage approach to the study of technology.

Two methods of historical inquiry—*nonhistorical analysis* and *contextual history*—broke the artifact-centered approach of the internalists in significant ways that have proven to drive the development of technology history to the present day. The nonhistorical analysts, interestingly, were often not historians, nor were they technologists. Instead, they tended to be economists and sociologists who were interested not so much in the artifacts of inventors, but more in

> the patterns of technological change at the heart of their analyses . . . [and] the relationship between new technology and societal values and structures. . . . For them, "technology" as a general socioeconomic force was more significant than individual "technologies." (Staudenmaier 11)

In order to measure such patterns and forces, their research thus tends to rely on quantitative and statistical analysis.

The *contextual historians*, as their name suggests, are interested in the connections between artifacts and the historical context of a given time period. Staudenmaier points to pre-SHOT historians like Lewis Mumford as the originators of this style of historical scholarship, and I believe that it would be fair to also claim philosophers such as Jacques Ellul and Martin Heidegger as inspirational to contextual research. This wide distribution of historical and philosophical scope probably accounts for the high interest in this form of historical method by present historians, philosophers, and even some sociologists of technology.

These three approaches to historical method, despite their differences, still have one thing in common: artifacts and their design. This may seem an unnecessary statement to make, but it is important to recognize that these three methods all rely upon the *design of artifacts* as being central. Stories of invention processes, "great" inventors, and the mechanical nuances of the artifacts form the basis for much of this research. Pushing the artifact and its inventors to the periphery was the consequence of yet a fourth approach—that of the *externalist* historian. In this method, research focuses on what Staudenmaier calls the "cultural ambiance" of technology (17), or what some of us might now term the "cultural context" or even "communities of discourse." Externalist researchers, thus, "study the ambiance of technology without analyzing the design characteristics of the technologies in question" (Staudenmaier 17).

The effects of externalist research have become increasingly widespread and have in recent years become common. Significant works done in the externalist vein are too numerous to name here, but two prime examples especially relevant to technical communicators are Ruth Schwartz Cowan's *More Work for Mother: Household Technologies from the Open Hearth to the Microwave*, and Pamela Long's investigations of sixteenth century mining, metallurgy, and the openness of knowledge. Cowan's book is an impressive analysis of the rather mundane technologies used by women, and the tremendous impacts these technologies have had upon the social order, work practices, and economic realities of women and their families. She focuses on larger social issues and primarily uses household technologies as points of reference or as evidence for her more global cultural concerns. Long, in turn, sketches the history of Renaissance metallurgy, not for the purpose of necessarily understanding mining processes, but instead to come to terms with the issue of knowledge ownership between the alchemists and mining barons. Of particular interest to technical communicators is Long's analysis of the role of instructional texts during this time of competition for knowledge of mining techniques and processes.

A fifth historical approach to technology is the *historiographical*. This is a meta-historical approach that critically analyzes the various methods of technology historians for the purpose of complicating, reflecting upon, and possibly even "correcting" the movement of the field. From a technical communicator's perspective, these historiographical discussions can prove most enlightening as they often reveal characteristics of the technology historian's approach that are often applicable to our own contexts.

For instance, a 1974 special issue of *Technology and Culture* devoted to defining the discipline of the history of technology contains an article by

Edwin Layton titled "Technology as Knowledge," where Layton lays out an argument concerning the epistemic nature of technology that is quite similar to critiques one might encounter in either rhetorical studies and/or technical communication. Layton makes the case that, throughout history, technology has always been epistemic, even though science has been perceived in modern times to have gained the upper hand in perceptions of knowledge creation. Layton also manages to invoke the issue of communal knowledge formation when he claims in his conclusion that

> if one sees the difference [between science and technology] in social terms, as values held by different communities, the result is a symmetric model of science-technology interaction. There is no contradiction involved in assuming that knowledge might flow from a community that values doing [technology] to one that values knowing [science]. In this view, technology and science might influence each other on all levels. . . . Even if scientists and technologists continue to value "knowing" and "doing," the precise significance of these values will change because of the changing context provided by other values and ideas. Such changes are interesting and important subjects of historical inquiry, but they have been rarely touched by historians of technology. (Layton 40–41)

Layton's conclusions are enlightening, and even surprising given the infant stage of research into notions of "community" in 1974. But beyond such interesting discoveries that one finds when exploring the history of technology it still remains to be asked: What might a technical communicator derive from these five historical methods? To begin, we might reflect on our use of "artifacts" as a focus of research. By that I mean, we should be conscious of how we use the artifacts of our profession's history—texts—when we conduct historical scholarship. We might ask, for instance, is our method internalist? If so, should that be our intent? What are the consequences of adopting such a purpose? One possible downside is that such research can lead us to a myopic vision of that artifact, a vision that could very well elide the cultural and ethical dimensions of the textual artifact. We might also be prompted to ask: If we portend to study technical texts contextually, are we apt to place the artifact in the center, or are we more concerned with getting at the "ambiance" within which the text resides? What, in other words, is the actual aim of the study we wish to pursue?

We also can learn something from the meta-historians, the historiographers. From Layton's article, for instance, there are direct applications to questions concerning the rhetorical study of technical communication—Where does knowledge reside? Who "owns" the knowledge? This is clearly a launching point for investigations of intellectual property.

Beyond this is potential for rethinking the entire enterprise of technical communication historical research *away from* the study of technical communication itself. What if we study not just the history of technical communication, but rather, we take a look at *history* from a technical communicator's perspective? What, for instance, could we learn of past agricultural practices, environmental history, or other technology-related phenomena by looking at those practices and events through the values and beliefs of technical communicators? More abstractly, what are our discipline's beliefs and values after all? What are our ethics? Can we use historical research to help define our discipline's motives and expectations? This might be an interesting way to get at critical questions of values and ethics that we seem to be increasingly drawn to as our profession reflects on its practice-oriented origins.

Investigating Technology as a Cultural Construct: The Sociologist's Approach

In the previous discussion of historical methods, we briefly encountered sociologists as they were involved, according to Staudenmaier's definition, in the "nonhistorical" analysis of technology history. These early journeys by sociologists and other social scientists into technology studies were important in the formation of investigative methods, but a more widespread involvement by sociologists didn't occur until the early 1980s, when a small group of researchers held several small conferences and workshops to explore the possibility of a "sociology of technology" (see Bijker, Hughes, and Pinch 1–6). During these early meetings, sociologists of science combined with those interested in technology to help write a definition of the sociology of technology. One early attempt that is most useful in understanding the methods of the sociologists is that of Donald MacKenzie and Judy Wacjman as they wrestled with a vocabulary for interpreting technology. They came up with three characteristics that can serve as a starting point in defining what it is that we mean by technology:

> First, there is the level of *physical objects* or *artifacts*, for example, bicycles, lamps, and Bakelite. Second, "technology" may refer to *activities* and *processes*, such as steel making or molding. Third, "technology" may refer to what people *know* as well as what they do; an example is the "know-how" that goes into designing a bicycle or operating an ultrasound device in the obstetrics clinic. (Bijker, Hughes, and Pinch 3–4, emphasis in original)

This definition of their subject of study had multiple purposes. It was meant, on one level, to move away from traditional approaches of studying technology. Specifically, they wanted to define their research as 1) *not* the study of individual inventors or geniuses, 2) *not* the analyses of technologically deterministic phenomena (many of these researchers see determinism as a socially constructed concept that can be "interpreted out" of existence) (I will not be discussing technological determinism in depth here as it is worthy of an entire discussion of its own. I will be mentioning it throughout this article, however, as it is a common theme that runs through most every discipline that critically investigates technology [for extended discussions of this concept, see Winner *Autonomous Technology*; Staudenmaier;

Smith and Marx]). A succinct definition offered by Staudenmaier will suffice for our purposes here:

> It [technological determinism] can best be understood in terms of two major premises and three corollaries. The first premise states that autonomous technology results from a disjunction between efficiency as a norm for judging technical success and all other cultural norms. The second premise argues that technological progress follows a fixed and necessary sequence through modern history. Three corollaries follow. First, the relationship of society to technological change is always adaptation. Second, the historiographic format most congruent with deterministic and progressive technology is the "technological success story." Third, the history of technology is, in fact, an account of the gradual triumph of Western science and technology over all other forms of human praxis. (135–36)

and 3) *not* as the study of discrete spheres of economic, technical, or political events, but rather as a combined network, or what they refer to as a "seamless web of society and technology" (Bijker, Hughes, and Pinch 3).

On another level, these researchers wanted to activate these definitions and concepts. Consequently, they developed some formal and fairly highly-structured research techniques in their effort to carry out their socially-centered analyses of technological artifacts and systems. These techniques are various, but most do revolve in one way another around concepts of social construction. The following is a brief example on one case study—the invention and early dissemination of the bicycle—that uses a sociological approach.

Social Construction Methodology and the Bicycle

Technology to social constructionists is a cultural construct that can be interpreted and reinterpreted depending upon the people involved; the context or situation in which it is designed, developed, or deployed; and the historical moment within it resides. Trevor Pinch and Wiebe Bijker use a rather formal method of analysis, which they term SCOT (or the Social Construction of Technological Systems). The overall goal of SCOT is to allow technical artifacts to be researched from a *multidirectional perspective*, something akin to the ethnographer's concept of triangulation, where several views of an environment are "captured" in order to provide a richer description. They argue that their method is a heuristic device derived from practical experience through case studies, as opposed to philosophical or theoretical foundations (39).

Instead of designating invention as the moment when the genius inventor succeeds in stabilizing an artifact, Pinch and Bijker turn to the concept of *relevant social groups* that played a role in the development and dissemination of an artifact. These groups can be formal, like existing institutions or organizations, or they can be informal groups whose bond is the result of some common aspect of the artifact's existence. In the case of the bicycle, they activate this method by first identifying large social groups, such as consumers or producers. Next, they narrow the definitions of the groups to provide a sharper focus for analysis. For instance, they examine women and men cyclists to see how they viewed the use of bicycles. They argue that women's clothing, and the social mores attached to the wearing of skirts and dresses, forced a bicycle design which was lower to the ground, thus keeping women's legs or undergarments from public view. For men, the riding of bicycles was seen as a "manly pursuit"—an attitude which for a time dissuaded the development of the inflated tire as these softer tires were not as dangerous, and therefore not as "manly."

In addition to the actual users of the bicycle, Pinch and Bijker point to non-users, or what they term in this case "anticyclists." During this period (1880–1900), informal groups reacted violently to the new two-wheeled artifact. Citing examples of riders having sticks and stones thrown at them and being chased out of town by angry citizens, the two researchers make the case that the anticyclists found meaning in the bicycle artifact, albeit a quite different meaning than that of the users (32). The anticyclists represented a Luddite-like segment of the population that defined bicycles in terms of fear: fear of technological innovation and the potential for cultural change brought about by an artifact. Such differences in meaning Pinch and Bijker define as *interpretive flexibility*, or the practice of using similar data but coming to quite different conclusions based upon various contextual constraints—a kind of relativistic tool, so to speak. For social constructionist advocates like Pinch and Bijker, interpretive flexibility is a mainstay of their approach to studying the development and impact of technological artifacts:

> the interpretive flexibility of a technical artifact must be shown. By this we mean not only that there is a flexibility in how people think of or interpret artifacts but also there is flexibility in how artifacts are *designed*. There is not just one possible way or one best way of designing an artifact. (40, emphasis in original)

Through this sociological approach to technology studies, advocates argue that set pathways of progress are constantly questioned, single interpretations of technological development are interrupted, and the potential for concentrating on consumers and users works counter to traditional ideas of the lone great inventor or genius developer. Technical communicators can certainly gain from both the findings of such research, as well as from the implementation of these methods into their own research. The sociological methods, in addition to claims of countering more traditional research methods, are very well defined. That is, these methods are discussed in some detail by the sociologists who develop them. Methodology is in many ways a paramount concern of these academic, and sometimes nonacademic, investigators (see, for instance, the work of Lucy Suchman or John Seely Brown and Paul Duguid at Xerox PARC, or that of the Scandinavian interface designers C. Floyd et al., or Pelle Ehn). This propensity to document the process of research can be quite helpful to technical communication faculty who are helping graduate students define methods for dissertation research. The methods are rigorous and sound, and because of the constructionist drive of the research, these methods are immediately applicable to research questions that technical communicators often ask regarding the social and cultural nature of discursive practices.

The SCOT model, and similar sociological approaches to technology studies, are not without critics, however. For instance, Pinch and Bijker appear to promote what might be called a classic view of "soft" determinism (see Smith and Marx): a methodological move that has been questioned by at least one scholar who believes that such a denial of determinism is merely an easy way to cover over the potential political and social ramifications of technology as a controlling enterprise (Winner, "Opening"). (I should mention that the work of John Law or Bruno Latour are two examples that go beyond some of limitations of sociological method mentioned here. Some feminist researchers, who I will mention in the end of this section on sociological methods, are likewise cognizant of these issues and are actively pursuing "corrective" research.) Put another way, almost as a turn to a social determinism that ignores its technological counterpart, SCOT tends to erase technological determinism—a methodological move that is possibly naive in that it only documents and describes, but fails to work actively toward institutional or cultural change.

Gender, Politics, and Power: A Feminist Sociological Approach

Potential methodological shortcomings such as those mentioned above are true of any discipline, and "correctives" are usually not far away. Feminist sociologists offer one strong avenue of research that promises to counter some these deficiencies. The feminist approaches cover a wide spectrum of interests, from medical and computer technologies (Hacker; Star), to household technologies (Cockburn), to workplace technologies (Suchman). Researchers of women and their encounters with technology share a fair amount of common ground with the sociologists discussed earlier. For instance, many of them have come from science studies to technology studies. They also are interested in countering issues such as technological determinism.

In addition to these common areas, however, the feminists offer an avenue into the arena of technology and politics that the other sociologists don't offer, at least much of the time. Specifically, the feminist approaches can move into the political dimensions of technology through what Wacjman terms "the missing gender dimension" in technology studies (22). Wacjman points out that feminist research in technology has pretty much been "at a general level" (22), but that movements to work more closely with gender in relation to technology could, among other things, help us to understand that "technology is not simply the product of rational technical imperatives. Rather, political choices are embedded in the very design and selection of technology" (22). Wedding traditional issues like determinism with sociological methods might help develop, through issues of feminist and gender-related research, understandings of the private and public technological spheres.

The ramifications of sociological method for technical communicators are clear at the level of ethnographic and case study methods. We have for quite a long time been interested in using these methods to understand the workplace and how people write, act, and think in nonacademic environments. We can also see, however, that the sociologists make some interesting connections between historical and sociological methods through their use of historical case studies, like the SCOT approach to the bicycle. Maybe this method is drawn from the sociologists' kinship with economics where historical case analysis has been prevalent for quite some time. Sociological approaches to technology are fruitful in many interesting and compelling ways. We should take heart in the possibility for picking some of these fruits and using them in cultivating our technical communication research methods.

Defining and Politicizing Technology: The Philosophical Approach

The philosophy of technology, similar in some ways to technical communication, is a discipline looking for an identity. This is ironic considering that philosophy as a discipline, in general, has a longevity at least as long as history's, and certainly longer than sociology's. Nevertheless, the philosophy of technology as a discipline has been somewhat slow to materialize.

I take issue with Pinch and Bijker, though, when they claim that the "literature on the philosophy of technology is rather disappointing. We [sociologists] prefer to suspend judgment on it until philosophers propose more realistic models of science and technology" (19). It is not the *literature* by philosophers of technology that is problematic. With philosophical research of technology conducted by the likes of Jacques Ellul, Jose Ortega y Gasset, and Martin Heidegger through the twentieth century, and most recently by Donald Ihde, Winner, and Carl Mitcham (to name only a few), it is difficult to claim that the literature is disappointing. Instead, it appears that the philosophers of technology have had a problem of negotiating a common ground of research upon which to clearly base a disciplinary research agenda in the same way chat historians or sociologists have. Carl Mitcham suggests that the philosophy of technology has had difficulties forming because it consists of two parts that he likens to "fraternal twins exhibiting sibling rivalry even in the womb" (17). The twins he refers to are the philosophy of technology as an engineering discipline and as a humanities discipline—one pro-technology, the other more critical. Consequently, a research consensus has not been established—a characteristic that Staudenmaier claims was essential for technology historians during the formative period of their discipline (see chapter one of *Technology's Storytellers*).

In this final discussion of disciplinary views of technology I will look at philosophical research from two influential strands of the philosopher's approach to technology studies. The first is an approach to *defining* what it means for a philosopher to study technology. For this I will draw primarily upon the work of Mitcham and his thorough account of the philosophy of technology. The second approach will be the philosopher in search of answers to questions of public life. The focus here will be on the work of Winner.

Mitcham's Taxonomies and "Being-With" Technology

In Mitcham's account of the development of the philosophy of technology (as mentioned above), he characterizes the field as being of two "minds" that I will describe as a theory-practice division. On the one side are humanities philosophers interested in theorizing technology and its relation to human action. On the other side are philosophers advocating engineering approaches concerned with the practical aspects of technology. Mitcham's overall division of two "minds" is indeed reductive, but it is far from another unreflective use of the "theory/practice split." Instead, he uses the binary as a backdrop for his greater purpose of demonstrating how a philosophy of technology can serve as a pathway between these two polar views of technological phenomena. (I want to point out that the binary that exists in the disciplines of philosophy between engineers and humanists is strikingly similar to the binary that I mentioned at the beginning of this article concerning "instrumental discourse" in technical communication. The more things change, the more they stay the same . . . just one more irony of disciplinarity.)

To elaborate this breaking of the binary, he describes the many ways that philosophers look at, and in Mitcham's terms "think through," technology. For instance, he divides the analysis of technology into four categories: technology as object, as knowledge, as activity, and as volition. Beyond these taxonomic devices of defining philosophical concepts in terms of technology, Mitcham also provides us with tools for approaching what he terms "being-with" technology. Coming from a historical perspective, he presents three ways that humans come to "be-with" technology. The first of these, ancient skepticism, centers on the ancients' love-fear relationship with technology that we often see in discussions of Greek *techne* (such as the Promethean myth of fire—beneficial, but at the same time dangerous). The second concept of "being-with" technology he calls Enlightenment optimism—the modern attitude of technology as a savior of humankind from the perils of Nature. The third and final concept, romantic uneasiness, presents the nineteenth and twentieth century skepticism (and fear) of technology as Frankensteinian: a monster out of control and operating of its own free will.

Mitcham's concepts of how humans have historically approached technology are highly useful as critical and analytical tools for technical communicators to dissect everything from technological artifacts to institutional systems to environmental ethics. For example, his discussion on the actions of making (under the larger category of technology as activity) can illuminate pathways to rhetorical issues of *techne* in rich ways. Mitcham places the actions of making on a spectrum that extends from cultivating on one end to constructing on the other:

> Cultivating involves helping nature to produce more perfectly or abundantly things that she could provide of itself, and includes the *technai* or arts of medicine, teaching, and farming. Construction entails reforming or molding nature to produce things not found even in rare instances or under the best of circumstances, as with carpentry. (211, emphasis in original)

He then uses this spectrum to speculate on the distinctions between alternative technologies that work in harmony with nature, and "hard or high" technologies that are removed from natural processes. To further complicate the distinction, he goes on to explain that the differences along the cultivating/constructing spectrum can be placed into historical relief:

> Premodern making was and is apt to see all making as a kind of cultivation, whereas engineering action virtually abandons concern with specific sensuous form in favor of methods of construction that can meet the needs of clients and users and thus reconceive even traditional cultivation as a kind of construction (witness production agricultural and biomedical engineering, as well as educational technology). . . . Indeed, perhaps it could be said that ancient making concentrated on cultivation in two dimensions, the natural and the human, whereas modern making becomes a construction of both the natural and the human. (214)

There are also direct applications of Mitcham's concepts to theories of use and usability, as Mitcham's definitions touch directly on often-neglected philosophical strands concerning the *use* of technology. According to Mitcham, the concept of *use* has been all but neglected by philosophers of technology (and even philosophy in general), so much so that "the concept of use is conspicuous by its absence as a theme in all major texts" (230). The research strands that a technical communicator could invent from this very statement would be grand in number. Not only does such a claim say something about the subordinate place of users on technological hierarchies, but it also provides historical rationale for explaining the less than glorious placement of technical communication on the disciplinary food chain.

Winner and the Politics of Technology

Winner's writings have been influential across all of the disciplines we have surveyed. He touches on issues (and sometimes nerves) that all disciplines concerned with technology must acknowledge as important. Above all, he concentrates on the political nature of technology throughout history. One need look no further than his first book, *Autonomous Technology: Technics Out-of-Control as a Theme in Political Thought*, to get a strong sense of his research focus. Nearly twenty years later, the emphasis on politics and technology can be seen as strongly as ever in his article from the infamous *Social Text* issue last summer where he described his own work as:

> expressing a desire to confront what I perceive to be a systematic disorder in modern life, a disorder manifest in certain technology-centered ways of living that I regard as unfriendly to any sane aspiration for human beings; and applying concepts and approaches of a particular discipline, political theory, to questions about the significance of technology for political life. ("Gloves Come Off" 84)

I imagine that the connections of Winner's research, and its concomitant relation to politics, is enough to demonstrate a relevance to technical communication. Problems of citizenship, ethics, and disciplinary relationships paint brightly colored illustrations of how technology can be questioned, yet preserved.

Such discussions of essential paradoxes of technology and human social order are fundamental to the growth of technical communication research. There is also an interdisciplinary thread in Winner's work that technical communicators might model. His reliance on political theory and technological issues allows him to weave stories that in some ways recall the narrative approach of the technology historians, a disciplinary community with which he shares some considerable allegiance. Additionally, his focus on topics such as environmental protection (see *The Whale and the Reactor*) and on participation in civic discourse (see "Citizen Virtues in a Technological Order") demonstrate clear parallels to research areas in our own field, including information technologies and interface design.

Shouldering the Borrowed Burden: Putting Comprehension to Work

The three disciplinary strands of technology studies discussed here—history, sociology, and philosophy—are interesting in themselves. There are many compelling stories told, and an equally rich display of methods from which one can choose. In the spirit of interdisciplinary research, though, it is important to incorporate these new understandings into our own research agendas. The burden of comprehension, in other words, becomes a burden of activation. In this concluding section, I will once again turn to the scholarship of interdisciplinary research for the purpose of activating these methods of technology studies in the realm of technical communication: an activity referred to in interdisciplinary circles as *translation*.

Klein offers George Steiner's four-stage "act of translation" to describe how one can bring multidisciplinary research into a commonly shared sphere of meaning. As Klein explains, Steiner's fourfold process consists of:

1. An *initiative trust* between the translator and the disciplines that are being translated;
2. An *incursive and extractive act* where the translator "invades and brings home";
3. An *act of incorporation*, where the extracted meaning is "assimilated and placed" into a new arena; and

4. A *compensatory act* of reciprocity that attempts to restore "balance while enhancing and even enlarging the stature of the original." (93–94)

This article has been an attempt to carry out the first three stages of translation. The initiative trust has been accomplished through a collegial and respectful act of translation that attempts to bring the knowledge of these three disciplines to technical communication, while at the same time maintaining a respect for the values and ideological contexts of those disciplines. Incursion and extraction have been accomplished through descriptions of the widely different disciplinary theoretical and methodological stances, and through attention to the contexts and histories of those disciplinary viewpoints. Much of this second stage has been done via the vehicle of example. I have brought particular moments forward from the three disciplinary contexts to illuminate their respective theories and methods. I have also extracted some elemental issues of debate (the "old chestnuts") to the surface so that the ideological assumptions of these disciplines are more visible. For instance, two key examples are the uneasy relationship between science and technology, and the slow but steady injection of cultural study into the study of artifacts.

The third stage, incorporation, has been attempted through speculation about how these methods might be used by technical communicators. In addition, I have used several references to the common theme of technological determinism and problems of human agency to show a link between these three disciplines and technical communication. Human agency is without a doubt one of the most probed issues in modern intellectual arenas, and for those who study technology, the issue of agency is most often discussed in terms of determinism. Technologies have a strong and defining influence upon whole complexes of cultural shifts that make the problem of locating agency difficult. When technologies accompany cultural changes it is often not clear as to who or what is controlling or influencing the change. This common thread of technological determinism is significant for us in technical communication; we have much to gain from those disciplines that have probed it to considerable depths.

The fourth and final stage—compensation—is beyond the scope of this article. Nevertheless, I will posit how such a reciprocity might occur between technical communicators and the greater arena of STS studies as this is possibly the most crucial aspect of interdisciplinary research. Without reciprocity, or the attempt to carry it out, we remain voiceless, passive observers peering through the disciplinary windows. In closing, I offer the following scenario as a way of describing how we might enter such an interdisciplinary dialogue.

Recently, I was sitting in my second floor office with the window open when I heard a small engine start up directly beneath me. I looked out and saw a grounds crew worker blowing leaves and grass cuttings from the sidewalk with a gasoline-powered blower. My immediate reaction was to shut the window; the blower was obnoxiously loud. As I shut the window, I noticed that the worker had a pair of headphone-like ear protectors draped around his neck. They were obviously not being used to block the sound that even at my distance appeared harmful.

The scene reminded me of a recent discussion in a technical communication graduate seminar regarding right-to-know information for workplace hazards. One of the students, a long-time employee of the National Institute for Occupational Safety and Health (NIOSH), mentioned that hearing loss is one of the most common threats to worker health. He went on to explain that there are many reasons for this, including reluctance by workers to wear uncomfortable headsets (especially on hot summer days), lack of inadequate information for workers regarding the danger of hearing loss, and a misperception in industry that many sounds are not as harmful as they seem. Another student remarked that her father, a highway worker for many years, had suffered hearing loss because of his reluctance to wear protection because it "got in the way of his work." She added that he once claimed the loss of hearing was a small price to pay for his job—a relatively high paying job in the rural, central Pennsylvania area where she had grown up.

As technical communicators, we might traditionally approach this problem of hearing protection through the development of clearly written and accessible documents that explain the hazards and how to avoid them. We also might design training workshops that orally provide similar information. In our boldest of moments, we might even attempt to persuade the designers of the headsets that the design is not usable, and that we would have some suggestions about how a re-design might improve the use of the product.

I believe that our knowledge of how to communicate and explain technology to other humans is indeed important. I am inclined to think that we could pique the interest of scholars in the greater sphere of STS with our own tales of technology: how people use it, how they learn about it, how they resist it. My own research into the interdisciplinary milieu indicates that few philosophers, historians, or sociologists of technology think about the instructional aspects of technology. We have much to discuss with them in this regard.

But I also think that technical communicators have an obligation to question technology—to approach it with a critical eye. For instance, we might ask: "Why does the grounds crew worker need to use a gas-powered blower at all?" What ideological, economic, and institutional pressures have called for the use of such devices: devices that not only cut costs (do they in the long-term really do so?), but that also needlessly cause hearing loss? Once we have pondered these beyond/before-the-documentation questions, then we can turn our gaze upon action: action that would be for the benefit of not just the immediate user (as important as that is), but also to the greater array of users who occupy the ethical space within which a given technological artifact or system operates. Because of our immediate involvement with the planners and developers of technologies, we are potentially in a unique position to affect such change—a position that few disciplines are privileged to occupy.

For this more critical and proactive approach we should borrow from the historians, the sociologists, the philosophers. We should enter the dialogue with our own values, ready to question our own approach while persuading them to question theirs. We should use this new dialogic space to realize our hidden potentials. It is this interdisciplinary space that we should enter as our discipline grows: a space where technical communicators can have the choice of becoming something other than scribes or instrumentalists. First, however, we must practice patience to comprehend what we borrow.

WORKS CITED

Bazerman, Charles. *Shaping Written Knowledge: The Genre and Activity of the Experimental Article in Science*. Madison: Wisconsin UP, 1988.

Bijker, Wiebe E., Trevor P. Hughes, and Trevor J. Pinch. *The Social Construction of Technological Systems: New Directions in the Sociology and History of Technology*. Cambridge, MA: MIT P, 1987.

Brown, John Seely, and Paul Duguid. "Borderline Issues: Social and Material Aspects of Design." *Human Computer Interaction* 9 (1994): 3–36.

Cockburn, Cynthia. *Machinery of Dominance: Women, Men and Technical Know-How*. London: Pluto P, 1985.

Cowan, Ruth S. *More Work for Mother: Household Technologies from the Open Hearth to the Microwave*. New York: Basic Books, 1984.

Doheny-Farina, Stephen. *Rhetoric, Innovation, Technology*. Cambridge, MA: MIT P, 1992.

Ehn, Pelle. *Work-Oriented Design of Computer Artifacts*. Stockholm: Arbetslivscebtrum, 1988.

Ellul, Jacques. *The Technological Society*. New York: Vintage Books, 1964.

Floyd, C., et al. "Out of Scandinavia: Alternative Approaches to Software Design and Development." *Human Computer Interaction* 4 (1989): 253–349.

Haas, Christina. *Writing Technology: Studies on the Materiality of Literacy*. Mahwah, NJ: Lawrence Erlbaum, 1996.

Hacker, Sally. *Doing It the Hard Way: Investigations of Gender and Technology*. Ed. Dorothy Smith and Susan Turner. Boston: Unwin Hyman, 1990.

Hagge, John. "Ethics, Words, and the World in Moore's and Miller's Accounts of Scientific and Technical Discourse." *Journal of Business and Technical Communication* 10 (1996): 461–75.

Heidegger, Martin. *The Question of Technology and Other Essays*. Trans. William Lovitt. San Franciso: Harper and Row, 1962.

Johnson, Robert R. *User-Centered Technology: A Rhetorical Theory of Computers and Other Mundane Artifacts*. Albany, NY: SUNY P, in press.

Klein, Julie T. *Interdisciplinarity*. Detroit: Wayne State UP, 1990.

Latour, Bruno. "Where Are the Missing Masses? The Sociology of a Few Mundane Artifacts." *Shaping Technology/Building Society: Studies in Sociotechnical Change*. Ed. Wiebe E. Bijker and John Law. Cambridge, MA: MIT P, 1992. 225–58.

Lauer, Janice M. "Composition Studies: Dappled Discipline." *Rhetoric Review* 3 (1984): 20–29.

Lauer, Janice M., and J. William Asher. *Composition Research: Empirical Designs*. New York: Oxford UP, 1988.

Law, John, ed. *A Sociology of Monsters: Essays on Power, Technology and Domination*. London: Routledge P, 1991.

Layton, Edwin. "Technology as Knowledge." *Technology and Culture* 15 (1974): 31–41.

Long, Pamela. "The Openness of Knowledge: An Ideal in Its Context in 16th-Century Writings on Mining and Metallurgy." *Technology and Culture* 32 (1991): 318–55.

MacKenzie, Donald, and Judy Wacjman. *The Social Shaping of Technology*. Philadelphia: Open UP, 1985.

Mitcham, Carl. *Thinking through Technology: The Path between Engineering and Philosophy*. Chicago: Chicago UP, 1994.

Moore, Patrick. "Instrumental Discourse Is as Humanistic as Rhetoric." *Journal of Business and Technical Communication* 10 (1996): 100–18.

Mumford, Lewis. *Technics and Civilization*. New York; Harcourt, Brace and World, 1934.

Myers, Greg. *Writing Biology: Texts in the Social Construction of Scientific Knowledge*. Madison: Wisconsin UP, 1990.

Pinch, Trevor J., and Wiebe E. Bijker. "The Social Construction of Facts and Artifacts: Or How the Sociology of Science and the Sociology of Technology Might Benefit Each Other." *The Social Construction of Technological Systems: New Directions in the Sociology and History of Technology*. Ed. Wiebe E. Bijker, Trevor P. Hughes, and Trevor J. Pinch. Cambridge, MA: MIT P, 1987. 17–49.

Ranney, Frances. "Reading, Writing, and Rhetoric: An Inquiry into the Art of Legal Language." Diss. Miami U, OH, 1997.

Reichert, Pegeen. "A Contributing Listener and Other Composition Wives: Reading and Writing the Feminine Metaphors in Composition Studies." *Journal of Advanced Composition* 16 (1996): 141–57.

Ross, Andrew. "Introduction." *Social Text* 14.1–2 (1996): 1–14.

Singer, Charles, et al., eds. *A History of Technology*, Vols. 1–5. Oxford, England: Clarendon P, 1954–58.

Smith, Merritt R., and Leo Marx, eds. *Does Technology Drive History? The Dilemma of Technological Determinism*. Cambridge, MA: MIT P, 1994.

Sokal, Alan. "A Physicist Experiments with Cultural Studies." *Lingua Franca* 6.4 (1996): 62–64.

———. "Transgressing the Boundaries: Toward a Transformative Hermeneutics of Quantum Gravity." *Social Text* 14-1–2 (1996): 217–52.

Star, Susan Leigh. "Power, Technologies and the Phenomenology of Conventions: On Being Allergic to Onions." *A Sociology of Monsters: Essays On Power, Technology and Domination*. Ed. John Law. London: Routledge, 1991. 25–26.

Staudenmaier, John. *Technology's Storytellers*. Cambridge, MA: MIT P, 1985.

Suchman, Lucy. "Working Relations of Technology Production and Use." *Computer Supported Cooperative Work* 2 (1994): 21–39.

Wajcman, Judy. *Feminism Confronts Technology*. University Park: Pennsylvania State UP, 1991.

Winner, Langdon. *Autonomous Technology: Technics Out-of-Control as a Theme in Political Thought*. Cambridge, MA: MIT P, 1977.

———. "Citizen Virtues in a Technological Order." *Inquiry* 35 (1992): 3–4.

———. "The Gloves Come Off: Shattered Alliances in Science and Technology Studies." *Social Text* 14.1–2 (1996): 81–93.

———. "Upon Opening the Black Box and Finding It Empty: Social Constructivism and the Philosophy of Technology." *Science, Technology, and Human Values* 18 (1993): 362–78.

———. The Whale and the Reactor. Chicago: Chicago UP, 1985.

Woolgar, Steve. "The Turn to Technology in Social Studies of Science." *Science, Technology, and Human Values* 16 (1991): 20–50.

3

Myths about Instrumental Discourse: A Response to Robert R. Johnson

PATRICK MOORE

In this response to Johnson's article, Patrick Moore takes issue with those teachers and scholars he labels "totalizing rhetoricians" (p. 47 in this volume). He addresses six claims about instrumental discourse, labeling them "myths." The two most essential claims he works to counter are Johnson's contention that advocates of "an instrumental approach to technical communication" are comfortable with or accept the definition of technical communicator as "mere scribe" (p. 48) and that a goal of technical communicator professors should be to complicate technology. Moore argues instead that they should "find creative, economical, and effective ways to integrate technology into [their] culture and [their] personal lives" (p. 53). Moore's portrayal of faculty who teach technical communication and the kinds of issues that he raises – issues of definition (e.g., technical communication, rhetoric); of obligations to students, users, and society; and of influence – are worth considering. Finally, it is worth noting that this debate is just one of several that Moore has participated in or begun in the past decade.[1]

In his Winter 1998 article in *TCQ*, "Complicating Technology," Robert Johnson says, among other things, that advocates of instrumental discourse (myself and John Hagge) limit technical communicators to the role of "mere scribe" and advocate "an uncomplicated, reductive stance" towards technical communication. Here is a fuller quotation of Johnson's comments:

> Instead of expanding the scope of the technical communicator, these arguments for an instrumental approach to technical communication illuminate vividly the profession's entrapment within, and comfort with, the role of the technical communicator as mere scribe (Moore; Hagge). To define narrowly the theoretical disposition of the profession as "instrumental" is to become defensively monodisciplinary. In so doing, we, unwittingly or not, pigeonhole ourselves as "nonrhetorical," "antihumanistic," or "pro-instrumental," and thus risk becoming subservient to

From *Technical Communication Quarterly* 8, no. 2 (1999): 210–23.

[1]References to other debates are included in the list of additional readings on p. 62.

> disciplines that occupy the other side, usually the power-side, of the binaries: disciplines that are unlikely to relinquish even the smallest vestige of influence.
>
> To become comfortable with such a narrow-gauge view of our profession is to become too comfortable—a complacency in part due to unproblematic attitudes toward the defining influence of our profession: Technology.
>
> An uncomplicated, reductive stance makes it far too simple to just perceive technology as an *is*: as something that predetermines our very thinking about who we are, what we do, and why we do what we do. (p. 25 in this volume)

In this passage, Johnson seems to trivialize and dismiss instrumental discourse, and in the process he expresses at least six myths about instrumental discourse, which I would like to rebut.

Before I introduce the myths, I shall review the definitions of instrumental discourse on which I have based my arguments. I repeat these definitions for readers who are not familiar with my earlier writings on this subject (see Moore, "Instrumental"; Moore, "Response"; Moore, "Rhetorical"). First, Stephen Toulmin, Richard Rieke, and Alan Janik say that instrumental discourse is "those utterances that are supposed to achieve their purpose directly, as they stand, without the need to produce any additional 'reasons' or 'supporting arguments'" (5). Second, Walter Beale defines the purposes of instrumental discourse as "the governance, guidance, control, or execution of human activities" (94).

How academics define technical communication is crucial because definitions influence curriculum design, classroom teaching strategies, financial expenditures, students' preparation for the workplace, and the heuristic power of theory. If technical communication is defined exclusively as rhetoric, then rhetoricians control the curriculum, heavily influence classroom teaching strategies, and dictate how departmental budgets are spent. That is, if rhetoricians control the definition of technical communication, then there will be a heavy reliance on rhetorical theory classes, fewer classes on applied technical communication, and less money spent on communication technologies and technical communication software. However, if the definition of technical communication is enlarged to include instrumental discourse, then there may be fewer rhetorical theory classes, more applied technical communication classes in online documentation, usability testing, project management, graphic design, and instructional design, and there will be more money budgeted in support of the hardware, software, and technical assistance needed for the applied technical communication curriculum.

How professors define technical communication determines whether students will be prepared effectively for competing for jobs in the workplace and whether practicing technical communicators will have much influence over what gets taught in the academy. As I later show in my discussion of Myth 1, many students who graduate with majors in technical or professional communication do not even write well.

How professors define technical communication also impacts the heuristic power of theory: the power of a theory to lead us to a better understanding of human behavior, especially, in this case, the communication behaviors of people in technological institutions and in a global communication economy. If all technical communication is defined as rhetoric, then rhetorical theorists have reduced the complexity of a broad range of behaviors to one purpose: persuasion. Such a reduction makes it difficult to create the just distinctions which form the basis of any effective theory. The pioneering French chemist Antoine Lavoisier (1743–1794) expressed a similar concern about how chemists of his time used the reductive concept or phlogiston:

> Chemists have made phlogiston a vague principle, which is not strictly defined and which consequently fits all the explanations demanded of it. Sometimes it has weight, sometime it has not; sometimes it is free fire, sometimes it is fire combined with an earth; sometimes it passes through the pores of vessels, sometimes they are impenetrable to it. It explains at once causticity and non-causticity, transparency and opacity, color and the absence of colors. It is a veritable Proteus that changes its form every instant! (qtd. in Meadows 104)

Substitute "Rhetoricians" for "Chemists" and "rhetoric" for "phlogiston" and you have the gist of my objection to defining all technical communication as rhetoric: such a definition is too vague, too Protean. Lavoisier and chemists after him tried to be more precise about defining chemical behavior, and some years later Mendeleev developed the periodic table of elements. One virtue of the periodic table of elements was its heuristic power: Mendeleev was able to predict the existence of other chemicals that had not yet been discovered. The periodic table of elements led the way to the discovery of many new elements. If instrumental discourse can gain some currency in the face of opposition from totalizing rhetoricians, then it has the potential to shed new light on communication relating to computer-human interfaces, gatekeeping, accessibility, and using discourse to accrue power when persuasion fails.

Trivializing instrumental discourse and defining technical communication broadly—and exclusively—as rhetoric is part of an academic power game which some faculty use to advance their political agendas within the profession and within their academic departments. But my experience suggests that many rhetoricians are open minded and ready to share the power in their departments. There are some distinguished technical communication programs in English, rhetoric, and humanities departments in American universities. Yet it is equally clear that some rhetoricians do not want to share the power with other faculty, because those rhetoricians value their own ideologies over the welfare of students, over the welfare of the corporations that are taxed to support public universities, and over adapting the theory of discourse analysis to suit the new technologies of communication and the new corporate, government, and international environments in which technical communication takes place. One purpose of this essay is to suggest how totalizing rhetoricians—those rhetoricians who believe that all discourse is directly or indirectly persuasive—attempt to accrue power by trivializing other approaches to discourse analysis, especially instrumental discourse.

Before I discuss the myths, I must say that I do not intend this discussion to be a personal attack on Robert Johnson, whom I have never met. Professor Johnson's attitudes towards instrumental discourse are shared by other rhetoricians, and I single him out only because he has expressed several myths about instrumental discourse in a very brief space.

Myth 1: Advocates of Instrumental Discourse Believe that a Technical Communicator Is a "Mere Scribe"

In my fuller definition of instrumental discourse, published in the May 1997 issue of *Technical Communication*, I explained that technical communicators had to manage resources, suitability, accessibility, and readability (167–72). I specifically said that "technical communicators do much more than write" (167). Among other things, effective technical communicators must be good information designers, writers, editors, graphic artists, project planners and managers, usability testers, politicians, and negotiators, and they must know a variety of hardware and software technologies. They must also be creative thinkers and rhetoricians if they are to be effective in the workplace. In no way do I believe that technical communicators are mere scribes.

Unfortunately, many technical communication faculty are so ineffectual that their students would encounter difficulties even if they *were* mere scribes. For years, professional technical communicators have expressed concern about the defects in academic theorizing and the teaching of technical communication (see Hayhoe et al.; Carliner; Casper).

But more complaints come out every year. Anne Coon and Patrick Scanlon from the Rochester Institute of Technology courageously surveyed 44 of the recent graduates of their professional and technical communication program and found "the results of both surveys emphasized the basics of writing and computer skills. The degree program alumni also expressed the desire for a 'more practical' curriculum that placed less emphasis on theory" (391). Again and again, Coon and Scanlon's former students said that they needed more emphasis on the fundamentals of writing. One former student said, "Through conversations with PTC [Professional and Technical Communication] grads and while recruiting others for possible roles in organizations I worked for, two things became VERY clear. One, the curriculum needs to focus on more practical skills. Secondly, writing—clean, polished, professional writing—needs further emphasis" (397). A second former student said, "I would recommend that the curriculum stress writing proficiency even more than it did when I completed the program" (396). A third student said, "I would include a class in advanced grammar and remedial spelling. PTC graduates are expected to be grammarians and excellent spellers and often are not" (397).

Although Peter Kent, a professional technical writer and author of *Making Money in Technical Writing*, lives across the country (i.e., in Texas) from

Coon and Scanlon, his experience in the workplace reinforces the comments of Coon and Scanlon's students: many technical communicators do not perform well. Kent has a section in the sales chapter of his book that deals with the objections that customers often have to hiring technical communicators: "The simple fact is that many of your prospective clients have very little respect for technical writers—and that includes you. As I discussed earlier in this book, the standards in technical writing are very low" (201). Kent does not specifically refer to technical communication educators, but the other people I cited do. Many practicing technical communication professionals are acutely aware that academic theorizing about technical communication takes important class time away from studying the fundamentals of writing and editing communication products.

Practitioners are probably less aware of other problems in the academy that contribute to the poor skills of recent graduates. Here are two brief examples of such problems: First, higher education has been overbuilt in America. As a result, there are too many colleges and universities pursuing too few qualified students. Virtually anyone who has passed the GED and can borrow money can get into college in America. Once public colleges admit students, they are reluctant to lose them—and their tuition, fees, and state-supported capitation subsidies. Thus many colleges emphasize retention, and two well-known ways to retain students are to inflate grades and dumb down classes. A second problem is finding qualified technical communication instructors. Professionals can make more money being a technical communicator than teaching the subject. Graduating students can make more money in their first jobs than their professors. It is well known in academic technical communication that almost anyone is allowed to teach the subject at many public colleges in the United States, in part because practitioners make more money and have better equipment.

Thus, the economic problems of American colleges and the emphasis on complicating and totalizing theories of rhetoric contribute to produce many technical communication graduates who are not good enough to be mere scribes. Because the tasks, audiences, and purposes or the workplace are so varied, college graduates must be able to do much more than merely write and edit. Unfortunately, however, many students are ill served by academic technical communication classes.

Myth 2: Advocates of Instrumental Discourse Believe the "Theoretical Disposition of the Profession" of Technical Communication Is Exclusively Instrumental

As I said in "Instrumental Discourse Is as Humanistic as Rhetoric," one of my goals was to develop "a definition of technical communication as both rhetorical *and* instrumental discourse" (102). Robert Johnson cites my article in his bibliography, but ignores my pluralistic approach to defining technical communication. Later in that essay I say, "Instrumental communications do not replace speeches, letters, and essays, and thus instrumental discourse theory certainly does not replace rhetorical theory or composition theory. Instrumental discourse theory complements existing theories of discourse by addressing certain purposes, situations, and technologies that those theories were never meant to address" (107). I do not believe that technical communication is exclusively instrumental.

Myth 3: Advocates of Instrumental Discourse Are "Defensively Monodisciplinary"

This statement is false. Much of academic technical communication theory seems to me to be out of touch with reality. I think discourse analysts should start over. That is, we should set traditional and contemporary rhetorical theories (i.e., that all discourse is persuasion) temporarily to the side, and then study all the genres, audiences, purposes, technologies, and contexts of discourse with an eye to what really happens when we communicate in our personal, artistic, academic, corporate, government, and electronic environments. My guess is that rhetorical theory and theories of artistic expression will prove very useful. But many kinds of communications in the academic, corporate, government, and electronic workplace are instrumental, and so I believe that we need a theory of instrumental discourse to complement rhetorical and artistic theories of discourse. Thus, my instrumental approach is not monodisciplinary or defensive. If anything, it is offensive, in several senses of the word.

For example, I am especially concerned about students who receive inappropriate and inadequate teaching (see my comments under Myth 1), and I am concerned about faculty and graduate and undergraduate technical communication programs which arrogantly waste students' time and money on totalizing and complicating theories of rhetoric. Students need more practice with the software technologies that technical communicators use in the workplace (i.e., graphics, desktop publishing, online help, and HTML programs), and students need more practice with the skills that practicing technical communicators use. David Hailey found in a survey of roughly 1,400 technical communication job postings that "The most sought after skills for the technical writer were copy editing (83 percent), writing (82 percent), publications management (60 to 80 percent, depending on how I interpreted the data), and visual design (66 to 86 percent, also depending on how I interpreted the data)" (27). But very few technical communication program curricula are built around addressing these skills and teaching students the software programs to apply them.

Professors typically respond to complaints that academic programs do not have enough software and hardware by saying that they do not have the money. But one reason they do not have the money is that corporations do not want to support academic technical communication programs that ignore workplace needs in favor of theory courses. Too many graduate and undergraduate programs waste students' time with curricula that do not help them solve important problems in the workplace. I think more technical communication faculty should take the offensive and change these conditions. Given the ideologies of many tenured faculty, however, my approach will offend them.

Where Johnson appears to be defensively multidisciplinary, I advocate an approach that combines an awareness of the disciplines that impact communication with a sensitivity to the needs of users. Because instrumental discourse is so pervasive—involving computer-human interfaces, instructions of all kinds, political manipulations, contracts, laws, forms, many kinds of graphics, indexes, and standards, to name a few—and because creating instrumental discourse involves working with so many different people—managers, graphic artists, engineers, sales people, subject matter experts, and local and international users, to name a few—practitioners must know as many relevant disciplines as possible, as I suggested in my discussion of Myth 1 above. But technical communicators and their professors must also study and understand what users need. The needs of users must be paramount. We should base our theories on what users need, not on theories from other academic specialties that are distantly related or unrelated to technical communication.

To that end, graduate and undergraduate technical communication programs should have more emphasis on user and task analysis, on mastering the standard software and hardware technologies, and on usability testing. I do not recommend abolishing all rhetorical theory courses, but I do recommend balancing the number of theory courses with courses in applied technical communication, especially applied courses that focus on defining user needs and then testing the resulting designs with users before the design is, as it were, chiseled in stone and distributed. Johnson never opposes practical courses in his essay, but he seems much more interested in academic research about historical, sociological, and philosophical aspects of technical communication, aspects which I believe will take our students even further away from serving users.

MYTH 4: ADVOCATES OF INSTRUMENTAL DISCOURSE ARE "ANTI-HUMANISTIC"

I devoted an entire article, "Instrumental Discourse Is as Humanistic as Rhetoric," to refuting Myth 4. Johnson cited the article in his essay, but apparently did not read it, and he certainly has not refuted it.

As I pointed out in that article, some people complain that instrumental discourse tries to control and coerce people. These instrumental purposes appear to some people to reduce our freedom and thus appear to be antihumanistic. But instrumental discourse controls and coerces in order to oppose the powers that try to destroy and dehumanize us. Those powers include nature, which arrays, among other things, hostile weather, infectious bacteria and viruses, and disease-carrying insects and animals against us. Those powers also include our fellow humans, who may try to harm us physically, steal or destroy our property, or violate our civil rights. Finally, our bodies also have powers over us: they demand nourishment, shelter, clothing, and safe living environments. Instrumental discourse is resoundingly humanistic when people use it to oppose these powers in order to live freer, happier, safer lives. But instrumental discourse, like rhetoric, is not humanistic when people use it to interfere with another person's attempt to gain freedom, safety, justice, and security.

Myth 5: Advocates of Instrumental Discourse "Risk Becoming Subservient to Disciplines that Occupy the Other Side, Usually the Power-Side, of the Binaries: Disciplines that Are Unlikely to Relinquish even the Smallest Vestige of Influence"

This statement more accurately describes the fate of totalizing and complicating rhetoricians like Johnson: by venturing farther and farther afield for approaches to complicate technology, such rhetoricians risk making their research irrelevant to practicing technical communication professionals. Patricia Goubil-Gambrell made a good point about this problem in her introduction to her special issue of *TCQ* in which Johnson's article appeared: "Technical communicators in the corporate world recognize the need for research, but don't seem to find much of what the academy produces very valuable" (6). I agree with this statement and I have cited evidence from technical communicators in my instrumental discourse articles, which supports Goubil-Gambrell's assertion.

One reason why Johnson's approach is not likely to solve the problem that Goubil-Gambrell has raised is implicit in his formulation of the problem, as quoted in Myth 5. Johnson seems worried about becoming subservient to the "other side, usually the power-side, of the binaries." Johnson sees himself (and technical communication professors) in conflict with the powers in the marketplace, when instead I think we (i.e., professors and practicing professionals) have more in common. We all want safe, usable, economical products and services, and we need to work together to get them. To do that, technical communication professors need to discover what practicing technical communication professionals and users need. Technical communication professors do not need to go shopping in other academic specialties such as philosophy, sociology, and history for their theories. We should talk to users, managers, technicians, decision-makers, and other users and developers of technology, and create theories based on that research.

Johnson's statement in Myth 5 also illustrates the key concern of his article: how do technical communicators "begin the long process of becoming more influential in technological planning and decision-making" (p. 25)? One way for some academic technical communication professors to become more influential is to realize that some of their theoretical assumptions are false. Two of those false assumptions are that (1) all discourse is rhetorical, and (2) instrumental discourse is anti-humanistic.

A third false assumption seems to be that ethical theories developed by one social group can be generalized to other groups. As David Russell has said, "Many, perhaps most, teachers of technical writing were (and are) trained as literary critics in departments of literature, which have for various reasons set themselves in opposition to commercial and technical interests" (86). Many literature professors are repelled by what they see as the materialism of the technological and business world, and they judge business, scientific, and technology professionals to be morally lacking by their literary standards. But, as Russell says,

> The current debate over ethics and practicality among professional communication teachers is in many ways a projection onto students of the discipline's own unresolved ethical conflicts, a way of maintaining the ethos (and values) instilled in instructors through their literary training while working in what is assumed by many in English departments to be an ethically compromising environment—an assumption that may be no more true of the institutional environment in business, technology, and science than the institutional environment of academic literary professionals, when critiqued from perspectives outside the hegemony of literary studies. (89)

Totalizing rhetoricians forget that all theories are local. That is, all theories begin in some specific set of conditions, and then they are elaborated and generalized from that initial focused locale to a larger context. But as those theories become more and more general, they lose their power to describe accurately. Beyond a certain level of description, they become useless. Shrewd theoreticians know the limits of their theories.

For Johnson, the road to becoming more influential in technological planning and decision-making is to learn better how to complicate technology. For me, and for other academics and practicing technical communicators I know, the road to greater influence with "the power-side, of the binaries" begins with recognizing that managers, engineers, customers, and users find technology too complicated already. To complicate technology further is overkill.

Thus the goal of technical communication professors should *not* be to complicate technology, but to find creative, economical, and effective ways to *integrate* technology into our culture and our personal lives. By complicating technology, Johnson and his supporters become less cooperative with users and they increase the chance that technical communication professors and their students will become more subservient and less influential in the workplace. They also increase the chances that academic technical communication will be ignored altogether by the powers in the workplace.

The way to avoid subservience to the powers in the workplace is to become better than those powers at inventing methods of integrating technology effectively into human life. By "effectively," I mean integrating technology economically, ethically, and safely into our lives. To use Johnson's words, the marketplace is "unlikely to relinquish even the smallest vestige of influence" (p. 25), but that is because too many academics advocate theories that are far-fetched and self-indulgent. To gain more power, professors of technical communication must learn to teach better the fundamentals of writing, information design, usability testing, graphic design, project management, and so on, and they must find better ways to cooperate with the people involved in technical planning and decision making—e.g., users, managers, engineers, technicians, and so on. We academics need to do more usability testing and user analysis of our own theories to see what the workplace needs to create safer, more economical, and more usable products and services.

Elsewhere in Johnson's article he advocates the importance of "the burden of comprehension" (p. 40). That is a good point, but the theories he has selected are precisely where Johnson's approach is weakest. In borrowing from histories of technology, from sociologists, and from philosophers, he forgets the contexts in which technical communicators actually work. Johnson should be borrowing from project planners, graphic designers, interface designers, usability testers, cognitive psychologists, and—*especially*—from actual users of technology: the everyday Joes and Janes who have to apply technology to solving their problems quickly, safely, and economically in order to create value for their organizations and themselves. Everyday users of technology do not want technology complicated. They want it integrated more effectively into their workplaces and their lives. Donald Norman says that one goal of manufacturers of technology should be "to move from the current situation of complexity and frustration to one where technology serves human needs invisibly, unobtrusively: the human-centered, customer-centered way" (ix). A fine recent book about how to integrate technology into the workplace is JoAnn Hackos and Janice Redish's *User and Task Analysis for Interface Design*.

MYTH 6: ADVOCATES OF INSTRUMENTAL DISCOURSE ENCOURAGE A "REDUCTIVE STANCE" TOWARDS TECHNOLOGY

In my "Response to Miller and Kreth" I argued that totalizing rhetoricians themselves were "reductive" (494). Much of my concern with totalizing rhetoricians is that they impoverish discourse analysis when they define all communication as rhetoric (i.e., persuasion). Discourse can have rhetorical, instrumental, *and* artistic purposes, and so can technical communication.

One of the problems with the term "reductive" is that it has positive and negative connotations. Totalizing rhetoricians apply "reductive" to instrumental discourse because one purpose of instrumental discourse is to divide the domain of discourse analysis into several areas—instrumental, rhetorical, and artistic—instead of one inclusive category called rhetoric. Strictly speaking, I do reduce the range of rhetoric in order to increase the precision and effectiveness of discourse analysis in technical communication. Johnson resists such a limitation and trivializes it by calling it reduction. I have returned the favor against totalizing rhetoricians in my own work. Since totalizing rhetoricians apply their god term to all genres of discourse, anyone who tries to set limits on their definition is open to accusations of being reductive. But reducing totalizing definitions can bring significant descriptive benefits, as I showed with my example of Lavoisier and the periodic table of elements in my introduction: using more precise definitions can open the field or discourse analysis to theories that are better designed to describe the communication behaviors involved in the contemporary corporate, government, and global information economy. The problem, however, is where the activity of reduction crosses the line from being constructive to trivial. I think that dividing the totalizing rhetorical definition of discourse into rhetorical (i.e., persuasion), instrumental, and artistic discourse is still far from "reduction" in the trivial sense of the word. But some totalizing rhetoricians may disagree. They insist that instrumental discourse is subordinate to rhetoric.

But if instrumental discourse is made subordinate to rhetorical theory, rather than equal to it, then that subordination cedes too much power to rhetoricians, just as defining women as subordinate to, rather than equal to men, cedes too much power to men. Lord Acton's saying about how power tends to corrupt is well known. As I have argued in my discussion of Myths 1 and 3, a totalizing definition of rhetoric has contributed, in part, to technical communication students being poorly prepared for the marketplace, to the overreliance on theory courses in some technical communication programs, to the scarcity of required applied technical communication classes in technical communication programs, and to the paucity of instruction in the software used by technical communicators.

As I see instrumental discourse, its goal is not to be reductive (in the trivializing sense) or to complicate technology, but to mediate between technology and users so that technology is better integrated with the needs of individuals, organizations, and the environment. To do that, people who design instrumental discourse must know what users need. Faculty who teach designers of instrumental discourse must base their theories on the needs of people who are close to the workplace, or—better still—on the needs of actual users themselves.

Conclusion

Johnson closes his essay with an appeal for patience: "we must practice patience to comprehend what we borrow" (p. 43). I agree with the spirit of that statement. I wish totalizing rhetoricians would exercise some patience with instrumental discourse, which they do not seem to understand, and I wish they would listen more productively to users in the workplace. I further wish that there could be a better balance of rhetorical and instrumental approaches to discourse analysis in technical communication programs.

Instrumental discourse has been a part of human communication since time immemorial. Using instrumental discourse, mothers and fathers taught their children to create, use, and maintain the artifacts that helped them harvest crops, hunt game, weave clothing, preserve food, cure hides, collect medicinal herbs, give birth to future generations, and preserve their cultures in troubling times. Ancient engineers, architects, and craftsmen who built aqueducts, pyramids, buildings, walls, tombs, statues, cranes, hoists, ships, and catapults used instrumental discourse to explain how they wanted their artifacts created. Lawmakers—religious and secular—have used instrumental discourse for millennia to govern people and to control destructive social behavior.

But instrumental discourse has been devalued for millenia by the cultural elites who found it beneath themselves to make their livings at the loom, in the kitchen, in the field, and at the forge. Similarly, instrumental discourse has been ignored by two thousand years of educators who aimed their teachings at ennobling and illuminating the spirit and not at developing, manufacturing, and maintaining material goods. More recently, instrumental discourse has been disparaged by professors who have seen it as the tool of capitalist oppression, existing for the purposes of profiteering, dehumanization, domination, and expediency.

During all that time, however, instrumental discourse helped people invent, develop, implement, revise, test, distribute, and maintain the technological artifacts—including books, clothing, communication technologies, medicines, food preservatives, transportation—that have helped so many generations live longer, safer, happier lives. During all that time, instrumental discourse has helped people create the laws and legal procedures which have led to more democratic political regimes in the world, which have reduced social oppressions and civil rights violations in many nations, and which have contributed to greater liberty, equality, and justice for more people in the world.

Obviously the job is not done. But our hopes for advancing political, social, scientific, and technological goals through oral, written, and electronic communication may be diminished if some critical theorists continue to trivialize and marginalize instrumental discourse in the academy. It is time to set aside the myths about instrumental discourse—and discourse in general—and invent better theories and better teaching practices.

WORKS CITED

Beale, Walter. *A Pragmatic Theory of Rhetoric*. Carbondale: Southern Illinois UP, 1987.

Carliner, Saul. "Finding a Common Ground: What STC Is, and Should Be Doing to Advance Education in Information Design and Development." *Technical Communication* 42 (1995): 546–54.

Casper, Rick D. "Teaching Technical Writing: Rethinking Our Approach." *Journal of Technical Writing and Communication* 25 (1995): 275–83.

Coon, Anne C., and Patrick M. Scanlon. "Does the Curriculum Fit the Career? Some Conclusions from a Survey of Graduates of a Degree Program in Professional and Technical Communication." *Journal of Technical Writing and Communication* 27 (1997): 391–99.

Goubil-Gambrell, Patricia. "Guest Editor's Column." *Technical Communication Quarterly* 7 (1998): 5–7.

Hackos, JoAnn T., and Janice C. Redish. *User and Task Analysis for Interface Design*. New York: Wiley, 1998.

Hailey, David E. "What You Need to Be Needed." *Intercom* 44.10 (1997): 26–29.

Hayhoe, George F., et al. "The Evolution of Academic Programs in Technical Communication." *Technical Communication* 41.1 (1994): 14–19.

Kent, Peter. *Making Money in Technical Writing*. New York: Macmillan, 1998.

Meadows, Jack. *The Great Scientists*. New York: Oxford UP, 1987.

Moore, Patrick. "Instrumental Discourse Is as Humanistic as Rhetoric." *Journal of Business and Technical Communication* 10 (1996): 100–18.

———. "A Response to Miller and Kreth." *Journal of Business and Technical Communication* 10 (1996): 491–502.

———. "Rhetorical vs. Instrumental Approaches to Teaching Technical Communication." *Technical Communication* 44.2 (1997): 163–73.

Norman, Donald. *The Invisible Computer*. Cambridge. MA: MIT P, 1998.

Russell, David. "The Ethics of Teaching Ethics in Professional Communication." *Journal of Business and Technical Communication* 7 (1993): 84–111.

Toulmin, Stephen, Richard Rieke, and Alan Janik. *An Introduction to Reasoning*, 2nd ed. New York: Macmillan, 1984.

4 *Johnson Responds*

ROBERT R. JOHNSON

Johnson's response is interesting for many reasons, not the least of which is his desire to situate it historically by citing the previous responses to Moore without elaborating on them. He addresses Moore's claims for the value and importance of "instrumental discourse" by returning to the source Moore uses to support that claim (the Toulmin, Rieke, and Janik text). More important, Johnson makes it clear that he is not embarrassed to claim an allegiance to rhetoric.

Many of the issues that Patrick Moore raises regarding instrumental discourse and its relationship to rhetoric already have been addressed most eloquently in previous responses to his arguments (see Kreth; Miller). Therefore, I will be brief.

I begin by placing my response into context. My *TCQ* article, "Complicating Technology: Interdisciplinary Method, the Burden of Comprehension, and the Ethical Space of the Technical Communicator," is, ironically, not meant to be a treatise on the importance of rhetorical approaches to technical communication. Much of my published work has been concerned with the histories and theories of rhetoric, and especially how the concepts of rhetorical arts are indispensable when it comes to developing practical solutions to usability methods, instructional document development, and pedagogical applications. In short, my overall research focus for the past decade has been to reach exactly those user-centered and student-centered goals that Mr. Moore seems to find at odds with my "complicated" approach to technology. For answers to many of Moore's questions regarding the relationships I see between rhetoric and technical communication, he might find it useful to review some of my work on these matters.

The central purpose of "Complicating Technology," however, is to explore the interdisciplinary milieu of technology studies and technical communicators' potential roles in this active and important realm of scholarship. Technology studies is a complex arena of scholarship that crosses virtually

From *Technical Communication Quarterly* 8, no. 2 (1999): 224–26.

every disciplinary boundary in and out of the academy. Within this arena of research is not only theory—a shortcoming Moore seems to suggest in his response. There are stories told by a wide variety of scholars, including historians, philosophers, sociologists, and anthropologists—researchers of different stripes who share the common experience of learning about humans as they wrestle with technology in everyday situations. There are researchers who share a multitude of methods for studying human-technology interaction in different corporations, nations, and cultures. There are even some who offer (gasp!) practical suggestions for living intelligently and productively with technology.

My primary reason for briefly mentioning instrumental discourse in this article was twofold. First, most disciplines (from the sciences to the social sciences to the humanities) perceive the term "instrumental" as, at best, a very narrow view of technology, and, at worst, as a view of technology that is simplistic to the point of being outright dangerous because it is an unreflective and naive approach to technology—an approach that I characterize in my article as one advocated by those who are afraid of biting the hand that feeds them. Thus, the concept of "instrumentalism" helped me to present a fine grain on a remote end of the technology studies spectrum that can be immediately understood both in and out of the academy.

Second, (and this is where I can thank Professor Moore for giving me the opportunity to expand on a point that would have been out of the scope of "Complicating Technology") I believe that Moore's interpretation of instrumental discourse takes the concept far beyond the point ever intended by the very people he relies upon. Most pointedly, Moore consistently quotes Stephen Toulmin, Richard Rieke, and Alan Janik's textbook, *An Introduction to Reasoning*, to present his rationale for instrumental discourse. Please listen (at some length) to the following lines that Moore quotes from their book *and* to the lines that I add which immediately precede and follow in their text (added lines are in italics):

> *To start with we may distinguish between instrumental and argumentative uses of language.* By instrumental uses we mean those utterances that are supposed to achieve their purpose directly, as they stand, without the need to produce any additional "reasons or supporting arguments." *We give orders, shout for joy, greet friends, complain of a headache, ask for a pound of coffee, and so on, and the things we say in these cases either work or fail to work, either achieve their purpose or fall flat, either have their intended effect or go astray, without giving rise to any debate or argument. By argumentative uses, by contrast, we mean those utterances that succeed or fail only to the extent that they can be "supported" by arguments, reasons, evidence, or the like and are able to carry the reader or hearer along with them only because they have such a "rational foundation."*
>
> *An order or a command, for instance, achieves its intended effect if it is obeyed or fails if it is disobeyed or ignored. It gives the person to whom it addresses only two options: either he can accept it and go along with it, or else he can reject it and/or disregard it. His understanding of it, and his assent to it, are shown in his direct response. A command represents an exercise of power through the use*

> *of language and takes the right to have that power for granted. So a command does not, as it stands, have to be "proved."*
>
> *By contrast, when people make most claims or assertions – scientific, political, ethical, whatever – they cannot expect to move other people directly. Instead, they have to appeal to the hearers' understanding and agreement by providing additional "support" for the original claims, and they seek in this way to enlist voluntary assent or compliance.* (5–6)

A clearer rationale for a rhetorical approach to technical communication would be hard to find. Toulmin, Rieke, and Janik purposely place instrumental discourse on a far end of the spectrum of language use. Instrumental language use is mentioned, but it is done strictly to point out that some utterances are taken at face value. Such utterances are important only in that they exist, and therefore they play the role of a marker at the end of the discursive playing field. I also want to note that this is the only reference to "instrumental" that I can find in their book (including its absence in the index). The remainder of the text is devoted to the much richer and complex range of discourses that constitute the multi-directional and often multi-interpretational acts of human communication.

These authors merely present instrumental discourse to demonstrate that there are moments of clear-cut understanding when the consequences of language use are limited by the power differential. From their examples of instrumental discourse, I gather that these utterances most often are found in cases of unquestioned one-way authority, such as orders given by commanding officers to recruits during times of war. No questions asked. "Yes, Sir!" This is certainly not the type of relationship I want to have, for instance, with the users I work with in usability evaluation and testing. Users should be part of the communication activity from the beginning to the end of development cycles (as I have advocated in a number of places – for instance see Johnson, *User-centered*; Johnson "Unfortunate").

Moore attempts to shore up his thin theory of instrumental discourse in his response to Carolyn Miller and Melinda Kreth when he admits that his definition of instrumental discourse "needs to be more elaborate" (500). He offers a short list of six areas of improvement, but even in this brief (instrumental?) listing it seems to me that his elaboration takes instrumental discourse far beyond any definition held by either Toulmin, Rieke, and Janik, or even Walter Beale. For example, he says that "rhetoric focuses on such persuasive genres as essays, reports, letters, memos, advertising, and so on. Instrumental discourse focuses on such genres as graphical user-interfaces, online documentation, procedures, quantitative graphs, indexes, and so on" (500). Further, in this present *TCQ* defense of instrumental discourse, Moore enlarges his scope to include "instructions of all kinds, political manipulations, contracts, laws" (p. 5).

Suddenly, instrumental discourse is laying claim to discourses that involve argument, affect, ethics, and legal actions. I believe this is the world of discourse that Moore wants to create, but to do so will take more than unsupported claims (see Toulmin, Rieke, and Janik). Maybe a more elaborate theory can be produced, although I see little evidence of this being done in this most recent defense by Moore of instrumental technical communication theory. Until a more satisfying theory and rationale for technical communication practice emerges, I'll stick with rhetoric.

Finally, I want to respond to Moore's assertions that technical communicators in the academy latch on to rhetoric in order to force a "power game . . . to advance their political agenda within the profession and within their academic departments." Further, he claims that we value our "own ideologies over the welfare of students, over the welfare of the corporations that are taxed to support public universities" (p. 47). I have thought long and hard about how these statements make me feel, and how I should respond. It has been difficult because I have had such a hard time even imagining a place where the discipline of rhetoric is so powerful that it controls the nature of students, curricula, public institutions, governmental agencies, and private corporations. I wonder, in fact, where such a land exists: a land where rhetoricians are held in such high esteem that they call all of the shots. If Professor Moore knows of such a place, then I would appreciate a map so that I can plan a visit. As it is, I can only wonder what it must be like there.

WORKS CITED

Beale, Walter. *A Pragmatic Theory of Rhetoric*. Carbondale: Southern Illinois UP, 1987.

Johnson, Robert R. "The Unfortunate Human Factor: A Selective History of Human Factors for Technical Communicators." *Technical Communication Quarterly* 3 (1994): 195–212.

———. *User-centered Technology: A Rhetorical Theory for Computers and Other Mundane Artifacts*. Albany, NY: SUNY P, 1998.

Kreth, Melinda. "Comment on 'Instrumental Discourse Is as Humanistic as Rhetoric.'" *Journal of Business and Technical Communication* 10 (1996): 482–86.

Miller, Carolyn. "Comment on 'Instrumental Discourse Is as Humanistic as Rhetoric.'" *Journal of Business and Technical Communication* 10 (1996): 476–82.

Moore, Patrick. "Instrumental Discourse Is as Humanistic as Rhetoric." *Journal of Business and Technical Communication* 10 (1996): 100–18.

———. "A Response to Miller and Kreth." *Journal of Business and Technical Communication* 10 (1996): 491–512.

Toulmin, Stephen, Richard Rieke, and Alan Janik. *An Introduction to Reasoning*, 2nd ed. New York: Macmillan, 1984.

ADDITIONAL READINGS

Darrah, Charles. "Skill Requirements at Work: Rhetoric versus Reality." *Work and Occupations* 21, no. 1 (1994): 64–84.

Hagge, John. "Ethics, Words, and the World in Moore's and Miller's Accounts of Scientific and Technical Discourse." *Journal of Business and Technical Communication* 10 (1996): 461–75.

Kreth, Melinda. "Comment on 'Instrumental Discourse Is as Humanistic as Rhetoric.'" *Journal of Business and Technical Communication* 10 (1996): 482–86.

Miller, Carolyn. "Comment on 'Instrumental Discourse Is as Humanistic as Rhetoric.'" *Journal of Business and Technical Communication* 10 (1996): 476–82.

Miller, Thomas P. "Treating Professional Writing as Social *Praxis*." *Journal of Advanced Composition* 11, no. 1 (1990): 57–73.

Mitchell, John H., and Marion K. Smith. "The Prescriptive versus the Heuristic Approach in Teaching Technical Communication." In *Technical Writing: Theory and Practice,* edited by Bertie E. Fearing and W. Keats Sparrow, New York: 117-27. MLA, 1989.

Moore, Patrick. "Instrumental Discourse Is as Humanistic as Rhetoric." *Journal of Business and Technical Communication* 10, no. 1 (1996): 100–18.

———. "A Response to Miller and Kreth." *Journal of Business and Technical Communication* 10, no. 3 (1996): 491–502.

———. "Rhetorical vs. Instrumental Approaches to Teaching Technical Communication." *Technical Communication* 44, no. 2 (May 1997): 163–73.

Redish, Janice. "Comments on 'Instrumental Discourse Is as Humanistic as Rhetoric.'" *Journal of Business and Technical Communication* 10 (1996): 486–90.

Ronald, Kate. "The Politics of Teaching Professional Writing." In *Landmark Essays on Advanced Composition,* edited by Gary A. Olson and Julie Drew, 183–89. Mahwah, NJ: Hermagoras P, 1996.

Smith, Robert E. "Rhetoric as Social Act: Cicero and the Technical Writing Model." *Journal of Writing and Technical Communication* 22, no. 4 (1992): 337–55.

Tebeaux, Elizabeth. "Technical Communication, Literary Theory, and English Studies: Stasis, Change, and the Problem of Meaning." *Technical Writing Teacher* 18, no. 1 (1991): 15–27.

CHAPTER TWO

Constructing a History of the Field

Chapter Two: Introduction

What is technical communication and when did people begin teaching it? These are two questions that anyone entering the field might ask. In this chapter, you will find readings that provide some essential background knowledge about the history of the field of technical communication. In addition, there are several discussions about definition, which, as Katherine Durack points out, is related to history: "How we define our profession influences where we look to find our past: definition, by function, tells us what is and what is not technical [communication]" (p. 100 in this volume). These articles should help you contextualize and define the field you are studying and propose to join.

In our scholarly work, thinking about and documenting what we do influences our actions. When people ask, "What is it you do?" you want to answer in a way that makes sense and will help them not only understand you but also value the work you do. As a teacher, defining the course you plan to teach and its goals is necessary in order to make the entire enterprise relevant to students. Without such relevance, students are likely to regard you and your course with suspicion if not hostility or resentment. They need to know what it is they're doing and why: they need a sense of purpose.

In addition, having a sense of history can be valuable for teachers. History helps us understand people and societies, particularly their values and beliefs. History also helps us to understand change and how the group or body we are members of came to be; it contributes to moral understanding, provides identity, helps us develop a sense of context and coherence while recognizing complexity and ambiguity, and gives us a broad perspective that enables us to possess the range and flexibility required in many work situations. While it may not necessarily be valuable on a day-to-day basis, having a sense of what has been tried and to what end will enable you to make better decisions about pedagogy. In addition, it is important to recognize what hasn't been documented. History is a *perspective* on the past, not the past.

Teachers who are reflective practitioners are able to explain and justify their work to students in ways that are understandable and make what they implicitly know explicit. They draw upon their experience, problem-solving skills, and historical knowledge to explain how they know something or why they have chosen a particular approach.

By thinking about how you will define the field you're entering and by examining its history critically, you will enhance your reasoning and decision-making abilities, develop skills for reflective practice, and deepen your understanding of and ability to substantiate that practice. More important, you'll prepare yourself to answer some of the toughest questions that students ask: 1) "Why am I taking this course?" and 2) "How will it help me prepare for my future job/profession?"

5 The Case Against Defining Technical Writing

JO ALLEN

In this classic statement about the issue of defining the discipline, Allen argues that we should, above all, recognize the problems and difficulties inherent in definition, making a case for "an extensive and flexible definition" (p. 75 in this volume) that will address current and future technologies and contexts. Allen demonstrates the potential problems for creating splits in the field by drawing on C. P. Snow's analysis of the split between science and humanities and by examining several dilemmas that practitioners have faced when they have attempted to create an all-encompassing definition. Demonstrating that "satisfactory" definitions have eluded the field so far, she makes a good case for putting more emphasis on other needs, such as a "theoretical framework" and "empirical evaluations" (p. 75).

> It is essential [to] understand that definitions are hypotheses and that embedded in each is a particular philosophical or political or epistemological point of view. It is certainly true that he who holds the power to define is our master, but it is also true that he who holds in mind an alternative definition can never quite be his slave.
>
> —Neil Postman, "Defending Against the Indefensible"

A recent issue of *Technical Communication* records the debate over whether a cookbook that was disqualified from the Twin Cities' Society for Technical Communication's (STC's) technical-publications competition because of its subject matter should, indeed, have been allowed as an entry. Arguing that the cookbook *is* technical writing, the author of the cookbook writes, "What can be more technical than a two-page description of the complete home process of making butter? . . . Or, how [to] make soap?" (Carlson 85). Defending the judges' decision to disqualify the cookbook because it is *not* technical writing, Mary Fae McKay responds:

> Those of us involved in the management of STC's competitions readily admit our difficulty in drawing the line between "technical" and nontechnical communications. . . . Would Stan Carlson's cookbook have been

From *Journal of Business and Technical Communication* 4, no. 2 (1990): 68–77.

> found technical if it had explained the use of a microwave oven to make such recipes or if it had included nutritional information? "Yes," say the organizers of the Twin Cities competition. . . . The basic criterion that the competition managers . . . have been using is the following: Is this the kind of document that STC members produce for pay and themselves regard as technical communication? (86)

In order to agree with the decision to disqualify the cookbook, we must conclude that STC's members do not write cookbooks—at least not for pay—and do not regard cookbooks as technical writing. I, for one, believe cookbooks are technical writing—regardless of whether they mention microwaves or nutrition and regardless of whether their authors get paid for the work. Would my volunteering to write—without pay—a software manual for a corporation disqualify the work as technical writing?

The judges of the Twin Cities' competition are not alone, however, in their frustrated efforts to define technical writing. Theorists and practitioners of the discipline have considered numerous components that such a definition should include; however, no definition of technical writing has emerged as universally acceptable. In fact, in 1989, STC's board members identified constructing such a definition as one of the objectives of their strategic plan for determining future goals of the organization. Ironically, the board members dropped this objective when differences about the definition could not be reconciled. According to William Leavitt, 1989 president of STC, the problem of constructing a definition will soon be referred to the academic branch of the Society.

The ongoing endeavors to construct this definition—or at least to identify the prominent characteristics that it should include—seem to insist that such a definition is possible, despite the history of foiled attempts to create one.

This article focuses on the issue of defining technical writing by, first, showing why a definition would be useful; next, discussing the most popular, previous definitions of the field; and, then, investigating the problems with defining technical writing. The final segment of the article focuses on the disadvantages of constructing this definition, arguing that we should abandon the search for one altogether.

Usefulness of Defining Technical Writing

Excellent reasons exist, beyond establishing guidelines for entries in publications competitions, for wanting to distinguish technical writing from other forms of writing. Certainly, for instance, some form of a definition would be useful in clarifying the bounds of our academic programs and our research. How, for instance, can we legitimately compare academic programs when we are not exactly sure what technical writing entails? Further, what topics are appropriate for researchers in technical writing to investigate within their field? The issue of definition may seem even more pressing when we consider the recent expansion of our field from a focus on individual writers and their writing to a focus on all the other technical-support personnel involved in the communication process and in nonwriting tasks, such as illustrations, communications management, public relations, editing, computer analysts and programming, researching, and so on. How does this expansion fit into a definition of technical writing?

Besides establishing boundaries for academic programs and research, a definition could provide the basis for establishing the professional status of technical communication. While much of the literature about professionalism and technical writing has focused on the issue of certification (see, for example, Malcolm; Harbaugh; Gordon), I would agree with those who suggest that true professionalism comes from dedicated service to the ideals of the profession—ideals that could be conveyed in a definition of technical writing, should we ever find one that could accommodate the variety of professional activities practiced by members of the profession.

Previous Definitions of Technical Writing

A review of the previous attempts to define technical writing reveals a universal problem: Each of these definitions focuses on a single aspect of technical writing, using this aspect as the basis for distinguishing technical writing from all other genres of writing. Some definitions stress only subject matter, some style, and some still other variables. Rather than catalog all prior definitions, I will point out just two articles valuable for their reviews of these definitions: W. Earl Britton's "What Is Technical Writing? A Redefinition" and David Dobrin's "What's Technical about Technical Writing?" (For representative essays on the definition of technical writing, see Dandridge; Harris; Hays; Hogan; Kelley and Masse; Limaye; Macintosh; Stratton; Walter, Zall.)

In his article, Britton reviews categories of definitions—those based on subjects, linguistics, thought processes, or purposes—calling each category "significant and useful," though he does not point out the weaknesses of the definitions (11). He then defines technical writing as communication that has "one meaning and only one meaning" (11). Britton's definition hinges on the notion of objectivity in writing—that precisely chosen words put together in precisely the right way will be interpreted by all readers to mean precisely the same thing. Those who argue against Britton's definition point out—quite obviously, I think—the unlikeliness of any utterance meaning exactly the same thing to all readers; after all, readers bring a wealth of experiences and background variables to their understanding of utterances that necessarily affect all their interpretations of meaning—as those who have attempted to create a mathematical language have found.

More recently, Dobrin also chronicles many of the previous attempts to define technical writing, noting their common offense:

> The definers of technical writing don't collect [information] systematically. Instead, they rely on a vast experience to govern the formulations they give us: they use a retrospective, intuitive, conservative procedure. They assume that something called technical writing exists, that it will

> change slowly, and that the bounds of their experience approximate the bounds of the corpus. They assume, in other words, that their experience is sufficient to comprehend . . . the texts they assemble and that those texts are in fact what technical writing is. But there is no reason to believe that their experience is complete, nor to believe that we can get at their experience in its totality with a few well-chosen words. So why should we depend on that experience for a definition? ("What's Technical" 229)

Later in his article, Dobrin creates his own definition: "Technical writing is writing that accommodates technology to the user" ("What's Technical" 242), a behaviorist definition that is flawed with the same kind of experience-based assumptions for which Dobrin has criticized others. Like the definitions he criticizes, Dobrin's definition stems from untested observations that present no evidence of any kind of systematic study. Further, there is little in Dobrin's article that makes his definition accessible since Dobrin's definition hinges on the explanation that "What is technical about technical writing is technology, to the extent that technology defines certain human behaviors among certain human beings and defines a group" ("What's Technical" 242). Finally, his arguments against using clarity, accuracy, and conciseness as requisites of technical writing are undermined by his own, often too complex, prose. The basic tenets of technical writing tell us, for instance, that in articulating a definition, writers should present straightforward ideas in straightforward terms. But Dobrin's definition is circular—the definition itself must be explained, and this explanation is as difficult as the original definition.

Problems with Defining Technical Writing

One of the problems with our attempts to define technical writing is the recognition that we cannot agree on the proper inflection of the term we are trying to define. Is it *technical* writing, implying that we write about technology as the sole subject matter, or is it technical *writing*, implying that we follow stringent rules in the practice of writing, regardless of subject matter?

This primary debate about the proper inflection of the term continues and, in fact, gives rise to a second problem: We cannot seem to agree on the parameters of the discipline. What, exactly, do the words *technical writing* mean—divorced from any attempt to explain the discipline? In other words, what would constitute the *technical* part and what would constitute the *writing* part of a definition?

The problem with inflection is clearly illustrated by the earlier example of the cookbook's exclusion from the technical-publications competition. The judges of the Twin Cities' STC's technical-publications competition, for example, chose to stress the word *technical*, depending etymologically on the word *technology*. These judges seem to require some kind of highly specialized subject matter—far more specialized, evidently, than making butter or soap—for a piece of writing to fit within their definition of technical writing. Other people, such as Carlson, stress the word *writing*; thus, if a writer writes about a subject in the same style and format and for the same purpose that a technical writer writes about a subject (e.g., writes a set of instructions in the imperative mood with consecutive, readable steps that give uninitiated readers the information necessary for performing a process), then that writer creates a piece of technical writing—regardless of whether the process or the subject concerns technology.

Interestingly enough, there are computer software programs, with their accompanying on-line documentation, that are cookbooks. *Dinner at Eight*™, for instance, gives recipes from famous restaurants in the Far East, France, Mexico, New York, San Francisco, and New Orleans—plus recipes for low calorie/low sodium dishes; ideas and recipes for dinner parties, foods to grill, intimate dinners, and fast-food dishes; discussions of wine; and conversions to and from US and metric measures (Johnston and Monaco). I could certainly be wrong, but I suspect that had Carlson presented his cookbook as such a documented software package, his writing would have been found acceptable for the Twin Cities' STC's technical-publications competition. If this is true, the issue concerning the *technical* part of the term may have as much or more to do with form than with content—a nasty little twist to the whole inflection question and one that Carlson recognizes.

More to the point, of course, a definition that is totally content dependent will invariably have to specify what content is technical and what content is not, and that dilemma will leave us no better off than we are now in trying to define technical writing. Further, a content-dependent definition would focus on what the writing is about (a focus that would lead to a stagnant definition) rather than on what the writing does (a focus that would lead to an active definition). Because technical writing is a recursive process—an ongoing relationship of messages created, formatted, sent, interrupted, received, evaluated, and responded to—it seems pretty clear that any definition of technical writing should focus on what the writing does and not on what the writing is about.

I do not mean to suggest that subject matter has no place in a definition of technical writing, but only that it cannot be used as the sole criterion for excluding works from the realm of technical writing—just as it would be absurd to use subject matter as the sole criterion for including works within the realm of technical writing. All writing about technology, after all, is certainly not technical writing. Even without a definition, we are astute enough to see that a short story describing the process a boy employs to care lovingly for his first car is not technical writing. Thus, subject matter clearly raises more questions than it resolves as a criterion for a definition.

In addition to disagreeing on the parameters of the *technical* part of the term, we also have problems with the *writing* part of the term as this part relates to style (clarity, accuracy, conciseness, objectivity) and purpose (to inform or to persuade). Most of us would agree, for instance, that Ernest Hemingway's style is dominated by clarity and conciseness, though we would hardly call him a technical writer. For obvious reasons, accuracy must be ignored in a consideration of Hemingway's fictive style, but it does not seem to be problems with accuracy that prevent us from calling Hemingway a technical writer. Hemingway's purpose for writing and the readers' purposes for reading, combined with the fictive understandings of the writer/reader relationship, keep us from thinking of Hemingway as a technical writer. Certainly, it is not because he wrote about nontechnical subject matter—wars and bullfights—that we have disqualified him as a technical writer.

Others have indicated their frustrations with style-dependent definitions of technical writing. Carolyn Miller, for instance, points out that using clarity as the sole touchstone for technical writing—relegating the entire issue of communication to clarity—necessitates a positivist perspective. Adopting, momentarily, this positivist perspective, Miller explains:

> Language provides a view out onto the real world, a view which may be clear or obfuscated. If language is clear, then we see reality accurately: if language is highly decorative or opaque, then we see what is not really there or we see it with difficulty. (p. 17 in this volume)

As important as clarity is, and it surely deserves a prominent place in our discussions of definitions of technical writing, Miller finds that communication requires a great deal more than only a clear windowpane. Communication also requires rhetorical savvy; invention strategies; appropriate points of view that accommodate different kinds of interactions with the subjects; and flexible senses of the writer/reader relationships that can be adapted to a variety of subjects, purposes, styles, and formats. These requirements for effective communication give the writer options rather than formulas for communicating (p. 18–20).

In "What's Difficult about Teaching Technical Writing," Dobrin also notes a paradox relating to style implicit in teaching technical writing: "The teacher of technical writing is teaching the student to perform for his or her peers in a particular technical community, a community of which the teacher is not . . . a member" (137). Thus, the teacher's understanding of the concept of clarity may conflict with the norms of the technical or scientific community for which the student will be eventually writing. Though techniques of style may clarify a topic for teachers or lay readers, certain techniques that are not suited to technical or scientific readers may actually impair these readers' understanding. Thus, clarity may be one of the essential components of a definition of technical writing, but a scientist's means of producing clarity may depend on field-specific conventions—appropriate uses of jargon, passive voice, and so on—that violate the technical-writing teacher's prescriptions.

As we have seen, attempts to define technical writing by style alone are problematic, and producing empirical research to support these attempts seems inherently troublesome because analyses of style require evaluation—measures of techniques that frequently lead to judgments about the goodness or badness of a piece of writing (p. 19). In other words, do we define technical writing by what it *should* be? Or do we define it by its most typical applications—in software documentation and income tax forms, for example—that are frequently poorly written? Consider, further, the difficulties with choosing texts to assess as examples of technical writing in empirical research. Can we analyze any piece of writing about technology as a representative sample of technical writing? Can we take any document written by a technical writer and presume it is suitably representative for our research?

These questions, unanswerable for now, simply lead to other equally disturbing questions. If we define technical writing only in terms of subject matter, how are we going to make necessary distinctions between good and bad technical writing? Is, for instance, a wordy, incoherent manual on installing computers still technical writing? According to those who define technical writing by subject matter only, the answer to this last question must be "yes." Some, perhaps, would argue that the answer is a qualified "yes," noting that the manual is a sample of *bad* technical writing.

In addition, distinguishing between good and bad technical writing according to whether it achieves its purpose is not a clear enough criterion for defining technical writing, since many poorly written manuals do eventually achieve their purposes but not before thoroughly irritating their readers. Is there, then, a time limit on how quickly the writer must accommodate the reader's needs? These issues are troubling, and they demonstrate the problems with basing definitions of technical writing on style.

The final problem with definitions of technical writing that emphasize the *writing* part of the term over the *technical* part of the term addresses the question of purpose. Initially, the issue of the writer's purpose seems to be less problematic with technical writing than with other forms of writing. For instance, we know that, in general, most technical writers write to communicate important information to readers who need this information. But what, exactly, is involved in the process of communication? We certainly have numerous models, or attempts at models, that try to explain communication; many of these models, however, are just as unsatisfactory as our attempts to define technical writing. Thus, we eventually whittle down the question of purpose to the role of purpose in specific works, but the possible answers to our question still degenerate into simplistic options: to inform or to persuade. Most of us would be hard pressed to give an example of a strictly informative piece of writing—one that has no tinges of persuasion.

Even if we do adopt the simplistic inform/persuade restriction on the technical writer's purpose, the biggest difficulty is that these two purposes are hardly exclusive to technical writing. Journalists inform; advertisers persuade. What kind of boundaries can we construct that will not overlap with these other areas? Even if we add something about "technological subject matter" to the equation, we still have to concede that journalists wrote quite ably about the technical aspects of the Challenger disaster. We must also concede that advertisers have done a pretty good job of describing some of the latest technological wizardry that has led to the comfort and performance of our new cars, while encouraging our desire to possess these cars.

Thus, we see that yet another criterion—the inform/persuade restriction—has vanished as the sole device for constructing a definition of technical writing. Combining criteria based on subject matter, style, and purpose seems most logical at this stage, but such a combination leaves us exactly where we are now: still arguing about what constitutes the components of the individual criteria.

DISADVANTAGES OF DEFINING TECHNICAL WRITING

At this point in our field's development and in our discussion, a satisfactory definition of technical writing eludes us. It strikes many as ironic—if not downright embarrassing—that a discipline that so frequently constructs definitions cannot muster one for its own enterprise. Before we continue with attempts to define technical writing, however, we should consider the potential disadvantages of doing so, beyond the problems already noted.

Primarily, definitions draw lines: *This* is and *that* isn't. We should be careful, in our earnest desire to create a definition, not to exclude or disenfranchise writing that falls outside our strict categories. I am thinking, in particular, about the cookbook incident and the potential for similar distinctions that serve no purpose other than to separate certain kinds of writing—and eventually writers—from the central core of technical writing, this core being concerned primarily with the creation of software documentation, instructions for building engines, and so on.

Where does cookbook writing fall in a continuum of writing? It does not fall within the fields of fiction, science writing, business writing, poetry, drama, editorial writing, advertising, press releases, reviews, or any other form of writing with which I am familiar. I am not suggesting that we should gather all forms of writing for which we do not have a specific category and place them within the field of technical writing. Rather, I am suggesting that we should reconsider works, like Carlson's cookbook, that fall so naturally in line with almost all the criteria we claim for technical writing before we exclude these works for violating a single criterion.

Further, some attempts at defining technical writing seem frighteningly reminiscent of the attitudes that led to the split between the sciences and the humanities—the two divergent spheres called "the two cultures" by C. P. Snow—because of the exclusionary tone that seems to accompany such distinctions: If you do not write about something that can be plugged into an electrical outlet or sold to the government, then you do not qualify as a technical writer—for which you can read, "one of us." Certainly, no one would argue that either the sciences or the humanities have benefited from their cultural separation from one another, and certainly a split in the discipline of technical writing engendered by our attempts to define the term would be just as harmful as previous cultural splits. It seems ironic, considering the role technical writing often plays as the bridge between the sciences and humanities, that we should be so close to creating, if not actively pursuing, our own split based on a restrictive definition of what we do.

Most telling of all, perhaps, is not the number of writing specialists concerned with defining the discipline, but the number who are *unconcerned* with this endeavor. I suspect that many technical writers recognize that they will continue to do the work they have always done regardless of the status of our attempts at a definition. However, other writing specialists have moved on to address more pressing needs of the genre, such as the need for a theoretical framework for technical writing (Moran and Journet ix), the need for empirical evaluations of the traditional do's and don't's we teach (Moran and Moran 313), and other theoretical and practical concerns (Smith).

At the risk of being called a naysayer, I must contend that no definition will adequately describe what we do. The historical problems surrounding any attempt at constructing a definition will continue to foil efforts to come up with the perfect definition of technical writing, and we have been doing our jobs for far too long without a definition to conceive of one that will accurately reflect all the activities we perform. Further, I think it's reasonable to predict that the past and present variations in our jobs are negligible compared to the variations the future will bring. How will a definition of technical writing accommodate new technology? Will hypermedia, on-line documentation, and other technological innovations be included or excluded from this definition? How will we decide?

It would be far better to keep our field intact—with our impressionistic, experience-based ideas of what technical writing encompasses—than to succumb to simplistic or exclusionary definitions that separate us from one another. Perhaps, therefore, we need to get over our embarrassment at not having a perfect definition and abandon the search for it altogether.

In the event I am wrong—in the event that some sort of definition is possible that will describe all we do while avoiding a disciplinary split—I predict that the definition will not be a handy one- or two-sentence catch-all. Rather, I think it will have to be an extensive and flexible definition that will represent the complexities and delicate balances of content, purpose, style, format, and all the other components of successful technical writing—not only the components of current technical-writing practices, but those of the twenty-first century as well.

REFERENCES

Britton, W. Earl. "What Is Technical Writing? A Redefinition." *The Teaching of Technical Writing*. Ed. Donald H. Cunningham and Herman A. Estrin. Urbana: NCTE, 1975. 9–14.

Carlson, Stan W. Letter. *Technical Communication* 36.1 (1989): 85–86.

Dandridge, Edmund P., Jr. "Notes toward a Definition of Technical Writing." *The Teaching of Technical Writing*. Ed. Donald H. Cunningham and Herman A. Estrin. Urbana: NCTE, 1975. 15–20.

Dobrin, David N. "What's Difficult about Teaching Technical Writing." *College English* 44.2 (1982): 135–40.

———. "What's Technical about Technical Writing?" *New Essays in Technical and Scientific Communication: Research, Theory, Practice*. Ed. Paul V. Anderson, R. John Brockmann, and Carolyn R. Miller. Farmingdale: Baywood, 1983. 227–50.

Gordon, Kenneth M. "Do We Deserve Professional Status?" *Technical Communication* 35.4 (1988): 268–74.

Harbaugh, Frederick W. "Professional Certification: To Be or Not to Be." *Technical Communication* 36.2 (1989): 93–96.

Harris, John S. "On Expanding the Definition of Technical Writing." *Journal of Technical Writing and Communication* 8.2 (1978): 133–38.

Hays, Robert. "What Is Technical Writing?" *Word Study* 36.4 (1961): 1–4.

Hogan, Harriet. "Distinguishing Characteristics of the Technical Writing Course." *Technical and Business Communication in Two-Year Programs*. Ed. W. Keats Sparrow and Nell Ann Pickett. Urbana: NCTE, 1983. 16–21.

Johnston, Dirk, and Jim Monaco. *Dinner at Eight*™. Vers. 1.03. Computer software. Starcor, 1985.

Kelley, Patrick M., and Roger E. Masse. "A Definition of Technical Writing." *The Technical Writing Teacher* 4.3 (1977): 94–97.

Leavitt, William D. Telephone interview. 31 Oct. 1989.

Limaye, Mohan R. "Redefining Business and Technical Writing by Means of a Six-Factored Communication Model." *Journal of Technical Writing and Communication* 13.4 (1983): 331–40.

Macintosh, Fred H. "Teaching Writing for the World's Work." *The Teaching of Technical Writing*. Ed, Donald H. Cunningham and Herman A. Estrin. Urbana: NCTE, 1975: 23–33.

Malcolm, Andrew. "On Certifying Technical Communicators." *Technical Communication* 34.2 (1987): 94–102.

McKay, Mary Fae. Reply to letter of Stan Carlson. *Technical Communication* 36.1 (1989): 86.

Miller, Carolyn R. "A Humanistic Rationale for Technical Writing." *College English* 40.6 (1979): 610–17.

Moran, Mary Hurley, and Michael G. Moran. "Business Letters, Memoranda, and Résumés." *Research in Technical Communication: A Bibliographic Sourcebook*. Ed. Michael G. Moran and Debra Journet. Westport: Greenwood, 1985. 313–49.

Moran, Michael G., and Debra Journet. Preface. *Research in Technical Communication: A Bibliographic Sourcebook*. Ed. Michael G. Moran and Debra Journet. Westport: Greenwood, 1985: ix–xv.

Postman, Neil. "Defending against the Indefensible." *Conscientious Objections: Stirring Up Trouble about Language, Technology, and Education*. New York: Knopf, 1988. 20–35.

Smith, Frank R. "The Challenges We Face." *Technical Communication* 35.2 (1988): 84–88.

Snow, C. P. "The Two Cultures." *The New Statesman and Nation* 6 Oct. 1956: 413–14.

Stratton, Charles R. "Technical Writing: What It Is and What It Isn't." *Journal of Technical Writing and Communication* 9.1 (1979): 9–16.

Walter, John A. "Technical Writing: Species or Genus?" *Technical Communication* 24.1 (1977): 6–8.

Zall, Paul M. "The Three-Horned Dilemma: Technical Writing, Business Writing, and Journalism." *The Practical Craft: Readings for Business and Technical Writers*. Ed. W. Keats Sparrow and Donald H. Cunningham. Boston: Houghton Mifflin, 1978. 14–21.

6 The Rise of Technical Writing Instruction in America

ROBERT J. CONNORS

Connors's foundational article outlines the growth of technical writing instruction. Beginning with a brief overview of engineering education prior to the Civil War, Connors explains how the growing technical needs of postwar America resulted in a demand for engineers, which ultimately led to a realization that engineers needed to be competent communicators (he documents a similar boom after World War II). Thus, in the beginning of the twentieth century, English faculty began to join the Society for the Promotion of Engineering Education (SPEE), and technical communication courses and textbooks were created to meet an expressed need. That said, Connors makes it clear that there has been (and remains to some extent) an uneasy tension between the two fields, some of which can be traced to the 'two cultures' split, with "engineers as soulless technicians . . . (and) English teachers as dreaming aesthetes" (p. 80 in this volume). Relying on the changes in textbooks primarily to outline the growth and transformation in the field, Connors brings the reader up to the early 1980s, and he, presciently, predicts that "technical communication will be an acceptable field of study . . . by the end of the decade" (p. 96).

I. The Early Years: 1895–1939

For as long as men have used tools and have needed to communicate with each other about them, technical discourse has existed. Scholarship has traced technical writing of a quite familiar sort back to the Sumerians, and we need come no farther forward in history than the Roman Empire to find technical writing as lucid and sophisticated as any that is done today. The tradition of technical writing is ancient, and, as Michael Connaughton's recent work shows, it can be traced historically. But systematic instruction in the methods of technical writing, though it is a relatively recent development and is thus not difficult to trace, has been the subject of few studies; for all that many technical writing teachers know, their discipline sprang full-blown from the brows of Mills and Walter in 1954. But now that technical writing has been

From *Journal of Technical Writing and Communication* 12, no. 4 (1982): 329–51.

accepted as an important part of the discipline of English and seems in many ways to have come of age, it deserves to know more about its own history and development at part of college curricula. In this article, therefore, I will trace instruction in technical writing from its beginnings in a few schools of engineering, through its lean times, when it was a poor cousin to literary studies in English departments, to its present eminence as a center of vital scholarly and pedagogic activity.

Engineering Education in the Nineteenth Century

It is only in the last century that technical writing courses have been taught in American colleges. To understand the genesis of these early courses, we must first understand the context from which they grew: the vast changes that took place in all American colleges during the period 1860–1900. Prior to the Civil War, colleges in America had been predominantly religiously based, usually fairly small, and reliant upon a classically descended curriculum. With the passage of the first Morrill Act in 1862, however, the foundations were laid for a revolution in American college study. The two Morrill Acts, in 1862 and 1877, founded and promoted the land-grant agricultural and mechanical colleges that were to make college education available in the later nineteenth century to a hugely increased percentage of the population, colleges that were to broaden and specialize the college curriculum in many ways.

In the last forty years of the nineteenth century, the traditional study of the classics of Greek and Roman philosophy and literature began to be supplemented by studies in mathematics, modern languages and literatures, liberal arts of all sorts, and by an ever-growing field of technical and applied specialties—chief among them engineering. The Civil War was largely responsible for this change in the status of the technical fields. During that conflict as never before, field engineers had been important figures, and with the burgeoning Industrial Revolution, the establishment of A & M colleges, and the growing technical needs of postwar America, the creation of schools and colleges of engineering (usually adjunct to the "arts" college in non–A & M schools) was a natural step. It was within these schools of engineering that the courses we now know as technical writing courses began.

These specialized upper-level courses in writing, however, hardly existed during the nineteenth century, and this rarity is explained by the manner in which engineering schools developed in America. Prior to 1870, the canon of established engineering materials was fairly small, and pre-1870 engineering curricula contained a large percentage of humanities-based courses as a result. Some of this coursework was classical, but much was relatively recent—modern languages, both English and foreign, freshman composition (which was itself a new course, at least in its modern form), and the "philological studies" of the early literary scholars, along with a few science courses, history courses, and varied electives. Before 1870 an engineer graduated with a good bit of knowledge of the "humane subjects." But the engineering discipline was rapidly being awakened by the fantastically rapid industrial development of the Gilded Age, and new engineering materials were not long in appearing in curricula. During the 1870s, courses in the humanities dropped almost completely out of sight in engineering schools. In a retrospective article published in 1932, H. L. Creek and J. H. McKee described what happened:

> The great decline in the amount of time given the humane subjects came between 1870 and 1885, the time at which the largest increase in the number of engineering colleges occurred, when more than one-third of the time given humane subjects disappeared from subject matter (1).

Losing ground most seriously during this period were the foreign and classical languages and literary study (2).

As we might expect, what were left after this rapid takeover of the engineering curriculum by technically based courses were the "old reliables" of language instruction—freshman English courses. Freshman composition requirements were almost universal, and the tacit assumption in engineering schools between 1880 and 1905 or so was that these first-year courses were all the introduction to writing that engineers needed. This period was, understandably, a rather dark time in the history of engineering education, a time when, by the schools' own later admissions, they turned out a large number of otherwise competent engineers who were near-illiterates.

Despite the fact that some freshman composition courses in engineering schools were specialized to the needs of technical students, there seem to have been no courses before 1900 that dealt with the needs of upperclassmen for knowledge of the writing demands of the engineering profession. Although engineering education itself became vastly more sophisticated as the nineteenth century drew to a close, it almost completely ignored the linguistic needs of its students. The Society for the Promotion of Engineering Education (SPEE) was founded in 1894, but it had no members from English departments until after 1905, and in general, engineering schools acted as if their students needed none but technical courses.

It took time, but a wave of reaction to this attitude began to build in the early twentieth century, and after 1903 or so there began to appear in the engineering journals and weeklies an increasingly bitter series of condemnatory articles about the illiteracy of engineering-school graduates. Letters and essays in most important professional organs decried the inability of the new men to write coherent engineering reports or even simple business letters. The *Engineering Record* spoke for many practicing engineers when it charged that "It is impossible, without giving offense to college authorities, to express one's self adequately on the English productions of the engineering students. . . . Most of them can be described only by the word 'wretched.' " (3)

The causes of the problem are not hard to trace. As pioneer technical writing teacher J. Martin Telleen explained in 1908, the standard freshman English course came too early in students' careers, it was too general in scope to be very helpful, it was not practically oriented enough, and there was almost no interdepartmental cooperation between English and engineering faculties (4).

Even as early as 1900 the familiar "two cultures" split had been established in colleges: English teachers saw engineers as soulless technicians, while engineers saw English teachers as dreaming aesthetes, promoting "refinement and culture" to the exclusion of reality (5). Clearly, though, some cooperation would have to be achieved if the problem that all admitted existed was to be solved, and technical writing courses in their earliest forms were the solution of choice.

Samuel Earle and Early Technical Writing Theory

The period 1900 through 1910 was the gestation period for technical writing courses. Although the surface of college life seemed quiet, at many schools there was furious activity that would soon come to fruition. Beginning around 1899, a number of engineering schools established separate English departments within themselves in order to serve the special needs of engineering students, the most famous of which still extant is the Department of Humanities at the University of Michigan. Initially these inhouse English departments taught only a specialized freshman and sophomore sequence, but they provided a natural climate for upper-level courses in specialized composition.

This activity was not long in producing prototypical technical writing materials. The first notable textbook devoted to technical writing was published in 1908: T. A. Rickard's *A Guide to Technical Writing*. This was a transitional text that dealt mostly with usage, meant more for practicing engineers than for college classes, but it sold well and was adopted at a number of schools. Rickard's 1908 book, though, was merely a precursor to the first genuine technical writing textbook written for use in college courses. The book was called *The Theory and Practice of Technical Writing*, and it was published in 1911 by a man who, more than any other, deserves the title of Father of Technical Writing Instruction: Samuel Chandler Earle of Tufts College.

The Theory and Practice was a genuinely new sort of textbook when it appeared, sharing only a few elements with the general composition texts of the early twentieth century. It grew out of courses in "engineering English" that Earle had been teaching at Tufts since 1904, courses that were perhaps the first recognizable technical writing courses. In addition to being the author of the first real text, Earle came to be the philosophical voice of the early technical writing movement as well. In an important article in 1911, he ably defended specialized composition for engineers, stating that although technical composition requires great specialized skill, "it has commonly been assumed that for such writing a course in general composition is enough." It was not enough, obviously, and Earle went on to describe the reforms he had instituted for engineering students at Tufts. "We have departed," he wrote, "from common practice mainly in three ways: in shaping the work in English more frankly and more completely for engineers; in giving systematic training in technical writing; and in adapting special means for increasing the efficiency of the work." (6)

Just as important as systematic technical writing training for students, in Earle's eyes, was the problem of the cultural split between English and engineering teachers. He condemned the attitude of English teachers that saw engineers as philistines, to be proselytised to about the superior virtues of culture and literature over engineering. In words that might be carved over the doorway of every Technical Writing Division office, Earle wrote in 1911,

> We find, as I believe everyone will who studies the case without prejudice, that for those who have already entered upon what is to be their life work, true culture comes not from turning aside to other interests as higher, but from so conceiving their special work that it will be worthy of a life's devotion (6, p. 35).

Such advice fell, unfortunately, on English department ears that were mostly deaf.

Earle's text is dissimilar to present day technical writing texts, due primarily to the fact that he approached his subject from a "modes of discourse" perspective which has since lost popularity. Technical writing for Earle was "narrative, descriptive, expository, or directive"; he did not cover any technical forms *per se*. *The Theory and Practice* included many examples of engineering writing (and it is important to remember that until the 1950s technical writing and engineering writing were synonymous), advocated only the plain style for engineers, and approached questions of audience in a surprisingly sophisticated way, but the book was a prototype and not a completely successful text. It found a ready audience, but it was superseded by other books in the early twenties.

Samuel C. Earle was a true educational ground breaker. "To him is largely due the present method of teaching English in engineering schools," said the obituary after his tragically early death in 1917 at the age of forty-seven, and though his passing was a loss to the profession he had helped to found, Earle's work gave direction and impetus to the "decade of great awakening" that followed the publication of his textbook (7). Between 1911 and 1920, the basic elements of technical writing courses as we now teach them were limned out at a number of schools around the country. The early centers of interest in technical writing were established by 1916—Tufts, the University of Cincinnati, Princeton, MIT, the University of Kansas, and Rensselaer Polytechnic Institute, to name the most active.

By 1916 the stream of professional complaints about technical school graduates had become a torrent, and engineering curricula began to change in an attempt to improve the situation. Writing in 1931 (and reflecting the fears and wishes of teachers of that period), J. Raleigh Nelson called the period 1915–1930 a time of "complete reaction" to the nonhumanistic training given to engineers during the period 1870–1910. Nelson saw a "unanimous demand for a more liberal and humanistic scheme of education" arise around 1915 (8). In actuality, the demand was for basic literacy in engineering graduates, but English teachers often put their own interpretation on the dissatisfaction with the older curricula. If engineering schools wanted English instruction, they would have to accept literature along with writing, because the English graduate schools of the time were not producing anything but literary graduate scholars—who wanted work. And thus grew up another problem in understanding between English and engineering faculties.

The essentially literary nature of nearly all available English teachers led throughout the early years of engineering education to real disagreements, both between engineering and English teachers and among English teachers themselves. On the east coast there grew up a movement led by Frank Aydelotte of MIT whose aim was frankly to "humanize the engineering student's character and his aims in life" through literary study. Aydelotte and his followers (who did *not* include Samuel Earle) claimed that the demand that engineering graduates "should be better able to write and speak their mother tongue is really a demand that they have better literary education." (9) Aydelotte's 1917 textbook, *English and Engineering,* was a reader of essays meant to "furnish some thing of the liberal, humanizing, and broadening element which is more and more felt to be a necessary part of an engineering education." (10)

Opposed to this "broad view of engineering education" (Aydelotte's term) was the "narrow view," which saw the promotion of reading and writing skills alone as the practical and proper goal. This position was most evident in the Midwest and far West, where English courses were taught most often by inhouse English departments working more closely with engineering faculty members. The A & M schools and schools of mines that grew up during 1900–1915 were especially uninterested in literary studies. In general, the more established the "arts college" at a school was, the more disagreement over the content of engineering English courses there would be.

During this period there were generally three sorts of English courses available for engineering students: the required freshman composition course, a sophomore literature sequence that was sometimes required, and the junior- or senior-level courses in "exposition for engineers" that were the prototypes of today's technical writing. This entire three-pronged sequence, however, was plagued from the beginning by certain problems. The most serious were the lack of interest in learning to write or read literature on the part of students, the quality and experience of many English teachers assigned to technical writing courses, and the lack of cooperation between English and engineering faculty members. Lack of student interest in English courses was in part a result of the way such courses tended to be taught. They were typically assigned to young and inexperienced faculty members who often looked down on engineering students as mere technicians and patronized them while preaching a gospel of literary sweetness and light. Engineering professors did not help either, often referring to English courses disparagingly as unrealistic and less worthy than technical courses. As an editorial in the *Engineering Record* stated in 1917, "Students usually regard the (English) courses as necessary evil." (11, p. 291)

The fact that technical writing courses were seen by English departments as second-rate and often staffed with younger faculty members or departmental fringe people meant that there was no glory and no real chance for professional advancement in technical writing. Thus the quality of technical writing courses was often low in the early days as departments rotated unwilling and uninterested teachers through them. Because of this second-class status given to engineering English, relations between English and engineering teachers ebbed. Engineering faculties had little patience with the stance of moral superiority assumed by many English teachers or with the idea that students must be "humanized" through English literature. In fact, when the English Committee of the SPEE conducted a survey in 1918, they found that although English as "training in thinking," "guarantee against illiteracy," and "a tool for use in technical work" got support from 72 per cent of engineering faculty members, the idea of English courses as "a cultural and recreational escape from the monotonous literalism of vocational study" (the English Committee's wording, not mine) was supported by only 5 per cent (12). Clearly the engineering faculty and the English faculty had different agendas.

THE FORMATION OF A DISCIPLINE

Despite the peripatetic wrangling over literature vs. vocationalism, the interest in technical writing grew apace. Prior to 1912, there had only been two English teachers in the SPEE, but seven more joined in that year. The English Committee had been formed by 1914 (chaired until his death by Samuel Earle), and by 1918 there were sixteen English teachers as SPEE members (13). The Mann Report on Engineering Curricula in 1918 recommended more time spent on English, and by 1920, 64 per cent of all engineering schools required some sort of technical writing course for their students (14). As J. Raleigh Nelson, whose technical writing course at Michigan began in 1914, suggests, it was during this period, 1915–1920, when the engineering-only hardliners threw up their hands and integrated English into the curriculum (8, p. 495).

As the twenties opened, technical writing was beginning to become self-aware. The amount of time devoted to it increased, new courses were proposed on both the freshman and upperclass levels, and new textbooks began to appear that were aimed specifically at the technical-writing student. T. A. Rickard published a new textbook in 1920, this one meant specifically for classroom use, but like his first text in 1908, Rickard's *Technical Writing* of 1920 was essentially concerned with good usage rather than with technical formats. A much more important step forward came in 1923, with the publication of the first "modern" technical writing textbook. It was called *English for Engineers,* and was the work of a tough-minded and professionally determined assistant professor at Ohio State University named Sada A. Harbarger. (The author was referred to in the book only as "S. A. Harbarger," perhaps because the publisher felt that many readers might resent a woman claiming to be able to teach technical writing.)

English for Engineers is the first textbook that is organized according to the "technical forms"—reports and letters—that still remain the basis for most textbook organization today. Chapters included treatments of many sorts of letters as well as explanations, abstracts, summaries, book reviews, editorials, articles, reports, and papers at meetings. But although this "forms" approach now seems natural to us, it was not immediately recognized as the best. Textbook organization by forms caught on slowly throughout the twenties, and Harbarger's text was not initially as popular as Rickard's non-forms text (though it outlasted Rickard by a decade, being reprinted last in 1943). Harbarger was extremely active in the SPEE, and her views of the profession as well as her textbook were to be influential in shaping technical writing instruction.

The mid-twenties saw two new developments in the profession, one of them practical and the other philosophical. The practical development was the introduction of technical writing texts that were concerned only with the writing of technical reports. Ralph Fitting's *Report Writing* of 1924 and the immensely popular and influential *Preparation of Scientific and Technical Papers* of Sam F. Trelease and Emma S. Yule (which lasted from 1925 to 1951) found immediate audiences in technical writing classrooms and their narrow-focus formal approach was to influence a whole generation of technical writers. Texts following Fitting and Trelease treated many different sorts of reports—preliminary, investigative, field work, recommendation, etc.—but seldom dealt with other technical writing tasks. They might be considered the apotheosis of the technical-forms approach to textbooks.

The philosophical development of the mid-twenties involved the rise of a younger group of technical writing teachers who defined themselves primarily as teachers of technical writing rather than as teachers of literature. The number of writing teachers grew slowly, of course—in 1926, J. Raleigh Nelson complained that "the little company of enthusiasts who have pioneered in this field the past twenty years do not see their ranks filling with recruits as rapidly as they might with"—but some of the younger technical writing teachers, seeing the doors of conventional literary departments closing to them, began to downplay the call for more literature for engineering students that had been part and parcel of the English lament for years (15). Bradley and Merwin Roe Stoughton made in 1924 the shocking statement that "the habit of creative literary imagination is a detriment to an engineer . . . Literary activity . . . is not desirable training for engineering students and does not help them present engineering data in brief and attractive form. . . . "(16)

This was still a minority position in the twenties, though; at that time most English teachers were fighting together to accomplish goals on a broad front. And there was evidence that these goals were being accomplished. A 1924 SPEE survey (the organization loved surveys) found that it was no longer necessary to urge the importance of English for engineers; the uproad over illiteracy since 1910 had done its work well. The survey also found that English requirements at engineering schools had doubled since 1914 and that more colleges were instituting technical writing courses each year (17). There was no question that by 1924 English was an important part of engineering education once again.

EXPANSION AND DEPRESSION

Changes continued within the discipline throughout the late twenties as new textbooks appeared, both traditional "usage" texts like Clyde Park's *English Applied in Technical Writing*, which enjoyed modest sales until the mid-forties, and the increasingly popular "technical forms" texts, the best-known of which was *Report Writing* by Carl Gaum and Harold Graves, which lasted well into the fifties. Technical writing courses of the period were gradually refining themselves, taking on the characteristics and beginning to teach some of the forms that we still use today. Most technical writing courses of the late twenties stuck to a few relatively rigid forms, though, and a contemporary description of an average course called it an "intensive study of the logical organization and effective presentation requirements of technical articles, reports, and business letters." (18)

This was a time of experimentation, as J. Raleigh Nelson was to say later, but the experimentation was conducted in an ever more secure atmosphere as English teachers realized how much they were needed. Another SPEE survey, in 1930, showed that of 1300 engineers and teachers, 95 per cent approved requirements in English composition, 75 per cent approved speech requirements, and 45 per cent approved literature requirements (8, p. 496). (This interest in speech, incidentally, was largely due to the vast influence of Dale Carnegie's books on *Public Speaking and Influencing Business Men* which were published in the late twenties. This first entrepreneur of self-improvement on a grand scale created a huge demand for speech courses in all technical fields. But that is another essay [19].)

Despite this acceptance, the early thirties were not a happy time for engineering English teachers. The Depression had hit engineering schools hard, and the professional publications of the time reflect a pervasive discontent, a feeling of compromise. Despite the demand for technical writing, most English teachers who made a specialty of it were still underpaid and little recognized in their own departments. Interest in composition teaching caused teachers to "lose caste" among their departmental peers and was seen as "professional suicide" by younger teachers (20). Engineering teachers still did not give English teachers the cooperation they felt was necessary, and engineering students often seemed to have little respect for the sorts of teachers being turned out by graduate schools in English. It was said in the thirties that many English teachers "appear to their critics as not of a sufficiently masculine type or of enough experience in the world outside their books to command the respect of engineering students" and they were called "effeminate" by some students. (One student was quoted in 1938 as calling his teacher "a budding pinko" [21].)

But in spite of these problems and discontents, in spite of the Depression, technical writing courses continued to fill. More sections were taught each year and new textbooks began to pour off presses at an ever-faster rate. (Would-be authors soon realized that the success ratio for technical writing texts was the highest for any type of composition text.) The most popular texts throughout the thirties were W. O. Sypherd and Sharon Brown's *The Engineer's Manual of English*, primarily a technical-forms text, and Thomas Agg and Walter Foster's *The Preparation of Engineering Reports*, which was a narrowly formal approach to report writing that practically led the reader step-by-step through writing a report.

There appeared in 1938 a study which showed the degree to which technical writing had come of age: a dissertation, later turned into a published report, called *A Study of Courses in Technical Writing* by Alvin M. Fountain. Fountain's exhaustive survey-and-interview study showed that of 117 engineering schools in America, seventy-six schools offered ninety-three different technical writing courses in 1937 (22). Fountain's study is an important diachronic slice of history, the only one extant; it covers the content of technical writing courses during the mid-thirties, the textbooks that were most popular, and the methods used by teachers of technical writing. The most important information in Fountain's study—and this is corroborated by the textbooks of the period—is that he shows how a technical-forms approach of a rigid and mechanical sort had become all but absolute by the late thirties. Fountain's study also indicated the range of forms taught at the time. Essentially, every technical writing course Fountain examined covered the report form; it seems to have been a *sine qua non* in such courses after 1935. Thirty of the ninety-three courses studied used "Reports" in their course titles, and more than one-third of the courses devoted the majority of the course time to report-writing. Fifty-one of the ninety-three courses also covered business letters of different sorts, usually of a technical nature, and only thirty-seven of the ninety-three reviewed fundamentals of usage—which was the hallmark of the fading older form of the upper-level technical-English course. In addition, thirty-three of the courses worked on technical articles, and oral presentations were important in many as well (22, pp. 83–98).

Fountain's report shows clearly that technical writing was a thriving industry in 1938, having produced its own authors, experts, and directors. The courses were more advanced and taught more forms. The study also showed, however, that little progress had been made on the professional front for teachers of technical writing. Conditions were still poor for many; there was still little chance for advancement, and the majority of technical writing courses was still staffed by instructors and assistant professors. At the same time the understanding gap between engineering and English teachers was widened, and by 1939 an important bastion of interdepartmental understanding was on the way out: a survey showed that of the more than two dozen departments of English that had once existed within engineering schools, only five remained (20, p. 412).

The dissatisfaction in the journal articles grew more shrill. Graduate schools still turned out nothing but literary scholars, and only the less talented of them gravitated to engineering English. After all the fruitless complaining of the past, little seemed likely to be done. In fact, technical writing pioneer W. O. Sypherd noted in a retrospective article in 1939 that "the prevailing notes are of uncertainty, discontent, and vague longing." Sypherd complained bitterly that literature courses were too few and too little to matter, that freshman courses were ineffective, and that lack of writing in other engineering courses, bad student attitudes, and no interdepartmental cooperation had brought engineering English to a critical pass. "I see little hope for any marked improvement," Sypherd concluded, "unless some radical upheaval should come to pass." (23)

That was in 1939, and a "radical upheaval" was certainly on the way. The first five years of the new decade brought activities that would result in a complete restructuring of engineering education and the beginnings of the final transformation of technical writing courses into the courses we still teach today. The World War, of course, was the greatest single factor in these changes, creating a new technological imperative that swept all before it, but back in the U. S. other forces were at work that would also transform the postwar engineering scene.

II. A Discipline Comes of Age: 1940–1980

Developments during World War II

On the surface, World War II brought the engineering English industry, at least as it appeared in journal articles, to an almost dead stop. In my research for this article, I found a huge hiatus in the production of articles of technical writing during the period 1940–1946—it is almost as if the concept of "engineering English" had dropped off the face of the earth. This journal silence, though, is not to be construed as meaning that the teaching of technical writing slowed or stopped during the war. It did not. Business in both technical schools and arts colleges went on much as usual despite lower enrollments. Technical writing courses continued to fill and new textbooks appeared, as did revisions of older books. (Notable texts of the period were J. Raleigh Nelson's *Writing the Technical Report* 1940 and new editions of Gaum and Graves in 1942 and Sypherd and Brown in 1943.) Sada Harbarger passed away in 1942 and was duly eulogized by the English Committee over which she had tyrannized for so long. In most ways, technical writing continued along a by now well-trodden path.

Despite the lack of journal articles, English teachers were not unoccupied during this period. They were responsible, in fact, for two wartime SPEE reports that, although they had no immediate effect, were to change the course of postwar engineering education in America. These were the reports of the SPEE Committee on the Aims and Scope of Engineering Curricula, produced in 1940 and 1944. The committee was chaired and directed by H. P. Hammond, and the works of his committee came to be known as the Hammond Reports. Both reports dealt with the same questions, and taken together they had an important effect.

The Hammond Report of 1940 brought together many of the fears and complaints that English teachers had been voicing throughout the previous decade in a new and powerful form. It condemned the narrow vocationalism of the engineering curriculum and put a stress on a proposed platform of "science, of humanities, and of social relationships rather than on the practical techniques of particular occupations or industries." (24) To this obviously Dewey-influenced pronouncement, the Report added a charge recommending "the parallel development of the scientific-technological and the humanistic-social sequences." These two "stems," as they became known, were at the heart of both Hammond Reports. There were, of course, already extant humanities requirements at most schools, but the Hammond Committee wanted more, and a second Hammond Report was issued in 1944, this one suggesting a complete four-year program that required 20 per cent or more of the student's time to be devoted to humanistic-stem courses—mostly literature, economics, history, and social studies. There was controversy about these reports during the late forties, but during the experimental period in education after the war the conception of the humanistic stem won out gradually, and by the early fifties the arm-twisting propaganda of the humanistic-stem proponents had achieved final victory.

What is interesting about this minor struggle in the history of engineering education is the fact that neither freshman composition nor technical writing courses were claimed or championed by either side. The engineering professor who saw no pressing need for curricular changes viewed composition courses as service adjuncts to his activities, not important to fight for, and the humanistic-stem supporters did not see writing courses as humanistic enough to be included under their rubric. As Paul Fatout said in a 1948 article on the growth of the humanistic stem, " . . . composition is not considered a legitimate offshoot of the humanistic stem." (24, pp. 715–716) There seemed to be no niche for technical writing in the controversy.

The Postwar Technical Writing Boom

In spite of the lack of champions, technical writing courses continued and even expanded, especially after the end of the war. Part of this expansion was due, of course, to the thousands of new students attending college on the GI Bill, but the striking growth of technical writing was also in part a result of the nature of WW II, the first truly technological war. During six years, necessity had mothered thousands of frightful and complex machines, and the need for technical communication had never been greater. (In 1939, British officers were ordered to prepare for the war by sharpening their swords—an eloquent example of how much technology had changed the world by the time of Nagasaki six years later.) Technical writers were in great demand during the war, for each new airplane, gun, bomb, and machine needed a manual written for it, and the centrality of the lucid explicator of technology was obvious as never before. As Jay R. Gould wrote later:

> WW II in an important date for the technical writing profession. . . . Reports had to be written for the men and the women who were inventing the machines and the electronic systems . . . much more importance was given to the technical writer, a man or woman who spent all of his

> time in communicating. . . . The need was so urgent that technical writers entered the profession from many sources (25).

For the first time, technical writing was more than an adjunct function of some other activity—it was a job in itself.

After the end of the war, technical writing finally became a genuine profession as wartime technologies were translated into peacetime uses. The giant technological corporations—General Electric, Westinghouse, GM—opened separate departments of technical writing after finding that it was no longer cost-effective to pay engineers both to design and write. The technical writing and editing profession became more aware of itself during these years, but in spite of these changes few colleges offered technical writing majors or structural changes in technical writing courses. Schools seemed to ignore the changing conditions of the field, and when the journals began to print technical writing articles again after war's end, the articles had subtly changed focus. Now they dealt with tasks and techniques within the teaching of technical writing rather than being concerned with the status and conditions of the teaching. It was during this time that the first "modern" technical writing articles were written and published, but what the profession gained in techniques it lost in self-awareness.

The postwar era was a demanding time for teachers of technical writing; the demand for their courses rose dramatically as the colleges were deluged with returning veterans after 1945. This was, as Alvin Fountain put it in a retrospective article, "the frantic era of the GI Bill, the quonset hut, the barracks classroom, and the tar paper apartment, infested by returning veterans armed with wives and children, a bunch of common sense, and a serious purpose." (26) Teachers tried to cope as best they could with this population explosion in their classrooms.

This period brought more complexity as well as more students to technical writing, and the late forties saw further expansion of the number of forms taught in typical courses. Initially, of course, the report had been central to courses in technical writing; only gradually had business letters been added, and before the war the technical article became a fairly common form as well. By 1951, however, these simple and basic forms had been heavily supplemented and diversified. A report of common forms taught in that year indicated that at least six different report forms were widely taught, and correspondence forms often proliferated until more than ten letter types were taught (27). As might be expected, manual-writing also became a popular skill to learn in postwar writing courses. This was partially a result of the military influence of the war, but it was also due to the increasing number of technically-based consumer products America was turning out.

A New Professionalism

The decade of the 1950s saw technical writing "grow up," assuming the essential form we know it in today. The profession of technical and scientific writing grew and matured during this period with the foundation of the

Society of Technical Writers and the establishment in 1958 of the influential *Transactions on Engineering Writing and Speech* (now *Transactions on Professional Communication*) of the Institute of Electrical and Electronics Engineers. During the fifties the importance of the profession of technical writing became apparent to industry, and colleges gave more serious consideration to turning out trained technical writers. The programs at MIT, the University of Michigan, and at Rensselaer Polytechnic Institute assumed during this decade the leading place they still have, and in 1958 RPI established the first master's degree in technical and scientific writing in the United States.

On most campuses the problems that had always plagued technical writing programs continued as usual, but in spite of them there was a continuing refinement and sophistication to the courses being offered (27, p. 176). Around the mid-fifties the humanistic-stem requirements that had been so heavily cried up during the immediate postwar era began to be replaced with technical writing requirements at some schools; this was largely the result of pressure from the engineering faculty and the continuing complaint of industry that new graduates still could not write well (28, 29). By 1957, nearly all colleges offered a technical writing course, and 64 per cent of engineering schools made such a course a requirement during the junior or senior year (30). The courses that were being required were often more carefully planned than technical writing courses had been in the past, and experimental methods of teaching became much more common during this period. The most successful experiments of the fifties were probably the cooperative courses that were team-taught by English and engineering teachers (31).

Textbooks throughout the fifties were still largely derivative of one another, but several stand out as being particularly popular and important. Joseph N. Ulman, Jr., and Jay R. Gould's *Technical Reporting* of 1952 was a conservative textbook that concentrated on the report (32), but its completeness has made it popular for over twenty years. Ulman and Gould represented a clear bridge to the traditional textbooks of the thirties, and many of the texts of the fifties followed its conservative lead. In 1954, however, there appeared a textbook which was not only extremely popular in its own time but which is arguably the single most important postwar technical writing text: Gordon Mills and John Walter's *Technical Writing* (33). Mills and Walter had begun working together in the late forties, and they determined to try to reinvigorate technical writing instruction by bringing it closer to the businesses and industries that actually used the forms that were taught. Mills and Walter conducted a survey of over 300 actual technical writing situations in industry, and from this survey came a number of changes in the approach that informed their textbook.

As Walter explained in 1973, two of the most important assumptions that he and Mills had gleaned from their survey had been these:

1. A rhetorical approach rather than the rigid "types of reports" approach that most texts used was best. Most reports are made up of several common processes: definition, description, explanation of process, etc.

2. The only good criterion for technical writing is "does it work?" This indicates that in technical writing as well as in other rhetorical forms, the writer-reader relationship is most important (34).

Technical Writing reflected these assumptions and went on to be the most popular and paradigmatic text of the fifties, pointing the way to a new rhetorical approach to technical writing that was to revivify what had been in danger of becoming a sterile and mechanical course (35).[1]

Mills and Walter were not alone in their concern with creating a sense of reader-writer relationship in technical writing instruction. A growing awareness that audience considerations had long been scanted in technical writing was one of the important developments of the 1950s. In a prescient article in the *Journal of Chemical Education* in 1951, James W. Souther mentioned this new awareness:

> . . . more and more, writers in industry are becoming aware of their readers' interests. They are placing conclusions, summaries, and recommendations at the beginning of the report because the administrators are most interested in such material. . . . The more widespread use of such devices as statements of purpose and background . . . is ample proof of the writer's growing awareness of the reader (36).

J. H. Wilson blasted college technical writing courses in 1955 for their traditional dismissal of audience considerations in the much discussed article "Our Colleges Can Teach Writing—If They Are Made To" (37).[2] And in 1959, Joseph Racker presented his influential concept of writing to audiences with different levels of technical expertise in his essay "Selecting and Writing to the Proper Level" (39).

Another important change that the fifties and the early sixties saw was the expansion of technical writing into fields other than engineering. Other applied sciences had long existed at many colleges, but only during this period did departments of agriculture, architecture, chemistry, pharmacy, even home economics begin to send their students in any numbers to technical writing. The course began to gain campus-wide recognition as a useful, no-nonsense addition to the curriculum of any serious student. Textbooks soon reflected this broadening of audience; Theodore Sherman's *Modern Technical Writing* of 1955 claimed that it was "appropriate to a wide range of subjects so that any technical writer, regardless of his field of specialization, will find the help that he needs." (40)[3] At this time, too, we find the first published mention of technical writing courses built around a single long project with a series of check-in assignments preceding the long report, a course arrangement that was to become widely popular in the sixties and seventies (41). Courses began to consider graphic presentations as well as verbal ones, due mainly to the effect of the Iowa State technical writing course, which provided a successful model (42).

Breakthroughs and Problems

By 1959, new textbooks were appearing in such profusion that even to list them would take too much space. Many technical writing texts from the late fifties are still in print (since the mortality rate for technical writing textbooks is still much lower than that for any other sort of composition text), and as the fifties drew to a close, more and more texts began to copy the rhetorical approach of Mills and Walter and the general-coverage approach of Sherman. But in spite of these successful new texts and the experimental advances, technical writing still had problems. Although technical writing had by this time a long and honorable history and was obviously in English departments to stay, it got as little welcome from literary departments in 1959 as it had in 1929. Still considered a low-level service course, technical writing was still assigned to graduate students and instructors.

After Sputnik was launched in 1957, an alarmed America began a war of technology with Russia that was to last into the early seventies, and as the sixties opened there was a serious shortage of technical writers in industry. Most English majors still saw technical writing as hack work and most engineers could do better if they remained specialized; as a result, industries engaged in bidding wars for those few technical writers extant. The Society of Technical Writers grew quickly and went through several name changes, emerging as today's thriving and influential Society for Technical Communication. As a group, technical writers advanced greatly in both pay and prestige during this period (43).

On college campuses, however, things were not so smooth. The 1960s were a time of disturbance and change for technical writing instruction as for so many other elements in American culture. Technical writing courses were struggling to define themselves; technical writing teachers were wrangling over what their jobs should entail; technical writing students were getting objectively more intelligent but were fewer and fewer in number as the decade proceeded. It was a confused time for American colleges and for technical writing instruction, but it was a period that prepared the ground for the great leap forward that was to come in the seventies.

A sort of critical self-examination and desire to define technical writing itself was an important element of the intellectual effort of technical writing teachers during the early and mid-sixties. As early as 1954, Mills and Walter had stated in the preface of their text that "nobody had ever seriously explored the concept of technical writing with the purpose of trying to say exactly what technical writing is." (33, p. vii) In the sixties, that investigation was taken up by a number of teachers. Robert Hays investigated the linguistic nature of technical writing in 1961 in a widely reprinted essay entitled "What Is Technical Writing?" (44). W. Earl Britton, in an article in *College Composition and Communication* in 1965, wrote what is probably the most comprehensive early definition of technical writing, defining it by subject matter, linguistic nature, thought processes involved, and purpose. Britton's conclusion was that technical writing is defined more than anything else by "the effort of the author to convey one meaning and only one meaning in what he says." (45)

This interest in the ultimate nature of technical writing was matched in the sixties by an awakening interest in the process of teaching it and the methods available for doing so. The first steps in the direction of empirical research into technical writing and the teaching of it were made during this period; for the first time, researchers were gathering and analyzing facts about technical writing in a scientific manner, obtaining results and conclusions that could not be dismissed as mere opinion. Several important early experiments were Harry E. Hand's 1964 study of the relative seriousness of different sorts of errors in technical writing papers and Richard M. Davis' massive investigation of the efforts of variables in the writing of a technical description in 1967 (46, 47).

In the midst of this growing professionalism and increasing self-consciousness, however, technical writing courses were still beset by the same old problems that had always dogged them. The ascent of literary studies throughout the sixties meant that the age-old battle raged on between those who wished to teach technical students to write and those who wished to teach them to read and appreciate great literature. Through the sixties many technical writing teachers continued to be graduate students and lower-level faculty members who had been dragooned into technical writing and whose primary interests remained literary studies. This split between interests and assignments came out strongly at a CCCC workshop on technical writing instruction in the early sixties, which was reported (rather ironically) thus:

> That this (technical writing course) is frequently thought of as a "service course" was recognized. Several expressed strong disapproval of the attitude, and stronger disapproval of admitting it. A few spoke in defense of the designation. Most confessed that the fact was inescapable, though the name was nauseous. . . .
>
> Some piously professed to see an encouraging resurgence of interest in and demand for the humanities. These strains, sweet to CCCC professional cars, played softly for the duration of the Workshop. . . . The Workshop believed, in the main, that recommended reading should be largely literary rather than scientific and technical.

The cosecretary of the workshop summed up her colleagues' responses this way:

> I sense that the Workshop members believe that technical writing must be about scientific matters in which they have no training and less interest. They see themselves doing grease monkey work on physics papers for spelling errors and would die first. . . . My minority opinion is that there is such a thing as technical presentation and reading and writing about literature doesn't teach it (48).

That was indeed a minority opinion in 1961, and although it came to be more widely held over the following ten years, literary studies continued to be the main interest of most technical writing teachers well into the seventies.

In terms of course content, the sixties were not a time of major change; the content and form of the reports and other forms traditionally taught continued to evolve as it always had, but only one new and important form emerged as a result of the expansion of the field of technical writing that the fifties had brought: the proposal. During the late fifties and early sixties, it was estimated that industry spent in excess of one billion dollars per year on the writing of proposals, and the importance of this new form soon became obvious to the writers of technical writing texts (49). The first textbook to seriously treat this form was published in 1962: Seigfried Mandel and David L. Caldwell's *Proposal and Inquiry Writing*. The book was popular and influential, prompting a reviewer to note that "At long last another relatively new and lustily growing American industry is beginning to have its folklore committed to writing . . . the 'technical-proposal generation' industry." (50) The proposal as a technical form quickly spread to all texts, partially because of the influence of Mandel and Caldwell, but also due to the influence of the second edition of Mills and Walter, which featured the proposal.

Retrenchment and a New Sense of Identity

As the sixties drew to a close, and well into the early seventies, there was a serious drop in the number of undergraduate students enrolled in engineering programs. In fall 1968 there were over 239,000 undergraduate engineering students, but by fall 1973 this number had fallen to fewer than 187,000—and this in a time of skyrocketing general enrollments (51). Enrollments in technical writing classes shrank accordingly, with the result that fewer unwilling conscripts were forced to teach the course. Still, though, many technical writing teachers were merely time-servers as the seventies opened. In a well-known experiment in 1970, Juanita Williams Dudley complained about the character of many technical writing classes in tones that are by now familiar: "Frequently the technical writing conscript regards his assignment as a humiliating, dehumanizing hairshirt that must be endured until advanced degrees and seniority confer upon him enough power to bargain for courses in literary criticism and creative writing." (52)

But a new day was dawning for technical writing instruction. Due in part to declining enrollments in courses, a solid core of committed technical writing professionals was forming by the late sixties, a growing number of teachers who considered technical communication their primary area of interest and expertise. In 1970 the *Journal of Technical Writing and Communication* was started, a journal which quickly became the most respected organ in the field of technical writing instruction. The journal reflected an ever-increasing sense of pride and self-consciousness on the parts of many experienced technical writing teachers who had served faithfully through the "lean years." Tools became more sophisticated; in 1971 Stello Jordan and his associates published a two-volume *Handbook of Technical Writing Practices* that was called "the most complete and sophisticated technical writing guide ever published . . . a true and important picture of the many-sided profession of technical writing, and an impressive, diversified explanation of why and how technical information is communicated." (53) In 1973 the Association of Teachers of Technical Writing was formed, and their journal, *The Technical Writing Teacher*, began publication in that year. Though early issues were somewhat crude, the journal underwent marked improvement throughout the decade and now ranks only behind *JTWC* in the opinions of many technical writing teachers.

Finally, in 1974, technical enrollments began once again to rise, and by the late seventies they were going up at a rate of more than 10 per cent per year at a time when general college enrollments were static. As the demand for courses in technical communication grew during the seventies, the demand for literature courses fell. Soon many chairmen of English departments became uncomfortably aware that the only thing supporting their sparsely populated Milton courses was the credit generated by the quondam poor relation, the Technical Writing Division. The Modern Language Association, which had for over fifty years refused to recognize technical writing as a legitimate function of English scholars caved in during the midseventies and gave technical writing belated recognition in 1976, when the first technical writing panel was presented at an MLA convention.

This demand was partially due to one thing that had not changed: the need for technical communications specialists in industry. A survey during the late seventies showed that over 50 per cent of an engineer's time was spent dealing with writing, and over 85 per cent of professional engineers polled said that a technical writing course should be required of all technical students (54). More and more departments, some of them only quasitechnical, began to require a technical writing course for their students as the good reputation of these courses became more widely known. As John Walter put it in 1977,

> The widespread emphasis on technical writing (coming primarily from students, I think) has led to considerable growth in the number of schools offering courses in technical writing and to increased enrollment in those schools which have offered the course for years. . . . We've come a long way, and more and more departments are compelled to recognize that technical writing is a legitimate concern of conscientious teachers, and one which must be rewarded when teachers do a good job (55).

Technical writing teachers were not always rewarded by their departments, but many found freedom and credit in the 1970s that had previously only been dreamt of. Their courses were crowded, and students had never been so eager to learn. Teachers of technical communication began to be tenured and promoted on the basis of their skills and publications within the field, a situation that had been rare prior to the seventies. Many found lucrative sidelines in consulting for industry, and such consulting nearly always rebounded to enrich the technical writing classroom with new insights into the contemporary world of industry. Each *MLA Job List* brought news of more and more tenure-track positions specializing in technical writing. Professionally, it was a satisfying decade.

Textbooks during the seventies grew ever more sophisticated and began to appear in versions aimed at two-year as well as four-year colleges. Old favorites such as Mills and Walter and Houp and Pearsall continued to sell well, but they were supplemented by a new sort of more rhetorically based text, exemplified by Andrews and Blickle's *Technical Writing: Principles and*

Forms and Lannon's *Technical Writing*. Perhaps the most influential—though not the most popular—text of the decade was Mathes and Stevenson's *Designing Technical Reports*, with its elegant audience-analysis procedure and its determined investigation into the purposes behind technical writing. A technical writing handbook appeared in the late seventies, giving teachers and students easy access to technical terms. It can truly be said that the seventies brought technical writing instruction to a state of efficiency and productive professionalism it had never known before.[4]

As the 1980s open, technical writing is not without problems, but its prospects have never been brighter. There are still arguments being made that the technical writing course should be taken out of the hands of English teachers, but these arguments are as old as technical writing instruction itself and will likely prove no more effectual now than they were in 1920 (56).[5] Technical writing scholarship is thriving, and there is a healthy tone of innovation and skepticism in the essays found in today's technical writing journals; the received wisdom is being tested against new situations and needs as never before, and the field is more vital than ever because of it. It now seems likely that technical communication will be an acceptable field of study for English graduate degrees in many schools by the end of the decade. The field has generated its own patriarchs and scholars, and some English departments have already begun to trade heavily on their technical-writing fame. There is finally evidence that many colleges see and appreciate the dedication of their technical writing staffs, and the technical writing division is no longer the repository of callow youths and second-raters that it once tended to be. In general the prospect is excellent for both teachers and students of technical writing. We have come a long way from 1939, when teaching technical writing was called "professional suicide," and, we can say with pride, an even longer way from 1915, when technical students' papers could be "described only by the word 'wretched.' " It has been a long road, but one well worth the traveling.

NOTES

[1]See for instance the complaint in Morris Freedman's "Technical Writing, Anyone?" (35).

[2]The problem was also addressed in John I. Mattill's "Writing as Communication: The Engineer Must Learn How to Reach His Constituents" (38).

[3]Much earlier, Sada Harbarger had tried with some Ohio State colleagues to expand the potential audience or technical writing texts with a 1938 textbook, *English for Students in Applied Sciences*. The profession was clearly not ready for it at the time. It bombed.

[4]Special thanks to Fabian Gudas and Barbara Sims of Louisiana State University for sharing with me their experiences of teaching technical writing during the period 1945–1980.

[5]This argument was most recently resurrected in J. C. Mathes, D. W. Stevenson, and P. Klaver, Technical Writing: The Engineering Educator's Responsibility (56). It brought, predictably, a rash of responses from English teachers and no action at all from engineering teachers.

REFERENCES

1. H. L. Creek and J. H. McKee, English in Colleges of Engineering, *English Journal, 21*, p. 819, 1931.
2. Anonymous, A Study of Evolutionary Trends in Engineering Curricula, *Proceedings of the Society for the Promotion of Engineering Education, 34*, p. 561, 1926.

3. English for Engineers, *Engineering Record*, p. 763, June 19, 1915.
4. J. M. Telleen, The Courses in English in our Technical Schools, *Proc. SPEE, 16*, p. 68, 1908.
5. H. R. O'Brien, Engineering English, *Engineering News*, p. 715, November 6, 1913.
6. S. C. Earle, English in the Engineering School at Tufts College, *Proceedings, SPEE, 19*, p. 33, 1911.
7. S. C. Earle, Obituary, *Proceedings, SPEE, 25*, p. 246, 1917.
8. J. R. Nelson, English, Engineering and Technical Schools, *English Journal, 20*, p. 495, 1931.
9. F. Aydelotte, Training in Thought is the Aim of Elementary English Course as Taught at M. I. T., *Engineering Record*, p. 300, February 24, 1917.
10. F. Aydelotte, *English and Engineering*, McGraw-Hill, New York, p. xiv, 1917.
11. A New Era in Teaching English to Engineers, *Engineering Record*, p. 291, February 24, 1917.
12. C. W. Park, Report of Committee #12, English, *Proceedings SPEE, 26*, p. 209, 1918.
13. G. R. Chatburn, The SPEE: A Survey of Its Past and A Reconnaissance of Its Future, *Proceedings SPEE, 27*, p. 187, 1919.
14. C. M. Park, Report of Committee #12, English, *Proceedings SPEE, 28*, p. 296, 1920.
15. J. R. Nelson, The English Department, *Proceedings, SPEE, 34*, p. 813, 1926.
16. B. Stoughton and M. R. Stoughton, Education in English for Engineering Students, *Proceedings, SPEE, 32*, pp. 144–147, 1924.
17. J. R. Nelson, The Department of English, *Proceedings, SPEE, 32*, p. 560, 1924.
18. A. V. Hall, English as an Essential Part of the Engineering Curriculum, *Proceedings, SPEE, 39*, pp. 419–420, 1931.
19. J. W. Parker, The Need for Speech Training for Engineers, *Proceedings, SPEE, 39*, pp. 226–228, 1931.
20. W. O. Birk, Organization and Conditions, *Proceedings, SPEE, 47*, p. 426, 1939.
21. H. L. Creek, Teachers of English in Engineering Colleges: Selection and Training, *Proceedings, SPEE, 47*, p. 301, 1939.
22. A. M. Fountain, *A Study of Courses in Technical Writing*, George Peabody College, Nashville, Tennessee, p. 82, 1938.
23. W. O. Sypherd, Thirty Years of Teaching English to Engineers, *Proceedings, SPEE, 47*, pp. 162–164, 1939.
24. P. Fatout, Growth of the Humanistic Stem, *Proceedings of the American Society for Engineering Education, 55*, p. 717, 1948.
25. J. R. Gould, *Opportunities in Technical Writing*, Universal Publishing, New York, pp. 12–13, 1964.
26. A. M. Fountain, Working with Electrical Engineers in Seminar, *Institute of Radio Engineers Transactions, on Engineering Writing and Speech, 2*, p. 47, June 1959.
27. M. L. Rider, Some Current Practices in Teaching Advanced Composition for Engineers, *Proceedings, ASEE, 58*, p. 177, 1951.
28. K. A. Kobe, What Colleges Are Doing To Train Chemists and Chemical Engineers in Technical Writing, *Journal of Chemical Education, 33*, pp. 55–57, 1956.
29. J. R. Pierce, The Challenging Field of Engineering Writing and Speech, *IRE Trans. on Engineering Writing and Speech, 1*, pp. 12–13, March 1958.
30. G. P. Wellborn, Is the Technical Student Short-Changed in College?, *College English, 21*, p. 394, 1960.
31. R. R. Rathbone, Cooperative Teaching of Technical Writing in Engineering Courses, *Proceedings, ASEE, 66*, pp. 126–130, 1958.
32. J. N. Ulman, Jr., and J. R. Gould, *Technical Reporting*, Dryden Press, New York, 1952.
33. G. H. Mills and J. A, Walter, *Technical Writing*, Holt, Rinehart and Winston, New York, 1954.
34. J. A. Walter, Confessions of a Teacher of Technical Writing, *The Technical Writing Teacher, 1*, pp. 5–6, 1973.
35. M. Freedman, Technical Writing, Anyone?, in *Technical and Professional Writing*, H. A. Estrin (ed.), Harcourt, Brace & World, New York, pp. 4–7, 1963.
36. J. W. Souther, Design That Report!, in *Technical and Professional Writing*, H. A. Estrin (ed.), pp. 225–229, 1963.
37. J. H. Wilson, Jr., Our Colleges Can Teach Writing—If They Are Made To, *Proceedings, ASEE, 62*, pp. 431–435, 1955.
38. J. I. Mattill, Writing as Communication: The Engineer Must Learn How to Reach His Constituents, *Proceedings, ASEE, 61*, pp. 476–479, 1954.
39. J. Racker, Selecting and Writing to the Proper Level, in *Technical and Professional Writing*, H. A. Estrin (ed.), Harcourt, Brace and World, New York, pp. 236–246, 1963.
40. T. A. Sherman, *Modern Technical Writing*, Prentice-Hall, Inc., Englewood Cliffs, New Jersey, p. v, 1955.
41. J. D. Thomas, Thwarting the Two-Day Term Report, *Proceedings, ASEE, 62*, pp. 138–139, 1955.

42. R. Sweigert, Jr., A Technical Writing Course That Works, *Proceedings, ASEE, 63,* pp. 262–266, 1956.
43. R. W. Smith, *Technical Writing,* Barnes and Noble, New York, Preface, 1963.
44. R. Hays, What Is Technical Writing?, *Technical and Professional Writing,* Harcourt, Brace and World, New York, pp. 64–69, 1963.
45. W. E. Britton, What Is Technical Writing?, *College Composition and Communication, 16,* pp. 113–116, 1965.
46. H. E. Hand, An Attempt to Measure Success in Technical Writing, *Proceedings, ASEE, 72,* pp. 70–72, 1964.
47. R. M. Davis, Experimental Research in the Effectiveness of Technical Writing, *IEEE Transactions on Engineering Writing and Speech, 10,* pp. 33–38, 1967.
48. K. Power, Special Problems of the C/C Course in Technical Schools, *College Composition and Communication, 12,* pp. 163–164, 1961.
49. R. Kendall, The Proposal Digest, *IEEE Transactions on EWS, 6,* p. 79, 1963.
50. W. E. Collins, Review of *Proposal and Inquiry Writing* by Mandel and Caldwell, *IRE Transactions on EWS, 5,* p. 31, 1962.
51. P. J. Sheridan, Engineering and Engineering Technology Enrollments, Fall 1978, *Engineering Education, 70,* pp. 58–63, 1979.
52. J. W. Dudley, Writing Skills of Engineering and Scientific Students, *IEEE Transactions on EWS, 14,* p. 42, 1971.
53. E. K. Schlesinger, Review of *Handbook of Technical Writing Practices,* S. Jordan et al. (eds.), *IEEE Transactions on Professional Communication, 16,* p. 45, 1973.
54. R. M. Davis, How Important Is Technical Writing?—A Survey of the Opinions of Successful Engineers, *The Technical Writing Teacher, 4,* p. 87, 1977.
55. J. A. Walter, Message From The President, *The Technical Writing Teacher, 5,* p. 2, 1977.
56. J. C. Mathes, D. W. Stevenson, and P. Klaver, Technical Writing: The Engineering Educator's Responsibility, *Engineering Education, 69,* pp. 331–334, 1979.

7 Gender, Technology, and the History of Technical Communication

KATHERINE T. DURACK

Relying on the groundbreaking work of historians of technology Ruth Schwartz Cowan, Autumn Stanley, and Judy Wajcman, Durack highlights the reasons that women have been "largely absent from our recorded disciplinary past" (p. 99 in this volume). Pointing toward cultural biases that have not valued the household, and by extension, women's tools, she points out the "cultural blinders" that have made it difficult to see women's contributions in the past. More important, she points out that, with the gradual disappearance of the "workplace," it is quite possible that the home and workshop, what Zuboff calls "principal centers of production as late as 1850" (p. 106), will again become such centers of production in the near future. Equally important is an recognition of the problems attached to definition and her willingness to offer an attempt at a flexible definition that both accommodates the past and takes future changes into consideration.

Women are largely absent from our recorded disciplinary past, whether as technical writers, as scientists, or as inventors or users of technology. There are a few notable exceptions from a handful of scholars: Elizabeth Tebeaux's work on Renaissance technical writing (see "Technical Writing" and sections of "Visual Language"), Tebeaux and Mary Lay's "Images of Women in Technical Books from the English Renaissance," Kathryn Neeley's "Women as Mediatrix: Women as Writers on Science and Technology in the Eighteenth and Nineteenth Centuries," a chapter on sewing machines in R. John Brockmann's *From Millwrights to Shipwrights*, and my own article on document design innovations in home sewing patterns ("Patterns for Success").

There are several possible explanations for the absence of women in the history of technical communication. One possibility is that women have contributed only very rarely to technical and scientific work (and, consequently, to technical and scientific communication). Indeed, Elizabeth Wayland Barber suggests that women's contributions to technological innovation have been hampered by their own productive (and reproductive) responsibilities: "The

From *Technical Communication Quarterly* 6, no. 3 (Summer 1997): 249–60.

only people who have the leisure to experiment with how to make new articles, or how to use new tools, are those *not* locked into basic subsistence production—people with time and/or cash to spare" (258). Because there are almost no cultures in which men bear the primary responsibility for child care, this task typically has fallen to women and influenced the variety and type of work they do (Brown 1075). We might agree then, that as scientific inquiry and technological innovation have been primarily the work of men, the contributions of women have consequently been subsumed, lost, or overlooked.

Yet another possible reason why the history of technical communication is so barren of women is that (as feminist scholars have noted about histories of technology) "the absence of a female perspective . . . was a function of the historians who wrote them and not of historical reality" (Cowan, "From Virginia Dare" 248). In our case, the omission arises not from the absence of women historians (after all, nearly one third of the articles named by Rivers in his 1994 bibliographic essay were authored by women), but instead can be attributed to the "peculiar set of cultural blinders" (Cowan, *More* 9) that make it difficult for us to see many of the ways in which women may have contributed to technical communication.

A "Peculiar Set of Cultural Blinders"

How we define our profession quite obviously influences where we look to find our past: definition, by function, tells us what is and what is not technical writing. While it is true that we have yet to agree upon what constitutes modern technical writing, popular definitions often exhibit either or both of two key characteristics: first, a close relationship (in subject matter or function) to *technology;* and second, an understanding that technical writing is associated with *work* and the *workplace.* An example of the former is David Dobrin's definition of technical writing as "writing that accommodates technology to the user" ("What's Technical" 242); an example of the latter is the premise proposed by Tebeaux and M. Jimmie Killingsworth to guide historical research, that "technical writing exists to help its readers to achieve work-related goals—to perform work; to solve problems in a work context" (7). It follows then, that "what counts" as technical writing is derived from what is considered *technology,* what we consider *work,* and where we understand the *workplace* to be.

The problem with regard to adding women to our disciplinary history lies in the assumption that *technology, work,* and *workplace* are gender-neutral terms, and that addressing gender and the history of technical communication is a simple matter of searching the annals of science and industry and tacking on articles about a few women who have distinguished themselves in scientific, medical, and technical fields. But as the work of feminist historians and scholars demonstrate, such terms represent contested ground, and such a simplistic view may be inadequate to fully address the elusive—and, as I suspect, frequently unintentional—biases that both define our past and govern our future.

History and Women's Work

Women's work has long escaped the notice of historians, leading feminist critics to assert that *his-story* itself is "deeply gendered" and "presented as a universal human story exemplified by the lives of men" (Scott 18; see Barber, Cowan, and Stanley as well). Most histories, including the history of technical communication thus far, focus primarily on the works of *great men*—Aristotle, Leonardo da Vinci, Galileo, Albert Einstein—and the *great works* of men—space travel, nuclear power, medical miracles, and the computer revolution. With the former, the focus is on *agency*—having identified persons who have contributed significantly to technical, scientific, or medical fields, we then seek samples of their writing to study. In contrast, the latter focuses on *products*—having identified artifacts of significant scientific, technical, or medical value, we seek to study ancillary texts associated with those artifacts and then the authors (when they can be identified). In both cases, there is a need to establish *significance,* which usually involves prerequisite location within the public sphere (allocated to men) rather than the private sphere (the realm of women). As Joan Wallach Scott (*Gender*) and Autumn Stanley (*Mothers* and "Women") each point out, history in general, and the history of technology in particular have tended to omit the activities of women in part by locating significance primarily in public and political activities and innovations, the very "realm[s] of social, political, and economic interaction" of such great interest today to researchers in technical communication (Cooper x). (See Kerber for an insightful discussion of the rhetoric of "separate spheres.")

Including women and women's work in a history of technical writing requires that we contest two assumptions that lead to their exclusion from our disciplinary story: First, (the assumption of agency) that women are not significant originators of technical, scientific, or medical achievement; and second, (the assumption of technological significance) that women's tools are not sufficiently technical, nor their work sufficiently important, to warrant study of their supporting texts.

Women as Significant Contributors to Science and Technology

Overcoming the assumption of agency first involves identifying women who have contributed significantly to science, technology, and medicine, then fitting their written works into our history: "gather[ing] evidence about women to demonstrate their essential likeness as historical subjects to men . . . [and] attempt[ing] to fit a new subject—women—into received historical categories" (Scott 18–19). The main difficulty facing the historian is the apparent lack of women's contribution to these fields. From the dawn of humanity, women, like men, have undoubtedly sought means for improving their work processes, yet we rarely conceive of women as technological innovators. Why is this the case?

In her search for women's technological achievements, Stanley determined that many women's inventive accomplishments are obscured by having been misclassified, trivialized, or attributed to men. Examples of these sometimes glaring obfuscations include:

- Harriet R. Strong's storage dam and reservoir system, which was "nearly built on the Colorado river during World War I [but in the patent record] is classified as a container for kitchen debris" (Stanley, *Mothers* xxx)
- Madeleine Vionnet's invention of the bias cut in dressmaking, which according to J.E. Gordon, "exploits the low shear modulus and high Poisson's ratio of certain square-weave fabrics in the 45-degree direction" (qtd. in Stanley, *Mothers* xxxii)
- The persistent debates over women's contributions to key inventions of the U.S. Industrial Revolution (Catherine Greene and the cotton gin, Elizabeth Howe and the sewing machine), plus documented instances where partial or total credit is given to men for women's inventions (such as the "Maltron" keyboard conceived by Lillian Malt, but known in England as "Stephen Hobday's keyboard") (Stanley, *Mothers* xxix)

Stanley contends that women's technological achievements have been routinely under-reported, at least in part, because "our sex-role stereotypes seek to confine that [feminine] creativity to such 'acceptable' areas as art, music, dance, writing, and cooking, whereas 'real' invention and technology have to do with weapons and machines and chemical compounds created in laboratories" (*Mothers* xx). Even when well-known women patent such "real" inventions of significance, they may not receive credit: screen actress Hedy Lamarr invented a secret communications system during World War II (and patented it, with composer George Antheil) yet "has never received either recompense . . . or due recognition," even though one of its key features—frequency hopping—"is the main anti-jamming technology used in today's billion-dollar defense systems" (Stanley, *Mothers* 383). Lamarr is far from the only woman to demonstrate that beauty and brains are not antithetical, but despite the fact that women have been receiving U.S. patents since 1809, as late as the 1970s librarians "did not even use *Women inventors* as a category for filing information" (Stanley, *Mothers* xviii).

Women's general absence from the patent record (and consequently, from histories of technology) is attributed by Stanley (*Mothers* xxviii–xxix) to several factors:

- Patents require disposable income and time, both resources of which women historically have had less than men
- Married women in the United States and Britain could not own their inventions or patents until after the Married Women's Property Acts passed (first in New York in 1848 and 1860; in Britain in 1870 and 1882)
- The technical and mathematical training necessary to build models of inventions and patent them was not available to women because of gender-segregated education
- Cultural stereotypes discourage women from claiming credit for their achievements
- These same stereotypes also encourage women to be generous and giving, resulting in sharing ideas rather protecting and profiting from them.

Judy Wajcman, like Stanley, observes that "we tend to think about technology in terms of industrial machinery and cars . . . ignoring other technologies that affect most aspects of everyday life" (137). Ruth Schwartz Cowan notes in *More Work for Mother*, her history of household technology, that we "do not ordinarily associate 'tools' with 'women's work'—but household tools there nonetheless are and always have been" (9). Stoves and spinning wheels are two such examples; the sewing machine is one such tool used in the household and in industry.

Furthermore, technologies that pertain specifically to women's biological functions and social roles have been essentially ignored by historians of technology. "The indices to the standard histories of technology . . . do not contain a single reference . . . to such a significant cultural artifact as the baby bottle," a technology that Cowan asserts has "revolutionized a basic biological process, transformed a fundamental human experience for vast numbers of infants and mothers, and been one of the more controversial exports of Western technology to underdeveloped countries" ("From Virginia Dare" 248). Such omission by categorization presents obvious problems for the researcher, who would find few women's technologies (such as horticulture, cooking, and childcare) in the standard indices of technology.

Women as Significant Users of Technology

With the first notion dispelled, that women do not contribute significantly to science and technology, we turn to the second assumption, that men's and women's experiences of technology are identical, thus relegating women to inferior technological roles. Addressing this second assumption—that women's traditional work is not technological—involves a different strategy: departing from conventional history to challenge existing definition, seeking "a new narrative" that focuses "on the causal role played by women in their history and on the qualities of women's experience that sharply distinguish it from men's experience (Scott 20). Men's and women's experiences of technology are quite different.

The industrial revolution brought with it not only great technological innovation, but increasing differentiation between appropriate work roles for men and for women (see Kerber; Oakley). "One of the most profound effects of industrialization was, and is, the separation of 'work places' from 'home places'—and the attendant designation of the former as the 'place' for men and the latter as the 'domain' of women," asserts Cowan (*More* 18). During the rise of industrial society and capitalism, "the modern concept of work, as the expenditure of energy for financial gain" (Oakley 4) came to further distinguish the stereotyped expectations of productive activity done by men and women.

In fact, Cynthia Cockburn points out that "Technological knowledge at the professional level, and technological know-how at the practical level, are sharp differentiators of men and women" (17–18). In her study of the sexual division of labor and technologies of production, Cockburn found that "a sexual division of labor in and around technology persists and survives" despite inroads women have made into many professions (8). "The consistent theme unfolding here is this: women are to be found in great numbers operating machinery . . . [b]ut women continue to be rarities in those occupations that involve knowing what goes on inside the machine" (Cockburn 11). As Cockburn puts it, "[w]omen may push the buttons but they may not meddle with the works" (12). The popular image of Rosie the Riveter and the fact of women's successes in all facets of industry during World War II testifies to women's technological competence; their immediate dismissal at the conclusion of the war punctuates the persistence of the view that a woman's place is in the home.

Both Cockburn and Wajcman observe technological competence is involved in establishing masculine and feminine difference. According to Wajcman, "skilled status has . . . been traditionally identified with masculinity and as work that women don't do, while women's skills have been defined as non-technical and undervalued" (38). She illustrates her point with the example of sewing: "It is not possible for anybody to sit down at sewing machine and sew a garment without previous experience. . . . Although this is one area where women are at ease with machines, this is seen as women's supposed natural aptitude for sewing and thus this technical skill is devalued and underpaid" (49). Women are accepted as users of machines, particularly those that are used for housework, but such knowledge is not considered as competence with *technology*.

Despite some changes in recent years, jobs remain sex-typed and the outcomes of technological activities—the production of goods and services—are typically associated with economic gain and the "workplace" rather than the household, where work is often unrecognized and generally unpaid or underpaid. Historical studies find women are excluded from *technology* as a consequence of the gender division of labor (see Rothschild, Cockburn, and Wajcman). Men remain predominantly the makers, repairers, designers, and users of what we typically consider technology. Wajcman observes that "technical competence is central to the dominant cultural ideal of masculinity and its absence a key feature of stereotyped femininity" (159) and that "the work of women is often deemed inferior simply because it is women who do it" (37). Hence the remarks of anthropologist George Murdock:

> The statistics reveal no technological activities which are strictly feminine. One can, of course, name activities that are strictly feminine, e.g., nursing and infant care, but they fall outside the range of technological pursuits. (qtd. in Stanley, "Women" 5)

Feminist critics of technology contend that women are excluded from that which we consider technological by definition: As Stanley puts it, technology is "what men do" rather than "what people do" ("Women" 5). The basis of this assertion lies in cultural views that:

- Deny women's identities as inventors and women's work aids as "tools"
- Deny women access to knowledge necessary for inventing and protecting tools and ideas

- Diminish the significance of women's technological skills in areas they are expected to have expertise
- Define women's unpaid labor as "not work"
- Define traditional women's work as not "technological"

The periodic submittal (and rejection) of texts such as cookbooks to the Society for Technical Communication's annual publications competition demonstrates the difficulty we have with considering as "work" a productive activity that is typically assigned to women and accomplished within individual households without benefit of financial compensation (see McKay for her response to the "Cookbook Caper"). John Harris' comments reveal the same subtle distinctions based on place and type of activity. Harris attributes his own success with teaching and practicing technical writing to his interest in mechanical devices of all sorts, including his mother's treadle sewing machine and the process of making root beer at home out of Hires Extract, sugar, and Fleischman's yeast. Yet, what Harris found remarkable about making root beer was not the productive activity itself, but rather the fact that it took place at home: "I suppose what impressed me was that we were doing at home what I would have considered industrial production," he comments (241). He reveals most explicitly a view of technology that excludes women near the end of the article as he laments the reduced stature of today's inventors:

> A few bodies of diehard inventors and tinkerers hang on. . . . We see them at the annual hot rod speed trials at Bonneville Salt Flats and at some power boat races and at bench-rest shooting matches and so on. (245)

Such gendered scenarios as hot rod speed trials and boat races encourage readers to conceive of significant inventions as the product—and playthings—of men and discount the many instances where (for example) kitchens double as chemistry labs for female entrepreneurs such as Bette Graham (who experimented with her formula for Liquid Paper® in her kitchen before enlisting the aid of a chemist to standardize the formula) (Stanley xviii).

The Household as a Setting of Consequence

Perhaps the greatest force working against the inclusion of women in the history of technical writing is the current focus on workplace writing. Defining technical writing as a type of writing geographically situated in the workplace fails to recognize the household as either a workplace or a "setting of consequence" at all (Cooper x, suggested by Ackerman and Oates). Certainly writers in organizations are more easily studied than writers within individual households: the researcher can identify more or less unified groups of individuals who face similar types of tasks to be accomplished through texts. Such practices (and groups) can also be identified (and therefore compared) among different organizations: most companies develop and publish policies and procedures, most write letters and send memos, many develop contracts, publish reports, and quite a few write software documentation for their own use or the use of their customers. Such comparisons are more difficult to make among individual households for various reasons, but ease of access for study should not be a reason to exclude from significance technical writing in and from the private sphere.

I believe there are significant instances of technical writing and the use of technical documentation that occur within the household. Many of the technologies produced by industry are targeted for home use; the associated documentation is used primarily within the household (by women *and* by men). Examples include instructions for computer hardware and software, but also those for vacuum cleaners, lawn mowers, blenders, and even coffee mills (note that Dobrin finds instructions for the coffee mill worthy of analysis; see "Do Not Grind"). Further examples of other types of technical communication that enter and are "consumed" within the household include credit card agreements, billing statements, and tax and insurance forms and documents. Daily life is not devoid of instances in which individuals might produce artifacts we would find worthy of study if they had originated within the "workplace": there are any number of situations in which private individuals must interact by text with organizations. Surely correspondence challenging billing errors or notifying insurance carriers of changes to personal information are as "significant" as intercompany correspondence and job postings.

An irony of our focus on workplace writing is that it comes at a time when the "workplace" itself is disappearing. To define technical writing by placing it strictly within the workplace denies the historical contributions of women, but in doing so it also denies a larger past—and future—where the household is a primary location for the economically productive activities of women and men. According to Shoshana Zuboff, "home and workshop continued to be the principal centers of production as late as 1850" (227); with the increase in computer technologies, the prevalence of two-income households, and the rise of an information economy, the separation of home space and work space blurs, and as Joan Greenbaum asserts, "the office of the future may be the home" (117). Many people (myself included) spend many of their productive hours working in a *home office*, connected to clients and coworkers by computer networks, fax, and phone. Barber welcomes these changes, and the increased flexibility they offer child-rearing members of our society: "We are looking forward into a new age, when women [and men?] who so desire can rear their children quietly at home while they pursue a career on their child-safe, relatively interruptible-and-resumable home computers, linked to the world not by muleback or the steam locomotive, or even a car, but by the telephone and the modem" (33).

Toward Inclusive Definitions

If we are to include the accomplishments of women in the history of technical communication, I believe we must challenge the dualisitic thinking that severs public and private, household and industry, and masculine and feminine labor. I do not know if it is possible to construct a single definition for *technical communication* that can flexibly accommodate past and future changes in the meaning and significance of *work, workplace,* and *technology,* but toward this end I offer the following observations.

- **Technical writing exists within government and industry, as well as in the intersection between private and public spheres.** Technical writing exists to accomplish something: as Cooper points out, it is a form of social action (x). This action can originate in a variety of settings and for many purposes; such action may occur as part of one's work for hire or arise from personal interaction with organizations. Although many forms of technical writing exist and are employed strictly within and among organizations, there are also significant instances of its use within and origination from individual households in their interactions with government and industry.
- **Technical writing has a close relationship to technology.** *Technical* writing *per se,* must have some logical relationship to *technology*. We have tended to employ a very narrow view of *technology,* and to conflate the term with *computer technology*. But as Wajcman points out, technology is more than just the latest computer hardware or software on the market. Technology refers equally to *knowledge, actions,* and *tools*: it is (for example) a network of constructed waterways, the knowledge of when and how to irrigate fields, and the entire set of human actions that comprise this method for farming. *Inventions,* as Stanley argues, therefore include innovations such as the prepaid health care plan (Jeanne Mance), social services in hospitals (Dr. Marie Zakrzewska), and flextime (Christel Kammerer) (*Mothers* xxxiii).
- **Technical writing often seeks to make tacit knowledge explicit.** When its purpose is to instruct persons in a new technology (whether using a tool or performing a process), technical writing seeks to make tacit knowledge explicit, bridging by way of text and graphics gaps in different ways of learning. Zuboff, Dorothy Winsor, and Wajcman all emphasize that knowledge is not just cognitive, but often tactile and visual as well, relying on cues from context on when to act and what to do. Such "action-centered skills" (to use Zuboff's term) are a hallmark of oral culture and transmission of knowledge. Both Renaissance patterns for laces (Tebeaux, "Technical Writing") and early instructions for home dressmaking (Durack) include scanty explanation and rely on the user to provide most of the relevant information necessary to complete the work. Transition to literate cultures, along with the rationalization of work processes, involves analysis of action-centered skills and their codification and standardization. This results in an increase in the need for a text to provide contextual cues and information for the user, hence increases in the level of detail in text and graphics as shown in the evolution of home sewing pattern design (Durack).

As Allen has pointed out, a hazard of definition is that we may "succumb to a simplistic or exclusionary [definition] that separate[s] us from one another" (76). The cultural link between science, technology, and masculinity combined with a bias that fails to find significance in productive activities that occur within the household and lack associated cash value has, I believe, resulted in an interpretation of "technical writing" that works to exclude the significant contributions of women. Articles, such as those in this issue, test our disciplinary boundaries—and blinders—to argue for the relevance and significance of texts that might otherwise be omitted from our history. As we construct this history, a major challenge will be to examine why we deem certain artifacts *technology*, their attendant activities *work*, their place of conduct *the workplace*, and therefore find reason to include associated writings within the corpus *history of technical writing*.

WORKS CITED

Ackerman, John, and Scott Oates. "Image, Text, and Power in Architectural Design and Workplace Writing." *Nonacademic Writing: Social Theory and Technology*. Ed. Ann Hill Duin and Craig J. Hansen. Mahwah, NJ: Lawrence Erlbaum, 1996. 81–121.

Allen, Jo. "The Case Against Defining Technical Writing." *Journal of Business and Technical Communication* 4 (1990): 68–77.

Barber, Elizabeth Wayland. *Women's Work: The First 20,000 Years*. New York: W. W. Norton, 1994.

Brockmann, R. John. *From Millwrights to Shipwrights to the Twenty-First Century: Historical Considerations of American Technical Communication*. Cresskill, NJ: Hampton, forthcoming.

Brown, Judith. "A Note on the Division of Labor by Sex." *American Anthropologist* 72 (1970): 1073–78.

Cockburn, Cynthia. *Machinery of Dominance: Women, Men, and Technical Know-How*. Boston: Northeastern UP, 1988.

Cooper, Marilyn M. Foreword. *Nonacademic Writing: Social Theory and Technology*. Ed. Ann Hill Duin and Craig J. Hansen. Mahwah, NJ: Lawrence Erlbaum, 1996. ix–xii.

Cowan, Ruth Schwartz. "From Virginia Dare to Virginia Slims: Women and Technology in American Life." *Science and Technology Today: Readings for Writers*. Ed. Nancy R. MacKenzie. New York: St. Martin's P, 1995. 247–58.

———. *More Work for Mother: The Ironies of Household Technology from the Open Hearth to the Microwave*. New York: Basic Books, 1983.

Dobrin, David. "Do Not Grind Armadillo Armor in this Mill." *Writing and Technique*. Urbana, IL: National Council of Teachers of English, 1989. 13–27.

———. "What's Technical about Technical Writing." *New Essays in Technical and Scientific Communication: Research, Theory, Practice*. Ed. Paul V. Anderson, R. John Brockmann, and Carolyn R. Miller. Farmingdale, NY: Baywood, 1983. 227–50.

Durack, Katherine T. "Patterns for Success: A Lesson in Usable Design from U.S. Patent Records." *Technical Communication* 44 (1997): 37–51.

Greenbaum, Joan. *Windows on the Workplace: Computers, Jobs, and the Organization of Office Work in the Late Twentieth Century*. New York: Monthly Review P, 1995.

Harris, John. "For Love of Machines." *Journal of Technical Writing and Communication* 22 (1992): 239–46.

Kerber, Linda K. "Separate Spheres, Female Worlds, Woman's Place: The Rhetoric of Women's History." *Journal of American History* 75 (1988): 9–39.

McKay, Mary Fae. Reply to letter of Stan Carlson. *Technical Communication* 36 (1989): 86.

Neeley, Kathryn A. "Woman as Mediatrix: Women as Writers on Science and Technology in the Eighteenth and Nineteenth Centuries." *IEEE Transactions on Professional Communication* 35 (1992): 208–16.

Oakley, Ann. *Woman's Work: The Housewife, Past and Present*. New York: Vintage Books, 1974.

Rivers, William. "Studies in the History of Business and Technical Writing." *Journal of Business and Technical Communication* 8 (1994): 6–57.

Rothschild, Joan. "Technology, Housework, and Women's Liberation: A Theoretical Analysis." *Machina ex Dea: Feminist Perspectives on Technology*. Ed. Joan Rothschild. New York: Teachers College P, 1983. 79–93.

Scott, Joan Wallach. *Gender and the Politics of History*. New York: Columbia UP, 1988.

Stanley, Autumn. *Mothers and Daughters of Invention: Notes for a Revised History of Technology*. New Brunswick, NJ: Rutgers UP, 1995.

———. "Women Hold Up Two-Thirds of the Sky: Notes for a Revised History of Technology." *Machina ex Dea: Feminist Perspectives on Technology*. Ed. Joan Rothschild. New York: Teachers College P, 1983. 3–22.

Tebeaux, Elizabeth. "Technical Writing for Women of the English Renaissance." *Written Communication* 10 (1993): 164–99.

———. "Visual Language: The Development of Format and Page Design in English Renaissance Technical Writing." *Journal of Business and Technical Communication* 5 (1991): 246–74.

Tebeaux, Elizabeth, and M. Jimmie Killingsworth. "Expanding and Redirecting Historical Research in Technical Writing: In Search of Our Past." *Technical Communication Quarterly* 1 (1992): 5–32.

Tebeaux, Elizabeth, and Mary Lay. "Images of Women in Technical Books from the English Renaissance." *IEEE Transactions on Professional Communication* 35 (1992): 196–207.

Wajcman, Judy. *Feminism Confronts Technology*. University Park: Pennsylvania State UP, 1991.

Winsor, Dorothy. "Writing Well as a Form of Social Knowledge." *Nonacademic Writing: Social Theory and Technology*. Ed. Ann Hill Duin and Craig J. Hansen. Mahwah, NJ: Lawrence Erlbaum, 1996. 157–72.

Zuboff, Shoshana. *In the Age of the Smart Machine: The Future of Work and Power*. New York: Basic Books, 1988.

8 The Social Perspective and Pedagogy in Technical Communication

CHARLOTTE THRALLS AND
NANCY ROUNDY BLYLER

In this article, Thralls and Blyler do for technical communication what Jim Berlin did for composition with his 1988 article entitled "Rhetoric and Ideology in the Writing Classroom": they argue that the shift toward a social perspective on writing has led theorists to develop new pedagogical strategies, and, more important, they provide a taxonomy of four primary orientations. These four orientations (social constructionist, ideologic, social cognitive, and paralogic hermeneutic) are explained in terms of both aims and classroom practices suitable to meeting those aims. Their goal is to outline implications for teachers and encourage teachers to reflect on the theoretical underpinnings of their pedagogy. In addition, because the paralogic hermeneutic pedagogy poses such significant challenges to institutional structures, they focus on some implications and possible alternatives for courses and programs.

Interest in socially based pedagogy has steadily increased since Lester Faigley's groundbreaking work ("Competing"; "Nonacademic") defining the social perspective and describing its major theoretical presuppositions. In this work, Faigley posits that a social view of writing is characterized by one basic tenet: "Human language (including writing) can be understood only from the perspective of a society rather than a single individual" ("Competing" 535). Thus, stresses Faigley, "communication is inextricably bound up in the culture of a particular society" ("Nonacademic" 236).

Influenced by this social perspective on writing, theorists and researchers have attempted to work out the implications of social theory for the classroom. The late 1980s and the early 1990s, for example, have seen greater use of techniques such as cases and collaboration, designed to give pedagogic shape to the connections social theory posits between communication and culture.

Although these techniques have certainly revitalized instruction in technical communication, enabling teachers to go beyond the positivistic

From *Technical Communication Quarterly* 2, no. 3 (1993): 249–69.

emphasis that characterized earlier discussions of the discipline (Rymer 179–80), the profession has tended to view socially based pedagogy as a unified classroom approach, informed by a single theoretical position. Profound differences, however, are now emerging among theorists endorsing a social perspective (Thralls and Blyler)—differences that are causing social theorists to interpret the links between writers and culture in radically alternate ways. As a result, we have an emerging menu of socially based pedagogies rather than a single social paradigm for writing instruction.

Our purpose in this essay, thus, is to assess these various pedagogies in order to illustrate how competing interpretations of the social translate into distinct classroom practices. More specifically, we will describe four socially based pedagogic orientations—the social constructionist, the ideologic, the social cognitive, and the paralogic hermeneutic—showing that, although all share a belief in the connections between writing and culture, each subscribes to a different pedagogic aim and recommends different practices for the technical communication classroom. Ultimately, we hope to show that these differences are rooted in competing philosophical notions about the nature of communication and the teachability of writing, with important implications for teachers and programs in technical communication.

Social Constructionist Pedagogy

Social constructionist pedagogy stresses the central role that communities play in both writing and writing pedagogy. To be more specific, social constructionists assert that communities shape and even determine the discourse of their members through communal norms (Freed and Broadhead; Lipson)—norms that include not only textual practices but also more abstract practices such as "the kinds of issues that the discipline considers it important to try to resolve, the lines of reasoning used to resolve those issues, and shared assumptions about the audience's role, the writer's ethos, and the social purposes for communicating" (Herrington 405).

Because community members share a belief in these norms, they are able to agree about what they will call knowledge. (Kenneth Bruffee ["Social"] discusses this agreement, which he terms consensus.) In addition, a shared belief in communal norms enables community members to produce what Bruffee—based on Richard Rorty's work—calls "normal discourse" ("Collaborative" 642–43).

Social constructionists' belief in communities and communal norms, then, influence constructionists' pedagogic aim.

Pedagogic Aim

Constructionist pedagogy focuses on acculturating students to the communities they wish to enter—a process that James Porter terms socialization (44) and that Chris Anson and L. Lee Forsberg call "social and intellectual adaptation" (201). Bruffee describes this process of acculturation or socialization as learning to produce normal discourse ("Social" 643) and to participate in the conversations of communities: learning to think in the ways community members think and write about topics that matter within those communities in ways that members endorse ("Collaborative" 638–41). Through this process of acculturation, students come to understand how a given community uses discourse to reach consensus about knowledge. Students also adopt the communal norms governing discourse practices, thus acquiring the tools to become what Bruffee terms "knowledgeable peers" ("Collaborative" 777).

To engage students directly in the conversations of communities, social constructionists advance the concept of collaborative learning, which Bruffee defines as "a process that constitutes fields or disciplines of study" ("Collaborative" 635). Collaborative learning is based on the rationale that the task of learning to think and write as a knowledgeable peer is not solely an individual and mental endeavor but instead occurs through interaction (Bruffee, "Collaborative" 640). In collaborative learning, then, interaction among students in the classroom "provides the kind of social context . . . in which students can practice and master the normal discourse exercised in established knowledge communities in the academic world and in business, government, and the professions" (Bruffee, "Collaborative" 644).

Constructionists' classroom practices focus on means for facilitating this process of acculturation through collaborative learning.

Classroom Practices

Constructionists believe that teachers can facilitate students' acculturation if the classroom mirrors the professional communities students will enter. Constructionists also believe that including collaboration in technical communication classes will enable collaborative learning to take place.

Mirroring Professional Communities. So that professional communities can be mirrored in the classroom, constructionists believe that teachers should base their classroom activities on research findings, such as Anson and Forsberg's, and Carol Berkenkotter, Thomas Huckin, and John Ackerman's findings concerning socialization and initiation, Anne Herrington's on the intellectual and social conventions demarcating two engineering courses, Rachel Spilka's on writer-reader interactions in the workplace, or Carol German and William Rath's on the rapidly changing environment of technical communication. Spilka underscores this concept of basing classroom activities on research when she suggests that her findings

> might cause technical communication instructors to question seriously what they have been asking novice writers to read in the textbooks about how to compose in the workplace, and to consider making adjustments in how they teach audience analysis and adaptation in their courses. (219)

Employing these findings from research, constructionists then advocate several kinds of activities for the technical communication classroom. One such activity involves the use of cases (e.g., Guinn; Hilton; Karis), which Barbara Couture and Jone Rymer Goldstein argue "give students problems in real-world communication set in organizational contexts that replicate in detail their technical and professional roles" (v). Among teachers, however, there may be concern about the ability of students to envision these roles adequately or about the lack of information provided in some cases (Butler). A second constructionist activity, therefore, involves the use of assignments asking students to construct cases using their experience or the research they conduct (Mahin). Finally, a third activity involves having students write within actual professional situations (Olds), at times provided by internship programs (Mahin). All of these activities, constructionists feel, enable realistic "conversations" among peers within communities to take place and thus facilitate students' acculturation. Collaboration, however, also enables conversation and acculturation.

Collaboration. Constructionists believe that classroom activities involving collaboration will best encourage collaborative learning and thus best facilitate students' acculturation to professional communities. John Beard and Jone Rymer, for example, assert that "scholars and researchers of collaboration . . . view learning as a cooperative, social enterprise, not only as a competitive, individual activity" (1).

So that students can be involved in learning through collaboration, constructionists endorse such classroom activities as peer review of documents (e.g., Bruffee, "Collaborative") and co-authoring and team writing, where students "gain experience with collaborative writing as it is used in the business and professional worlds" (Morgan et al. 20). In such co-authoring and team writing, however, teachers are cautioned to reflect practice in professional fields by using writing tasks that "(1) are large enough to require a division of labor, (2) benefit from a breadth of specialized skills, or (3) need to represent the synthesis of divergent views" (Morgan et al. 20). In addition, computer-aided instruction is providing new means for supporting collaborative activities that mirror "most business people's work today" (Easton et al. 34). Annette Easton and her colleagues, for example, describe the software that supports collaborative work. This software includes both systems that writers do not use simultaneously—such as word processing, computer conferencing, electronic mail, and group authoring systems—and systems that writers do use simultaneously. Ann Hill Duin and Mary Elwart-Keys and Marjorie Horton then discuss particular tools for computer-aided collaboration: software that functions as "an interactive learning and productivity tool" (Duin, "Terms" 46), and the "Capture Lab" or computer-supported conference room (Elwart-Keys and Horton).

Classroom activities such as those enabling the teacher to mirror professional communities in the technical communication classroom and those involving collaboration will, constructionists believe, provide the pedagogic apparatus necessary to support and encourage collaborative learning, engagement in communal conversations, and thus acculturation to professional communities. Pedagogy influenced by the ideologic critics of social construction, however, views classroom activities differently, as means for rectifying some of the more negative aspects of acculturation that ideologic critics claim social constructionists have ignored.

Ideologic Pedagogy

Ideologic—or liberatory—pedagogy has been most currently articulated by composition scholars—James Berlin, Patricia Bizzell, Greg Myers, Carolyn R. Miller, John Trimbur, John Schilb, John Clifford, James Sledd—who, in turn, have been influenced by Aristotle as well as such cultural and education theorists as Jurgen Habermas, Michel Foucault, Henry Giroux, and Paulo Freire. Although important differences exist among these scholars, they generally share key assumptions in constructionist theory. These scholars tend to agree, for example, that reality, discourse communities, and the self are social constructions; and that language is processed within a framework of community norms—conventions of grammar, style, logical development, rules of evidence, and so forth—which authorize notions of effective communication.

Ideologic critics depart sharply from constructionists, however, on how the discourse norms of communities should inform the focus and aim of writing instruction. For ideologic critics, the fact that community norms govern knowledge and notions of good writing within discourse groups is no reason to valorize those norms in the classroom. For example, C. Miller, T. Miller, Myers, and Trimbur assert that when we uncritically teach students the discourse norms that will enable them to function in their profession as social workers, engineers, or lawyers, we downplay the hierarchical structures of authority that privilege and protect "normal" ways of knowing and speaking within communities. By Myers' account, "consensus in usage, although it seems democratic, ignores the conflicts that characterize language change, and leaves the authority of certain types of language unquestioned" (160).

Holding that constructionists' acculturative pedagogy downplays this link between community norms and authority structures, ideologic critics are primarily interested in raising questions about the political implications of community norms: How do conventions of discourse come to be codified as normal within academic and professional communities; how does this privileging impact on individuals and the larger social good? More specifically, whose interests are protected and reproduced through community norms in disciplinary, professional, and other social groups? What voices and interests are silenced, suppressed, or marginalized when the good, the normal, and the possible are encoded and prescribed through community norms?

Pedagogic Aims

For ideologic critics, these questions translate into writing pedagogy aimed not at acculturation but at resistance, which Joy S. Richie defines as "the process of critiquing and intervening in oppressive ideologies," helping students "see where they are located within ideology and within the interplay of conflicting ideologies and their own experience" (117). Resistance thus is emancipatory, involving a transformation of critical consciousness. For Giroux, this transformation is expressed in terms of "theoretical opportunities for self-reflection and struggle in the interest of *self*-emancipation and *social*-emancipation" (109; emphasis ours). Self-emancipation encompasses both students and teachers, as students move toward what Berlin calls their "full humanity" (490; see also Shor), and as teachers develop what Myers describes as "awareness" and "belief"—"awareness that one's course is part of an ideological structure that keeps people from thinking about their situation, but also a belief that one can resist this structure and help students to criticize it" (169). Social emancipation then follows, because students and teachers are empowered to act as agents of social change, controlling rather than being controlled by normalized social arrangements in educational, professional, and governmental institutions.

Although scholars advocating liberatory pedagogy see resistance as the pedagogic aim of writing classrooms, they are reluctant to assert that resistance actually constitutes a method of instruction—Myers prefers the term "stance" (169). Scholars do seem to believe, however, that this stance can be facilitated through classroom practices designed to demystify and transform relations of power.

Classroom Practices

Advocates of liberatory pedagogy in the technical communication classroom believe that problematizing discourse and social interaction are two classroom practices that can reveal to students the ideological work of discourse conventions and promote opportunities for more ethical and egalitarian social relations.

Problematizing Discourse. Problematizing discourse entails any type of rhetorical analysis that situates language conventions within ideology for the purpose of identifying privileged or dominant systems, including the way social systems reproduce themselves while, at the same time, they dissimulate the fact of domination. In the technical communication classroom, problematizing activities can focus on either written or visual conventions in professional documents. For written discourse, for example, students might emulate M. Jimmie Killingsworth and Dean Steffens' analysis of environmental impact statements or Susan Wells' analysis of instructional manuals in order to see how seemingly objective conventions construct a subject position for readers that protects a dominant group's way of talking and knowing. For graphic elements, students might deconstruct the innocence of maps, following, for example, Ben F. Barton and Marthalee S. Barton, to see how visual arrangements often position readers to view information from the perspective of a dominant order.

Because such analyses encourage students to take a critical perspective on the structures and signs that are traditionally employed in technical documents, liberatory pedagogy shifts the classroom agenda away from acculturation. Instead of helping students adopt the normative conventions of professional communities, problematizing activities lead students to reevaluate rhetorical principles—such as objectivity and unity—valued in much technical writing, and then to experiment with alternate discourses, such as narration (Brodkey) or visual strategies that denaturalize the act of reception (Barton and Barton).

For those advancing an ideologic orientation, problematizing activities also shift the skills orientation away from a mastery of normative rhetoric for fitting into communities and toward "deliberative" or "prudential judgment," which C. Miller defines as "the ability (and willingness) to take socially responsible action" (23; see also Sullivan 381). Because technical communicators should promote the larger community good within which the corporation operates rather than merely reproduce private or corporate interests, students should be encouraged to consider technical rhetoric, Miller maintains, "as a matter of arguing in a prudent way toward the good of the community rather than constructing texts" (23). Problematizing community discourse facilitates this process by giving students a way to identify and challenge the authority claims implicit in community norms.

Social Interaction. Like problematizing activities, social interaction, as interpreted within an ideologic orientation, entails strategies for revealing ideology and promoting more responsible social relations. Although constructionist pedagogy also stresses social interaction in the classroom in the form of collaborative learning and writing, liberatory pedagogy emphasizes social interaction as a way to challenge traditional authority structures and even advocate alternate social relations.

Advocates of liberatory pedagogy believe, for example, that collaborative activities in the technical communication classroom can change relations among students by drawing attention to these relations and thus revealing entrenched patterns of class, race, gender, and authority. For Lisa Ede and Andrea Lunsford and for Elizabeth A. Flynn and her colleagues, collaborative activities can require students to develop nonhierarchical or asymmetrical relations of power; for Mary Lay, collaborative groups can foster androgynous modes of interaction; for Rymer, having students view a videotape of their collaborative interactions can heighten their awareness of how groups privilege or suppress members' voices. For those endorsing liberatory pedagogy, the computerized classroom can offer further opportunities for egalitarian interactions among students. For example, researchers exploring network theory—Duin ("Computer-Supported"); Sara Kiesler, Jane Seigel, and Timothy McGuire; Cynthia L. Selfe and Billie J. Wahlstrom; Thomas T. Barker and Fred O. Kemp—see teleconferencing, which eliminates many cues of status and authority, as a way of fostering more democratic social interchanges.

In terms of the social interactions between students and teachers, proponents of liberatory pedagogy believe the computerized classroom has the further potential to forge new patterns of shared responsibility for learning. Because computer labs are typically incompatible with a presentation mode of instruction—with the teacher as the center of attention—the lab can be used to create a more student-centered classroom, with teachers serving as editors, collaborators, mentors, and problem posers.

Classroom activities that problematize discourse and enable more socially responsible interaction can, ideologic critics suggest, help students understand and resist the authority structures in professional communities. Like the constructionists and their ideologic critics, social cognitive pedagogy is interested in "the social and ideological forces that circumscribe thought and action" (Greene 152). Social cognitivists, however, add a cognitive dimension to this interest.

Social Cognitive Pedagogy

Social cognitivists unite their concern for social and ideologic forces with their traditional area of study: the mental processes of individual writers. By joining these two interests, social cognitivists view themselves as correcting a deficiency in other social theories about writing. More specifically, social cognitivists believe that because constructionists focus on the power of communities to determine—rather than simply facilitate—communication, constructionists have not fully accounted for the role human agency plays in communication. (See, for example, Greene 150–54; Flower, "Cognition" 282–87.) Social cognitivists wish, then, to redress this imbalance. As Linda Flower says, "I want a framework that acknowledges the pressure and the potential the social context can provide, at the same time it explains how writers negotiate that context" ("Cognition" 284).

In keeping with this dual focus on the social and the cognitive, social cognitivists assume that communication is shaped in two ways. First, social cognitivists subscribe to the constructionist concept of discourse communities, believing that systems of norms help community members create knowledge and communicate. Thus, Sarah Warchauer Freedman and her colleagues posit that "learning to write . . . is learning to enter into discourse communities which have their own rules and expectations" (3). Similarly, in a study of reading-to-write, Flower views her students as "*attempting to enter a new discourse community posed by college*" ("Negotiating," 222; emphasis in original). In this new discourse community, students have "to learn the textual conventions, the expectations, the habits of mind, and the methods of thought that allow one to operate in an academic conversation" (Flower, "Negotiating" 222). These conventions, expectations, and methods of thought then, in Ackerman's words, "strongly influence," but do not determine, community members' discourse (173).

Second, however, social cognitivists believe that the conventions, expectations, and methods of thought that mark specific communities are internalized by individuals as mental constructs or schemata that influence the way people comprehend writing tasks. These schemata "provide procedures for acting in accordance with cultural and contextual expectations" (Ackerman 176), thus facilitating communication. By viewing communal conventions, expectations, and methods of thought as internalized constructs, social cognitivists are able to integrate their belief in community norms with their focus on cognition.

This integration is clear in social cognitivists' concept of strategic knowledge, which Flower defines as "*the goals writers set for themselves, the strategies they invoke, and the metacognitive awareness they bring to both these acts*" ("Negotiating" 222; emphasis in original). To social cognitivists, strategic knowledge is not merely individual and mental. Instead, it is doubly social: it is both drawn from the socially based schemata that writers have internalized and—as Flower claims—"geared for action within a specific context" where a writer sets goals and calls on certain strategies in "response to the social and rhetorical context as the writer interprets it" ("Negotiating" 222).

Social cognitivists believe that this strategic knowledge, which both expert and novice writers exhibit, can be examined and described. The strategic knowledge of experts, however, becomes the standard to which novices should aspire, because this knowledge enables experts to produce more effective documents than novices are capable of doing. Social cognitivists' belief in the power of expert writers' strategic knowledge then influences their pedagogic aim.

Pedagogic Aim

Because strategic knowledge can be taught to novices whose repertoire of thinking strategies may be unsuitable for particular communities and contexts, social cognitive pedagogy has an integrated, dual aim: both adaptation to communities and negotiation of new writing situations (Flower, "Negotiating" 227–30). Social cognitive pedagogy seeks to accomplish this dual aim through a growth in metacognitive awareness, which—according to Flower—"*means an increased sense of rhetorical options and an expanded power to direct one's own cognition*" ("Negotiating" 229; emphasis in original). Metacognitive awareness, thus, allows students to represent more accurately to themselves the demands of writing tasks and increases their strategic knowledge about their rhetorical options for a given writing task (Flower, "Negotiating" 243). Social cognitivists' classroom practices are intended to further this dual process of adaptation and negotiation.

Pedagogic Practices

Social cognitivists believe that teachers can facilitate adaptation and negotiation through classroom practices that enable students to reflect on their writing processes and that model the strategic knowledge of expert writers. Both types of practices, cognitivists believe, will help technical communication students expand their metacognitive awareness.

Reflecting on Writing Processes. To engage students in reflection on their writing processes, social cognitivists advocate such activities as the use of protocols and self-studies, where students tape-record their thoughts while they are performing a writing task and then analyze the protocols they generate (Ackerman 191; Flower, "Negotiating" 8). Through such analyses, social cognitivists believe, technical communication students can better understand their writing processes and critique what they do. A related activity involves audio-taping collaborative writing groups, so that students can be alerted to the collaborative strategies they employ and can alter these strategies if they are ineffective (Burnett 11–12).

Modeling the Strategic Knowledge of Expert Writers. In order to model the strategic knowledge required in various professional communities, social cognitivists advocate basing classroom practices on research that investigates both the larger social contexts in which writing takes place and the thinking strategies used in those contexts. Concerning larger social contexts, for example, Ackerman and Kathleen McCormick describe the cultural and ideologic roots of reading-to-write as an academic task, finding these roots in the legacy of schooling that students have internalized. Concerning thinking strategies, Flower and her colleagues use such methodologies as think-aloud protocols, blind ratings of the quality of texts, and interviews to study the strategies that both expert and novice writers in academe use (*Reading*).

In social cognitivist pedagogy, research such as this then serves as a foundation for classroom activities modeling the strategic knowledge of expert writers. Technical communication teachers can, for example, employ on-line computer aids, heuristics, and—in the case of collaborative strategies—role-playing, as prompts for effective strategies (Burnett 11–13; Flower et al., *Planning* 48). These activities, social cognitivists believe, will enable students to incorporate into their own repertoires the strategic knowledge exhibited by expert writers. In doing so, novice writers may enhance their metacognitive awareness, gaining greater control over their writing processes and their responses to writing tasks in various professional communities and contexts.

To sum up our discussion thus far, then, constructionist, ideologic, and social cognitivist pedagogies all embrace the idea that a system of norms enables communication within communities and thus links writers, writing, and culture. All three orientations, however, offer a unique spin on these norms as they function in technical communication pedagogy: for social constructionists, acculturating students to norms; for ideologic critics, demystifying structures of power that regulate these norms; and for social cognitivists, enabling students to internalize the norms as cognitive strategies for negotiating communities and contexts. Although these different emphases are acknowledged by advocates of paralogic hermeneutics, paralogic theorists suggest that the differences among the constructionist, ideologic, and the social cognitive orientations are less significant than their shared beliefs about the nature of communication and the sense in which writing is teachable. By challenging these shared beliefs, paralogic hermeneutic pedagogy thus poses a radical departure from the other socially based pedagogies.

Paralogic Hermeneutic Pedagogy

The most recent of the socially based orientations to emerge in composition and technical communication pedagogy, paralogic theory has been articulated most fully by Thomas Kent ("Paralogic Hermeneutics"; *Paralogic Rhetoric*) and Reed Way Dasenbrock, who draw on an anti-Cartesian tradition in linguistics and philosophy, including most directly the work of Donald Davidson. Pedagogy informed by this orientation is based on the idea that communication is a hermeneutic skill refuting codification and therefore that writing must be taught as an unsystematic and paralogic (uncodifiable) activity. Paralogic theorists see the other three socially based pedagogies as holding an antithetical view: that communication is a systemic process that can be codified and taught according to certain internal structures or schemes.

To explain these oppositional claims, paralogic theorists posit the existence of two theoretical camps: an internalist camp, which would include the three socially based pedagogies we have discussed thus far; and an externalist camp, which would include paralogic hermeneutic pedagogy. According to Kent (*Paralogic Rhetoric*), the internalist camp holds that a split exists between the mind and reality—a split mediated by some internal scheme that makes knowledge of the world possible. In terms of language and communication, this emphasis on a mediating scheme means that language is always processed within a systematic, codifiable framework—community norms for constructionists, structures of power that control community norms for ideologic critics, and certain thinking processes for social cognitivists. Because meaning and understanding are always relative to these authorizing schemes, the schemes themselves are what allow people to communicate. Some kind of scheme, according to Kent, is at the heart of all internalist pedagogies, for all "presuppose that discourse production can be reduced to a process that represents, duplicates, or models" these schemes (*Paralogic Rhetoric* 101). In internalist pedagogies, learning to write thus consists of mastering a particular scheme.

Kent and other paralogic theorists reject internalist-driven pedagogies because they believe that internalism cannot explain how communication operates as a social phenomenon. They also believe that internalist schemes attempt to impose control on a communication process that defies such control. To counter what they see as flaws in internalism, paralogic theorists advance an externalist position which holds that meaning and understanding do not derive from internalized schemes that structure language: Neither communal norms, nor the exclusionary power of norms, nor again cognitive strategies based on norms make communication possible. From an externalist perspective, meaning and understanding derive from on-the-spot interpretations people make as they communicate. As an external and social act, communication requires that we interpret the language of others in the give and take of an interaction in an attempt to arrive at understanding. In Kent's words, "Discourse production . . . always embodies interpretation, for in order to produce discourse that will be comprehensible to others, we must first interpret the other's code before we can attempt to match ours to it" ("Paralogic Hermeneutics" 26).

Because externalists assert that this interpretation is never codifiable or systematic, they reject the idea that writing is teachable as a formalized process involving norms as an authorizing scheme. For externalists like Kent, "no formal pedagogy can be constructed to teach the act of writing or critical reading" ("Paralogic Hermeneutics" 36) and thus writing is teachable only as an uncodifiable negotiation of interpretive moves. This emphasis on unsystematic interpretation informs the aim of a paralogic pedagogy.

Pedagogic Aim

For those endorsing a paralogic hermeneutic orientation, writing courses should aim to reveal to students the external, social, interpretive, and unsystematic nature of communicative interaction. Under this pedagogic orientation, students would come to understand, for example, that communication is always fluid and indeterminate because norms and cognitive strategies do not themselves stabilize meaning. Thus, writers who are steeped in their own interpretive codes must try to ascertain the codes of prospective readers or other language users. Because these codes of writers and readers, which Davidson labels "prior theories" (442), never match perfectly, writers must engage in what Kent calls "hermeneutic guessing" ("Paralogic Hermeneutics" 29), the development of provisional assumptions about the meanings readers might have for certain words. Readers undergo a similar process in discourse analysis, as they try to ascertain what writers mean by their words. The result of this guessing is a "passing theory" (Davidson 442), a concept that denotes the contingent hermeneutic strategy that writers and readers develop to understand one another. When writers and readers come to share a passing theory, they have reached understanding, although this understanding is itself temporary because additional interactions will lead to further guesses and adjustments among communicants.

Because, for paralogic theorists, writing is a matter of this guessing about another's interpretive strategies, these theorists believe that the acculturative, resistive, and adaptive/negotiative aims of the other three socially based pedagogies are possible only if framed within the larger conception of writing as an open-ended dialogue—the hermeneutic interplay of prior and passing theories. Regarding the aim of resistance, for example, paralogic theorists would embed issues of empowerment—confronting and overturning communal norms—within specific dialogic interactions. For these theorists, it is through our efforts to understand one another and arrive at a passing theory that we are drawn out, in Dasenbrock's words, "of the prisonhouse of our beliefs and prior theories" and led "to a new understanding or passing theory."

In as much as paralogic hermeneutic pedagogy stresses writing as an open-ended dialogue resisting codification, advocates of this orientation envision classroom practices that bring students into dialogic interaction with others.

Classroom Practices

Paralogic theorists challenge classroom practices in technical communication that attempt to systematize the language of communities or expert writers. More specifically, paralogic theorists oppose the idea that classroom practices designed to mirror the conventions of communities, problematize these communities' conventions, or expand metacognitive awareness can ever guarantee that students will learn to write. From a paralogic perspective, these practices may help students develop useful background knowledge, but this background knowledge—be it community norms or thinking strategies based on norms—cannot be reduced to a process that students then can apply to subsequent writing projects in order to assure effective communication.

For paralogic theorists, students learn by "entering into specific dialogic and therefore hermeneutic interactions with others' interpretive strategies" (Kent, "Paralogic Hermeneutics" 37). To facilitate this learning, paralogic pedagogy would create activities in the technical communication classroom that engage students in dialogic conversations and in student/teacher interactions.

Dialogic Conversations. Both Kent and David Russell, who have explored the implications of paralogic/dialogic pedagogy, emphasize immersing technical communication students in conversations that occur within their disciplines. Through such conversations about actual problems in their fields, students would bring their knowledge of a discipline into the fluid give and take of actual dialogue, learning firsthand that communication requires active interpretive interaction with another.

For Russell, disciplinary writing is essential if students are to understand this dialogic process: "Students may learn to parrot the phrasing or structure of some genre, but unless they are then involved (directly or vicariously) in the problems, the activities, the habits of those who found a need to use writing in those ways, the discourse is meaningless—except as a requirement of a powerful institution" (194). For Kent, such disciplinary writing argues against the use of cases in the technical communication classroom. Writing generated from cases, according to Kent, promotes monologic instead of dialogic writing: Such writing "never affects the world in the sense that it engages the other in a dialogic/collaborative way, for in order to engage the other, the writer obviously must possess a conception of the other's identity which is impossible to grasp in the case study approach" ("Paralogic Hermeneutics" 38). This emphasis on dialogue also informs a paralogic perspective on student/teacher interaction in the classroom.

Student/Teacher Interactions. Paralogic theorists question that, as a method, collaboration will acculturate students to community norms, help students to critique the authority implicit in those norms, or help students internalize expert writers' strategic knowledge. Instead, paralogic pedagogy advances student/teacher interactions as a model of dialogic discourse. As one who grasps the paralogic/dialogic nature of writing, the technical communication teacher would model the hermeneutic interactions with another that must take place in discourse production. By working one-on-one with students—discussing students' writing and making suggestions—teachers would show students that communication is actively linked, in a Bakhtinian sense, to others who have preceded a writer and to others whose responsive reactions a writer anticipates (Bakhtin 91–93). The teacher would help sensitize students to this complex interplay, helping them to "adapt their discourses to the discourses of others" (Kent, "Paralogic Hermeneutics" 40) and thus to understand the paralogic nature of communication.

In describing the paralogic hermeneutic, constructionist, ideologic, and social constructionist pedagogies, we have attempted to point out how differently theorists have interpreted the link between communication and culture and thus envisioned the aims and practices of the technical communication classroom. In the last section, we explore how these differences speak to our concerns as teachers and administrators as we try to sort out socially based pedagogies and consider their implications for technical communication courses and programs.

Implications of Diverse Social Pedagogies

Clearly, the differences among pedagogic orientations within the social perspective have implications for technical communication teachers as they design their classroom practices. These differences, however, also have broader institutional implications for technical communication courses as they are currently configured in the academy.

Implications for Teachers

One implication of these differences concerns the degree to which the aims and pedagogic practices of various orientations can be melded in the technical communication classroom. Can teachers, for example, mix the aim and activities of one pedagogic orientation—say the paralogic hermeneutic—with those of the other orientations? Although this question merits lengthier study, we are skeptical that such melding is possible.

Most obviously, because the paralogic positron on the nature of communication and the teachability of writing are antithetical to what paralogic theorists characterize as the internalist position, the aims and practices of paralogic pedagogy would seem to be incompatible with social constructionist, ideologic, and social cognitive approaches in the classroom. More specifically, because paralogic theorists believe that communication is an uncodifiable hermeneutic activity and therefore that writing must be taught within the framework of dialogic interactions, paralogic pedagogy cannot be integrated with a focus on communal norms as the authorizing force behind communication or the basis of writing instruction. For example, although paralogic theorists advocate a form of collaboration in the classroom, the dialogic cast that this pedagogy gives to student/teacher interactions makes the paralogic version of collaboration fundamentally different from the acculturative acts of collaboration that social construction endorses, the resistive forms of collaboration that ideologic theorists espouse, or the adaptive and negotiative strategies for collaboration—as evidenced by expert writers—that social cognitivists advance. It would seem, then, that technical communication teachers cannot, at one and the same time, espouse a paralogic hermeneutic and a constructionist, ideologic, or social cognitive approach to pedagogy.

On a less obvious level, however, the superficial agreement among social constructionist, ideologic, and social cognitive theorists about the influence on the writing of communities and their norms may mask a basic incompatibility as well. It is difficult to imagine, for example, how ideologic theorists' focus on resistance to communal norms can be joined with constructionists' focus on acculturation. Because ideologic theorists' problematizing practices are intended to lead students to question their roles as writers in professional settings, these practices appear to undermine the very basis of acculturation. Similarly, although constructionists and social cognitivists agree that acculturation or adaptation to communities is a pedagogic aim, social cognitivists' interest in expanding students' metacognitive awareness leads to classroom practices that position social concerns within the sphere of mental activity. Given social construction's announced opposition to cognitive principles (e.g., Bruffee, "Social" 776–79), such a positioning would seem to signal—at the very least—an incompatibility concerning the focus of pedagogy as it directs classroom teaching.

If, as we suggest, these four socially based pedagogies appear to be incompatible in their aims and classroom practices, technical communication teachers should consider the theoretical underpinnings of their pedagogical practices in order to ensure that these practices will achieve the objectives teachers have set. On the plus side, however, understanding the pedagogic aims that underlie certain classroom practices may assist inexperienced teachers in clarifying for themselves possible objectives for a technical communication class and the ways those objectives might be reached.

In addition to these implications for the technical communication teacher, the differences we describe among pedagogic orientations also have broader institutional implications for technical communication programs.

Institutional Implications

Given that, of the four socially based pedagogies, only the paralogic hermeneutic rejects the assumption that writing is teachable via a scheme or formalized method, paralogic pedagogy poses the most significant challenge to our institutional structures for teaching technical communication. In its most radical form, we could interpret the paralogic position to mean that we abandon technical communication courses as they are envisioned within internalist pedagogies. From a paralogic perspective, the fact that technical communication cannot be taught through a formalized process based on norms renders internalist-driven writing courses untenable. Such courses can never fulfill their objectives—teaching students to write—and thus there can be little reason to support such courses in the academy.

As an alternative, paralogic theorists would support technical communication courses that are externalist driven. Even with these courses, however, the responsibility for writing instruction would not be the exclusive domain of English departments or writing faculty. Rather, as Kent suggests, writing instruction would be integrated throughout the disciplines: "When we view writing and reading as paralogic/hermenetuic acts, we come to see that writing and reading instruction resides at the very center of every student's academic curriculum," with every instructor "responsible for providing information about discourse production and analysis" ("Paralogic Hermeneutics" 39–40).

Finally, a more modest, though still controversial, implication of the paralogic orientation has to do with the size of college and university courses. The intense one-on-one dialogue between students and teachers required by paralogic pedagogy argues for smaller teacher-to-student ratios than are conventional in most university and technical communication classrooms, and certainly argues against large lecture sections for engaging students in the conversations of their disciplines.

Although we have touched on only a few implications of diverse socially based pedagogies for technical communication teachers and programs, a more detailed discussion is beyond the scope of what we can reasonably address here. Given, however, the growing complexity of the social perspective, we urge the profession to pursue in a vigorous way the discussion we have begun in order to debate the impact of socially based pedagogies and to clarify competing visions of the social perspective for technical communication.

WORKS CITED

Ackerman, John. "Translating Context into Action." *Reading to Write: Exploring a Social and Cognitive Process*. Ed. Linda Flower et al. New York: Oxford UP, 1990. 173–93.

Anson, Chris M., and L. Lee Forsberg. "Moving Beyond the Academic Community. Transitional Stages in Professional Writing." *Written Communication* 7 (1990): 200–31.

Bakhtin, Mikhail M. *Speech Genres and Other Late Essays*. Trans. Caryl Emerson and Michael Holquist. Austin: U of Texas P, 1986.

Barker, Thomas T., and Fred O. Kemp. "Network Theory: A Postmodern Pedagogy for the Writing Classroom." *Computers and Community*. Ed. Carolyn Handa. Portsmouth: Boynton/Cook, 1989. 1–28.

Barton, Ben F., and Marthalee S. Barton. "Ideology and the Map: Toward a Postmodern Visual Design Process." *Professional Communication: The Social Perspective*. Ed. Nancy Roundy Blyler and Charlotte Thralls. Newbury Park: Sage, 1993. 49–78.

Beard, John D., and Jone Rymer. "The Contexts of Collaborative Writing." *The Bulletin of the Association for Business Communication* 53 (1990): 1–3.

Berkenkotter, Carol, Thomas N. Huckin, and John Ackerman. "Conventions, Conversations, and the Writer: Case Study of a Student in a Rhetoric PhD Program." *Research in the Teaching of English* 22 (1988): 9–44.

Berlin, James. "Rhetoric and Ideology in the Writing Classroom." *College English* 50 (1988): 477–94.

Brodkey Linda. "Writing Ethnographic Narratives." *Written Communication* 4 (1987): 25–50.

Bruffee, Kenneth A. "Collaborative Learning and the 'Conversation of Mankind.'" *College English* 46 (1984): 635–52.

———. "Social Construction, Language, and the Authority of Knowledge: A Bibliographic Essay." *College English* 48 (1986): 773–90.

Burnett, Rebecca E. "Benefits of Collaborative Planning in the Classroom." *The Bulletin of the Association for Business Communication* 53 (1990): 9–17.

Butler, Marilyn S. "A Reassessment of the Case Approach: Reinforcing Artifice in Business Writing Courses." *The Bulletin of the Association for Business Communication* 48 (1985): 4–7.

Couture, Barbara, and Jone Rymer Goldstein. *Cases for Technical and Professional Writing*. Boston: Little, Brown, 1984.

Dasenbrock, Reed Way. "A Response to 'Language, Writing, and Reading: A Conversation with Donald Davidson.'" *Journal of Advanced Composition*, forthcoming.

Davidson, Donald. "A Nice Derangement of Epitaphs." *Truth and Interpretation: Perspectives on the Philosophy of Donald Davidson*. Ed. Ernest LePore. New York: Blackwell, 1986. 544–46.

Duin, Ann Hill. "Computer-Supported Collaborative Writing: The Workplace and the Writing Classroom." *Journal of Business and Technical Communication* 5 (1991): 123–50.

———. "Terms and Tools: A Theory and Research-Based Approach to Collaborative Writing." *The Bulletin of the Association for Business Communication* 53 (1990): 45–50.

Easton, Annette, et al. "Supporting Group Writing with Computer Software." *The Bulletin of the Association for Business Communication* 53 (1990): 34–37.

Ede, Lisa, and Andrea Lunsford. *Singular Texts/Plural Authors: Perspectives on Collaborative Writing*. Carbondale: Southern Illinois UP, 1990.

Elwart-Keys, Mary, and Marjorie Horton. "Collaboration in the Capture Lab: Computer Support for Group Writing." *The Bulletin of the Association for Business Communication* 53 (1990): 38–44.

Faigley, Lester. "Competing Theories of Process: A Critique and a Proposal." *College English* 48 (1986): 527–42.

———. "Nonacademic Writing. The Social Perspective." *Writing in Nonacademic Settings*. Ed. Lee Odell and Dixie Goswami. New York: Guilford, 1985. 231–48.

Flower, Linda. "Cognition, Context, and Theory Building." *College Composition and Communication* 40 (1989): 282–311.

———. "Introduction: Studying Cognition in Context." *Reading to Write: Exploring a Social and Cognitive Process*. Ed. Linda Flower et al. New York: Oxford UP, 1990. 3–32.

———. "Negotiating Academic Discourse." *Reading to Write: Exploring a Social and Cognitive Process*. Ed. Linda Flower et al. New York: Oxford UP, 1990. 221–61.

Flower, Linda, et al. *Planning in Writing: The Cognition of a Constructive Process*. Technical Report #34. Berkeley and Pittsburg: U of California and Carnegie Mellon, 1989.

Flower, Linda, et al. *Reading to Write: Exploring a Social and Cognitive Process*. New York: Oxford UP, 1990.

Flynn, Elizabeth A., et al. "Gender and Modes of Collaboration in a Chemical Engineering Design Course." *Journal of Business and Technical Communication* 5 (1991): 444–62.

Freed, Richard C., and Glenn J Broadhead. "Discourse Communities: Sacred Texts and Institutional Norms." *College Composition and Communication* 38 (1987): 154–65.

Freedman, Sarah Warchauer, et al. *Research in Writing: Past, Present, Future*. Technical Report #1. Berkeley and Pittsburg: U of California and Carnegie Mellon, 1987.

German, Carol J., and William R. Rath. "Making Technical Communication a Real-World Exercise: A Report of Classroom and Industry-Based Research." *Journal of Technical Writing and Communication* 17 (1987): 335–46.

Giroux, Henry A. *Theory and Resistence in Education: A Pedagogy for the Opposition*. South Hadley: Bergin, 1983.

Greene, Stuart. "Toward a Dialectical Theory of Composing." *Rhetoric Review* 9 (1990): 149–72.

Guinn, Dorothy Margaret. "The Case for Self-Generated Cases." *The Bulletin of the Association for Business Communication* 60 (1988): 4–10.

Herrington, Anne J. "Classrooms as Forums for Reasoning and Writing." *College Composition and Communication* 36 (1985): 404–13.

Hilton, Chad. "Campus and Community: Sources for Writing Cases that Work." *The Bulletin of the Association for Business Communication* 49.2 (1986): 30–31.

Karis, Bill. "Climbing the Corporate Ladder: Becoming Aware of the Rungs." *Journal of Business and Technical Communication* 5 (1991): 76–87.

Kent, Thomas. "Paralogic Hermeneutics and the Possibilities of Rhetoric." *Rhetoric Review* 8.1 (1989): 24–42.

———. *Paralogic Rhetoric: Writing and Reading as Hermeneutic Acts*. Lewisburg: Bucknell UP, 1993.

Kiesler, Sara, Jane Siegel, and Timothy McGuire. "Social Psychological Aspects of Computer-Mediated Communication." *Computer-Supported Cooperative Work*. Ed. Irene Greif. San Mateo: Morgan Kaufmann, 1988. 657–82.

Killingsworth, M. Jimmie, and Dean Steffens. "Effectiveness in the Environmental Impact Statement: A Study in Public Rhetoric." *Written Communication* 6 (1989): 155–80.

Lay, Mary. "The Androgynous Collaborator: The Impact of Gender Studies on Collaboration." *New Visions of Collaborative Writing*. Ed. Janis Forman. Portsmouth: Boynton/Cook, 1992. 63–81.

Lipson, Carol. "A Social View of Technical Writing." *Journal of Business and Technical Communication* 2 (1988): 7–20.

Mahin, Linda. "Replies to Marilyn S. Butler's Article 'A Reassessment of the Case Approach: Reinforcing Artifice in Business Writing Courses.'" *The Bulletin of the Association for Business Communication* 49 (1986): 2–4.

McCormick, Kathleen. "The Cultural Imperatives Underlying Cognitive Acts." *Reading to Write: Exploring a Social and Cognitive Process*. Ed. Linda Flower et al. New York: Oxford UP, 1990. 194–218.

Miller, Carolyn R. "What's Practical about Technical Writing?" *Technical Writing: Theory and Practice*. Ed. Bertie E. Fearing and W. K. Sparrow. New York: MLA, 1989. 14–24.

Miller, Thomas P. "Treating Professional Writing as Social Praxis." *Journal of Advanced Composition* 11 (1991): 57–72.

Morgan, Meg, et al. "Collaborative Writing in the Classroom." *The Bulletin of the Association for Business Communication* 50 (1987): 20–26.

Myers, Greg. "Reality, Consensus, and Reform in the Rhetoric of Composition Teaching." *College English* 48 (1986): 154–73.

Olds, Barbara, "Beyond the Casebook: Teaching Technical Communication through 'Real Life' Projects." *The Technical Writing Teacher* 14 (1987): 11–19.

Porter, James E. "Intertextuality and the Discourse Community." *Rhetoric Review* 5.1 (1986): 34–47.

Richie, Joy S. "Resistance to Reading: Another View of the Minefield." *Journal of Advanced Composition* 12 (1992): 117–36.

Russell, David R. "Vygotsky, Dewey, and Externalism: Beyond Student/Discipline Dichotomy." *Journal of Advanced Composition* 13.1 (1993): 173–97.

Rymer, Jone. "Collaboration and Conversation in Learning Communities. The Discipline and the Classroom." *Professional Communication. The Social Perspective*. Ed. Nancy Roundy Blyler and Charlotte Thralls. Newbury Park, Sage, 1993. 179–95.

Selfe, Cynthia L., and Billie J. Wahlstrom. "Computer-Supported Writing Classes: Lessons for Teachers." *Computers in English and the Language Arts*. Ed. Cynthia L. Selfe, Dawn Rodriques, and William R. Oates. Urbana: NCTE, 1989. 257–68.

Shor, Ira. *Critical Teaching and Everyday Life*. 1980. Chicago: U of Chicago P, 1987.

Spilka, Rachel. "Studying Writer-Reader Interactions in the Workplace." *The Technical Writing Teacher* 15 (1988): 208–22.

Sullivan, Dale L. "Political-Ethical Implications of Defining Technical Communication as a Practice." *Journal of Advanced Composition* 10 (1990): 375–86.

Thralls, Charlotte, and Nancy Roundy Blyler. "The Social Perspective in Professional Communication. Diversity and Directions in Research." *Professional Communication. The Social Perspective*. Ed. Nancy Roundy Blyler and Charlotte Thralls. Newbury Park: Sage, 1993. 3–34.

Trimbur, John. "Consensus and Difference in Collaborative Learning." *College English* 51 (1989): 602–16.

Wells, Susan. "Habermas, Communicative Competence, and the Teaching of Technical Discourse." *Theory in the Classroom*. Ed. Cary Nelson. Urbana: U of Illinois P, 1986. 245–69.

APPLIED THEORY

9 Researching the History of Technical Communication: Accessing and Analyzing Corporate Archives

HENRIETTA NICKELS SHIRK

In this short piece, Shirk argues that studying history, particularly at the personal and local levels (e.g., company and corporation), can lead to significant benefits for technical communicators and their organizations. Not only can technical communicators use historical information to "negotiate[e] the rhetorical and social constructions of meaning in their field (p. 137 in this volume)," but they also can use it to make decisions about their work, learning to choose appropriate techniques or strategies to avoid mistakes and create "an enhanced sense of self-identity and tradition" (Brockmann, qtd. on p. 137). Especially useful are Shirk's discussions of history as tool, analogy, and heritage, as well as her discussion of the value and uses of archives.

STUDYING THE HISTORY OF TECHNICAL COMMUNICATION

It is often remarked that every profession has a history, and that having a history is part of what truly makes a profession a profession. However, if most technical communicators were asked to discuss the history of their field, there would be little consensus about when it began and most likely vehement disagreement about whether such a concern is even important in the fast-paced changing environment of today's workplace.

Although definitive responses to these major issues are beyond the scope of this paper, it does suggest several directions and a rationale for technical communicators to engage in historical research techniques within corporate environments. When the study of history is undertaken by technical communicators at a personal and local level, it becomes relevant in terms of organizational contexts. The organizations in which practitioners work have their own histories (and sometimes mysteries) waiting to be explored by the curious and determined.

Knowing why, what, where, and how to look for historical corporate information can contribute to ongoing career successes. Equally important is

From STC Conference 2000 Proceedings. http://www.stc.org/proceedings/ConfProceed/2000/PDFs/00079.PDF.

knowing what to do with historical information once it is located – that is, how to apply it to current workplace situations.

Why Should You Study the Past?

The folklore of the field of technical communication generally assumes that the field began with the writing of technical manuals that resulted from the increased uses of military technologies during World War II. Historical researchers know that this is not true and that there is actually a long tradition of communicating about technical and scientific subject matter that goes back to the ancient Egyptians and Greeks. My assumptions in addressing several aspects of researching the history of technical communication are that:

- It is intellectually significant and emotionally meaningful for all technical communicators to become informed concerning the origins and history of their profession.
- Knowledge about such historical information is not the sole prerogative of scholars in academic settings, but is rather information that can and should be accessed (and assessed) by practitioners.
- Information about the history of technical communication can be used in practical ways within corporate settings to better inform and justify present and future standards and practices.

In terms of corporate histories, it is generally documents of one sort or another that constitute the official records of the organization. There are economic and practical reasons for such preservation of records, in addition to their historical significance. Business historian Donn C. Neal has remarked that "an organization profits when its records having lasting fiscal, legal, evidential, historical, and administrative value are preserved and managed so that the essential information in them can be brought to bear upon the organization's current needs and future planning" (1, p. 1).

The past can frequently inform the present—it can tell us where we have been, and it can provide information upon which to make decisions about where we might go in the future. It can also give us a clearer understanding of the present (how it came to be what it is).

The study of corporate archives provides three possible perspectives on the uses of history—diagnosis, analogy, and heritage. These perspectives have been described by Smith and Steadman (2), who have extensively studied corporations to determine what types of historical investigation are the most useful and legitimate for a company's purposes. I will summarize their major findings here and demonstrate how these findings might be applied by practicing technical communicators.

History as a Diagnostic Tool. Most corporate employees have a need for a history of their company that is larger than their own experience, in order to direct and/or cope with necessary changes. For technical communicators, using corporate history as a diagnostic tool can assist them in seeing beyond their own immediate experiences in order to understand their audiences more completely and how current publications evolved to be the way they are. This knowledge can provide a foundation for proposing and implementing changes in existing publications to enable them to communicate more effectively with their intended audiences.

History as Analogy. While all organizations develop their own peculiar histories and cultures, different organizations often face similar problems and issues. Corporate histories, especially of older companies with continuity in single industries, often contain analogues to contemporary concerns that can illuminate truths and reveal lost lessons about the fundamental nature and operations of particular industries.

For example, knowing how a particular software company has evolved its user documentation over the course of time can demonstrate the effectiveness of changing delivery media to meet market requirements within certain budgetary constraints. History, of course, never repeats itself exactly, and it is dangerous to rely uncritically on the past to predict the future. Even so, lessons are there to be learned. Sometimes a history's relevance lies in pointing out the irrelevant. Sometimes finding out why and how major publications decisions were made reveals not only their latent significance or comparative value but also their pertinence to the present.

History as Heritage. Resurgent interest in corporate cultures has led students of organizational behavior to serious study of the role traditions play in the life of a company. Every company, even a new one, has a heritage and a body of tradition. If a company's heritage is the whole of its discoverable history, then technical communicators can define tradition as the selective transmission of that heritage. In other words, tradition can be thought of as the company's surface memory—the folklore, ritual, and symbols that represent the company's sense of its origins, purpose, and identity over time.

Company tradition is passed on formally through orientation programs, written histories, tangible symbols, policies, and corporate publications. It is also informally transmitted through stories and routines that people accept as standard practices. Even the technical publications process is a kind of history. All traditions are embedded in the past but are alive in the present. For this reason, their history is vital to the technical communicator.

Perhaps all of these three uses of history are best summarized by Kenneth Burke in his book *Attitudes Toward History*, when he comments that "even in the 'best possible of worlds,' the need for symbolic tinkering would continue. One must erect a vast symbolic synthesis, a rationale of imaginative and conceptual imagery that 'locates' the various aspects of experience" (3, p. 179). Burke goes on to explain that symbolism guides social purpose by providing one with "cues" as to what is important and how one should pursue or not pursue what is valued.

How Do You Study the Past?

The practical question of how technical communicators should best approach the study of their past suggests a variety of possible actions, ranging from defining exactly what kinds of information and materials one is looking for, to deciding what to look at and where it might be located. These activities could include academic research among business document collections in traditional libraries, as well as research in corporate file rooms, company records storage warehouses, and electronic storage repositories.

Regardless of where various forms of technical communication are to be found, all of these approaches involve locating and analyzing collections of materials called "archives."

Defining Corporate Archives

What, then, is an archive? The essential meaning of the word has been rhetorically described by Derrida as the simultaneous naming of a "commencement and a commandment" (4, p. 1). Or, stated another way, an archive is both the place where information commences physically (that is, has physical presence in the public arena where it can be accessed), and the place where authority and social order are exercised in maintaining security and organization concerning the collected material. Derrida also observes that archives are characterized by "domiciliation," a kind of house arrest in the place in which they permanently reside.

In more prosaic and corporate terms, an archive is a collection of unpublished documents that are the result of the chance survival of some of the documents and the corresponding chance loss or deliberate destruction of others (5, 6). Although typically unexplored, the history of an organization or corporation can be an important and helpful resource for technical communicators.

There are eight basic types of archival information that practicing technical communicators might look for and use in gaining knowledge of a corporation's history. These categories are loosely based on the types of documents described in the book *Business Documents: Their Origins, Sources and Uses in Historical Research* by Armstrong and Jones (7), although the perspective of these authors is focused on business documents in Great Britain, not those in the United States.

Letters, Memos, and Journals

Business letters and memos are typically archived documents, especially from pre-digital technology times, and they can provide rich sources of historical material for technical communicators. An additional source of information might also come from job journals, sometimes kept by people involved in keeping financial records, tabulating data, or recording procedures or heuristics for accomplishing tasks. Drawings and sketches may also be a part of this record keeping. Technical communication researchers can use these kinds of materials to reconstruct information about the daily operations of a particular corporation.

Prospectuses, Ads, and Proposals

Documents that attempt to induce the public to buy stocks in a particular company or that propose that the public purchase various goods and/or services from the organization often reveal much about not only corporate interests, but also about corporate attitudes towards various customers and publics. Marketing materials provide information for rhetorical analyses of the persuasive techniques used by a corporation. Technical communicators can use this kind of information to assess how a corporation has persuaded its many publics in the past, and thereby view their own work in comparison to both effective and ineffective past practices. They may even use the best of past persuasive approaches to justify a creative new approach that combines both old and new techniques.

Articles of Incorporation

Although a very formal type of document, articles of incorporation specify in legal terms the limits and purposes of a company and how its affairs should be conducted. They are, in theory, a tool for the shareholder to use in controlling the directors of the company, if they should step outside the specified limits. However, as detailed specifications of the parameters within which the company has agreed to operate, the rules and regulations concerning its running, and the powers of authority of the directors, they provide a historical framework from which technical communicators can view a company and begin to see how it accomplishes its vision.

Minutes of Meetings

Corporations are typically run by meetings, and well-run corporations have the requirement to keep minutes of all meetings of the board of directors as well as those minutes of important work groups and committees within the organization. These minutes are typically filed and stored "for the permanent record." Meeting minutes can reveal much about the social construction of knowledge within a corporate entity and the functioning (or lack thereof) of teamwork within project groups and committees. They are an important source for technical communicators to understand the corporate culture within any organization in which they might be employed, and how best to function within it.

Annual Reports

Corporate annual reports provide a rich source of historical information. Not only do they provide an annual financial statement in the form of a certified balance sheet, but they also give a report (usually with text and graphics) of the status of the company's efforts. Annual reports typically provide a brief statement from the chairman of the board of directors that draws attention to one or two salient points of the company's activities during the past year. These documents are typically kept in corporate archives, and they can provide yet another method for viewing a company's past performance over time, as it is viewed from the perspective of management communicating to their shareholders and even to the general public (as potential shareholders).

Financial Records and Reports

Companies, of course, are required by law to keep financial records, for tax and government regulatory purposes, as well as for internal documentation about how well or poorly they are performing financially. For those who know how to "read" such documents, they can provide a fascinating glimpse into the details of the daily running of the corporation, and they can provide some perspectives on how corporations allocate their resources (money, people, and equipment). For example, a technical publications manager may be able to determine the past history of a particular company's investment in documentation, because there will be financial records (receipts and invoices) that provide written evidence of the publications services purchased in the past. Such information can be useful in justifying the status quo or in implementing change.

Patents, Trademarks, and Copyrights

Patents, trademarks, and copyrights, as well as related kinds of legal documents can provide glimpses into the technological or scientific research and development characteristics of an organization. The professional work of engineers, scientists, communicators, and others that is valued by the company and important to its financial successes is recorded in such documents. Like other kinds of legal documents, patents, trademarks, and copyrights will be carefully archived by most corporations. In the event of the loss of such "official" documents, there is usually a record of them in the archives of the agencies which granted them. All of these documents can be used by technical communicators to research information about the past development efforts of a particular company. Knowing what has been created and valued in the past can contribute to the generation and implementation of current new ideas and designs for products and services.

Licenses and Agency Agreements

Licenses and agreements are a final category of legal documents typically archived by corporations. Generally, a license is merely a granting of permission to do something, typically between two entities. The original purpose of a license was to create a legal document, binding on both parties, which would stand up in a court of law in case of any dispute between the two companies, for example. In a somewhat related legal situation, agency agreements between two companies allow one company to delegate part of its business operations to another. In a sense, this relationship is a kind of subcontracting in which the main company appoints another to act on its behalf and the specific agreement is a legal document which defines the extent of the delegation and the fees to be paid for the services performed. Continuing relationships with subcontractors for publishing or providing distribution support for documentation is an example of this kind of document. Such historical information can assist technical communicators in better understanding past publications practices and relationships.

Finding Corporate Archives in Established Libraries

In addition to the types of archives that may be found in workplace settings, there are also a number of archival repositories that could be of interest to many technical communicators, depending on their areas of historical research. The following four types of resources offer some general directions for locating such archives.

Widely Available Reference Books

Reference librarians can be very helpful for helping historical researchers locate archives. Two of the standard reference works found in most libraries are:

- *Documents of American History*, 2 vols., edited by Henry Steele Commager and Milton Cantor, Prentice-Hall, Englewood Cliffs, NJ, 1988.
- *Historic Documents*, an annual serial publication published by the Congressional Quarterly, Inc., Washington, DC.

Relevant Internet Sites

The Internet is filled with many resources for business researchers. Some useful starting places on the Web are:

- Links for Business Historians: http://www.history.ohio-state.edu/buslinks.htm
- Business History Archives: http://www.history.ohio-state.edu/bus-arch.htm
- WWW Virtual Library (has a variety of links dealing with business history): http://www.iisg.nl/~w3vl/

Libraries with Business Archives

For historical research in the United States, technical communicators can check various reference books on sources such as Philip Hamer's *A Guide to Archives and Manuscripts in the United States* (8). The Library of Congress and the National Archives in Washington, DC, are also places to begin historical research projects.

Other helpful contacts might be:

- The Business Archives Affinity Group, Society of American Archivists, 330 S. Wells Street, Suite 810, Chicago, Illinois 60606.
- Baker Library, Harvard Business School, Soldiers Field, Boston, Massachusetts 02163.

Finally, local libraries at both universities and within states, counties, and townships sometimes have available materials of regional, state, or local historical interest for technical communicators.

Museums with Business Archives

There are several museums with corporate archives that provide access (and monetary support through fellowships) to visiting researchers. Foremost among these resources are:

- The Hagley Museum and Library, P. O. Box 3630, Wilmington, Delaware 19807-0630.
  Website: http://www.hagley.lib.de.us

  The Hagley is an independent research library whose holdings include more than 30,000 linear feet of manuscripts, one million photographs, and 200,000 imprints. It has an active program of conferences, seminars, and lectures and is the administrative center for the Business History Conference.
- Additional museums may be located in *The Official Museum Directory*, an annual serial publication published by the American Association of Museums and National Register Publishing Co., Inc.

ACCESSING AND USING CORPORATE ARCHIVES

The specific techniques for accessing and using archives have been well-documented by authors such as Brooks (9), Frick (10), Hedlin (11), and Hill (12). The logistics of getting into archives, communicating with archivist librarians, taking notes, and organizing one's findings are straightforward and easy to learn.

Frequently, what is not so easy to understand is the reasons why particular archives came into existence and why they are organized in a particular manner. In *Doing Rhetorical History*, Kathleen Turner defines rhetorical history as "a social construction not only in the sense that rhetorical processes constitute historical processes but also in the sense that historical study constructs reality for the society in which and for which it is produced" (13, p. 8). Archives possess the potential to assist technical communicators in re-constructions of business realities.

The construction and organization of corporate archives is also frequently a re-creation of the economic, social, and even ethical and personal dimensions of the business entity represented in the archives. Decisions about what to keep in the archives and what to throw away are always based on certain attitudes and assumptions about the value of what has occurred in the past and the value of the records that provide evidence of past events.

In his introduction to a series of articles on "Archivists with an Attitude" in *College English*, John C. Brereton has cautioned scholars in the field of rhetoric and composition "to begin asking what is missing from the archive and how it can get there. And we can also ask some questions while there is still time to act: Are there things we should be working to preserve right now? What can we do now to make sure current practices and materials will be accessible in the archives of the future?" (14, pp. 474–5). These same questions also apply to technical communicators. While they cannot be answered within the scope of this paper, they are certainly worth pondering.

Likewise, when technical communicators access corporate archives for the purpose of learning something from the history of the organization in order to better inform their current work, they must be aware of the limitations of selectivity (the corporation's and their own) in relation to their research endeavors. It is easy to look for only what one wants to find and ignore other, perhaps equally relevant and contributory, materials.

For example, my recent experiences in conducting historical research in the DuPont Corporation's archives on the topic of cancer research was initiated by my interest in tracing aspects of the rhetorical history of this corporation's contributions to environmental pollution that resulted in possible causes of cancer. Initially, I searched the archives for all references to cancer at DuPont during the early to mid-twentieth century. With this focus in mind, I found much evidence in internal reports and statistical compilations about the disease of cancer among DuPont employees who worked at various DuPont dye plants where they had contact with toxic chemicals.

This archival evidence seemed to point to the unquestionable guilt of DuPont as a corporate entity contributing to mid-twentieth century concerns about contaminating the environment with cancer-causing toxic chemicals. Regulatory legislation in the 1970s began the first efforts at forcing corporations like DuPont to "clean up their act" and to stop polluting the environment. However, there was more to this corporate history, and I was only able to discover it by broadening the focus of my research in the DuPont archives.

Rather than confining my search only to the official DuPont corporate records, I began looking at some of the personal papers of two of DuPont's corporate leaders who were in charge of the company during the first half of the twentieth century. There I have found evidence (both corporate and personal) of significant funding of various cancer research efforts outside of the DuPont Corporation, as well as a continued effort to downplay publicizing these very sizeable monetary contributions.

Although I am still gathering and interpreting my findings about DuPont, I have now modified my previous conclusions about DuPont's uncaring attitudes toward environmental pollution. As a result of the expansion of my view of the DuPont archives, I have been able to add some new dimensions to my study of the rhetoric of cancer research funding and of environmentalism.

Applying the Past to the Present

Historical corporate information may be used by technical communicators in the process of negotiating the rhetorical and social constructions of meaning in their field. One of the things that studying the past can do for technical communicators is to provide them with the tools to consider evolving patterns of rhetorical strategies. As historian Carl Schorske describes this activity, "the historian pursues the analysis of the object's particularity . . . only to the extent that he or she can appropriate it as an element in weaving a plausible pattern of change" (15, p. 6).

Such plausible patterns of change need to be part of the repertoire of information and skills available to technical communicators as they make daily decisions about their work. Choices about appropriate techniques to use for communicating with various audiences in terms of media delivery selection, organization, writing style, and visual presentation should be considered from within the patterns established by their historical backgrounds, from within particular corporations, and from within the profession of technical communication itself.

According to John Brockmann, technical communicators need to know the history of their profession for four reasons. First, historical perspectives can provide a basis for answering questions about standards, education, and future directions of the profession. Second, as technical communicators create new "documents" such as online hypertexts and websites, they need to appreciate the style and techniques of their forebears' "documents." Third, even if technical communicators do not know past styles and techniques, they can learn from examining their inadequacies and avoid repeating such problems in the future. Fourth, developing a historical perspective in technical communication can help create an enhanced sense of self-identity and tradition, both prerequisites for the establishment and continuance of any profession (16). Obviously, technical communicators can benefit from being "historically literate" about their corporations and about their field in general.

Corporate archives possess both a resource and a challenge for technical communicators. In *Uses of the Past,* Herbert Muller reminded us that we have a "continued need of an adventurous spirit—of still more creative thought, bold, imaginative, experimental, self-reliant, critical of all 'infallible' authority" (17, p. 349). Corporate archives do not provide infallible authority for technical communicators, but they do offer some previously untapped resources that can help to better inform current workplace practices. For those who are curious and adventurous enough to explore them, many corporate archives are waiting to be discovered.

REFERENCES

1. Neal, Donn C., "Introduction," in Arnita A. Jones And Philip L. Cantelon, *Corporate Archives and History: Making the Past Work*, Krieger Publishing Company, Malabar, FL, 1993, pp. 1–4.
2. Smith, George David, and Steadman, Laurence E., in "Present Value of Corporate History," in Arnita A. Jones and Philip L. Cantelon, *Corporate Archives and History: Making the Past Work*, Krieger Publishing Company, Malabar, FL, 1993, pp. 163–76.
3. Burke, Kenneth, *Attitudes Toward History*, 3rd Ed., University of California Press, Berkeley, CA, 1984.
4. Derrida, Jacques, *Archive Fever: A Freudian Impression*, trans. Eric Prenowitz, The University of Chicago Press, Chicago, 1996.
5. Evans, Richard J., *In Defense of History*, W. W. Norton & Company, New York, 1999.
6. Chesebro, James W., and Bertelsen, Dale A., *Analyzing Media: Communication Technologies as Symbolic and Cognitive Systems*, The Guilford Press, New York, 1996.
7. Armstrong, John, and Jones, Stephanie, *Business Documents: Their Origins, Sources, and Uses in Historical Research*, Mansell Publications, New York, 1987.
8. Hamer, Philip M., *A Guide to Archives and Manuscripts in the United States*, compiled for the National Historical Publications Commission, Yale University Press, New Haven, CT, 1961.
9. Brooks, Philip Coolidge, *Research in Archives: The Use of Unpublished Primary Sources*, University of Chicago Press, Chicago, 1969.
10. Frick Elizabeth, *Library Research Guide to History: Illustrated Search Strategy and Sources*. Pierian Press, Ann Arbor, Michigan, 1980.
11. Hedlin, Edie, *Business Archives: An Introduction*, Society of American Archivists, Chicago, 1978.
12. Hill, Michael R., *Archival Strategies and Techniques*, Sage Publications, Inc., Newbury Park, CA, 1993.
13. Turner, Kathleen J. (ed.), *Doing Rhetorical History: Concepts and Cases*, The University of Alabama Press, Tuscaloosa, AL, 1998.
14. Brereton, John C., "Rethinking Our Archive: A Beginning," *College English*, Vol. 61, No. 5, May 1999, pp. 474–576.
15. Schorske, Carl E., *Thinking with History: Explorations in the Passage to Modernism*, Princeton University Press, Princeton, NJ, 1998.
16. Brockmann, R. John, *From Millwrights to Shipwrights to the Twenty-First Century: Explorations in a History of Technical Communication in the United States*, Hampton Press Inc., Cresskill, NJ, 1998.
17. Muller, Herbert J. *The Uses of the Past: Profiles of Former Societies*, Oxford University Press, New York, 1952.

ADDITIONAL READINGS

Berlin, James. "Rhetoric and Ideology in the Writing Classroom." *College English* 50 (1988): 477–98.

Blyler, Nancy. "Theory and Curriculum: Reexamining the Curricular Separation of Business and Technical Communication." *Journal of Business and Technical Communication* 7, no. 2 (1993): 218–45.

Britton, W. Earl. "What Is Technical Writing: A Redefinition." In *The Teaching of Technical Writing*, edited by Donald Cunningham and Herman A. Estrin, 9–14. Urbana, IL: NCTE, 1975.

Brockmann, R. John. *From Millwrights to Shipwrights to the Twenty-First Century: Explorations in a History of Technical Communication in the United States*. Cresskill, NJ: Hampton Press, Inc., 1998.

Connors, Robert J. "The Rhetoric of Explanation: Explanatory Rhetoric from 1850 to the Present." *Written Communication* 2 (1985): 49–72.

Couture, Barbara. "Categorizing Professional Discourse: Engineering, Administrative, and Technical/Professional Writing." *Journal of Business and Technical Communication* 6, no. 1 (1992): 5–37.

Dobrin, David. "What's Technical about Technical Writing?" In *Writing and Technique*, 29–58. Urbana, IL: NCTE, 1989.

Durack, Katherine T. "Researching Opportunities in the U. S. Patent Record." *Journal of Business and Technical Communication* 15, no. 4 (2000): 490–510.

Forman, Janis. "Business Communication and Composition: The Writing Connection and Beyond." *The Journal of Business Communication* 30, no. 3 (1993): 333–52.

Grego, Rhonda Carnell. "Science, Late Nineteenth-Century Rhetoric, and the Beginnings of Technical Writing Instruction in America." *Journal of Technical Writing and Communication* 17, no. 1 (1987): 63–78.

Halloran, Stephen M. "Classical Rhetoric for the Engineering Student." *Journal of Technical Writing and Communication* 1 (1971): 17–24.

Halloran, S. Michael, and Merrill D. Whitburn. "Ciceronian Rhetoric and the Rise of Science: The Plain Style Reconsidered." In *The Rhetorical Tradition and Modern Rhetoric*, edited by James J. Murphy, 58–72. New York: MLA, 1982.

Hays, Robert. "What Is Technical Writing?" In *The Teaching of Technical Writing*, edited by Donald Cunningham and Herman A. Estrin, 3–8. Urbana, IL: NCTE, 1975.

Killingsworth, Jimmie M. "Technical Communication in the 21st Century: Where Are We Going?" *Technical Communication Quarterly* 8, no. 2 (1999): 165–74.

Kynell, Teresa C. *Writing in a Milieu of Utility*. Norwood, NJ: Ablex, 1996.

Kynell, Teresa C., and Michael G. Moran, eds. *Three Keys to the Past: The History of Technical Communication*. Stamford, CT: Ablex, 1999.

Longo, Bernadette. *Spurious Coin: A History of Science, Management, and Technical Writing*. Albany: State U of New York P, 2000.

Miller, Carolyn R. "Learning from History: World War II and the Culture of High Technology." *Journal of Business and Technical Communication* 12, no. 3 (1998): 288–315.

Paradis, James. "Bacon, Linneaus, and Lavoisier: Early Language Reform in the Sciences." In *New Essays in Technical and Scientific Communication: Research, Theory, Practice*, edited by Paul V. Anderson, R. John Brockmann, and Carolyn R. Miller, 200–24. Farmingdale, NY: Baywood, 1983.

Polanyi, Michael. *The Tacit Dimension*. New York: Doubleday, 1967.

Reynolds, John Frederick. "Classical Rhetoric and the Teaching of Technical Writing." *Technical Communication Quarterly* 1, no. 2 (1992): 63–76.

Rivers, William E. "Studies in the History of Business and Technical Writing: A Bibliographic Essay." *Journal of Business and Technical Communication* 8 (1994): 6–57.

Rutter, Russell. "History, Rhetoric, and Humanism: Toward a More Comprehensive Definition of Technical Communication." *Journal of Technical Writing and Communication* 21, no. 2 (1991): 133–53.

Staples, Katherine. "Technical Communication from 1950–1998: Where Are We Now?" *Technical Communication Quarterly* 8, no. 2 (1999): 153–64.

Sullivan, Dale. "Political-Ethical Implications of Defining Technical Communication as a Practice." *Journal of Advanced Composition* 10, no. 2 (1990): 375–86.

Sullivan, Patricia A., and James E. Porter. "Remapping Curricular Geography: Professional Writing in/and English." *Journal of Business and Technical Communication* 7, no. 4 (1993): 389–422.

Tebeaux, Elizabeth. "The Voices of English Women Technical Writers, 1641–1700: Imprints in the Evolution of Modern English Prose Style." *Technical Communication Quarterly* 7, no. 1 (1998): 125–52.

Walzer, Arthur E. "Ethos, Technical Writing, and the Liberal Arts." *The Technical Writing Teacher* 8 (1981): 50–53.

Whitburn, M. D., M. Davis, S. Higgins, L. Oates, and K. Spurgeon. "The Plain Style in Scientific and Technical Writing." *Journal of Technical Writing and Communication* 8, no. 4 (1978): 349–58.

CHAPTER THREE

Laying a Foundation for Ethical Praxis

Chapter Three: Introduction

As teachers, we face a number of difficult decisions when it comes to choosing topics to cover in class, including how or even whether to introduce the topic of ethics. If we choose to address this topic, one very straightforward way involves the use of cases or scenarios. The workplace is often seen as an environment rife with everyday ethical difficulties, both simple (e.g., the use of office equipment for personal use) and complex (e.g. whistle blowing), and scenarios that ask students to examine dilemmas and respond with solutions are often effective teaching strategies. More difficult cases, those involving injury or death (e.g., the Space Shuttle Challenger, Three Mile Island, Firestone and Ford), questionable or unfair business practices (e.g., the case involving Microsoft and Netscape), or copyright infringement or intellectual property concerns (e.g., Napster), which require the close analysis of texts, are also useful. Texts presenting these kinds of cases are readily available, and using these kinds of cases is an effective way to help students compare reactions, learn interpretative strategies, and become more thoughtful members of their communities.

Other strategies that address issues of ethics include those, such as service-learning, that put students to work in their communities. Doing so lays the groundwork for the kinds of tasks they will actually face and prepares them for potential problems and complications involved in working with others. Johnson argues for such "direct involvement," claiming that a "user-centered approach" provides a sense of agency, demonstrates the "ill-defined nature of actual situations," and, finally, highlights the problem of time when trying to solve problems (162–63). And, in terms of the issue of ethics, this pedagogical strategy addresses tensions between "organizations and clients, workplace preparation and civic literacy, and . . . can be a bridge or a path toward virtue . . . [helping to] create orators and citizens who put their knowledge and skills to work for the common good" (Dubinsky 62).

However, before you can make decisions about whether or not you should teach ethics, and if so, which strategies to use, you need to address an a prior question or issue: What are your beliefs about both the role of ethics in the discipline and the social responsibilities of technical communicators?

To address that question and lay the groundwork for helping you to come to knowledge about your beliefs, this chapter presents a number of angles on the issue of *praxis,* which is more than just the act of doing; it also involves informed and committed action. For Aristotle, praxis means being guided by a moral disposition to act truly and rightly; a concern to further human well-being and the good life. Praxis involves what the Greeks called *phronesis* and requires an understanding of other people.

Beginning with a foundational piece (Quintilian's *Institutio Oratorio*) to establish the connection between working for the public good and speaking (or communicating well) and building on that connection with the works of Miller and Russell, you will have the opportunity to reflect upon and come to some opinion about the nature of this field and its practitioners, and to decide how you feel about the social nature of the work you do, the professional obligations inherent in the field, if any, and the connection between what you do in the classroom and what students will do in the workplace and community. In so doing, you will lay the foundation for your own praxis, which, as Miller claims, is indeed a "matter of conduct" (163). Just as Miller's article focuses on how we understand what it means to be a technical communicator, this chapter, as a whole, asks you to think about what it means to be a technical communicator's teacher.

WORKS CITED

Dubinsky, James. "Service-Learning as a Path to Virtue: The Ideal Orator in Professional Communication." *Michigan Journal of Community Service Learning* 8, no. 2 (2002): 61–74.

Johnson, Robert R. "Technical Communication, Ethics, Curricula." In *User-Centered Technology.* Albany, NY: SUNY Press, 1998. 153–68.

10 From The *Institutio Oratorio, Book XII,* Chapter I

QUINTILIAN

TRANSLATED BY THE REVEREND JOHN SELBY WATSON

In this chapter from Book XII, Quintilian claims that he has "arrived at by far the most important part of the work which [he] had contemplated," a statement he explains by saying that he hopes to "attempt to define the orator's moral character, and to prescribe his duties" (p. 146 in this volume). To do so, he outlines the conditions for an orator, whom he defines "quoting Cato" as "a good man skilled in speaking" (p. 146). Being "good," for Quintilian, means being "entirely free from vice" (p. 147), unwilling and unable to "utter words at variance with his thoughts" (p. 151), and capable of discerning when it might be necessary to mislead those whom he addresses if the goal is worthy. Another essential condition is that of study: "no man will ever be thoroughly accomplished in eloquence, who has not gained a deep insight into the impulses of human nature, and formed his own moral character on the precepts of others and on his own reflection" (418). Reading Quintilian, you will begin to see not only the roots of our field in classical rhetoric but also the complex nature of the work we do. If we argue that our job is to be skilled communicators (and perhaps even orators), we need to consider what, if any, obligations come with that ability. One of the difficult tasks associated with this discipline is contemplating the civic responsibility associated with our work.

INTRODUCTION

1. I have now arrived at by far the most important part of the work which I had contemplated. Had I imagined, when I first conceived the idea of it, that its weight would have been so great as that with which I now feel myself pressed, I should have earlier considered whether my strength would be able to bear it. But, at the commencement, the thought of the disgrace that I should incur if I did not perform what I had promised, kept me to my undertaking; and afterwards, though the labor increased at almost every stage, yet I

The Rhetorical Tradition. Eds. Patricia Bizzell and Bruce Herzberg. 2nd. ed. Boston: Bedford/St. Martins, 2001. 412–18.
From *Institutes of Oratory*, Quintilian Book XII, chapter 1. Trans. Rev. John Selby Watson.

resolved to support myself under all difficulties, that I might not render useless what had been already finished. 2. For the same reason at present, also, though the task grows more burdensome than ever, yet, as I look towards the end, I am determined rather to faint than to despair.

What deceived me, was, that I began with small matters; and though I was subsequently carried onwards, like a mariner by inviting gales, yet, as long as I treated only of what was generally known, and had been the subject of consideration to most writers on rhetoric, I seemed to be still at no great distance from the shore, and had many companions who had ventured to trust themselves to the same breezes. 3. But when I entered upon regions of eloqouence but recently discovered, and attempted only by very few, scarcely a navigator was to be seen that had gone so far from the harbor as myself; and now, when the orator whom I have been forming, being released from the teachers of rhetoric, is either carried forward by his own efforts, or desires greater aid from the inmost recesses of philosophy, I begin to feel into how vast an ocean I have sailed, and see that there is

> —*Cælum undique et undique pontus.*
> On all sides heaven, and on all sides sea.

I seem to behold, in the vast immensity, only one adventurer besides myself, namely Cicero; and even he himself, though he entered on the deep with so great and so well equipped a vessel, contracts his sails, and lays aside his oars, and contents himself with showing merely what sort of eloquence a consummate orator ought to employ. But my temerity will attempt to define even the orator's moral character, and to prescribe his duties. Thus, though I cannot overtake the great man that is before me, I must, nevertheless, go rather than he, as my subject shall lead me. However, the desire of what is honorable is always praiseworthy, and it belongs to what we may call cautious daring, to try that for failure in which pardon will readily be granted.

Chapter I

A great orator must be a good man; according to Cato's definition, § 1, 2. A bad man cannot be a consummate orator, as he is deficient in wisdom, 3–5. The mind of a bad man is too much distracted with cares and remorse, 6, 7. A bad man will not speak with the same authority and effect on virtue and morality as a good man, 8–13. Objections to this opinion answered, 14–22. A bad man may doubtless speak with great force, but he would make nearer approaches to perfect eloquence if he were a good man, 23–32. Yet we must be able to conceive arguments on either side of a question, 33–35. A good man may sometimes be justified in misleading those whom he addresses, for the attainment of some good object, 36–45.

1. Let the orator, then, whom I propose to form, be such a one as is characterized by the definition of Marcus Cato, *a good man skilled in speaking*.

But the requisite which Cato has placed first in this definition, that an orator should be *a good man*, is naturally of more estimation and importance than the other. It is of importance that an orator should be good, because, should the power of speaking be a support to evil, nothing would be more pernicious than eloquence alike to public concerns and private, and I myself, who, as far as is in my power, strive to contribute something to the faculty of the orator, should deserve very ill of the world, since I should furnish arms, not for soldiers, but for robbers. 2. May I not draw an argument from the condition of mankind? Nature herself, in bestowing on man that which she seems to have granted him preeminently, and by which she appears to have distinguished us from all other animals, would have acted, not as a parent, but as a stepmother, if she had designed the faculty of speech to be the promoter of crime, the oppressor of innocence, and the enemy of truth; for it would have been better for us to have been born dumb, and to have been left destitute of reasoning powers, than to have received endowments from providence only to turn them to the destruction of one another.

3. My judgment carries me still further; for I not only say that he who would answer my idea of an orator, must be good man, but that no man, unless he be good, can ever be an orator. To an orator discernment and prudence are necessary; but we can certainly not allow discernment to those, who, when the ways of virtue and vice are set before them, prefer to follow that of vice; nor can we allow them prudence, since they subject themselves, by the unforeseen consequences of their actions, often to the heaviest penalty of the law, and always to that of an evil conscience. 4. But if it be not only truly said by the wise, but always justly believed by me vulgar, that no man is vicious who is not also foolish, a fool, assuredly, will never become an orator.

It is to be further considered that the mind cannot be in a condition for pursuing the most noble of studies, unless it be entirely free from vice; not only because there can communion of good and evil in the same breast, and to mediate at once on the best things and the worst is no more in the power of the same mind than it is possible for the same man to be at once virtuous and vicious; 5. but also, because a mind intent on so arduous a study should be exempt from all other cares, even such as are unconnected with vice; for then, and then only, when it is free and master of itself, and when no other object harasses and distracts its attention, will it be able to keep in view the end to which it is devoted. 6. But if an inordinate attention to an estate, a too anxious pursuit of wealth, indulgence in the pleasures of the chase, and the devotion of our days to public spectacles, rob our studies of much of our time, (for whatever time is given to one thing is lost to another,) what effect must we suppose that ambition, avarice, and envy will produce, whose excitements or so violent as even to disturb our sleep and our dreams? 7. Nothing indeed is so preoccupied, so unsettled, so torn and lacerated with such numerous and various passions, as a bad mind; for when it intends evil, it is agitated with hope, care, and anxiety, and when it has attained the object of its wickedness, it is tormented with uneasiness, repentance, and the dread of every kind of punishment. Among such disquietudes, what place is there for study, or any rational pursuit? No more certainly than there is for corn in a field overrun with thorns and brambles.

8. To enable us to sustain the toil of study, is not temperance necessary? What expectations are to be formed, then, from him who is abandoned to

licentiousness and luxury? Is not the love of praise one of the greatest incitements to the pursuit of literature? But can we suppose that the love of praise is an object of regard with the unprincipled? Who does not know that a principal part of oratory consists in discoursing on justice and virtue? But will the unjust man and the vicious treat of such subjects with the respect that is due to them?

9. But though we should even concede a great part of the question, and grant, what can by no means be the case, that there is the same portion of ability, diligence, and attainments, in the worst man as in the best, which of the two, even under that supposition, will prove the better orator? He, doubtless, who is the better man. The same person, therefore, can never be a bad man and a perfect orator, for that cannot be perfect to which something else is superior.

10. That I may not seem, however, like the writers of Socratic dialogues, to frame answers to suit my own purpose, let us admit that there exists a person so unmoved by the force of truth, as boldly to maintain that a bad man, possessed of the same portion of ability, applications, and learning, as a good man, will be an equally good orator, and let us convince even such a person of his folly.

11. No man, certainly, will doubt, that it is the object of all oratory, that what is stated to the judge may appear to him to be true and just; and which of the two, let me ask, will produce such a conviction with the greater ease, the good man or the bad? 12. A good man, doubtless, will speak of what is true and honest with greater frequency; but even if, from being influenced by some call of duty, he endeavors to support what is fallacious, (a case which, as I shall show, may sometimes occur,) he must still be heard with greater credit than a bad man. 13. But with bad men, on the other hand, dissimulation sometimes fails, as well through their contempt for the opinion of mankind, as through their ignorance of what is right; hence they assert without modesty, and maintain their assertions without shame; and, in attempting what evidently cannot be accomplished, there appears in them a repulsive obstinacy and useless perseverance; for bad men, as well in their pleadings as in their lives, entertain dishonest expectations; and it often happens, that even when they speak the truth, belief is not accorded them, and the employment of advocates of such a character is regarded as a proof of the badness of a cause.

14. I must, however, notice those objections to my opinion, which appear to be clamored forth, as it were, by the general consent of the multitude. Was not then Demosthenes, they ask, a great orator? yet we have heard that he was not a good man. Was not Cicero a great orator? yet many have thrown censure upon his character. To such questions how shall I answer? Great displeasure is likely to be shown at any reply whatever; and the ears of my audience require first to be propitiated. 15. The character of Demosthenes, let me say, does not appear to me deserving of such severe reprehension, that I should believe, all the calumnies that are heaped upon him by his enemies, especially when I read his excellent plans for the benefit of his country and the honorable termination of his life. 16. Nor do I see that the feeling of an upright citizen was, in any respect, wanting to Cicero. As proofs of his integrity, may

be mentioned his consulship, in which he conducted himself with so much honor; his honorable administration of his province; his refusal to be one of the twenty commissioners; and, during the civil wars, which fell with great severity on his times, his uprightness of mind, which was never swayed, either by hope or by fear, from adhering to the better party, or the supporters of the commonwealth. 17. He is thought by some to have been deficient in courage, but he has given an excellent reply to this charge, when he says, *that he was timid, not in encountering dangers, but in taking precautions against them;* an assertion of which he proved the truth of his death, to which he submitted with the noblest fortitude. 18. But even should the height of virtue have been wanting to these eminent men; I shall reply to those who ask me whether they were orators, as the Stoics reply when they are asked whether Zeno, Cleanthes, and Chrysippus, were wise men; they say that they were great and deserving of veneration, but that they did not attain the highest excellence of which human nature is susceptible.

19. Pythagoras desired to be called not *wise,* like those who preceded him, but a *lover of wisdom.* I, however, in speaking of Cicero, have often said, according to the common mode of speech, and shall continue to say, that he was *a perfect orator,* as we term our friends, in ordinary discourse, *good and prudent men,* though such epithets can be justly given only to perfectly wise. 20. But when I have to speak precisely, and in conformity with the exactness of truth, I shall express myself as longing to see such an orator as he himself also longed to see; for though I acknowledge that Cicero stood at the head of eloquence, and that I can scarcely find a passage in his speeches to which anything can be added; however many I might find which I may imagine that he would have pruned, (for the learned have in general been of opinion that he had *numerous excellences* and *some faults,* and he himself says that he had cut off most of his *juvenile exuberance,*) yet, since he did not claim to himself, though he had no mean opinion of his merits, the praise of perfection, and since he might certainly have spoken better if a longer life had been granted him, and a more tranquil seasons for composition, I may not unreasonably believe that the summit of excellence was not attained by him, to which, notwithstanding, no man made nearer approaches. 21. If I had thought otherwise, I might have maintained my opinion with still greater determination and freedom. Did Marcus Antonius declare that *he had seen no man truly eloquent,* though to be eloquent is much less than to be a perfect orator; does Cicero himself say that *he is still seeking for an orator,* and merely conceives and imagines one; and shall I fear to say that in that portion of eternity which is yet to come something may arise still more excellent than what has yet been seen? 22. I take no advantage of the opinion of those who refuse to allow great merit to Cicero and Demosthenes even in eloquence; though Demosthenes, indeed, does not appear sufficiently near perfection even to Cicero himself, who says that he *sometimes nods,* nor does Cicero appear so to Brutus and Clavus, who certainly find fault with his language even in addressing himself, or to either of the Asinii, who attack the blemishes in his style with virulence in various places.

23. Let us grant, however, what nature herself by no means brings to pass, that a bad man has been found, endowed with consummate eloquence, I should nevertheless refuse to concede to him the name of orator, as I should not allow the merit of fortitude of all who have been active in the field, because fortitude cannot be conceived as unaccompanied with virtue. 24. Has not he who is employed to defend causes need of integrity which covetousness cannot pervert, or partially corrupt, or terror abash, and shall we honor the traitor, the renegade, the prevaricator, with the sacred name of orator? And if that quality, which is commonly called *goodness*, is found even in moderate pleaders, why should not that great orator, who has not yet appeared, but who may hereafter appear, be as consummate in goodness as in eloquence? 25. It is not a plodder in the forum, or a mercenary pleader, or, to use no stronger term, a not unprofitable advocate, (such as he whom they generally term a *causidicus*) that I desire to form, but a man who, being possessed of the highest natural genius, stores his mind thoroughly with the most valuable kinds of knowledge; a man sent by the gods to do honor to the world, and such as no preceding age has known; a man in every way eminent and excellent, a thinker of the best thoughts and a speaker of the best language. 26. For such a man's ability how small a scope will there be in the defense of innocence or the repression of guilt in the forum, or in supporting truth against falsehood in litigations about money? He will appear great, indeed, even in such inferior employments, but his powers will shine with the highest luster on greater occasions, when the counsels of the senate are to be directed, and the people to be guided from error into rectitude. 27. Is it not such an orator that Virgil appeals to have imagined, representing him as a calmer of the populace in a sedition, when they were hurling firebrands and stones?

Tum pietate gravem et meritis si forte virum quem
Conspexere, silent, arrectisque auribus adstant,
Then if perchance a sage they see, rever'd
For piety and worth, they hush their noise,
And stand with ears attentive.

We see that he first makes him *a good man*, and then adds that he is *skilled in speaking*:

Ille regit dictis animos, et pectora mulcet,
With words
He rules their passions and their breasts controls.

28. Would not the orator whom I am trying to form, too, if he were in the field of battle, and his soldiers required to be encouraged to engage, draw the materials for an exhortation from the most profound precepts of philosophy? for how could all the terrors of toil, pain, and even death, be banished from their breasts, unless vivid feelings of piety, fortitude, and honor, be substituted in their place? 29. He, doubtless, will best implant such feelings in the breasts of others who has first implanted them in his own; for simulation, however guarded it be, always betrays itself, nor was there ever such power

of eloquence in any man that he would not falter and hesitate whenever his words were at variance with his thoughts. 30. But a bad man must of necessity utter words at variance with his thoughts; while to good men, on the contrary, a virtuous sincerity of language will never be wanting, nor (for good men will also be wise) a power of producing the most excellent thoughts, which, they may be destitute of showy charms, will be sufficiently adorned by their own natural qualities, since whatever is said with honest feeling will also be said with eloquence.

31. Let youth, therefore, or rather let all of us, of every age, (for no time is too late for resolving on what is right,) direct our whole faculties, and our whole exertions, to this object; and perhaps to some it may be granted to attain it; for if nature does not interdict a man from being good, or from being eloquent, why should not some one among mankind be able to attain eminence in both goodness and eloquence? And why should not each hope that he himself may be the fortunate aspirant? 32. If our powers of mind are insufficient to reach the summit, yet in proportion to the advances that we make towards it will be our improvement in both eloquence and virtue. At least, let the notion be wholly bannished from our thoughts, that perfect eloquence, the noblest of human attainments, can be united with a vicious character of mind. Talent in speaking, if it falls to the lot of the vicious, must be regarded as being itself a vice, since it makes those more mischievous with whom it allies itself.

33. But I fancy that I hear some (for there will never be wanting men who would rather be eloquent than good) saying "Why then is there so much art devoted to eloquence? Why have you given precepts on rhetorical coloring, and the defense of difficult causes, and some even on the acknowledgment of guilt, unless, at times, the force and ingenuity of eloquence overpowers even truth itself? for a good man advocates only good causes, and truth itself supports them sufficiently without the aid of learning." 34. These objectors I shall endeavor to satisfy, by answering them, first, concerning my own work, and, secondly, concerning the duty of a good man, if occasion ever calls him to the defense of the guilty.

To consider how we may speak in defense of what is false, or even what is unjust, is not without its use, if for no other reason than that we may expose and refute fallacious arguments with the greater ease; as that physician will apply remedies with the greater effect to whom that which is hurtful is known. 35. The Academicians, when they have disputed on both sides of a point of morality, will not live according to either side at hazard; nor was the well known Carneades, who is said to have argued at Rome, in the hearing of Cato the Censor, with no less force against the observance of justice than he had argued the day before in favor of it, an unjust man. But *vice*, which is opposed to *virtue*, shows more clearly what virtue is; *justice* becomes more manifest from the contemplation of *injustice*; and many things are proved by their contraries. The devices of his adversaries, accordingly, should be as well known to the orator, as the stratagems of an enemy in the field to a commander.

36. Even that which appears, when it is first stated, of so objectionable a character, *that a good man, in defending a cause, may sometimes incline to withhold the truth from the judge,* reason may find cause to justify. If any one feels surprised that I advance this opinion, (though this is not mine is particular, but that of those whom antiquity acknowledged as the greatest masters of wisdom,) let him consider that there are many things which are rendered honorable or dishonorable, not by their own nature, but by the causes which give rise to them. 37. For if *to kill a man* is often an act of virtue, and *to put to death one's children* is sometimes a noble sacrifice; and if it is allowable to do things of a still more repulsive nature when the good of our country demands them, we must not consider merely what cause a good man defends, but from what motive, and with what object he defends it. 38. In the first place, every one must grant me, what the most rigid of the Stoics do not deny, that a good man may sometimes think proper to tell a lie, and occasionally even in matters of small moments, as, when children are sick, we make them believe many things with a view to promote their health, and promise them many which we do not intend to perform; 39. and much less, is it forbidden to tell a falsehood when an assassin is to be prevented from killing a man, or an enemy to be deceived for the benefit of our country; so that what is at one time reprehensible in a slave is at another laudable even in the wisest of men. If this be admitted, I see that many causes may occur for which an orator may justly undertake a case of such a nature, as, in the absence of any honorable motive, he would not undertake. 40. Nor do I say this only with reference to a father, a brother, or a friend, who may be in danger, (because even in such a case I would allow only what is strictly lawful), though there is then sufficient ground for hesitation, when the image of justice presents itself on one side, and that of natural affection on the other; but let us set the point beyond all doubt. Let us suppose that a man has attempted the life of a tyrant, and is brought to trial for the deed; will such an orator as is described by us, be unwilling that his life should be saved? and, if he undertake to defend him, will he not support his cause before the judge by the same kind of misrepresentation as he who advocates a bad cause? 41. Or what if a judge would condemn a man for something that was done with justice, unless we convince him that it was not done; would not an orator, by producing such conviction, save the life of a fellow-citizen, when he is not only innocent but deserving of praise? Or what if we know that certain political measures are in contemplation, which, though just in themselves, are rendered detrimental to the commonwealth by the state of the times, shall we not adopt artifices of eloquence to set them aside, artifices which, though well-intended, are nevertheless similar to those of an immoral character?

42. No man, again; will doubt, that if guilty persons can by any means be turned to a right course of life, and it is allowed that they sometimes may, it will be more for the advantage of the state that their lives should be spared than that they should be put to death. If, then, it appear certain to an orator, that a person against whom true accusations are brought, will, if acquitted, become a good member of society, will he not exert himself that he may be acquitted?

43. Suppose, again, that a man who is an excellent general, and without whose aid his country would be unable to overcome her enemies, is accused of a crime of which he is evidently guilty, will not the public good call upon an orator to plead his cause? It is certain that Fabricius made Cornelius Rufinus, who was in other respects a bad citizen, and his personal enemy, consul, by voting for him when a war threatened the state, because he knew him to be a good general; and when some expressed their surprise at what he had done, he replied, that *he had rather be robbed by a citizen than sold for a slave by the enemy*. Had Fabricius, therefore, been an orator, would he not have pleaded for Rufinus even though he had been manifestly guilty of robbing his country?

44. Many similar cases might be supposed, but even any one of them is sufficient; for I do not insinuate that the orator whom I would form should often undertake such causes; I only wish to show that if such a motive as I have mentioned should induce him to do so, that definition of an orator, *that he is a good man skilled in speaking*, would still be true.

45. It is necessary, too, for the master to teach, and for the pupil to learn, how difficult cases are to be treated in attempting to establish them; for very often even the best causes resemble bad ones, and an innocent person under accusation may be urged by many probabilities against him; and he must then be defended by the same process of pleading as if he were guilty. There are also innumerable particulars common alike to good and bad causes; as oral and written evidence, and suspicions and prejudices to be overcome. But what is probable is established or refuted by the same methods as what is true. The speech of the orator, therefore, will be modeled as circumstances shall require, uprightness of intention being always maintained.

11 What's Practical about Technical Writing?

CAROLYN R. MILLER

In this foundational article, Miller builds on her earlier piece ("A Humanistic Rationale for Technical Writing") by expanding the "need to promote both competence and critical awareness" with what she calls "prudential judgment" or "the ability (and willingness) to take socially responsible action" (p. 163 in this volume). Her discussion of the meaning and value of being "practical," for which she relies upon Richard Bernstein's discussion of the "high" and "low" senses of the word, opens up questions between "what is" and "what ought to be" and offers readers insight into the function and roles that universities, and by extension, curricula, play in society. According to Miller, "prudential reasoning" concerns "both universals and particulars" and "applies knowledge of human goods to particular circumstances" (p. 162). Thus "practical rhetoric is a matter of conduct rather than of production, as a matter of arguing in a prudent way toward the good of the community" (p. 163), and as such, enables teachers and program developers in our field to shift our focus beyond the utilitarian and the purely economic to the good of the larger community within which both the academy and the institutions where our students may find employment lie.

The Meaning of "Practical"

Most immediately, the practical seems to be concerned with getting things done, with efficient and effective action. Furthermore, efficiency and effectiveness seem more important for some types of action than for others; that is, some actions themselves have practical aims (rather than aesthetic or ritual ones), actions concerned with the material necessities of making a living or managing a household. One can thus *be* practical (or impractical) *about* practical action. *Being* practical suggests a certain attitude or mode of learning, an efficiency (or goal-directedness) that relies on rules proved through use rather than on theory, history, experience, or general appreciation. Practical rhetoric therefore seems to concern the instrumental aspect of discourse—its potential for getting things done—and at the same time to invite a how-to, or handbook, method of instruction. Technical writing partakes of both these dimensions of practical rhetoric.

From *Technical Writing: Theory and Practice,* edited by Bertie E. Fearing and W. Keats Sparrow, 14–24. New York: MLA, 1989.

The rhetoric of the early Greeks also involved both dimensions. They emphasized that rhetoric was an art (or techne). This meant (to Aristotle, at least) that rhetoric was conceptualized and teachable (not a knack, as Plato had feared) but neither certain nor absolute (not a science, as Plato had hoped). Greek rhetoric thus initiated both a handbook tradition of instruction and a counterposed theoretical appreciation for the multiplicity of relations between means and ends.

Richard Bernstein has suggested that there are both "low" and "high" senses of "practical," two senses that parallel the handbook and theoretical traditions of rhetoric. It is the low sense, Bernstein says, that calls to mind "some mundane and bread-and-butter activity or character. The practical man is one who is not concerned with theory (even anti-theoretical or anti-intellectual), who knows how to get along in the rough and tumble of the world" (x). The high sense, which derives from the Aristotelian concept of praxis and underlies modern philosophical pragmatism, concerns human conduct in those activities that maintain the life of the community. One of the many reasons for the discrepancy between these two senses of the practical highlights the dilemma of technical writing, which is usually called practical in the low sense (by both its friends and its enemies, incidentally). This reason has to do with the social structure of the Greek city-state, which permitted the free citizen to be concerned with the good of the polis without being much concerned with bread-and-butter activities. The reason, of course, is the institution of slavery. Manual labor and most commercial activity were performed by noncitizens—slaves, foreigners, women. These activities were "preconditions" to the fulfillment of human potential in self-government, according to Nicholas Lobkowicz: "One would almost be tempted to say that the Greeks considered all 'prepolitical' activities prehuman and that only in the political life were they able to see a way of life which transcended the animal realm" (22). Technical writing, the rhetoric of "the world of work," of commerce and production, is thus associated with what were low forms of practice from the beginning. In a world in which it is more dishonorable to own slaves than it is to work for a living, we might question whether this association should prevail.

A Conceptual Contradiction

Before trying to suggest what it might mean to apply the higher sense of practical to technical writing, I want to indicate some difficulties in accepting the low sense uncritically, as many technical writing teachers have. These difficulties are revealed by a contradiction within the self-justifying discourse of technical writing pedagogy: the attempt to hold both that nonacademic rhetorical practices are inadequate (and therefore need improvement through instruction) and that they serve as authoritative models (and therefore define goals for instruction). We seem, that is, uncertain about where to locate norms, about whether the definition of "good writing" is to be derived from academic knowledge or from nonacademic practices. Most teachers will recognize the contradiction in the familiar dilemma of having to admit to students the discrepancy between practices that are supposed to be effective and those that are actually preferred and accepted.

The first side of the contradiction is the familiar justification for teaching technical writing. We teach it because when students graduate and begin writing on the job, they do not do very well. In the technical writing textbook I use, the first chapter, "Why Study Technical Communication?" documents the "inadequate communication skills of many technical professionals" (Olsen and Huckin 7). For example, it quotes a survey about recently graduated civil engineers showing that writing and speaking are the areas of competence most important to civil-engineering practice but that about two-thirds of recent graduates are judged "inferior" in these areas; results for mechanical and electrical engineers are similar. Complaints about technical writing from senior officials in science and industry include "foggy language," failures of emphasis and coherence, illogical reasoning, poor organization—a familiar litany. Most technical writing textbooks begin with the same rationale, that nonacademic rhetorical practices are wanting. The justification for academic instruction is that academics know something that can help improve professional practices.

The second side of the contradiction derives from the research that interested faculty members have begun to do on rhetorical practices in business, industry, and science. This research is justified not only by the academic assumption that knowledge is a good thing but also (and often primarily) by the belief that knowledge of nonacademic practices is necessary to define goals for teaching practical rhetoric. As Paul Anderson puts it, "We [educators] must first understand the profession, then design our curricula accordingly. Only if we understand intimately the job we intend to prepare our students to perform can we create effective professional programs" ("What Technical" 161).

One of the favorite research projects is the survey, which can show what kinds of work-related writing the population surveyed does, how important it seems to be, what its common problems are, and what qualities and features are valued. In reviewing selected surveys, Elizabeth Tebeaux notes discrepancies between instructional assumptions and industrial practices and concludes that "several curricular changes are clearly mandated" in order to "meet the communication needs of writers in industry" (422). Anderson reviewed fifty surveys, because they can provide "teachers with important insights they can use as they design courses in business, technical, and other forms of career-related writing" ("What Survey" 4). Many surveys, such as those by Marcus Green and Timothy Nolan and by Bill Coggin, have been proffered as authoritative sources of information about what a curriculum should accomplish for its graduates. Ethnographic research has also been justified in instructional terms: according to Stephen Doheny-Farina, for example, "By learning more about nonacademic contexts for writing, we are learning more about the kinds of rhetorical demands faced by many of our college graduates," and this knowledge "can inform the teaching of writing" (159).

Major national grants have gone to researchers engaged in work justified in these same ways, a clue to the institutionalization of this line of reasoning, as well as to its extension from technical writing to composition in general. The Fund for Improvement of Post-Secondary Education (FIPSE) sponsored a project on writing-program evaluation at the University of Texas; the project produced a report saying that "before any college writing program can be judged effective or ineffective, we must know first if what it teaches has value to its graduates in later life. Like any educational program, the overall effectiveness of writing programs must be judged according to the needs of the population they serve" (Faigley et al. 1–2). Another FIPSE grant went to Wayne State for a university-industry collaborative effort on research and curriculum development in professional writing. The researchers present cooperation between academics and practitioners as the way to "ensure that students are prepared for the diverse communication tasks outside the university" (Couture et al. 392–93). FIPSE has also sponsored research on collaborative writing in the workplace by Lisa Ede and Andrea Lunsford, who cite as a major problem "the dichotomy between current models and methods of teaching writing . . . and the actual writing situations students will face upon graduation"; this dichotomy results, in part, from "our lack of detailed understanding about on-the-job writing" ("Research" 69). The National Institute of Education earlier sponsored work by Lee Odell and Dixie Goswami on writing in nonacademic settings; their study also suggests that our ability to teach writing will be "enhanced" by more complete understanding of how people come to write successfully on the job ("Writing" 257).

Practice as Descriptive or Prescriptive

In its eagerness to be useful—to students and their future employers—technical writing has sought a basis in practice, a basis that is problematic. I do not mean to suggest that academics should keep themselves ignorant of nonacademic practices; indeed, much of the research I cited above has been extremely illuminating. But technical writing teachers and curriculum planners should take seriously the problem of how to think about practice. The problem leads one to the complex relation between description and prescription. Odell warns against mistaking one for the other: "we must be careful not to confuse *what is* with *what ought to be*. . . . We have scarcely begun to understand how organizational context relates to writing, and we have almost no information about which aspects of that relationship are helpful to writers and which are harmful" (278). Anderson also warns us about this mistake: in presenting a model of the technical writing profession for use in designing curricula, he cautions that the model "represents an ideal. It is built around the *best* practices of the profession, not around *common* practice—or malpractice" ("What Technical" 165). He gives as examples usability testing (not common but good) and readability formulas (common but bad). Neither Odell nor Anderson, however, gives us much help in understanding what is helpful and what is harmful, what is good practice and what is malpractice. Even David Dobrin's discussion of the contradictions involved in teaching to the standards of employers, although it recommends both curricular and corporate reform, relies finally on accepting practices of the workplace on their own terms; teachers should "make people at work better able to deal with others" ("What's the Purpose" 159).

At this point, it is worth recalling an earlier (unfunded) study of writing in nonacademic settings, "Writing, Out in the World," a chapter of Richard Ohmann's *English in America*. Ohmann avoids the contradiction of taking practice as both imperfect and authoritative by positing a wider perspective from which to make such judgments; he requires, as Odell and Anderson and Dobrin do not, a basis for evaluating a practice other than that of the practice itself. The nonacademic writing Ohmann examined is that of futurists and forecasters, of foreign-policy analysts, and of the government officials who wrote the memorandums we call "The Pentagon Papers." Ohmann sought to establish, not that academic writing is different from writing in the workplace, but that they are dangerously similar: he concludes that academic instruction in writing "has helped, willy nilly, to teach the rhetoric of the bureaucrats and technicians" (205). He claims that the

> writing of the powerful and influential shares some characteristics with the required writing of their college-age sons and daughters; that these characteristics are fairly important to the style of thinking and planning that guides the most powerful country in the world; and that this style has some systematically dangerous features when it operates not in the classroom but on the stages of history. (173)

A similar and more direct charge has been made recently by Susan Wells, who claims that "the ideology of technical writing explicitly assents to its instrumental subordination to capital; the aim of the discipline as a whole is to become a more responsive tool" (247). Being useful is not necessarily good, according to these Marxist critics, but little in the discourse of technical writing allows for this conclusion or explores its consequences. Because the Marxist critique features practical activity as a central concept, it raises questions that are particularly germane to technical writing, questions about whose interests a practice serves and how we decide whose interests should be served.

Practice and Higher Education

The uneasy relation between nonacademic practice and academic instruction has been part of academic discussions about technical writing from their beginnings in the late nineteenth century, as Robert Connors's historical work has shown. Connors documents recurrent debates over whether practical or humanistic goals should prevail in technical writing courses (or, as they were commonly called, "engineering English"), whether, that is, such study should prepare technical students for work or for leisure. Moreover, these debates reflect a larger debate in American higher education, about the appropriate relation between vocational preparation and cultural awareness. In mid-nineteenth century, this debate transformed the American college curriculum, according to the educational historian Frederick Rudolph, who points specifically to the Morrill Act of 1862 and the founding of Cornell in 1866. The first president of Cornell, Andrew White, "confronted all the choices that had been troubling college authorities: practical or classical studies, old professions or new vocations, pure or applied science, training for culture and character or for jobs" (117). White opted for pluralism, for providing many courses of study in preparation for many kinds of lives: "the Cornell curriculum . . . multiplied truth into truths, a limited few professions into an endless number of new self-respecting ways of moving into the middle class" (119). In a similar vein, Laurence Veysey's study of the emergence of the American university in the nineteenth century traces the development of "utility" as a basis for education. During this period, according to Veysey, "America was a scene of vocational ambition," both in terms of individual aspirations and in terms of the desire for public service. At the same time, the notion of public service broadened to include practical and technical occupations, not just the gentlemanly occupations for which earlier education had been preparatory. "Vocational training," says Veysey, "directly affected the undergraduate curriculum of the new university" (66).

Other commentators have emphasized that the relation between instruction and practice is part of a more general condition, the subsistence of higher education in a socioeconomic matrix. Clark Kerr, in *The Uses of the University*, says that "the life of the universities for a thousand years has been tied into the recognized professions in the surrounding society, and the universities will continue to respond as new professions arise" (111). (This view, of course, implies that the classical curriculum served as preparation not for leisure but for the upper-class vocations of law, politics, and the ministry.) John Kenneth Galbraith has noted that "it is the vanity of educators that they shape the educational system to their preferred image. They may not be without influence, but the decisive force is the economic system"(236). More specifically, in his critique of nonacademic writing. Ohmann comments that

> the constraints upon English from the rest of the university and especially from outside it are strong. . . . [T]he writers of the textbooks and the planners of courses . . . can hardly ignore what passes for intellectual currency in that part of the world where vital decisions are made or what kind of composition succeeds in the terms of that part of the world. (206)

Current enthusiasm for "industry-university collaboration" in applied research and development is perhaps the most recent manifestation of this general and necessary relation. But there is also a repertoire of accepted mechanisms for channeling the relation—internships, advisory councils, certification of graduates, and procedures for justifying and accrediting programs. These mechanisms are used in educational programs for the established professions, like law, medicine, engineering, and teaching, as well as in several areas of practical rhetoric with relatively long curricular histories, like journalism and public relations. For the most part, the channels these mechanisms create are one-way: influence flows primarily from nonacademic practices to the academy. The gradient is reflected in the language at the industry-university interface, which includes, on the one hand, "demand," "need," "value," and, on the other, "response," "service," "utility." My own university, a land-grant institution, provides a case in point. Its "Mission Statement" declares that the university "has responsibility for the academic, research, and public service programs in areas of primary importance to the State's economy." University policies concerning proposals for new degree programs require statements concerning the proposed program's relation to the institutional mission, to student demand, and to "manpower" needs in the state.

Teachers of technical writing have advocated applying the mechanisms of nonacademic influence to their new programs, using the same kinds of language. Internship programs should be adopted in technical communication programs, according to a recent review of literature, because they encourage students to relate their study of theory to practice, permit faculty members to "keep in touch with" current practices, and enable employers "to influence college programs" (Gloe 18–19). Advisory councils are advocated because they "integrate the endeavors of the two worlds [academic and business-industrial] directly and in a[n] . . . effective manner" (Brockmann 137). (Certification has been discussed within the Society for Technical Communication, but there is insufficient consensus in the profession to arrive at standards ["Certification" 6]; accreditation is now being investigated by the society [*Strategic Plan*].)

Such language echoes the discourse of other professional programs, programs that have provided precedents for technical communication.

> **Library science**
> It is widely believed and reported that a chasm of mutual ignorance and indifference separates librarians and library educators from one another. . . . All sectors of practice regularly and strongly express a desire for more influence over the content and character of professional education. (Clough and Galvin 2)
>
> **Public relations**
> Practitioners and educators must act in concert to guide public relations in the direction of professionalism. (Commission on Graduate Studies in Public Relations 5)
>
> **Information science**
> Lack of communication between the employers of information professionals and the institutions that educate and train them is one reason that educational institutions are not meeting needs and demands of the changing environment and new technologies. (Griffiths, abstract)
>
> **Business**
> MBA curricula must be reevaluated and, perhaps, restructured if they are to meet business expectations, and—from the point of view of business—if they are to better prepare students for the real world in which they will build their careers. (Jenkins and Reizenstein 24)
>
> **Journalism**
> What training and preparation do radio and television journalists consider important for a career in their field? Answers . . . should contain valuable insights for the broadcast journalism educator. (Fisher 140)
>
> **Training and development**
> Training activities involve a wide variety of skills, abilities, knowledge, and information. . . . An interdisciplinary approach to T&D preparation is important, given the range of competencies required. (Reed 11)

This discourse is infected by the assumptions that what is common practice is useful and what is useful is good. The good that is sought is the good of an existing industry or profession, with existing structures and functions. For the most part, these are tied to private interests, and to the extent that educational programs are based on existing nonacademic practices, they perpetuate and strengthen those private interests—they do indeed make their faculties and their students "more responsive tools." As the minutes of one meeting of the advisory council to the School of Engineering at my university indicate, regular contact between the university and industry "makes students more valuable to industry."

PRAXIS AND TECHNE

My discussion so far has relied on a set of related oppositions that pervade the discourse of higher education:

theory	versus	practice
academy	versus	industry
ivory tower	versus	marketplace
idle speculation	versus	vocationalism
inquiry	versus	action
gentleman-scholar	versus	technician-dupe
contemplation	versus	application
general	versus	particular
knowing-that	versus	knowing-how
science	versus	knack

In this form the oppositions are probably unresolvable, and the best we can hope for is Anderson's notion that they should form a "creative tension" (Introd. 6).

Another approach is to suspect the worst: that a dichotomy so widespread must be (at least partly) false. And in fact, Aristotle's characterization of rhetoric as an art, rather than a science or a knack, cuts through these oppositions with a middle term—techne. As he defines it in the *Nicomachean Ethics*, "a productive state that is truly reasoned" (VI, iv), techne requires both particular and general knowledge, both knowing-how and knowing-that; techne is both applicable and conceptualized. Donald Schön's recent critique of professional education relies on the same middle term: it is "art," he says, that professionals display in practice, and it is art that unifies theory and application in a process he calls "reflection-in-action." Aristotle's *techne rhetorike*, or treatise on rhetorical art, joins theory and practice by deriving knowing how from knowing that, prescription from description. Although positivist philosophy claims that this derivation is fallacious ("you can't get 'ought' from 'is' "), one of the major insights of Marx, according to Bernstein, is to deny the positivist fallacy. Marx (as well as Aristotle) is able to derive from description of existing social practices the shape of human need and potential which provide the basis for prescription.

But to understand Aristotle's *Rhetoric* only as a techne is to miss what Aristotle himself has to say about practice. Understood as techne, Aristotle's treatise would fall within the handbook tradition, as a set of instructions that helps one produce texts. Such a treatise would concern productive knowledge, or *episteme poietike*, one of three kinds of knowledge in Aristotle's system: theoretical (concerned with knowing for its own sake), practical (concerned with doing), and productive (concerned with making). According to George Kennedy, Aristotle does not make the connection between rhetoric and productive knowledge (as he does for poetics) but treats rhetoric as theoretical knowledge concerned with "discovering" the available means of persuasion (63).

The remaining alternative—that Aristotelian rhetoric is practical, rather than theoretical or productive—has been argued by Richard McKeon, and its implications have been explored by Eugene Garver. To see rhetoric as practical, in Aristotle's system, is to emphasize action over knowledge or production; rhetoric becomes a form of conduct, like the related practical realms of ethics and politics, which are constant background presences in the *Rhetoric*. Aristotle distinguishes carefully in the *Nicomachean Ethics* between production and practice, poiesis and praxis: as distinct from "science," or theoretical knowledge, both concern the variable, or that which can be other than it is; but they differ in that production "aims at an end other than itself," the product, and practice aims at its own performance, at "doing well." The reasoning appropriate to production takes the form of techne, art or technique, and the reasoning appropriate to performance, or conduct, takes the form of *phronesis*, prudence; for Aristotle there can be no art, or technical knowledge, of conduct. Prudence is the reasoning that makes one "capable of action in the sphere of human goods" (*NE* 6: v). Like techne, prudential reasoning is situated to undermine the oppositions that plague discussions of professional education, for it necessarily concerns both universals and particulars: it applies knowledge of human goods to particular circumstances (*NE* 6: vii; Garver 64). Unlike techne, however, which is concerned with the useful (that is, with the quality of a product given a set of expectations for it), prudence is concerned with the good (that is, with the quality of the expectations themselves).

Aristotle's concept of praxis has also informed some recent thinking about human action. As the central concept in Marx, praxis highlights the way in which the human person "is the result of his [or her] own work" (Bernstein 39; see also Lobkowicz 418–20). Human belief structures and social relations are understood to be based in practical relations between human beings and objects. Schön's account of professional practice emphasizes the "knowing inherent in intelligent action" (50). Moreover, practices, as Alasdair MacIntyre has insisted, create not only knowledge but their own goods, and because practices are necessarily social, these goods require "subordinating ourselves within the practice in our relationship to other practitioners" (191). The insights for the academic are that practice creates both knowledge and value and that the value thus created comprehends the good of the community in which the practice has a history.

Understanding practical rhetoric as a matter of *conduct* rather than of production, as a matter of arguing in a prudent way toward the good of the community rather than of constructing texts, should provide some new perspectives for teachers of technical writing and developers of courses and programs in technical communication. For example, it provides a reasonable basis for the necessary combination of academic and nonacademic contributions to curriculum. If praxis creates knowledge, academics should indeed know about nonacademic practices. But the academy does not have to be just a receptacle for practices and knowledge created elsewhere. The academy itself is also a set of practices, including those of observation, conceptualization, and instruction—practices that create their own kind of knowledge. Such knowledge allows the academy to provide a standpoint for inquiry into and criticism of nonacademic practices. We ought not, in other words, simply design our courses and curricula to replicate existing practices, taking them for granted and seeking to make them more efficient on their own terms, making our students "more valuable to industry"; we ought instead to question those practices and encourage our students to do so too. Wells's "pedagogy for technical writing" suggests that we should aim "to work within the structures of technical discourse so that students can negotiate their demands but also be aware of the limited but real possibility of moving beyond them" (264). My own earlier sketch of a new pedagogy similarly suggested the need to promote both competence and critical awareness of the implications of competence ("Humanistic" 617). I might now supplement critical awareness with prudential judgment, the ability (and willingness) to take socially responsible action, including symbolic action.

An understanding of practical rhetoric as conduct provides what a techne cannot: a locus for questioning, for criticism, for distinguishing good practice from bad. That locus is not the individual or any particular set of private interests but the human community that is created through conduct; this community is the basis for practice in Bernstein's "high" sense. While the good that praxis in this higher sense creates may include the interests of individuals and industry, it is larger and more complex; the relevant community is not the working group or the corporation but the larger community within which the corporation sells its products, pays taxes, hires employees, lobbies, issues stock, files lawsuits, and is itself held accountable to the law.

Through praxis we make ourselves and each other in interaction: Aristotle emphasizes the political dimension of this interaction, Marx the economic. But whether our everyday activities are primarily those of governing a community or those of making a living, they have both political and economic dimensions. If technical writing is the rhetoric of "the world of work," it is the rhetoric of contemporary praxis. In teaching such rhetoric, then, we acquire a measure of responsibility for political and economic conduct.

WORKS CITED

Anderson, Paul V. "What Technical and Scientific Communicators Do: A Comprehensive Model for Developing Academic Programs." *IEEE Transactions on Professional Communication* PE-27 (1984): 161–67.

———. "Introduction" to Special Issue on Education. *Technical Communication* 31.4 (1984): 4–8.

———. "What Survey Research Tells about Writing at Work." Odell and Goswami, *Writing* 3–83.

Aristotle. *Rhetoric.* Trans. Lane Cooper. Englewood Cliffs: Prentice, 1932.

———. *Michomachean Ethics.* Trans. J. A. K. Thompson. New York: Penguin, 1955.

Bernstein, Richard J. *Praxis and Action.* U of Pennsylvania P, 1971.

Brockmann, R. John. "Advisory Boards in Technical Communication Programs and Classes." *Technical Writing Teacher* 9 (1982): 137–46.

Clough, M. Evalyn, and Thomas J. Galvin. "Educating Special Librarians: Toward a Meaningful Practitioner-Educator Dialogue." *Special Libraries* 75 (1984): 1–8.

Coggin, Bill. "Better Educational Programs for Students of Technical Communication." *Technical Communication* 27.2 (1980): 13–17.

Commission on Graduate Studies in Public Relations. *Advancing Public Relations Education: Recommended Curriculum for Graduate Public Relations Education.* New York: Foundation for Public Relations Research and Education, Inc., 1985.

Connors, Robert. "The Rise of Technical Writing Instruction in America." *Journal of Technical Writing and Communication* 12 (1982): 329–52.

Couture, Barbara, et al. "Building a Professional Writing Program through a University/Industry Collaborative." Odell and Goswami, *Writing* 391–426.

Dobrin, David N. "What's the Purpose of Teaching Technical Communication." *The Technical Writing Teacher* 12 (1985): 146–60.

Ede, Lisa, and Andrea Lunsford. "Research into Collaborative Writing." *Technical Communication* 32.4 (1985): 69–70.

Faigley, Lester, et al. *Writing after College: A Stratified Survey of the Writing of College-Trained People.* Technical Report No. 1. FIPSE Grant No. 6008005896, 1981.

Fisher, Harold A. "Broadcast Journalists" Perceptions of Appropriate Career Preparation," *Journalism Quarterly* 55 (1978): 140–44.

Galbraith, John Kenneth. *The New Industrial State.* 2nd ed. New York: New American Library, 1971.

Garver, Eugene. "Teaching Writing and Teaching Virtue." *Journal of Business Communication* 22.1 (1985): 51–73.

Gloe, Esther M. "Setting up Internships in Technical Writing." *Journal of Technical Writing and Communication* 13 (1983): 7–27.

Green, Marcus, and Timothy D. Nolan. "A Systematic Analysis of the Technical Communicator's Job: A Guide for Educators." *Technical Communication* 31.4 (1984): 9–12.

Griffiths, J. M. "Competency Requirements for Library and Information Science Professionals." *Information Science Abstracts* 20 (1985) 85–2017.

Jenkins, Roger L., and Richard C. Reizenstein. "Insights into the MBA: Its Contents, Output and Relevance." *Selections* (Graduate Management Admissions Council) 1 (1984): 19–24.

Kennedy, George A. *Classical Rhetoric and Its Christian and Secular Tradition from Ancient to Modern Times.* Chapel Hill: U of North Carolina P, 1980.

Kerr, Clark. *The Uses of the University.* New York: Harper, 1966.

Lobkowicz, Nicholas. *Theory and Practice: History of a Concept from Aristotle to Marx.* Notre Dame: U of Notre Dame P, 1967.

Maclntyre, Alasdair, *After Virtue.* 2nd ed. Notre Dame: U of Notre Dame P, 1984.

McKeon, Richard. "Aristotle's Conception of Language and the Arts of Language." *Critics and Criticism.* Ed. R. S. Crane. Chicago: U of Chicago P, 1952. 176–231.

Miller, Carolyn R. "A Humanistic Rationale for Technical Writing." *College English* 40 (1979): 610–17.

Odell, Lee. "Beyond the Text: Relations between Writing and Sect. 1 Context." Odell and Goswami, *Writing* 249–80.

Odell, Lee, and Dixie Goswami. "Writing in a Nonacademic Setting." *New Directions in Composition Research.* Ed. Richard Beach and Lillian S. Bridwell. New York: Gullford, 1984. 233–58.

———, eds. *Writing in Nonacademic Settings.* New York: Guilford, 1985.

Ohmson, Richard. *English in America.* New York: Oxford UP. 1976.

Olsen, Lesllie A., and Thomas N. Huckin. *Principles of Communication for Science and Technology.* Newyork: McGraw, 1983.

Reed, Jeffrey G. "Preparing the Training and Development Professional: Skills and Knowledge Essential for Practice." *Journal of Business Education* 60.1 (1984): 8–13.

Rudolph, Frederick. *Curriculum: A History of the American Undergraduate Course of Study Since 1636.* San Francisco: Jossey, 1977.

Schön, Donald. *The Reflective Practitioner: How Professionals Think in Action.* New York: Basic, 1983.

Socitey for Technical Communication. *Strategic Plan 1986–1990.* [Washington, DC: Society for Technical Communication, 1986].

Society for Technical Communication, Ad Hoc Committee on Certification. "Certification of Technical Communicators." *Technical Communication* 27.1 (1980): 4–6, 15.

Tebeaux, Elizabeth. "Redesigning Professional Writing Courses to Meet the Communication Needs of Writers in Business and Industry." *College Composition and Communication* 36 (1985): 419–28.

Veysey, Laurence R. *The Emergence of the American University.* Chicago: U of Chicago P, 1965.

Wells, Susan. "Jurgen Habermas, Communicative Competence, and the Teaching of Technical Discourse." *Theory in the Classroom.* Ed. Cary Nelson. Champaign: U of Illinois P, 1986. 245–69.

12 The Ethics of Teaching Ethics in Professional Communication: The Case of Engineering Publicity at MIT in the 1920s

DAVID R. RUSSELL

Russell's article, aimed primarily at teachers of the service course, many of whom he believes will have some, if not extensive, background in literary criticism, focuses on answering two central questions: 1) "To what extent, if any, should business and technical writing courses serve the pragmatic needs of business and industry, and to what extent, if any, should those courses teach the concerns of literary studies?" and 2) "What is the responsibility, if any, of the instructor of these courses to teach ethics?" (p. 165–66 in this volume). To answer these questions, he examines two very different positions from the field of technical/professional communication (Miller, "Practical"; Rentz and Debs), as well as pedagogical methods used in the early 1920s at MIT in their engineering program. Finding that both current positions seem less than ideal, Russell examines the historical, pedagogical response of MIT's Engineering Publicity Program from the 1920s, which sought to prepare engineers for "the ethos of the professional and business world they would enter" (p. 177). Relying on this historical example, Russell concludes that it is possible for teachers to meet what he considers their responsibility "to promote ethical behavior" and teach students practices of "critical reflection" (p. 166). His synthesis or solution falls under what he calls the "kairos of critique" (p. 182), which relies primarily on a full understanding of rhetorical situation and context (historical, professional, and curricular). Relying on contexts rather than methods, he argues that teachers can help students "negotiate the distance between 'the two cultures'" and help "students learn to be more responsible professionals" (p. 183–84).

In recent years, two questions have received a good deal of attention in the field of business and technical writing, or professional communication, as I will call it. One question is old and one new, but both are closely related—at least to professional communication teachers and researchers who are trained in the profession of literary criticism. The first question is as old as technical and business writing courses, dating back to the 1910s: To what extent, if any, should business and technical writing courses serve the

From *Journal of Business and Technical Communication* 7, no. 1 (January 1993): 84–111.

pragmatic needs of business and industry, and to what extent, if any, should those courses teach the concerns of literary studies?[1] The second question is relatively new, but it has received a great deal of attention in recent years: What is the responsibility, if any, of the instructor of these courses to teach ethics?[2] The two questions are related in complex ways because, for some teachers in the field of professional communication, putting business and technical writing courses at the service of business and industry is viewed as ethically suspect, and there have been a number of articles recently that argue or suggest that business and technical writing courses for students majoring in science, technology, and business should ask those students to critique the ethical basis of science, business, and industry from what is essentially the perspective of literary studies, as we shall see.[3]

Let me say from the outset that I believe all teachers—and all professions and all institutions and indeed all human beings—have a responsibility to promote ethical behavior. So, too, every profession, institution, and human being ought to engage in critical reflection at times. The question is not whether teachers, courses, disciplines, professions, and institutions should promote ethical behavior and critical reflection but how, when, and for what purposes they should be promoted. These are far more complex questions, and they cannot be answered without instructors considering their methods, timing, and motives for raising ethical issues. In this article, I want to point out some potential difficulties—what are essentially ethical difficulties—in literature-trained faculty teaching ethics in professional communication courses, and I will warn against a too-hasty—uncritical, if you will—pursuit of certain kinds of critical reflection as a goal of these courses.

First, I will examine the historical and an institutional context of my two central questions and look at two recent answers to them. Then I will turn to an obscure chapter in the history of business and technical communication—the teaching of "engineering publicity" at Massachusetts Institute of Technology (MIT) in the early 1920s—to see the unusual answer of one institution to these questions at a crucial point in its history. Finally, I will suggest why I believe that answer is worth serious consideration by those of us involved in writing instruction and curricular planning for students who will enter business and professional communities, both outside and within academia (for we must remember that academics—even those in literary studies—are professionals as well).

The "Two Cultures" Meet: Historical and Institutional Contexts

I begin with two assumptions. If writing is *not*—as has often been supposed—merely the recording of preexisting, fully formed, value-neutral facts but a complex social (and often political) process involving the assumptions, values, and interests of one or more communities, then, at bottom, writing instruction is about helping students learn to produce the kinds of texts necessary to those social (and political) processes, to internalize and negotiate those values and interests in their writing. The second assumption is related.

We know that professional communities are by their very nature exclusionary. They guard their expert knowledge in various ways to exert influence and, at times, wield power (Abbott). To survive and accomplish its tasks, each professional community must teach its future members the ethos of the profession, the *professional manner*, as it is sometimes called: those values, those rules of conduct—tacit or explicit—that create and maintain the professional community, that give it its "integrity," its identity (see Miller, "Technology"). In other words, professional communities must initiate new members and teach them to make the rhetorical choices that will project the image that serves the profession.

This is true not only of scientists, engineers, and business managers but also of academic literary professionals. Throughout my analysis, I will attempt to view the profession of the academic literary critic as one profession among many and thus try to put into institutional perspective the conflict between "the two cultures," in C. P. Snow's famous phrase. Professional teachers of literature, represented by their professional organization, the Modern Language Association (MLA), have their own ethos, their own values and interests, which they project and defend—and pass on to future members as they are trained (socialized) into the profession. In the process of this socialization, future literary professionals often acquire deep loyalties to the values and perspectives of their discipline, which they will represent in their careers, just as future engineers and managers often acquire deep loyalties to the values and perspectives of their profession.

Many, perhaps most, teachers of technical writing were (and are) trained as literary critics in departments of literature, which have for various reasons set themselves in opposition to commercial and technical interests. From the turn of the century, academic literary professionals felt alienated from "real-world" matters, and indeed cultivated that alienation as a virtue, setting themselves apart from business and industrial concerns and upholding values they took to be higher than those of what they viewed as philistine commercial interests (Veysey 114). Literary critics, as Gerald Graff puts it,

> expressed a reaction against American materialism that would continue . . . to be a powerful theme in American criticism. Yet their social criticism led for the most part to a defeatist feeling that the world had passed them by, that the spirit of vulgar materialism had taken over higher education itself and rendered their very lives a contradiction. (93; see also Fish 354–55)

That contradiction is perhaps felt most deeply by business and technical writing teachers, who were (and in large measure still are) poised between the "two cultures." As Thomas Wilcox wrote in 1973, from the perspective of English departments, business and technical writing courses

> are frankly identified as service courses . . . and the values they foster are those of the profession they serve. Members of the departments who teach in these programs are often an embattled band who see themselves slighted and their courses depreciated by their literary colleagues. (qtd. in Sullivan 6)

Wilcox went on to point out that the conflict was so strong that some institutions dealt with it by moving business and technical writing courses to another department or college. Looked down on by scientists as not being scientific and by their literary colleagues as representing alien and hostile values, some professional communication instructors simply left—or were forced out of—English departments, and some engineering and business colleges set up their own writing—or even humanities—programs (Michigan and Washington are perhaps the most visible examples) (Russell, *Writing* 122). Others dealt with the conflict in values by remaining loyal to their disciplines and attempting to foster the English department's professional values in their students from science, engineering, and business departments to humanize them or make them well-rounded. MIT, for example, has vacillated between humanities-based and technical-based writing programs over the past 100 years (Russell, *Writing* 107–28; Caldwell; "Course").

Given this institutional context, the two questions we began with—those of practicality and ethics in professional communication courses—are best viewed first of all as questions of ethos, of conflicting professional cultures. Because professionals are ordinarily socialized in one field, they tend to see the world in terms of that field and to see other professional cultures (and their values) as somehow suspect (McClosky). Outside of the humanities, it would be difficult to argue that the humanities disciplines (or faculty or students) are more or less ethical than disciplines (or faculty or students) in the sciences, technologies, or social sciences, even if one could find a measure of ethics all could agree on. The few extant empirical studies on the ethics of college students suggest that business students, for example, are no less ethical than nonbusiness students (Arlow). The historical record provides little help either. There have been great saints and great scoundrels from all fields. Virtue—and vice—seem to know no disciplinary boundaries.

Neither is academic expertise in ethics confined to English departments, of course. The *Business Index* listed some 132 books and articles on business ethics in 1991 alone, with 22 related terms, from accounting ethics to telemarketing ethics. That year there were 36 articles on the study and teaching of ethics, including subheads for articles on business ethics instruction in Asia, Europe, and South America. The *Philosopher's Index* listed 87 books and articles on business ethics that same year. There are three academic journals and two newsletters devoted to business and professional ethics and a wide range of other journals that regularly publish articles in the field. There are endowed chairs of business ethics and even a Society for Business Ethics, affiliated with the American Philosophical Association. Unfortunately, the discussion of ethics in professional communication has largely ignored or dismissed this very broad and complex academic debate.[4]

Moreover, within the scientific, engineering, and business communities there is an ongoing critical examination of their own professional ethics at many levels, including research institutes on ethics, corporate ethics programs, associations for the advancement of ethics, and so on—a critical examination that the discussion of ethics in professional communication has also largely ignored or dismissed (Brenner).[5] These ethical discussions and critiques are not confined within a profession or discipline but are often carried on among disciplines, as with the business-philosophy discussions that produce the leading journal in the field, *Journal of Business Ethics*. This allows individuals, professions, and businesses to test their own ethical stances against other positionings.

Finally, within college curricula there is also much interest in ethics within scientific, engineering, and business disciplines. Many business colleges even require of their majors a course in business ethics. Indeed, it seems to me that there is more self-critical discussion of professional ethics in these professions than in the humanities. I know of no English department in any institution that requires its majors to take a course on the ethics of literary studies, despite a number of widely publicized cases that have recently raised issues of humanists' professional ethics.[6] At any rate, one need not import an ethical discussion or critique from literary studies; scientific, technical, and business professions contain their own lively ethical discussions and critiques. As an outsider, one can engage the ongoing discussion in those professions by bringing one's own perspective to them—publishing in their periodicals, attending their meetings, and inviting them to do the same in one's own field—or one can ignore their discussions and critiques in favor of one's own perspective.[7] I think the former alternative is healthier, more useful, and more likely to result in that kind of consensus sometimes called the truth or, at least, in that chief virtue of pluralist democracies, tolerance.

In any case, from an institutional perspective, the debate over teaching ethics in business or technical writing courses for non-English majors does not arise because students majoring in science, engineering, and business have a unique need to be taught ethics. Nor does it arise because technical and business departments ask professional communication instructors to shoulder the burden of teaching ethics. It arises, I believe, because of a conflict in professional ethos among (or even within) teachers and researchers in professional communication, because those teachers and researchers were socialized or acculturated in one discipline, usually literary studies, with one set of values and assumptions, yet they are teaching courses that serve programs with different sets of values and assumptions. It is first of all the faculty who have the value conflict, not the students; it is first of all the faculty who need to critique and examine their own ethics and their own ethos, as well as those of the other academic "cultures." The current debate over ethics and practicality among professional communication teachers is in many ways a projection onto students of the discipline's own unresolved ethical conflicts, a way of maintaining the ethos (and values) instilled in instructors through their literary training while working in what is assumed by many in English departments to be an ethically compromising environment—an assumption that may be no more true of the institutional environment in business, technology, and science than the institutional environment of academic literary professionals, when critiqued from perspectives outside the hegemony of literary studies.

A Mirror for Literary Professionals

I want to examine two versions of the argument that professional communication courses should have an English department perspective and should critique the ethics of business and industry from that perspective: Carolyn R. Miller's "What's Practical about Technical Writing?" and Kathryn C. Rentz and Mary Beth Debs's "Language and Corporate Values: Teaching Ethics in Business Writing Courses."[8]

Carolyn Miller criticizes the widespread view that writing instruction should serve professional communities in a practical way by merely training students to be more useful to industry, a more skilled work force, or "more responsive tools" in the service of an industry or a profession. She calls for a "higher" sense of the practical: "not some mundane and bread-and-butter activity or character" but rather in a broader and deeper sense of that which "concerns human conduct in those activities that maintain the life of the community" (p. 155 in this volume). After quoting appeals from several fields for more curricular "relevance," she concludes:

> This discourse is infected by the assumptions that what is common practice is useful and what is useful is good. The good that is sought is the good of an existing industry or profession, with existing structures and functions. For the most part, these are tied to private interests, and to the extent that educational programs are based on existing nonacademic practices, they perpetuate and strengthen those private interests—they do indeed make their faculties and their students "more responsive tools." (p. 161).

I agree that these assumptions underlie the arguments that professional communication courses should be practical, although I would hardly use the word *infected*. I see nothing sinister in the desire of industries and professions for curricula to train students who will further the interests of those industries and professions and, inevitably, the interests of private individuals associated with them. The profession of literary studies, for example, surely wants its graduate (which is to say professional) programs to train students who will do good literary criticism when they become professional academics, and the MLA expends some effort on improving that training. That this will further the interests of the profession—including the private interests of those associated with it (professors, administrators, granting agencies, editors, publishers, authors, and so on)—is surely not objectionable in and of itself. Perpetuating and strengthening an industry or profession (and, as it often happens, the private interests associated with it) is laudable—to the extent that an industry or profession serves the public good. Academic practices (as opposed to the "nonacademic practices" that Miller refers to) do not necessarily serve the public good, either, but may instead serve private or professional interests at the expense of the public good.

Indeed, one of the recurring criticisms of professional humanists in academia—particularly literary critics—is that they ignore the practical to the detriment of the public good. The literary critic's Arnoldian stereotype of the philistine commercial enterprise ignoring the higher things of life to the detriment of society has its counterpart in the business person's stereotype of literary critics pursuing research that serves the interests of professional specialists while ignoring their responsibility to teach reading, writing, and a broader cultural perspective to students (see, for example, Fish). As we shall see, the histories of both literary study and of engineering suggest that there is more than a kernel of truth in both stereotypes. Fortunately, however, individuals and professional groups can and usually do serve their own interests and the public interest at the same time. If they did not, modern societies would disintegrate. Doctors may often gouge their patients and ignore the medical needs of those without means, but they also often cure illnesses and so further the public good. Academic literary critics may often feed at the public trough and ignore illiteracy to pursue their arcane specialisms, but they also often teach reading, writing, and literature and so further the public good. Individuals further their own private interests as they climb the professional career ladder, reaping the rewards the profession offers for service. In doing so, individuals further the special interests of the profession. Finally, a profession furthers the common good in society at large to the extent that the interests of the profession are in accord with the public interest, the common good. There is sometimes conflict between the interests of professions and the common good, just as there is between the interests of an individual and the common good. Groups and individuals find it difficult to make sacrifices for others. Sometimes these inevitable conflicts are resolved by the exercise of power through violence or the threat of it, but usually they are resolved by the very human, very rhetorical exercise of power through persuasion and negotiation—through legal proceedings, political or economic pressure, the media, alliances with others, and so on. How one views the teaching of ethics in professional communication courses depends a great deal on one's view of the nonviolent means of conflict resolution, the nonviolent exercise of power—one's view of rhetoric, in other words.

Miller points out that Greek culture initiated two traditions of rhetoric: a handbook tradition and a counterpoised theoretical tradition. She suggests that the study and teaching of professional communication ought to have more to do with the theoretical tradition, particularly the tradition of thoughtful practice or *phronesis*, practical wisdom, as opposed to mere production or technical competence (the high sense rather than the low sense of the term *practical*). But as George Kennedy points out, there was a third tradition in Greek rhetoric, the sophistic tradition. Unlike Plato and Aristotle in the theoretical or (to use Kennedy's term) *philosophical* tradition, who posited a final good above human social interactions, the sophistic tradition assumed that competing interests must negotiate the good in a very social, very human, very rhetorical process that Cicero called *controversia*. This is a pragmatic view, which does not locate truth or knowledge of the common good in any transcendent ideal or any single individual or group but in the social—and largely rhetorical—processes of negotiation.

To ally oneself with other organizations that have similar interests, whether a political party, corporation, labor union, or professional association (including the MLA), to learn its discourse and values, to participate in its service to society and reap the rewards, material and immaterial, that society offers for that service—this is a crucial way that individuals serve society as well as themselves, a way they become empowered. And it is through the controversia of public discourse, the negotiation of competing special interests, that we as a society arrive at the public good (or, of course, ill). No person or profession has absolute knowledge of the public good—an ethical calculus—although some act as if they did.

From this sophistic rhetorical perspective, the most important duty of teachers of professional communication is to encourage such empowerment: teaching students the discourses of the social groups the students have chosen to be part of, helping students become socialized into roles within those communities, and aiding students as they internalize and negotiate those values and interests.

I agree with Miller that a goal of professional communication courses must be thoughtful practice and practical wisdom (phronesis), which "concerns human conduct in those activities that maintain the life of the community," as opposed to mere production or technical competence. But from a sophistic perspective, the "life of the community" is not a single entity whose common good is self-evident to those not blinded by self-interest (p. 155). The "life of the community" is a complex polity made up of many communities—political, social, entrepreneurial, professional, and so on—with many different and often competing interests, which together negotiate the common good. But unless an individual is allied with one or more of those communities, alienation and powerlessness are the result.

Thus the goal of a professional communication course might well be to teach thoughtful practice in one or more of those professional communities as a way of helping students find empowerment through participating effectively in the discourse of those professions and thus in the community as a whole. When a professional communication instructor trained in the humanities stands outside the professions his or her students have chosen to enter and critiques the ethics of their chosen professions, one must ask whether the critique serves the interests of the instructor's profession at the expense of the student's own professional—or indeed human—development.

Kathryn C. Rentz and Mary Beth Debs also assume that professional communication courses should critique professional practice from what is essentially the perspective of the academic literary critic. They extend the argument beyond the ethics of specific actions to include the ethics of an organization's ethos as projected in the documents it produces. Rentz and Debs criticize typical approaches to teaching business ethics that suggest that

> an observer can sufficiently determine the ethical code of an organization by studying its official explicit code of ethics. Students are not directed toward sources that reveal the "unofficial" ethos of the organization's culture, as exhibited through its predominant metaphors and ways of expressing itself. . . . To say things in a particular way is to advance a particular way of seeing—a way based upon particular values. Indeed, "any

> utterance," as Richard M. Weaver has written, "is a major assumption of responsibility." (38)

I wholeheartedly agree that any reading of the world has ethical import. But there is a certain irony, perhaps an ethical ambiguity, in the pedagogy they advance. Rentz and Debs illustrate their classroom method with an analysis of a sales letter for a business magazine. They employ analytical and pedagogical methods of literary criticism to critique values they find revealed in the letter. They argue that the letter creates "a distinct version of the business world" through "key metaphors," and they ask students to

> spin out the implications. Business is an aggressive, even violent environment where one's very existence is threatened by the enemy (other business persons). . . . Furthermore, war is actually kind of fun—almost like baseball or chess—as long as you are winning. (40)

Rentz and Debs as well as their students found the letter ethically questionable to the extent that it "might unduly play on the fears of the readers, in the sense that the readers' freedom to choose another way of seeing was being too severely limited," that "an antisocial and antihuman scheme of values was being promoted" (40).

The ethical difficulties Rentz and Debs found in (or, one might argue, projected onto) this magazine sales letter reflect the criticisms of business that have been commonplace in literary studies since that discipline became professionalized in academia in the late nineteenth century. They critique the letter from the perspective of the literary professional. In other words, they themselves "advance a particular way of seeing—a way based upon particular values," and their utterance, we might conclude, is also "a major assumption of responsibility." Following their assumption to its logical conclusion, then, we might ask: What is the "'unofficial' ethos" of the literary professional, and how is it revealed in the discourse of literary criticism?

For the sake of illustration, let me turn the tables and imagine an undergraduate English course—say, an introduction to literary criticism required of all English majors preparing to teach literature at the secondary and tertiary levels—which had as a central goal what Rentz and Debs say should be a central goal of professional communication courses: "to enable students to perceive the values underlying word choices and to consciously assess them" (41). Let us imagine further that the instructor engaging the introductory literature class in this critique of the motives and ethics of literary criticism was not trained in literary criticism but in business or engineering, an instructor whose values were those of a different professional culture.

Following the procedure of Rentz and Debs, students would presumably read pieces of literary criticism—the texts produced by the professional community the students are preparing to enter—and discover the underlying professional and private agendas in order to assess the ethical lapses of the profession of literary studies and how the language of literary criticism masks those lapses. The instructor might help students discover how professors of literature enrich themselves (private interests) by publishing Marxist critiques of society while ignoring the growing illiteracy of the nation's young (public good). Or students might read Lawrence Veysey's historical analysis of the humanities in academia to understand the elitist and defensive posture that the humanities habitually take in regard to American business and industry (ch. 4).

Or students might read Jeanne Fahnestock and Marie Secor's "The Rhetoric of Literary Criticism" to learn how the language of literary criticism reveals the institutionalized norms of the profession, such as its "assumption of despair over the condition of courses of modern society," disclosed in the pervasive *contemptus mundi* topos in literary criticism. Fahnestock and Secor conclude their analysis of conventional rhetorical topoi in literary criticism:

> Ultimately all the topoi we have discussed reduce to one fundamental assumption behind literary inquiry: that literature is complex and that to understand it requires patient unraveling, translating, decoding, interpreting, and analyzing. Obviously, here we stumble on an endless circularity in literary criticism, the characteristic which creates the complexity which justifies it. We are led to ask, "Do we have literary criticism because literature is complex, or is literature complex because we have literary criticism?" (89–90)

Following Rentz and Debs's lead, the instructor might then ask his or her students to consider the ethical questions these uses of language by literary critics raise. Does this approach to literature primarily serve the profession by providing research for more and more literary critics instead of more teaching, which holds lower status in the profession (*churning* is the pejorative term used in some professions)? Or does all this effort spent on complexity further the public good somehow? Is it moral for America to pay hundreds of millions of dollars a year to professional academic literary critics to discover (or create) difficulty in literature when 27 million functionally illiterate adult Americans cannot read the documents on which their future depends or write well enough to defend their own interests? Is it ethical for a professor to produce yet another interpretation of a literary work for specialists instead of teaching another course to increase the literacy of the public? When is a piece of literary criticism a contribution to the public good, and when is it merely self-serving for the professor and/or the special interests of the profession of literary studies? And does the rhetoric of literary criticism mask these assumptions to the extent that students of literature are discouraged from raising these ethical issues?

I offer this counterexample not to propose that undergraduate literature surveys have this sort of ethical critique as a central component—quite the opposite. To structure an undergraduate course in literature in this way would be a terrible introduction to the profession and its discourse. It would call into question the values and activities of literary criticism before students have even had a chance to learn those values and practice those activities. At the undergraduate level, it would, in short, be counterproductive for the students, the profession, and ultimately for society at large. This kind of radical critique might be appropriate, even healthy, at the graduate level and in discussions within the literary studies, particularly because that profession trains far more literary critics than it can place in full-time positions within the profession, creating what some believe is another conflict between the public good and professional interests (large graduate programs provide high-status graduate teaching for literary professionals and provide cheap labor in low-status first-year composition courses). But even in discussions at these higher levels, such radical self-criticism is difficult, precisely because professions tend to see the world in their own terms and quite naturally resist attacks on their culture, their values, and, of course, their interests. Indeed, if professions spent much of their time examining their fundamental assumptions and discourse, they would have precious little time for their work, as well as a permanent identity crisis.

I offer this counterexample to suggest that most professions, including literary study, wisely exclude radical critiques of their culture and discourse until neophytes have had a chance to learn something of the professional culture and discourse. And most professions expect those who teach those courses to be members of the community and represent its values. Even seasoned professionals tend to engage in this radical self-examination only when their professional culture and values are challenged by outside forces and interests in that ongoing social dialogue out of which the public good is constructed. Professions are reluctant self-critics for good reason. Because there is no omniscient perspective, no final appeal except to the ongoing social dialogue, constant criticism can be paralyzing, an endless series of Chinese boxes, if it is not balanced by affirmation, acceptance, collective identity, and collective action. But unless one has become a member of a group, unless one has a social identity and role, unless one has interests to defend (as well as critically examine), one cannot effectively enter that public dialogue out of which public good (or ill) is constructed. One must remain an alienated individual, relatively powerless. Although the pose of the alienated individual, the critical outsider, has been cultivated by academic literary critics for almost a century, it is only a pose—and not a particularly useful one, I would argue, although that is another matter. College students must be socialized into some group(s), play some social role(s) to find a social identity and the empowerment—or potential empowerment—that come from collective action, whether that group is professional business managers, engineers, academic literary critics, or any other.

The Case of Engineering Publicity at MIT in the 1920s

The history of any profession provides examples of conflicts between professional or personal interests and the public good (if only because the public good is defined in so many conflicting ways by the many competing interests that negotiate it). If we examine the history of the profession that most business and technical writing teachers were socialized in, academic literary criticism, there are many such conflicts. There was the desire for professional status (and lower teaching loads and higher compensation that accompanied that status) attained through research in the modern university versus the commitment to undergraduate teaching (especially of rhetoric) in the old college (the MLA entirely disbanded its pedagogical section in 1903 [Stewart]). There was the desire to be accepted as professionals within the new secular, scientific-oriented university versus the commitment to moral improvement as a goal of rhetoric in the old college (the profession generally opted for a "New Criticism" that placed rigorous analysis and aesthetic interpretation of texts above moral improvement) (Veysey 203–12; Graff 145–47). And, of course, there was the desire for large graduate programs (another bearer of status and its accompanying benefits) to train more literary professionals versus the claims of writing instruction (the profession opted to use lower-paid graduate students and temporary instructors to teach composition, thus supporting graduate programs) (Parker, "Where Do English Departments Come From?").

Technical writing instruction posed another ethical challenge to the professional interests of English departments, as I noted earlier, and this produced the historical conflicts this article treats (see for example, Connors; Russell, *Writing* ch. 4). One response was to uphold the values of the literary studies in the alien environment of a classroom full of business or engineering students, to *humanize* these students or make them *well-rounded* as defined by the literary professionals. However, there were other alternatives to the teaching of professional ethics, alternatives that were responses to the conflicts within the technologies rather than within the humanities.

One of these was the experimental Engineering Publicity program at MIT in the early 1920s, where the peculiar values and interests of the engineering profession consciously shaped engineering curricula and technical writing instruction. By the very nature of its work—applying science to industry—American engineering is poised between science and business, between a commitment on the one hand to the scientific values of knowledge for its own sake and service to the discipline (and through it to humanity, broadly conceived) and on the other hand to the business values of profit and loyal service to the company. As Edwin T. Layton convincingly argues in his classic history of the American engineering profession, *The Revolt of the Engineers*, professionals in engineering have been divided between their need to establish themselves as an autonomous profession independent of business interests (with the status and independence that autonomy brings to a profession) and their practical need to work within large bureaucratic structures (in America, profit-seeking corporations) that provide the financial and organizational means that engineers need to do their work—designing and building large, expensive, complex machines and systems of machines. Like other professional organizations, engineers guarded their expert knowledge through rigid controls on membership and publication and, at times, by overt censorship of members who wished to bring sensitive professional matters to the attention of the public or the government. In the late 1910s, as engineers became prominent in the war effort, the profession confronted not only the question of its ethics but also the importance of its ethos, or *engineering publicity*, as it was called—the power of projecting an image of themselves to government and the public through the press and also, no less significantly, the importance of projecting an image of the profession to their corporate employers.

Let me turn now from this all-too-broad sketch of the sociopolitical forces within engineering during the 1910s to an all-too-brief sketch of MIT's pedagogical response, its Engineering Publicity program. How does this program answer the two questions with which I begin this article? First, the Engineering Publicity program defined *broadening* in a very different way than literary professionals defined it. The program clearly viewed writing as a social (and often political) process, not simply the clear recording of value-neutral facts, and the courses directly attempted to teach students to make rhetorical choices based on the values and interests of the profession (and the industries the profession served). The program attempted to initiate neophyte engineers into the ethos of the professional and business world they would enter by employing Deweyan pedagogical methods. And the program addressed the whole person, treating language—reading, writing, listening, and speaking—as an integrated whole, not as a set of technical skills. Engineering Publicity taught the ethos of the profession by consciously bringing students into the discourse community, by directly teaching the community's ethos, its rules of conduct its professional manner. The curriculum empowered students, teaching them to play social roles that carried power. Second, the program's director, Archer T. Robinson, saw no obligation to critique the ethics of engineering from a liberal arts perspective; instead, he presented a series of professional issues with ethical import and showed students how professionals in the field approached those issues. He then let the students discuss the issues among themselves and with the professionals. Finally, they wrote about the issues from the perspective of an engineering professional (in a report or memorandum to an engineer), not from the perspective of an academic humanist (in a critical essay written to a professor).

MIT had had a long history of progressive composition instruction. Indeed, the institute was founded on progressive educational principles—*mens et manus* its motto says; the mind is linked to the hand, the theoretical to the practical.[9] And from 1889 when its first composition director, George Carpenter, was hired until 1916, faculty had eschewed lectures in favor of student-centered pedagogy, using conferences (consultations, as MIT called them), group work, class chairmen to lead discussions, class criticism of papers, and so on. Students were free to write on technical subjects, and there was a much-praised program for encouraging writing across the curriculum (Russell, "Composition"). But in 1916, in response to outside critics' complaints that MIT's students were not well-rounded enough, MIT hired a literary scholar as department head, Frank Aydelotte, who required students' compositions to be on literary and historical topics and insisted that

> in the education of this broader engineer, whom society so badly needs, the study of the mother tongue must be more than the acquirement of facts or a superficial accomplishment; it must be a training in thought,

> the influence of which is to clarify and humanize the student's character and his aims in life. ("Training" 302)

By "training in thought," Aydelotte meant the perspective of the literary professional (clearly, faculty in science, business, and engineering think and teach students to think). He edited a textbook entitled *English and Engineering* that contained belletristic essays on scientific topics, the first in a long line of literary technical writing readers that extends to the present. Aydelotte's story is a familiar one in the history of technical writing, repeated several times at MIT and countless times at other institutions as the curricular pendulum swung from "utility" to "well-roundedness" and back (Russell, *Writing* ch. 4)

Unfortunately for Aydelotte and the professional interests he represented, the engineering students were not much interested in having their characters and aims of life humanized in Aydelotte's way, and they chafed at the literary instruction. When Aydelotte left three years later to become president of Swarthmore, an old department hand, Archer T. Robinson, proposed a series of "contact courses," as he called them, "designed to establish a contact between [the students'] engineering and scientific interests and the broader world" ("Contact Courses" 1).[10] The contact courses would humanize the neophyte engineers in a different way than the traditional liberal arts lecture course. "A certain portion" of MIT's students, says Robinson in his course proposal, "are prepared to benefit" from a literary education:

> By some accident of training or association they have already approached some problem of literature, psychology, history, or pure science, and are thus naturally disposed to further study. For such men these [traditional] courses may be broadening, because they begin with natural interests and lead outward. The majority, however, find their concerns rather closely limited to professional development and material success. Any broadening which is possible for these men must begin with these material considerations and must lead from them outward to an interest in the rest of the universe. This, it seems to me, is the logical approach from engineering to what we sometimes call culture. (1)

This is an extraordinary rationale. Robinson specifically problematizes the concept of culture—it is more than the usual American liberal arts formulation of the genteel tradition, more than "high culture." And he evokes Deweyan assumptions: that student interest is central, that it is aroused by problem solving, and that students move from their own experience to "the rest of the universe." This is progressive education, *mens et manus*—but applied to professionalization.

The three contact courses Robinson introduced were The Engineering Field, The Human Factor in Business, and Engineering Publicity. The methods he used were firmly Deweyan, uniting experience and reading, personal investigation and writing. Students did oral and written reports "based on investigation, as often as the time and subject permit, and on reading" (note that reading is secondary to experience) ("Contact Courses" 2). Class discussions were led not by the instructor but by a class chairman elected for the period by the class (5). Most important, Robinson brought the world into the classroom—but it was the world according to engineering. Working engineers and corporate executives with engineering backgrounds visited the class, spoke about their work—usually presenting a problem—and the class then discussed the situation or problem and wrote on it.[11]

Robinson was clearly choosing his speakers to give students a broad picture of the engineering profession. He brought in 42 speakers in 1920–21 representing some 25 different industries. They spoke on a vast range of topics—none of them directly technical—such as safety, corporate organization, labor-management problems, consulting, writing for engineering journals, job analysis, and scientific management. Clearly, these courses would be broadening for engineering students fed on a steady diet of technical courses. Students apparently got a wide view of the issues and problems facing engineers in business. But students apparently got only one point of view on those issues and problems—that of upper-level engineers, many of whom had gone into management (a typical career path then as now). As far as I am able to tell, none of the 42 speakers represented labor or government; only one represented supervisory-level management (a foreman). The other 41 were established engineers and/or executive-level managers. By listening to and talking with successful engineers (successful by the profession's standards), by writing about the issues relevant to engineers from the perspective of engineers, the students were doubtless absorbing the ethos—and the ethics—of the profession (Robinson, "Executive Committee").

The syllabus for Engineering Publicity makes this goal of initiation abundantly clear. The goal of the course is "to give some notions of how to sell services and ideas." The first topic is "professional ethics and self-advertising." Note the pairing. Ethics is paired with ethos, virtue with its projection, *vir bonus dicendi peritus*. If the first duty of an engineer is loyalty to the company, then professional ethics has profit as its highest goal. Even if the first duty of the engineer is to uphold the profession, then the way the profession is presented to the public—and the employer—is crucial, although it must be handled subtly by professionals. As the catalog description puts it, the course taught "professional ethics and *indirect* [italics mine] publicity"—presumably the only kind proper to an engineering professional. The other contact course, The Human Factor in Business, discussed "the principal executive problems which an engineer is likely to be called upon to solve in organizing and handling men"—such things as hiring and training, of course, but also "housing, feeding, welfare . . . morals," and "securing cooperation" (a management euphemism for dealing with labor unrest). This course also frankly acknowledged the usual career path of engineers—those students "looking forward to the possible executive control of the enterprises in production or construction that an Institute graduate would naturally enter" (*MIT Bulletin*).

For me, Robinson's answers to the two questions I take up in this article raise complex questions for professional communication teachers and researchers, questions not only of our ethos but also of our professional ethics. Is it the responsibility of a technical writing instructor, helping students to learn the discourse of a community and thus become a part of that community, to teach a different set of ethics, or to problematize, critique, or otherwise challenge or resist the ethos and perhaps the ethics students are learning as part of their initiation into a professional community, as some in our discipline argue?[12] I sometimes wonder how professional humanists would react if business or engineering colleges insisted that English majors should be required to take a business or engineering course that had as one of its aims to humanize English majors by teaching them the values of laissez faire capitalism or the virtues of technocracy?[13] And as I suggested earlier, literature professors rarely problematize the literary study by introducing a radical critique of their own professional interests, values, and ethics. Those of us who have taught in writing-across-the-curriculum programs or worked closely with business or engineering faculty in professional writing programs can remember the sociocultural conflicts we felt, and we can appreciate the conflicts our students feel as they are socialized into a new discipline. Our profession, teachers and researchers in professional communication, has historically handled the problem by viewing writing as a value-neutral set of skills, independent of disciplinary values, or by adopting Aydelotte's solution and compartmentalizing: teaching imaginative literature on the assumption that it would somehow humanize students entering other professional communities in a superior way to the humanizing they get as part of their professional training. But now that our profession (like many professions in both the sciences and the humanities) is beginning to see knowledge—and writing acquisition—as bound up with the ethos (and ethics) of individual communities, we face new questions of our own ethos and ethics. We must decide, as individual teachers and ultimately as a profession, how we will present ourselves to other professional communities and to those students who have chosen to enter those communities, students who are often struggling with questions of their identity, their humanity.

On Tolerance as an Academic Virtue: The *Kairos* of Critique

The MIT technical writing program in the early 1920s chose to consciously, systematically initiate students into the writing (and with it the ethos and ethics) of the engineering profession as it was then structured. It would be easy—too easy, I think—to dismiss the MIT program as moral compromise, as selling out to the mercantile values of business and industry, as narrow and dehumanizing. In a complex, pluralist, specialist-driven society—what some are calling a postmodern society—the moral high ground is often very hard to take firm footing on. Perspectives are manifold and shifting. Allow me some personal thoughts for a moment from my perspective as an instructor of professional communication at Iowa State University of Science and Technology.

At Iowa State, I have seen working-class and minority students, first-generation college students, struggling mightily to become engineers. Engineering professors tell me that most of these students drop out. I have seen young women—all too few of them—who have chosen to overcome the immense obstacles society puts in their way as they try to realize their human potential as members of the engineering profession. It is a tough fight, and many drop out.

For me, the first ethical question is, How can I, as a professional teacher of writing—and as a human being—best respect a student in her life choice and help her in her struggle? Is it my task, as her technical writing teacher, to pose an outsider's fundamental critique of the engineering profession at the very moment she is struggling with all her might to learn to speak and write and act and think like an engineer, to get through the program, to realize her dream? She needs to know how to write successfully as an engineer. I believe it is my central task to help her learn to do that, to respect and support the decision she has made about how she will "humanize [her] character and [her] aims of life" (Aydetotte, "Training" 302).

I do not mean that we should never raise ethical issues in the technical writing classroom. If we teach writing as more than mere recording of value-neutral facts (and I hope we do), then ethical issues will inevitably arise. We bring our personal values through the classroom door every day, along with our humanity. And in professional schools today, as at MIT in 1920, technical writing (and the engineering profession itself) inevitably intersects nontechnical issues, questions of safety, welfare, housing, feeding, morals, and conversation, to use terms from progressive-era engineering, or of environmental protection, resource allocation, and affirmative action, to use terms from today's engineering profession. In my classroom, as in many technical writing classrooms, my students and I discuss documents that raise ethical issues: for example, memos relating to the *Challenger* tragedy and to Three Mile Island. We discuss these in terms of the engineering profession and its corporate, governmental, and social contexts to answer such questions as, How can engineers communicate more effectively and responsibly to prevent these disastrous aberrations?[14]

But I do not take it on myself to attack, from a perspective drawn from academic literary criticism, the fundamental values of the discipline that students are struggling to enter, to radically problematize the ethical status of the work they have chosen to devote their lives to. Every working-class person, every person of color, every woman studying engineering is a walking critique of the engineering profession. Each student, of whatever background, in a professional communication course is a living problematic—a human being striving to enter a profession, to create a new life with that community. And every faculty member who teaches these students should be sensitive to that critique and to the unique struggles these students have, not only with their studies but with their very identities.

For some students, radical critique is necessary and even inevitable. And if that critique grows out of the life experience of the student, out of his or her situation in the institution, out of his or her struggle, then I think we should welcome it and support it. But I also think we have an obligation to critique other professions in such a way that students will understand that we are informed of the virtues as well as the vices of the other's—and of our own—profession, that we have taken the time to learn something of the profession's ethical issues and its struggles to resolve them. Preaching with missionary zeal the latest indictment of science, technology, or business fashionable among literary critics may, as Paul Dombrowski has pointed out, "damage our ethos as professors and do a disservice to students" (1).

Insensitive or ill-informed critique, however well-meaning, can undercut the credibility of the critic. However powerless, marginalized, and alienated academic literary professionals may be (or perceive themselves to be), as instructors, they still have the power of the grade over students. The result of a facile or closed-minded critique may well be resentment against the instructor or, worse, reinforcement of the stereotype of academic literati as hopelessly impractical and irrelevant. Indeed, the marginalization of literary studies in the university may in part be due to its hanging on to a version of humanism that saw itself as isolated, alienated, and inevitably oppositional. By failing to engage in a dialogue with professionals in science, technology, and business, literary studies may be missing an opportunity to influence students, educational institutions, and the wider culture—to gain its own empowerment.

As professional business and technical writing teachers, we ought to consider what might be called the *kairos* of critique. When is the moment ripe for critiquing the structures and values of the community that an individual student is struggling to enter? And when is the moment ripe for affirming the decision a student has made, by helping him or her to enter that community through its discourse? I think we ought to take these questions very seriously, as seriously as our students take their career choices, their hopes, and their plans for the future.

Of course this kairos of critique will be different for every discipline, instructor, class, and even student. Finding the ripe moment, the right way, is difficult in almost any educational situation, more difficult still when the instructor and the students are simultaneously insiders and outsiders to a profession, between two worlds. There is no formula, but I want to conclude by suggesting that, as in any ethical situation, respect for those who have less power—students, in this case—is at the heart of finding that kairos. And as in any rhetorical situation, genuine respect and timely dialogue are more likely when one understands the context. Here are several contexts worth exploring:

1. *Historical context*. Learn something of the history of the disciplines one's students come from—the history of both "cultures"—to formulate for oneself (and at the same time collectively for one's profession) an ethos that is responsible to both cultures. Studies of the history, sociology, and rhetoric of the professions are proliferating. These offer multiple perspectives on questions of ethos and ethics that students—and their instructors—face in negotiating professional interests and the public good. And a chat with a senior professor in a business or technical discipline might provide a historical perspective on a field (or one's institution) that standard histories—often written by outsiders—may not provide.

2. *Professional context.* Learn something of the critical discussions of ethics going on in the disciplines one serves—again from both cultures—so that one can bring to students (and gain from students) an informed critique when critique is appropriate. What steps are being taken to make more humane the disciplines and enterprises one's students are striving to enter? What steps are being taken to make the humanities more humane—and more tolerant of other professional communities with different interests? Where is dialogue going on between the two, and how can one further it? For example, one might invite a faculty member from engineering to a discussion of the Three Mile Island memos and videotape the discussion. Or one might study the mission statements of companies or talk with employees to get a sense of institutional dynamics in which ethical decisions are made (see, for example, Rogers and Swales).
3. *Curricular context.* Learn something of the ethical discussions that students have been involved in through the curriculum, whether those discussions were a deliberate part of a curriculum or informal responses among peers to issues that the curriculum, faculty, and society at large inevitably raise. (I have found students to be very sensitive and articulate about ethical issues, although perhaps not about the issues I perceive and raise.) Many programs require students to take a course in ethics. And almost all students in scientific, business, and technical programs take several humanities courses in college or have taken several in secondary school. What have they learned from these about ethics? What attitudes have they formed about the conflicts between the "two cultures"?

I only propose contexts; I do not prescribe methods. But I do suggest one rule of thumb for teaching ethics in professional communication courses where students are from scientific, technical, and business majors: Teach ethics to these students as you would have instructors from other disciplines teach ethics to English majors. I see this not as a commandment or a categorical imperative but as a very pragmatic way of coming to terms with ethical and pedagogical issues in a heterodox institution within a pluralist society.

The temptation is to take sides and foreclose dialogue, to assume that one's own professional perspective must represent the public good. This is especially dangerous because instructors in professional communication courses often have a captive audience, particularly where the courses are required for a degree program. And if faculty are not sensitive to the kairos of critique, attempts at empowerment may lead instead to resentment, from students and from disciplines. The history of business and technical writing instruction is replete with examples of programs that came to be housed not in English departments but in departments of business or engineering because the conflict in values could not or would not be negotiated.

But if we foster a mutually respectful dialogue with professionals in the disciplines our students are preparing to enter, and if professionals interested in ethical issues can bring their perspective to bear on our discourse and in the process bring ours to their deliberations, then the study and teaching of professional communication may clarify its own professional identity and ethos, its own ethical conflicts, and in doing so help students learn to be more responsible professionals in whatever fields they have chosen and more humane participants empowered to enter a public discourse in which the literary professional is only one voice.

Teachers of professional communication have a unique interdisciplinary perspective and thus a unique responsibility. They can—indeed they must—daily negotiate the distance between "the two cultures." C. P. Snow, who coined the phrase, was both a physicist and a man of letters, and it is salutary to recall that his famous essay (perhaps more cited than read) is not an indictment of the ethical position of scientific "culture," but just the opposite. Writing to his fellow literati, he says, "the greatest enrichment the scientific culture could give us is . . . a moral one." Snow praises scientific "culture" for its commitment to human improvement manifested in active involvement. Snow takes to task the other culture, the "mainly literary" one, for an ethical complacency "made up of defeat, self-indulgence, and moral vanity," a complacency to which "the scientific culture is almost totally immune." And he concludes, "It is that kind of moral health of the scientists which, in the last few years, the rest of us have needed most; and of which, because the two cultures scarcely touch, we have been most deprived" (414). Both cultures have changed much in the four decades since Snow published his essay, but perhaps each culture still has much to learn from the other, even about ethics.

NOTES

1. The conflict began shortly after the first business and engineering writing courses and textbooks appeared (see, for example, Faith Maris). For historical overviews of the traditional tension between pragmatic and humanistic concerns in professional communication courses, see Russell *Writing* ch. 4 and Connors. For more recent discussion, see, for example, Harris; Miller, "Humanistic Rationale"; Tebeaux; Zappen.

2. The importance of the topic in the field of professional communication instruction is suggested by the recent issue of *Journal of Business Communication* devoted to ethics, by the regular column on ethics in the Society for Technical Communication (STC) newsletter, *Intercom* (Brockmann), and by the number of articles on the subject in professional communication literature. For an overview of ethics research in business communication, see Reinsch.

3. Here and throughout I am speaking of business and technical writing courses for students outside professional communication programs that train specialists in communication. With the growth of professional communication as a field, there are courses for students majoring in business and technical writing, students who will go on to be writing or communication specialists in science, business, industry, and government. The ethics of teaching ethics to these students poses a different (although related) set of problems, which I will not broach in this article.

4. See, for example, Lewis and Speck's characterization of this discussion as "a piecemeal and/or mechanical attempt to understanding ethics that emphasizes utilitarianism" (217).

5. Two notable exceptions are Priscilla S. Rogers and John M. Swales's analysis of Dana Corporation's policies document, which discusses the literature on ethics statements in both corporate and academic circles, and James E. Porter's study of the legal and ethical issues of disclosure ("Ideology"; "Role"; "Truth"). See also Reinsch's critique of the nonpedagogical articles in the professional communication literature on ethics (267).

6. See, for example, the Paul de Man case (Hamacher, Hertz, and Kenan) and the Jamie Sokolow case (Mallon).

7. An excellent step toward dialogue was the appointment of a special review panel that included experts in business ethics to select articles for the issue of the *Journal of Business Communication* (27.3: 1990) devoted to ethics.

8. See also Miller's "A Humanistic Rationale for Technical Writing."

9. On the relation between progressive education and MIT, see Cremin 25–26.; Russell, "Composition"; Russell, *Writing* ch. 4.

10. This account of the contact courses is drawn from Robinson's papers in the MIT archives. My thanks to archival assistant Bridgit P. Carr Blagboroug.

11. This method is quite similar to the case study methods in use at the nearby Harvard Graduate School of Business Administration (indeed, some of Robinson's speakers were from that school or also presented cases there) (see Russell, *Writing* 129–32).

12. In recent years, critiques from English department faculty of professional communication courses sometimes have been reinscribed in a Marxist or *Marxisant* vocabulary and emphasize the role of the technical writing teacher in *resistance*, or a radical critique of the political structures and values of a profession or of professionalization itself (see, for example, Susan Wells).

13. Engineering has a tradition (although erratic) of systematically teaching its own ethos and ethics (see, for example, Jackson and Jones; King). At some institutions, such as Carnegie Mellon University, there is a required course for engineers on the relationship between technology and society. It is taught by engineering faculty. However, at other institutions, such as Georgia Institute of Technology, there is a humanities program specifically for engineers taught by humanities faculty. And in recent years engineering schools have sometimes taught engineering ethics directly in special courses. See, for example, Schaub and Pavlovic for an anthology designed for such courses.

14. The ethical case studies in the STC newsletter, *Intercom*, are interesting as well.

REFERENCES

Abbott, Andrew. *The System of Professions: An Essay on the Division of Expert Labor*. Chicago: University of Chicago Press, 1988.

Aydelotte, Frank, ed. *English and Engineering*. 2nd ed. New York: McGraw-Hill, 1923.

———. "Training in Thought as the Aim of Elementary English Course as Taught at MIT." *Engineering Record* 24 Feb. 1917: 300–02.

Brenner, Steven N. "Ethics Programs and Their Dimension." *Journal of Business Ethics* 11 (1992): 391–99.

Brockmann, John R. "Ethical Case for Discussion." *Intercom* 4 (1988): 4–5.

Caldwell, Robert G. "The Humanities of Technology." *Technology Review* 42 (1941): 210–28.

Connors, Robert J. "The Rise of Technical Writing Instruction in America." *Journal of Technical Writing and Communication* 12 (1982): 349–54.

"Course XXI—A History." Unpublished manuscript. MIT Archives, Cambridge, n.d.

Cremin, Lawrence A. *The Transformation of the School: Progressivism in American Education*. New York: Vantage, 1961.

Dombrowski, Paul M. "The Ethos of Science in the Technical Communication Classroom." Conference of College Composition and Communication. Cincinnati, 19 Mar. 1992.

Fahnestock, Jeanne, and Marie Secor. "The Rhetoric of Literary Criticism." *Textual Dynamics of the Professions: Historical and Contemporary Studies of Writing in Professional Communities*. Ed. Charles Bazerman and James Paradis. Madison: University of Wisconsin Press, 1991. 76–96.

Fish, Stanley. "Profession Despise Thyself." *Critical Inquiry* 10 (1983): 349–64.

Graff, Gerald. *Professing Literature*. Chicago: University of Chicago Press, 1987.

Hamacher, Werner, Neil Hertz, and Thomas Kenan, eds. *Responses: On Paul de Man's Wartime Journalism*. Lincoln: University of Nebraska Press, 1989.

Harris, Elizabeth. "In Defense of the Liberal Arts Approach to Technical Writing." *College English* 44 (1982): 628–36.

Jackson, Dugald C., Jr., and W. Paul Jones, eds. *The Profession of Engineering*. New York: Wiley, 1929.

Kennedy, George. *Classical Rhetoric and Its Christian and Secular Tradition from Ancient to Modern Times*. Chapel Hill: University of North Carolina Press, 1980.

King, W. J. *The Unwritten Rules of Engineering*. New York American Society of Mechanical Engineers, 1944.

Layton, Edwin T. *The Revolt of the Engineers*. Cleveland, OH: Case Western Reserve University Press, 1971.

Lewis, Phillip V., and Henry E. Speck III. "Ethical Orientations for Understanding Business Ethics." *Journal of Business Communication* 27 (1990): 213–32.

Mallon, Thomas. *Stolen Words: Forays into the Origins and Ravages of Plagiarism*. New York: Ticknor, 1989.

Maris, Faith. "Shall the Teaching of English be Commercialized?" *Educational Review* 58 (1919): 70–72.

McCloskey, Donald N. "Why Academics Criticize Each Other." Project on the Rhetoric of Inquiry Seminar. Iowa City, IA, 12 Dec. 1991.

Miller, Carolyn R. "A Humanistic Rationale for Technical Writing." *College English* 40 (1979): 610–17.

———. "Technology as a Form of Consciousness: A Study of Contemporary Ethos." *Central States Speech Journal* 29 (1978): 228–36.

———. "What's Practical about Technical Writing?" *Technical Writing: Theory and Practice*. Ed. Bertie E. Fearing and W. Keats Sparrow, New York: Modern Language Association, 1989. 14–24.

MIT Bulletin. Cambridge, MA: MIT Archives, 1920.

Parker, William Riley. "Where Do English Departments Come From?" *College English* 28 (1967): 339–51.

Porter, James E. "Ideology and Collaboration in the Classroom and the Corporation." *Bulletin of the Association for Business Communication* 53 (1990): 18–22.

———. "The Role of Law, Policy, and Ethics in Corporate Composing: Toward a Practical Ethics for Professional Writing." Conference of College Composition and Communication. Boston, 21 Mar. 1991.

———. "Truth in Technical Advertising: A Case Study." *IEEE Transactions on Professional Communication* 30 (1987): 182–89.

Reinsch, N. L., Jr. "Ethics Research in Business Communication: The State of the Art." *Journal of Business Communication* 27 (1990): 251–72.

Rentz, Kathryn C., and Mary Beth Debs. "Language and Corporate Values: Teaching Ethics in Business Writing Courses." *Journal of Business Communication* 24.3 (1987): 37–48.

Robinson, Archer T. "Memorandum for the Executive Committee." 16 Mar. 1921. Archer T. Robinson Papers. MIT Archives, Cambridge, MA.

———. "Memorandum in Regard to Proposed Contact Courses." 5 May 1919. Archer T. Robinson, Papers. MIT Archives, Cambridge, MA.

Rogers, Priscilla S., and John M. Swales. "We the People? An Analysis of the Dana Corporation Policies Document." *Journal of Business Communication* 27 (1990): 293–313.

Russell, David R. "Composition for the Culture of Professionalism: Writing and Industrial Relations in the Progressive Era, 1895–1920." *Rhetoric and Ideology: Compositions and Criticism of Power*. Selected Proceedings of the Rhetoric Society of America. Ed. Charles Kneupper. Arlington: University of Texas at Arlington Press, 1989.

———. *Writing in the Academic Disciplines, 1870–1990: A Curricular History*. Carbondale: Southern Illinois University Press, 1991.

Schaub, James H., and Karl Pavlovic. *Engineering Professional and Ethics*. New York: Wiley, 1983.

Snow, C. P. "The Two Cultures." *New Statesman* 6 Oct. 1956: 413–14.

Stewart, Donald C. "The Status of Composition and Rhetoric in American Colleges, 1880–1902: An MLA Perspective." *College English* 47 (1975): 734–46.

Sullivan, Patricia. "Competing Meanings for Professional Writing: Implications for Discipline Formation." Conference of College Composition and Communication. Boston, 21 Mar. 1991.

Tebeaux, Elizabeth. "Let's Not Ruin Technical Writing, Too: A Comment on the Essays of Carolyn Miller and Elizabeth Harris." *College English* 41 (1980): 822–25.

Veysey, Laurence R. *The Emergence of the American University*. Chicago: University of Chicago Press, 1965.

Wells, Susan. "Jürgen Habermas, Communicative Competence, and the Teaching of Technical Discourse." *Theory in the Classroom*. Ed. Cary Nelson. Urbana: University of Illinois Press, 1986. 245–69.

Wilcox, Thomas W. *Anatomy of Freshman English*. San Francisco: Jossey, 1973.

Zappen, James P. "The Discourse Community in Scientific and Technical Communication: Institutional and Social View." *Journal of Technical Writing and Communication* 19 (1989): 1–11.

APPLIED THEORY

13 The Exercise of Critical Rhetorical Ethics

JAMES PORTER

By examining three cases ("Newsgroup Intervention," "Free Speech on the Listserv Group," and "Harassment in Cyberspace") that shed light on how "members of a class who can be victimized by the electronic speech of others," Porter considers the obligations of a teacher to "encourage [students] to be responsible, fair, and ethical" writers (p. 188 in this volume). Adopting a position similar to Russell's, Porter explains that a "critical rhetorical ethics does not generate specific answers" but instead "suggests heuristics" (p. 188). Because one of his goals is to develop an "ethical standpoint toward issues involving the rights of electronic citizens" (p. 188), Porter posits that teachers should consider developing a "critical rhetorical ethics, . . . a praxis*" that inquires and is willing to judge and act when necessary (p. 188). In addition to his focus on positions for teachers, Porter relies on the work of Dussel, Horkheimer, and Feenberg (among others) to explain that cyberwriters, too, have to negotiate positions from what he labels as "competing frames," a legal frame and the ethics for "internetworked writing," which he defines earlier in his book as "computer-based electronic writing that makes synchronous or asynchronous links to remote participants or databases [referring specifically] to the creation, design, organization, storage, and distribution of electronic information via wide-area networks" (2), in order to be "rhetorical" and, therefore, ethical. Ultimately, in the larger work in which this chapter is situated, Porter seeks a "postmodern rhetorical ethics" – that recognizes and respects differences in rhetorical situations (194), "calls for more active advocacy of users" (210), emphasizes the study of situated contexts (198), and involves a commitment to improving conditions for learning (199).*

> Bringing ethics into rhetoric is not a matter of collapsing spectacular diversity into universal truth. Neither is ethics only a matter of radical questioning of what aspires to be regarded as truth. Lyotard insists that ethics is also the obligation of rhetoric. It is accepting responsibility for judgment.
>
> — FAIGLEY, 1992, p. 239

From *Rhetorical Ethics and Internetworked Writing*, by James Porter, 133–47. Greenwich, CT: Ablex, 1998.

My perspective looks at the issue of ethics on computer networks from the point of view of rhetoric. In taking the perspective of the writer (or rhetor), rhetoric focuses on the issue of the writer's (and writers') responsibility toward readers. The questions of interest pertain not so much to what the writer *can* do (what is *legally permissible*) as to what the writer *should* do (what is *ethically obligated*). My primary professional role—that of writing teacher—places me in a specific ethical standpoint toward issues involving the rights of electronic citizens. What obligations do I have as the teacher of a writing class toward members of a class who can be victimized by the electronic speech of others? What obligations do I have as a teacher of writing to encourage members of my class to be responsible, fair, and ethical electronic writers?

My heart lies with postmodernist approaches to addressing ethics . . . but, like Lyotard and Thébaud (1985), I am nervous about the problematic politics of taking the postmodern *ironic* position. It is too easy to stand and smirk in the middle and point out that emperors and empresses have no clothes, but *then* what? What do you *do*? How do you justify any ethical or political stand? The issue for rhetorical ethics is to deal with the plurality and contingency of choices—and yet at the same time to be able to take a firm stand when it is necessary to do so.

So what do we do? Where do we position ourselves? Overall I am advocating ethics. A critical rhetorical ethics does not generate specific answers. It suggests heuristics, tactics for exploring what "right answers" might look like in any particular case. . . . It offers procedural criteria for determining how ethical decisions might be made in the particular case. (Procedural criteria themselves are never innocent or neutral, of course; they should not pretend to universality. Procedural criteria are situated.) A critical rhetorical ethics is a *praxis* occupying the position on the border. It *inquires in a nomadic fashion*, but recognizes that at some level at some point *practical judgment is necessary*: the ability to inquire and then *to act in the manner necessary*. We might consider this position as that of *postmodern commitment* (as opposed to the kind of ludic postmodernism, which, in its extreme forms, can lack the capacity for decision and choice).

I do not think, however, that everyone needs to occupy the same position. There is simply not enough room for us all to stand in the same place, even if it were a good idea. We will inevitably have different inclinations based on our backgrounds, our passions, our characters as they have developed, and our life-world experiences, which lead us in different directions. We may have different positions when we occupy different roles: As a writing teacher using the network I have different responsibilities and obligations to students than I would have as a LISTSERV moderator or as a web site developer.

Personally, I tend to float in the lower right section of the rhetorical/ethical grid, with Paulo Freire and Iris Marion Young and, to a lesser extent, with Kenneth Burke: strong inclination toward the situated and the communitarian, but sympathetic to the postmodern critique and (with Irigaray) positing difference as a fundamental principle. My position is that problems are best worked out in terms of a situated and kairotic rhetorical ethics, which grants ethical authority to local practice and the conventions of particular communities, which accounts for the specific nature of the electronic medium, and which invokes a discourse ethic that is relatively pluralistic in its constitution and heuristic and rhetorical in its methodology. [T]he sources of this discourse ethic can be found in various postmodern ethical systems: critical and feminist ethics, liberation communitarian ethics, and casuistic rhetorical ethics. Politically, this position can certainly be viewed as leftist, but it differs sharply from the political postures advocated by groups such as the Electronic Frontier Foundation, which promotes network policies based on legal principles of Enlightenment liberalism. Attempts to settle issues invoking some grand metanarrative of the self or of Universal Principles alone (e.g., Habermas) are not likely to address either the pluralistic nature of electronic communities or the situated nature of writing acts and so will be unlikely to settle the sorts of practical problems that are now arising on the networks.

Occupy the border, and be ready to move, nomadically, when necessary. At some level, *phronesis*, or practical judgment, is required to do what is necessary and just. As a writer or writing teacher, you have to recognize that your rhetorical action of taking a position involves an authority and responsibility and, yes, a power that *cannot* be evaded or redistributed. What you can do is use that power wisely and responsibly—or try. As Foucault (1987) says, the power cannot be dissolved "in the utopia of a perfectly transparent communication" (p. 18); rather, we can work to develop in ourselves and to encourage our students to develop "the rules of law, the techniques of management, and also the ethics, the *ethos*, the practice of self, which would allow these games of power to be played with a minimum of domination" (p. 18).

The message here is that teachers should not try to control their students' writing, but that in their effort to avoid control they should not give up their role as interveners, their role as teachers of commitment. Of course, writing teachers should not presume to dictate absolutely what ethical writing practices consist of in every given case, but they should also not surrender their responsibility to promote ethical writing practices. Foucault (1984e) himself warns against the danger of opposing consensuality: "Perhaps one must not be for consensuality, but one must be against nonconsensuality" (p. 379). The danger of consensuality is that it can threaten difference, but the far greater danger is that in the fear of obliterating difference we become advocates of nonconsensuality—that is, we fail to recognize the importance of common ground, of judgment, of commitment, of responsibility. As Faigley (1992) says,

> Bringing ethics into rhetoric is not a matter of collapsing spectacular diversity into universal truth. Neither is ethics only a matter of radical questioning of what aspires to be regarded as truth. Lyotard insists that ethics is also the obligation of rhetoric. It is accepting responsibility for judgment. (p. 239)

A postmodern rhetorical ethic, of course, opposes any effort to insist on the absolute dominance of rules (what Faigley refers to as "collapsing spectacular diversity" into universalist hegemony), but in this opposition it does not satisfy itself *only* with celebrating the absence of rules (in the kind of "radical questioning" that can lead to uncommitted pluralism or relativism). A committed postmodern rhetorical perspective focuses, rather, on the "invention of rules" (Steuerman, 1992, p. 112); *what* rules—and how constituted?

CASE 1: NEWSGROUP INTERVENTION, OR BEING COMMITTED WITHOUT BEING A BULLY

Let us start with some actual cases and use them to work toward an understanding of what I mean by the praxis of critical rhetorical ethics. Several years ago, a graduate teaching assistant at Purdue set up an electronic newsgroup for his technical writing class discussions. Because of my interest in the course, I read the postings on that newsgroup from the beginning of the class.

During the first week of class, a male computer science student posted a list of jokes, some of them anatomically and sexually explicit, about what he called "dumb blondes" (by which he meant women with blonde hair). The posting was written assuming as implied audience a set of like-minded male fraternity brothers who could appreciate a good joke about dumb women, but in fact there were several women, and several blonde women, in the class. Before any of them had a chance to post, they were already typecast on the newsgroup as occupying a subject position as ignorant sexual toys. If you are familiar with newsgroups, then you know that this sort of thing is fairly common, if not endemic. However, this was not a typical newsgroup, as it was tied to a nonvirtual academic community.

So what do *you* do if you are the teacher or a lurking faculty member reading this newsgroup? To write or not to write?—that is the question.

I will tell you what I did, *not* because I think it represents *the right answer*, but because it represents *the answer that was right for me at that time in those circumstances*. I predict that many will disagree with the response I took to the case, deciding either that I made a big deal out of nothing, was too impulsive, or lacked political conviction. Yet the right or wrong of the ultimate decision is not the issue here, and I do not think that rhetorical ethics answers that question anyway. What I am interested in, and what I hope to illustrate, is *the process of rhetorically interrogating the writing situation from a rhetorical ethical standpoint*.

I applied a kind of ethical stasis procedure to the problem. The first determination was "How important is this?" Is a list of jokes something to get angry about, or should I simply do what Howard Rheingold and others in the Electronic Frontier Foundation say is the right thing to do in cases of electronic boorishness: Ignore it? That was an easy question for me: I see the electronic network as an ethical frontier where it is particularly important for people (and maybe especially people with some measure of power) to step forward and actively participate in constructing the network as a place that encourages open discussion from diverse participants. Yes, it is worth countering messages that dominate and exclude, that make the network a hostile place.

OK, this kind of stupidity should be opposed, but the second question is: Should *I* be the one to do it? I contemplated my several selves. As a lurker and an outsider (in the class), I wondered if I had the *right* to say anything. As a faculty member at Purdue, as a teacher, and as a concerned electronic citizen, I wondered if I had the *obligation* to say something. Like a good sophist I found compelling arguments for both sides. I decided to wait (sophists end up doing a lot of waiting, the problem with having an overdeveloped sense of irony) to see if the teacher or others in the class would do anything, thinking that my position as an outsider and possibly an intruder made my *ethos* in the matter suspect. Clearly it would be preferable if the teacher responded, or the women in the class. Being a white male faculty member further disabled me: Would this be an unfair use of power? The big faculty bully coming in to lay the law down to students and a graduate teaching assistant? Or worse, white knight syndrome—that is, hero knight saving damsel in distress—not roles I coveted.

Could this constitute interference on my part with the teacher's authority in the class? (I decided that this would not be a particular problem with *this* teacher, as he and I had participated on each other's class discussions before. It would be with others.) Could my intruding in the group create a chilling effect on the discussion? (Well, actually, I did want to have a chilling effect on blonde jokes.)

Partly my response to the case was situated in the material fact that this was a newsgroup rather than a LISTSERV or other more private electronic forum. A newsgroup is a relatively public forum (it does not have a subscribed membership as such). It is a more free-wheeling forum. Its membership is not closed or private. Given its more public nature, I would say that comments from those outside the class are far more appropriate than they would be on a LISTSERV class group where I might be an invited member.

I waited two days, but since no one else responded to the jokes, I decided to.

Part of figuring out *whether* to become involved is related to deliberations about *what* to say and *how*. How do I construct myself and my relations with the others in the newsgroup? Do I identify myself as a Purdue faculty member—or simply respond as a reader? Do I give a long and elaborate apology, post a rude flame, or give a short personal reaction?

I finally posted a two-sentence remark that did not identify me as a faculty member, saying in effect that I thought the jokes were not harmless fun, but were rather an instance of promoting an unfair stereotype. I said that the jokes were offensive and "demeaning" and that others might think so, too, particularly women.

At this point two things happened, one of them predictable, one of them perhaps not. In response to my implied advice to "get a sense of audience," the student replied back with a post that said, in effect, "get a sense of humor." (I decided to let that one pass—but I was also relieved: I need not have worried about intimidating anyone with my writing.) Then, a woman in the class wrote to me privately thanking me for saying something because it encouraged her to post something to the newsgroup, which she did a day later, telling the joke poster that his message made the class environment less comfortable for her. After this point, there was no further response or discussion of the issue on the newsgroup, and no further blonde jokes. Discussion moved in other directions.

My guess about this incident is that the computer science student had learned a style of locker-room conversation from his male peers that was also probably reinforced on the mostly male technology newsgroups he inhabited. He carried this style into a forum where there were women (surprise), and he did not think carefully enough about a basic rhetorical/ethical principle—"know your readers, and respect them"—or else he just did not care. Should his email account be revoked? Of course not. Should he be ignored? No, because ignoring such acts constitutes tacit approval of them. Should he be challenged? Yes, I strongly believe so. Here is an instance that points up the difference between ludic postmodernism (which would have a hard time justifying any such intervention) and the postmodern *commitment*, which I am advocating—which is not "rule bound," but which does make some attempt to construct a negotiated position considering the competing ethical principles and rules that comprise the situation.

Should I have spoken at all? Am I guilty in this instance of what Spivak (1988) cautions against as an act of imperialism: white men saving women from other men? Well, perhaps. But then I am a white man. What am I supposed to do? Silence is tacit approval, collusion; speech is imperialism. Take your pick.

To see this as an either-or choice is to simplify the rhetoric of the scene. Rhetoric points out in the first instance that there are different ways to speak and different forms of silence. The *how* is complicated. Looking at the scene from a rhetorical frame (something Spivak does not do) can be helpful here. There is a way in which effecting political action/change in this scenario calls for a man speaking to other men. Would the oppressor males even hear the lone female student voice? Cannot a man speaking to other men make some difference here? It might perhaps take someone from within the oppressor group to effect the change—or at least to serve as a catalyst for eventual change. The oppressor group will not see or hear the subaltern speaking. As a stage in a process of change it might require an insider "speaking for" the subaltern. Spivak dismisses such a subject position out of hand (in her critique of Foucault, for instance). But I am suggesting here that such a subject position might serve a pragmatic purpose, might in fact be required as a stage in a process of change.

Case 2: Free Speech on the Listserv Group

In the early 1990s, Paul Trummel was infamous on Listserv groups in rhetoric and professional writing for distributing an online publication, Contra Cabal, in which he excoriated a rhetoric/writing doctoral program he was formerly enrolled in. He accused administrators at the university of gross malfeasance and the faculty of drunkenness. He argued that this program trampled on his rights as a student—and has continued to threaten his right to free speech, by which Trummel meant his right to distribute electronic attacks on the program.

The ethical issue of interest to me is not Trummel's grievance against his former program, but rather his insistence on posting CONTRA CABAL to numerous electronic groups in rhetoric and professional writing, even though these groups have made it clear to Trummel that they are not interested in his postings and do not see CONTRA CABAL as relevant to the themes and topics defining the groups. However, if a particular LISTSERV group does not exercise an editorial screening of messages—and many do not—then there is nothing from preventing Trummel's postings from going out to all members of the list. Trummel can be refused as a subscriber, but he can still post to these lists.

A consensus that seems to be emerging on the nets and in discussions of network freedoms is that indiscriminate "mondo posting" is unethical and should be discouraged, if not disallowed. The "Yahweh is God" message, which went out to thousands of lists in 1993, is one example. An advertisement for replacements for the pentium chip (posted in 1994) is yet another. Generic messages, advertisements, lists of jokes, and off-topic stupidities waste bandwidth—and are clear examples of unethical mondo posting.

Do Trummel's postings fall into the same category? From one viewpoint, they are slanderous and unsupported attacks that damage the reputation of a university. However, Trummel casts these attacks in the form of a political questioning of an entire set of academic and institutional practices, representing them as a set of secret and powerful efforts to defraud students and taxpayers. Trummel's postings are not "mondo" in one sense, they are directed specifically at rhetoric and writing groups.

CONTRA CABAL is clearly unwanted on most of these groups, and the question is: What should the response to this be? Some LISTSERV administrators complained to the systems administrators of the university to which Trummel transferred to see if his activities violated that university's acceptable use policy. (Apparently they did not because the university was unwilling to act in the matter.) Other LISTSERV owners wrote Trummel personal messages asking for his cooperation: In one case, the manager said that Trummel could certainly advertise CONTRA CABAL on the group, but she asked him to please stop posting it directly to the group. None of these avenues effected any change: In 1994 and 1995, Trummel continued to post CONTRA CABAL.

The rhetorical and pragmatic viewpoint I am developing here would not begin by invoking a rights First Principle—such as "free speech" or "the good of the community"—to be applied algorithmically as a formula to solve the problem; rather, it would begin by looking at the rhetorical and technological circumstances of the case. It is not possible for LISTSERV listowners to stop Trummel from posting to their lists unless they are willing to implement an editorial screening procedure. Personally, then, I would advise LISTSERV owners to balance the furor over and inconvenience of Trummel's postings versus the trouble involved in setting up editorial screening. Editorial screening of messages will also have the side-effect of changing the personality and dynamic of the list: No matter how quickly the editor works, the spontaneity of postings will be lost.

How much trouble is Trummel? That is a question that can only be answered in terms of specific lists. Trummel posts to several lists of which I am a member: His postings might amount to one per month per list, but the postings by other members protesting his postings frequently quadruple that. (There are no doubt numerous personal postings to the LISTSERV moderator as well; see Howard, 1992, 1993.) LISTSERV managers have to balance the trouble of Trummel's presence against the trouble of ridding the list of CONTRA CABAL.

The response to the question of what to do is also determined by one's particular role in the case. A LISTSERV manager has a certain obligation to the members of the list: to serve their interests. He or she also has some obligation to protect innocent parties from unwarranted attacks. (Legally, of course, the LISTSERV manager might also incur some liability for libel.) Yet the issue for any LISTSERV manager in this case is to balance the needs of the many and the few. What if the desires of the many threaten the legitimate rights of a single member?

What if I am not the LISTSERV manager, but am simply a participant on the list? Should I write a message of complaint or stew quietly at home? At what point do I decide that I should write something? And if I decide to write, to whom? If Trummel's lengthy messages cost me download time, then I am likely to take a far less tolerant view of unwanted mail. I could write a private note of complaint to the list manager or to the systems administrator at Trummel's home university. I could write a private note to Trummel. I could write a public note to the entire list. (I could write a book using the Trummel case as a case involving the ethics of electronic writing.) The choice of whether to write, and where to post it, is part of the rhetorical ethics of the situation. What if I am a faculty member at the university that Trummel attacks? Should I defend my program and myself against his unfair assaults? Or would such an act simply call further attention to Trummel's slander—and perhaps even serve to instantiate his self-proclaimed status as victim? Is ignoring him the best policy?

There are different writing roles and relations vis-à-vis Trummel and distinct members of particular lists. A "one-size-fits-all" approach to network ethics fails to account for the distinctness of these particular roles and relations. A rhetorical ethics *begins* with this distinctness, with the differences in rhetorical situations—that is, with the particular alignment of sites, writers, and readers.

Complaining to the list compounds Trummel's off-topic postings by adding more off-topic postings. Writing Trummel himself would seem to be a reasonable ethical starting place, as the one LISTSERV manager realized. That response gives Trummel the benefit of the doubt and asks for cooperation (rather than merely demanding it or expecting it). It is a response that assumes a dialogic ethic of caring, that is, it respects the personhood of the

Other, essentially by turning the Other (the interloper, the intruder, the irritant on the list) into a Thou. The strategy apparently did not work in this instance, but that is not to criticize the strategy as a starting point for rhetorical/ethical inquiry.

CASE 3: HARASSMENT IN CYBERSPACE

Let us up the stakes a bit. Let us look at what might be the most famous piece of electronic student writing ever: the story written by University of Michigan student Jake Baker and posted on January 9, 1995, on the Internet newsgroup alt.sex.stories. Baker's story described in vivid detail the torture of a woman with a hot curling iron and her mutilation and sodomization while gagged to a chair (Lewis, 1995a).

The story itself would have probably passed into oblivion, but for two extenuating circumstances: (a) the woman's name in the story was the same as that of a University of Michigan woman who was in one of Baker's classes—and her name was actually used in the subject line of the posting; and (b) in an email exchange with a virtual friend, "Arthur Gonda" (whom authorities were unable to locate), Baker said that he was ready to "really" do what he describes in the story, that writing about it was not good enough anymore. These two points moved the story out of the realm of fiction—at least as interpreted by the courts and by the University.

For this offense, Baker was jailed and held without bond for 29 days, charged with the federal crime of transporting threatening material across state lines (because Internet postings cross state lines). He was also expelled by the University of Michigan (Branam, 1995; Branam & Bridgeforth, 1995).

After Baker was released from jail, the government dropped the charges related to his writing the fantasy story on alt.sex.stories. The prosecution's case against Baker will be based entirely on the e-mail exchange with "Arthur Gonda," which, they will argue, constitutes a specific threat (Cain, 1995).

Baker's defense lawyer tried to present his client's position in these terms: Big Government and a Powerful State University are in collusion to censor the individual expression of an individual. Baker's lawyer calls the story and the email exchange with Gonda as simply a "fantasy," the act of an "active imagination." The ACLU and the Electronic Frontier Foundation are defending Baker's writing as a type "acceptable under the community standards" of alt.sex.stories (Lewis, 1995a; see Shade, 1996).

We can look at Baker's original act in another light. Catharine MacKinnon sees his rape/torture fantasy as *itself* an act of aggression and intimidation against women as well as against a particular woman (the University of Michigan student whose name Baker used in the story). From this view, the law's entrance is not designed to stifle an individual, but rather to protect a student who is also a member of a group that has been historically marginalized.

The legal judgment in such a case has to consider the degree of harm involved (in this case, how much aggression? how much intimidation? how likely is the suspect to commit the acts he describes in his story?). Aside from that determination, MacKinnon would argue that the act itself constitutes a harm: The posting is not "only words," but is itself an act of aggression. The First Amendment is not a First Principle: It is rather one principle to be balanced against many others and to be applied with consideration of the particular circumstances that comprise each and every case (including the relational status of the parties involved).

I believe, based on what I have read about the case, that Jake Baker did not understand the complexity of his writing situation—and this is an indictment of an educational system that never helped him to understand it. Baker did not understand that writing has *force,* that it has the capacity for harm, and that his writing mattered in a way that he could not imagine *for readers* that he did not think about. He is rhetorically and ethically illiterate, although maybe after his 29 days in jail that is no longer true.

A mitigating circumstance in the case is that the story he wrote was well within the standards of the electronic community he inhabited. Part of his ethical illiteracy, however, was not recognizing that such a newsgroup is not a closed and isolated community. What he posts there is public: It can be read by people not in agreement with community standards; it can be copied and reposted in communities with a less tolerant view of his writing; and it has real implications for people outside that closed community. This failure to be aware of "audience," his failure to understand the rhetorical dynamic of the technology; and his blurring of the fiction/nonfiction boundary are all components of his particular brand of ethical illiteracy. (In fact, the Internet and the World Wide Web may blow apart the entire notion of a selective audience; although electronic documents might *address* one or another particular audience, in terms of distribution potential, anyone with Internet access could potentially read the posting. In other words, the vast distribution potential of the electronic network poses something of a problem for print notions of audience, which tend to be more exclusive constructs tied to more limited distribution potential.)

In *Only Words* (1993), Catharine MacKinnon points out that the First Amendment was originally developed to protect the powerless from the powerful (the U.S. government or Government generally). Increasingly, the First Amendment is being used in defense of continued discrimination against the less powerful, as both MacKinnon (1993) and Stanley Fish (1994) have noted.

MacKinnon implies that the free speech principle should have built into it a preferential option for the marginalized. That is, it should allow the marginalized, oppressed, or silenced a chance to speak against the majority, the dominant, the hegemonic, but it should not be applied to further discrimination against the marginalized, oppressed, and silenced (p. 39). In any particular case, of course, one has to determine the degree of possible harm to those involved. Usually it is the weaker, the oppressed, and the marginalized who bear the greater burden of risk in such cases—although not always. (Acts of terrorism—for instance, the bombing of the federal building in Oklahoma

City—show quite vividly how any individual or small group can, through an act of ultimate extremity, cause some harm to the more powerful. The futility of such acts, however, is that the terrorist attempt to harm the powerful usually ends up harming individuals while leaving the system of domination intact.) Essentially, MacKinnon is urging us toward a kind of affirmative action ethic in such cases.

The other implication—more mine than that of MacKinnon—is that the First Amendment is not a rule, but a principle to be applied heuristically. Yes, it represents a deeply held value—but in any given case it may conflict with other deeply held values, in which case some kind of careful judgment is necessary. (MacKinnon argues that in cases such as Baker's, the First and Fourteenth Amendment, which mandates equal protection for all citizens, ought to be placed in a kind of binary tension—although the courts typically do not do that.)

The Electronic Frontier Foundation takes the position that all network discourse should absolutely be protected by the First Amendment (Rheingold, 1994). I consider this as a presumptive position, but they advocate it as an absolute rule. To advocate such a position is, to me, to underestimate the power of an individual's use of language, its capacity to do harm, and, especially on electronic networks, its capacity to shut down communities. Yes, the presumption lies with the individual because the individual is usually the weaker entity, but the controversy of the position I am advocating is that it says that in some situations it is the community that needs protection (Riddle, 1990).

There is yet another position that says that teachers are responsible for promoting, and maybe even legislating, ethical writing practices. Should not respect for audience be a requirement of "good" writing?

TOWARD A CRITICAL RHETORICAL ETHICS

So what are we left with? Where is this critical rhetorical ethics of internetworked writing?

Developing his theory out of the framework of liberation theology (a frame of reference he shares in common with Paulo Freire, 1970/1993), Enrique Dussel (1988) draws a sharp distinction between the legal and the ethical. He sees the legal as representing the minimal norms of behavior established by the consensus of society. These norms are by no means adequate in guiding human action because the consensus of society can be, and often is, oppressive, stultifying, unfair, and just plain wrong. Do not look for morality in inscribed law, in the social order, in majority consensus, or in governmental strictures and institutions (Althusser, 1971). Dussel, instead, argues the necessity of developing an ethical/moral counterauthority, which is necessary to critique social norms and conventions as established through law. This counterauthority is, for Dussel, a higher authority—and no resistance is possible without the existence of some ethic that provides criteria for challenging the domination of law. Maybe U.S. law grants you the right to read your employees' private email and electronic files under the aegis of system administration. That does not mean it is ethical to do so.

The cyberwriter must negotiate a position among at least two competing frames. One frame, the legal frame, derives chiefly from a world of modernist assumptions and print expectations. In saying this I do not want to suggest that this world has no value, is impotent, or can be safely ignored—hardly. This set of assumptions constantly insists on affirming its value and its power (if not domination) over the realm of electronic discourse. It is a force to be reckoned with.

Yet it might also be a force to be resisted. A second frame, what I am constructing as a rhetorical ethics for internetworked writing, is a set of assumptions and practices that constitute a kind of cyberspace common law whose contours we can only dimly see. To negotiate this second frame, I am suggesting that the cyberwriter must develop a *critical rhetoric* that is also an ethical rhetoric. I am calling for an electronic ethics, a critical positioning that serves as a place for critique of the dominant legal realm. But what is meant by a *critical* rhetorical ethic (Porter, 1997)?

When I use the term *critical* I am invoking Horkheimer's distinction between critical and traditional theory. Horkheimer (1972) criticizes the traditional approach to theory because it *decontextualizes* (Feenberg, 1991), it separates knowledge and action in the pursuit of knowledge for its own sake. Critical theory, on the contrary, articulates a liberatory aim—"emancipation from slavery" (Horkheimer, 1972, p. 246). Critical theory *contextualizes*, considering the relationship of the individual to the society in terms of a situated web of relations, including historical factors, the system of labor and production involved, and the class implications of such relations (Deetz, 1994; Geuss, 1981; Hoy & McCarthy, 1994; Luke, 1991; Poster, 1989; Simons & Billig, 1994).

In invoking the term *critical* I am invoking a particular tradition—that of the Frankfurt School—but Patricia Sullivan and I (Porter, 1996; Porter & Sullivan, 1996; Sullivan & Porter, 1997) are moving toward a version of *critical* that merges more conventional critical theory with several other areas: the social postmodernism of Foucault (1979, 1984a, 1984b), postmodern geography (e.g., Soja, 1989; Sullivan & Porter, 1993a), and feminist theory, especially as regards methodology (e.g., Lather, 1991; Stanley, 1990a, 1990b; Stanley & Wise, 1990) and ethics (e.g., Benhabib, 1992; Card, 1991; Young, 1990). Of course, "critical" does not simply mean attack, negative commentary, undermining, or ludic deconstruction of, but critical in the sense of critical reflection on, challenge, and then positive action. It is closer to what Lather (1992), Ebert (1991), and others have referred to as "resistance postmodernism." It may, in fact, be more appropriately described as "postcritical" (Lather, 1992; see also Luke & Gore, 1992).

This rhetorical ethics borrows from diverse theoretical positions, including critical Marxism (Feenberg, 1991), feminist communicative action (Benhabib, 1992; Young, 1990), and rhetorical casuistry (Jonsen & Toulmin, 1988). This ethic focuses particularly on ethics as situated praxis, as central to human relations, and as particularly sensitive to the role of rhetoric (and language) in determining ethical action. It is an ethic of situated relations, that is, of situated rhetorical relations and of composing processes. It draws on both feminist and neopragmatic discussions in focusing on ethics as a rhetorical process and on rhetoric as an ethical process of constituting relations given the spatial and material conditions that define power.

The realm of cyberspace can become a realm of domination, unless writers are willing to adopt the role of "cyborgs" (Haraway, 1991) and resist the rigid formulation of legal realities. Timothy Luke (1991) calls for a critical theory that "must be essentially reflective, reflexive, and ironic rather than positive, objective, and methodologically formalistic" (p. 21). The goal of this critical theory is "human emancipation." Luke uses this theory to articulate a critical agenda for cyberwriters:

> Power in hyperreality derives from controlling the means of simulation, dominating the codes of representation, and managing the signs of meaning that constitute what hyperreality is taken as being at any particular time. By setting the limits of what is hyperreal, and therefore at least temporarily "real," the managers of media, movements, and displays can set agendas, determine loyalties, frame conflicts, and limit challenges to the prevailing organization of what is or is not taken as being real. (p. 20)

The central aim of critical rhetoric is clear: It posits as its goals liberation of the oppressed (Dussel, 1988; Freire, 1970/1993); improved communicative relations (Habermas, 1990); the improvement of social conditions, including the quality of work life (Zuboff, 1988); and, in academic contexts, the improvement of learning conditions. For cyberwriters, this critical rhetoric translates into an ethic of advocacy for one's electronic audiences—users, browsers, electronic readers—that aims to improve their conditions of learning and ease their conditions of oppression or dominance within institutional settings (see Cushman, 1996; Kleinman, 1995).

Critical rhetorical ethics has several emphases: First, the dominant views of writing have tended to see writing as mainly or only a product, that is, a text that floats in cyberspace. The first step in taking a critical point of view is to recognize writing as a social action with legal and ethical implications. It is a doing as well as a making. So critical rhetoric is conscious of how acts of writing constitute acts of *power* within an already dynamic set of power relations; it raises the political and ethical questions pertaining to the nature of power relations: To whose benefit am I working/writing? To whose advantage/disadvantage?

Second, critical theory reminds us that writing resides in an economic system (Eagleton, 1976). Writing is a commodity, and U.S. law seems to be increasingly viewing writing, and especially internetworked cyberwriting, as *private property to be protected,* rather than as *social resource to be shared and distributed* and, therefore, as a *means of enabling broader, more active citizen participation.*

Third, critical theory points to the necessity of "rhetoricizing" one's writing actions, understanding them as situated in a network of human relations involving multiple writers and multiple readers engaged in overlapping communities of discourse. It is politically dangerous to hold to a simplified view of the writing process as I Writer producing My Text to be read by You Reader. It is dangerous, especially in cyberspace writing, to presume that your writing will have a limited and well-defined audience. (When Jake Baker was indicted for posting a pornographic story on the newsgroup alt.sex.stories, his story was "appropriate" given the standards and conventions of that newsgroup; however, what he failed to appreciate was that a newsgroup, although existing as a community with its own standards, is not totally sealed off from other communities, including the U.S. legal community.)

"Being rhetorical" means attending to situated contextual features that form, maintain, and constrain discursive relations, such as examining one's position at a participant in a network of relations in which the goals of liberation and freedom must be situationally negotiated through discourse; recognizing the role of power in human relations (including but by no means limited to the variables of class, gender, sexual orientation, race, economics, and labor status); and acknowledging the role of technologies, institutions, disciplines, and other modes of system and production in constituting and constraining human relations.

The Second Cybernetic and Writing the Interface

On a daily basis, the cyberwriter will be working at the point of the technological interface, working *at* the interface and also working *at the design* of interface. By *interface* I am not talking about screen design elements only (trash cans and such), but rather larger space (what Foucault, 1986b, might call a heterotopia) in which the screen intersects with situated uses of the technology in the classroom, community, and workplace—a contextualized interface, in other words.

Unlike the rationalist and systems-oriented approach, a critical approach to cyberwriting is against viewing computer technology in a detached, decontextualized way and in favor of seeing technology as created by, situated in, and constitutive of basic human relations. This critical view of technology is affiliated with the so-called "second cybernetic," a philosophical movement in computer theory that "looks at the world [and technology] from the standpoint of the involved subject rather than from that of the external observer" (Feenberg, 1991, p. 106; see also Johnson-Eilola, 1995; Lyytinen, 1992; Suchman, 1987; Winograd, 1995; Winograd & Flores, 1986). It sees technology not as abstracted or decontextualized systems, but rather as involving real people using human-designed machines for situated purposes.

Andrew Feenberg (1991) is one of the leading theorists of this second cybernetic. Feenberg's "critical theory of technology" aims to counter the modernist notion of technology that ends up installing in technology "the values and interests of ruling classes and elites" (p. 14). Far from seeing technology as a neutral tool (which the rationalist supposes) or as inherently bad (which the Romantic "substantist" supposes), Feenberg argues for viewing the tool in its context design and use. He rejects the decontextualizing move of High Theory and philosophy toward formal abstraction and offers instead the contextualizing move of critical theory, which historicizes, situates, and personalizes technology: "Critical theory shatters the illusion [of neutrality] by recovering the lost contexts and developing a historically concrete understanding of technology" (p. 181). (For a fuller discussion of Feenberg's critical theory, see Sullivan and Porter, 1997. Chap. 5.)

Feenberg's theory is affirmed by Zuboff's (1988) distinction between uses of technology that "informate" versus those that "automate." Automation "displace[s] the human presence" (p. 10) by computerizing activities in a way that either eliminates the human presence altogether or reduces it to a lesser status (cognitively, institutionally) in some production process. However, computer technology that "informates" enhances the status of the human presence in the production process, perhaps by engaging people in new ways or by allowing them to collect new types of information or in some cases actually producing a new "quality of information" (p. 10). Informating "sets into motion a series of dynamics that will ultimately reconfigure the nature of work and the social relationships that organize productive activity" (p. 10–11). Thus, Zuboff's distinction calls attention to the importance of social relations in network space. She says that better relations, enhanced status for workers, should be the primary goal of technology applications in the workplace (i.e., as opposed to reducing worker status or eliminating workers altogether). Zuboff's goal of informating provides a criterion for cyberwriters who are developing interface designs and web sites.

Selfe and Selfe's (1994) study of "The Politics of the Interface" is an example of research that applies critical theory directly to interface design. Their study articulates a clear agenda for technological change in the direction of liberating users. They notice, for instance, that the Macintosh interface, which represents the virtual world in terms of a desktop metaphor, presents "reality as framed in the perspective of modern capitalism, thus, orienting technology along an existing axis of class privilege" (p. 486). Furthermore, they note how this metaphor aligns with "the axes of class, race, and gender" (p. 487). Entry in this interface signals to users that they are entering a certain world, and that to attain the power that this world represents requires adopting the "values of white, male, middle- and upper-class professionals" (p. 487). The hypothesis that Selfe and Selfe develop is that computer interfaces are not neutral, but assert cultural value and in so doing practice a power.

Selfe and Selfe are speaking to teachers, but their call applies to cyberwriters as well: They want teachers and writers to move in the direction of influencing the design of computer spaces, certainly the design of the screen, but also the design of computer classrooms, workspaces, and other technological arrangements. In this respect, their political agenda instantiates the proactive goals of the second cybernetic, which calls for more active advocacy of users (see Johnson-Eilola, 1996; Kleinman, 1995; Mirel, 1996). A critical rhetorical ethic calls for writers to take a direct stand in constructing a less oppressive and more liberated electronic network.

REFERENCES

Althusser, Louis. (1971). Ideology and ideological state apparatuses. In Louis Althusser, *Lenin and philosophy and other essays* (B. Brewster, Trans.). New York: Monthly Review Press.

Benhabib, Seyla. (1992). *Situating the self: Gender, community and postmodernism in contemporary ethics*. New York: Routledge.

Branam, Judson. (1995, February 3). U-M expelling student for Internet fantasy. *The Ann Arbor News*, pp. A1, A14.

Branam, Judson, & Bridgeforth, Arthur, Jr. (1995, February 10). Internet writer arrested. *The Ann Arbor News*, pp. A1, A12.

Cain, Stephen. (1995, March 16). Grand jury sets new indictments against writer. *The Ann Arbor News*, pp. A1, A18.

Card, Claudia. (Ed.). (1991). *Feminist ethics*. Lawrence: University Press of Kansas.

Cushman, Ellen. (1996). The rhetorician as an agent of social change. *College Composition and Communication, 47*, 7–28.

Deetz, Stanley. (1994). The new politics of the workplace: Ideology and other unobtrusive controls. In Herbert W. Simons & Michael Billig (Eds.), *After postmodernism: Reconstructing ideology critique* (pp. 172–199). London: Sage.

Dussel, Enrique. (1988). *Ethics and community* (Robert R. Barr, Trans.). Maryknoll, NY: Orbis Books.

Eagleton, Terry. (1976). *Marxism and literary criticism*. Berkeley: University of California Press.

Ebert, Teresa L. (1991). The "difference" of postmodern feminism. *College English, 53*, 886–904.

Faigley, Lester. (1992). *Fragments of rationality: Postmodernity and the subject of composition*. Pittsburgh: University of Pittsburgh Press.

Feenberg, Andrew. (1991). *Critical theory of technology*. New York: Oxford University Press.

Fish, Stanley. (1994). *There's no such thing as free speech, and it's a good thing, too*. New York: Oxford University Press.

Foucault, Michel. (1979). *Discipline and punish: The birth of the prison* (Alan Sheridan, Trans.). New York: Vintage.

Foucault, Michel. (1984a). Panopticism. In Paul Rabinow (Ed.), *The Foucault reader* (pp. 206–13) New York: Pantheon.

Foucault, Michel. (1984b). Space, knowledge, and power. In P. Rabinow (Ed.), *The Foucault reader* (pp. 239–256). New York: Pantheon.

Foucault, Michel. (1984c). Politics and ethics: An interview. In Paul Rabinow (Ed.), *The Foucault Reader* (pp. 373–380). New York: Pantheon.

Foucault, Michel. (1986). Of other spaces. *Diacritics, 16*, 22–27.

Foucault, Michel. (1987). The ethic of care for the self as a practice of freedom (J. D. Gauthier, S. J., Trans.). In James Bernauer & David Rasmussen (Eds.), *The final Foucault* (pp. 1–20). Cambridge, MA: MIT Press.

Freire, Paulo. (1993). *Pedagogy of the oppressed* (Rev. ed., Myra Bergman Ramos, Trans.). New York: Continuum. (Original work published in 1970).

Geuss, Raymond. (1981). *The idea of a critical theory: Habermas and the Frankfurt school*. Cambridge, UK: Cambridge University Press.

Habermas, Jürgen. (1990). *Moral consciousness and communicative action* (Christian Lenhardt & Shierry Weber Nicholsen, Trans.). Cambridge, MA: MIT Press.

Haraway, Donna. (1991). *Simians, cyborgs, and women: The reinvention of nature*. New York: Routledge.

Horkheimer, Max. (1972). *Critical theory: Selected essays* (Matthew J. O'Connell & others, Trans.), New York: Herder and Herder.

Howard, Tharon W. (1992). *The rhetoric of electronic communities*. Unpublished doctoral dissertation, Purdue University, West Lafayette, IN.

Howard, Tharon W., (1993, April). *E-mail ethics: Confessions of a listowner*. Paper presented at the Conference on College Composition and Communication, San Diego. CA.

Hoy, David Couzens, & McCarthy, Thomas. (1994). *Critical theory*. Cambridge, MA: Blackwell.

Johnson-Eilola, Johndan. (1995, March). *Little machines: Rearticulating hypertext users*. Paper presented at Conference on College Composition and Communication, Washington, DC.

Johnson-Eilola, Johndan. (1996, March). *Out of bounds: The politics of technology*. Paper presented at Conference on College Composition and Communication, Milwaukee, WI.

Jonsen, Albert R., & Toulmin, Stephen. (1988). *The abuse of casuistry: A history of moral reasoning*. Berkeley; University of California Press.

Kleinman, Neil. (1995). Don't fence me in: Copyright, property, technology. *Readerly/Writerly Texts, 3*, 9–50.

Lather, Patti. (1991). *Getting smart: Feminist research and pedagogy with/in the postmodern*. New York: Routledge.

Lather, Patti. (1992). Post-critical pedagogies: A feminist reading. In Carmen Luke & Jennifer Gore (Eds.), *Feminisms and critical pedagogy* (pp. 120–137). New York: Routledge.

Lewis, Peter H. (1995a, February 11). Writer arrested after sending violent fiction over Internet. *New York Times*, p. 10.

Luke, Carmen, & Gore, Jennifer. (Eds.). (1992). *Feminisms and critical pedagogy*. New York: Routledge.

Luke, Timothy W. (1991). Touring hyperreality: Critical theory confronts informational society. In Philip Wexler (Ed.), *Critical theory now* (pp. 1–26). London: The Falmer Press.

Lyotard, Jean-François, & Thébaud, Jean-Loup. (1985). *Just gaming* (W. Godzich, Trans.). Minneapolis: University of Minnesota Press.

Lyytinen, Kalle. (1992). Information systems and critical theory. In Mats Alvesson & Hugh Willmott (Eds.), *Critical management studies* (pp. 159–180). London: Sage.

MacKinnon, Catharine A. (1993). *Only words*. Cambridge, MA: Harvard University Press.

Mirel, Barbara. (1996, March). *Writing for problem-solving aspects of computer literacy: Theories to guide practice*. Paper presented at Conference on College Composition and Communication, Milwaukee. WI.

Porter, James E. (1996, February). *Professional writing as postmodern work: Toward a postmodern/critical rhetoric*. Paper presented at Business and Technical Writing Lecture, Department of English, University of Wisconsin-Milwaukee, Milwaukee, WI.

Porter, James E. (1997). Legal realities and ethical hyperrealities: A critical approach toward cyberwriting. In Stuart C. Selber (Ed.), *Computers and technical communication: Pedagogical and programmatic perspectives*. Greenwich, CT: Ablex.

Porter, James E., & Sullivan, Patricia. (1996). Working across methodological interfaces: The study of computers and writing in the workplace. In Patricia Sullivan & Jennie Dautermann (Eds.), *Electronic literacies in the workplace: Technologies of writing* (pp. 294–322). Urbana, IL: NCTE and Computers and Composition.

Poster, Mark. (1989). *Critical theory and poststructuralism: In search of a context*. Ithaca, NY: Cornell University Press.

Rheingold, Howard. (1994, April 5). Why censoring cyberspace is futile. *San Francisco Examiner*, p. 27.

Riddle, Michael H. (1990). *The electronic pamphlet – computer bulletin boards and the law*. <http://www.eff.org/pub/Legal/bbs_and_law.paper>

Selfe, Cynthia L., & Selfe, Richard J., Jr. (1994). The politics of the interface: Power and its exercise in electronic contact zones. *College Composition and Communicate, 45*, 480–504.

Shade, Leslie Regan. (1996). Is there free speech on the net? Censorship in the global information infrastructure. In Rob Shields (Ed.), *Cultures of Internet: Virtual spaces, real histories, living bodies* (pp. 11–32). London: Sage.

Simons, Herbert W., & Billig, Michael. (1994). *After postmodernism: Reconstructing ideology critique*. London: Sage.

Soja, Edward W. (1989). *Postmodern geographies: The reassertion of space in critical social theory*. London: Verso.

Spivak, Gayatri Chakrovorty. (1988). Can the subaltern speak? In Cary Nelson & Lawrence Grossberg (Eds.), *Marxism and the interpretation of culture* (pp. 271–313). Chicago: University of Illinois at Chicago Press.

Stanley, Liz. (Ed.). (1990a). *Feminist praxis: Research, theory, and epistemology in feminist sociology*. London: Routledge.

Stanley, Liz. (1990b). Feminist praxis and the academic mode of production: An editorial introduction. In Liz Stanley (Ed.), *Feminist praxis: Research, theory, and epistemology in feminist sociology* (pp. 3–19). London: Routledge.

Stanley, Liz, & Wise, Sue. (1990). Method, methodology and epistemology in feminist research processes. In Liz Stanley (Ed.), *Feminist praxis: Research, theory and epistemology in feminist sociology* (pp. 20–60). London: Routledge.

Steuerman, Emilia. (1992). Habermas vs. Lyotard: Modernity vs. postmodernity? In Andrew Benjamin (Ed.), *Judging Lyotard* (pp. 99–118). London: Routledge.

Suchman, Lucy A. (1987). *Plans and situated actions: The problem of human-machine communication*. Cambridge, UK: Cambridge University Press.

Sullivan, Patricia A., & Porter, James E. (1993). Remapping curricular geography: Professional writing in/and English. *Journal of Business and Technical Communication, 7*, 389–422.

Sullivan, Patricia, & Porter, James E. (1997). *Opening spaces: Writing technologies and critical research practices*. Greenwich, CT: Ablex.

Winograd, Terry, & Flores, C. Fernando. (1986). *Understanding computers and cognition: A new foundation for design*. Norwood, NJ: Ablex.

Winograd, Terry. (1995). Heidegger and the design of computer systems. In Andrew Feenberg & Alastair Hannay (Eds.), *Technology and the politics of knowledge* (pp. 108–27). Bloomington: Indiana University Press.

Young, Iris Marion. (1990). *Justice and the politics of difference*. Princeton, NJ: Princeton University Press.

Zuboff, Shoshana. (1988). *In the age of the smart machine: The future of work and power.* New York: Basic Books.

ADDITIONAL READINGS

Atwill, Janet M. "Instituting the Art of Rhetoric: Theory, Practice, and Productive Knowledge in Interpretations of Aristotle's *Rhetoric*." In *Rethinking the History of Rhetoric: Multidisciplinary Essays on the Rhetorical Tradition*, edited by Takis Poulakos, 91–118. Boulder, CO: Westview Press, 1993.

Brown Stuart C. "Rhetoric, Ethical Codes, and the Revival of Ethos in Publications Management." In *Publications Management: Essays for Professional Communicators*, edited by O. Jane Allen and Lynn H. Deming, 189–200. Amityville, NY: Baywood, 1994.

Caher, John M. "Technical Documentation and Legal Liability." *Journal of Technical Writing and Communication* 25 (1995): 5–10.

Cicero. *De Oratore, Book I*, chapters II–VI, XIV–XV. Translated by E.W. Sutton and H. Rackham. Edited by Patricia Bizzell and Bruce Herzberg, *The Rhetorical Tradition*. 98–99, 290–92. 2nd ed. Boston: Bedford/St. Martins, 2001.

Clark, Gregory. "Ethics in Technical Communication: A Rhetorical Perspective." *IEEE Transaction on Professional Communication* 30, no. 3 (1987): 190–95.

Dombrowski, Paul. "Can Ethics Be Technologized? Lessons from *Challenger*; Philosophy and Rhetoric." *IEEE Transactions on Professional Communication* 38, no. 3 (1995): 146–50.

———. "Challenger and the Social Contingency of Meaning: Two Lessons for the Technical Communication Classroom." *Technical Communication Quarterly* 1, no. 3 (1992): 73–86.

———. *Ethics in Technical Communication*. Boston: Longman, 2000.

Dragga, Sam. "Ethical Intercultural Technical Communication: Looking through the Lens of Confucian Ethics." *Technical Communication Quarterly* 8, no. 4 (1999): 365–81.

———. "A Question of Ethics: Lessons from Technical Communicators on the Job." *Technical Communication Quarterly* 6, no. 2 (1997): 3–29.

Dragga, Sam, and Dan Voss. "Cruel Pies: The Inhumanity of Technical Illustrations." *Technical Communication* 48, no. 3 (2001): 265–74.

Faber, Brenton. "Gen/Ethics? Organizational Ethics and Student and Instructor Conflicts in Workplace Training." *Technical Communication Quarterly* 10, no. 3 (2001): 291–318.

———. "Intuitive Ethics: Understanding and Critiquing the Role of Intuition in Ethical Decisions." *Technical Communication Quarterly* 8, no. 2 (1999): 189–202.

Garver, Eugene. "Teaching Writing and Teaching Virtue." *Journal of Business Communication* 22, no. 1 (1985): 51–73.

Gates, Rosemary L. "Understanding Writing as an Art: Classical Rhetoric and the Corporate Context." *Technical Writing Teacher* 17, no. 1 (1990): 50–60.

Grabil, Jeffrey, and Michele Simmons. "Producing Citizens: Toward a Critical Rhetoric of Risk Communication." *Technical Communication Quarterly* 7 (1998): 415–42.

Gurak, Laura J. *Persuasion and Privacy in Cyberspace: The Online Protests over Lotus Marketplace and the Clipper Chip*. New Haven, CT: Yale U.P, 1997.

Herndl, Carl G. "Teaching Discourse and Reproducing Culture: A Critique of Research and Pedagogy in Professional and Non-Academic Writing." *College Composition and Communication* 44 (1993): 349–63.

Herrington, TyAnna K. "Ethics and Graphic Design: A Rhetorical Analysis of the Document Design in the Report of the Department of the Treasury on the Bureau of Alcohol, Tobacco, and Firearms Investigation of Vernon Wayne Howell, also Known as David Koresh." *IEEE Transactions on Professional Communication* 38, no. 3 (1995): 151–57.

Katz, Steven. "Aristotle's Rhetoric, Hitler's Program, and the Ideological Problem of Praxis, Power and Professional Discourse." *Journal of Business and Technical Communication* 7 (1993): 37–62.

———. "The Ethic of Expediency: Classical Rhetoric, Technology, and the Holocaust." *College English* 54, no. 3 (1992): 255–72.

Kynell, Teresa C., and Wendy Krieg Stone. *Scenarios for Technical Communication*. Boston: Allyn & Bacon, 1999.

Miller, Thomas P. "Treating Professional Writing as Social Praxis." *Journal of Advanced Composition*, 11, no. 1 (1991): 57–72.

Ornatowski, Cezar M. "Between Efficiency and Politics: Rhetoric and Ethics in Technical Writing." *Technical Communication Quarterly* 1, no. 1 (1992): 91–103.

Rentz, Kathyrn C., and Mary Beth Debs. "Language and Corporate Values: Teaching Ethics in Business Writing Courses." *Journal of Business Communication* 24, no. 3 (1987): 37–48.

Sims, Brenda. "Linking Ethics and Language in the Technical Communication Classroom." *Technical Communication Quarterly* 2, no. 3 (1993): 285–300.

Smith, Howard T., and Henrietta Nickels Shirk. "The Perils of Defective Documentation: Preparing Business and Technical Communicators to Avoid Products Liability." *Journal of Business and Technical Communication* 10, no. 2 (1996): 187–202.

Stone, Mary Specker. "In Search of Patient Agency in the Rhetoric of Diabetes Care." *Technical Communication Quarterly* 6, no. 2 (1997): 201–17.

Sullivan, Dale. "Political-Ethical Implications of Defining Technical Communication as a Practice." *Journal of Advanced Composition* 10, no. 2 (1990): 375–86.

Sullivan, Dale, and Michael S. Martin. "Habit Formation and Story Telling: A Theory for Guiding Ethical Action." *Technical Communication Quarterly* 10, no. 3 (2001): 251–72.

Tillery, Denise. "Power, Language, and Professional Choices: A Hermeneutic Approach to Teaching Technical Communication." *Technical Communication Quarterly* 10, no. 1 (2001): 97–116.

Tyler, Lisa. "Ecological Disaster and Rhetorical Response: Exxon's Communications in the Wake of the *Valdez* Spill." *Journal of Business and Technical Communication* 6 (1992): 149–71.

Walzer, Arthur E. "The Ethics of False Implicature in Technical and Professional Writing Courses." *Journal of Technical Writing and Communication* 19, no. 2 (1989): 149–60.

Wells, Susan. "Jürgen Habermas, Communicative Competence, and the Teaching of Technical Discourse." In *Theory in the Classroom*, edited by Cary Nelson, 245–69. Champaign, IL: U of Illinois P, 1986.

Whitburn, Merrill. "The Ideal Orator and Literary Critic as Technical Communicators: An Emerging Revolution in English Departments." In *Essays on Classical Rhetoric and Modern Discourse*, edited by Robert J. Connors, Lisa S. Ede, and Andrea Lunsford, 226–47. Carbondale and Edwardsville, IL: Southern Illinois UP, 1984.

CHAPTER FOUR

Following User-Centered Design Practices

Chapter Four: Introduction

In "Not Just for Idiots Anymore," the third chapter of *User-Centered Technology*, an NCTE award-winning book written to help readers understand users, technical communication, and the user-centered design process, Robert R. Johnson tells a story about how a team of technical communicators from the University of Washington helped the city of Seattle solve a traffic problem by studying drivers instead of traffic. The point he makes is that the engineers who had been working on the problem prior to the technical communicators had been collecting data about traffic patterns and focusing on the artifacts, but they had lost sight of the fact that the data and those artifacts all involved people.

Johnson tells this story to encourage technical communicators to include users as "active participant[s] in the social order that designs, develops, and implements technologies" (64). His story and conclusion are relevant for technical communication classrooms for several reasons, not the least of which is the fact that many of your students will come from engineering and other technical backgrounds and may well come into your class with a perspective similar to that of the traffic engineers in Seattle. They will most likely want to solve problems by gathering data and using quantitative techniques, and they will have the impulse to look for answers that provide templates, formulas, and grids that they can overlay and apply in many situations. As a result, they will find it difficult, at first, to understand that they will need to study situations and the people in them in order to find the most effective and efficient responses to problems that involve people.

One of the essential points that teachers of technical communication need to make early on is that the writing (or designing) that their students will do will be done for others to use. Thus, if students desire to be successful (and they do), they need to think about the people who will use what they write/design and the ways in which those artifacts will be used. Understanding and, if at all possible, involving the users in the design process will help to ensure success.

In this chapter, you will learn about information design and the centrality of user-centered practice. Beginning with the most basic critical question (what is information design?) and concluding with a demonstration of the implications for corporations when such user-centered design is employed, you will learn that the writer or designer's goal involves meeting needs, enhancing others' ability to "understand, learn, use or retrieve information" (Schriver, 320). Focusing on users is a fundamental principle that underlies most technological innovation and problem solving, and, once they understand this principle and develop strategies for its use, technical communicators have the potential to add value to any project or operation by offering their expertise as both designers and project leaders.

WORKS CITED

Johnson, Robert R. "Not Just for Idiots Anymore." In *User-Centered Technology*. Albany: SUNY Press, 1998. 43–67.

Schriver, Karen. "Document Design from 1980 to 1989: Challenges that Remain." *Technical Communication* 36, no. 4 (1989): 316–31.

14 *What Is Information Design?*

JANICE C. REDISH

In this short, informative piece, Redish, a former director of the Information Design Center and one of the foremost usability experts in the country, defines information design *as both the "overall process of developing a successful document" and the presentation of information on page and screen (p. 212 in this volume). In addition, she offers a model of the information design process and a brief history of the term* information design, *focusing on its roots in the Document Design Project. Finally, she outlines the significance of information design for technical communicators in the future, focusing on page and Web design and single sourcing, a concept that involves a database and chunks of information that may be used many times for many different purposes, saving time and money. In so doing, she emphasizes an essential point about technical communicators: they don't just create information for information's sake; they design and present information to* people to be used, *and, as a result, they need to focus on learning about and understanding those users.*

Introduction

STC's Special Interest Group on Information Design was founded in 1997. A scant 3 years later, it has over 2,700 members. That astonishing and rapid growth is testimony to the widespread interest in the topic and is deeply gratifying to those of us who have thought of ourselves as information designers for many years.

What do those 2,700 SIG members mean by *information design*? As Beth Mazur says about plain language in her article in this issue, "Ask 10 people and you'll get 10 different answers."

In part, the differences in those answers may reflect the backgrounds of the people answering the question. Information design, like many other aspects of technical communication, draws on many research disciplines and many fields of practice, including anthropology and ethnography,

From *Technical Communication* 47, no. 2 (2000): 163–66.

architecture, graphic design, human factors and cognitive psychology, instructional design and instructional technology, linguistics, organizational psychology, rhetoric, typography, and usability.

The Two Meanings of Information Design

In part, the differences in definitions may reflect an ambiguity between using *design* in a very broad sense and, at the same time, in a narrower sense (see Redish 1999). I and—I suspect—many others within the Information Design SIG use *information design*, perhaps at different times, to mean

1. The overall process of developing a successful document
2. The way the information is presented on the page or screen (layout, typography, color, and so forth)

Using the same term for the whole and a part of that whole violates a guideline of good writing, but the fact is that the term *information design* means both. (A little later in this commentary, I briefly describe a historical reason for this dual usage, at least within the North American technical communication community.)

Information Design as the Overall Process

My definition of *document design* or *information design* has always been, first and foremost, the "whole." Information design is what we do to develop a document (or communication) that works for its users. Working for its users means that the people who must or want to use the information can

- Find what they need
- Understand what they find
- Use what they understand appropriately

This definition comes with two additional points that information designers must always remember:

- Most of the time, most users of functional information are using that information to reach a personal goal—to answer a question or to complete a task.
- The users, not the information designer, decide how much time and effort to spend trying to find and understand the information they need.

To develop a successful document (or any other type of product, such as a Web site, software application, or hardware device) requires a process that starts with understanding what you are trying to achieve, who will use it, how they will use it, and so on.

When I drew a model (flowchart, job aid) for that process in 1978, I called it the "document design process." Today it might well be called the "information design process." The model has been updated many times over the years based on experience, conversations with colleagues and clients, and changes that make it more appropriate for different media, but many characteristics have remained through all the permutations of the model, especially:

- The importance of the planning questions and of the front-end analysis
- The role of iterative evaluation
- The interaction and equal importance of writing and presentation (the other, narrower, meaning of information design)
- The fact that the specific guidelines that one uses depend on the answers to the planning questions (That is, there is no one best design for all situations.)

Figure 1 is an example of a recent version of this model.

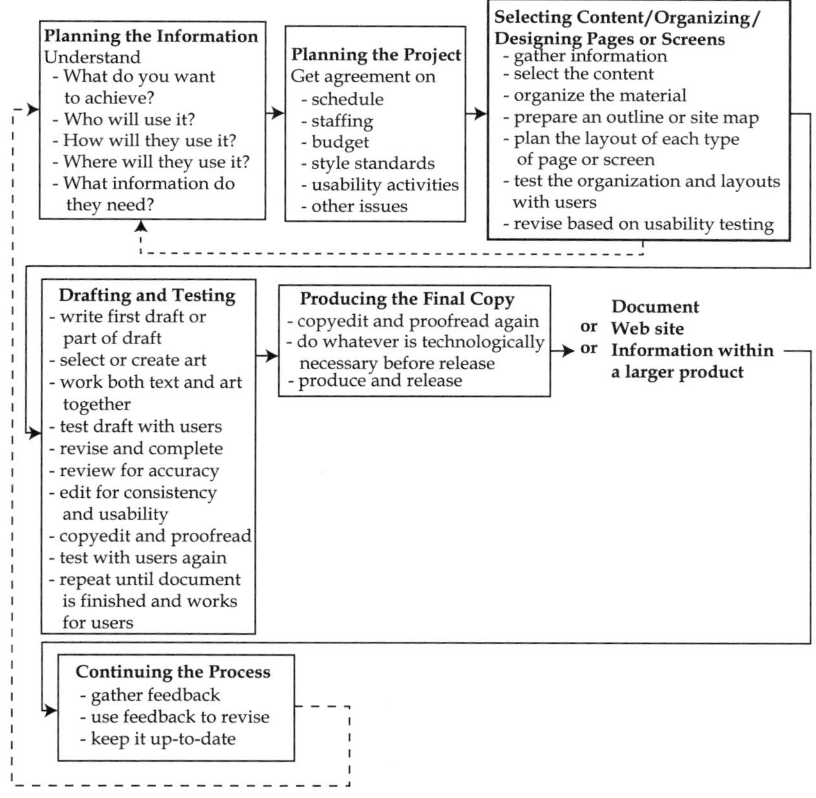

FIGURE 1 *A model of the information design process. This is a visual of information design in the broad sense of doing what is necessary to develop information that works for users. The dotted arrows indicate that the process is iterative, not strictly linear. A dotted arrow should also connect the Drafting and Testing box back to the box on Selecting Content/Organizing/Designing Pages or Screens. Model © 1999, Janice C. Redish, based on versions of a similar model developed between 1978 and 1999 at the American Institutes Research and at Redish & Associates, Inc.*

Information Design as the Presentation on Page or Screen

Information design in the narrower meaning of the way the information is presented on the page or screen is a part of the larger information design process. In this sense, information design encompasses layout, typography, color, relationship between words and pictures, and so forth.

The two meanings of information design are intertwined. Clear presentation on the page or screen is critical. However, the presentation that works for users is not just a matter of aesthetics. The best presentation for a specific communication depends on the situation—on the answers to the planning questions that the broader definition makes us think through.

Information design on the level of page or screen also depends on doing a good job of other parts of the broader process, such as selecting the right content and organizing so users can find what they need quickly. Information design as whole and as part must work together.

A Bit of History

How did I (and others) come to use *information design* in both the broad and narrow meanings? I can think of two reasons:

- Many STC people come to information design from a background in rhetoric and technical communication, which take the broad view, stressing users, content, organization, and writing, as well as presentation.
- The U.S. federal government funded a broad-view project and called it the Document Design Project.

For an excellent treatise on the first of these reasons, read Karen Schriver's *Dynamics in Document Design* (1997). I elaborate a bit here on the second reason because many readers of *Technical Communication*, especially those who have joined the field recently, may be unaware of this history.

The Document Design Project

My own involvement in the field that I have on different occasions called "document design," "information design," "plain language," and "technical communication" began in the late 1970s. The National Institute of Education (NIE), which was then part of the U.S. Department of Education, funded a project to find out why most public documents are difficult to use and to find out what could be done to make them better. The group at NIE named the project they were asking for the Document Design Project.

NIE was clearly not concerned only with the layout of public documents. By "document design," they meant the entire process of developing the document. In fact, because they were primarily linguists and reading specialists, they were most concerned with the content, organization, and writing of the documents.

My colleagues and I at the American Institutes for Research (AIR), a not-for-profit research firm in Washington, DC, wrote the winning proposal to conduct the Document Design Project for NIE. We did that in collaboration with Carnegie Mellon University and the New York information design firm of Siegel & Gale.

The Document Design Center and the Communications Design Center

A year into the project (1979), we at AIR expanded the project into the Document Design Center, which I directed through the 1980s. The project staff at Carnegie Mellon University expanded their part of the project into the Communications Design Center. We both used "Design" in our Centers' names in part to reflect the continuity of the original project. Both Centers practiced information design in both the broad and narrow meanings. That is, we followed the model in Figure 1 on all projects, and we paid as much attention to page or screen design as we did to writing.

Karen Schriver was part of the Communications Design Center (CDC), and the projects described in her book carry on the dual meaning of information design that was a hallmark of the CDC. When Susan Kleimann became director of the Document Design Center in 1993, she renamed it the Information Design Center—still with the dual meaning of both whole and part.

From 1979 to 1989, through its newsletter, *Simply Stated,* the Document Design Center reached about 18,000 people 10 times a year, espousing the process of document design in the broad sense; and the process with its name was picked up by many people who were and are part of STC. Document design or information design in the narrower sense of presentation on page or screen was always a necessary but not sufficient aspect of the process that the Document Design Center and the Communications Design Center used in their work.

Plain Language as Another Term for Information Design—In the Broad Meaning as Overall Process

A side note (related to Beth Mazur's article in this issue): We also used the term "plain language" primarily in the same broad meaning. As I have written elsewhere (1985, 1996, 1999), a document in plain language is one that works for its users. To develop a document that works for its users requires the entire process shown in Figure 1, not just a few guidelines for sentences and words.

The Importance of Information Design in Both Meanings in the Future

As technical communicators, we do all the parts of the process that I show in Figure 1. We may specialize or call on colleagues who specialize in helping us with aspects of the process, such as user and task analysis, usability evaluations, copyediting, and proofreading. If we think of ourselves as primarily "word" people, we may call on others to collaborate with us on the "design" (here, design in the more narrow meaning of page or screen layout, typography, and so forth)—or vice versa, if we think of ourselves as primarily "visual" people, we may rely more on colleagues to review our writing.

However, we are all going to need to understand both information and design and how they relate to each other even more in the future. Whichever way you have come to technical communication, I urge you to spend time learning the aspects you feel least comfortable with now. At least two critical trends in technical communication require us to think even more about information design. They are

- The Web, which requires us to make information even more visual than in other media
- Single-sourcing, in which technical communicators prepare information that can be reused in different formats

Information Design for the Web

The Web requires information design in the broad sense of the entire process described in Figure 1. We must not let excitement over technical possibilities or the super-rapid pace of development eliminate the front end of the process. To develop a successful Web site, you must first consider the planning questions in the process, select the relevant content, and organize it into an appropriate hierarchy for ease of navigating quickly to the right place.

The Web also requires information design in the narrower sense of paying great attention to the mix of text and pictures and to presentation on the screen. Technical communicators know that for information on a page to be accessible, it must be chunked into small pieces, and the different page elements (such as headings, instructions, notes, screen shots) have to be clearly visible, separable, and easily identified. That's even more true on the screen where the amount of space available is smaller, where reading from the screen is slower and more difficult than from paper, where people have come to expect less text and more visuals. Learning to turn text into visual presentations (lists, tables, maps, pictures, fragments) is one of the most important skills for a technical communicator turned Web designer.

Single-Sourcing—Planning Information for Multiple Uses

Single-sourcing means creating a database of pieces of information (chunks of content) that can be used in different situations. The mantra of single-sourcing is "Write once, use many times." The goals of single-sourcing are to save time and money; to ensure consistency and accuracy; and to allow technical communicators to spend more time on aspects of developing information that have perhaps been neglected, such as user and task analysis, content, and evaluation.

Although developing Web pages brings writing and page/screen design closer together, single-sourcing separates them. The content resides in the database, sometimes tagged with conditions that indicate that one version of the content is for paper and another for online help, or that one version is for Model 35 and another for Model 36, or that one version is for novices and another for experts. The formatting for different outputs (information design in the narrower sense) is contained in document definitions. A document definition indicates, for example, the font, size, placement, and color of each level of heading for that particular type of output (paper, online help file, PDF file, Web page, and so forth).

Despite this separation of writing and page/screen design, anyone planning on single-sourcing must pay close attention to information design in both the broad and narrow meanings. First, whether assembling a document from pieces in a database or writing the document from scratch, the technical communicator must start from the beginning of the information design process (information design in the broad sense as in Figure 1), understanding the business goals, the users, the ways users will work with the documents, and so on. Second, successful single-sourcing requires highly structured documents in which the writing style and the output formats have been carefully planned. (Schriver [1997, pages 341–357] describes how to plan the output format based on a detailed analysis of the types of content in the document.) Technical communicators who work in a single-sourcing system, even though they may not determine the output format for their documents, need to know what those formats are, and technical communicators need to be involved in planning them.

REFERENCES

Redish, J. C. 1996. "Defining plain English." *Australian language matters* (July/August/September): 3.

Redish, J. C. 1999. "Document and information design." In *Encyclopedia of electrical and electronics engineering*, J. Webster, ed. New York, NY: John Wiley & Sons, vol. 6, pp. 10–24.

Redish, J. C. 1985. "The plain English movement." In *The English language today: Public attitudes toward the English language*, S. Greenbaum, ed. Elmsford, NY: Pergamon Press, pp. 125–38.

Schriver, K. A. 1997. *Dynamics in document design*. New York, NY: John Wiley & Sons.

15 *Advancing a Vision of Usability*

BARBARA MIREL

Barbara Mirel's essay focuses on the overall process of information design as she makes a case that technical communicators need to assume a leadership role in the information design process. Concentrating on the software industry, which is where many technical communicators will find work, she presents a short case from a hospital that demonstrates the need for "designing for usefulness" *(p. 220 in this volume). Answering questions such as "What is usability?" and outlining the importance of "usefulness" for "complex tasks," she asks both those practitioners in the field and those who teach future members of the field to think more strategically by focusing on both problem solving and enacting new foundations and frameworks (p. 236). Advocating new approaches to task analysis and development processes, Mirel states that it will be these new approaches that will take the usability field forward rather than "simply [having it] continue to run in place" (p. 238).*

A nurse on an acute care hospital floor wheels her medication cart into a patient's room, careful not to jostle the laptop and radio frequency scanner that sit on top of the cart. She parks her cart, taps the icon on the touch screen of the computer that opens the bar code medication program, and logs into the program. She then scans the patient's identification number and, in response, the bar code medication program displays the patient's record—a list of his prescribed drugs for this scheduled medication pass. One by one, the nurse takes the patient's drugs from a cart drawer and scans the bar code of each. As soon as a bar code matches a prescription for this patient ID, the system "bings," marks the drug approved on the screen, and documents the match, presuming it to be an accurate and successful drug administration. All eight medications for this patient "bing" positively. The nurse fills a cup with water, gives it to the patient along with his pills, and closes his record. The process took moments; the right patient got the right drugs at the right time and place; and the nurse moves on.

From *Reshaping Technical Communication*, edited by Barbara Mirel and Rachel Spilka, 165–88. Mahwah, NJ: Lawrence Earlbaum, 2002.

In this situation, the bar code medication software is highly efficient, effective, and usable. The program readily opens to the patient's record; the screen provides quick and easy access to the drug names, times, dosages, and approval markings. The user signs on, then opens and closes the record simply. The functionality for administering and documenting all and only the right drugs seems comprehensive; and, true to its objective, the program guards against human error and assures patient safety.

This usability picture grows dim, however, once patient cases are not textbook perfect. When the slightest deviation occurs, the software frustrates rather than supports nurses in their work. One such case involves a patient who cannot swallow easily so that the nurse needs to crush the pills and mix them with applesauce. This patient has 13 pills scheduled for the morning medication pass. All goes well at first. When scanned, all 13 drugs "bing" positively. The nurse begins feeding the patient the applesauce mixture but the patient is only able to swallow a quarter of it. Now usability takes a nosedive. The nurse has to edit the record documenting the drug administration to undo the automatic entry for successfully giving medications that the program entered for each positive scan. But to edit, the nurse must access the documentation from a centralized patient record system that runs on a different operating system and that interfaces with a different program. The nurse spends 5 minutes logging into the other program, hung up by a painfully slow and underfunded hospital network. Once in the other program, she has to edit each of the 13 medications separately, another time-consuming process. It is exceptionally long because each entry requires overriding the predefined editing options to note that in this unusual case, the patient took some but not all of each pill.

Other cases introduce different complications, each requiring its own set of interactions. One patient, for example, has a tapered dosage, meaning that the nurse must clinically judge the amount to give based on 72-hour-long patterns that she has seen in the patient's pain levels, vital signs, and cumulative prior dosages. The nurse has to gather this information from at least three sources, one within the bar code medication program and two outside of it. Retrieving the necessary information requires many navigation steps and query procedures, but it is only one part of what quickly becomes an excessively difficult task. Most taxing are the actions and memory load required for copying relevant data into one display, arranging it for easy interpretation, and deriving the totals needed for a diagnosis.

These "exceptional cases" are more common in everyday nursing than are the textbook perfect cases. Yet the bar code medication program does not accommodate them readily. The problem is not omission. The bar code medication program has the functionality, features, and interface controls to enable users ultimately to get the information and commands that they need. But nurses are not willing to go through the extensive processes that the program and other related information systems demand. They object to the many scattered and piecemeal actions required for putting together what to them is a single "chunked" task—for example, analyzing vital sign history. They object to the inordinate amount of time spent working the tool and remembering data. It compromises the efficiency on which they are judged in their performance evaluations, and it takes away from the time that they can spend on the personalized bedside care that motivated them to go into nursing in the first place. Faced with a program at odds with their professional culture, organizational practices, and technology infrastructure, many nurses devise workarounds or cut corners that unintentionally can introduce new risks to patient safety. As a result, poor usability due to a mismatch with actual work practices and needs can truly be a life-and-death matter.

This case with the bar code medication program is not atypical of software design for complex problem solving. Unfortunately, it is not some isolated incident of design gone amiss. What happens in software production contexts to cause this large disconnect between usability in letter-perfect situations and in situations that are messy, conditional, or idiosyncratic? Questions such as this are gaining urgency as software companies increasingly become customer- rather than technology-driven and realize that software must fit the messy realities of users' complex work-in-context. Software development teams often are unsure about what it means to build for this kind of usability or what it should look like. As a result, usability specialists rapidly are being brought onto software projects. However, positive as this trend is, it is not enough to assure a lead role for usability in enhancing the success of a product. To assume and exert leadership, usability specialists need to be agents of change, a role they have not yet assumed in most workplace contexts.

As technical communicators increasingly move into usability roles—in the software industry and elsewhere—they could readily assume this leadership. They are trained, perhaps as are no other specialists in human-computer interaction, in the rhetorical perspectives necessary for effectively matching the media and design of software support to particular audiences, purposes, activities, and contexts. Yet, in many companies usability leadership is sorely lacking.

In this chapter, I argue that as leaders, usability specialists have to introduce a new vision of what it takes to support complex work-in-context, discussed in more detail later as *designing for usefulness*. In particular, if usefulness is to take center stage, a shift is needed in analyzing and designing for complex tasks. This shift involves moving from task- and even user-centered designing to designs centered on use-in-context. Making this shift depends on strong usability leadership because it requires new ways of thinking and doing. Usability leaders have to bring about innovation and change in task analysis, task representations, and development processes.

This chapter examines the vision, approaches, and changes involved in designing for usefulness in one type of environment—contexts that produce software for complex tasks. The bar code medication software mentioned earlier is one such program. Others include programs that support, for example, product planning, analysis of profitability, or allocation of resources. In these environments and for this end of supporting users' complex work, the chapter examines issues relevant to bringing usability leadership to bear on the design and development of the software.

WHAT IS USABILITY?

> "We're user-centered but we're pretty vanilla about it—you know, the usual interface improvements—because of constraints. We figure it's still better than it might have been."
>
> —USABILITY DIRECTOR, BUSINESS-TO-BUSINESS WEB DEVELOPMENT FIRM

Fifteen years ago, Gould and Lewis (1985, p. 300) defined usability, arguing that "any system designed for people to use should be easy to learn (and remember), useful, . . . contain functions people really need in their work, and be easy and pleasant to use." Usability specialists since have elaborated on the qualities identified in this definition, but the scope of what usable programs should do has not changed from this succinct description. Usability, as Gould and Lewis note, involves multiple dimensions—ease of use, ease of learning, pleasantness, and usefulness; all combined, they provide users with a positive work experience. Each dimension is equally necessary for assuring that users seamlessly integrate a program into their ongoing work. All are intricately intertwined. None is independent of the others.

Yet, in many development contexts, a comprehensive vision of interrelated usability dimensions gets broken apart. Each dimension—ease and efficiency of use, learnability, enjoyment, and usefulness—becomes a separate objective. The comprehensive whole becomes a pick list of options. Design and development teams choose to build for some dimensions while neglecting others based on project deadlines, resources, and other constraints (Grudin, 1991). From a pick list perspective, team members are likely to accept without question a rationale for designing the bar code medication program that might go something like the following: The program should read in and display patients' vital signs from other programs. But we do not have the architecture or headcount to build that cross-program integration into this release and ship on time. So we will be user-centered in the interface and provide menu options and buttons that will let users easily access the path that they have to take to get out of our program and into another to get the data that they need.

Despite such expressed user-centered intentions, actual users in context are hardly grateful for such make-do ease of access, and they are hard pressed to find these programs user-centered. Rather, they get exceedingly frustrated with the program. Put simply, it does not do what users want for the work that they have to do.

In these and other similar cases, design choices and rationales are out of sync with users' holistic experiences of usefulness. This phenomenon is one of the core issues that usability leaders must raise and counter. In the midst of doing their work, users experience usability as a component of the total program quality. Designers, by contrast, often treat usability as a set of discrete parts, ready to be traded off without resistance as soon as the "too costly" behemoth rears its head. Cowed by budget or personnel constraints, development teams routinely forgo hard but useful solutions without debate and opt for "vanilla" ease-of-use interface designs such as navigation buttons. They rationalize that by offering improved ease of access at the interface, they are delivering user-centered programs.

Usability leaders must distinguish between ease of use and usefulness. Ease of use involves being able to work the program efficiently and easily, usefulness involves being able to use the program to do one's work-in-context effectively and meaningfully. Stripping usefulness from ease of use and focusing primarily on the latter is an incomplete recipe for usability or user-centeredness.

Tradeoffs are inevitable in design and development, but they require critical assessment and debate (Rosson & Carroll, 1995). They require posing and answering such questions as: Is a sacrificed or neglected capability negotiable from a user's point of view or is it critical to integrated work practices? Is it better in the long run to invest more in development now and release later, than to provide only make-do solutions in order to release now?

To adequately position usability in these debates, strong leaders are needed. They need to overcome teammates' piecemeal notions of usability and show that partial usability is no more favorable to users than partial system performance. To do so, usability leaders need to bring in empirical data on users' needs, practices, and boundaries of tolerance. To build a convincing case from these data, however, leaders first need to lay a groundwork. They need to clearly show how the dimensions of usability are related to each other for a given product and what this relationship implies for software design for complex tasks.

The Primacy of Usefulness for Complex Tasks

> "Requirements are discovered through the contingencies of everyday use."
>
> —Suchman, 1997, p. 56

> "A designer who is thinking, 'how do I decrease the number of keystrokes,' often ends up finding and improving lots of little problems with all these improvements adding up to little. By contrast, a designer who tries to craft an interface that elegantly fits a user doing the task often ends up sidestepping many more problems in one fell swoop by neatly eliminating the task actions in which those problems lived."
>
> —Dayton, quoted in Strong, 1994, p. 17

The ways in which the dimensions of ease of use and usefulness relate to each other vary by product and by the work, users, contexts, and purposes that are supported by the product. In software for complex work, this relationship needs to give primacy to usefulness. Complex tasks characteristically vary with context; the same task is rarely if ever performed the same way twice. In complex tasks the means for performance are not entirely known at the outset. They emerge and become more specified as people explore conditional factors relevant to the task. Knowing what to do next requires coordinating, arranging, and relating relevant factors. Typically, several renditions of acceptable arrangements exist. Similarly, the rules, heuristic strategies, or trials-and-error that people apply lead to processes that allow for several outcomes. Complex tasks, therefore, cannot be formalized into fixed procedures and rules. Programs cannot presuppose rules and map formulaic steps onto program features and commands. Rather, software for complex tasks has to be flexible enough to "lean on" the knowledge and frames of reference that users bring to it and to adapt to a range of situational factors, emergent conditions, goals, and moves (Agre, 1997). Designing for this flexibility and variation in work-in-context is designing for usefulness. For complex tasks, usability leaders need to work with program designers and developers to understand and figure out how to support the range of users' possible approaches in context. Correspondingly, they need to understand the ways in which various configurations of contextual factors and relationships shape the range of actions that are possible and the choices that people make in a given instance. Designing for usefulness assures that the right sets and structures of interactivity will be in place for the right users to perform the right possible actions for the right situations. When software is effectively designed for usefulness, it provides and displays a framework for task performance that is consonant with the goals and situational "markers" that trigger users to conduct their work in specific ways. After this framework is established, making interactivity easy, quick, accessible, understandable, enjoyable, and navigable falls into place. To do otherwise—that is, to address ease of use first without initially assuring usefulness—increases the risk of making the wrong model of a workspace easy to use and, therefore, of little pragmatic value.

Unfortunately, designing for usefulness is usually given short shrift in production contexts. Design teams are prone to jumping prematurely to detailed specifications and ease-of-use concerns. One reason may be competitive pressure. Teams hurry to establish features and operations so that they can get on with coding and usability testing and ship before competitors do. Even if competition were not a factor, however, foregrounding usefulness is more the exception than the rule because it runs counter to several solidly rooted, conventional design practices. These include teams' tendencies (a) to analyze and design for tasks at a low level of detail; (b) to assume a procedural or operational orientation to representing and supporting user tasks; and (c) to exclude usability from the critical junctures in the development cycle in which decisions are made that either leave open or close later design possibilities for usefulness.

Each of these three tendencies is inappropriate and counterproductive for building the support that users need for complex tasks. Each needs to be addressed and redressed by usability leaders. I now turn to new approaches and challenges associated with each.

Designing for Usefulness: Approaches to Task Analysis

> "There is a tremendous difference between designing for function and designing for humans."
>
> —Cooper, 1999, p. 89

> "We're all smart people here. We don't need to go out and do all these studies. We know what to build."
>
> —Chief Technology Officer at a Project Team Meeting

As noted earlier, in software contexts at present, a common approach to analyzing and designing for users' tasks is to break them down to their smallest parts and rules. At this unit level, tasks are the simplest actions that users can handle without going into problem-solving mode and that require no control structure to accomplish (Green, Schiele, & Payne, 1988). By decomposing performance and its rules and resources, analysts can represent users' activity as a hierarchical flow of goal-driven actions and knowledge down to the smallest set of tasks. At this low level of analysis, they can design, specify, and implement corresponding program features and objects. These programs represent users' work by representing its composite parts. The underlying assumption is that the whole of users' activity equals the sum of its parts.

Increasingly, many design teams are resisting a formal decomposition method of task analysis and design (Bever & Holtzblatt, 1998; Kies, Williges, & Rosson, 1998; Rudisill, Lewis, Polson, & McKay, 1996; Wixon & Ramey, 1996). Bever and Holtzblatt (1998), for example, suggest five frameworks for representing contextual inquiry findings that capture relationships among work processes, social roles, environmental dynamics, and physical arrangements. These researchers' representations take the form of workflows, task sequence and goal diagrams, models of artifact use, cultural dynamics models, and physical layouts of the work environment. Yet these and other researchers' representations often end up unintentionally designing for unit tasks. These teams pursue alternate contextual and ethnographic methodologies and represent tasks as interrelated user cases, user profiles, and models of workflows, task sequences, and communications and culture. However, when these teams move from contextual descriptions to object-oriented design and programming, such factors as situational influences, contingencies, and high level conditional interdependencies become too hard to capture in design. Teams end up focusing instead primarily on separate elements of the work, ultimately mapping them in one-to-one fashion to program features and controls. Contextually oriented designers struggle with finding methods to use to move from task descriptions to design without ending up with a focus on discrete, context-free, low level actions (Wood, 1998). As detailed in the next section, it is unlikely that any methodology will achieve this end unless designers first change the framework of the task representations that they compose.

In regard to level of detail in task analysis, usability leaders need to continue to promote a contextual vision and ensure that this vision does not devolve into designing for dissociated low level operations. To do so, they first must reveal why the dynamics of complex tasks necessitate against summing parts to a whole. They then need to compose task representations that do not readily lend themselves to being dissected into elemental actions. This section addresses why summing unit tasks is inappropriate for complex tasks. The next section examines ways to compose task representations.

Regardless of how a unit-level focus occurs, complex tasks can neither be supported nor conducted as a sum of unit parts. Usability leaders need to argue that complex tasks are complex because they are not comprised of well-defined, rule-based, serial steps that cumulatively and predictably sum to the whole of a task. Rather, they are emergent and dynamic. As noted earlier, many components interact with and adapt to one another—cognitive, behavioral, situational, and technological components—creating problem spaces in which a number of moves are possible. Interdependencies across components and unexpected side effects from their interactions make it impossible to sum parts to a whole. At any given point, people choose some moves and not others. These choices reconfigure arrangements between components, setting into play new constraints, interactions, and effects. In computer-supported complex tasks, much of the difficult processing needed for resolving a task or problem has to take place on the screen and be controlled by users rather than going on invisibly "beneath the hood." Users have to process and interact with displayed information to gain the insights needed for transferring knowledge to similar tasks and to shape analysis as they like. Or, another way to view it is that, in complex tasks, users need to learn to fish, not simply be fed the fish.

For example, a marketing analyst for a coffee manufacturer, analyzing the potential of a new product, needs to view, process, and interact with the data directly. To break into the high-end espresso market with a new product, the analyst examines as many markets, espresso products, and attributes of products as is deemed relevant to the company's goals and analyzes as many as available technical tools and cognitive limits permit. Looking at these products, the analyst moves back and forth between big picture and detailed ("drill-down") views. The analyst assesses how espresso has fared over past and current quarters in different channels of distribution, regions, and markets, and imposes on the data the analyst's own knowledge of seasonal effects and unexpected market conditions. For different brands and products—including variations in product attributes such as size, packaging, and flavor—20 factors or more might be analyzed, including sales revenue, volume, market share, promotions, and customer demographics and segmentation. The analyst arranges and rearranges the data to find trends, correlations, and two- and three-way causal relationships, and then filters data, brings back part of them, and compares different views. Each time, the analyst gets a different perspective on the lay of the land in the "espresso world." Each path, tangent, and backtracking move helps to clarify the problem, the goal, and ultimately the strategic and tactical decisions. In such complex tasks, instead of people attending temporally to a stable territory and clearly mapped action sequences, they spatially survey an unstable territory of complexity, understand its structure, and repeatedly manipulate arrangements and relationships. All the while, they progressively are reducing uncertainty.

Inherently, complex tasks embody uncertainty. Goals for complex tasks are often broad, vague, and revised as inquiries and insights emerge. Problem spaces are not well bounded. Relevant information may be spread across many problem spaces and resources of knowledge at once. Relevant information, moreover, is conditional, multidimensional, and multiscaled. It takes on different meanings depending on the perspectives that people take, and, in complex tasks, people take several perspectives because they have to account for contingencies and conditional relationships. Courses of action are dynamic and emergent, exploratory and opportunistic. At decision points, people face contending legitimate moves, and within the degrees of freedom that they have, they choose based on situational and subjective criteria. As these traits of complex tasks suggest, the structure of complex work is more a dynamic feedback mode than serial behaviors with clearly defined starting, stopping, and decision rules.

Task analyses and designs that attempt to represent complex tasks as linear, decomposed unit actions and rules misrepresent these tasks. In doing so, they often lead to programs that undercut people's abilities to do their work effectively and productively. For complex tasks to succeed, users must have optimal control over information, perspectives, paths, possible actions, and criteria for choosing. Programs diminish this control when they represent complex tasks as a composite of discrete unit tasks without integrating actions and situational arrangements or without calling forth relationships between resources. Such programs overdetermine interactivity, underestimate the scope of people's work, underrepresent important contextual dynamics, and underdevelop the strategies and interactions that people use for getting "from here to there," monitoring progress, and managing emerging knowledge. Usability leaders need to argue against developing programs that model complex work through a built-in prepackaging of means and ends. Ideally, their arguments are based on empirical data from user sites.

Some usability professionals may blame a piecemeal approach to design on the dominance of engineering in a production context and its object-oriented programming. Admittedly, a low-level, unit orientation is needed once product development moves to the stages of detailed specifications and programming. Object-oriented programming does require attributing elemental properties and events to low-level objects, be they things or acts. Yet the constraints of object-oriented programming and design do not force usability specialists or designers down a slippery slope of designing principally for discrete low-level actions and operations. In fact, object orientation emphasizes giving users support in taking whatever actions and order of actions that they want while maintaining a focus on the primary task (Pancake, 1995). Equally important to properties and events in object technology is the need to carefully construct appropriate relationships within and across classes of objects.

The meaning of complex tasks and task actions lies in relationships. If object-oriented designers and programmers lapse into assuming that whole task meanings are deduced from the sum of properties inherent in component objects, this assumption is not intrinsic to object technology. Object orientation does not foreclose a software team's opportunities to design for situated tasks and integrated actions.

In fact, constraints inherent in object technology are less an obstacle to maintaining an integrated and situated view of complex work during design than is the composition of task representations. Ultimately, object-oriented designing and programming take shape from the task representations that usability specialists bring to the design table and the interpretations drawn from them.

Usability leaders need to assure that these representations are framed around task structure and the structure of functional relationships and interactions. Framed in this way, task representations provide an organizing structure that signals socially shared repertoires of moves and intentions for a given type of problem in a particular time, place, and set of circumstances. Structurally framed task representations are spatial. They emphasize the arrangements and patterns of actions, rules, objects, and interactions that cannot be severed from one another and distilled into discrete parts if users are to see in the program their notions of their work and conduct it seamlessly. Current contextual models do not guard well enough against this severing and distillation.

Promoting and implementing a structural framework for task representations is likely to meet resistance. Usability leaders are apt to find that this orientation challenges assumptions that many people in a production context have about what it means to support users' tasks.

Designing for Usefulness: Approaches to Supporting and Representing Tasks

> "As developers, we're freaks. Ordinary people don't think like us. Our users don't think like us. We have to learn how they think."
>
> —Vice President of Development in a Software Firm at a Development Group meeting

The preceding sections stressed that conventional models for representing tasks and the software designs derived from them are inadequate for users' complex problem-solving activities. Whether in task models or in resulting interface designs, aiming for a set of prepackaged actions that are tied to precomputed plans does not support users' critical needs for inquiring into open-ended, ill-defined problems. Complex problem solvers need and expect leeway in choosing from available options the best courses of action for their purpose, time, and place, and they need to control the actions that they choose and the information with which they work. To capture and design for the interactive forces in problem solvers' workspace—forces that condition the degrees of freedom and control needed at various points in problem solving—usability leaders need to apply a conceptual framework that encourages and sustains such a view of complex tasks and leads to adequate support for them.

Structural versus Procedural Frameworks for Representing and Supporting Tasks

Software designers and developers may support users' tasks in three main ways. First, they may build in the units and categories of action that move people closer to a solution or goal. Second, they may display the structure of users' tasks and problems. Finally, they may construct some combination of these two approaches, a blend of procedures and structures. Of these possible approaches, the first—building in categories of action and procedures for solution—is more often than not the default position, presumed by most developers and designers to be the most appropriate support for users' tasks. Even when software combines procedural and structural support, procedural support predominates.

As noted earlier, procedural support is typically low level. It rests on building in functions and operations for unit tasks such as search, select, and sort and enabling users to access and execute them through interface commands or direct manipulations. In addition, procedural support includes features and user interface interactions for moving from one program state or mode to another and knowing its allowable interactions. It also includes support for controlling window behaviors and keystrokes and for verifying the contents of a screen display and its history.

Importantly, providing procedural support is appropriate for many tasks. In general, it is advantageous for tasks that are well structured and that have clearly defined goals. In these tasks, because hierarchies of task actions and knowledge are determinate, procedural support is best for helping users readily identify unknowns, find and relate relevant factors, and plainly see their actions in relation to the whole of their task (Rasmussen, Pejtersen, & Goodstein, 1994). A bibliographic program exemplifies tasks that benefit from a procedural emphasis in task representations. Most tasks supported by a bibliographic program have the clear goal of producing a standard reference list or bibliography. The scope, form, and parameters of acceptable entries for authors, titles, and other data are well defined. Users primarily need procedural support to know required entries and their formats, processes for entering data, and shortcuts for reusing data. Conformity to set procedures is necessary for activating the behind-the-scenes "task work" that the program does in order to produce the desired reference list or bibliography.

It is not that procedural representations ignore the structures that occasion user activities, especially representations developed from contextual and ethnographic stances. But it is a matter of emphasis, of figure and ground, of what is dominant and what is in the background. When foregrounded, actions—even contextually grounded actions—lend themselves to dissection into discrete operations. By contrast, structurally framed task representations foreground and underscore the indivisibility of configurations, interactions, and relationships among elements in users' problem and situation workspace.

Structural support has proven most advantageous for open-ended tasks in which processes and strategies emerge during performance and vary by individuals' knowledge, roles, social and domain practices, and organizational resources and constraints (Rasmussen et al., 1994). When workspaces are indeterminate, structural support helps people discover the task components and information that are relevant, construct trials and exploratory paths, and evaluate actions and their effects incrementally.

An example is the nursing task presented earlier involving the rejected applesauce-and-pills mixture. Had the bar code medication program been structurally oriented to the complexity of this work, it would have represented and fostered interface designs that displayed a nurse's workspace as the full range of resources involved in effective patient care during medication, not simply as elements of a medication record required to assure that a drug's barcode and a patient ID match safely. This patient-care workspace would have included medication documentation, a patient's full health record and care plan, and nursing control over indicating whether a drug was administered successfully or not. Structurally, the nurse's workspace would have embodied the opportunity to work at once in several data displays about the patient, possibly with dynamic linking across displays. For example, it would have represented access to data on the patient's condition and opportunities to configure the information as needed so that the nurse could check the potential effects of refused medications. To complete the task, the structure of the workspace would have embodied the relationship between one nurse's experiences with a patient and experiences of nurses on the next shift who need to seamlessly continue the patient's bedside care and medication.

Rasmussen et al. (1994) and Vincente (1999) comprehensively discuss what is needed for framing task representations structurally and spatially. To summarize, these researchers stress that structural representations are not decomposed functions of individual structural elements. Rather, they capture functional relationships and regularities of behaviors associated with various constraints. Representations may consist of a series of displays to capture complex task workspaces and overlapping boundaries. A single display may embody several separate yet related structures, for instance, different graphic representations of the same information for taking multiple perspectives.

The structures highlighted in task representations suggest possibilities for action, define workspace boundaries or constraints, and account for emergence. They capture patterns or regularities in performers' task behaviors for a certain type of complex inquiry and tie them to the work-related features, roles, conditions, and contingencies that shape them. They depict the numerous boundaries that constrain these work activities—organizational, professional, cultural, cognitive, and technological. For example, possible actions for a certain complex inquiry are bounded professionally by the work practices that are deemed acceptable in a given profession. When, in the applesauce-and-pills example, the nurse encountered a representation of work in the interface that had no immediately discernible possibilities for controlling the information documented about the pills, she was pushed to the limits of her professional responsibilities. Professionally acceptable work for her includes fully managing a patient's medication and assuring that the next shift gets accurate information about it, but the technological aspects of her work did not support this professional accountability.

The closer people have to move to the borders of their responsibilities or capabilities because of technological constraints, the more confusion and difficulty they experience in conducting their work (Rasmussen et al., 1994). Structural representations of problem solvers' work-in-context provide powerful renditions of their work because they call attention to all of the boundaries of users' work and show compatibilities, for instance, between professional and technological conditions. These representations make it possible to see if model of work that are built into a program are mismatched with users' social, cognitive and organizational dimensions of their work-in-context. Finally, to do justice to the dynamism of complexity, structural representations have to present both the changes in a workspace during task performance and the adaptations of patterns.

To promote and encourage this structural approach to design, usability leaders may liken structural task representations to genres of performance. Genres are an apt metaphor because they underscore the situated, social, and dynamic nature of complex tasks. Genres are "dynamic rhetorical forms that are developed from actors' responses to recurrent situations and that serve to stabilize experience and give it coherence and meaning" (Berkenkotter & Huckin, 1995, p. 4). They are embedded in social practices, roles, and interactions and signal norms and shared ways of knowing. As such, they fulfill vital functions within professions and institutions. They embrace and evoke a sense of what content is appropriate for a particular purpose and situation at a specific point in time. All of these qualities define complex task performance.

In evoking a genre of performance, a structural representation of a complex task gives people "a template—or organizing structure—for social action" (Orlikowski & Yates, 1994, p. 542). Drawn from users' situated work experiences, spatial and structural representations signal to users that a given complex task is a distinct type of work with associated patterns of action and thought that fulfills a recognized function and purpose within their domain and social and organization context. Without scripting actions into standard steps, structural representations instead organize performance. They suggest or call forth shared performance goals for a given context and circumstance. They reveal possibilities for action and offer performers ample latitude in specific behaviors based on their roles, arrangements of labor, infrastructure constraints, and the like.

Like genres, structural task representations rest on descriptions of recognizable patterns, that is, on the pragmatic patterns of people's work-in-context. Pragmatic patterns of work are different from the patterns that many software developers and interface specialists discuss as either software patterns or human-computer interaction patterns. Software patterns present coding and under-the-hood integration routines that help programmers to achieve such difficult goals as portability or scalability (Coplien & Schmidt, 1995; Gamma, Helm, Johnson, & Vlissides, 1995). Human-computer interaction patterns capture combinations of screen objects, dialogues, window manipulations, and keystrokes that support users' low-level interactions, for instance, combining a filtering mechanism with a list to facilitate finding items in the list (The Pattern Gallery). Software and interface patterns focus at too low a level in design to help much with usefulness.

By showing crucial interactions and arrangements in many aspects of problem solvers' workspaces, pragmatic patterns at once address the situational, cognitive, and technological dynamics that shape people's problem-solving behaviors. That is, these pragmatic patterns express a relationship between a work context, problem, and solution. As Alexander et al. (1977) note, "A pattern describes a problem which occurs over and over again in our environment, and then describes the core of the solution to that problem, in such a way that you can use this solution a million times over, without ever doing it the same way twice" (p. x).

Complex tasks are indeterminate, but they still embody regularities and relationships—genre-like (not context-free) practices and structures used to solve recurring problems. Representations of pragmatic patterns for complex tasks are accurate and complete when they are coherent with the full range of approaches typifying people's work-in-context, when they fully account for relevant systemic interactions, when they logically account for every connection for getting "from here to there," when performance as a whole is seamless, and when patterns have an inner consistency that is true to the internal forces of the system of work (Alexander, 1979).

Making a Case for a Structural Framework

The shift to structurally representing and designing for complex problem solving is a critical change from project teams' habitual assumptions. Implicit in the structural shift is a move from orienting design toward tasks or users' activities—an action emphasis—to work-in-context with an emphasis on the structure of situated work and how it sets and constrains possibilities for action. A structural orientation shifts the focus or unit of analysis to the context of work. This focus, in some ways, resembles the spotlight on the activity system that typifies other contextual orientations, but it differs from the common contextual orientation insofar as it highlights structural relationships in the activity system more than the actions that occur between its components. It highlights interactions between conditions and constraints in problem solvers' interdependent social, organizational, cognitive, and technological contexts of work along with the actions that are made possible by these conditions and constraints. It also emphasizes contextually determined patterns of inquiry for various types of problems. This focus on structural relationships, interactions, and work-in-context patterns encourages the higher level analysis of tasks discussed in the previous section. It also gives form to a socially and cognitively open architecture that "leans on" and trusts in the domain expertise and control that users bring to their complex work (Agre, 1997).

This difference in emphasis—between structure and action—may seem slight, but it is not trivial. Team members may resist this change in orientation, not the least because it does not offer the same closure that procedural orientations do. Usability leaders need to show their teams why and how taking one emphasis or another in task representations matters. They have to stress that how problem solving is modeled affects how designers interpret what problem solvers do and why, and guides how they design for it. Designs created from structural representations are likely to lead to structurally framed interfaces; procedural task representations similarly reproduce themselves in screen displays.

A procedural or structural emphasis moves from task representation to interpretation to interface design, and it ultimately affects users and their work. By and large, a procedural representation, first in a task model and then in an interface design, is interpreted by "readers" as a single act (Rasmussen et al., 1994). No matter how many times someone "reads" the representation, he or she reads it the same way each time and responds with the same standard actions. This single act is appropriate if the program being designed is a bibliographic program. One set of actions is sufficient for entering bibliographic information in a way that produces a desired reference list.

By contrast, a structural representation leads to a multiplicity of interpretations, a far more appropriate interpretation for complex tasks. Each reading and rereading produces many understandings due to the complex of actions that may be realized through the task structure. A structural rendition also limits its own multiplicity. Its form and content trigger people to recognize this construction as a particular genre of performance, and the conventions of the genre themselves set limits on the domain, focus, and actions (Pentland & Rueter, 1994).

In proposing a shift in emphasis from actions to structures in task representations, usability leaders introduce the need to design for flexibility and adaptation. Interfaces alone cannot single-handedly bring about program flexibility or adaptive computing. They can go no farther in evoking genres of performance than the program scope, architecture, and features allow. For example, the bar code medication program discussed earlier frustrates users because its scope is too narrow—safety procedures rather than patient care—and because its architecture lacks the "plumbing" for reading and writing data across multiple programs and platforms.

Usability leaders need to move usability concerns beyond interface design. They must assure that these concerns inform program scope, architecture, and feature lists, as well. To bring usability into these front-end decisions, usability leaders need to induce changes in the processes of the development cycle.

Designing for Usefulness: Approaches to Development Processes

> "Why can't we just design first and think of the problems we're solving later?"
>
> —Market-Facing System Engineer at a Design Team Meeting

Whether software development cycles follow a waterfall, iterative, or extreme programming model (discussed later), they all fit usability into fairly similar phases and roles. Conventionally, usability efforts start after the conclusion of such front-end processes as deciding the optimal product for the market, building a business case and scope for it, and assuring that it is technically and architecturally feasible. Therefore, they occur after or at best concurrent with decisions about product scope and architecture. In addition, before user research findings are brought to the design table, a high proportion of the program features and priorities are also set. Customer input that informs these front-end decisions comes primarily from market researchers, business strategists, and account managers.

Generally, usability specialists enter the development process by conducting user research and task analysis for design. Findings feed the design of interactivity. This design deals largely with user interfaces but in the process also extends to some new choices and refinements of features relevant to users' tasks. After design, in such formal development cycles as the waterfall model (still common in modified form in many organizations), usability efforts that involve direct contact with users often stop for a while. Engineering phases kick in. In these phases, detailed specifications are written, development begins in earnest, and usability assessments with users do not occur until after developers produce an alpha or beta version for usability testing. During the engineering phase, the usability of prototypes or of portions of the program is gauged largely through processes that do not involve user performance, such as expert reviews or heuristic evaluations.

By contrast, in more spiraled, iterative development models, usability specialists often continue to gather user input after initial user research and task analysis. In these development approaches, designing and prototyping often merge. Usability specialists may take evolving prototypes to users for feedback as often as every week. They may elicit feedback on usefulness; more often than not, however, they focus primarily on ease-of-use issues, for example, comparing one design for choices and layouts of interface controls and dialogues to another to find the quickest and most intuitive option. In extreme programming, user participation and partnerships in prototyping processes may supplant the presence of usability specialists (Beck, 1999).

At some point, regardless of the model of development that project teams follow, features and user interfaces freeze and no more changes are made. Often this freeze occurs before usefulness is assured or fully designed for; often, usability experts have little say in the decision. Whether usefulness is assured or not, the focus of usability now turns to running usability tests to assess from users' performance of various tasks how easy and efficient it is to operate the program. In many contexts, usability specialists who conduct usability tests are not the same individuals who conduct the user research and task analysis.

Finally, in the midst of engineering and testing, some teams begin to plan for the next version of the product. Next-version planning, for instance, may run parallel to the beta piloting and usability testing of the current product. Ideally, although rarely the case in reality, usability specialists at this point assess and inform the next version with improvements needed for usefulness while plenty of time is still available to undertake difficult solutions.

As this admittedly simplified overview shows, regardless of development model, at decision points that affect delivering support for usefulness, usability specialists are notably absent. They come into the picture after decisions are made about product scope, architecture, and features. They rarely participate in determining the readiness to freeze, especially to freeze features. And in usability testing, usability specialists focus predominantly and, at times, exclusively on ease-of-use improvements instead of using the opportunity of in-context use in beta sites to gather and bring to the next version empirically based recommendations for improving usefulness.

Giving little heed to usability at these critical junctures in the development cycle is not surprising because designing for usefulness is given little heed in the first place. Without placing high priority on usefulness, project teams overlook the very real consequences of architecture and scope decisions in terms of opening or forever closing later possibilities to support users' actual work-in-context. Usability leaders' efforts to situate usability in front-end development processes and next-version decisions are therefore part and parcel of getting teams to see the significance of usefulness for complex tasks.

Summary

Developing useful software for complex work-in-context requires a program of innovation and change. It needs to start with a view of usability that is somewhat new to many development teams. Teams need to view usability as a holistic experience that, for complex tasks, turns first and foremost on the experience of usefulness. Usability leaders are needed for articulating the primacy of usefulness and for shifting the unit of analysis for design and development from task actions to task structure—to the structural arrangements and relations between people, resources, and contextual conditions for a given task or problem.

Understanding what it takes to design for usefulness goes hand-in-hand with understanding the nature of complex tasks. Complex tasks, by definition, are not linear, rule-driven, or formulaic. Software will not offer useful support for these tasks if its design, as is often the case, presupposes these task traits. Similarly, complex tasks are greater than the sum of their parts; therefore, software will not be useful if its design is based on another common tendency, to decompose work into unit tasks, implement these unit tasks as program operations, and assume that cumulatively these operations total to the whole. Even contextual orientations to task and user analyses, by foregrounding actions, may devolve unintentionally to this focus on elemental actions and produce less than useful programs.

Users find software support for complex tasks useful when it provides them with flexibility, control, and adaptability. The software needs to cue the patterns or genres of performance that are fit for a given type of work, job role, set of situational conditions, and purposes. Software for complex tasks is useful for people's actual work if they are able to pursue the actions that they value from a range of possibilities and tap into and relate various resources relevant to their work purposes. Usefulness also derives from users being able to relate actions to conditional factors, to arrange and configure the resources and conditions of work as they see fit, and to plan as they go based on emergent opportunities and constraints.

Contextual perspectives on user-centered or activity system-centered design embody the goals and spirit of designing for usefulness and make some strides in this direction. However, they neither highlight the distinctive demands and patterns of complex work nor strive to usher in the shift in emphasis that helps guard against design devolving into a procedural focus on discrete low-level tasks.

This shift demands a different view of what lies at the center of analysis and design. Software, usability, and documentation professionals have variously put at the center the technology, users, information, tasks, actions, activity systems, or interactions. Although wildly different from one another in some aspects, all of these "-centricities" have the common theme of highlighting procedures and actions, whether they are the actions that systems perform, that users in context perform, or that users perform via interfaces. The shift that is necessary is one toward highlighting the structure of work-in-context. This focus places attention in analysis and design on a problem in a certain context and on ways in which the problem space evokes various behaviors, knowledge, relationships between people and things, strategies, and rules of thumb. To reinforce a contextual and pragmatic orientation to complex work, task representations for design purposes need to center on the arrangements and configurations of problems and workspaces that cue, condition, and constrain certain socially constructed patterns of performance.

This new orientation requires practical approaches to design that challenge many conventional methods. Design teams need to analyze tasks and design at a higher than unit-task level, focusing on the integrated sets of relations and actions that in users' notions of their work signify a "single task." Designing for usefulness also involves framing task representations around structure rather than action so that they are organized to evoke genres of performance, and it involves changing the points at which usability concerns come into the development cycle. Issues of usefulness need to inform front-end processes of defining scope, architecture, and features, and they need to be brought in early for next-version planning.

Looking Ahead

This program for innovation and change will be a major undertaking. It will be a program for the next decade, not for the next year. I have explored the usability needs of software for complex tasks in order to exemplify initiatives that need to be tackled over time. In sum, these initiatives include:

- Creating, justifying, and disseminating a vision of what it takes to design useful products.

- Bringing about a shift in focus for analyzing user needs for complex problem solving and designing for them.
- Becoming efficacious leaders of usability concerns.

Usability professionals in industry and academia alike have a stake in bringing about the new ideas and practices implicit in these initiatives. Both worlds will strengthen and grow in status if specialists in usability become centrally positioned in front-end decisions and design representations and methodologies. Both worlds will further a shared professional commitment to integrate social and technical systems in ways that support and enhance human initiative, wonder, satisfaction, and ease.

Professionals in industry and academia may have strong interests in furthering these initiatives. However, recognizing that they share these interests does not answer the question of how, if at all, the two worlds might jointly direct their talents and strengths to bring these initiatives to fruition. That is, what are the most important complementary efforts that industry practitioners and academics may make to strengthen and advance the long-term project of placing a top priority on "holistically usable" software?

These efforts have to differ from the usual approaches taken for university-industry partnerships. The usual approaches are mostly about "doing" something together or building bridges for better relationships and more relevance between the worlds. Efforts for usability innovations and changes for the future, by contrast, need to be less about tactical projects and more about strategically defining and enacting new foundations and frameworks. Together, professionals in industry and academia need to define new foundational problems. Purposes of investigations in scholarship and industry projects have to be grounded in seminal problems that are meaningful no matter where one's paycheck comes from. Industry practitioners and academics also need to devise new frameworks for the questions implicit in these problems so that a long-term integrated agenda is apparent. The questions need to call forth contributing roles and inquiries for members of both worlds and embody an integrative sense of how the various parts fit to the whole.

For example, as positive as curricular changes and industry-based workshop courses are for building bridges, there is no class per se that can teach the ability to create a vision of usability and usefulness, to earn and assert leadership, or to make and influence paradigmatic shifts. Similarly, although "collaboratories," hybrid professional institutes, and other cooperative ventures between the two worlds can create important synergies and inculcate vital skills in "speaking different languages," setting up more of them without changing leadership structures on software teams or promulgating a vision is not likely to advance forward-looking usability initiatives any more than existing ventures do today. Finally, although striving for a freer flow of academic research and industry white papers across worlds and to the lay public is good for cross-fertilization, the "solutions" of making academic research more accessible for practitioners or framing industry research in ways that do not compromise its proprietary dimensions beg the question. If the given research is based on assumptions and practices that reinforce approaches that run counter to designing for work-in-context, then a wider dissemination of this research will not directly advance the innovations and change needed for usability initiatives.

To advance these initiatives, mentoring technical communicators to make transitions into expanded career roles and responsibilities is a beginning. This would encourage the mindsets and strategies needed for identifying foundational problems and inquiry frameworks (Anschuetz & Rosenbaum, chapter 9, this volume). And a start has been made in articulating thorny pragmatic problems that require a long-term agenda of investigation in academic research and industry projects alike. Many of them surround the issue of designing usefulness into software for complex-problem solving. Another example is the problem of describing and designing support for learning as well as use in wholly new products for wholly new task domains (Borland, chapter 11, this volume). By focusing on foundational problems and inquiry frameworks, industry and academia will indeed be "doing" something together of great significance. They will be creating new ways of thinking about and expressing the purposes, core investigative areas of the field, and orientations to usability. In doing so, they will be working toward innovating software for greater usefulness and changing the relevant organizational forces of production.

The foundational problems as well as the frameworks, level of detail, and content of the questions still need to be worked out. At present, the main questions that drive inquiries in both academia and industry generally are detached from real-world situations and their underlying large and persistent problems. Academic questions such as "What are the relationships among cognitive, social, and cultural factors in document design?" are framed in ways that do not evoke pragmatic problems. Industry inquiries focus on concrete situations to discover "What do I do on the screen tomorrow?" but often are not tied to an underlying problem. Perhaps the best-trod investigative meeting ground for academic and industry professionals at present has been inquiries into guidelines—handbook strategies and techniques for such questions as "At what points in the development process are particular evaluation methods most useful?" Unfortunately, though, this meeting ground will do little to advance the conceptual reorientations and practical changes associated with the usability initiatives proposed in this chapter.

The problem of developing effective and efficient support for complex work requires a large agenda of investigative questions. For example, what types of complex tasks or problems do people perform with what patterns of inquiry? For various patterns, what relationships and resources should interfaces display and how should they display them? How should interfaces be designed so that users may interact with the layers of information relevant to their task and know where they are at all times? What aspects of users' work need some form of intelligent assistance and what form should it take? The same questions may be answered differently for distinct types of software, domains, users, work activities, and work contexts, but the questions all feed into resolving an overarching, pragmatic problem so that people who pursue different inquiries can recognize and draw on the relatedness of their work. They jointly and incrementally can build a body of knowledge that has pragmatic significance, even when they work separately in their own worlds or areas of strength. They can depend on each other to answer a mutually shared problem, even if they do not participate in some formal joint program or institute.

It will be a difficult project to identify and disseminate the hard problems that warrant joint investigative agendas and to frame pragmatic and interrelated questions for inquiring into them. It will be a project of synthesis and invention. It will involve extensive efforts in examining existing investigations and future aspirations, inferring patterns, categorizing, debating, and building consensus. It will demand a great deal of professional dedication and communication. But it must be done. At a certain point, new tools and techniques for bringing about improvements in usability can go no farther than the underlying and prevailing system of thought allows. Unless the field diligently works to think in new ways and articulate and advance the resulting visions, it will simply continue to run in place.

REFERENCES

Agre, P. (1997). *Computation and human experience.* Cambridge: Cambridge University Press.

Alexander, C. (1979). *A timeless way.* New York: Oxford University Press.

Alexander, C., Ishikawa, S., & Silverstein, M., with Jacobson, M., Fiksdahl-King, I., & Angel, S. (1977). *A pattern language.* New York: Oxford University Press.

Anschuetz, L., & Rosenbaum, S. (2002). Expanding roles for technical communicators. In B. Mirel & R. Spilka (Eds.), *Reshaping technical communications: New direction and challenges for the 21st century* (pp. 149–63). Mahwah, NJ: Lawrence Erlbaum Associates.

Beck, K. (1999). *Extreme programming explained: Embrace change.* New York: Addison-Wesley.

Berkenhotter, C., & Huckin, T. N. (1995). *Genre knowledge in disciplinary communication: Cognition/culture/power.* Hillsdale, NJ: Lawrence Erlbaum Associates.

Bever, H., & Holtzblatt, K. (1998). *Contextual design: Defining customer-centered systems.* San Francisco: Morgan Kaufman Publishers.

Borland, R. Tales of Brave Ulysses. In B. Mirel & R. Spilka (Eds.), *Reshaping technical communication: New directions and challenges for the 21st century* (pp. 189–201). Mahwah, NJ: Lawrence Erlbaum Associates.

Cooper, A. (1999). *The inmates are running the asylum.* Indianapolis, IN: SAMS Publishing.

Coplien, J., & Schmidt, D. (Eds.). (1995). *Pattern languages of program design.* New York: Addison-Wesley.

Gamma, E., Helm, R., Johnson, R., & Vlissides, J. (1995). *Design patterns.* New York: Addison-Wesley.

Gould, J. R., & Lewis, C. (1985). Design for usability—Key principles and what designers think. *Communications of the ACM, 28,* 300–11.

Green, T., Schiele, F., & Payne, S. (1988). Formalizable models of user knowledge in human–computer interaction. In G. Van der Veer, T. Green, J. Hoc, & D. Murray (Eds.), *Working with computers: Theory vs. outcome* (pp. 1–41). London: Academic Press.

Grudin, J. (1991). Systematic sources of suboptimal interface design in large product development organizations. *Human–Computer Interaction, 6,* 147–96.

Kies, J., Williges, R., & Rosson, M. B. (1998). Coordinating computer-supported cooperative work: A review of research issues and strategies. *Journal of the American Society for Information Science, 49,* 776–91.

Orlikowski. W., & Yates, J. (1994). Genre repertoire: The structuring of communicative practices in organizations." *Administrative Science Quarterly, 39,* 541–574.

Pancake, C. (1995). The promise and cost of object technology: A five year forecast. *Communication of the ACM, 38,* 33–49.

Pattern Gallery, The. Available: *http://www.cs.ukc.ac.uk/people/staff/saf/patterns/gallery.html*

Pentland, B., & Rueter, H. (1994). Organizational routines as grammars of action. *Administrative Science Quarterly, 39,* 484–510.

Rasmussen, J., Pejtersen, A., & Goodstein, L. P. (1994). *Cognitive systems engineering.* New York: John Wiley.

Rosson, M. B., & Carroll, J. M. (1995). Narrowing the specification–implementation gap in scenario-based design. In J. M. Carroll (Ed.), *Scenario-based design* (pp. 247–78). New York: John Wiley.

Rudisill, M., Lewis, C., Polson, P., & McKay, T. (Eds.). (1996). *Human–computer interface design: Success stories, emerging methods, and real-world context.* San Francisco: Morgan Kaufman.

Strong, G. W. (1994). *New directions in human–computer interaction: Education, research, and practice.* Washington, DC: National Science Foundation.

Suchman, L. (1997). Centers of coordination: A case and some themes. In L. Resnick, R. Saljo, C. Pontecorvo, & B. Burge (Eds.), *Discourse tools and reasoning: Essays on situated cognition* (pp. 41–62). Berlin: Springer-Verlag.

Vincente, K. (1999). *Cognitive work analysis: Toward safe, productive, and healthy computer-based work.* Mahwah, NJ: Lawrence Erlbaum Associates.

Wixon, D., & Ramey, J. (Eds.). (1996). *Field methods casebook for software design.* New York: John Wiley.

Wood, L. (Ed.). (1998). *User interface design: Bridging the gap from user requirements to design.* New York: CRC Press.

16 *Teaching Text Design*

ROBERT KRAMER AND STEPHEN A. BERNHARDT

Kramer and Bernhardt's essay addresses and exemplifies Redish's second definition of information design – "the way information is presented on the page or screen" (p. 212 in this volume). Their very pedagogical piece sets out to enact the principles of design they espouse. Pragmatic and immediately useful, this essay demonstrates the benefits for users when writers "exercise control over rhetorical design" (p. 243). Especially useful are their explanations and illustrations of principles such as presenting the page as a grid and creating a "typeset look" (p. 243).

Since the introduction of personal publishing tools first made available through the coupling of the personal computer and the laser printer, we have found ourselves in possession of the means for not merely typing essays but designing text. In recognition of the power and possibilities of these tools, the fields of rhetoric and technical communication have begun to construct a rhetoric based on the design of texts that display their meanings through visual/verbal integration. In all corners of our culture, visually informative texts are on the ascendancy, and it is crucial that we continue to map the principles of visual design and that we pursue principled methods for learning to become text designers. In this essay, we suggest a scope and sequence of text design skills and knowledge as a contribution toward a curriculum that helps writers become text designers. In a spirit of playfulness that is true to our subject, we attempt to create an object lesson here that demonstrates through display. We will struggle throughout to not only *tell* but *show* the principles we are discussing, beginning with our "student essay" text on the next three pages—then to a designed text.

From *Technical Communication Quarterly* 5, no. 1 (Winter 1996): 35–60.

Robert Kramer, Stephen A. Bernhardt
Designing Text
English 101

Designing Text

We will begin this article with a visual distinction between designed, rhetorically active text, and the texts that our students are most familiar with: essays.

Students of technical and professional writing often come directly from introductory composition classes, where they may have been expected to do very little work with text design. The prevailing composition aesthetic is a strict, almost puritanical functionalism, meant not for readers but for the teacher who will annotate the text. Students are taught to create pages with flat surfaces: long, double-spaced paragraphs punctuated only by the occasional half-inch or five-space indent; generously wide and symmetrical, one-inch margins all around; and a simply-typed page number in the upper right corner of following pages.

Writers would begin to understand the rhetorical design principles of professional documents, as well as increase their software skills, if they were to immediately jettison this clunky design. Changing our perception of the page as a *writing* space to the page as a *design* space propels us to think beyond the confines of the semantic and lexical constructions of words alone and toward the shape of text and our authorial control over its useful readability.

The contrast of these two "school essay" pages with the rest of this journal suggests how much information is communicated through a few simple design elements. The page grid on these facing pages says little except "block of text." The consistent double spacing, desired presumably for interlinear annotation, wastes the potential of white space to convey meaning in active ways. The white space is spread passively, indiscriminately, between every line. Similarly, the monospaced one-inch-all-around margins cause the writer to miss opportunities for using indentation for meaningful effects. In general, there is little in the design that reflects an understanding of the crucial distinction between *active* and *passive* white space.

Headings that would signal text divisions are conspicuous only in their absence, and the particularly unattractive and tiring Courier font make for pages with little appeal.

Understanding that text is a surface, layered in its meaning, and most successful when its design is both helpful and intuitive to the reader are important starting places for writers as they begin to exercise control over rhetorical design.

We began making a few simple but significant changes at the page break. We reintroduced the facing page headers that identify us as authors on the left (with a somewhat redundant acronym TCQ) and identify the journal on the right with the page numbers on the outside margins where they are most useful. More obviously, we went to single-spaced paragraphs, using space breaks between paragraphs, instead of double spacing every line. Interparagraph space breaks are not the practice in this journal, but it is a style that makes sense for many kinds of memos, reports, and correspondence. The space breaks start to divide the piece into meaningful units instead of spreading ink uniformly across the page.

We then switched fonts to a 10 point Palatino. This change is significant, since it increases the typeset quality by substituting for the monospaced Courier font (where each letter gets the same space, whether an i or an m) a proportional font (where letters take different widths depending on their shape). Since proportional fonts carry intersentential spacing with them (a little extra space break after a period), we went from double-spacing between a period and capital letter to single-spacing (not an easy adjustment for those of us drilled in touch typing). We adjusted the paragraph indents from a one-half inch tab to a one-quarter inch, in keeping with the more modern look of the journal. Finally, we allowed ourselves to introduce a heading on the next page (in a larger, bold, sans-serif font) to begin to further segment the text into meaningful subsections and to provide signposts to busy readers.

Each of these adjustments reflects small but significant changes brought about by the transition from typewriter to desktop tools for producing paper texts. To summarize our changes as design guidelines:

- See the page as a grid.
- Use active whitespace.
- Use text structures to guide the reader.
- Create a typeset look through appropriate use of proportional fonts and spacing.
- Control the document through features such as style definitions.

We will take up each of these principles in the following sections, moving in each section from basic understandings toward more sophisticated. These guidelines are simple enough to be learned in any class, whether composition or technical writing, whether in English or in the disciplines. Writers can work to gradually refine and advance their understanding of text design and their competence with the tools.

See the Page as a Grid

A first principle of page design is to think of the page as a grid that organizes communicative elements. Lay shows how grids create unity, balance, and proportion in documents (Lay 73). Others have pointed out that page design cues various gestalts: groupings, progressions, beginnings and endings, digressions (Bernhardt; Moore and Fitz). We can think of grids as ways of organizing the space of a page. Readers need to know where they are in a document, where they are going, and how they can get there. They need to know what sort of information is in what predictable place. Grids bring predictability; readers use the grid to know how to read the page.

Pages are spaces comprised of defined areas and boundaries. When a grid overlays a page, text and graphic elements are placed in the resulting rectangular spaces. Page design software and more sophisticated word processors provide grids that are variable in granularity and visible on screen, although they do not print. The alignment of textual and visual elements to a grid ensures consistency between parallel text elements, and creates a defined and recognizable look. In highly functional documents, such as computer documentation, a grid helps define and separate explanation from cautions, from steps in a procedure, from tips for experts. In other documents, such as ads or brochures, a grid contributes to a balanced, aesthetically pleasing page design. Grids are a powerful design tool.

The *TCQ* grid is fairly simple: 4.5″ x 7.5″ blocks of print. Headers and (first page only) footers break out of the block, and the headings are outdented from the block. Lists and extended quotations are block indented an extra quarter inch. The narrow page width leads to a readable line length (about 65 characters) for a publication that is meant to be read seriously.

We can easily imagine other grids that might inform other texts, page designs derived from making intentional choices of layout for given communicative tasks. A play-script layout, with one-third/two-third vertical columns, as on the following pages, proves to be highly pleasing and useful for a wide variety of publications.

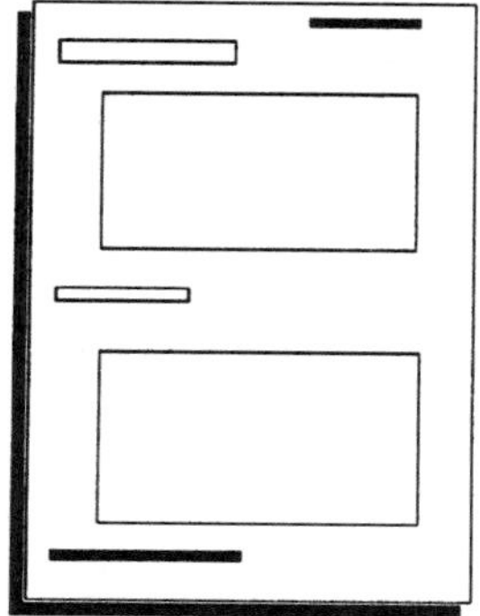
The TCQ Grid

We have seen grant proposals in this format that were simply beautiful, with call-outs, highlight points, and compelling graphs and data displays fitting nicely into the left column. The design prevents long, hard-to-scan lines, and uses plenty of white space to create an open look. Visuals can occupy any of the thirds, spanning the columns to take two-thirds or the whole width of the page.

Many publications use a "play script" format, with a one-third/two-thirds grid. It is a flexible design that allows marginalia – commentary, headings, graphic elements – to float beside the text.

Grids make great planning tools, as publications can be roughed out with pencil and paper as thumbnails or storyboards before executing the actual design and investing time at the computer. Books on desktop publishing have much to say about designing with grids, and they provide great examples from both popular media and from serious graphic design artists. Some good sources include Shushman and Wright; Brown; Bivens and Ryan; Parker; and White. Planning on the grid also encourages the designer to consider facing pages as the unit of composition, rather than single pages.

As in any art, grids provide stability and constraint. Once the grid is in place, the artist can violate it, break the frame, work to his or her own vision. The temptation for beginning page designers is to imagine grid spaces as symmetrical, rectangular and right angled to the page orientation. While such thinking makes a good starting point, most experienced designers love to play with the grid, break its constraints, and layer objects across and on top of the spaces of the grid.

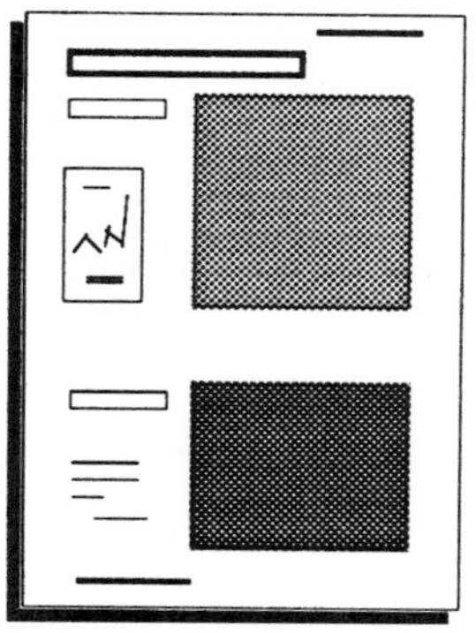
A One-Third/
Two-Thirds Grid

An activity that gets writers thinking about grids is to produce a simple essay or review in two-column format. A writer might prepare

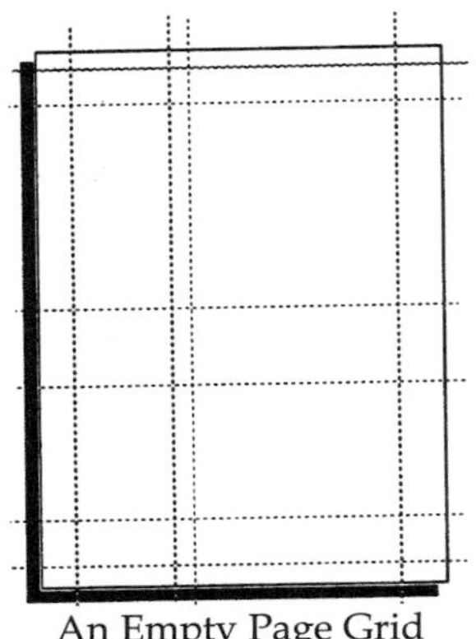
An Empty Page Grid

a movie review to look exactly as it would if it appeared in the feature pages of the local paper, complete with headline, teaser, and mug shot. A more complicated task would be to set up a résumé on two different, contrasting grids, perhaps with one purposefully over-designed. Such experiments help a writer learn to contrast serious grids with playful ones and gain control over the rhetoric of design.

Use Active White Space

Any discussion of the rhetoric of practical documents must encompass the language of visual design"
— Kostelnick

Designers begin to use white space actively when they start to see both the positive (ink-filled) and negative (white) spaces on the page. White space conveys a lot about a document: what type it is, how it should be approached, and what must be read and what can be skipped.

White space can be either active or passive: passive white space is defined incidentally by the space left over as the text takes shape. Active white space, in contrast, intentionally defines the shape, organization, progression, and readability of the text itself. Passive is accidental; active is intentional.

We recognize a memo by its heading, perhaps a company logo or letterhead, the arrangement of its To-From-Date-Subject introduction, and its block-style text body and signature. Our recognition is largely a case of recognizing a form as it is defined by the shape of the text. The text shape, in turn, is defined by the page space around it, or its (sometimes not white) white space.

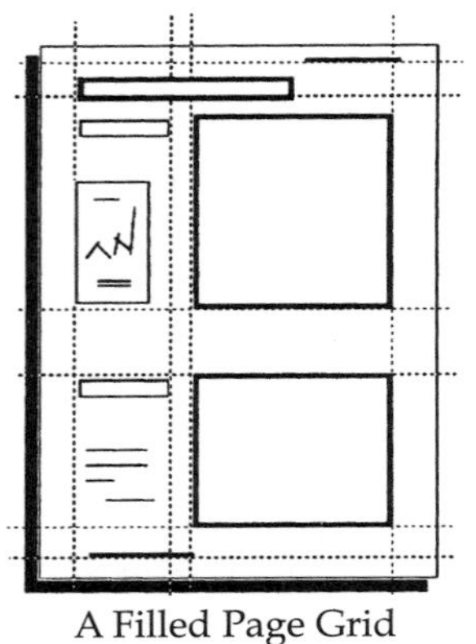
A Filled Page Grid

On the following page, the text is set to conform fully to the *TCQ* format, with an indent to mark paragraphs and no space break between paragraphs. To aid readability and signal organization, we might choose to separate paragraphs in a memo with a space break because it makes the paragraphs easier to read as specific points or makes those points distinct from other content and easy to reference. *TCQ* also uses two spaces after a period.

White space can also act as a stylistic tool (Kostelnick 26). The arrangement and style of textual elements on a page can either inhibit or invite readers into a document. An inviting document tends to be open and expansive, with text defined into blocks by white space, headings that are separated by spacing, text that is set with a little extra space between each line, and visual elements that are bordered by white space. Many readers avoid intimidating, dense texts. In a journal such as this, readers are present on their own volition, out of a sense of intellectual curiosity, with plenty of motivation to read pages, even if they are a bit dense (the pages, not the readers) in their ink to white space ratio.

Designers tend to see blocks of text as shapes in space, not necessarily as something to be read. Page design programs frequently provide mumbo-jumbo filler text in a meaningless "Greek" filler (lorum ipsit), so the designer can concentrate on shape and not be distracted by meaning. Text blocks become design elements in balance and juxtaposition with other graphic elements.

In many kinds of text, there really is no need to cover the page with ink. Much designed text has an ink-to-space ratio of less than 50%. As writers develop their design styles, they can become more aware of white and black as defining elements of the page and begin to use white space actively to structure their ideas, invite readers into the text, and show them how it can be read. Writers need to recognize the truth in the huckster's maxim, "If you don't get'em into the tent, they ain't going to see the show." A visual style, with plenty of white space on an attractive grid, is the ticket.

Use Text Structures to Guide the Reader

Design is functional insofar as it shows readers how to read a text: what the structure and progression is, what can be read or skipped, what is more important or less important. Page composition programs provide a wide range of tools to help writers show structures. Such displayed structures ideally complement the internal, logico-semantic meanings created within the text.

Margins, Justification, and Indentation

The use of white space for margins, justification, and indentation deserves special consideration. The one-third/two-thirds grid that organized the previous facing pages can be thought of as providing a wide left margin, but a special sort of margin that can include visual and textual elements. Some texts, especially those being bound, benefit from a wide, empty inner margin. Other texts benefit from a wide right margin, especially those that will be annotated. Functional design challenges the default settings: one inch all around and a half-inch indent on each paragraph.

Business writing classes have traditionally experimented with block styles, with and without indentation, some with full justification, some with left justification.

This text is **flush left**.

This text is flush right.

This text is centered.

We have set this page to full justify to show the effect. The journal carries a "ragged right" margin, meaning that the text is not flush to the right margin. This is consistent with some marginally compelling research on readability that suggests that readers use the ragged right to track the text and keep their place. It also helps avoid "rivers" of white space that result when the extra word spacings of full justification form noticeable alignments—rivers—of white space that run down the page. Tight hyphenation zones can help control such accidental effects, though for most texts, it is best to keep the hyphenation off or set loose so not too many words are broken at line ends.

Some texts look better and work better in full justified block paragraphs, without any paragraph indent, especially texts with small column width: brochures, newspaper-style columns, and some flyers. Narrow columns of print just cannot support the indentation without the overall look being ragged. Sometimes the design decisions are motivated more by aesthetics than strict criteria of legibility or readability. There's no good reason, for example, to indent a paragraph following a heading; such following paragraphs actually look better without the indent.

Understanding and controlling left, right, center, and full justification is by no means intuitive. Particularly with right justification, writers need to experiment to see how it works, what happens when lines wrap, and how text lines up on a return. A little time might well be spent investigating the ruler bar, which typically offers easy control of margins and indents. Some of the settings are hard for many to grasp, for example, the two little triangles that control the left indents on the the first and following lines of paragraphs. Distinguishing and manipulating decimal, center, and right tabs can be hard for others to understand. Many relatively advanced users of a program like Word have not necessarily discovered the control of details afforded by the ruler bar. For example, double-clicking on a tab allows the user to set the tab to carry leader dots (as in a table of contents) or a leader line (useful for drawing a rule across a page). The ruler bar from Microsoft Word for Macintosh shown below is the type of tool writers need to develop a skilled awareness of:

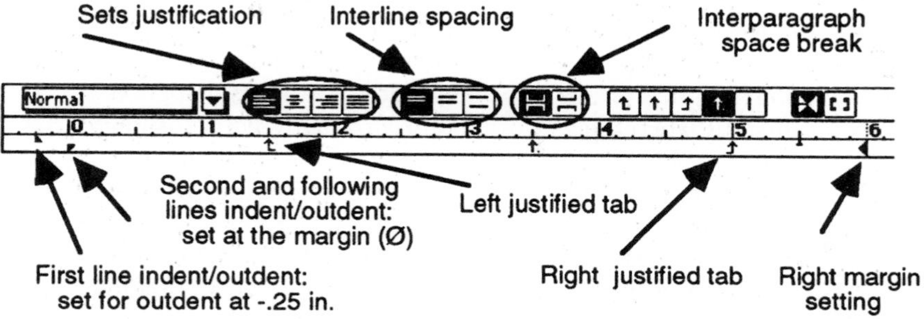

In many kinds of technical texts, the really important information conveyed by indentation is not paragraph breaks, but structural levels in the document hierarchy.

Two or three levels of subordination can be signaled by text that is block indented from the left.

The levels of indent correspond to the patterns of indent in a traditional outline.

Any indent pattern that goes beyond two levels of indent is probably useless to readers.

They are likely to lose track across pages of the level they are on.

A structural cue that is understood by the author and that confuses or is unnoticed by readers is no structural cue at all. Writers, especially technical writers, need a good understanding of how left block indents signal document structure, and how white space can be used in general to signal divisions and hierarchies.

Tabs and Columns

Nothing is more frustrating than working with a highly formatted document that someone has produced using the space bar and forced returns instead of tabs. Tabs are related to tables, of course, and controlling information in a multiple-columned format is made possible through some combination of tab settings and a page that is set up either in columns or as a table. Tabs, tables, and columns allow the designer to place and manipulate text within the space of the page, rather than simply having text appear within the preset margins.

Every working writer needs to know how to design simple tables for text and data. Doing so is made increasingly simple by word processing software that automates table formatting. Formatting tables still requires that one pay attention to internal margins in the table cells and to the use of borders on cells, and that one understand how a right tab works to keep text or data flush right. There is no excuse for formatting with spaces and forced returns, and as one quickly discovers, with proportional fonts, it is impossible to get text to line up vertically using the space bar. The text may look accurately aligned on the screen, because most fonts display in monospacing, but when the text prints proportionally, columns lined up with the space bar will all be off.

Learning to work with text in columns is an important layout skill. Page composition programs (like PageMaker or Quark or Framemaker) are designed to treat text and graphics as independent blocks, objects that can be moved around and placed on the page. Tabs, margins, and indents can be set independently within the different text blocks that compose the page. Word processors treat text a bit differently and require more finagling with the text to work in columns. Word processors handle columns just fine in newspaper style, when continuous text snakes from the bottom of one column to the top of the next. When the page design requires independent columns of text, as in our one-third/two-thirds pages, a word processor works best when the text is placed inside a table, which is what we did. The two facing pages of our play script format are actually two tables, each with two columns and one row per page and no borders on the cells. We had to futz with the layout a lot to get it to fill the pages and break in the right places, but we were able to do it. Setting tabs is useful any time one needs to line up information in opposing columns of print; creating a table is useful when the text in columns is a bit complicated or when the columns do not correspond line by line.

The ability to handle text (and graphics) as an object that can be placed in a window on a page and moved about is the real advantage of composition programs as opposed to word processors. But the differences are disappearing as programs like Word for Windows 6.0 or WordPerfect 6.0 for Windows incorporate most page composition features, including grids and 'snap to grid.' In such programs, the writer can place text in a box that can be moved and dropped into place, even over other text or graphic objects. The text can also be made to flow around the frames of graphic objects.

Headers and Footers

Most printed texts use page tops and bottoms for orienting information called *headers* and *footers*. Page numbers, author names, publication information (volume and issue), dates and titles are often found in these areas of the page. These lines of text are separate contextually from the body, riding above and below the running content of the pages themselves, and act as quick reference points, always in the same place, and always saying the same thing in the same way.

TCQ uses alternating headers at the top left and top right of facing pages. The left header has the page number outdented, followed by TCQ: Author Name. The right header spells Technical Communication Quarterly, followed by a page number that is flush with the right page margin. Both headers are in 9 pt. Helvetica to distinguish them from the body text. Outdenting the even page header follows the *TCQ* grid of outdenting headings from the page margin. Odd page headers are flush right. A footer on the initial page of an article, outdented again, identifies the year, volume, volume number and pages of the article, convenient for keeping track of the source document for photocopies.

We used a different header design on these two pages, placing the page numbers in a footer with alternating author and title lines. The headers have been moved to the inside margins, and the footers to the outside, with the even pages outdented to follow our grid. Whether or not this makes a significant difference is a matter of reading habit. We are used to page numbers in the upper left and right in this type of journal. Magazines place page numbers, if at all, in the footer, often on the inside margins where they are difficult to find. The headers and footers frame the text on the diagonal. Such framing effects are enhanced in some texts by the addition of a rule (a straight printed line in a variable point width) either above or below the header, or by boxing the header and printing the header in inverse (white type on a black background) or with a screen (some ink proportion less than 100% to give a shaded effect). These are small details, but depending on the document and the audience a writer is designing text for, they could become important.

Word processing programs like Microsoft Word and WordPerfect will create headers and footers in separate windows, and then place them in a document in defined areas, automatically appearing on and numbering each page. Content is linked in these text structures, so that changes made to a single header or footer will change all headers and footers on all pages, hence the terms "running head" and "running footer." This is a control feature that allows this part of a text to be set up once, and then essentially ignored, while it adds important orientation to the reader. Students have always been expected to put at least a page number on all following pages of a document. It is good practice to learn to think about information in headers and footers and to make good use of navigational areas of the page.

Headings

Headings break up continuous text into visually coherent parts. They cue the reader to content structure without disrupting the flow of reading, and they partially eliminate the need for paragraph-level transitions. Headings make promises about the content of subsections, and they allow busy readers to find information quickly and to scan documents for information.

When written to be highly specific and directive, headings can carry much more information than paragraph indentations or space breaks. This section is about headings, as indicated by its sub-heading **Headings**. Our entire section on text structures is comprised of a single heading and five sub-heads. Our headings state topics, but in other documents, headings might ask or answer questions, identify actions, or list steps in a process. Careful attention to heading wording and design can make a document navigable and efficient for readers who come to a text to complete a specific task. Readers can approach the text with varied reading strategies, either to read from beginning to end, or to reference specific points in almost the same way they would look at indexed subjects in a catalogue, reference volume, or hypertext book. Headings are an easy and powerful way to make text less linear and to improve its rhetorical flexibility.

Designers know that headings need to be made visually distinct through some combination of typeface and style features. *TCQ* changes its typeface (to Helvetica from their body type Goudy), point size (to 14 point for a top-level heading in the text and to 12 point for a sub-heading), and type style, going to bold to contrast with the normal body type. Readers have a hard time distinguishing a single point difference in type, but they can usually distinguish a two-point difference, and can certainly do so when the point shift is coupled with other changes (as in normal to bold). The *TCQ* designers add extra spacing around the headings, more before than after, to logically and visually structure the heading with what follows rather than with what came before. The articles don't go below a sub-heading, so there are two levels of descension in the hierarchy. Readers might have trouble with a system of greater subtlety. In headings, designers achieve a lovely melding of form and function, with variables of size, weight, and space signaling the logical hierarchy of the text. A text with problems of global coherence can often be mended with some attention to the structure of sections and their headings. Headings force writer-designers to make promises they actually keep as the document finds a working organization.

Lists

Lists are highly visual and ordered text structures. When buried list structures are extracted from sentences and paragraphs and represented in an indented list, spaced from the body text and numbered or bulleted, they become instantly accessible to the reader. What headers do for whole sections of text, lists do for specific points in a text: they organize parallel ideas into easily referenced and readable forms. We make lists everyday for various purposes, and are accustomed to reading information in list form:

Milk

Olives

Toilet Paper!

Soap

It is hard not to imply precedence through a visual list. Our grocery list has several items, but the user need not purchase milk first, then olives, then toilet paper (though the more obsessive among us order our shopping lists this way, imagining the store layout). The hierarchical arrangement, though, forces the impression of order of importance.

Some lists reflect chronology:

1. lower the blade guard
2. unlatch the blade lock
3. engage the blade with the clutch lever

Visual cues like numbers make the order of the sequence in this list unquestionable.

We used a carefully formatted bulleted list in this article, indenting our bullets one-quarter inch and tabbing the list items another one-quarter inch:

- See the page as a grid.
- Use active white space.
- Use text structures to guide the reader.
- Create a typeset look through appropriate use of proportional fonts and spacing.
- Control the document through features such as style tags, templates, and links.

To keep the look clean, when a bulleted item wrapped at the end of a line, we lined up the following line on the left indent of the first. This list mirrors the order of both first mention of each of these topics in our introduction and the sequence of discussion that structures the whole text. Each item from this initial list became its own section heading.

We indulge a brief confession here. When we first wrote the introductory section where this list of design principles appears, the individual items were buried inside paragraphs and spread across a page. Our design instincts recognized a list buried in the linear prose structure and urged us to pull the separate points out into a vertical list, bullet them, and bring them into parallel verb/complement structures. Once we had done so, we saw them as the structure that could hold the whole essay together and so created section headings from the list. The design of the whole grew from a local design principle: if information is list-like, make it a visible list. This is a liberating moment for writers: when they recognize a list that is buried in a paragraph and decide to make the logical structure visible.

Create a Typeset Look

Typography as a design concept includes the selection of typefaces: family, size, and spacing on a page (Shushman and Wright 14). The writer facing the blank page must be able to make decisions about what sort of typographic design is appropriate given a specific rhetorical situation. Decisions can be based on what type is best suited to the purpose and audience, what is most readable, what styles best cue the content, and what type offers the most aesthetic face without sacrificing legibility.

Type in its simplest clothing is a graphic element comprised of widths and lengths, spacing and subtle shapes, its meaning displayed by the controlled spread of ink on a page. To ignore the visual value of a typeface is to ignore the single most important feature affecting the readability and design of a text.

Page design software and sophisticated word processors grant authorial control over text size, shape, style, color, spacing, width, and proportion. Type treatments such as bold, italics, and underline provide additional levels of meaning to a font without changing its family, an important consideration: font changes in documents should be used to signal new content through structures like headings and call-outs. By using different type families and type styles, writers can create multiple levels of meaning and visual cues in a document while contributing to its readability.

Controlling Line Length, Leading, and Kerning

Line length, called *measure*, is a factor in text readability. Generally, shorter lines mean easier tracking for the reader and fewer instances of losing one's place. A rule of thumb that is frequently violated is that lines should be about 1 1/2 to 2 alphabets long (≈40–60 characters). A good actual line length for a specific text is dependent on how closely spaced the font is and how large the point size is. With larger point type, lines can be made longer.

Leading (pronounced "ledding" after the name of the metal slugs that separated lines of set type) provides interlinear space. Type can be set tight or open, with very little space from the bottom of the characters on one line to the top of the characters on the next or with extra space to open up the text. All word processors provide gross adjustments to leading through single, space-and-a-half, or double-spaced line settings, a system inherited from the typewriter. Sophisticated word processors allow the type designer to control leading more exactly. This paragraph is set as 10 point Palatino on 14 point leading, a little open.

Leading is measured in points (a point is approximately 1/72 of an inch; 12 points≈1 pica; 6 picas≈1 inch). The leading of a text is described in terms of point size of type on leading. This paragraph is set in Avant Garde 12/20, giving a very open look that might work for ad copy, marketing information, or highly designed annual reports. *TCQ* sets its body type as Goudy 11 point type on 11.5 point leading (expressed "11 on 11.5"). This is a bit tight. Setting the leading to **AUTO** would generally result in 9-point text set 9/11, or 10-point as 10/12, with about two extra points of leading, spread proportionally above and below the line of type. With larger font sizes, less leading is needed. Leading can also be set negatively, so lines of type actually touch or overlap. Shushan and Wright, and Brown both provide technical discussions of these issues and provide good examples.

Kerning is an advanced design tool that allows the typesetter to adjust for the spacing between letters to approximate a hand-set look. Kerning refers to the space between letters, which can be open or tight. All proportional fonts do some automatic kerning, so an A and a V would be set a little tight to accommodate their shapes, which are not strictly rectangular but oblique. A little kerning with the eye on a display text, like a poster or flyer, can make a difference in the professional look. A series of lines beginning with capital letters, for example, will not line up to the eye on the left margin because of the different letter shapes, but can be kerned into an alignment that pleases the eye.

Line length (or measure), leading, and kerning are design tools that allow for careful copy-fitting. While controlling these features is not necessary in many ordinary texts, they can provide for special effects or contribute to the design of texts that must be highly readable.

Understanding the Face of Type

Writers accustomed to writing essays with flat text surfaces and undistinguished type find themselves loose in a candy store when they discover the typographic variation available today on most word processing systems. Our network offers a choice of well over 200 fonts in various styles and the invitation to experiment is irresistible. Any number of fonts may end up in a document as students begin to explore the possibilities of playing with type:

• **Now Available** •
T Y P O g r A p h y
Hundreds of styles
I n s t a n t A c c e s s to
Voice *Tone* **E x p r e s s i o n**
All at your FINGERTIPS
You've Never Seen
Anything Like This!!

While writers discover how to use software to manipulate type features, they also develop awareness of typography's role as both an aesthetic and structural element. As they learn to talk type on its own terms, they gain respect for its influence on the page.

For our sample "essay" pages, we chose Courier, a particularly rigid and under-designed font that is associated with typewritten text. Courier lacks variability in both letter width (it is monospaced, with no kerning) and stroke: the lines that form the characters are of uniform thickness. Courier does have the virtue of being robust under abuse: it can be repeatedly photocopied or faxed and hold its defining shapes well. Courier is a sturdy but boring font.

Typographers have a whole language for talking about type, some of which is displayed in this diagram:

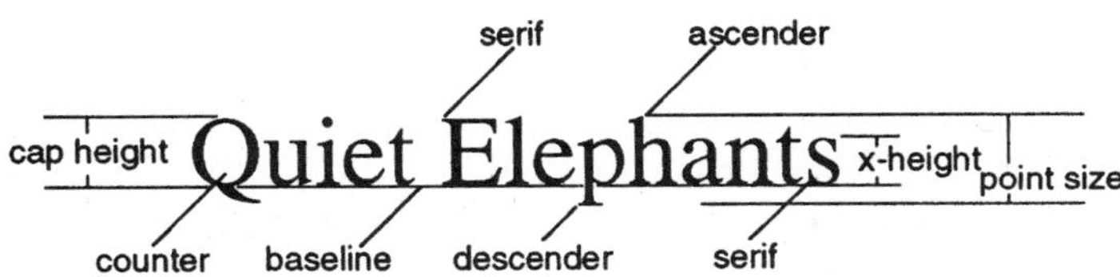

adapted from Shushman and Wright, 1991

A typeface is a graphical image, its details highly refined and carefully designed to be unique from font to font. It is a conditioned habit to look right through the typeface to the words of the text, and not see type as a graphically rich design element. While modern type does not have the graphic texture derived from being stamped onto a page by a small, letter-shaped brick attached to a levered arm, the ink or toner is spread precisely as if brushed, and meaning *is* created by the combination of intricate graphic details forming identifiable design characteristics.

The differences in many of the features indicated in our display of Quiet Elephants (below) are what define different type families. A type family is the sum of all the variations of a single typeface (Shushan and Wright, 21). These variations include widths, *slant* and styles like **bold**, regular, underline, and light. The most identifiable changes in type families occur in serifs, x-height, and counters. Our Quiet Elephants take on different appearances on these subtle levels when the typeface is changed:

Quiet Elephants	14pt. Palatino
Quiet Elephants	14pt. Times
Quiet Elephants	14pt. Bookman
Quiet Elephants	14pt. Bernhard Modern

These four lines are all set in 14 point type, but vary widely in measure. Bookman has a large counter (the open space in closed letter forms like a, o, p, g, and q) and requires significantly more line length per word. Its x-height is roughly the same as Palatino, yet its counters are horizontally oval rather than round. Font designers find pleasure in adding high detail to certain letters: the Q is highly unique in these faces. (While we are on the subject of Qs, allow yourself to linger on the gorgeous Q on the cover of this journal. It is a fine example of type as a design element.)

Lines in Bookman appear almost stretched lengthwise as they spread across a page; our article would be several pages longer in this font. Bookman is also considerably heavier in stroke than Palatino or Times. Large text bodies like those in this article would not be difficult to read, but the space consumed by this heavy, open font makes it a poor choice for an academic article. It remains a favorite of children's book designers.

Times has a taller x-height than Bookman, but is more compressed, or tighter, on its baseline than Bookman and Palatino. It is a highly efficient typeface for columns and grids that require a great deal of compressed text. Newspapers make excellent use of Times, and some of the many variants of this font family are at use in all sorts of academic texts. Our article would be significantly shorter in this font, but not as easily read. Times is an extremely popular body font, available on all laser printers, and always a good choice for serious text. These four fonts are also called serif or Roman fonts; each point on each letter has a flourishing stroke.

Often, the only way to decipher a type's readability and appropriateness is to see it in action. It is very difficult to distinguish immediately between typefaces like Palatino and Times unless seen side by side; not so difficult with Bernhard Modern. Setting the same text in different typefaces and then discussing the effects is a good way to start to pay attention to type design. A writer might first print a memo in Courier, then in Palatino. Seeing the very obvious differences will begin to train the designer to make sense of the candy store options. Try for a moment to distinguish between *TCQ*'s use of Goudy in this journal, and our use of Palatino. Another useful exercise is to print samples of a variety of fonts and discuss people's impressions about which fonts would be suitable for what types of documents (party invitations, newspapers, lab reports, computer documentation, and so on).

Invitation Party brochure **banner**

Newspaper screen document

Poster

Type Styling

Type can be styled to add meaning without changing the font family. Styles can include **bold**, *italic*, CAPS, SMALL CAPS, underlined, double-underlined, shadow, ~~strikethru~~, and hidden.

Both of the following sentences are in 10 point Helvetica. The second has style treatments that add important dimensions to its meaning and effectiveness:

> Press the red button prior to initiating the grinding roller.

> Press the **red** button PRIOR to initiating the grinding roller.

Writing instructions using one or two fonts are good style assignments. Writers increase their rhetorical skills by using style, instead of point size and different type families, to guide the reader carefully through a text that *could* have serious consequences if not read correctly: like not pressing the **red** button.

The threat of these styles is that novice designers sometimes end up producing texts that look like ransom notes. A careful book designer decides on a specific use for each type style: for example, **bold** for action steps, *italic* for emphasized words, single quotes for words as linguistic examples, underline for titles of published works, and SMALL CAPS for glossary terms. Carefully defining functions for each style and resisting the temptation to overuse the styles leads to effective use.

Choosing for Function: Display/Body/Legibility

Most students would not have trouble discerning which of the two memorandums following would be the more effective document:

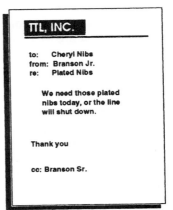

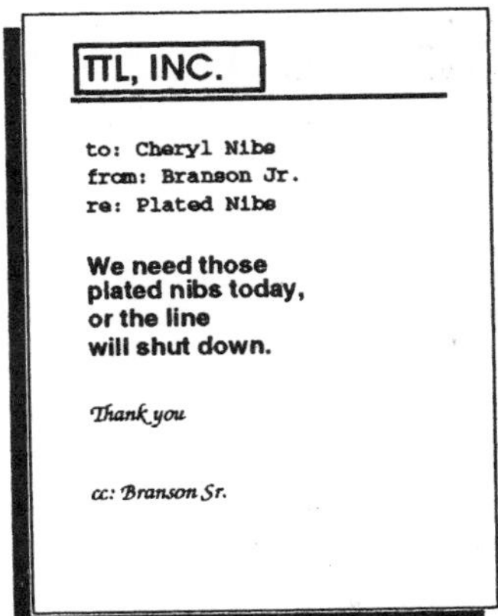
TTL, INC.

to: Cheryl Nibs
from: Branson Jr.
re: Plated Nibs

We need those
plated nibs today,
or the line
will shut down.

Thank you

cc: Branson Sr.

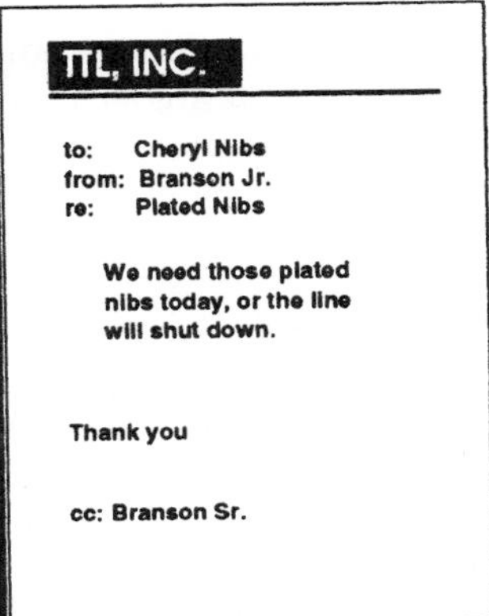
TTL, INC.

to: Cheryl Nibs
from: Branson Jr.
re: Plated Nibs

We need those plated
nibs today, or the line
will shut down.

Thank you

cc: Branson Sr.

The first memo uses a display font, Castellar MT, for both the memo's letterhead and its body, Courier for its heading, and a script font, Zapf Chancery, for its signature line. It is nearly impossible to get a sense of tone or professionalism from its display, and it is distracting to read. The second memo uses a sans serif font for both heading and body, a successful choice because of the short length of the memo. A larger body might have warranted a serif font like Palatino.

It is important to recognize that some font families were designed for screen displays only and never meant to be printed. Apple Computer created fonts and assigned city names (Geneva, Chicago, Monaco) that would look very large and distinct and readable on screen. But they do not make good choices for printed documents. Within the last couple of years, we have seen the development of font families that erase the distinction between screen font and printer font. The older font families had separate files for each point size and for both screen and printer. The new scalable typefaces are vector-defined, so the whole range of point size is defined mathematically. The newer fonts go by names like TrueType on the Macintosh and ATM (Adobe Type Manager) within Windows.

Sans serif, or Swiss/Gothic typefaces are uniform and do not have finishing strokes at the end of each form. Common sans serif fonts include the standard Helvetica as well as Univers, Futura, and Arial. Some of the these fonts, like the Avant Garde of this paragraph, are so round that they make better display fonts, or at best detract from the "serious" look of a text. Avant Garde usually makes a poor choice for body text.

The bold styles of Helvetica are a favorite of many designers for headings, as is the case in this journal. Nobody, however, would want to read much body text in a bold Helvetica. It is a matter of debate whether sans serif fonts slow readers down. It may just be a matter of our being used to seeing body text set in serif.

The absolute default setting in current practice favors a bold Helvetica font for headings and a Times-Roman font for body type (a look similar to this journal). Such a pairing is undoubtedly conservative, but never wrong. It represents a starting point and type can be designed from there, with various and subtle effects.

Some Fine Points on Type

Gaining control of a few typographic details can lend an element of professional design to a document:

- Since proportional fonts build in extra spacing after end punctuation, it is not necessary to space twice after periods, exclamation points, question marks, and colons. Though not extinct, double spacing is a holdover from the typewriter era.

- Quotation marks and apostrophes are designed elements of a type family (called *typographer's quotes* or *smart quotes*). Some software has a setting to turn on typographer's quotes; in other software, combination keystroke commands will display them. They look much better than the all-purpose variety ("these" vs. "these").
- Dashes and hyphens are distinguishable in typeset text. Dashes are available through certain keystroke combinations or through special character maps. Picky people can further distinguish n-dashes from the slightly longer m-dashes (named for their width, which corresponds to the letters *n* and *m*).
- Advanced word processors have equation editors for writing formulas. Students of science, math, and engineering in particular appreciate learning how to insert $\sqrt{1/5} \geq \bar{x}$.
- Character maps or Key-Caps provide special characters that can be quite useful, beginning with bullets, but also symbols such as ©, ø, ∧, ✔, and ❻. Where these symbols reside and how they are inserted in documents varies, but they are not difficult to master.

Control the Document

A final design skill involves using the advanced tools of the word processor or composition program to ensure consistency in the elements of layout and typography discussed above. Everything we have discussed here can be done "on the fly" with text marked up and formatted as one composes. Indeed, we had to do a lot of formatting on the fly, since we have tried to demonstrate so many variables of layout and typography. For most documents, however, *style sheets* allow for much better design control than designing on the fly. Style sheets (sometimes called *style formats* or *style tags*) allow the text designer to define and tag each structural element of the composition. Style sheets are a sort of mark-up language, similar to SGML (Standardized General Markup Language) used in many kinds of technical publications or HTML (Hypertext Markup Language) used to format hypertexts.

A style sheet for a document defines the various elements of composition. In this text, we have defined our heading levels, headers, body paragraphs, bulleted lists, and bibliographic entries within the style sheet of the word processor. Our style definition for the top level heading in this article stipulates:

> Normal + Font: B Helvetica Bold 18 Point, Indent: Left – 0.25 in First 0 in. Space Before 24 pt After 12 pt, Keep With Next

The definition inherits the defining features of Normal (the definition of our body paragraph), but changes the font, indents it negatively (outdents), provides 24 points of white space before the heading (to drop it away from the last line of the previous body paragraph), inserts 12 points of white space below the heading, and keeps the heading with the following paragraph (so as not to widow the heading at the bottom of a page). Not evident in the definition is its singular association with the heading text; after typing it and pressing return, the next paragraph is defined as normal (body text). Any formatting element (tabs, indents, spacing, type style, justification) can be embedded in the style definition.

Style sheets can be created for different types of documents: memos, proposals, personal letters, forms, lab reports. Then a new file can be opened with the template that is governed by the appropriate style sheet. Style sheets can also be used to govern the "look" of a company's documents, so that people working on different projects will produce documents that have a similar corporate identity.

Once defined, any change to a style definition ripples through a document and all the elements with that tag change consistently. Thus, if the designer decides to open up the body paragraph by introducing a little extra leading, going say from 12 auto to 12/14, the change would take place on every other body paragraph in the text. Further, if other elements in the style sheet are "based on" the definition of the body paragraph, those would change, too. So if the designer wanted to change the font from Palatino to Times, and all style definitions were based on the body paragraph definition, then all the definitions would change based on a single change to the font for body paragraphs.

Many word processors provide additional tools for document control. Some allow one to avoid leaving widows (the first line or two of a paragraph or a header that is left behind at a page break) and orphans (a line that is pushed to the next page at the break). Others allow for flexible hyphenation zones. Some allow text to be defined so that it is not separated from what follows, or so that a group of lines stays together, or so it always starts at the top of a column or the beginning of a new page. All such features begin to automate document design and control the design from the top level, so decisions are not made locally.

It is hard to convey why this high-level document control is important until one starts working with long and complexly formatted documents. But as documents grow longer and as formatting grows more complex and subtle, keeping the formatting decisions consistent across the text becomes increasingly difficult. Style sheets provide extremely powerful and reliable tools for doing so. Learning to use style sheets in a word processor also prepares one for using them in other applications: in composition programs, in hypertext authoring languages, or in scripting languages.

Designing Documents

All of the elements discussed above are brought into play as writers design working documents. Writers can begin by thinking of the page as a grid and seeing the space as divisible into areas of ink and white space. The white space itself can be considered an active design element, used to separate content, to open up the page, and to cue the reader to the progress of the document. Areas of the page can be designed to contain orienting information in the form of headers and footers, and the logical organization of the text can be cued through headings that signal the hierarchy and content.

An attractive and readable design can be further encouraged by controlling line length and leading, making sure these elements are in balance with the appropriate font. The font can be chosen and sized with regard for the function of the document and its audience. Internally, the designer can choose body fonts for readability and display fonts for headings. All the elements can be defined and controlled through style sheets, with the careful definitions evolving into templates or master pages for certain documents that are produced more than once.

We have touched on some basics of text design in this article. Any of these elements can be extended, their subtleties played upon, the use of typographic tools developed and refined. We have discussed primarily text, but beyond text lie the important areas of designing and incorporating visuals (Tufte) and architecting whole publications. Developing control over the elements of layout and typographic design leads one naturally to begin thinking about designing documents with multiple pages. The challenge of design becomes an issue of how to lead readers into documents and how to direct their reading processes once the document has their attention. Facing pages can be designed as single design units, information can be emphasized or de-emphasized, and the page can gain texture from elements that are central or peripheral, verbal or visual.

Some may object that the kinds of learning we are describing here are superficial, launching the old challenge that we are modern sophists, more concerned with form than context, with display over truth. But we think not. Seeing is thinking (Arnheim, Horowitz).

Thinking about design is thinking about structure, function, and aesthetics. Making decisions about layout and text structures is one powerful way a writer brings organization and coherence to a text. Controlling documents with the sophisticated tools of word processing and page composition is no simple matter, but goes directly to the issue of capable control over hardware and software, a skill increasingly critical for all those of us who are surrounded by machines. Seeing a text at the top level and watching the many design decisions filter down through the actual printing of the text—being in control of the software and the text—grants a powerful feeling of mastery of language and machine. These kinds of learning are worth developing, through the classes we teach and take, and through our personal struggles to control the tools well enough to design the texts we envision.

WORKS CITED

Arnheim, Rudolf. *Art and Visual Perception*. Berkley: University of California P, 1954.

———. *Visual Thinking*. Berkeley and Los Angeles: University of California P, 1969.

Bernhardt, Stephen A. "Seeing the Text." *College Composition and Communication* 37 (1986): 66–78.

Bivens, Thomas, and William E. Ryan. *How to Produce Creative Publications: Traditional Techniques and Computer Applications*. Lincolnwood, IL: NTC Business Books, 1991.

Brown, Alex. *In Print*. New York, NY: Watson-Guptill Publications, 1989.

Horowitz, Mardi Jon. *Image Formation and Cognition*. New York: Appleton-Century-Crofts. 1970.

Kostelnick, Charles. "Visual Rhetoric: A Reader-Oriented Approach to Graphics and Design." *The Technical Writing Teacher* 16 (1989): 77–88.

Lay, Mary. "The Non-Rhetorical Elements of Design." *Technical Writing, Theory and Practice*. New York: MLA. 1989.

Moore, Patrick, and Chad Fitz. "Using Gestalt Theory to Teach Document Design and Graphics." *Technical Communication Quarterly* 2.4 (1993): 389–413.

Parker, Roger. *The Makeover Book: 101 Design Solutions for Desktop Publishing*. Chapel Hill. NC: Ventana P. 1989.

Shushman and Wright. *Desktop Publishing by Design*, 2nd Edition. Redmond, WA: Microsoft Press. 1991.

Tufte, Edward R. *Envisioning Information*. Connecticut: Graphics P, 1990.

White, Jan V. *Graphic Design for the Electronic Age*. New York: Watson-Guptill Publications, 1988.

APPLIED THEORY

17 The Rhetoric of Design: Implications for Corporate Intranets

LISA ANN JACKSON

Jackson's essay demonstrates, through a number of excellent examples, that user-centered design is both a process involving problem solving and a method of presentation. In essence, her discussion of the importance of designing intranets so that they enable users to "perform work-oriented tasks with the greatest efficiency and least effort" (p. 271 in this volume) and add functionality illustrates the principles presented by both Redish and Mirel. Her discussions of elements of design on the Web also substantiate Kramer and Bernhardt's points about simplicity, consistency, and standardization. In summary, her article illustrates that design should begin and end with the user's point of view. Otherwise writers/designers/ developers run the risk of creating something that will not be used or will not be used to its fullest capacity.

Companies often use rhetorical tricks to persuade employees to become users of a corporate intranet. At Novell, e-mail messages with live links to new pages and features go out to every employee; at Microsoft, the travel services department posts vacation and airline specials to the intranet (Braley 1997). At Reading and Bates, the intranet administrator takes candid snaps of employees and posts them on bio pages (Melendez 1997). At Walker & Associates, intranet administrators have hosted an intranet scavenger hunt complete with prizes (McIntosh 1997). And at Flowserve, the intranet team gave a t-shirt to anyone who found a cartoon surfer during the intranet's roll-out (Turner 1998). The rhetorical elements of intranet development range from methods like these designed to catch user attention, to well-crafted proposals written to convince corporate decision makers of the fundamental need for an intranet. However, an often overlooked persuasive device available to intranet developers is the subtle effectiveness of good design.

The rhetoric of design includes both esthetic appeal and organizational structure. Navigational structure integrated with visual aids can determine whether employees make the intranet an integral part of their work processes

From *Technical Communication* 47, no. 2 (2000): 212–19.

or consciously avoid the intranet until paper forms, manuals, or directories go out of print. A poorly designed intranet can quickly frustrate and disillusion users, sending them back to previously learned methods of accomplishing tasks (Albers 1997). But an effectively designed intranet can become a valuable medium for facilitating work processes and communication throughout a company.

Some intranet developers mistakenly assume that the value of an intranet lies in merely making information available online, in whatever form, and that users will turn to an intranet simply because a body of facts exists there. However, this perspective

> assumes that . . . a "fact" is an indivisible construct that is self-evident to all observers. And it assumes that documents, as well as other forms of communication, exist primarily to provide conduits or conveyor belts for moving facts along from one brain to the next. . . . If we proceed on this assumption, then we can visualize ranks of pigeon holes into which we can file the data and from which, if we specify the data we are looking for accurately enough, we can retrieve them without error or ambiguity. (Ramey 1997, p. 385)

Ramey argues that this is precisely not the case, that facts cannot stand alone and have real value. Rather they combine to create information, which in turn combines to create messages and communication. An intranet needs to be designed, both aesthetically and navigationally, to facilitate the creation of information and messages from the body of facts that reside on servers and in databases.

Therefore, sound structure and visual appeal are as important in attracting users to an intranet as is the content itself because organization and visual guideposts will allow users to navigate the site effectively and find the information they seek. Therefore, by employing sound design principles, intranet developers can turn facts into information and information into communication, thus helping the intranet achieve its purpose as a new medium for communicating in an organization. If an intranet is thoughtfully and strategically designed, it can become the "one-stop shopping for all kinds of information" that developers envision (Hample 1996, p. 32).

To help developers achieve this goal, this article examines form as a result of function, audience needs and wants, and structural and visual design principles. Because the members of intranet development teams represent a variety of skill sets—too often not including basic communication skills—it is becoming increasingly important for professional communicators to review basic communication concepts in light of intranet development and design so they can contribute expertise to their company's intranet development.

Form and Function

In planning and creating effective design, form is dictated by function. The specific functions of an intranet vary from business to business, but in general terms, an intranet functions as a medium for gathering, submitting, and creating information. Because intranets exist in an environment where employees want to make their work processes simpler and where businesses want to make work processes more efficient, the form an intranet takes needs to reflect that efficiency. "Intranets need to function. It's like your car dashboard. Where's the turn signal?" (Bantsari 1997, p. 27).

But even a totally functional dashboard can contribute to the visual appeal of a car. Too often in the flurry to create functionality, form is de-emphasized or ignored. According to Mullet and Sano, "[Some] design disciplines—including most branches of engineering— . . . tend to focus largely or even exclusively on functional issues, often at the expense of aesthetics" (1995, p. 1). With estimates that roughly half of all intranets are created and maintained in a company's management information systems department (Holtz 1998), technology engineers are often the decision makers in intranet projects, from deciding navigational flow to selecting esthetic elements. Often these engineers are primarily concerned with function and not form.

At the Springville, UT, office of a large multinational corporation, the intranet was designed and created by a systems administrator in the information systems department. With degrees in engineering and business administration, his focus for the development of the intranet was on "functional issues" and the result has, in many ways, been "at the expense of aesthetics." Speaking of the intranet, this project manager said, "The intranet doesn't need to have all kinds of graphics or animated GIFs; that's not what an intranet is for. It's for getting information. That's it" (Turner 1998).

While the purpose of an intranet clearly *is* to provide and gather information, by focusing exclusively on functional issues, this project manager misses perhaps one of the most valuable tools available in making an intranet functional: design. Visual rhetoric can play a vital role not only in drawing curious novices to the intranet, but in helping them glimpse the impact such an information vehicle can have.

Form and function do not need to be at odds in intranet design. "Good design defuses the tension between functional and esthetic goals precisely because it works within the boundaries defined by the functional requirements of the communication problem" (Mullet and Sano 1995, p. 11). The functional requirements of an intranet do allow for better form than is often used. Yes, design must reflect function, but "fortunately, there is almost always a wide latitude for esthetic expression within these bounds, and experienced designers realize that solving a problem in a manner that is uniquely appropriate brings an esthetic satisfaction all its own" (Mullet and Sano, p. 11).

CONSIDERING AUDIENCE

Before solving the problem of form, developers first need to clearly define the intranet's function and goals. Corcoran says, "To realize an intranet's strategic potential, companies must have a vision of what they want to accomplish and a central plan to carry it out. Once they have an objective, companies can then decide how to logically organize information so users can find it efficiently" (1997, p. 86).

In determining the objectives of an intranet, only three things matter: audience, audience, and audience. Shortsighted developers will begin designing after having satisfactorily defined their own goals for the intranet but before having addressed their audiences' needs and wants (Ramey 1997, p. 389). Although user-centered writing and design are concepts fundamental to communicators, because a large percentage of intranets are being developed by information technology departments (Holtz 1998), it is easy to see that audience analysis may elude some developers untrained in structuring communication issues.

But for an effective and profitable intranet, these issues cannot remain elusive. Ramey cautions, "Don't start the design of a communication from the 'source' point of view. Instead, begin the design from the 'user' point of view" (1997, p. 389). Without considering the user's perspective, developers run the risk of designing an intranet that cannot fully exploit the communication possibilities they envision.

To illustrate the need for user-oriented design, Ramey speaks of her phone book search for the address of Seattle's hazardous waste facility. Based on the information she had (the name of the facility, what waste it handled, and her assumption that it was a city-run office), she first turned to the yellow pages. When they yielded nothing, she turned to the government pages. They also yielded nothing, so she gave up and phoned a friend who had been to the facility before. When she went to the facility, she discovered that it was county-run, not city-run. When she got home, she looked again and found the facility's address in the county government pages. Her point: "I am not saying that it doesn't make any sense to list facilities and services under the governmental units that run them. I am only saying that doing so may not communicate the facts to the intended consumer" (p. 388).

Hackos offers another example of source-based design. She tells of the instructions that came with her cellular phone: "The instructions appear to be written by an expert and assume that I know all about the inner workings of a cellular phone. . . . Such documentation is typical of an organization that has its development engineers write the manuals. It focuses on the inner workings, the system functions, rather than on what users want to do" (1997, p. 100). She concludes that "well-designed and -written online information focuses on the users and what they are trying to accomplish. . . . If we design and write online information with a user focus, rather than a system focus, our users will be able to recognize answers to their questions" (pp. 100–01).

While neither of these examples specifically addresses an intranet, the underlying theory applies. If intranet developers proceed without considering how employees will use the intranet, the intranet's design and organization will reflect that negligence and may hinder use rather than encourage it, particularly as the intranet compels users to learn new business processes and develop new working mindsets. As Albers points out, people will tend toward the familiar, reducing the cognitive strain involved in learning new tasks: "People . . . economize on cognitive resource allocation and attempt to produce satisfactory output with minimal effort. To relieve additional cognitive strain, they ignore options or use inefficient but familiar methods of accomplishing the task. Learning new methods requires mental exertion. If users feel pressed, they choose to perform a task in a known way. The result is that users don't consistently exploit new features" (1997, p. 2). He continues, citing system design as the root of the problem:

> When the system gives minimal guidance and requires users to figure out how to solve the task, they quickly become overloaded. The easiest way to reduce their cognitive load is to stop. . . . Rather than devising ways to efficiently handle the cognitive load, users often simply reduce cognitive strain by dumping parts of the problem and reverting to previously learned conventions. (p. 2)

If intranet developers do not devote sufficient time and research to designing a user-friendly, user-oriented intranet, as Albers notes, they may discourage users from turning to the intranet rather than encouraging them.

Albers' theme echoes Carroll's in his long-term research about design and usability issues: "Our interpretation of our subjects' struggles was that they were actually making rather systematic attempts to think and reason, to engage their prior knowledge and skill, to get something meaningful accomplished. They did not seem to be getting the appropriate guidance from the systems and documentation they were using, even though they were being presented with a huge amount of information through these channels" (1997, p. 28). Therefore, the "huge amount of information" inherent in an intranet must be deliberately organized through user-oriented design to reduce the cognitive strain on users and encourage them to work with the new medium.

The form of an intranet's function will be vital in convincing employees to become committed intranet users; therefore, audience should play a vital role in determining form because audience members are integral to an intranet's function (Moeller 1997, p. 110). At EDS Communications, intranet developers recently redesigned their intranet, and of the nine months it took to develop and deploy the new intranet, seven of those months were used to conduct user surveys and focus groups and to elicit user input. "We are using classic communications models—understanding the needs of an audience and delivering a message that the audience wants," says intranet administrator Jerry Stevenson, whose background is in communications and journalism and who has been cross-trained in systems engineering at EDS. The result of the extensive user studies? "We know users want what we provide before we even give it to them" (Stevenson 1998). It is important to conduct user studies to determine audience needs and wants, as well as to confirm the effectiveness of the intranet design. As intranet developers meld corporate goals with user needs in the design of the intranet, they will accomplish the fundamental goal of encouraging users to turn to the intranet for information and communication, which in turn speaks to the bottom line of more efficiently using company resources.

User-Oriented Design

Once functionality has been addressed by determining corporate goals and user needs, the form can begin to take shape. According to Rand, "To design is much more than simply to assemble, to order, or even to edit; it is to add value and meaning, to illuminate, to simplify, to clarify, to modify, to dignify, to dramatize, to persuade, and perhaps even to amuse" (1993). As intranet developers consider users in designing the structure of the intranet and the visual support of that structure, they will create a corporate medium that adds value and meaning, which in turn will ultimately persuade employees to become users. This section provides a specific discussion of those structural and visual issues—how to give form to the intranet's function.

Navigational Structure

"Navigational structure" refers to the organization of an intranet: what information is found where, how users move from page to page, and what is the overall hierarchy of the structure. Web-based communication has introduced several new dimensions to the architecture of information. I will examine points that are key to effective online information design.

Rethinking Print. One of an intranet's biggest selling points is that it can reduce paper and printing costs by replacing materials that are typically printed, such as directories, manuals, newsletters, memos, and brochures. However, with this advantage comes the inevitable temptation to lift "documents wholesale from another medium . . . and publish them as is on the site in HTML format" (Bocchi 1998, p. 10). Because word processors and desktop publishing programs can save documents as HTML files with the click of the mouse, some misguided organizations save otherwise paper-based documents in HTML and post them directly to the intranet with no attempt taken to reformat for the medium (Hackos 1997, p. 99). The result is lengthy pages through which to scroll and sometimes even unnecessary and cumbersome graphic representations of text. It can also mean that online content is as "flat" as it is on paper, losing the "web" feature of the new medium and its ability to intertwine relevant information spatially rather than linearly. When print documents are merely "posted" to an intranet, there is no value added to the online document, and often the print document is easier to use, a fact that compels users to revert to previously learned methods of performing their work.

When transferring print documents to an intranet, developers have to rethink the design of the document. "We can no longer assume that information written for paper can be transferred without change into online forms. . . . Using new design methods, we have the opportunity to provide information that is more useful, less frustrating, less voluminous, and less expensive" (Hackos 1997, p. 99). Bocchi suggests that "ideally, the web editor/administrator should ensure that . . . documents are redesigned and edited for navigability" (1998, p. 10).

The navigability comes with the "webbed" nature of an intranet, which allows for a level of dynamics impossible to obtain on a static page. Information can be layered and connected through active links, providing a way for a user to determine the depth of information he or she chooses to obtain.

For example, when an employee looks up someone on the intranet's company directory, rather than being presented with a lengthy alphabetized list through which to scroll, the employee uses a search engine to find the entry for the individual he or she seeks. That entry might include a name, title, department, address, phone number, and e-mail address. But should the user choose to seek more information, there could be a link to the person's bio page, department page, and e-mail. These added layers provide the user with the ability to obtain a greater depth of information and functionality than would be available in a static directory; they also allow the user to determine how much information to obtain. If the user simply needs a phone number or an e-mail address, then the top layer provides the needed information. But if the user is seeking further contact with the department for which the individual works, then the listing allows the user to explore further.

With information enriched by the additional layers, intranet users will find that in many cases, an intranet proves more useful and informative than a printed document. But only through the careful planning and redesigning of printed documents published online will users be convinced of the effectiveness of the intranet.

Imposing Structure. The intranet team at Amoco boasts of the lack of corporate-imposed structure to its intranet. Growing from a grassroots movement, the intranet has evolved into a structure that could be termed eclectic at best (Greenberg 1998). While administrators are beginning to take a more active approach to structure, Amoco's unregulated intranet structure has resulted in difficult-to-find information and dead-end searches. "There's not just one way to find what you want; it takes some searching, some intuitive linking" (Greenberg 1998). But with hundreds of pages strewn across the intranet and only "intuitive" links binding them, users whose intuition differs from that of a page's author can quickly become frustrated and disillusioned by the intranet and its lack of navigability.

In addition, Amoco's lack of cohesive structure has resulted in mounds of information through which users have to dig to find what they seek. "The information is presented with a lot of context. . . . That way, you can come from a number of different angles" (Greenberg 1998). Unruly structure misses the essence of an intranet, however. The purpose is to help users find information and perform work-oriented tasks with the greatest efficiency and least effort. Making users endure drawn out searches for information and then making them wade through that information in all its context defeats the purpose of the intranet, will likely discourage frequent use, and ultimately defeats the bottom-line goals of conserving employees' time and the company's resources. Rather, a degree of regulatory structure will help those publishing to the intranet better design their contributions, helping reduce and eliminate unclear navigational structure and facilitating more efficient intranet use.

To determine an effective intranet structure, Corcoran suggests that developers "figure out who is communicating and what information they are exchanging. Chances are this won't be reflected in the organizational chart, which does not mirror the flow of information in a company or a company's business processes" (1997, p. 86). By addressing how potential users are already communicating with each other, intranet developers can structure the intranet around that natural flow of information while adding the multiple dimensions of the interactive medium. Corcoran notes that at "Silicon Reef, information is grouped according to what employees want to do [on the intranet], not by department (Corcoran 1997, p. 86). While this specific structure may not be appropriate for every company, it is appropriate to determine a structure—as broad and generalized as the structure might be—and impose it so that users can quickly gain a familiarity with the intranet and how it is organized.

Creating Macro/Micro Design. Separating pages by macro and micro distinctions can also aid in structuring an intranet. In Tufte's structural design principles, "Micro/macro design is a critical and effective principle of information design that applies to every type of data because it enables readers to understand complex content by giving them an overview while at the same time presenting immense detail" (Zimmerman 1997, p. 310). The hierarchy of a well-organized intranet is inherently macro/micro. Pages should be made accessible to users based on audience needs: pages relevant to everyone are considered macro and are given the most prominent place on the intranet; next are pages relevant to many; and then pages relevant to few. For example, the home page links users to various department pages, which in turn link users to topical pages, which in turn link users to increasingly specialized pages.

Visual Guideposts

When designing the structure of an intranet, Sano says the "primary goal . . . in the design process is to communicate the organizational framework structure to the user. . . . The problem of users when lost in cyberspace is usually a symptom of an unclear, maze-like structure or web pages that all look the same without any emphasis to communicate hierarchy to the user" (1996, p. 143). Visual elements must serve as guideposts throughout the intranet to help users understand site structure and hierarchy, as well as to help them navigate the intranet efficiently and effectively.

Visual Precedents. Visual elements allow intranet developers to identify various information groups and assign them levels of precedence within the hierarchy of the site. "When pages are designed well, users are able to scan rapidly across the web page, with the most important information visually salient, providing the necessary cues to access further information or perform the required user interaction" (Sano 1996, p. 144). Visual precedents can be set by separating layers of information through the "distinctions of texture, weight, shape, value, size, or color" (Zimmerman 1997, p. 311). Says Horton, "The arrangement of elements on the page is the biggest factor in determining what people notice and read—or whether they abandon the page" (1996, p. 403).

A typical page arrangement, for instance, is one that includes common "action items" placed in a small navigation bar across the top of the screen, including elements such as "login," "e-mail," "stock price," or "tech support." In a column on the side of the screen runs another navigation bar or list that includes the broad categories of the intranet: for example, human resources, sales, engineering, and accounting. Finally, the balance of the page is comprised of content.

Within the content, visual precedents are set by creating headings and subheadings that differ in size and weight so the user can scan the page for information pertinent to him or her, by adding recognizable graphic elements to represent repeated categories such as home page or the company newsletter, and by placing information that needs particular attention in a call-out box. By setting visual precedents on the page, developers reinforce the hierarchical structure of the intranet, enabling users to navigate more easily. The result will be users who know to look at the top of the page to "do" something, to go to the side of the page to browse by category, and to scroll down to scan the main points of the content.

Consistency and Standardization. With the sheer magnitude of some corporate intranets and the number of people and departments from various locations contributing to those intranets, consistency and standardization can be difficult to manage and may be disregarded. For example, on the Amoco intranet, "At a business unit level, a common look and feel was never forced, and we developed a natural way to construct our intranet. . . . Design, to us, is not as important as making information available to people who might need it" (Greenberg 1998). The result of ignoring design in the name of "natural construction," however, is that the information may actually become less available rather than more available to those who need it. Without clear visual guideposts for a worker trying to accomplish a task, uncertainty is inevitable and can quickly persuade the user to go elsewhere for information.

Microsoft expressed a similar problem with their external Web site. With 300,000 pages contributed by more than 300 different groups (Dukay 1997, p. 321), Microsoft's Web site is at least as large as entire intranets at some companies, and is much larger than others. As the site grew and developed, team members overseeing the site elicited response from users. Typical of the responses was the following:

> I think you should have more consistency in the pages. All have good layout design, like the front page and the games page . . . but they're not consistent. This matter may not be important to everyone, but I think it would improve on the orientation of the site. (p. 324)

Similarly, when Sun Microsystems did usability tests of their large external Web site, they reported,

> Users across the board cited lack of consistency as a major problem in their use of the site. The difficulties in navigating through a large information site like Sun's and the lack of consistency in organization/presentation of information are major usability problems cited by all users. (Lau 1997, p. 150)

By including standard and consistent elements in the design of an intranet, developers can better facilitate employees' use of the intranet and guide them to the information they seek. "The intranet embodies a grand vision of corporate communication and cooperation. For this vision to be fully realized, it is essential that the intranet, taken as a whole, have a consistent and coherent design-without imposing Draconian restrictions on the individual departments" (Kreitzberg 1997, p. 63). Corcoran agrees that intranet administrators do not necessarily need to dictate so many rules that they stifle creativity and delay publication, "but it's good to standardize on a few elements such as a navigation bar for every page and icons for e-mail and chatting, . . . that way you establish basic 'grammar' for visual communication that everyone can understand" (1997, p. 87). Providing employees who are publishing to the intranet with a "grammar book" or a style guide—or even basic page templates—can help ensure consistency and standardization.

Simplicity and Personality. While intranet design should be visually appealing and even alluring to potential users, the function does not necessarily call for flashy or complex design. Rather, simplicity couched in clean design and corporate personality will better serve corporate purposes and user needs. "Consider simplicity and directness as a central, overall objective to help ensure clarity and understanding. The page design should enable, and not get in the way of, the user through the required task flow sequences" (Sano 1996, p. 149).

Fundamental to simple and clean design is eliminating extraneous elements. As Zimmerman notes, "Elements of the page must be designed to accomplish an overall goal" (1997, p. 310). Those elements might include a company logo, navigational bar, background image or color, and other graphical cues. If there are elements that do not contribute to achieving the goal of the page specifically and the intranet in general, they can be considered unnecessary and expendable. Examples might be animated graphics or other bells and whistles. That is not to say there is no place on an intranet for indulgent extras; indeed the multimedia nature of an intranet warrants enriching information by providing such things as 3-D images of building plans or by offering a ticker to track corporate stock prices. When designing pages for the intranet, however, developers need to be sure that the visuals contribute to the intended impact of the site and to the users' ability to navigate it.

CONCLUSION

Winsor notes,

> If persuasion is defined as changing the way someone else thinks or acts, then persuasion is at work [in electronic media], although it takes a somewhat different form than traditional notions of persuasion might suggest: It is interactive, multidirectional, and ongoing rather than a force that is exercised on one person by another in a single, discrete encounter. (1996, p. 70)

A large element of this rhetoric is found in the deliberate and subtle nature of navigational and visual design. Ultimately, if all the "facts" each contributor wants to publish to an intranet can be ordered, structured, and visually supported in such a way as to combine those loose facts into information that can then be communicated through networks and browsers, then an intranet is accomplishing its primary purpose: to facilitate communication among employees. And if better communication is taking place and work processes are refined in the electronic environment, then the company can look forward to experiencing the reduced costs, increased return on investment, and knowledge sharing that intranet champions promise will come with the deployment of a corporate intranet.

REFERENCES

Albers, Michael J. 1997. "Cognitive strain as a factor in effective document design." *The 15th Annual International Conference on Computer Documentation proceedings*. New York, NY: Association for Computing Machinery, pp. 1–6.

Bantsari, Lea Anne. 1997, "Elemental intranets, part 2." *Interactivity* (July).

Bocchi, Joseph. 1998. "Technical editing in transition: Editors wanted for intranet site development." *IEEE transactions on professional communication* 41: 5–15.

Braley, Sarah J. F. 1997. "Internal affairs: Planners tapping into corporate intranets to reach out to meeting-goers online." *Meetings and conventions* (August).

Carroll, John M. 1997. "Reconstructing minimalism." *The 15th Annual International Conference on Computer Documentation Conference proceedings*. New York, NY: Association for Computing Machinery, pp. 27–34.

Corcoran, Cate T. 1997. "Hack through the tangle of the corporate intranet." *InfoWorld* (11 August): 85–56.

Dukay, Kristin. 1997. "Unifying a large corporate Web site: A case study of www.microsoft.com," *IEEE International Professional Communication Conference proceedings*. Piscataway, NJ: IEEE, pp. 321–27.

Greenberg, Ruth. 1998. "Intranet introspective." *CIO WebBusiness Magazine* (August).

Hackos, JoAnn T. 1997. "Online documentation: The next generation." *The 15th Annual International Conference on Computer Documentation Conference proceedings*. New York, NY: Association for Computing Machinery, pp. 99–130.

Hample, Scott. 1996. "Intra-networking." *American demographics* (November/December): 28–32.

Holtz, Shel. 1998. Phone interview with Lisa Ann Jackson, 2 October.

Horton, W., L Taylor, A. Ignacio, and N. Hoft. 1996. *The Web page design cookbook: All the ingredients you need to create 5-star Web pages*. New York, NY: John Wiley and Sons.

Kreitzberg, Charles. 1997. "Intranet design takes planning." *Communications Week* (28 July): 63.

Lau, Teresa. 1997. "Toward a user-centered Web design: Lessons learned from user feedback." *IEEE International Professional Communication Conference proceedings*. Piscataway, NJ: IEEE, pp. 149–66.

McIntosh, Tera. 1997. E-mail to Lisa Ann Jackson, 7 October.

Melendez, Tony. 1997. E-mail to Lisa Ann Jackson, 8 October.

Moeller, Elizabeth Weise. 1997. "Designing a winning (and usable) Web site." *IEEE International Professional Communication Conference proceedings*. Piscataway, NJ: IEEE pp. 109–121.

Mullet, Kevin, and Darrell Sano. 1995. *Designing visual interfaces*. Mountain View, CA: SunSoft Press.

Ramey, Judith. 1997. "Fact, context, communication: The value added to data by communication design." *IEEE International Professional Communication Conference proceedings*. Piscataway, NJ: IEEE, pp. 385–392.

Rand, Paul. 1993. *Design: Form and chaos*. New Haven, CT: Yale University Press.

Sano, Darrell. 1996. *Designing large-scale Web sites*. New York, NY: Wiley Computer Publishing.

Stevenson, Jerry. 1998. E-mail to Lisa Ann Jackson, 13 October.

Turner, Cory R. 1998. Interview by Lisa Ann Jackson, 25 September.

Winsor, Dorothy A. 1996. "The textual negotiation of corporate 'reality,'" *Writing like an engineer*. Mahwah, NJ: Lawrence Erlbaum, pp. 69–86.

Zimmerman, Beverly B. 1997. "Applying Tufte's principles of information design to creating effective Web sites." *The 15th Annual International Conference on Computer Documentation Conference proceedings*. New York, NY: Association for Computing Machinery, pp. 309–17.

ADDITIONAL READINGS

Allen, Nancy. "Ethics and Visual Rhetoric: Seeing's Not Believing Anymore." *Technical Communication Quarterly* 5, no. 1 (1996): 87–105.

Bailey, Edward P. Jr. *The Plain English Approach to Business Writing*. New York: Oxford, 1990.

Barton, Ben F., and Marthalee S. Barton. "Ideology and the Map: Toward a Postmodern Visual Design Practice." In *Professional Communication: The Social Perspective*, edited by Nancy Roundy Blyler and Charlotte Thralls, 49–78. Newbury Park: Sage, 1993.

———. "Simplicity in Visual Representation: A Semiotic Approach." *Journal of Business and Technical Communication* 1, no. (1987): 9–26.

———. "Toward a Rhetoric of Visuals for the Computer Era." *The Technical Writing Teacher* 12 (1985): 126–45.

Beene, Lynn. "How Can Functional Documents Be Made More Cohesive and Coherent?" In *Solving Problems in Technical Writing*, edited by Lynn Beene and Peter White, 108–29. Oxford UP, 1988.

Bernhardt, Stephen A. "Seeing the Text," *College Composition and Communication* 37, no. 2 (1986): 66–78.

Carliner, Saul. "Physical, Cognitive, and Affective: A Three-Part Framework for Information Design." *Technical Communication* 47, no. 4 (2000): 561–76.

Coe, Marlana. *Human Factors for Technical Communicators*. New York: Wiley, 1996.

Coney, Mary B. "Technical Readers and their Rhetorical Roles." *IEEE Transactions on Professional Communication* 35, no. 2 (1992): 58–63.

DeJong, Menno, and Peter Jan Schellens. "Reader-Focused Text Evaluation," *Journal of Business and Technical Communication*, 11 (1997): 402–32.

Duin, Ann Hill. "Factors that Influence How Readers Learn from Text: Guidelines for Structuring Technical Documents." *Technical Communication* 36 (1989): 97–101.

Hart-Davidson, William. "On Writing, Technical Communication, and Information Technology: The Core Competencies of Technical Communication." *Technical Communication* 48, no. 2 (2001): 145–55.

Horton, William. "The Almost Universal Language: Graphics for International Documentation." *Technical Communication* 40 (1993): 682–93.

———. "Pictures Please: Presenting Information Visually." In *Techniques for Technical Communicators*, edited by Carol M. Barnum and Saul Carliner, 187–218. New York: Macmillan, 1993.

Huckin, Thomas. "A Cognitive Approach to Readability." In *New Essays in Technical and Scientific Communication: Research, Theory, Practice*, edited by Paul V. Anderson, R. John Brockmann, and Carolyn R. Miller, 90–108. Farmingdale, NY: Baywood, 1983.

Hughes, Michael. "Rigor in Usability Testing." *Technical Communication* 46, no. 4 (1999): 488–94.

Kaufer, David S. "From *Tekhne* to Technique: Rhetoric as a Design Art." In *Rhetorical Hermeneutics*, edited by Alan G. Gross and William M. Keith, 247–78. Albany: SUNY P, 1997.

Keyes, Elizabeth. "Typography, Color, and Information Structure." *Technical Communication* 40 (1993): 638–54.

Kinross, Robin. "The Rhetoric of Neutrality." In *Design Discourse: History, Theory, Criticism*, edited by Victor Margolin, 131–43. Chicago: U of Chicago P, 1989.

Kintsch, Walter, and Teun A. van Dijk. "Toward a Model of Text Comprehension and Production." *Psychological Review* 85 (1978): 363–94.

Kostelnick, Charles. "Conflicting Standards for Designing Data Displays: Following, Flouting, and Reconciling Them." *Technical Communication* 45, no. 4 (1998): 473–82.

———. "From Pen to Print: The New Visual Landscape of Professional Communication." *Journal of Business and Technical Communication* 8 (1994): 81–117.

———. "Supra-Textual Design." *Technical Communication Quarterly* 5, no. 1 (Winter 1996): 9–33.

Kumpf, Eric. "Visual Metadiscourse: Designing the Considerate Text." *Technical Communication Quarterly* 9, no. 4 (2000): 401–24.

Lewis, James R. "Introduction: Current Issues in Usability Evaluation." *International Journal of Human-Computer Interaction* 13, no. 4 (2001): 343–49.

Markel, Mike. "Using Design Principles to Teach Technical Communication." *Journal of Business and Technical Communication* 9, no. 2 (1995): 206–18.

Markel, Mike, and Kevin Wilson. "Design and Document Quality: Effects of Emphasizing Design Principles in the Technical Communication Course." *Technical Communication Quarterly* 5, no. 3 (1996): 271–94.

Mirel, Barbara. "Applied Constructivism for User Documentation: Alternatives to Conventional Task Orientation." *Journal of Business and Technical Communication* 12, no. 1 (1998): 7–49.

Nielsen, Jakob. *Designing Web Usability: The Practice of Simplicity*. Indianapolis: New Riders, 1999.

Porter, James E., and Patricia A. Sullivan. "Repetition and the Rhetoric of Visual Design." In *Repetition in Discourse: Interdisciplinary Perspectives*, volume 2, edited by Barbara Johnstone, 114–29. Norwood, NJ: Ablex, 1994.

Redish, Janice C. "Reading to Learn to Do." *IEEE Transactions on Professional Communication* 32 (1989): 289–93.

———. "Understanding Readers." In *Techniques for Technical Communicators*, edited by Carol M. Barnum and Saul Carliner, 14–41. New York: Macmillan, 1993.

Redish, Janice, Robbin Battison, and Edward Gold. "Making Information Accessible to Readers." In *Writing in Nonacademic Settings*, edited by Lee Odell and Dixie Goswami, 129–53. New York: Guilford P, 1985.

Rubens, Philip M. "A Reader's View of Text and Graphics: Implications for Transactional Text." *Journal of Technical Writing and Communication* 16 (1986): 73–86.

Schriver, Karen A. *Dynamics of Document Design*. New York: John Wiley & Sons, 1997.

———. "Taking our Stakeholders Seriously: Re-Imagining the Dissemination of Research in Information Design." In *Reshaping Technical Communication*, edited by Barbara Mirel and Rachel Spilka, 111–33. Mahwah, NJ: Lawrence Erlbaum, 2002.

Spiekermann, Erik, and E. M. Ginger. *Stop Stealing Sheep & Find Out How Type Works*. Mountain View, CA: Adobe P, 2000.

Spinuzzi, Clay. "'Light Green Doesn't Mean Hydrology!': Toward a Visual-Rhetorical Framework for Interface Design." *Computers and Composition* 18, no. 1 (2001): 39–53.

Sullivan, Patricia A. "Beyond a Narrow Conception of Usability Testing." *IEEE Transactions on Professional Communication* 32 (1989): 256–64.

Tebeaux, Elizabeth. "Visual Language: The Development of Format and Page Design in English Renaissance Technical Writing." *Journal of Business and Technical Communication* 5, no. 3 (1991): 247–74.

———. "Writing in Academe; Writing at Work: Using Visual Rhetoric to Bridge the Gap." *Journal of Teaching Writing* 7, no. 2 (1988): 215–36.

Tufte, Edward R. *The Visual Display of Quantitative Information*. Cheshire, CN: Graphics Press, 1983.

Wagner, Brian J. "An Easy Outlining Approach for Producing Solidly Structured, Audience-Driven Reports." *Journal of Business and Technical Communication* 8, no. 4 (1994): 475–82.

Williams, Robin, and John Tollett. *The Non-Designer's Web Book*. 2nd ed. Berkeley CA: Peachpit Press, 2000.

Williamson, Jack H. "The Grid: History, Use, and Meaning." In *Design Discourse: History, Theory, Criticism*, edited by Victor Margolin, 171–86. Chicago: University of Chicago P, 1989.

Wright, Patricia, Audrey Hall, and Deborah Black. "Integrating Diagrams and Text." *Technical Writing Teacher* 17 (1990): 244–55.

CHAPTER FIVE

Learning on the Job

Chapter Five: Introduction

One of the long-standing criticisms of the discipline of technical communication (usually voiced by other faculty in the humanities) is that its courses consist primarily of vocational training. At the heart of this criticism is the belief that courses in technical communication are not about knowledge for knowledge's sake; instead they help to prepare students for the workplace. What the faculty members who make the complaints don't understand, however, is that the task of preparing students for the workplace is no easy one. The workplace is not a monolithic entity, and the tasks that technical communicators will face in their workplaces are many. Providing a series of handouts consisting of templates or prescribed rules will not suffice. Nor will generic models of problem solving or information transfer. Making the pedagogical problem even more complex is the fact that the tasks writers face involve people, deadlines, and the challenge of making information accessible, often across a number of boundaries (e.g., time, space, culture).

To better understand the worlds of writing that technical communicators will enter, researchers, particularly those in cognitive science and qualitative inquiry, have made considerable progress in a number of areas, including ethics (see chapter 3), information design (see chapter 4), and intercultural studies (see chapter 6). Often relying on qualitative studies of workplace environments, which include the various genres of communication used in those environments, researchers have opened up the field, helping practitioners understand the complex situations they will encounter.

In this chapter, you will learn about this research in cognitive science and naturalistic inquiry, some of which can be (and often is) conducted in teachers' own classrooms. The essay from an award-winning volume by Carol Berkenkotter and Thomas Huckin presents a theoretical framework for genre and counters the notion of a static, template-driven environment. Two pieces about the role of genres and the nature of situated learning and communication competence in several different activity networks (Freedman and Adam; Spinuzzi) will demonstrate the difficulties involved in creating courses that can actually assist students in making the transition from university to workplace. Finally, the last two articles present qualitative studies from the workplace and two different collaborations between the classroom and the working world, to help you appreciate the complexity of the tasks before you. These studies focus on specific contexts in specific organizations, the difficulty of maintaining identity and authority amid social change, and the importance of recognizing what should be obvious, but often is overlooked: the workplace and the classroom are not the same, and strategies that work in one will not often work in the other. As you read these essays, you will learn that professional success depends on many things, including an understanding of the genres of communication in one's discipline or workplace, the social and cultural negotiations required to effect practical or material outcomes, and the importance of creating a "rich discursive context" (Freedman and Adam, p. 319 in this volume) to guide or facilitate both learning and "authentic participation" (p. 324).

18 *Rethinking Genre from a Sociocognitive Perspective*

CAROL BERKENKOTTER AND THOMAS N. HUCKIN

Berkenkotter and Huckin provide an important overview of genre theory to illustrate that an understanding of the genres in one's field is essential to success in that field. Building on the work of Bakhtin and others, they demonstrate that genres represent the way language is used in context, and as such, are dynamic. Their theoretical framework of five principles (dynamism, situatedness, form and content, duality of structure, and community ownership) is presented as a synthesis toward a sociocognitive theory. As students and teachers of technical communication, you will find their work useful for a number of reasons, not the least of which is the insight you will gain about the very heart of the courses we teach (the genres we ask our students to learn and replicate). Thinking about these genres not as static or historically frozen but as active, living "intellectual scaffolds on which community-based knowledge is constructed" (p. 304 in this volume) will enable you to open up your students' eyes to the kinds of learning they will need to do not only in class but also when they transition into the workplace.

> *The significance of generic categories . . . resides in their cognitive and cultural value, and the purpose of genre theory is to lay out the implicit knowledge of the users of genres.*
>
> —Ryan (1981, p. 112)

> *. . . the shapes of knowledge are ineluctably local, indivisible from their instruments and their encasements.*
>
> —Geertz (1983, p. 4)

Written communication functions within disciplinary cultures to facilitate the multiple social interactions that are instrumental in the production of knowledge. In the sciences and humanities, maintaining the production of knowledge is crucial for institutional recognition, the development of subspecialities, and the advancement of scientists' and scholars' research

From *Genre Knowledge in Disciplinary Communication*, Hillsdale, NJ: Lawrence Erlbaum, 1995. 1–25.

programs. Scientific and scholarly productivity are also the criteria by which careers are assessed, tenure given, and grants awarded. Knowledge production is carried out and codified largely through generic forms of writing: lab reports, working papers, reviews, grant proposals, technical reports, conference papers, journal articles, monographs, and so on. Genres are the media through which scholars and scientists communicate with their peers. Genres are intimately linked to a discipline's methodology, and they package information in ways that conform to a discipline's norms, values, and ideology. Understanding the genres of written communication in one's field is, therefore, essential to professional success.

A great deal has been written about the literary genres, and in rhetorical studies, genre theory have had a healthy resurgence since the late 1970s. Much of this material can be seen as various attempts to develop taxonomies or classificatory schemes or to set forth hierarchical models of the constitutive elements of genre (for reviews, see Campbell & Jamieson, 1978; Miller, 1984; Swales, 1990). This taxonomical scholarship and theory building has been based largely on analyses of the features of written or oral texts. Although such an approach enables one to make generalizations about what some writers refer to as a genre's *form, substance, and context* (see, e.g., Yates & Orlikowski, 1992), it does not enable us to determine anything about the ways in which genre is embedded in the communicative activities of the members of a discipline. Nor does a traditional rhetorical approach enable us to understand the functions of genre from the perspective of the actor who must draw upon genre knowledge to perform effectively.

Bakhtin (1981) argued that genres and other forms of verbal communication are sites of tension between unifying ("centripetal") forces and stratifying ("centrifugal") forces. "The authentic environment of an utterance, the environment in which it lives and takes shape, is dialogized heteroglossia, anonymous and social as language, but simultaneously concrete, filled with specific content and accented as an individual utterance" (p. 272). Genres are "typical forms of utterances" (Bakhtin, 1986, p. 63), and as such, they should be studied in their actual social contexts of use. In particular, analysts should pay attention to ways in which genre users manipulate genres for particular rhetorical purposes. Bakhtin (1981) argued that this "intentional dimension" can only be fully understood and appreciated by observing "insiders":

> For the speakers of the language themselves, these generic languages and professional jargons are directly intentional—they denote and express directly and fully, and are capable of expressing themselves without mediation; but outside, that is, for those not participating in the given purview, these languages may be treated as objects, as typifactions, as local color. For such outsiders, the intentions permeating these languages became *things*, limited in their meaning and expression. (p. 289)

To date, very little work on genre in rhetorical studies has been informed by actual case research with *insiders*. Instead, there has long been a tendency among genre scholars to reify genres, to see them as linguistic abstractions, and to understate their "changeable, flexible, and plastic" (Bakhtin, 1986, p. 80) nature.[1]

In this chapter we argue for an alternative way of looking at the genres of academic cultures, focusing on the ways in which writers use genre knowledge (or fail to use such knowledge) as they engage in such disciplinary activities as writing up laboratory experiments, judging conference proposals, negotiating with reviewers over the revisions of a research report, reading the drafts of a scientific article, or creating a new forum for scholarly publication. Our thinking is based on 8 years of rhetorical and linguistic analyses of case study data that foreground individual writers' language-in-use; this approach has led to our present view that writers acquire and strategically deploy genre knowledge as they participate in their field's or profession's knowledge-producing activities.

Our thesis is that genres are inherently dynamic rhetorical structures that can be manipulated according to the conditions of use, and that genre knowledge is therefore best conceptualized as a form of situated cognition embedded in disciplinary activities. For writers to make things happen (i.e., to publish, to exert an influence on the field, to be cited), they must know how to strategically utilize their understanding of genre. Their work must always appear to be on the cutting edge. This means that they must understand the directions in which a field is developing at any given time and possess the rhetorical savvy necessary for positioning their work within it. An academic writer needs to possess a highly developed sense of timing: At this moment, what are the compelling issues, questions, and problems with which knowledgeable peers are concerned? What is the history of these issues in the field? In the humanities, and the social and natural sciences especially, knowing what winds are blowing in the intellectual zeitgeist is essential to good timing (Miller, 1992).

The theoretical view we espouse here is *grounded* (Glaser & Strauss, 1967; Lincoln & Guba, 1985) in our observations of the professional activities of individual writers, specifically in the data that we have been collecting since 1984 on adult writers in disciplinary communities. Our method, however, has not been purely inductive. Over the last several years our perspective has been informed by a number of disciplines and by various writers' theoretical constructs. These include structuration theory in sociology,[2] rhetorical studies,[3] interpretive anthropology,[4] ethnomethodology,[5] Bakhtin's theory of speech genres (1986), Vygotsky's theory of ontogenesis,[6] and Russian activity theory[7] as it has shaped the movement in U.S. psychology called *situated* or *everyday cognition*.[8] From our research and from this literature we have developed five principles that constitute a theoretical framework:

- *Dynamism*. Genres are dynamic rhetorical forms that are developed from actors' responses to recurrent situations and that serve to stabilize experience and give it coherence and meaning. Genres change over time in response to their users' sociocognitive needs.
- *Situatedness*. Our knowledge of genres is derived from and embedded in our participation in the communicative activities of daily and professional life. As

such, genre knowledge is a form of "situated cognition" that continues to develop as we participate in the activities of the ambient culture.

- *Form and Content*. Genre knowledge embraces both form and content, including a sense of what content is appropriate to a particular purpose in a particular situation at a particular point in time.
- *Duality of Structure*. As we draw on genre rules to engage in professional activities, we *constitute* social structures (in professional, institutional, and organizational contexts) and simultaneously *reproduce* these structures.
- *Community Ownership*. Genre conventions signal a discourse community's norms, epistemology, ideology, and social ontology.

In the sections that follow we explicate each of these principles in detail, referring to a number of constructs in the literature mentioned earlier. We are not so much articulating a fully developed sociocognitive theory of genre as we are *working toward one* by integrating concepts from a number of fields. Thus we present a synthesis of perspectives and constructs from which a sociocognitive theory of genre can be developed.

Dynamism

Genres are dynamic rhetorical forms that are developed from actors' responses to recurrent situations and that serve to stabilize experience and give it coherence and meaning. Genres change over time in response to their users' sociocognitive needs.

This principle is derived from contemporary rhetorical examinations of genre (as reviewed by Campbell & Jamieson, 1978; Miller, 1984) and is perhaps best exemplified by Bitzer's (1968) discussion of recurrent rhetorical situations:

> From day to day, year to year, comparable situations occur, prompting comparable responses; hence rhetorical forms are born, and a special vocabulary, grammar, and style are established. . . . The situations recur and, because we experience situations and the rhetorical responses to them, a form of discourse is not only established but comes to have a power of its own—the tradition itself tends to function as a constraint upon any new response in the form. (p. 13)

Although Bitzer did not use the term *genre*, his notion of rhetorical forms emerging in response to recurrent situations sparked several scholarly discussions of rhetorical genres. A number of scholars invoked Bitzer's notion of recurring rhetorical responses to situational exigencies to characterize genre (Campbell & Jamieson, 1978; Harrell & Linkugel, 1978; Miller, 1984; Simons, 1978). And recently in an essay that examines the genres of organizational communication, Yates and Orlikowski (1992) treated Bitzer's claim as a concept symbol (Small, 1978) to mean that "genres emerge within a particular sociohistorical context and are reinforced over time as a situation recurs. . . . These genres, in turn, shape future responses to similar situations" (p. 305).

In a widely cited essay that reconceptualizes rhetorical views of genre from a sociological perspective, Miller (1984) proposed that "recurrence" does not refer to external conditions (a realist view) but rather, is socially constructed: "What recurs cannot be a material configuration of objects, events, and people, nor can it be a subjective configuration, a 'perception,' for these too are unique from moment to moment and person to person. Recurrence is an intersubjective phenomenon, a social occurrence, and cannot be understood on materialist terms" (p. 156).

Miller's major contribution to the discussion of genre was to take the notion of genre as recurrent response to a rhetorical situation and link it to Schutz and Luckmann's (1973) construct of "typification" as a socially construed meaning-making process. Our "stock of knowledge," Miller (1984) argued, following Schutz and Luckmann, is based on types:

> useful only insofar as [this knowledge] can be brought to bear on new experience: the new is made familiar through the recognition of relevant similarities; those similarities become constituted as a type. . . . It is through the process of typification that we create recurrence, analogies, similarities. What recurs is not a material situation (a real objective factual event) but our construal of a type. The typified situation, including typifications of participants, underlies typification in rhetoric. Successful communication would require that the participants share common types; this is possible insofar as types are socially created. (pp. 156–157)

Miller's social constructionist view of genre, which incorporates Schutz and Luckman's notion of typification, has been significant to rhetorical studies of genre for a number of reasons. First, it has influenced scholarship in the rhetoric of science (e.g., Bazerman, 1988; Swales, 1990). Second, it has provided scholars with an interpretive framework for dealing with the thorny issue of the relationship between socially determined human communicative activity and agency.[9] Finally, Miller's application of the construct of typification—grounded as it is in Schutz's sociological perspective of actors' behaviors in the life-world, in contrast to previous rhetorical and literary notions of genre—extricates the concept from its moorings in Aristotelian and literary classification systems, relocating it in a more microlevel understanding of the generic communicative behaviors of actors in everyday life. As she stated:

> To consider as potential genres such homely discourse as the letter of recommendation, the user manual, the progress report, the ransom note, the lecture, and the white paper, as well as the eulogy, the apologia, the inaugural, the public proceeding, and the sermon, is not to trivialize the study of genres; it is to take seriously the rhetoric in which we are immersed and the situations in which we find ourselves. (Miller, 1984, p. 155)

Miller's insistence that considerations of genre encompass the typifications of the agora as well as those of the senate has been important to studies in technical and organizational communication (see e.g., Devitt, 1991; Herndl,

Fennell, & Miller, 1991; Miller & Selzer, 1985; Yates & Orlikowski, 1992). And in locating genre in the social actions and practices of everyday life (in the professions and other social institutions such as the school), Miller's essay anticipates the interest in Bakhtin's construct of *speech genres*, which will figure importantly later in this discussion.

But just as language itself has to accommodate both stability and change, genres must do more than encapsulate intersubjective perceptions of recurring situations. They must also try to deal with the fact that recurring situations resemble each other only in certain ways and only to a certain degree. As the world changes, both in material conditions and in actors' collective and individual perceptions of it, the types produced by typification must themselves undergo constant incremental change. Furthermore, individual actors have their own uniquely formed knowledge of the world; and socially induced perceptions of commonality do not eradicate subjective perceptions of difference. Genres, therefore, are always sites of contention between stability and change. They are inherently dynamic, constantly (if gradually) changing over time in response to the sociocognitive needs of individual users. This dynamism resembles that found in other aspects of language acquisition, including, for example, the negotiated learning and use of individual words (cf. Huckin, Haynes, & Coady, 1993; Pinker, 1984), and to a lesser extent, the construction of sentences via "emergent" grammar (Goodwin, 1979; Hopper, 1988).

An example of this internal dynamism can be found in Huckin's study of 350 scientific journal articles published between 1944 and 1989 (chap. 2). In this study, Huckin analyzed formal patterns and interviewed a number of working scientists who regularly read and contribute to the literature. The scientific journal article has long been thought of as a conservative, relatively static genre, especially on the formal level, yet Huckin found that it had actually undergone significant changes over this 45-year period. For example, he found experimental results increasingly being foregrounded in titles, abstracts, introductions, and section headings, but methods and procedures sections increasingly being relegated to secondary status. The interviews with scientists revealed perhaps the main reason for these changes, namely, that in this age of information explosion, readers of scientific journals cannot keep up with the literature and are forced to skim journal articles the way many newspaper readers skim newspapers. These scientist readers are also writers, and their individual reading behavior affects their writing strategies. Inasmuch as they also belong to a scientific community, they find themselves responding in similar ways to similar communicative pressures. Thus, on both a communal and individual (i.e., sociocognitive) level, scientists shape the genre to better serve their needs. The result is a continually evolving, not static, genre.

SITUATEDNESS

Our knowledge of genres is derived from and embedded in our participation in the communicative activities of daily and professional life. As such, genre knowledge is a form of "situated cognition" (Brown, Collins, & Duguid, 1989) that continues to develop as we participate in the activities of the culture.

From a sociocognitive perspective, genre knowledge of academic discourse entails an understanding of both oral and written forms of appropriate communicative behaviors. This knowledge, rather than being explicitly taught, is transmitted through enculturation as apprentices become socialized to the ways of speaking in particular disciplinary communities. Because it is impossible for us to dwell in the social world without repertoires of typified social responses in recurrent situations—from greetings and thank yous to acceptance speeches and full-blown, written expositions of scientific or scholarly investigation—we use genres to package our speech and make of it a recognizable response to the exigencies of the situation.

Bakhtin's (1986) distinction between "primary" and "secondary" speech genres is a useful framework for helping us to distinguish between those forms of response that we use in daily communicative activities (greeting our children after school, making love, calling a colleague to ask for a favor) and those that are removed from the contexts of activities in which "primary genres" are embedded (e.g., scholarly and scientific articles, written forms of organizational communication, summons, subpoenas, patents). These "secondary genres" codify activity in situations occurring over time and in distant locales.[10] For this reason Bakhtin called the secondary speech genres "complex." The primary speech genres, in contrast, are "simple"; it is not the formal characteristics that are foregrounded but rather the particular communicative activities in which these genres are embedded. For example, young children, when they enter public school (or even preschool programs), learn the ways in which space and time in the classroom are configured during the school day and year and by association they learn the various forms of talk appropriate to a particular time of day and spacial configuration (e.g., sharing circle, reading groups, drawing and painting, etc.). Thus, children's accumulation of *school* genre knowledge begins very early in public school as they learn the patterned responses or "participation structures" (Cazden, 1986) associated with various school temporal/spatial activities, such as "sharing time"—which take place in the sharing circle.[11]

The sharing circle or "show and tell," like every other classroom language event, is governed by rules of interaction. Children leave their desks or tables and go to an open area in the classroom where they sit on the floor as a group. In the center of this group is the teacher, who most often sits on a child's chair. In this setting children make presentations to the group about some experience they have had outside of school. When a child's language behavior is not appropriate—interrupting while other children or the teacher is talking, taking the floor without raising a hand—the teacher gives strong negative cues (verbal and nonverbal) to child and peers. Time and space configurations are, therefore, an intrinsic part of primary speech genres. From this perspective, school days in school classrooms can be seen to consist of series of contiguous time/space/speech events: reading time, storytime, writing time, sharing circle, and so forth, as can be seen in Fig. 1.1. Through repeatedly carrying out

FIGURE 1.1 Structuration of School Days through Recurrent Events (e.g., "show and tell time," "spelling time," "nap time")

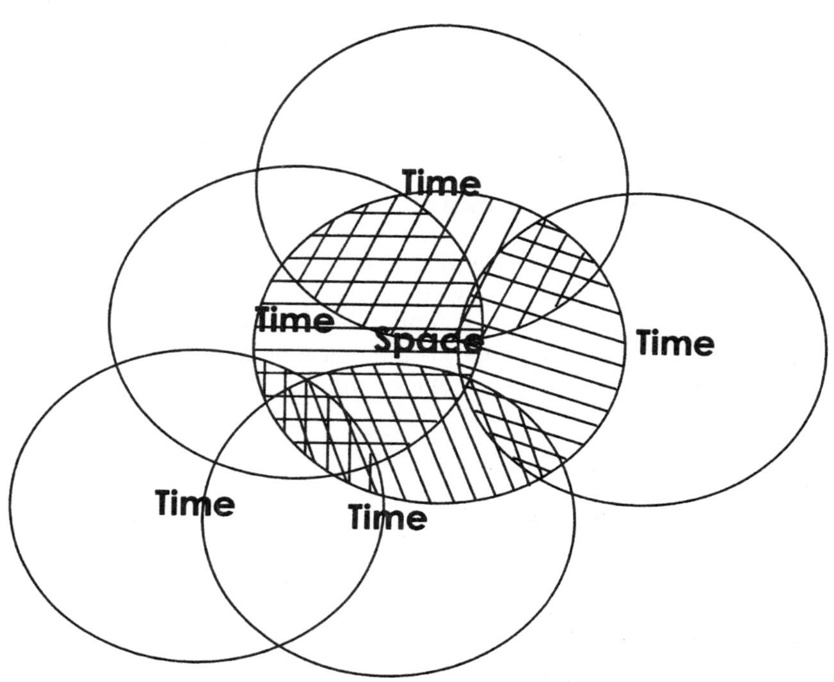

these activities, children come to learn what are situationally appropriate generic behaviors. Although Bakhtin does not elaborate his concept of primary speech genres in such detail, we would argue that the given characterization is entirely consistent with Bakhtin's view that the primary genres are to be found in the local communicative activities of everyday life.

Whereas primary genres are embedded in the milieu in which they occur, secondary speech genres are removed from their instantiation. Bakhtin (1986) put the matter this way:

> Secondary (complex) speech genres—novels, dramas, all kinds of scientific research, major genres of commentary, and so forth—arise in more complex and comparatively highly developed and organized cultural communication (primarily written) that is artistic, scientific, sociopolitical, and so on. During the process of their formation they absorb and digest various primary (simple) genres that have taken form in unmediated speech communion. These primary genres are altered and assume a special character when they enter into complex ones. They lose their immediate relation to actual reality and to the real utterances of others. For example rejoinders of everyday dialogue or letters found in a novel

> retain their form and their everyday significance on the plane of the novel's content. They enter into actual reality only via the novel as a whole, that is, as a literary, artistic event and not as everyday life. (p. 62)

Bakhtin's theoretical formulation seems prescient in light of recent research in the sociology of science (Gilbert & Mulkay, 1984; Latour, 1987; Latour & Woolgar, 1986) that suggests that the experimental article reifies archetypal experiential activities (such as scientists' lab experiments) by transforming them into seamless accounts of scientific activity. Thus Bakhtin's notion of secondary genres as forms of organized cultural communication helps us to see a basic and major difference between the genres of everyday life and their more culturally complex cousins. It is not possible in these latter forms to discern the embedding of tangible activities in the genre as we are able to in the case of the genre-in-activity of the elementary school classroom. Yet Bakhtin maintained that even though the secondary speech genres reflect complex cultural communication, it is the primary genres that "legislate permissible locutions in lived life and secondary genres made up out of these . . . constitute not only literary but all other text types (legal, scientific, journalistic) as well. In fact, what distinguishes one human undertaking from another, one science from another is the roster of genres each has appropriated as its own" (Holquist, 1986, pp. xv–xvi).

Bakhtin's perspective, grounded as it is in his concept of the dialogical nature of *all* oral and written communication, is one way of resolving the thorny issue of what kinds of communicative acts should be accorded "genre status," as Swales (1990) put it. This latter view is most often espoused by scholars in literary studies, rhetorical studies, and discourse analysis who focus on the formal characteristics of texts (written and oral) rather than on the activities or practices in which genres are embedded.[12] Their view rests on what Brandt (1990) called "strong text" (formalist) assumptions rather than a dialogical view of language-in-interaction (see also Nystrand & Wiemelt, 1991). This latter perspective is more common among sociolinguists and educational psychologists who share Bakhtin's (and Vygotsky's) view that social interaction is at the center of language and concept learning.

For Bakhtin (1986) the "responsive utterance" is the basic unit of analysis of human communication. The utterance is a rejoinder made in response to the other (which may also be internalized). Thus communication, oral *or* written, is constituted by a series of turns:

> Sooner or later what is heard and actively understood will find its response in the subsequent speech or behavior of the listener. In most cases, genres of complex cultural communication are intended precisely for this kind of actively responsive understanding with delayed action. . . . Any utterance—from a short, single-word rejoinder in everyday dialogue to the large novel or scientific treatise—has, so to speak, an absolute beginning and absolute end: its beginning is preceded by the utterance of others, and its end is followed by the responsive utterances of others. (pp. 68–69, 71)

From a Bakhtinian dialogical perspective, academic—or any other institutional—discourse can be seen to take place on a "conversational continuum" that inevitably for the language user involves a transition from naturalistic conversational turns to turns that are extended and monological. Along similar lines, Bergvall (1992) argued that:

> Academic discourse takes place on a variety of levels: casual hallway chats, lectures, conversations between teachers and students in and out of class, e-mail, memos, scholarly papers, books. Each of these is a form of academic "conversation," with a variety of levels of formality, personal involvement, number of participants, etc. The length of turns ranges from the quick exchanges of informal, intense conversation to the extended monologues of writing. Usually conversation is a natural pattern learned in childhood, but the appropriate use of the voice in academic conversation, particularly the monologic style, requires extensive training, and enculturation into the modes of conversation sanctioned by academic discourse communities. New members must learn style, vocabulary, citation format, organization, and length of texts or talk, etc. (p. 1)[13]

This view that actors' knowledge of academic discourse in its various permutations grows out of their enculturation to the oral and written "forms of talk" of the academy brings us to our next point—that genre knowledge is a form of *situated cognition*, in other words, knowledge that is indexical, "inextricably a product of the activity and situations in which it [is] produced" (Brown, Collins, & Duguid, 1989, p. 33). Learning the genres of academic discourse, like other forms of concept learning, evolves "with each new occasion of use because new situations, negotiations, and activities inevitably recast it in a new, more densely textured form" (Brown, Collins, & Duguid, 1989, p. 33).[14] As we have seen in our own research and that of others dealing with "cognitive apprenticeship" (Collins, Brown, & Newman, 1989), generally the enculturation into the practices of disciplinary communities is "picked up" in the local milieu of the culture rather than being explicitly taught. As Brown, Collins, and Duguid (1989) suggested:

> Given the chance to observe and practice *in situ* the behavior of members of a culture, people pick up the relevant jargon, imitate behavior, and gradually start to act in accordance with its norms. These cultural practices are often recondite and extremely complex. Nevertheless, given the opportunity to observe and practice them, people adopt them with great success. Students, for instance, can quickly get an implicit sense of what is suitable diction, what makes a relevant question, what is legitimate or illegitimate behavior in a particular activity. (p. 34)

Brown, Collins, and Duguid's argument here is based on their own as well as other studies of situated or everyday cognition (Engstrom, 1987; Lave, 1977, 1988a, 1988b; Lave & Wegner, 1991; Rogoff, 1990; Rogoff & Lave, 1984; Scribner, 1984). These studies owe a debt to the work of Russian activity theorists such as Vygotsky, Leontiev, and others, which has also influenced recent educational research (see Cazden, 1989; Clay & Cazden, 1990; Cole, 1985, 1990; Daiute, 1989, 1990; Dyson, 1987, 1988, 1990; Gallimore & Tharp, 1990; Wertsch, 1991). We believe that these latter studies are also relevant to our inquiries concerning the nature of genre knowledge.

Wertsch (1991) observed that Bakhtin and Vygotsky held a number of ideas in common:

> First [they shared] the assertion that to understand human mental action one must understand the semiotic devices [such as language] used to mediate such action. . . . Second [they held] the assumption that certain aspects of human mental functioning are fundamentally tied to communicative practices . . . that human communicative practices give rise to mental functioning in the individual. (pp. 12–13)

These views undergird much of what has recently been written about the situated nature of individual concept development. For example, Brown, Collins, and Duguid (1989) argued that acquiring conceptual knowledge, like learning the use of tools, is "both situated and progressively developed through activity" (p. 33):

> People who use tools actively rather than just acquire them . . . build an increasingly rich, implicit understanding of the world in which they use the tools and of the tools themselves. The understanding, both of the world and of the tool, continually changes as a result of their interaction. . . . The culture and the use of a tool act together to determine the way that practitioners see the world; and the way the world appeals to them determines the culture's understanding of the world and of the tools. Unfortunately, students are too often asked to use the tools of a discipline without being able to adopt its culture. To learn to use tools as practitioners use them, a student, like an apprentice, must enter the community and its culture. (p. 33)

An activity-based theory of genre knowledge would therefore locate our learning of academic genres in the processes that Vygotsky described as "socially distributed cognition," occurring in the situated activities of a practitioner-in-training. Genre knowledge, as we have seen in our own research, is very much a part of the conceptual tool kit of professional academic writers, linked to their knowledge of how to use the other tools of their trade: the biologist's lab assay, the literary historian's knowledge of how to synthesize information from archival microfiche, the psychologist's use of statistical procedures to determine degrees of freedom, the metallurgist's knowledge of the workings of the electron microscope. This is what we mean when we claim that genre knowledge is a form of situated cognition, inextricable from professional writers' procedural and social knowledge. *Social knowledge,* as we use the term here, refers to writers' familiarity with the research networks in their field (Kaufer & Geisler, 1989). It is the knowledge they draw on to create an appropriate rhetorical and conceptual context in which to position their own research and knowledge claims. Genre knowledge, procedural knowledge (which includes a knowledge of tools and their uses as well as of a discipline's methods and interpretive framework), and social knowledge are acquired incrementally as students progress through a period of apprenticeship, generally at the graduate level.

Learning the genres of disciplinary or professional discourse would therefore be similar to second language acquisition, requiring immersion into the culture and a lengthy period of apprenticeship and enculturation (cf. Freedman, 1993). In contrast, undergraduate university students, like secondary school students, learn many institutional, or curriculum, genres. Following Brown, Collins, and Duguid's (1989) line of reasoning, we would contend that many of these pedagogical genres contain *some* of the textual features and *some* of the conventions of disciplinary genres but that they are also linked to and instantiate classroom-based activities such as reading, writing, solving decontextualized math problems, or conducting simple experiments of the kind found in lab manuals. This view has a number of important implications for current notions of the teaching of disciplinary discourse. It may be the case, for example, that writing-across-the-curriculum programs should try to sensitize faculty in the disciplines to the fact that, in contrast to the specialized rhetorics they routinely use in their professional writing, the genres of the undergraduate curricula are characterized by quite different textual features and conventions, given their classroom-based contexts and rhetorical functions.

Form and Content

Genre knowledge embraces both form and content, including a sense of what content is appropriate to a particular purpose in a particular situation at a particular point in time.

If genres are dynamic rhetorical structures and genre knowledge a form of situated cognition, it follows that both genres and genre knowledge are more sharply and richly defined to the extent that they are *localized* (in both time and place). Traditional generic classifications are pitched at such a broad level of generality that they can describe only superficial parameters of form or content. For example, "the business letter," as discussed in traditional writing textbooks, is depicted in largely formal terms with only vague comments about content. By contrast, more localized genres like "a letter from a Utah bank promoting a new savings program" can be more fully described, with reference made to specific aspects of content (e.g., subtopics such as interest rates, security, tax benefits, etc. discussed in ways that are relevant to people from Utah). In the dynamic, grounded view of genre that we advocate here, what constitutes true genre knowledge is not just a knowledge of formal conventions but a knowledge of appropriate topics and relevant details as well.

Recent studies of academic discourse contain numerous examples of how deeply content is implicated in genre knowledge. For instance, Marshall and Barritt (1990), in their study of *American Educational Research Journal* articles, explained how this particular genre is strongly affected by philosophical considerations. They noted that "the forms of argument, in other words the rhetoric, used by scholars who publish in *AERJ* continue to be influenced by the objectivist tradition of research that owes so much to the analogy between natural and social events" (p. 605). They showed how this positivist stance manifests itself in particular textual features, such as the way in which reference is made to teachers, students, and parents. For example:

> Parents' decisions and opinions, when they are considered at all, are dismissed as economically motivated or as the result of intimidation rather than treated as genuine reflections of alternative beliefs about schools, education, or their own children. . . . It would be possible for the rhetoric of these articles to acknowledge parents as most often genuinely concerned about their children's well being. Parents could be constituted as adults who have perceptions different from those of teachers or researchers but whose views are no less accurate, complete, or complicated. . . . Yet such a shift in the rhetoric would necessitate attention to the role of the experience, common sense, reflection, relationship, perception, and motivation of parents as well as of researchers; a different rhetoric that would negate the authority of the researcher as expert knower. (p. 603)

The clear implication is that anyone wishing to publish in *AERJ* would do well to not give parents the same voice or status as researchers and, more generally, to avoid any methodology not adhering to positivistic norms. (For some other examples of how basic philosophical differences between social science research and humanistic scholarship reveal themselves in textual features, see Hansen, 1988; MacDonald, 1987, 1989, 1992.)

Another aspect of content that should be considered in defining a genre is background knowledge, that is, knowledge (of the world, of a particular community, of a discipline, etc.) that readers of that genre are assumed to have. A recent study by Giltrow (1992) provides a good example. Giltrow collected all newspaper reports of sentencing for violent crime that appeared in a major Canadian daily over a 2-month period in 1950 and over a 3-month period in 1990. She then analyzed and compared these two sets, focusing on how textual coherence is maintained via unstated assumptions of background knowledge. For example, in the following excerpt from a 1991 article about a child molester, a naive reader might wonder how the third sentence is related to the first two:

> The judge agreed with prosecutor Wendy Sabean that Blakemore, 31, of Georgetown "poses a real threat to the safety of others." The judge was told that Blakemore has confessed to sexually assaulting at least 17 boys and girls ranging in age from 6 to 10. Blakemore wants his mother, father, and Sunday school teacher charged for abusing him when he was a child, court was told. (*Toronto Star*, Jan. 3, 1991, p. A9)

Giltrow noted that the reporter who wrote this article was apparently assuming that a typical reader of this particular newspaper in 1991 would know (or believe, at least) that "a widely observed cause of adult violence is childhood experience of abuse by family members and/or respected members of the community" (p. 7). Indeed, as Giltrow showed, this assumption is embedded in the genre, enabling those readers who are familiar with the genre to move smoothly through the article. By contrast, such an assumption was apparently *not* part of the background knowledge expected of readers in 1950. The family was seen then, according to Giltrow, not as a corrupting influence but as a corrective one. Hence, in 1950 the excerpt quoted above would not have had the coherence it had in 1991. In addition to showing how background knowledge bears on genre knowledge, this example indicates how genres can, indeed must, change over time as community knowledge itself changes.

Closely related to background knowledge is the concept of surprise value or novelty, which can also play a role in definitions of genre and genre knowledge. In writing up news reports, for example, a journalist is expected to have a keen sense of what aspects of a story are most "newsworthy." Indeed, newsworthiness is the primary factor in the use of the so-called inverted-pyramid text schema (van Dijk, 1986). An appreciation of novelty is also important in academic disciplines. Bazerman (1985), Huckin (1987), and Kaufer and Geisler (1989), among others, showed how scholarly articles are expected to be at the "cutting edge," to make an original and novel contribution to disciplinary knowledge. The two philosophers in Kaufer and Geisler's study, for example, based their composing strategies on proposing novel knowledge claims and showing how these claims went beyond the consensual knowledge, or "framework knowledge," of the field. Their rhetorical expertise contrasts sharply with the inexpert behavior of two undergraduate students, who merely summarized the framework knowledge in one case and ignored it in the other. Kaufer and Geisler (1989) observed that:

> Despite significant differences between them, both freshmen, we submit, lacked the concept of novelty as a design strategy for academic argument. What exactly did they lack? They lacked the knowledge or skill to interplay two competing impulses: the impulse to account for the information one inherits from a cultural community (represented in sources) and the impulse to move beyond these givens by breaking a consensus within them (even if the consensus is only "As of yet, no one has"). Writers who successfully orchestrate both impulses design for newness. (p. 297)

In Berkenkotter and Huckin (1993a), we presented a case study showing how an experienced microbiologist uses the peer review process to orchestrate these two impulses.

Another aspect of content that should be taken into account in much academic writing (as well as in journalism and other fields) is that of *kairos*, or rhetorical timing. A good illustration of this strategy can be seen in the history of the discovery of DNA, as discussed in Miller (1992). DNA was first theorized by Avery and two colleagues in 1944. Nine years later its structural properties were described by Watson and Crick, who received much greater acclaim than did Avery, as well as the Nobel Prize. Halloran (1984) attributed these differences in reception partly to differences in the way the two teams wrote their reports. Avery's report of his discovery (published in the *Journal of Experimental Medicine*) is very cautious in style: long-winded, depersonalized, and dense with technical details; Watson and Crick's famous *Nature* report is short, elliptical, and coy. Halloran implied that Watson and Crick simply made better use of the genre than did Avery. In a strong counterargument, however, Miller observed that the rhetorical conditions for the two reports were vastly different. Avery was far ahead of his time, breaking new ground at a pace for which the scientific community was unprepared. Watson and Crick, by contrast, were riding the crest of a wave long in the making and well known to many observers. "Avery was working at one end of a 9-year 'revolution' in the understanding of genetic mechanisms. Watson and Crick at the other. The *kairos* in each case was quite different" (Miller, 1992, p. 311). In Giltrow's terms, the background knowledge that each writer could assume of his audience was very different. Thus, Avery was compelled to painstakingly lay out his methodology and findings and carefully situate his work in the larger body of scientific knowledge, whereas Watson and Crick could rush into print with only the sketchiest of details. Indeed, as Miller (1992) noted, "We might suspect that the two papers belong to quite different genres, which are defined in part by the rhetorical action achievable within the differing scientific situations" (p. 318).

In these examples, we can see how matters of content—epistemology, background knowledge, surprise value, kairos—influenced the selection and use of formal features in the instantiation of particular genres. Considerations of audience and situation are fundamental to these determinations, underscoring the rhetorical nature of genre knowledge and genre use. This is especially apparent in more "localized" cases where the characteristics of the audience and the situation are more sharply delineated. But this raises an interesting question: Is there some point at which a piece of communication becomes so localized that it ceases to be generic? In other words, is there some "threshold" of genericness? At the beginning of this section we suggested that "a letter from a Utah bank promoting a new savings program" could be considered a localized genre. But what if it is a new kind of savings program, and it is being promoted by only one bank via only one letter? Would such a letter constitute a genre? We feel that genericness is not an all-or-nothing proposition and that there is not a threshold as such. Instead, communicators engage in (and their texts reveal) various degrees of *generic activity*. No act of communication springs out of nothing. In one way or another, all acts of communication build on prior texts and text elements, elements that exist on different levels, including words, phrases, discourse patterns, illustrations, and so on. If texts arise out of discursive differences, as Bakhtin, Kress, and many others argued, such texts can be expected to embody different kinds of *recurring rhetorical responses* in different ways. Thus, rather than taking a holistic, normative approach to genre, as is done in traditional studies, we feel it makes more sense to take a more articulated approach in which individual texts are seen to contain heterogeneous mixtures of elements, some of which are recognizably more generic than others.[15]

Duality of Structure

In our use of organizational or disciplinary genres, we *constitute* social structures (in professional, institutional, and organizational contexts) and simultaneously *reproduce* these structures.

To make this principle clear, we need to introduce the concept of *duality of structure* that is at the center of structuration theory in sociology, as developed mainly by Giddens (1979, 1984). Traditional conceptions (Parsons, Althusser) maintain a clear separation between social structure and human action. Giddens (1984) noted that according to this view, "structure" is seen as "external to human action, as a source of constraint on the free initiative of the independently constituted subject" (pp. 6–17).

Such frameworks leave little conceptual space for a reflexive agent. Rather, the social actor is seen as something of a sociological dope who knows little of the institutions working in the background and whose values he or she is producing and reproducing. Giddens faults these schools of sociological thought because they discount people's reasons for their actions and assume that the only "real" stimuli for people's actions are institutional forces.

In contrast, Giddens (1984) argued that:

> The knowledge of social conventions, of oneself and of other human beings, presumed in being able to "go on" in the diversity of contexts of social life is detailed and dazzling. All competent members of society are vastly skilled in the practical accomplishments of sociology and are expert "sociologists." The knowledge they possess is not incidental to the persistent patterning of social life, but is integral to it. (p. 26)

According to this perspective, human agency and social structure can be seen to be implicated in each other rather than being opposed (Swales, 1993).

In place of dualisms such as the individual and society, or subject and object, Giddens (1979) proposed a single conceptual move, the *duality of structure*. Through this concept Giddens argued that social life was essentially recursive: "Structure is both medium and outcome of the reproduction of practices. Structure enters simultaneously into the constitution of the agent and social practices, and 'exists' in the generating moments of this constitution" (p. 5). Reproduction, it should be noted, does not mean simple replication; Giddens sees reproduction as allowing for changes and evolution within it. Duality of structure is akin to Bourdieu's (1987) concept of "double structuration," though Bourdieu put more emphasis on agents' struggle and on the use of strategies rather man rules.

As might be expected with the spread of such concepts through academic culture, a number of researchers and scholars in various fields have begun invoking Giddens' duality of structure concept to argue for a reciprocal relationship between social structure and rule-governed communicative activity. For example, in the field of conversation analysis, Wilson (1991) contended that:

> Traditionally, sociology seeks to describe and explain social phenomena in terms of notions such as status, role, class, religion, positionally determined interests, attitudes, beliefs, values, and so on. Although these may represent quite different substantive theoretical commitments, they share

> the fundamental Durkheimian assumption that social structure is exterior to and constraining on individuals and their actions and, consequently, *is an independent causal factor that can be adduced to explain social phenomena*. . . . The actor is portrayed as a judgemental dope, whose sense-making activities, if any, are treated as epiphenomenal, since the relations between categories and rules, on the one hand, and their concrete instances, on the other, are assumed for theoretical purposes to be transparent and unproblematic. (pp. 26–27, italics added)

The problem with this formulation is, acccording to Wilson, that it does not account for actors selecting the social–structural contexts that are most relevant to their communicative activity in a particular setting at a particular time—what Giddens (1984) described as actors' monitoring of their behavior. "Consequently," Wilson suggests, "parties to a concrete interaction must address who they relevantly are and what it is they are about on any given occasion. . . . This is an irremediable circumstance facing the participants, and the [conversation] analyst cannot settle the issue on their behalf by invoking some theoretical scheme or interpretation of the situation" (p. 25).

In contrast to the conventional view of social structure, conversation analysts such as Garfinkel, Goffman, Zimmerman, Wilson, and Mehan, who subscribe to the principle of relevance as developed from ethnomethodological research on microlevel social interactions, depict social structure as consisting of:

> Matters that are described and oriented to by members of society on relevant occasions as essential resources for conducting their affairs and at the same time, reproduced as external and constraining social facts through that same interaction. Thus, we must abandon any standard Durkheimian conception of social structure that takes externality for granted as a methodological stipulation. Rather, externality and constraint are members' accomplishments, and social structure and social interaction are reflexively related rather than standing in causal or formal definitional relations to one another. (Wilson, 1991, p. 27)

What does this alternative conception of social structure—derived from structuration theory and grounded in the findings of ethnomethodological research—have to do with rhetorical discussions of genre and, in particular, with our approach to genre from the perspective of actors' genre knowledge? Wilson's characterization of the reflexive, reciprocal relationship between social structure and social interaction is based on microlevel research on conversational interactions. Our perspective on genre, as we have indicated, is similarly based on several years of microlevel (although not ethnomethodological) investigations of academic researchers' meaning-making processes as they try to communicate with an audience of fellow professionals.[16] We have repeatedly observed such individuals drawing on genre knowledge to meet the requirements of a particular rhetorical moment. We would argue, with Wilson (1991), that "the fundamental justification for a classification of occasions must be that the participants orient to it [the occasion] as a type of situation, and moreover, orient to the present interaction as an instance of that type" (p. 39). People appear to orient to genre as situationally appropriate and relevant to a particular cultural framework.

A related perspective is taken by Mehan (1991), who, as a conversation analyst investigating oral classroom interactions, argued that:

> A second position on macro-micro relationships denies that the phenomenal aspects of society are merely reflections of large scale institutional forces. Instead they are contingent outcomes of people's practical activity (Giddens, 1979). Researchers in this constructionist tradition attempt to locate social structure in social interaction. . . . The constructionist line of investigation, as I see it, studies the situated artful practices of people and the ways in which these are employed to create an objectified everyday world without losing sight of institutional and cultural context. In this line of work, everyday practices are examined for the way in which they exhibit, *indeed, generate* social structure. The practices which generate the social structures are treated as endogenous to the work domains in which they occur and which they constitute. (p. 75, italics added)

To borrow from Mehan, then, our use of rhetorical genres is both constitutive of social structure (as it is instantiated through our observing a genre's rules-for-use or conventions) and generative as situated, artful practice.

Two researchers in the field of organizational communication, Yates and Orlikowski (1992), have attempted to capture this complex interrelationship in their discussion of the evolution of an institutional genre as a result of changing technological and demographic conditions.[17] They contended that social structures emerge from historical, institutional contexts constituted by the collaborative work of people adjusting to changing times and technologies. They suggested that one can best understand the development of organizational genres such as the business letter and the memo as "communicative action[s] situated in a stream of social practices which shape and are shaped by it" (p. 22). In their case history of the evolution of the office memo as a form of internal business correspondence away from the business letter genre of external correspondence, Yates and Orlikowski attempted to demonstrate that a reciprocal relationship exists between the changing textual features of a new genre and concomitant rules for use that are determined by people responding to a changing technological and demographic climate.

For example, the appearance of the typewriter and the vertical file (which dramatically increased the production and storage of inter- and intraoffice documents) can be seen to have led to the need for textual features and conventions that would help workers distinguish the office memo from formal business correspondence. With the appearance of the typewriter, which was adopted by businesses in response to the growth in correspondence and which increased the production of all correspondence, there emerged conventions such as underlining, subheads, and the use of all capital letters to facilitate readability. When tab stops were added to typewriters at the outset of the twentieth century, it became possible for the writer to easily make columns, including the columns comprising the typical To–From–Subject–Date heading. With the advent of typewriter technology there also appeared a need for a new occupational group, typists, to serve as operators of this new technology. Typists acted as agents of standardization and served to stabilize the document format within and across firms. Thus, according to Yates and Orlikowski's account of the evolution of the office memo, technological development acted in concert with demographic changes to influence the practices of a new population of office workers—all of which combined to influence the development of the genre's distinctive features and conventions. To paraphrase Giddens (1984) paraphrasing Marx, it is the social actors that are the agents of change (in this case, change in the structural features and conventions that come to distinguish internal correspondence from the business letter), but not through conditions of their own making.

In attempting to characterize the reciprocal character of the evolution of textual features and conventions of the interoffice memo, Yates and Orlikowski were among the first in organizational communication to draw on Giddens' (1984) structuration theory (see also Contractor & Eisenberg, 1990; Manning, 1989; Poole & DeSanctis, 1990). Their contribution to our understanding of the institutional dynamics of genre, building as it does on Bazerman's (1988) studies of the evolution of the experimental article, has important implications for scholars in rhetorical studies interested in the textual dynamics of the professions.

Community Ownership

Genre conventions signal a discourse community's norms, epistemology, ideology, and social ontology.

Asserting a relationship between the concept of genre and that of "discourse community" is a slippery proposition because neither concept refers to a static entity. Nevertheless, recent research in composition studies and discourse analysis supports our view that studying the genres of professional and disciplinary communication provides important information about the textual dynamics of discourse communities. For example, Swales' work on the conventions of the experimental article (Swales & Najjar, 1987) and more recently on the genres of academic writing (Swales, 1990) makes a strong case for understanding the functions of genre in terms of the discourse communities that "own" them (pp. 25–27).[18]

Similarly, Bazerman's (1988) study of the development of the experimental article in the natural sciences establishes an important connection between the formation of a scientific discourse community and the development of appropriate discursive strategies for making claims about experiments which, in turn, reveal the inner workings of the natural world. In examining the evolution of the experimental article in the natural sciences (in the first scientific journal, the *Philosophical Transactions of the Royal Society of London*), Bazerman demonstrated a fruitful historical methodology for understanding the emergence of a genre's textual features and rhetorical conventions in relation to disciplinary community formation. His study of the development of the features and conventions of scientific writing between 1665 and 1800 reveals how the increasingly complex interactions of an emergent argumentative community of natural scientists is tied to the appearance of genre conventions.

Our own research on discourse communities has led to our growing attention to the ways in which the genres of academic writing function to instantiate the norms, values, epistemologies, and ideological assumptions of academic cultures. Over the last several years we have had many opportunities to observe how writers and readers convey, through their textual practices, the beliefs and value systems of the disciplinary cultures in which they participate. In one study (Berkenkotter, Huckin, & Ackerman, 1988, 1991), for example, we observed a graduate student's socialization into a field of study and noted the extent to which his acquiring discipline-specific text conventions was connected to his learning a research methodology. Although the assumptions, norms, and values underlying the empirical methodology that he learned were not made fully explicit to this student during his training, he nonetheless assimilated the rationalist–realist epistemology that constitutes empiricist inquiry in the social sciences.

A study by Berkenkotter (1990) of the formation of a disciplinary subspecialty in literary studies, as seen through the evolution of a scholarly journal, reveals how disciplinary norms and values are codified as the forum becomes professionalized. In this case study, an emergent community of literary specialists interested in reader-response theory, criticism, and pedagogy organized a newsletter as a forum for exchanging ideas. The early issues of the newsletter contained a number of informal personal statements expressing the discontent of young professors with the norms of scholarly writing. These writers specifically inveighed against the elaborate style of professional discourse with its jargon, convoluted syntax, and pedantic authorial persona. A number of the contributors to the newsletter declared themselves to be members of a vanguard interested in transforming conventional academic writing with its underlying elitist, hegemonic value system. Despite this concern, as the newsletter evolved into a scholarly journal, it incorporated the formal textual features and conventions of literary scholarship and thereby demonstrated its movement into the disciplinary mainstream. The contributors' increasing use of the standard conventions of formal scholarly discourse with its overt intertextual mechanisms suggests that, despite a short period of rebellion, the textual instantiation of the values of the academy was an inevitable outcome of the institutionalization of the journal. What counted as knowledge had to be couched in the formal discourse of the literary scholar.

A third example of how genre conventions instantiate a discourse community's values and ideology can be seen in our study of a biologist's revisions of an experimental article (chap. 3 & 4). The biologist, who had published considerably in the field of immunology, submitted for review a paper with an underdeveloped introduction; instead of the standard literature review, she attempted to justify her present study by citing her own prior research, including an unpublished manuscript. Reviewers of the manuscript insisted that she position her study and her findings in the context of related scientific activity in the field. In the biologist's subsequent attempts to accommodate her reviewers, we see evidence of the ways in which genre conventions instantiate the scientific community's values and epistemology. In the final draft of the biologist's manuscript there appears a constructed narrative (what the biologist called a "phony story"), a chronology of events in other labs leading to, and therefore justifying, the present study. Such a narrative, which the reviewers agreed was essential for publishing local findings, reinforces a view of scientific activity as collective, inductive, and cumulative. As Lewontin (1991) suggested:

> Most natural scientists, and especially biologists, are really positivists. They rely heavily both on confirmation and falsification, and they believe that the gathering of facts, followed by inference rather than the testing of theories, is the primary enterprise of science. At times they speak highly of "strong inference," by which they mean something close to a Popperian falsification criterion, but this is not the modal form of biological work. . . . Whatever the popularity of notions about "normal science" and "paradigm shifts," the ideal of the "critical experiment" and "strong inference" remain the chief epistemological commitments of scientific ideology. (pp. 141–142)

This view of science is reinforced, Lewontin suggested, by scientists' daily reading and writing. The four-part structure of the scientific paper and the content within each of the four parts functions to reinforce the normative view just described of how science gets done. Learning the schema of the four-part structure of the scientific report (which for most students occurs at the graduate level as they write with their senior professors) means that young professionals assimilate the epistemology of their discipline as they learn the conventions of writing science. As we noted earlier, this was the case with the graduate student in educational research whom we observed learning the conventions of the social science research report (which is modeled on the experimental article in the natural sciences). To the extent that epistemological assumptions are embedded in the conventions of a genre, it seems reasonable to infer that many of this student's assumptions regarding empirical research in education studies were linked to the formal means of communication in which he regularly engaged.

Conclusion

When we speak of genre knowledge in disciplinary and professional cultures, we refer to knowledge that professionals need in order to communicate in disciplinary communities. Our perspective is both structurational, that is, based on our reading of Giddens (1979, 1984), and sociocognitive, compatible we believe with much recent research on language-in-activity coming from such diverse fields as sociolinguistics, cognitive psychology, educational anthropology, and conversation analysis. In our discussion of the five principles that undergird our understanding of genre, we have attempted to present a synthesis of some of this recent work. We then integrated these concepts with those that have emerged from our empirical studies to produce a framework for a sociocognitive theory of genre. We wish to underscore the relevance of structuration theory because we consider it a rich and exciting body of theory for insight regarding the relationship between available patterns for communicative utterances (Ongstad, 1992) and people's ability to alter or modify such patterns.

As social actors, we constantly monitor our actions and recognize the available patterns through which we might act at any given moment, yet we are capable of modifying those patterns to accommodate our reading of the rhetorical moment. We determine, for example, when a colleague offers a "Good morning. How are you?" those occasions when what is called for is a short, conventional reply, and those occasions (given our relation to that colleague), when it is appropriate for us to unburden ourselves of the rage we felt when we could not start the car because it was $-10°$ outside. We have the linguistic and rhetorical repertoires to choose our comments *artfully* in light of our reading of the occasion and of our relation to our interlocutor as we conceive it through both retrospective and prospective structuring of other occasions. It is through our constitution of many such encounters as they are enacted across time and space that we construct our social worlds.

Full participation in disciplinary and professional cultures demands a similarly informed knowledge of written genres. Genres are the intellectual scaffolds on which community-based knowledge is constructed. To be fully effective in this role, genres must be flexible and dynamic, capable of modification according to the rhetorical exigencies of the situation. At the same time, though, they must be stable enough to capture those aspects of situations that tend to recur. This tension between stability and change lies at the heart of genre use and genre knowledge and is perhaps best seen in the work of those who are most deeply engaged in disciplinary activity. Fully invested disciplinary actors are typically well aware of the textual patterns and epistemological norms of their discourse community, but are also aware of the need to be at the cutting edge, to push for novelty and originality. As the intellectual content of a field changes over time, so must the forms used to discuss it; this is why genre knowledge involves both form *and* content. In using the genres customarily employed by other members of their discourse community, disciplinary actors help constitute the community and simultaneously reproduce it (though, as we noted earlier, not in a simple replicative way). Thus, genres themselves, when examined closely from the perspective of those who use them, reveal much about a discourse community's norms, epistemology, ideology, and social ontology.

NOTES

1. This so even in cases where the theorist cites some case-study research. For example, Swales (1990) briefly mentioned the anthropological research of Knorr-Cetina, Latour, and Woolgar, and Gilbert and Mulkay, but otherwise relied heavily on his own text-based analyses. Schryer's (1993) description of a veterinary medical record system draws heavily on her own ethnographic research, but not in a way that enables her to capture the rhetorical dynamism

posited by Bakhtinian theory; instead of showing bow insiders manipulate and modify the genre for rhetorical purposes, her account emphasizes its more stable and normalizing aspects.

A noticeable exception is Myers (1990), who tapped substantial insider knowledge in depicting the struggles of practicing biologists to make the best use of certain scientific genres.

2. See Giddens (1984), Bourdieu (1987), and Bryant and Jary (1991).

3. See Bitzer (1968), Miller (1984), Yates and Orlikowski (1992), and especially the rhetoric of science (Bazerman, 1988; Swales, 1990).

4. See Geertz (1973, 1983), Clifford (1983), and Clifford and Marcus (1986).

5. See Garfinkel (1967).

6. See Vygotsky (1978, 1986).

7. See Wertsch (1981, 1991).

8. See Brown, Collins, and Duguid (1989) and Rogoff and Lave (1984).

9. For example, Bazerman (1994) extended Miller's notion of typification in some important ways, rescuing agency from an overly deterministic reading of typification as socialization into categories of response independent of individuality:

> ... such typification of moments goes hand in hand with learning genres of responses: this is the time for such-and-such kind of comment. Moreover, this typification helps us develop our set of characteristic social actions. We are learning how to recognize not only categories of social moments and what works rhetorically in such moments but also how we can act and respond ...
>
> *Nonetheless given the great variety of our biographies, we develop different constructs of moments and appropriate responses* [italics added]. ... Each [of us] perceives the moment as a different kind of occasion, calling on a different repertoire of responses. Each individual's characteristic sense-making and action patterns contribute to what we call *personality*. (p. 178)

10. Although be did not use the term *genre*, Giddens' (1984) concept of the reciprocal, reflexive character of structuration possesses an interesting resemblance to Bakhtin's notion of the textual dynamics involved in actors' creation of secondary genres:

> Repetitive activities located in one context of time and space have regularized consequences unintended by those who engage in those activities, in more or less "distant" time–space contexts. What happens in this second series of contexts then, directly or indirectly, influences the further conditions of action in the original context. To understand what is going on no explanatory variables are needed other than those which explain why individuals are motivated to engage in regularized social practices across time and space, and what consequences ensue. (p. 14)

11. For studies of the ways in which teacher–student interactions are controlled through the teacher's contextualization cues, see McHoul (1978) and Dorr-Bremme (1990).

12. For discussions of criteria that should be applied to determine which typifications can be considered genres, as opposed to pre-genres, forms, or appropriate level of abstraction, see Miller (1984), Swales (1990), and Yates and Orlikowski (1992). For critiques of this approach, see Derrida on the law of genre (1981) and Bennett (1990).

13. A number of linguists whose work is associated with the systemic–functional school of linguistics (pioneered by M. A. K. Halliday) have written extensively on the importance of making explicit to children the conventions of the primary and secondary speech genres found in different disciplinary settings, such as *talking science* (see Lemke, 1990). The best known of these neo-Hallidayans is Kress (1982, 1987, 1989, 1993a, 1993b), whose work on the social semiotics of school language learning calls attention to the ways in which childrens' and adolescents' social identities are situated in the multiple discourses they acquire through reading, writing, listening, and speaking. Other noted members of the "genre school" include Christie, Martin, and Rothery. This group's research and writing have provoked a heated debate in the United Kingdom over whether or not teachers should be trained to explicitly teach curriculum genres, that is, the genres of speaking and writing that are appropriate to different disciplinary contexts such as science, history, and literary study. The issues that this debate has raised can be found in Reid (1988).

14. Learning the genres of academic discourse thus involves learning both spoken and written modes, as mediated by the technologies entering the culture such as e-mail and electronic conferences. Because technology alters genres, producing blurred genres (see, e.g., Ferrara, Brunner, & Whittemore, 1991; Yates & Orlikowski, 1992), part of one's apprenticeship involves becoming fluent in various communicative media.

15. Swales (1990) also argued against a definitional approach to genre in favor of a "family resemblance" approach according to which "exemplars or instances of genres vary in their prototypicality" (p. 49). We share Swales' endorsement of prototype theory, but we are using it somewhat differently, namely, to describe generic elements at all levels rather than just unitary texts.

16. Our studies are not ethnomethodological in the sense that Garfinkel (1967) used the term in referring to studies of "the formal properties of commonplace, practical common sense actions 'from within' actual settings as ongoing accomplishments of those settings" (p. viii). Although his definition is applicable to recent work on conversation analysis (see, e.g., Boden & Zimmerman, 1991), we think that would be stretching a point to refer case study data as ethnomethodological, although our research aims coincide.

17. Yates and Orlikowski (1992) attempted to express the reciprocal relationship between social structure and human action in the following way:

> Structuration theory is centrally concerned with the reproduction and transformation of social structures, which are enacted through generalizable techniques or social rules. These rules shape the action taken by individuals in organizations, while at the same time by regularly drawing on the rules, individuals affirm and reproduce the social structures in an ongoing, recursive interaction. . . . The approach we develop . . . draws on the notion of structuration to capture the reciprocal and recursive relationship between genre and organizational communication, and to position the role of communication media within it. (pp. 4–5)

18. Swales (1990) characterized a relationship between discourse communities and the generic forms of communication that they produce, suggesting that:

> Discourse communities are sociorhetorical networks that form in order to work toward sets of common goals. One of the characteristics that established members of these discourse communities possess is familiarity with the particular genres that are used in the communicative furtherance of those sets of goals. In consequence, genres are the properties of discourse communities; that is to say, genres belong to discourse communities, not individuals, other kinds of grouping, or to wider speech communities. (p. 9)

REFERENCES

Bakhtin, M. (1981). *The dialogic imagination: Four essays by M. M. Bakhtin* (C. Emerson & M. Holquist, Trans.; M. Holquist, Ed.). Austin: University of Texas Press.

Bakhtin, M. (1986). *Speech genres and other late essays* (V. W. McGee, Trans.; C. Emerson & M. Holquist, Eds). Austin: University of Texas Press.

Bazerman, C. (1985). Physicists reading physics: Schema-laden purposes and purpose-laden schema. *Written Communication*, 2(1), 3–23.

Bazerman, C. (1988). *Shaping written knowledge: The genre and activity of the experimental article in science*. Madison: University of Wisconsin Press.

Bazerman, C. (1994). *Constructing experience*. Carbondale: Southern Illinois University Press.

Bennett, T. (1990). *Outside literature*. London: Routledge.

Bergvall, V. (1992, April). *Different or dominant? The role of gender in the academic conversation*. Paper presented at the annual meeting of the American Educational Research Association, San Francisco, CA.

Berkenkotter, C. (1990). *Evolution of a scholarly forum: Reader*, 1977–1988. In G. Kirsch & D. Roen (Eds.), *A sense of audience in written communication* (pp. 191–215). Newbury Park, CA: Sage.

Berkenkotter, C., & Huckin, T. N. (1993a). You are what you cite: Novelty and intertextuality in a biologist's experimental article. In N. R. Blyler & C. Thralls (Eds.), *Professional communication: The social perspective* (pp. 109–127). Newbury Park, CA: Sage.

Berkenkotter, C., Huckin, T. N., & Ackerman, J. (1988). Conventions, conversations, and the writer: Case study of a student in a rhetoric Ph.D. program. *Research in the Teaching of English*, *22*, 9–44.

Berkenkotter, C., Huckin, T. N., & Ackerman, J. (1991). Social contexts and socially constructed texts: The initiation of a graduate student into a writing research community. In C. Bazerman & J. Paradis (Eds.), *Textual dynamics of the professions: Historical and contemporary studies of writing in academic and other professional communities* (pp. 191–215). Madison: University of Wisconsin Press.

Bitzer, L. (1968). The rhetorical situation. *Philosophy and Rhetoric*, *1*, 1–14.

Boden, D., & Zimmerman, D. H. (1991). *Talk and social structure: Studies in ethnomethodology and conversation analysis*. Berkeley: University of California Press.

Bourdieu, P. (1987). *Choses dites* [Things said]. Paris: Les Editions de Minuit.

Brandt, D. (1990). *Literature as involvement: The acts of writers, readers and texts*. Carbondale: Southern Illinois University Press.

Brown, J. S., Collins, A., & Duguid, P. (1989). Situated cognition and the culture of learning. *Educational Researcher, 18*, 32–42.

Bryant, C. G. A., & Jary, D. (Eds.). (1991). *Giddens' theory of structuration: A critical appreciation*. London: Routledge.

Campbell, K. K., & Jamieson, K. H. (1978). Form and genre in rhetorical criticism: An introduction. In K. K. Campbell & K. H. Jamieson (Eds.), *Form and genre: Shaping rhetorical action* (pp. 9–32). Falls Church, VA: Speech Communication Association.

Cazden, C. (1986). Classroom discourse. In M. Wittrock (Ed.), *Handbook of research on teaching* (pp. 432–463). New York: Macmillan.

Cazden, C. (1989, March). *Vygotsky and Bakhtin: From word to utterance and voice*. Paper presented at the annual conference of the American Educational Research Association, San Francisco, CA.

Clay, M. M., & Cazden, C. B. (1990). A Vygotskian interpretation of Reading Recovery. In L. C. Moll (Ed.), *Vygotsky and education: Instructional implications and applications of sociohistorical psychology* (pp. 206–222). Cambridge, MA: Cambridge University Press.

Clifford, J. (1983). On ethnographic authority. *Representations, 1*, 118–146.

Clifford, J., & Marcus, G. E. (Eds.). (1986). *Writing culture: The poetics and politics of ethnography*. Berkeley: University of California Press.

Cole, M. (1985). The zone of proximal development: Where culture and cognition create each other. In J. V. Wertsch (Ed.), *Culture, communication and cognition: Vygotskian perspectives*. Cambridge, MA: Cambridge University Press.

Cole, M. (1990). Cognitive development and formal schooling: The evidence from cross-cultural research. In L. C. Moll (Ed.), *Vygotsky and education: Instructional implications and applications of sociohistorical psychology* (pp. 89–110). Cambridge, MA: Cambridge University Press.

Collins, A., Brown, J. S., & Newman, S. E. (1989). Cognitive apprenticeship: Teaching the craft of reading, writing, and mathematics. In L. B. Resnik (Ed.), *Knowing, learning and instruction: Essays in honor of Robert Glaser* (pp. 453–494). Hillsdale, NJ: Erlbaum.

Contractor, N. S., & Eisenberg, E. M. (1990). Communication networks and new media in organizations. In J. Fulk & C. W. Steinfield (Eds), *Organizations and communication technology* (pp. 143–172). Newbury Park, CA: Sage.

Daiute, C. (1989). Play as thought: Thinking strategies of young children. *Harvard Educational Review, 59*, 1–23.

Daiute, C. (1990). The role of play in writing development. *Research in the Teaching of English, 24*, 4–45.

Derrida, J. (1981). The law of genre. In W. J. T. Mitchell (Ed.), *On narrative* (pp. 51–77). Chicago: University of Chicago Press.

Devitt, A. (1991). Intertextuality in tax accounting: Generic, referential, and functional. In C. Bazerman & J. Paradis (Eds.), *Textual dynamics of the professions: Historical and contemporary studies of writing in professional communities* (pp. 336–357). Madison: University of Wisconsin Press.

Dorr-Bremme, D. (1990). Contextualization cues in the classroom: Discourse regulation and social control functions. *Language and Society, 19*, 379–402.

Dyson, A. H. (1987). The value of "time off task": Young children's spontaneous talk and deliberate text. *Harvard Educational Review, 57*(4), 396–420.

Dyson, A. H. (1988). Negotiating among multiple worlds: The space-time dimension of young children's composing. *Research in the Teaching of English, 22*(4), 355–391.

Dyson, A. H. (1990). The word and the world: Reconceptualizing written language development; or Do rainbows mean a lot to little girls? *Research in the Teaching of English, 25*(1), 97–119.

Engstrom, Y. (1987). *Learning by expanding*. Helsinki: Orienta-Konsultit Oy.

Ferrara, K., Brunner, H., & Whittemore, G. (1991). Interactive written discourse as an emergent register. *Written Communication, 8*(1), 8–34.

Freedman, A. (1993). Show and tell? The role of explicit teaching in the learning of new genres. *Research in the Teaching of English, 27*, 222–251.

Gallimore, R., & Tharp, R. (1990). Teaching mind in society: Teaching, schooling, and literate discourse. In L. C. Moll (Ed.), *Vygotsky and education: Instructional implications and applications of sociohistorical psychology* (pp. 175–205). Cambridge, MA: Cambridge University Press.

Garfinkel, H. (1967). *Studies in ethnomethodology*. Englewood Cliffs, NJ: Prentice-Hall.

Geertz, C. (1973). *The interpretation of cultures*. New York: Basic Books.

Geertz, C. (1983). *Local knowledge: Further essays in interpretive anthropology*. New York: Basic Books.

Giddens, A. (1979). *Central problems in social theory: Action, structure and contradiction in social analysis*. London: Macmillan.

Giddens, A. (1984). *The constitution of society: Outline of the theory of structuration.* Berkeley: University of California Press.

Gilbert, G. N., & Mulkay, M. (1984). *Opening Pandora's box: A sociological analysis of scientists' discourse.* Cambridge: Cambridge University Press.

Giltrow, J. (1992, April). *Genre and the pragmatic concept of background knowledge.* Paper presented at the International "Rethinking Genre" Conference, Carleton University, Ottawa, Canada.

Glaser, B. G., & Strauss, A. L. (1967). *The discovery of grounded theory: Strategies for qualitative research.* New York: Aldine de Gruyter.

Goodwin, C. (1979). The interactive construction of a sentence in everyday conversation. In G. Psalthas (Ed.), *Everyday language: Studies in ethnomethodology* (pp. 97–122). New York: Irvington.

Halloran, M. (1984). The birth of molecular biology: An essay in the rhetorical criticism of scientific discourse. *Rhetoric Review, 3,* 70–83.

Hansen, K. (1988). Rhetoric and epistemology in the social sciences: A contrast of two representative texts. In D. Jolliffe (Ed.), *Writing in academic disciplines* (pp. 167–210). Norwood, NJ: Ablex.

Harrell, J., & Linkugel, W. A. (1978). On rhetorical genre: An organizing perspective. *Philosophy and Rhetoric, 11,* 262–281.

Herndl, C. G., Fennel, B. A., & Miller, C. R. (1991). Understanding failures in organizational discourse: The accident at Three Mile Island and the shuttle Challenger disaster. In C. Bazerman & J. Paradis (Eds.), *Textual dynamics of the professions: Historical and contemporary studies of writing in professional communities* (pp. 279–305). Madison: University of Wisconsin Press.

Holquist, M. (1986). Introduction. In M. M. Bakhtin, *Speech genres and other late essays* (V. W. McGee, Trans.; C. Emerson and M. Holquist, Eds., pp. ix–xxii). Austin, TX: University of Texas Press.

Hopper, P. (1988). Emergent grammar and the *a priori* postulate. In D. Tannen (Ed.), *Linguistics in context: Connecting observation and understanding* (pp. 117–134). Norwood, NJ: Ablex.

Huckin, T. (1987, March). *Surprise value in scientific discourse.* Paper presented at the 38th annual meeting of the Conference on College Composition and Communication. Atlanta, GA.

Huckin, T., Haynes, M., & Coady, J. (1993). *Second language reading and vocabulary learning.* Norwood, NJ: Ablex.

Kaufer, D. S., & Geisler, C. (1989). Novelty in academic writing. *Written Communication, 6,* 286–311.

Kress, G. (1982). *Learning to write.* London: Routledge & Kegan Paul.

Kress, G. (1987). Genre in a social theory of language: A reply to John Dixon. In I. Reid (Ed.), *The place of genre in learning: Current debates.* Geelong, Australia: Deakin University Press.

Kress, G. (1989). *Linguistic processes in sociocultural practice.* Oxford: Oxford University Press.

Kress, G. (1993a). Against arbitrariness: The social production of the sign as a foundational issue in critical discourse analysis. *Discourse & Society, 4,* 169–192.

Kress, G. (1993b). Genre as a social process. In B. Cope & M. Kalantzis (Eds.), *The powers of literacy: A genre approach to teaching writing* (pp. 22–37). Pittsburgh, PA: University of Pittsburgh Press.

Latour, B. (1987). *Science in action.* Cambridge. MA: Harvard University Press.

Latour, B., & Woolgar, S. (1986). *Laboratory life: The social construction of scientific facts.* Princeton, NJ: Princeton University Press.

Lave, J. (1977). Tailor-made experiments and evaluating the intellectual consequences of apprenticeship training. *The Quarterly Newsletter of the Institute for Comparative Human Development, 1,* 1–3.

Lave, J. (1988a). *Cognition in practice.* Boston, MA: Cambridge University Press.

Lave, J. (1988b). *The culture of acquisition and the practice of understanding* (IRL Report No. 88–00087). Palo Alto: CA: Institute for Research on Learning.

Lave, J., & Wegner, E. (1991). *Situated learning: Legitimate peripheral participation.* Cambridge, MA: Cambridge University Press.

Lemke, J. (1990). *Talking science: Language, learning, and values.* Norwood, NJ: Ablex.

Lewontin, R. C. (1991). Facts and the factitious in natural sciences. *Critical Inquiry, 18,* 140–154.

Lincoln, Y. S., & Guba, E. G. (1985). *Naturalistic inquiry.* Beverly Hills, CA: Sage Publications.

MacDonald, S. P. (1987). Problem definition in academic writing. *College English, 49,* 315–330.

MacDonald, S. P. (1989). Data-driven and conceptually driven academic discourse. *Written Communication, 6,* 411–435.

MacDonald, S. P. (1992). A method for analyzing sentence-level differences in disciplinary knowledge-making. *Written Communication, 9,* 435–464.

Manning, P. K. (1989). *Symbolic communication.* Cambridge, MA: MIT Press.

Marshall, M. J., & Barritt, L. S. (1990). Choices made, worlds created: The rhetoric of *AERJ. American Educational Research Journal, 27,* 589–609.

McHoul, A. (1978). The organization of turns at formal talk in the classroom. *Language and Society, 7,* 183–213.

Mehan, H. (1991). The school's work of sorting students. In D. Boden & D. H. Zimmerman (Eds.), *Talk and social structure: Studies in ethnomethodology and conversation analysis* (pp. 71–90). Berkeley: University of California Press.

Miller, C. R. (1984). Genre as social action. *Quarterly Journal of Speech, 70,* 151–167.

Miller, C. R. (1992). *Kairos* in the rhetoric of science. In S. Witte, N. Nakadake, & R. Cherry (Eds.), *A rhetoric of doing: Essays honoring James L. Kinneavy* (pp. 310–327). Carbondale: Southern Illinois Press.

Miller, C. R., & Selzer, J. (1985). Special topics of argument in engineering reports. In L. Odell & D. Goswami (Eds.), *Writing in nonacademic settings* (pp. 309–341). New York: Guilford.

Myers. G. (1990). *Writing biology: Texts in the social construction of scientific knowledge.* Madison: University of Wisconsin Press.

Nystrand, M., & Wiemelt, J. (1991). When is a text explicit? Formalist and dialogical conceptions. *Text, 11,* 25–41.

Ongstad, S. (1992, April). *The definition of genre and the didactics of genre.* Paper presented at the International "Rethinking Genre" Conference, Carleton University, Ottawa, Canada.

Pinker, S. (1984). *Language learnability and language development.* Cambridge, MA: Harvard University Press.

Poole, M. S., & DeSanctis, G. (1990). Understanding the use of group decision support systems: The theory of adaptive structuration. In J. Fulk & C. W. Steinfield (Eds.), *Organizations and communication technology* (pp. 195–219). Newbury Park, CA: Sage.

Reid, I. (Ed.). (1988). *The place of genre in learning: Current debates.* Geelong, Australia: Deakin University Press.

Rogoff, B. (1990). *Apprenticeship in thinking: Cognitive development in social context.* New York: Oxford University Press.

Rogoff, B., & Lave, J. (Eds.). (1984). *Everyday cognition: Its development in social context.* Cambridge, MA: Harvard University Press.

Ryan, M. L. (1981). Introduction: On the why, what and how of generic taxonomy. *Poetics, 10,* 109–126.

Schryer, C. (1993). Records as genre. *Written Communication, 10,* 200–234.

Schutz, A., & Luckmann, T. (1973). *The structures of the life-world* (R. M. Zaner & H. T. Engelhardt, Jr., Trans.). Evanston, IL: Northwestern University Press. (Original work published 1975)

Scribner, S. (1984). Studying working intelligence. In B. Rogoff & J. Lave (Eds.), *Everyday cognition: Its development in social context* (pp. 9–44). Cambridge, MA: Harvard University Press.

Simons, H. W. (1978). "Genre-alizing" about rhetoric: A scientific approach. In K. K. Campbell & K. H. Jamison (Eds.), *Form and genre: Shaping rhetorical action* (pp. 33–50). Falls Church, VA: Speech Communication Association.

Small, H. G. (1978). Cited documents as concept symbols. *Social Studies of Science, 8,* 327–340.

Swales, J. M. (1990). *Genre analysis: English in academic and research settings.* Cambridge, UK: Cambridge University Press.

Swales, J. M. (1993). Genre and engagement. *Revue Belge de Philologie et d'Histoire, 71,* 687–698.

Swales, J. M., & Najjar, H. (1987). The writing of research articles: Where to put the bottom line? *Written Communication, 4,* 175–191.

van Dijk, T. (1986). News schemata. In C. Cooper & S. Greenbaum (Eds.), *Studying writing: Linguistic approaches* (pp. 155–185). Beverly Hills, CA: Sage.

Vygotsky, L. S. (1978). *Mind in society: The development of higher psychological processes* (M. Cole, V. J. Steiner. S. Scribner, & E. Souberman, Eds.). Cambridge, MA: Harvard University Press.

Vygotsky, L. S. (1986). *Thought and language* (A. Kozulin. Trans. and Ed.). Cambridge, MA: MIT Press.

Wertsch, J. V. (Ed.). (1981). *The concept of activity in Soviet psychology.* Armonk. NY: M. E. Sharpe.

Wertsch, J. V. (1991). *Voices of the mind: A sociocultural approach to mediated action.* Cambridge, MA: Harvard University Press.

Wilson, T. P. (1991). Social structure and the sequential organization of interaction. In D. Boden & D. H. Zimmerman (Eds.), *Talk and social structure: Studies in ethnomethodology and conversation analysis* (pp. 22–43). Berkeley: University of California Press.

Yates, J. A., & Orlikowski, W. J. (1992). Genres of organizational communication: A structurational approach. *Academy of Management Review, 17,* 299–326.

19 *Learning to Write Professionally: "Situated Learning" and the Transition from University to Professional Discourse*

AVIVA FREEDMAN AND CHRISTINE ADAM

Freedman and Adam's essay, which relies on theories of "situated learning" or "practical cognition" (p. 311 in this volume) as well as on recent work in genre theory, outlines some important differences between how people learn to write in the university and in the workplace. Drawing on two qualitative, naturalistic studies (three students in an upper-division finance course and seven graduate students working as interns), they argue for a slight reformulation of the theories currently labeled "guided participation" and "legitimate peripheral participation." They propose "facilitated performance" *and* "attenuated authentic participation," *which are, in their own words, "more specialized and possibly narrower" formulations (p. 314). The distinctions they make are based upon the contexts they describe: disciplinary classrooms have a richness resulting from the focused lectures, relevant readings, and what they call "extraordinarily elaborated semiotic signs" (p. 320) that result in a slightly different overall experience than "guided participation." In addition, the workplace context, because of focused goals ("institutional action"), creates an environment that is slightly different than the apprenticeships described as* "legitimate peripheral participation" *(p. 313). As you read their essay, you will note that there is much to be learned from the ways in which learning is facilitated and performance enhanced by teachers or mentors. Equally important are their findings that students need to learn to learn again (p. 334) when they leave their university, and the emphasis on the importance of "attenuation," which involves improvisation and "guider-learner roles."*

Over the past four years, we have been part of a team involved in a large-scale research project comparing discourse written by university students and practicing professionals within the same fields.[1] Our specific task has been to compare the writing of students in public administration programs with the writing of public servants employed in government or government-related work.

In the course of this project, we have found that the kinds of writing elicited at universities differ in many ways from the kinds expected in the workplace. Even in courses where the instructor is directly simulating a

From *Journal of Business and Technical Communication* 10, no. 4 (1996): 395–427.

workplace task through a factually based case study, the nature of the writing is fundamentally different because of the radical differences between the two rhetorical contexts (cf. Freedman, Adam, and Smart). In this article, we wish to make a separate, although related, point: When students move from the university to the workplace, they not only need to learn new genres but they also need to learn new ways to learn these genres.

To illuminate the differences in the kinds of learning experienced, we draw on the growing literature on theories of situated learning, or practical cognition. And an incidental purpose of this article is to reveal the usefulness of these theories for illuminating what happens in both university and workplace settings as members of both communities set out on the business of writing and learning to write.

To make our argument, we first contextualize our discussion theoretically—briefly explaining our use of the term *genre* and, at greater length, describing the newly developing field of situated learning that has provided us with the framework for differentiating between the two kinds of genre learning observed in the two sites: the university and the workplace.

We then present some of our research, focusing in detail on two settings: (1) a fourth-year course in financial analysis in which students were asked to simulate workplacelike reports in response to actual case histories and (2) an internship program, where novices were called upon to learn and perform the normal writing-related duties of that workplace. Our primary aim is to illustrate and clarify the nature of the differences—not so much between the genres elicited but rather between the kinds of learning experienced in, and necessitated by, the two settings.

Theoretical Background: Genre and Situated Learning

In the past few years, the notion of genre has been reconceived. Rather than referring simply to sets of textual regularities or text types, genres have come to be seen, in the words of Carolyn Miller's seminal 1984 article, as social action or "typified rhetorical actions based in recurrent situations" (151). It is not that textual regularities do not exist but rather that these textual regularities have come to be seen as correlates or indications of larger contextual regularities—social, cultural, ideological, political. This notion of genre has also proved to be particularly consonant with the theories of situated learning that are described here and that have guided our analysis.

In the past decade, a new field in psychology has emerged, variously called situated learning, socially shared cognition, everyday cognition, or situated experience. A primary focus of this new field has been on knowing and learning, but these terms have been redefined so that they carry very different meanings from those held within traditional studies of cognition. In fact, this new field is not so much cognitive science as a response to cognitive science as currently conceived. Fundamental to this work is the notion that knowing is social—not in the sense that one mind transmits knowledge to another but rather in the Vygotskian sense that the source of intrapersonal cognitive functioning is the interpersonal (*Thought, Mind*).

Nevertheless, the field of situated learning is not unitary. Although the importance of both social and collaborative performances in learning is commonly recognized, scholars and researchers conceive many of the key notions differently. The commonalities underlying this field are these: Learning and knowing are context specific, learning is accomplished through processes of coparticipation, and cognition is socially shared.

Given these commonalities, however, there are different streams within the literature. Jean Lave has specified three different theories of "situated experience." In the first, the "cognition plus view," researchers simply "extend the scope of their intraindividual theory to include everyday activity and social interaction. . . . Social factors become conditions whose effects on individual cognition are then explored" ("Situating Learning" 66).

The second, the "interpretive view," "locates situatedness in the use of language and/or social interaction" ("Situating Learning" 63). Furthermore, "language use and, thus, meaning are situated in *interested,* intersubjectively negotiated social interaction" (67, emphasis added). Individuals work together hermeneutically, through (largely verbal) interactions, toward a shared understanding, within contexts where they are each or all actively engaged.

Both the first and second theories are limited, according to Lave, in that they "bracket off the social world" and thus "negate the possibility that subjects are fundamentally *constituted in* their relations with and activities in that world" ("Situating Learning" 67). The third theory, "situated social practice" or, where appropriate, "situated learning," includes the interpretive perspective along with an insistence that "learning, thinking, and knowing are relations among people engaged in activity *in, with, and arising from the socially and culturally structured world*" ("Situating Learning" 67). A qualified version of this latter perspective informs our analysis.

Fundamental to that perspective is the recognition of the degree to which human activity is mediated through tools—especially that most powerful semiotic tool, language. In his discussions, James Wertsch ("Sociocultural," *Voices*) emphasizes the need to complement situated learning with Bakhtinian notions. Wertsch emphasizes in particular the way in which speakers "ventriloquate" portions or aspects of their ambient social languages in attempting to realize their own speech plans. All our words are filled with, and are echoes of and responses to, others' words. (To quote Bakhtin, "No one breaks the eternal silence of the universe" ["Problem" 69].) Our utterances are dialogic responses to earlier utterances as well as anticipations of our listeners' responses. The relations are multiple, complex, shifting, and dynamic. They demand and reward engagement and attention—and involve notions of complex interplay between an individual's free speech plans and the speech genres available, between an individual's own utterances and the ambient social languages.

The literature about situated learning has produced (at least) two analytic perspectives from which such learning can be viewed: Barbara Rogoff's "guided participation" (*Apprenticeship*, "Social") and Jean Lave and Etienne Wegner's "legitimate peripheral participation." Although these two perspectives have not been developed as alternatives to each other, they do, in fact, foreground different aspects of the learning process.

Rogoff uses the term *guided participation* to describe the learning process or cognitive apprenticeship that primarily middle-class children experience within their homes:

> Guided participation involves adults or children challenging, constraining, and supporting children in the process of posing and solving problems through material arrangements of children's activities and responsibilities as well as through interpersonal communication, with children observing and participating at a comfortable but slightly challenging level. The processes of communication and shared participation in activities inherently engage children and their caregivers and companions in stretching children's understanding and skill . . . [and in the] structuring of children's participation so that they handle manageable but comfortably challenging subgoals of the activity that increase in complexity with children's developing understanding. (*Apprenticeship* 18)

This perspective echoes notions like "scaffolding" and Lev Vygotsky's "zone of proximal development" (*Mind* 84–91): that space in which a learner can perform an action (cognitive or rhetorical) *along with* a skilled practitioner but not alone. The assumption is that, by so performing the act along with the practitioner, the child will later be able to operate alone: The intersubjective will become intrasubjective.

Guided participation can be contrasted with the learning that Lave and Wenger call *legitimate peripheral participation*, a process that characterizes various forms of apprenticeship—from that of Vai and Goan tailors to Yucatan midwives to butchers' apprentices to newcomers in Alcoholics Anonymous. Central to all these forms of apprenticeship is their focus on something other than learning. Apprentices and masters—or rather newcomers and old-timers—are both involved in activities that have a purpose above and beyond the initiation of newcomers. The tailors learn by becoming involved in making real garments. In all the instances, the activity as a whole has an end other than the learning of its participants.

In both processes, however, the newcomers do learn. The two processes are similar in very important respects;

1. Both are based on the notion of learning through performance or engagement—"learning through doing," as one of the instructors in our research kept repeating, as opposed to earlier cognitive notions of learning through receiving bodies of knowledge. "The individual learner is not gaining a discrete body of abstract knowledge (s)he will then transport and reapply in later contexts. Instead, (s)he acquires the skill *to perform by actually engaging in the process*" (Hanks 15, emphasis added).
2. Both processes are social—instructors and learners collaborate, in a broad sense, and one result is that learners are able to do something at the end that they were unable to do before.

3. In both, learning is achieved through sociocultural mediation of tools and especially linguistic and other semiotic signs. Also, in both kinds of learning the learners do not fully participate. The conditions for performing are attenuated; only some of the task is given over to the learner, and this attenuation (generally a subtle and highly nuanced attenuation) allows for the learning.

On the other hand, there is at least this radical difference between the two processes: In guided participation the goal of the activity itself is learning; in legitimate peripheral participation the learning is incidental and occurs as part of participation in communities of practice, whose activities are oriented toward practical or material outcomes. This difference has important consequences, as we shall see.

We have chosen to use the terms *facilitated performance* and *attenuated authentic participation* to differentiate between the two kinds of situated learning we observed. The echo in the names is intended to acknowledge their sources; the difference in wording is intended to reflect the fact that we use these terms in more specialized and possibly narrower ways than those intended by the originators.[2]

Research

Our goal in this article is to differentiate the processes of novices learning to write in the workplace from the processes of students learning new genres in their university courses. However, we focus primarily on the novices, comparing them to the students whose processes we have already described in other studies (cf. Freedman, "Learning," "Reconceiving"; Freedman and Adam; Freedman, Adam, and Smart).

University Courses

The university course we used for this study was an upper-level undergraduate semester course in financial analysis, where students responded to case studies (Freedman, Adam, and Smart). We selected this course because the instructor intended the writing assignments to be more like workplace writing than typical academic essays. In other words, we selected course writing that was as similar as possible to that of the workplace in order to highlight the contrasts. These findings have been corroborated and refined in the course of the larger project by more extensive observation of several different courses and classes in our business and public administration programs. The findings are also consonant with those of an earlier intensive case study focusing on an undergraduate course in law (Freedman, "Learning," "Reconceiving," "Argument").

Of the 25 students in the finance course, 3 students volunteered for close observation. These students provided us with the following: (1) the drafts of, and notes for, all written assignments; (2) papers written for other courses; (3) extensive retrospective interviews focusing on their composing—at the beginning, middle, and end of each of the three major assignments; and (4) tape recordings of segments of their joint composing sessions.

Before, during, and after the course, we interviewed the instructor, using open-ended questions to get at his goals, expectations, and ongoing reactions to the course and the writing assignments. He provided us with the course outline as well as the guidelines and task specifications for all assignments. The instructor also performed reading protocols in response to students' assignments. In classes we observed and recorded field notes on both the instructor's lectures and students' presentations. We collected written essays and case studies from all students in the class and observed oral case presentations.

The case study writing involved simulations based on actual case histories in which students were asked to write reports, as though they were managers or consultants to boards of directors of real companies, suggesting courses of action for the beleaguered companies at particular historical moments of crisis. Students were expected to write their reports using a workplace format, with an executive summary at the beginning and the format that one might expect in a business setting; at the same time, they were required to deliver oral summaries of their written reports, dressed like consultants and using professional accoutrements, such as overheads and briefcases.

Novices or Interns

The novices we observed were graduate students involved in full-time internships. The internships were organized by the School of Public Administration specifically for students in the midst of their MA studies. The internships were neither compulsory nor graded as part of the curriculum: They were opportunities for students to spend one or more semesters working in paid, full-time public sector jobs—the kind that they might aspire to upon graduation. The school facilitated the hiring procedure by advertising potential placements, collecting résumés from students, and providing a locale for interviews. The potential employers interviewed and hired interns using their own criteria.

We followed seven interns, each assigned to different government agencies, over the course of at least one semester. They presented us with copies of all their written work (and with all drafts of that work, including notations and responses by supervisors and peers). We interviewed the interns regularly, visited some work sites, interviewed superiors, and observed and taped work in progress on-site.

Analysis

Our observational data consisted of field notes taken during class presentations and work-site visits; notes based on the tape-recorded and transcribed interviews with the instructor, students, supervisors, and interns; notes based on the tape-recorded and transcribed compoting sessions; and the actual audiotapes and transcriptions. We analyzed our notes and transcriptions for recurrent themes and then cross-referenced and triangulated these themes with findings from the textual data. Working alone and cross-checking our observations with each other, we sought informant corroboration whenever possible (see Goetz and LeCompte).

Our underlying orientation throughout has been naturalistic; that is, our goal has been to elicit and value the participants' own constructions of the meaning of the discursive practices and on that basis to point to patterns in the richly textured, socially constructed realities of each discursive context.

FINDINGS

In keeping with the naturalistic orientation of this research, we organized the findings thematically, largely according to the theoretical models of situated learning described earlier—which themselves were constantly cross-checked and refined throughout the observations and analyses. The first subsection focuses on how the students learned to write the genres elicited in the university classes we observed. The second focuses on the differences in the two settings and, in the course of doing so, clarifies further the distinctive nature of the learning in the university as well as the workplace. The third subsection points to some of the problems that arise when university graduates accustomed to one mode of learning are placed in a context that requires another.

Facilitated Performance: Learning to Write at School

The theoretical frame that accounts for how students learned to write in the university classes we observed is best captured by the term *facilitated performance*. Our argument is that this frame, based on Rogoff's guided participation, accounts for how university students learn discipline-specific writing in the classes that we observed in much the same way as guided participation accounts for early child language acquisition or cognitive apprenticeship in middle-class homes (*Apprenticeship*).

The most salient commonality is that the guide in both cases, caregiver and instructor, is oriented entirely to the learner and to the learner's learning. In fact, the activity is undertaken primarily for the sake of the learner. (Presumably, parents do not read *Mother Goose* to themselves any more than instructors deliver lectures to themselves.) The guide's concentration is focused and centered on the learner and the activity—which is quite different from what we will see in the instances of workplace-based learning (and also quite different from what Rogoff ["Guided"] reported, as did Shirley Brice Heath in non-middle-class child rearing).

Not only is the guide's attention focused on the learner but the whole social context has been shaped and organized by the guide for the sake of the learner (recognizing that each such context is itself located in some larger institution whose goals are also at play—family, university, capitalist society, etc.). The caregiver organizes the storytime experience, and the instructor orchestrates the course (within certain temporal, spatial, organizational constraints): Readings are set, lectures delivered, seminars organized, working groups set up, assignments specified—all geared toward enabling the learners to learn certain material.[3]

Further, students did not, in the courses we observed, learn to write new genres on the basis of explicit direction by their guides (the instructors and teaching assistants), except in the crudest terms with respect to format, length, and subject matter (Freedman, "Show"). Nevertheless, the writing was shaped, constrained, and orchestrated from the first meeting of the course—that is, from its specification on the course outline and, more significantly, from the first words uttered by the instructor.

Our observations of these classes, and the students composing for them, revealed that learning new genres in the classroom came about as a result of carefully orchestrated processes of collaborative performance between the course instructor and students: Students learned through doing, specifically through performing with an attuned expert who structured the curriculum in such a way as to give the students increasingly difficult tasks. The instructor both specified the task and set that task within a rich discursive context. Both the collaborative performance and the orchestration of a richly evocative semiotic context enabled the acquisition and performance of the new genres—whether these were traditional academic essays about political theory, analyses of legal cases according to appropriate statutes of interpretation, simulations of workplace proposals, or feasibility studies.

Collaborative Performance. At the beginning of the course in financial analysis, for example, the instructor assigned cases to be written up at home, and then in class he modeled appropriate approaches to the data, identifying key issues and specifying possible recommendations for action. As they attempted to write up the cases themselves at home, the students were "extremely frustrated" because "[they had] to do a case before [they had] the tools to know how to do it." As one student described it, "It's like banging your head against a wall." However, after the instructor modeled appropriate approaches in class—especially *in the context of the students' struggles to find meaning in the data themselves*—the students were gradually able to make such intellectual moves themselves. As one of the students said, "[At the beginning,] when he would tell us the real issue, we're like—'Where did that come from?'" "[Then,] when you're done and he takes it up in class, you finally know how to do it!"

Modeling what the students would later do themselves, the instructor presented a number of cases at the beginning of the course. Like the mother with the storybook, the instructor showed the students first where to look and then what to say, picking out the relevant data from the information in the case, very often in the form of questions:

- "What's the significance of [items] 7 and 8 in the text? Did it add to your thinking about this case?"

- "At what market share restriction would that growth strategy not work?"
- "Assuming best-case scenario, what will this company look like in five years?"

He constructed arguments using the warrants of, and based on the values and ideology valorized in, the discipline. Drawing on the simulated purposes for the case, he pointed to the importance of looking at and presenting information in particular ways:

- "As a consultant to the bank, is this a critical value to know?"
- "In real life, you have to quantify this relationship between business risk and financial risk."

And as he moved from modeling the performance to having the students present the cases themselves orally in class, he provided corrective feedback:

- "Walk people through how you thought about the problem."
- "Let people know what the agenda is and your role."

Gradually, students were inducted into the ways of thinking, that is, the ways of construing and interpreting phenomena, valued in that discipline.

We see here many of the elements that Wood, Bruner, and Ross (1976) specified as functions of the tutor in scaffolding. The tutor defines the task, demonstrates an idealized version of the act to be performed, and indicates or dramatizes the crucial discrepancies between what the child has done and the ideal solution (qtd. in Rogoff, *Apprenticeship* 93–94). The element of motivation in scaffolding is unnecessary in the university setting because the institution of schooling itself, with its accreditation process, provides sufficient motivation for learning.

Discursive Context. These processes of collaborative performance offer part of the answer to how the students teamed to write the genres expected of them. In addition, the instructor set up a rich discursive context—through his lectures and through the readings—and through the mediation of these discourses, the students were able to engage appropriately in the tasks set.

Wertsch, drawing on Bakhtin, talks of the power of "dialogism" and of echoing (or "ventriloquating") social languages and speech genres. The students we observed responded—"ventriloquistically"—to the readings and the instructor's discourse, as they worked through the tasks set for them ("Sociocultural," *Voices*). Initially, they picked up (and transformed in the context of their preexistent conversational patterns) the social language or register they had heard. Here are oral samples culled from students' conversations as they worked on producing their case study:

> MIKE: I figured this is how we should structure it. . . . First, how did they get there is the first thing.

JUDY: So that's . . .

MIKE: business versus financial risk or operations versus debt, whatever. . . . Then . . . like we will get it from the bankers' perspective.

JUDY: Yeah, that's pretty much like what I was thinking too.

MIKE: So, right now I have their thing before 78. How do you want it, pre-78 post-78? This is what I did. I went through all. . . .

JUDY: internal comparison and stuff.

MIKE: I guess the biggest thing is the debt-to-equity ratio. Notice that? X has way more equity. If you look at Y, their equity compared to their debts is nowhere near, it's not even in the ballpark.

JOE: Which company is it that took a whole bunch of short-term debt?

Then, as the students wrote their papers, the conversational syntax lexicon, and intonational contours of their earlier conversations disappeared, and they reproduced discipline-specific terms in the context of academic written English, achieving thus the written social register of a financial analyst designated by their instructor (see Freedman, Adam, and Smart). In the final draft of a case study, we find the following:

> Short-term debt restructuring is a necessity. The 60% ratio must be reduced to be more in line with past trends and with the competition. This will be achieved by extension of debt maturities, conversion of debt to equity, reduction of interest rates, as well as deferral of interest payments.

In other words, through the mediation and appropriation of the social languages provided by the instructor's lectures and the readings, students created the new genres expected of them.

Findings from Other Undergraduate Courses. We have focused on this course in financial analysts because its writing was primarily intended to be most like that of the workplace, hence making differences particularly salient. To buttress our argument, however, we should add that analyses of learning to write in other academic courses revealed a similar pattern with the following qualification: In the other academic courses, there was typically far less collaborative scaffolding or modeling of problems to be solved; rather, facilitation was realized primarily in the carefully orchestrated and highly cued discursive context, established by the instructor(s) through lectures and readings, to which the students were expected to respond.

To repeat what has been reported elsewhere, learning to write the appropriate genres, in the courses we observed, was not achieved through *explicit* direction from instructors. The writing, nevertheless, was powerfully shaped and constrained by the instructor from the first meeting of the course. From the instructor's first words, a rich discursive context was created in the courses—through the lectures, seminars, and readings—a context that was clearly demarcated and differentiated from the wider-ambient discourse environments of the students' lives by its time slots, spatial location, and specification in course outlines. Students responded "dialogically" and "ventriloquistically" (to use Bakhtin's and Wertsch's terms) to this discursive context, when responding to the questions posed in the assignments.

To be more specific, the discursive context of the course—created through intonation, repetition, and other forms of cueing in the instructor's words and the words in those readings the instructor deemed relevant—shaped and constrained the writing in the following ways: The lexicon was echoed through the specialized usage of both the terminology of each field and common words appropriate to that field. Certain kinds of modalities were echoed; syntactic relations were modeled (e.g., clauses of condition or concession in law papers, clauses of qualification and causation in others). Lines of reasoning were modeled, and thus students learned which warrants were appropriate, the kinds of evidence they might (and might not) draw on, the degree of certainty to assign to different kinds of evidence, and the kinds of backing that might be necessary and when to use them. The instructors thus collaborated with the students and facilitated the production of each paper by providing this thickly textured and highly cued discursive context and then defining the kinds of questions in the assignments that encouraged the students to draw on the lines of argument and use the lexicon and syntax modeled in the classes.

From the perspective of situated learning, the disciplinary classes provided the same kind of "guided participation" that Rogoff describes (*Apprenticeship*). The guide or instructor shapes the context in such a way that the learner learns through performing activities elicited in this context. Our research revealed that, through being immersed in the rich discursive contexts provided in disciplinary classrooms—where instructors lectured to students for three hours a week, with these lectures often accompanied by a seminar of one or two hours and certainly accompanied by relevant readings—students began to be able to ventriloquate the social language and respond dialogically to the appropriate cues from this context. Their learning was mediated through extraordinarily elaborated semiotic signs—that shaped, constrained, and enabled their responses to the tasks that were set.

Attenuated Authentic Participation: Learning to Write Again

The interns we observed learning the genres appropriate to the government agencies to which they were assigned went through processes that, in some ways, were fundamentally similar to those engendered by the university settings. In both instances, learning resulted from collaboration, in the widest sense, or shared social engagement, as well as through the mediation of sociocultural tools (primarily, but not solely, linguistic signs). There were important differences, however, that are all the more significant for being tacit and implicit, complicating the transition into the workplace. Both the commonalities and the differences are suggested in the scene described next.

The following scene from one of our internship observations captures many of the significant features of the learning we call attenuated authentic participation. Any extended analysis and commentary is in square brackets. Douglas is the learner and Richard is his mentor or supervisor.

> Douglas and Richard are observed as they respond to a sudden request to prepare a briefing note on the state of a particular set of negotiations for a new minister.
>
> [Political events such as the appointments of new ministers often interrupt the anticipated flow of business in government offices. Mentors or supervisors must improvise if they are to include the learners in the new tasks. Both mentors and learners must be agile.]
>
> Douglas and Richard are standing in front of a desk that has a pile of previous briefing notes and reports on these negotiations. Their task is to develop a new document, summarizing succinctly what the new minister needs to know.
>
> The two discuss the potential content in global terms, brainstorming on a whiteboard, and then they sit down to write. Richard suggests that they work collaboratively. Douglas understands this to mean dividing up the task in two, with each taking responsibility for one half.
>
> [Presumably this reflects his notion of collaboration, based on what passed for collaboration as it was undertaken in his university courses.]
>
> Richard corrects this misconception, explaining that he means that they will actually produce the whole text together—the two of them sitting together to generate and compose text, with one person assigned to do the actual inputting. There is some joking and jockeying about who will do the inputting, but Richard decides that Douglas's superior expertise in word processing (he can use *Windows*) warrants his taking the seat in front of the computer.
>
> [It is not untypical in the workplace for novices to display superior expertise in relevant skills.]
>
> The two proceed to formulate and reformulate text together, with Richard taking the lead and providing feedback to each of Douglas's suggestions but at the same time constantly eliciting suggestions and listening carefully to Douglas's comments about his own suggestions. The two respond to each other conversationally in a series of half-sentences, which reveal the highly interactive nature of the interchange. Each half-sentence responds to, and builds on, the previous, so that the product becomes more and more jointly generated.
>
> [This kind of interactive generating and composing between a guide and learner is hard to imagine in a school context—even in a tutoring center. The coparticipation often reaches a flow at which it is difficult to determine who is suggesting which words.]
>
> Complicating this interactiveness is a tacit interaction with, or mediation through, already extant texts. Specifically, the suggestions for text are all based on the briefing notes and reports that are already available in the documents in front of them—with the words and phrases being modified,

echoed, reaccentuated, qualified. These earlier texts are cultural artifacts, which have been shaped by, and encode, the cultural practices and choices of the organization as it has evolved to that point. [In Bakhtin's terms, the words in the new evolving documents are being echoed from the earlier ones and reaccentuated in light of the current "speech plan" ("Problem" 76) so that the words become reinfused with slightly different meanings. This dialogism and mediation through cultural artifacts is true of university writing and hence learning as well but without the complicating factor of the intersubjective activities of guide and learner.]

In other words, the scene shows persons in activity with the world as mediated through the technological tools (word processors and software) and the cultural artifacts available. It depicts a hermeneutical grappling with notions, making it sometimes difficult to discover where one thinker's processes end and the other's begin and where the new speech plan begins and the older cultural artifacts end.

To sum up, this typical scene reveals learning as taking place through active processes (in this case, writing), guided by mentors, and mediated through cultural tools. In that respect, the learning parallels that of the university setting. The differences are the nature of the interactive coparticipation and collaboration between mentor and learner, the improvisatory nature of the task, the task's authenticity and ecological validity within a larger context (the institution and indeed society as a whole), and the varied and shifting roles played by mentor and learner. Furthermore, no conscious attention is paid to the learner's learning; all attention is directed to the task at hand and its successful completion. Table 1 summarizes these differences, which will be fleshed out in the discussions to follow.

TABLE 1 Differences between Facilitated Performance and Attenuated Authentic Participation

	Facilitated Performance	*Attenuated Authentic Participation*
Setting	University	Workplace
Goal of writing	Writer's learning *therefore*	Institutional action *therefore*
	Learning task sequenced by the guide	Improvisatory quality of learning occasions
	Context and task simplified	
Guide-learner role	Static and fixed	Shifting and multiple
Evaluation	Quality of texts determined by guide's grade Individualistic culture	Quality of texts determined by rhetorical success Collaborative culture
Learning site	Most guidance takes place before text is completed	Much guidance takes place, through extensive iterative collaboration after draft is completed

Goals of the Writing Task. The most striking difference between the learning that takes place in the university and the workplace—one with far-reaching implications—is that the goal of the writing task in the school context is clearly and explicitly for students to learn (with learning to write as a route to, or specialized instance of, learning). In contrast, the workplace operates as a community of practice whose tasks are focused on material or discursive outcomes and in which participants are often unaware of the learning that occurs.

Freedman, Adam, and Smart illustrate the degree to which learning and the learner are the foci of the writing tasks assigned in a university class (even when these tasks were presented as simulations of workplace situations, and the reports elicited ended with recommendations for action). As that study shows, the real goal of the writing was neither action nor policy but rather the demonstration that students knew the appropriate arguments to make in order to ground appropriate claims in the relevant arenas (as circumscribed by the course content). Both students and instructors understood that this demonstration of learning was the writing goal. We contrasted the university's writing goals with the action or policy orientation of workplace writing produced in the research unit of a government institution.

Our own research in the workplace and that of others have repeatedly shown that one consequence of this difference in writing goals is that it is often unclear to newcomers *that* they must learn, let alone *what and how* they must learn, and *from whom* they can learn. In the government agencies we observed, newcomers often asserted that they did not think that they would need to learn to write differently (see also MacKinnon). And when the supervisors were asked whether they considered the novices' learning to be one goal of the tasks they assigned them, their response was an unequivocal: "Hell, NO! They can learn on their own time." (As it turned out, these very supervisors were expert masters and mentors; they simply did not think of learning as implicated in the enterprise because it was not their explicit task goal.)

Role of Authenticity. Another way of illuminating this difference in orientation is suggested by the following: A key criterion of success in an internship relates to the degree to which the learner sees the task as authentic—that is, one that has consequences in its context. One intern we observed expressed his frustration over being assigned a "make-work project"—one that his coworkers did not see as relevant to the operations of the office and whose ultimate audience was as undefined for his supervisor as it was for him. This intern characterized the situation not as a loss in learning opportunities but rather as an obstacle to his ability to function legitimately as a member of that workplace community. Anthony Paré, a colleague in our larger project, has reported on a social work intern's disaffection toward a supervisor who provided him with thoughtfully invented simulations as opposed to a supervisor who gave the intern an authentic task, even though the simulations involved taking ownership of the whole task, whereas his involvement in the authentic task was necessarily limited because of his status. In contrast, any task in the university context is seen as authentic insofar as the instructor assigns it. From the perspective of the classroom, simulations are as authentic as academic essays, lab reports, or book reviews.

Attenuation. Assigning appropriate attenuated authentic tasks to newcomers requires mentors' skill, subtlety, tact, and imagination, especially given the complex and multifaceted nature of the work environments we observed. Not every mentor met that challenge. Sometimes, newcomers were given routine tasks at the outset, much to their frustration. At other times, however, tasks considerably below the ability and professional orientation of novices were assigned as a way of allowing them enough time to observe the complex operation. More imaginative mentors provided interns with authentic and more challenging tasks from the start—tasks that were within the competence of very green newcomers and that engaged them in processes that ultimately enabled fuller participation. For example, one intern was asked to take minutes at a round of negotiations; the task was authentic and necessary, was within her ken, and allowed her to observe the complex dynamics of the negotiating process as well as gave her an overview of the whole activity in which her work was to play a part. Observing the negotiations helped her understand how the different parts of the task she would be involved in related to the whole. It also opened her eyes to the dynamics of negotiating as well as to the competing value of systems at play.

Reflecting on this initial task in her placement, the intern emphasized the value of the experience in that it was relatively easy, familiarized her with a "government format" (e.g., "notes to file"), emphasized the importance of accuracy, "showed them [she] kn[e]w when to ask for help," and provided an opportunity to find out about the context of the meetings. A second intern was asked to compare in detail different sets of land claim agreements. The point-for-point, careful (and later collaboratively performed) comparisons introduced the newcomer to the whole activity—and engaged the newcomer in thinking through and reorganizing the relevant issues by operating on the discourse that was one material outcome of the activity.

The necessity to involve newcomers in attenuated authentic tasks, however, has certain consequences for the nature of the involvement—consequences that sharply distinguished such learning from school learning. These include (a) the improvisatory quality of the learning opportunities in the workplace in contrast to the carefully sequenced curriculum possible in the classroom and (b) the relative messiness of the workplace context in comparison with the simplified and facilitated context of the classroom.

Improvisatory Quality of Learning Opportunities. One consequence of the necessity for authentic participation that Lave and Wegner have noted and that we observed frequently in our work is the highly improvisatory character of the interns' tasks (as opposed to those in the classroom, where a curriculum can be more or less planned in advance—allowing for some degree of improvisation and responsiveness to learners). For example, we saw the intern from the scene we described earlier being pulled away from one task to prepare a briefing note for a newly elected minister.

A negative consequence of the opportunistic quality of learning in the workplace is that, because the tasks are authentic and respond to external demands unrelated to a learner's needs, the delicate apportioning of parts of the task at times must be truncated, and—even in the best internships—the master must take over. Sometimes, deadlines need to be met; at other times, the supervisor suddenly finds herself short-staffed. And often, the supervisor cannot be certain that the intern can operate under the added pressure. As one intern reflected, "He [the supervisor] would always think about it first before he would ask for my involvement—to see if he thought that I could function under that pressure. And if he thought I couldn't, he would do it himself alone." Even the best workplace guides find themselves having to fulfill responsibilities other than the apportioning of newcomers' tasks. One of the interns we observed described how his otherwise very successful internship had a rough start in that, for the first week after he arrived at the workplace, his supervisor was out of town. No one knew what work to give him, and so he was given "joe-jobs" (photocopying and filing) until his supervisor returned.

To put it another way, unlike the course curriculum, workplace tasks cannot possibly be carefully sequenced and designed. The institution of schooling gives instructors a degree of control, allowing them to sequence activities and to simplify tasks. (For example, in an undergraduate law course, we were struck by the sophisticated sequencing of the tasks, such that—among other things—the textual analyses showed increasing degrees of syntactic complexity and genre realization over the course of the year [see Freedman, "Learning," "Argument"].)

Messiness of Workplace Context. As suggested in an earlier study (Freedman, Adam, and Smart), the workplace context simulated in a university course, even when case studies are used and even when the case studies are not invented but based on actual histories, is enormously simplified and abstracted from the untidy realities experienced in the everyday work world. No matter how much irrelevance and ambiguity these case histories include, they are still abstractions from the experience of the workplace—abstracted to facilitate learning. In other words, the noise is removed and the task is simplified; something like Carl Bereiter and Marlene Scardamalia's procedural facilitation is taking place.

The tasks cannot be so simplified in the workplace. It is true that mentors will often model their thinking about issues in such a way as to reveal to the apprentices how to limit and define the problems, and newcomers may be assigned only a part of the task. The task itself, however, cannot be simplified.

For example, social and political relations in the workplace context are considerably more complex. Tensions among employees must be discerned and then navigated. Some of the complexities of relations are evident in the following extract where a supervisor explains to an intern why they have been having such a difficult time obtaining feedback on a document from a superior. "She was not too concerned, because she was ticked off that she wasn't invited to the meeting. That's why she wasn't consistent. . . . So that was an obstacle to my getting out of [her] what I was looking for." In fact, novices not only have to determine whom to trust as a guide (as we will see) but they also must learn to make that choice without alienating other would-be guides.

Guide-Learner Roles. A further difference between the two kinds of learning derives from the differences in the roles of, and interactions between, guides and learners in the two settings. The roles are more clearly defined in the university setting. The instructor is designated as the authority for the duration of the interaction (which is recognized to be relatively short). In apprenticeship situations, roles are more fluid and indeterminate: There are new old-timers and old old-timers, fresh newcomers and more-seasoned newcomers. Furthermore, newcomers are expected to become old-timers.

In the workplace novices must learn to discern (a) what their role is to be and (b) from whom they can learn. We observed in a number of settings that novices or interns resisted their would-be or could-be guides. Because no clearly sanctioned institutional teaching authority was vested in their superiors and because their supervisors were often less-than-seasoned old-timers, interns often resisted and consequently missed opportunities for learning. One intern, for example, refused to acknowledge the opportunities for learning offered by his supervisor because of her relative "greenness." That is, he incorporated her revisions to his draft of a document because he had to, but he refused to acknowledge the appropriateness of, and hence learn from, such editing changes as "land claims" to "land claim agreements"—which to us he insisted were really synonymous and merely a matter of idiosyncratic personal style.

Furthermore, as the different terms connote, the relations between old-timers and newcomers are far more complex, subtle, shifting, and nuanced than the relatively stable and straightforward relations between instructors and students. To quote William Hanks:

> Legitimate peripheral participation is not a simple participation structure in which an apprentice occupies a particular role at the edge of a larger process. It is rather an interactive process in which the apprentice engages by simultaneously performing in *several roles*—status subordinate, learning practitioner, sole responsible agent in minor parts of the performance, aspiring expert, and so forth—each implying a different sort of responsibility, a different set of role relations, and a different interactive involvement. (23)

We observed one intern taking on a range of these roles, all within one morning: With respect to the use of technology, he was the expert; however, when time constraints forced his supervisor to take control of the whole task, the intern's status as a subordinate was clear. For most of the morning, he operated as a learning practitioner, working collaboratively, but in an attenuated role, with his supervisor; at other points, he was named sole responsible agent for specific tasks (e.g., finding and contracting work out to a mapmaker). Later, in an interview with us, his supervisor kept stressing the degree to which he, as mentor, learns from newcomers—not only the most current academic theory but also different approaches to complex internal social and political relations.

Evaluation. Earlier we emphasized the fact that university writing is learning- and learner-oriented. To be fair, one must acknowledge the equally pressing institutional reality: University writing is also oriented toward evaluating and hence ranking students. The instructor's basic goal is that her students learn, but that goal is limited by the equally pressing need to grade and rank. Thus, in the end, the university instructor has a vested interest in a quality spread—which necessarily qualifies and limits the degree and the nature of the mentoring and collaborative performance. The guide-learner roles in the university are affected by the fact that, in the end and at every point, the guide evaluates the learner.

In the workplace, both newcomer and old-timer share the goal of producing the best work possible. There is some evaluation in the workplace, of course, but it is far less frequent and pervasive; more significantly, for specific tasks, newcomer and old-timer are often on the same side—they are working together on a task that will be evaluated by some outsider, usually in terms of its rhetorical or material success—in persuading others, in effecting action.

Consequently, there is no use of tests and grades in the workplace, and sparse use of praise and blame. Performance is evaluated by the overall success of the endeavor—the success of the writing, for example, as a rhetorical or social action. One of the interns recognized that his success in producing an initial document earned him his supervisor's trust and resulted in more significant tasks. "So," the intern claimed, "it was a big test." The reward for success was that the novice was entrusted with more responsibility and riskier tasks.

Learning Sites. Perhaps the most striking difference, however, is that the learning sites in the two settings are distinct. Consequently, when students move from university to workplace (or, in some cases, those experienced in the workplace move to the university), they do not necessarily recognize the opportunities for learning in the new setting because they are used to the way they learned in the old setting.

In the classrooms we observed, the performance was always guided by a great deal of careful stage managing of the prompt, task, and discursive context. The writing itself took place either alone or sometimes in collaboration with peers—with an occasional visit to the instructor or teaching assistant for advice. The students' final submission of their papers almost always meant the end of their involvement with the task.

In the workplace, the initial task itself was less controlled and shaped by the guide; typically, it was initiated and constrained by external sources. There was some collaborative interpretation of the task and often collaborative performance of the task at some stages of the writing. The most significant difference, however, was that completion of the draft began a long process of iteration. The most important learning site in the workplace, as a result, comes during the kind of extensive feedback James Paradis, David Dobrin, and Richard Miller described as "document cycling": "the editorial process by which [supervisors] helped staff members restructure, focus, and clarify their written work" (285). Graham Smart describes the typical process in a government agency that we observed:

> In all genres, composing processes are structured by a similar cycle of writer/reviewer collaboration. Typically [after composing a draft for review], the writer incorporates rounds of spoken and written feedback from the supervisor, into successive revisions until the latter is satisfied. At this point, another round of collaboration usually occurs, involving the writer, the supervisor, and a more senior reviewer. As the collaborative cycle continues, unnecessary technical detail is filtered out, key concepts are defined, and the argument becomes increasingly issue-centered, coherent, and succinct. When the chief of the department decides the text has been refined sufficiently, it is sent to its executive readership. (131)

The intensive and extensive nature of the feedback offered at each writing stage is described by a senior executive at a government financial institution we observed:

> When you do things at [this agency], it's a process that someone writes a paper (and it's an important paper—other than a one-pager or two-pager). When they write you a paper, you read it first from a high level—find out if the ideas are there, are the arguments consistent. So, when someone does something for me, I say, "Well, yeah, you're kinda on the right track." And I say, "Go back and try this, try that." So, it doesn't get down to the nitty-gritty of the writing at this point. You're still at the, almost the methodological stage, trying to deal with the question that's being posed. And so you go through *a number of iterations*. The person will come back with the paper answering a different question or adding another question to the analysis, and it's not until the very end that we'll say, "Now I know all the ideas are there. Now I'm going to read it from the perspective of how it's written. Are the ideas now expressed clearly?"

Another way of looking at the differences between the two settings is this: In the university context, most of the contextual shaping and coparticipation takes place *before* the preparation of the first draft. In the workplaces we observed, although some collaboration took place during the generating and planning, a long and intense process of responding and revising—a process during which attuned learners could intuit the expectations of the genre within that context and institution—began *after* the draft was handed in to the supervisor. The important point is that all the comments provided on drafts are collaborative, not evaluative. The revising itself is an intense period of coparticipation where learning can and should take place. But newcomers often do not recognize this as a potential occasion for learning.

Complicating the fact that the learning site is different—especially at the revision stage—is the interference from their previous learning patterns that suggests that anything written in response to a text by a grader is evaluative and final. Because novices in the workplace are typically not accustomed to *using* these comments for further revision, they hit a roadblock when a supervisor returns a draft to them with comments that the supervisor expects to be incorporated into a revised draft. For these novices, then, the comments written on their drafts mean negative evaluation and thus evoke resistance rather than recognition of opportunities for learning (and further collaborative performance).

Learning to Learn Again

We found considerable evidence in our research (Freedman, "Learning," "Reconceiving"; Freedman, Adam, and Smart) and that of others (Herrington; McCarthy; Walvoord and McCarthy) that university students are expected to learn new genres as they move from class to class. Such learning is both so inevitable and so naturalized that students hardly commented on it (Freedman, "Learning"). Consequently, as students move to the workplace, they seem to hold the same expectation: They may need to learn new genres, but the modes of learning will be the same (see initial assurance expressed in Anson and Forsberg). However, after some time on the job, the novices commonly reported feelings of disjuncture and anxiety not experienced in their schooling (Anson and Forsberg; MacKinnon; Freedman and Adam).[4] We claim that these feelings are not so much due to the need to learn new genres (such as memos, briefing notes, reports)—something they have been doing regularly throughout their schooling—but rather to the need to learn new ways to learn such genres.

Ronald Popken writes about the particular problems associated with learning new written genres, or "discourse transfer" (3). We observed a related problem: inappropriate transfer of learning patterns. Many novices did not think that they would have to learn at all—and certainly not in new ways.

For example, one intern, Julie, viewed each task as though it was set in a university context, with its clearly defined beginning and end and its clearly demarcated occasions for learning (in class and through assignments). Consequently, she consistently insisted on "getting on with her work" rather than availing herself of the learning opportunity offered her twice each day by the supervisor who invited her to take a short walk with him and another intern. Every day she refused the opportunity for shared reflection on, and learning about, what had been happening in the complex political and social rhetorical context of their workplace. During these walks the other intern learned how to read and interpret meetings and other interactions as an insider.

Julie consistently missed opportunities for learning, misconstruing them as new assignments, rather than as occasions for learning. "I didn't know I was expected to go to that meeting," she said resentfully, when she was called into a meeting that, although one she was not required to attend, would have given her a broader picture of the activity as a whole and thus have clarified her specific task. "Was I *supposed* to come?" she asked under her breath in annoyance. In other words, Julie was still mentally situated within the school context—where specific tasks are set out in clearly defined ways, within the context of clearly defined discursive environments (i.e., the assigned readings and the three or four hours a week of lecture, seminar, or both).

Other interns failed to learn from their supervisors' comments for revising drafts of their work, dismissing these comments as simply matters of personal stylistic preference. Rather than learning from these suggested revisions—changed wordings that often signified a great deal about how that particular culture viewed the world and the distinctions that were important there—the interns chose to see these changes as idiosyncratic personal preferences that they were being forced to accept but that they could resist learning from. When asked about what she had learned from her supervisor's comments, one intern reflected:

> I don't feel so much that it's the government way versus my way. It's just my way and Gill's way and Sandra's way. And my way isn't wrong, and when I'm the Director, I'm gonna write the memo however I want to.

One fundamental difference in the two contexts studied is the value placed on individualism in the university culture as opposed to the more collaborative ethos of the government agencies. (A negative take substitutes the words *anonymous* or *leveling* for *collaborative*.) In the end, all university students are graded individually, even when they collaborate on specific assignments.

Novices' transfer of this individualist ethos sometimes interferes with their ability to do the kind of collaboration necessary for performing and learning in the workplace. In our early interviews, interns displayed a kind of egotism: "It's my style. Why should I have to change it?" This egotism is exacerbated by the fact that students rarely revise their drafts in response to their instructor's written comments accompanying the grade. The comments serve to justify the grade, and although the instructor has the right to give a "B−," the students have the right to maintain their ideas and language.

Furthermore, the nature of the ownership is different. At least in theory, students' ideas belong to them, and instructors are berated for plagiarizing from students in a way not conceivable within a workplace. As suggested in Freedman, Adam, and Smart, employees in the government workplaces we have been observing rely heavily on intertextual references to each other's work (sometimes cited, sometimes not). Employee writing is kept on file, often for frequent consultation; student writing is filed, if at all, at home, and rarely consulted thereafter.

Summary

To sum up, in both contexts the learners learn new genres. The two processes of learning are similar in very important respects: Both are based on the notion of learning through performance or engagement—"learning through doing" (as one of the instructors kept repeating) as opposed to earlier cognitive notions of learning through receiving bodies of knowledge. What is entailed for the "teacher" in each setting is, in Hanks's words, "not giving a discrete body of abstract knowledge . . . instead . . . the skill to perform by actually engaging in the process" (14).

That is, students learn through activity and through social engagement: Instructors and learners collaborate, in a broad sense, and as a result learners are able to do something at the end that they have not done or been able to do before. In addition, learning is also achieved through sociocultural mediation of tools—especially linguistic and other semiotic signs.

Common to both processes as well is the notion of less than full participation by the learners. In each case, the conditions for performing are attenuated: In the university the curriculum is sequenced in terms of order of difficulty; in the workplace only some of the task is given over to the learner, and it is this attenuation (which is generally subtle and highly nuanced) that allows for the learning or fuller participation.

On the other hand, the two processes do differ radically. In the university, through processes of facilitated performance, the goal of the activity itself is learning; in the workplace, through processes of attenuated authentic participation, the learning is incidental and occurs as an integral but tacit part of participation in communities of practice, whose activities are oriented toward practical or material outcomes.

As a result, the guide-learner relations are different. In the workplace, the terms used are *old-timers* and *newcomers* (or *masters* and *apprentices*), and different people represent varying degrees of each (relative old-timers and relative newcomers); there is the further expectation that the newcomers will become old-timers. In the classroom, the instructor remains the instructor throughout, and the learner remains the learner. The roles are more static and fixed, and power is more clearly distributed—which is augmented by the fact that the instructor is also the evaluator and consequently has extra dimensions of authority and power, and hence alienation from the learner.

In the workplace, newcomers and old-timers typically work together on the same side for specific tasks (although not always—tensions of a different kind are possible there). In the classroom, however, the instructor has a vested interest in a quality spread of performance among students, causing a different kind of built-in tension between instructors and students, and among students.

In the classroom, the instructor has enormous latitude and authority in setting up the learning environment. Consequently, the curriculum is often sequenced and tasks are simplified, and most of the classroom activities are explicitly designed to enable learning. This sequencing and simplification is largely replicable from one course offering to the next. In the workplace, however, although a number of regular activities are built around institutional schedules, a considerable amount of spontaneity allows for reacting to unforeseen events and their resulting activities.

Finally, the learning sites are different in the two environments. In the university context, most of the contextual shaping and coparticipation takes place before the preparation of the first draft; in the workplace, learning takes place primarily through collaborative composing and revising, especially after a first draft is produced.

Discussion

The distinction we have been making between facilitated performance and attenuated authentic participation can begin to blur. Thus, if we focus only on the relationship between, and the activities of, newcomers and old-timers in the work setting, we may very well find a kind of collaborative guidance through performance that is at least broadly similar to that in the university setting.[5] Alternatively, one can find examples of university interactions that attempt to approximate more closely those of related communities of practice, where the learning is intended to be like that found in instances of legitimate peripheral participation or attenuated authentic participation (see Gutierrez; Rogoff, "Models"). These are classes in which tasks with real-world consequences are selected and where students work in collaborative groups of peers. Without denying the value of such experiments or the possibility of seeing interactions that resemble facilitated performance in some mentor-novice relations in the workplace, our claim is that it is very useful to continue considering facilitated performance and attenuated authentic participation as distinct in important ways—in ways that privilege neither one nor the other but rather reflect the institutional constraints and societal needs expressed in each.

For example, we must acknowledge that the institutional realities of schooling militate against a total appropriation of the apprenticeship model. A pervasive goal of schooling (not the only goal, but an inevitable one) is to rank or slot students. Susan Hubboch and Joseph Petraglia have each commented on our discipline's deep discomfort with that reality—but denial is a poor refuge. This requirement to grade and evaluate contaminates the relationship between students and instructors, at least to some degree. We may be locked in Peter Elbow's "embracing contraries," but at least one pole of the contraries pushes against the kind of collaboration and shared intention possible in the workplace.

On the other hand, although we may chafe at these constraints and seek different kinds of interactions, we should acknowledge as well the advantages of schooling, which also have become normalized through their tacitness. Schools do offer the opportunity for an uncontaminated focus on learning and the learner (uncontaminated by concerns for results or material outcomes) that allows for a kind of teaching—involving sequencing of curriculum and close attunement to the learner's pace—perhaps not possible in the workplace.

Our choice of the terms *performance* versus *participation* has allowed us to highlight an important contrast. Schools indeed do provide occasions for students to perform, with the attendant implications of display and attention. We must remember, though, that the attention is directed to the learner and the learning—so much so, in fact, that the nature and the degree of facilitation and orchestration are often invisible, even to researchers.

In contrast, the workplace privileges participation—collaborative engagement in tasks whose outcomes take center stage and where the learning is often tacit and implicit. A subtly different alignment and attunement is at play. Guides and learners play different roles, with differently nuanced strategies for the necessary attenuation of tasks.

Our task, as a profession and discipline, is not to jettison one in favor of the other by aiming to replicate the processes of attenuated authentic participation in the classroom[6]—a tendency that has been heightened by the identification of the modes of language use and learning in schooling with those of the middle class (Heath; Rogoff, "Guided"). This is neither possible nor necessarily beneficial. Our task, as a discipline, is to consider and weigh carefully (after considerably more research has been amassed) the advantages and implications of each kind of learning and its match with each kind of setting.

Our first step must be a sensitive anthropological analysis—perhaps even archaeological excavation—of each learning site, as it now stands, assuming a certain ecological wholeness. But ecology can be a limiting metaphor too in that it implies conservation, and hence conservatism (see Freedman and Medway, "New Views"). After the first stage of archaeological unearthing, critical analysis must be brought to bear and, with it, consideration of the alternatives.

In the meantime, it is important to acknowledge that in the two kinds of settings we observed, as they now stand, there are important differences in the learning of new genres. Our research has led us to posit a continuum within the general frame of situated learning—with facilitated performance at one end and attenuated authentic participation at the other.

Of course, we must acknowledge, even stress, the fact that there are occasions in which the university does allow for, and even encourages, workplace processes and products. Some practicums situate students directly in the workplace, and even within some communication courses, students are sometimes encouraged to bring writing that they may be doing for the workplace into the classroom (e.g., as part of a co-op placement). Elsewhere, we describe a fourth-year practicum in systems analysis in which the students become engaged collaboratively in authentic workplace tasks with their instructor serving throughout as a kind of mentor (Freedman and Adam, "Proving"). Our conclusion to that study, however, is that this kind of crossover program tends to be exceptional almost by its nature and that its exceptionality proves the rule that we have been arguing here about the necessary divergence between the two learning settings.[7]

The upshot is that, on the whole, when students leave the university to enter the workplace, they not only need to learn new genres of discourse but they also need to learn new ways to learn such genres. The two kinds of processes, although sharing certain fundamental features, are different enough that the transition from one setting to the other poses particular problems for students, eliciting feelings of disjuncture, anxiety, or displacement. These feelings, so commonly cited in the research literature and in anecdotal evidence, are inevitable, given the differing nature of the institutions, and not signs of student or school failure.

NOTES

1. Two teams of researchers at Carleton University, Ottawa, and McGill University, Montreal, are conducting the project with the aid of a grant by the Social Sciences and Humanities Research Council of Canada. Although the areas under investigation are social work, architecture, business, and government, our particular focus has been writing in government agencies and in related university preparatory programs.

2. Wertsch ("Sociocultural") distinguishes between approaches to socially shared cognition that focus primarily on social interchanges and those that focus on sociocultural mediation; Rogoff ("Apprenticeship") has focused largely on the former. Our use of the term *facilitated performance* involves far more mediation through sociocultural signs—a mediation at least partially orchestrated by the guide. We follow Wertsch's lead to include such Bakhtinian concepts as dialogism and addressivity as well as the Bakhtinian notion that individual utterances are ventriloquated through speech genres and social languages.

3. In contrast to the child-caregiver model of guided participation referred to here, school-situated guided participation is affected, and affected profoundly, by its institutional setting, one of whose pervasive and dominant goals is to sort and especially *rank* students. It is true that the ranking is primarily based on the degree to which students have succeeded in learning (or adopting the way of construing reality modeled in that classroom and discipline); nevertheless, evaluation is omnipresent (although often so naturalized as to be invisible to the participants) and frequently in conflict with the impulse to nurture and engender learning implicit in the guided participation model.

4. If students' moves within the university involve a particularly wide stretch intellectually—as in the move from undergraduate to graduate school (Berkenkotter and Huckin)—they may have feelings of disjuncture and anxiety as well. The differences between learning university and workplace genres (e.g., learning to write academic essays versus briefing notes) do not seem to involve greater intellectual challenge. Hence we believe that the strength of the workplace novices' feelings of anxiety is due to other factors, and specifically to the need to find new ways to learn.

5. Of course, this would provide us with a very simplistic view of what actually happens in attenuated authentic participation. For example, in the instances that Lave and Wegner present of legitimate peripheral participation, much of the learning takes place through collaboration among near peers rather than through direct interactions between masters and apprentices.

Furthermore, the analytic unit is the activity as a whole as constituted by persons in activity with the socially/culturally mediated world. Thus, although the task environment as a whole can be conceived as an environment facilitated by the old-timers, the environment, in fact, has only partly been created and mainly inherited by them.

6. We do not mean to diminish those pedagogical reforms that aim at increasing epistemic effectiveness through creating communities of practice or collaborative interactions within the classroom contort. Our point is that the criterion for reform should relate to the goal of the institution.

7. To provide only one reason, teachers in such practicum situations must be allowed to give up what is a primary role of schooling: the ranking of students. If the school and the instructor are to continue a successful collaboration with the workplace, all students must be allowed to, even expected to, receive "A's."

REFERENCES

Anson, Chris M., and Lee L. Forsberg. "Moving Beyond the Academic Community: Transitional Stage in Professional Writing." *Written Communication* 7 (1990): 200–31.

Bakhtin, Mikhail M. "The Problem of Speech Genres." *Speech Genres and Other Late Essays*. Ed. C. Emerson and Michael Holquist. Trans. V. W. McGee. Austin: University of Texas Press, 1986. 60–102.

Bereiter, Carl, and Marlene Scardamalia. *The Psychology of Writing*. Hillsdale, NJ: Lawrence Erlbaum, 1987.

Berkenkotter, Carol, and Thomas Huckin. "Rethinking Genre from a Socio-Cognitive Perspective." *Written Communication* 10 (1993): 475–509.

Elbow, Peter. *Embracing Contraries: Explorations in Learning and Teaching*. New York: Oxford University Press, 1986.

Freedman, Aviva. "Argument as Genre and Genres of Argument" *Perspectives on Written Argumentation*. Ed. Deborah Berrill. Norfolk, NJ: Hampton, 1996.

———. "Learning to Write Again." *Carleton Papers in Applied Language Studies* 4 (1987): 95–116.

———. "Reconceiving Genre." *Texte* 8/9 (1990): 279–92.

———. "Show and Tell? The Role of Explicit Teaching in Learning New Genres." *Research in the Teaching of English* 27 (1993): 222–51.

Freedman, Aviva, and Christine Adam. "Learning and Teaching New Genres: New Literacies, New Responsibilities." Conference of College Composition and Communication. Washington, DC. 23–25 Mar. 1995.

———. "Proving the Rule: Situating Workplace Writing in a University Context." Unpublished manuscript.

Freedman, Aviva, Christine Adam, and Graham Smart. "Wearing Suits to Class: Simulating Genres and Simulations as Genre." *Written Communication* 11 (1994): 193–226.

Freedman, Aviva, and Peter Medway. "New Views of Genre and Their Implications for Education." *Learning and Teaching Genre*. Ed. Aviva Freedman and Peter Medway. Portsmouth, NH: Boynton/Cook HEINEMANN, 1994. 1–22.

Goetz, Judith, and Margaret LeCompte. *Ethnography and Qualitative Design in Educational Research*. New York: Academic Press, 1984.

Gutierrez, Kris. "Laws of Possibility: Reconstituting Classroom Activity for Latino Children." American Educational Research Association Conference. New Orleans. 4–8 Apr. 1994.

Hanks, William F. Foreword. *Situated Learning: Legitimate Peripheral Participation*. Ed. Jean Lave and Etienne Wenger. Cambridge, Eng.: Cambridge University Press, 1991. 11–21.

Heath, Shirley Brice. *Ways with Words: Language, Life, and Work in Communities and Classrooms*. New York: Cambridge University Press, 1983.

Herrington, Ann. "Writing in Academic Settings: A Study of the Contexts for Writing in Two College Chemical Engineering Courses." *Research in the Teaching of English* 19 (1985): 331–61.

Hubboch, Susan. "Confronting the Power in Empowering Students." *The Writing Instructor* 9.2–3 (1989–90): 35–44.

Lave, Jean. "Situating Learning in Communities of Practice." *Perspectives on Socially Shared Cognition*. Ed. Lauren Resnick, J. Levin, and S. Teasley. Washington, DC: American Psychological Association, 1991. 63–83.

Lave, Jean, and Etienne Wegner. *Situated Learning: Legitimate Peripheral Participation*. Cambridge, Eng.: Cambridge University Press, 1991.

Mackinnon, James. "Becoming a Rhetor: Developing Writing Ability in a Mature, Writing Intensive Organization." *Writing in the Workplace: New Research Perspectives*. Ed. Rachel Spilka. Carbondale: Southern Illinois University Press. 1993. 41–55.

McCarthy, Lucille P. "Stranger in Strange Lands: A College Student Writing across the Curriculum." *Research in the Teaching of English* 21 (1987): 233–65.

Miller, Carolyn. "Genre as Social Action." *Quarterly Journal of Speech* 70 (1984): 151–76.

Paradis, James, David Dobrin, and Richard Miller. "Writing at Exxon ITD: Notes on the Writing Environment of an R&D Organization." *Writing in Nonacademic Settings*. Ed. Lee Odell and Dixie Goswami New York: Guilford, 1985. 281–308.

Petraglia, Joseph. "Spinning Like a Kite: A Closer Look at the Pseudotransactional Function of Writing." *Journal of Advanced Composition* 15.1 (1995).

Popken, Ronald. "Genre Transfer in Developing Adult Writers." *Focuses* 5 (1992): 3–17.

Rogoff, Barbara. *Apprenticeship in Thinking*. New York: Oxford University Press, 1990.

———. "Guided Participation of Children and Their Families." American Educational Research Association Conference. Atlanta. 12–16 Apr. 1993.

———. "Models of Teaching and Learning: Development Through Participation." American Educational Research Association Conference, New Orleans. 4–8 Apr. 1994.

———. "Social Interaction as Apprenticeship in Thinking: Guided Participation in Spatial Planning." *Perspectives on Socially Shared Cognition*. Ed. Lauren Resnick, J. Levine, and S. Teasley. Washington: American Psychological Association, 1991. 349–64.

Smart, Graham. "Genre as Community Invention: A Central Bank's Response to Its Executives' Expectations as Readers." *Writing in the Workplace: New Research Perspectives*. Ed. Rachel Spilka. Carbondale: Southern Illinois University Press, 1993. 124–40.

Vygotsky, Lev. *Mind in Society*. Cambridge, MA: Harvard University Press. 1978.

———. *Thought and Language*. Trans. E. Hanfmann and G. Vakar. Cambridge, MA: MIT Press, 1962.

Walvoord, Barbara, and Lucille McCarthy. *Thinking and Writing in College: A Naturalistic Study of Students in Four Disciplines*. Urbana, IL: National Council of Teachers of English, 1993.

Wertsch, James. "A Sociocultural Approach to Socially Shared Cognition." *Perspectives on Socially Shared Cognition*. Ed. Lauren Resnick, J. Levine, and S. Teasley. Washington, DC: American Psychological Association, 1991. 85–99.

———. *Voices of the Mind: A Sociocultural Approach to Mediated Action*. Cambridge, MA: Harvard University Press, 1991.

20 Pseudotransactionality, Activity Theory, and Professional Writing Instruction

CLAY SPINUZZI

In this article, Spinuzzi examines the problem of pseudotranactionality, *a term coined by Joseph Petraglia that refers to writing designed to meet the needs of the teacher or class and not designed to help students engage in a transfer of information or demonstrate mastery of material (qtd. on p. 338 in this volume). This problem may occur in any class, but the potential for it happening in technical communication classes is very real. Teachers, hoping to address the students' needs to learn genres in context, often try to replicate the actual workplace environment, or what Spinuzzi terms an "*activity network *(AN)" (p. 340). Unfortunately, because "classrooms are not workplaces," and, complicating the problem further, each classroom and workplace is a different AN (p. 341), students often get confused or they recognize the disjunction. Regardless, the result is that they choose a path of least resistance: they write to the teacher. Reading this article will help you better understand both the Bakhtinian conception of communication that influences genre theory and the Vygotskian-influenced concept of activity theory. More important, it will suggest a starting place for pedagogical strategies that you'll want to consider in order to help students learn about genres so that they can learn to write transactionally, and in doing so accomplish goals for others.*

Probably all teachers of professional writing have a dozen stories about *pseudotransactional writing*—that is, writing that is patently designed by a student to meet teacher expectations rather than to perform the "real" function the teacher has suggested. Let me begin this article by sharing such a story.

A few semesters ago, I asked students in my junior-level business communication class to write actual request letters to be sent to a genuine nonacademic audience. Students were given broad latitude in what they could write about: some chose to ask for information about a product, others wrote to realtors asking about the availability of housing, and so forth. The students were to hand in two copies of the letter along with a stamped, addressed envelope; I was to mail one copy of the letter to the audience and grade the

From *Technical Communication Quarterly* 5, no. 3 (1996): 295–308.

other copy. The assignment was, of course, designed to be transactional—after all, it involved a "real" audience—yet as I graded the papers I was disappointed to see that the letters were a mix of transactional and pseudotransactional voices. The letters requesting product information, for instance, nearly all contained copious praise for those products. The letters requesting realty information explained in great detail *why* the students needed the information. In short, the letters tended to concentrate on verbal display at the expense of the brevity that usually characterizes such requests.

It is ironic that a supposedly transactional assignment brings out excesses of pseudotransactionality in students' papers. Yet, in retrospect, I suppose I should have expected it. In "Spinning Like a Kite: A Closer Look at the Pseudotransactional Function of Writing," Joseph Petraglia defines *transactional writing* as "that which does not pretend to function in any way other than it does" and *pseudotransactional writing* as "solely intended to meet teacher expectations rather than engage in a transference of information for the purposes of informing the uninformed or demonstrating mastery over content" (21). Petraglia sets up two poles here; my students' papers are situated somewhere in between them, but closer to the pseudotransactional pole than I would like.

Pseudotransactionality is a particular problem for professional writing instructors. After all, few students are expected to write a comparison-contrast essay or a theme on a controversial topic after they graduate. But students quite often have to be prepared to write professional documents during internships and in their post-graduation jobs. Most writing teachers want them to be prepared to write transactionally, just as future employers expect them to be prepared.

In this article, I explore the problem of pseudotransactionality through the lens of two related theoretical approaches, Bakhtinian genres and Vygotskian activity theory. The first part of this article elaborates on the two approaches and uses them to discuss why pseudotransactionality appears in the first place. The second part suggests how we can deal with pseudotransactional writing as we teach our students to write for their future workplaces.

Bakhtinian Genres

A growing number of scholars from various theoretical camps have embraced M. M. Bakhtin's concept of communication as sociohistorical rather than structural (e.g., Cole; Morson; Emerson; Wertsch; Berkenkotter and Huckin; Kent, "Hermeneutics"; Brady). For instance, externalists such as Thomas Kent view communication as "a hermeneutic guessing game" that cannot be reduced simply to a "grammar or theory of cognition" (*Paralogic Rhetoric* 158). Kent sees in Bakhtin's concept of genre a way to describe this uncodifiable activity (166), since genres "cannot be reduced to a set of conventional elements that function together as a structural or organic whole" ("Hermeneutics" 295). Similarly, sociocognitivists Carol Berkenkotter and Thomas N. Huckin view genres as "dynamic rhetorical forms" that "change over time in response to their users' sociocognitive needs" (4) and must be evaluated in terms of those needs.

In the Bakhtinian conception, genres evolve under pressure from two forces: history and addressivity. *History* influences the genre because each genre evolves from a previous genre (see, for instance, Voloshinov 68, 86, 93), and that previous genre exerts some pressure on what the new genre looks and acts like, even if the individual writers are unaware of the history of the genre (Ritva Engeström 202).

Addressivity also influences the genre: each genre evolves to fit a new activity that might be similar to yet different from the activity that the old genre responded to (Medvedev/Bakhtin 132; Kent, "Hermeneutics" 299). The genre cannot be separated from the activity to which it responds; it only makes sense in localized "spheres of human activity and communication" (Bakhtin 64; see also 65). Genres clue us in to what hermeneutic strategies we might successfully employ to understand an utterance *in a particular activity* (Kent, "Hermeneutics" 301–02).

Thus, genre is formed by the meeting of history—the past genres from which the present genre evolved—and addressivity—the changes that language users make to the genre in response to events. As Charles Bazerman puts it, "the regularities that appear in the genre come from the very historical presence of the emerging genre," but "each new text produced within a genre reinforces or remolds some aspect of the genre" (8) because each new text responds to a localized set of circumstances and a localized activity, and that response itself becomes a part of the genre's history. Berkenkotter and Huckin also stress the role of activity: "both genres and genre knowledge are more sharply and richly defined to the extent that they are *localized* (in both time and place)" (13–14). That is, although genres are influenced by the general features that their histories provide them, those features might be dropped or altered in localized instances of the genres because of the localized events to which they respond. (See Yates and Orlikowski for an example of how one genre, that of the memorandum, has evolved since its inception in response to various events.)

To analyze how genres evolve, then, we—and students—need a sociohistorical approach to analyzing particular workplaces, one that allows us to see how both history and addressivity shape genres within those workplaces. One suitable approach is activity theory.

Activity Theory

Activity theory has its roots in L. S. Vygotsky's circle in the 1920s and was further developed by Vygotsky's colleagues A. N. Leont'ev and A. R. Luria (Raeithel 396). Although activity theory has its roots in Marxism, it also was apparently influenced by the non-Marxist ideas of the Bakhtinian circle: the contemporaries Vygotsky and Bakhtin never cite each other, but some commonalities are evident (Emerson 27), and many scholars have connected the Bakhtinian concept of genre with activity theory (Davydov and Radzikhovskii; Emerson; Ritva Engeström; Yrjö Engeström, *Interactive Expertise*;

Morson; Prior; Wertsch). Among the commonalities are, of course, an awareness of history and of social interaction.

Activity theory uses a unit of analysis that I will term an *activity network* (AN). In an activity network, one or more *subjects* use a *tool* to achieve an *object(ive)* (Russell) that results in an *outcome*. The activity itself is the cyclical transformation of an object (Yrjö Engeström, *Learning* 78). Perhaps the best way to explain this unit of analysis is through an extended illustration (figure 1).

In figure 1, the *subjects* are the people who are engaged in the AN, that is, those who carry on the activity of the institution. Although they perform different jobs and thus different actions—for instance, programmers generally program and janitors generally clean—those actions contribute to the institution's *object(ive)*: software (Russell 53). The object(ive) has a double meaning, because it refers both to the object to be transformed and to the objective of transforming it, an objective that elicits different actions from different people within the AN. As the institution transforms the object (in this case, by developing and releasing new versions of a particular software package), it achieves a continually occurring *outcome*. Here, outcomes might include accrual of market share and profits.

The subjects mediate the transformation of the object through their use of *tools*. Here, the tools are both physical (computers, office supplies, briefcases, mops) and semiotic (written words, voices, computer graphics). And just as physical tools have evolved to address certain activities, so have semiotic tools. "Variance in semiotic tools" stabilized through typical use, Russell suggests, "may be called *genre*" (54).

Like variance in other kinds of tools, genres have evolved under the pressure of history and addressivity. History can be seen both as institutional

FIGURE 1 The Activity Network of a Software Development Company

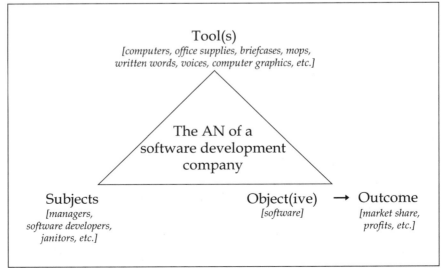

(the way an AN's genres have evolved) and individual (how a person's experience with particular genres has shaped that person's use of the genres). Addressivity can similarly be seen as institutional (the strategies an institution employs to handle recurring events) and individual (how an individual adapts a genre to address particular needs). Different ANs can use the same tools in their different activities, but those tools will be used differently and will tend to evolve differently to meet the different needs of the subjects.

Naturally, a genre that has evolved in a particular AN—our mythical company, for instances—will differ significantly from a similar genre in another AN, such as that of a professional writing classroom.

Classroom and Workplace Activity Networks

Professional writing classrooms tend to attempt to replicate the activity network of the workplace through various means: having students participate in simulations (Freedman et al.); asking students to write in response to extended case studies (Driskill 42; Rozumalski and Graves); asking industry professionals to set assignments, give lectures, lead field trips, and evaluate papers (Hart and Glick-Smith); and engaging students in actual writing opportunities (Mansfield; Hill and Resnick; MacKinnon; Anson and Forsberg; Lutz). The latter sometimes results in documents that might even be used in industry (Reither 202–3).

Nevertheless, many agree that these efforts have limited success, primarily because for the students, classrooms are not workplaces (Reither 205; Mansfield 72; Freedman et al.). Each classroom and each workplace is a different AN. We cannot replicate "the workplace" because each workplace is different, just as each class is different. Granted, some of these ANs are parts of larger activity networks and therefore share some similarities—for instance, software development companies tend to use tools similarly because they belong to the same industry—and they may use tools in ways similar to the ways participants in computer science classes do, since those students are pursuing the object(ive) of entering the software development AN. Figure 2 shows a simplified relationship between the activity networks of a computer science classroom and a future employer; if we wanted to pursue a broader analysis, we could conflate these two into a larger activity network (that of "software development") in which a more diverse set of subjects uses a more diverse set of tools to transform a more general object(ive).

As Anne Herrington points out, "each classroom presents a community in its own right, situated at once in two larger communities: a school and a disciplinary community" (333). Yet our professional writing classrooms attempt to teach future engineers, foresters, architects, botanists, and chemists as well as future computer science students. Each of these students is trying to join a community or AN that has evolved "standard" genres that meet its particular needs and reflect its particular history. That AN may contain several other AN whose tools differ to meet *their* particular needs and reflect *their* particular genres.

FIGURE 2 Two Activity Networks—The Student's Program of Study and Future Employer

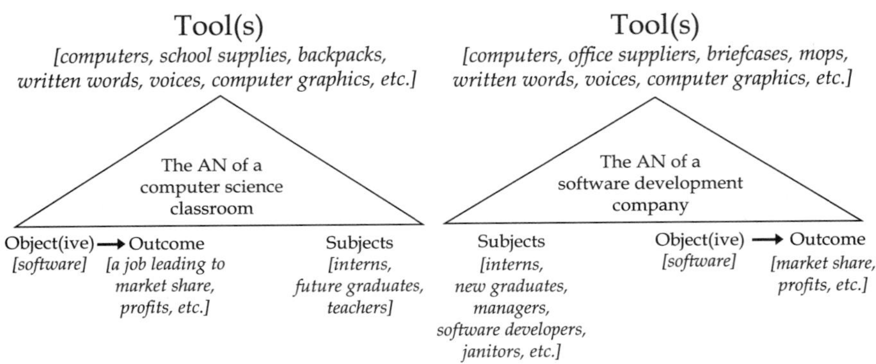

To their credit, many if not most professional writing teachers realize that their students' future workplaces are too diverse to imitate in a single course, but they sometimes have trouble helping their students grapple with learning another AN's tools in a way meaningful to the ANs that those students are trying to enter.

One result is pseudotransactionality, which can be seen as a sort of overarching genre developed to facilitate certain object(ive)s of the writing course AN. Pseudotransactionality, to put it another way, can be conceived as a bundle of habits that a writer uses to achieve an object(ive). When a writer attempts to learn a new genre composed of a new set of habits, the old habits can interfere, as in the case of an engineering student who found himself writing in a workplace setting during an internship:

> Jason evidently anticipated an audience that would evaluate his text based upon its correctness. That is, he saw a writer/audience relationship that echoed a common student/teacher relationship. Partly this was because Mark was to some degree functioning like his teacher. But partly it was also because until this point he had probably seldom or never written for anyone who wasn't a teacher. His entire experience of writing fit into that mode. (Winsor 25)

The student's past encounters with a genre and awareness of the teacher's goals cannot help but affect the genre's form. What results is a genre adapted for meeting the object(ive)s of the particular classroom AN in which the student writes, not the object(ive)s of a particular workplace. And, as the quote above points out, such a genre can take some time to unlearn.

Researchers have long recognized that classroom ANs tend to have object(ive)s that are quite different from those of workplace ANs. For instance, Freedman et al. claim that "classroom writing" and "workplace writing" have four basic differences (Table 1).

Typically, a workplace writer's documents are for multiple audiences within an organization (Forsberg 46); they are part of a dialogue with a

TABLE 1 Differences between Classroom and Workplace Writing, According to Freedman et al.

Classroom Writing	*Workplace Writing*
Epistemic: For its own end.	*Instrumental*: For a separate end.
Writer-oriented: Focused on the writer's knowledge or skill. A rhetorical display.	*Reader-oriented*: Focused on how it affects the reader.
Ephemeral: Exists/is used only for a brief time.	*Continued*: Exists/is used indefinitely.
Evaluated: The reader has no stake in the document's success and therefore merely evaluates the document.	*Collaborated on*: The reader has a stake in the document's success and therefore collaborates with the writer.

community of peers (Odell 19). In marked contrast, students' writing is clearly shaped by a very different relationship with a single reader (Freedman et al. 202, 204; Forsberg 45; Petraglia 24) and is primarily epistemic, that is, aimed towards producing tangible evidence of the students' competence as measured by the teacher's criteria (Reither 201–02). And students know that teachers typically will attempt to evaluate them all using the same static set of criteria—something that is usually not true in the workplace. This is not to deny that some writing assignments can include all of the characteristics of workplace writing, but we must be aware that students are *also* addressing the activity of classroom writing, and that activity inevitably affects the forms of their utterances. The resulting versions of the genre are pseudotransactional: they have evolved to accomplish the goals of a specific classroom rather than those of the workplace that the classroom supposedly emulates.

Although teachers may be able to spot the characteristics of pseudotransactionality in a particular document, they might not be able to accurately predict what writing strategies will work better for a workplace AN. In fact, students are in many ways better prepared to evaluate their workplace genres than their teachers because of their interaction with related ANs. Dorothy Winsor, for instance, finds that her four research subjects "learned to write like engineers at work largely by trying to function within the engineering community" (19) during their internships.

Even within their coursework, however, students are learning how to function within their "communities" or ANs. Students studying computer science, for instance, are studying to enter that particular discipline or AN, an AN that encompasses both classes and workplaces. This AN has certain object(ive)s that shape its tools. For instance, the needs of this AN have produced the genre of the software development plan, a genre that tends to be telegraphic, have a highly articulated outline, and use visual genres such as finite state diagrams. This genre tends to be quite concise and organized compared to many other workplace genres.

Now suppose that an English teacher unfamiliar with the computer science AN tries to help a computer science student with a proposal, which includes a software development plan. The teacher is probably not familiar with the genre the student is using or the AN that most strongly influences the student's document, and may thus tend to give advice that will not be as successful. For instance, the teacher might advise the student to elaborate on a certain section, or to be less obvious about the document's structure. In a classroom AN, this unfamiliarity with workplace ANs may lead to nothing more than the student shrugging her or his shoulders and revising the document to make the teacher happy—sort of a rhetorical detour in the student's education, something that may not actually hurt (although it probably will not help either).

If, on the other hand, the student takes the advice to heart—and judging by the number of people who are unwilling to break meaningless rules about placing conjunctions at the beginning of a sentence or splitting infinitives, this is a real danger—then that student could be negatively affected by the teacher's advice. The advice becomes part of the student's personal history with the genre; it becomes a habit that the student will have to unlearn as she or he continues in the computer science AN.

To sum up, although a teacher may have greater knowledge of *general* hermeneutic strategies (or at least what the AN of technical writing instruction constructs as general hermeneutic strategies), she or he knows less about the student's AN, and therefore may give advice that directly *contradicts* the object(ive)s of the AN.

Encouraging Students to Enter Workplace Activity Networks

If we accept the claim that genre evolution is constrained (although never fully determined) by addressivity and history, pedagogical implications follow. Below, I attempt to outline a few ways to encourage students as they write within various activity networks.

First, as Reed Way Dasenbrock suggests (29), we should teach the various systemic elements of communication, the common habits that are often collected into professional writing genres, descriptively rather than prescriptively—that is, sociohistorically. I am thinking specifically of *genre habits that are rhetorically effective in most relevant ANs*—habits such as including certain information in the heading of a memorandum, for instance, or inserting an abstract at the beginning of an experimental article. We should be able to explain not just *what* the habits associated with a common professional genre are, but also *why* those habits have historically built up and *why* they have evolved differently for different ANs. Resources here might include sociohistorical research on the genre, such as Yates and Orlikowski's research on the memorandum or Bazerman's on the experimental article. As we teach genres as collections of habits, we should append the caveat that they are *similar* to the genres writers might use in certain activities, not templates that writers *universally* follow or that are automatically successful. That is, we should continue to require of the students the actions of evaluating and writing that they traditionally perform in our classroom, but encourage them to examine the specific object(ive)s that are addressed by *their* disciplines' genres.

Second, we can ask students to take part in an AN outside of the English classroom, perhaps as apprentices, interns, or participants in a workplace (see Mansfield; Hill and Resnick; MacKinnon; Anson and Forsberg; Lutz) or as students in a program of professional education in their chosen field (Ackerman; Berkenkotter, Huckin, and Ackerman; Bazerman; Britt et al.; Herrington; Kent, *Paralogic Rhetoric*; McCarthy). The particular AN is not necessarily important: the point is not for the students to learn general "writing" skills, but rather to learn how to examine and appropriate localized genres and how to understand their uses in that AN. They should not expect to pick up merely a list of conventions. Rather, they should analyze the sociohistorical actions within that AN, because those actions strongly influence the genres that are used within those ANs. Such an analysis might involve shadowing workplace professionals; interviewing writers; recounting particular incidents found relevant to their writing; examining previous documents to determine why they were or were not successful; ferreting out the object(ive)s of the AN and of related ANs; and determining how the student's own documents address those object(ive)s.

Such analyses can benefit not only the individual students but also the entire class: students can share their experiences, as various scholars have suggested (see Anson and Forsberg; Spilka). Thus, students can learn from each other how their activity networks shape the genres used within them. By reflecting on and sharing their experiences, students can demonstrate to each other the variations within workplaces, and as a result may begin to see genres as vital and evolving.

Finally, students can rhetorically analyze the workplace documents that they and others produce within their workplace ANs, explaining their rhetorical choices. Such rhetorical analyses would be transactional, because they do not pretend to be other than what they are. Additionally, rhetorical analyses fall within the focus of the teacher's field: the collection of habits into genres, the forming of utterances. Such an arrangement lets the teacher off the hook. No longer does the teacher have to judge the workplace document, a document whose genre addresses an AN that the teacher does not fully share and therefore cannot fully evaluate.

Implications

Some readers may be wondering at this point whether I view professional writing as something that must be learned entirely within the AN for which it is intended. Not at all. As Anson and Forsberg demonstrate in their study of interns, participating in an AN does not necessarily teach one the skills necessary to succeed within it. Simply immersing a student in a workplace AN is a bit like the old method of teaching a child to swim by throwing him or her in a lake: the method might often work, but the price of failure could be quite high. At the same time, the traditional approach of teaching students generalized communication strategies without reference to localized ANs will not help much either, as Thomas Kent takes pains to demonstrate in the last chapter of *Paralogic Rhetoric*.

In this article, I have argued that students should join other ANs and use the professional writing classroom as a forum for discussing them and as an opportunity to examine their practices. By involving students in a localized AN, we can encourage them to write transactionally and to learn *how to learn* genres.

WORKS CITED

Ackerman, John M. "The Promise of Writing to Learn." *Written Communication* 10 (1993): 334–70.

Anson, Chris M., and L. Lee Forsberg. "Moving Beyond the Academic Community: Transitional Stages in Professional Writing." *Written Communication* 7 (1990): 200–31.

Bakhtin, M. M. "The Problem of Speech Genres." *Speech Genres and Other Essays*. Ed. Caryl Emerson and Michael Holquist. Trans. Vern W. McGee. Austin: U of Texas P, 1986. 60–102.

Bazerman, Charles. *Shaping Written Knowledge: The Genre and Activity of the Experimental Article in Science*. Madison: U of Wisconsin P, 1988.

Berkenkotter, Carol, and Thomas N. Huckin. *Genre Knowledge in Disciplinary Communication: Cognition/Culture/Power*. Hillsdale, New Jersey: Erlbaum, 1995.

Berkenkotter, Carol, Thomas N. Huckin, and John Ackerman. "Conventions, Conversations, and the Writer. A Case Study of a Student in a Rhetoric Ph.D. Program." *Research in the Teaching of English* 22 (1988): 9–44.

Brady, Laura A. "A Contextual Theory for Business Writing." *Journal of Business and Technical Communication* 7 (1993): 452–71.

Britt, Elizabeth C., Bernadette Longo, and Kristin R. Woolever. "Extending the Boundaries of Rhetoric in Legal Writing Pedagogy." *Journal of Business and Technical Communication* 10 (1996): 213–38.

Cole, Michael. "Preface." *The Concept of Activity in Soviet Psychology*. Ed. James V. Wertsch. Armonk, NY: M. E. Sharpe, 1981. 7–10.

Dasenbrock, Reed Way. "The Myths of the Subjective and the Subject in Composition Studies." *Journal of Advanced Communication* 13 (Winter 1993): 21–32.

Davydov, V. V., and L. A. Radzikhovskii. "Vygotsky's Theory and the Activity-Oriented Approach in Psychology." *Culture, Communication, and Cognition: Vygotskian Perspectives*. Ed. James V. Wertsch. New York: Cambridge UP, 1985. 35–65.

Driskill, Linda. "Understanding the Writing Context in Organizations." *Writing in the Business Professions*. Ed. Myra Kogen. Champaign, IL: National Council of Teachers of English, 1989. 125–45.

Emerson, Caryl. "The Outer World and Inner Speech: Bakhtin, Vygotsky, and the Internalization of Language." *Bakhtin: Essays and Dialogues on His Work*. Ed. Gary Saul Morson. Chicago: U of Chicago P, 1986. 21–40.

Engeström, Ritva. "Voice as Communicative Action." *Mind, Culture, and Activity* 2.5 (1995): 192–214.

Engeström, Yrjö. *Interactive Expertise: Studies in Distributed Working Intelligence*. Helsinki: U of Helsinki, 1992.

———. *Learning, Working, and Imagining: Twelve Studies in Activity Theory*. Helsinki: Orienta-Konsultit Oy, 1990.

Forsberg, L. Lee. "Who's Out There Anyway? Bringing Awareness of Multiple Audiences Into the Business-Writing Class." *Journal of Business and Technical Communication* 1 (September 1987): 45–69.

Freedman, Aviva, Christine Adam, and Graham Smart. "Wearing Suits to Class: Simulating Genres and Simulations as Genres." *Written Communication* 11 (April 1994): 193–226.

Hart, Hillary, and Judith L. Glick-Smith. "Training in Technical Communication: Ideas for a Partnership Between the Academy and the Workplace." *Technical Communication* 41 (August 1994): 399–405.

Herrington, Anne J. "Writing in Academic Settings: A Study of the Contexts for Writing in Two College Chemical Engineering Courses." *Research in the Teaching of English* 19 (1985): 331–59.

Hill, Charles A., and Lauren Resnick. "Creating Opportunities for Apprenticeship in Writing." *Reconceiving Writing, Rethinking Writing Instruction*. Ed. Joseph Petraglia. Mahwah, NJ: Erlbaum, 1995. 51–77.

Kent, Thomas. "Hermeneutics and Genre: Bakhtin and the Problem of Communicative Interaction." *The Interpretive Turn: Philosophy, Science, Culture*. Ed. David R. Hiley, James F. Bohman, and Richard Shusterman. Ithaca: Cornell UP, 1991. 282–303.

———. *Paralogic Rhetoric: A Theory of Communicative Interaction*. Lewisberg: Bucknell UP, 1993.

Lutz, Jean. "Understanding Organizational Socialization: The Role of Internships in Helping Students Acquire Strategies for Writing Effectively in Organizations." *Establishing and Supervising Internships*. Ed. William O. Coggin. St. Paul, MN: ATTW, 1989. 78–89.

MacKinnon, Jamie. "Becoming a Rhetor. Developing Writing Ability in a Mature, Writing-Intensive Organization." *Writing in the Workplace: New Research Perspectives*. Ed. Rachel Spilka. Carbondale, IL: Southern Illinois UP, 1993. 195–206.

Mansfield, Margaret A. "Real World Writing and the English Curriculum." *College Composition and Communication* 44 (February 1993) 69–83.

McCarthy, Lucille Parkinson. "A Stranger in Strange Lands: A College Student Writing Across the Curriculum." *Research in the Teaching of English* 21 (1987): 233–65.

Medvedev, P. N./M. M. Bakhtin. *The Formal Method of Literary Scholarship: A Critical Introduction to Sociological Poetics*. Trans. Albert J. Wehrle. Baltimore: Johns Hopkins UP, 1978.

Morson, Gary Saul. "Introduction to Extracts from 'The Problem of Speech Genres." *Bakhtin: Essays and Dialogues on His Work*. Ed. Gary Saul Morson. Chicago: U of Chicago P, 1986. 89-90.

Petraglia, Joseph. "Spinning Like a Kite: A Closer Look at the Pseudotransactional Function of Writing." *Journal of Advanced Composition* 15 (1995): 19–33.

Prior, Paul. "Response, Revision, Disciplinarity: A Microhistory of a Dissertation Prospectus in Sociology." *Written Communication* 11 (1994): 483–533.

Raeithel, Arne. "Activity Theory as a Foundation for Design." *Software Development and Reality Construction*. Ed. Christiane Floyd, Heinz Zullighoven, Reinhard Budde, and Reinhard Keil-Slawik. New York: Springer-Verlag, 1991.

Reither, James A. "Bridging the Gap: Scenic Motives for Collaborative Writing in Workplace and School." *Writing in the Workplace: New Research Perspectives*. Ed. Rachel Spilka. Carbondale, IL: Southern Illinois UP, 1993. 195–206.

Rozumalaski, Lynn P., and Michael F. Graves. "Effects of Case and Traditional Writing Assignments on Writing Products and Processes." *Journal of Business and Technical Communication* 9 (January 1995): 77–102.

Russell, David R. "Activity Theory and Its Implications for Writing Instruction." *Reconceiving Writing, Rethinking Writing Instruction*. Ed. Joseph Petraglia. Mahwah, NJ: Erlbaum, 1995. 51–77.

Spilka, Rachel. "Influencing Workplace Practice: A Challenge for Professional Writing Specialists in Academia." *Writing in the Workplace: New Research Perspectives*. Ed. Rachel Spilka. Carbondale, IL: Southern Illinois UP, 1993. 195–206.

Voloshinov, V. N. *Marxism and the Philosophy of Language*. Trans. Ladislav Matejka and I. R. Titunik. New York: Seminar P, 1973.

Wertsch, James V. *Voices of the Mind: A Sociocultural Approach to Mediated Action*. Cambridge: Harvard UP, 1991.

Winsor, Dorothy. *Writing Like an Engineer: A Rhetorical Education*. Mahwah, NJ: Erlbaum, 1996.

Yates, Joanne, and Wanda J. Orlikowski. "Genres of Organizational Communication: A Structurational Approach to Studying Communication and Media." *Academy of Management Review* 17 (1992): 299–326.

21 Bridging the Workplace and the Academy: Teaching Professional Genres through Classroom-Workplace Collaborations

ANN M. BLAKESLEE

Blakeslee's award-winning work, drawing on work in genre and situated learning as well as recent work in activity theory, examines ways teachers can use collaborations with the workplace as vehicles to teach professional genres and to begin to enculturate students into the activity systems they'll encounter as professionals. Relying on two qualitative studies of her own classrooms at two different institutions, Blakeslee illustrates the advantages of teacher-research methodology as a scholarly activity. Her findings are not unexpected: students involved in these collaborations value their exposure to the workplace, but recognize that the projects are not complete or "authentic" replications of workplace experiences. That said, they learn much about audience and writing as a technê *and a praxis. Finally, this essay points to the value of these experiences "as a bridge between school and work": students engage in workplace activities and are "exposed to the cultural knowledge" of the workplace (p. 361 in this volume). Reading this piece in conversation with the Freedman and Adam essay will provide a rich continuum of possible strategies and open up some interesting questions about what kinds of assignments to use and for what purposes.*

In recent years, rhetorical scholars have shown how newcomers to a domain learn its genres through immersion and participation in the activities of the domain (e.g., Berkenkotter and Huckin; Berkenkotter, Huckin, and Ackerman; Blakeslee; Doheny-Farina; Freedman and Adam; Freedman, Adam, and Smart; Freedman and Medway; Haas; Prior; Russell; Swales; Winsor, *Engineer*). However, such processes, which generally occur gradually (see Blakeslee), call into question whether we can teach such genres effectively in the classroom, where both the amount of time and the opportunities to immerse students in actual situations are limited. In other words, recent findings in genre studies raise important questions about how we teach genres in our technical and professional writing classes.

Technical and professional writing instructors often use two types of assignments to simulate workplace practice and to teach professional

From *Technical Communication Quarterly* 10, no. 2 (2001): 169–92.

genres: case studies or client projects. However, few scholars have examined the effectiveness of such assignments for achieving these objectives. Lynn Rozumalski and Michael Graves' and Gregory Wickliff's studies address the benefits and value of both case studies and client-based assignments. Aviva Freedman, Christine Adam, and Graham Smart, who examine cases, point to some important shortcomings of these kinds of assignments. These scholars suggest that differences in the contexts of school and work constrain teachers' attempts to simulate and teach workplace genres. They contend that case study writing performed in the classroom differs in significant ways from workplace writing and, therefore, does not fully convey important features of professional genres, such as the rhetorical contexts and the social actions entailed by them (221). They conclude that students exhibit a limited awareness of audience with such assignments, continuing to write to display their knowledge to the instructor (203–06).

Those of us who teach technical and professional writing may read Freedman, Adam, and Smart's findings and end up feeling that our efforts to simulate workplace writing and to teach workplace genres in our classrooms are at best unreliable and at worst futile. However, client assignments that involve actual workplace projects are different from the case study assignments that these scholars examined. Such assignments, which ask students to complete workplace projects provided by clients, potentially preserve more of the culture of the workplace, while also allowing students to address a variety of audiences. Their differences from cases suggest that we also should assess their effectiveness in teaching students professional genres.

In this article I report on two studies of classroom-workplace collaborations where students solved workplace problems as part of an academic course requirement. Drawing on genre and professional writing research, I identify and explore four issues—exposure, authenticity, transition, and response—that may help in assessing the effectiveness of such assignments. These four issues shed light on what students may learn from classroom-workplace collaborations and how they learn it. They also shed light on the ways in which we can use such collaborations to teach professional genres. For example, my research suggests that these collaborations may act as useful transitional experiences that bridge classroom and workplace contexts for students and expose them gradually to workplace practices and genres.

Issues and Research Questions

Research on genres is fairly consistent in its conclusions about how individuals learn genres. This research suggests that individuals must be immersed in a community, interact with the members and artifacts of the community, participate in and adapt to the social actions of the community, and appropriate the routinized tools-in-use of the community (Anson and Forsberg; Berkenkotter and Huckin; Blakeslee; Burnett; Doheny-Farina; Freedman and Adam; Freedman, Adam, and Smart; Miller; Russell; Spinuzzi; Winsor, "Writing Well"). While our classrooms seldom permit the level of immersion these scholars say is needed, they may still provide a certain amount of it. In assessing classroom-workplace collaborations, we thus should consider how these collaborations may immerse students in or expose them to workplace practices and genres, and what students learn from this exposure.

A second issue that may shed light on classroom-workplace collaborations is authenticity, or students' perceptions of how similar the activities are to actual workplace projects. In using this term, I am cognizant of Joseph Petraglia's cautions about the frequent vagueness and contradictions that often attend discussions of authenticity in our field (2). As Charles Bazerman points out, what is key is not what is real in an absolute sense, but what our students perceive as real, and as motivating (x). Petraglia says, "From a rhetorical perspective, authenticity is a judgment rather than a characteristic inhering in a learning situation. . . . In sum, judging something to be authentic entails an intricate balancing of knowledge and belief" (131).

Some of the researchers I cited above also show a concern with this issue of authenticity, but they relate it to the particular types of assignments they study. The scholars who studied cases, for example, were concerned with how closely cases match the actual writing that occurs in the workplace. Rozumalski and Graves' main research question was "Do our teaching strategies and assignments successfully simulate authentic contexts and real audiences to bridge academic and nonacademic settings?" (78). They argued that cases recreate on-the-job situations and make students more sensitive to audience and context (77, 80, 92). This likeness to workplace situations and heightened awareness of audience, they claim, are what motivate and make the students more effective writers.

Freedman, Adam, and Smart, who also studied cases, arrived at a somewhat different conclusion. Questioning whether case study writing simulates and provides useful preparation for workplace writing, they conclude that such simulations do not convey adequately the rhetorical contexts and social actions of the workplace. They say,

> The reader/writer relations, the social roles adopted, the reading practices, the collaborative composing processes, and, above all, the social motive governing the production of the genre of case-study writing were all fundamentally distinct from those in the parallel workplace. (221)

Finally, Wickliff, whose research is most similar to my own in focus, wondered if the skills students acquire in client-based group projects are ones they also will need and use in the workplace. He concludes that such projects provide skills that are valued in the workplace, but that the classroom setting and agenda often fail to simulate the workplace (171). All of this research suggests considering whether the tasks students undertake in our classes are similar to those carried out in the workplace. We also should consider students' perceptions of these tasks and whether, and in what ways, they find them motivating.

The issues of exposure and authenticity also have bearing on a third issue that I explored in my research, transition. The question of how students move from the contexts of schooling to those of the workplace has been explored by a number of scholars (e.g., Anson and Forsberg; Blakeslee; Freedman and Adam; Winsor). Generally, these scholars agree that students have difficulties with such transitions, and they attribute these difficulties to the differences between the two contexts. Chris Anson and Lee Forsberg, for example, detail the disorientation, frustration, and double binds students experience when encountering new contexts and genres (214). Freedman and Adam argue that the processes by which learning occurs in these contexts are different enough to pose problems for students when moving between them (395, 424). Dorothy Winsor addresses how the co-op students she studied valued workplace practice over classroom explanations of how to write ("Writing Well" 164). Another scholar, however, has begun to explore and theorize the connections between the two settings. David Russell, who is concerned with constructing a model of the ways in which classroom writing is linked to writing in wider social practices, addresses how newcomers learn a profession's genres:

> Through continued interaction with others in the activity system, the ways of using the tool . . . becomes a routine operation, often unconscious. Moreover, as an individual appropriates (learns to use) the ways with words of others, they may (or may not) also appropriate the object/motive, and subjectivity (identity) of the collective, of a new activity system. The process of learning (to write) new genres is a part of a process of expanding one's involvements with activity systems. (516)

This latter idea, which is influenced by Yrjö Engeström's work, suggests that individuals move into new activity systems gradually. It also suggests that students or newcomers may benefit from experiences that bridge the two contexts and that facilitate this gradual entry.

Russell's and these other scholars' work suggests examining how workplace projects may facilitate students' transitions from the classroom to the workplace, or, how they may enable students to expand their involvements in new activity systems. This work also encourages considering the ways in which the projects may bridge school and the workplace. All of these considerations suggest examining the experiences students have with these projects, including the kinds of structure provided with them and the support that students receive.

Finally, many of the scholars who have addressed the transition issue also have discussed how response may differ in workplace and classroom contexts: response tends to be less evaluative in the workplace and readers respond in ways that reflect a different stake in the writing (e.g., they may respond in a more collaborative manner and/or take a more active role in revision because of the greater personal stake they have in the document) (Anson and Forsberg; Burnett; Freedman and Adam; Freedman, Adam, and Smart). Freedman and Adam say that in university settings a contextual shaping and coparticipation occurs that supports the development of a draft. In workplace settings, on the other hand, a long and intense process of responding and revising occurs, but not until after a draft is handed over to a supervisor (418). This research suggests additional questions for assessing classroom-workplace collaborations. For example, how and by whom is students' work evaluated with these projects? Also, how useful do students find the feedback they receive, and what value do they assign it? Whose response do students value most?

Studies of Classroom-Workplace Collaborations

To begin investigating these issues, I carried out two case studies of classroom-workplace collaborations where students completed workplace projects that were provided by clients (e.g., professionals in industry or academia). I performed the first case study at a large, state-supported research university (subsequently referred to as Univ A), and the second at a large, regional, state-supported teaching university populated largely by commuter and nontraditional students (subsequently referred to as Univ B). Over 30,000 students were enrolled at the first university and approximately 25,000 students were enrolled at the second. Many of the students enrolled at Univ B work 30 to 40 hours a week in addition to taking a full class load. Some of the students from this university also were working already in their professional fields, a factor that may have influenced their experiences with and responses to these activities, since they generally were more accustomed to workplace environments than the students at Univ A.

At Univ A, I studied an introductory (300-level) technical communication course taken primarily by civil engineering majors (only one student had a different major, which was technical communication). At Univ B, I studied a class on computer documentation (400-level) taken by both undergraduate and graduate students. All of these students were pursuing degrees in technical communication. I was the instructor in both classes. (Both studies received human subjects approval from the institutional review boards at the universities.)

Before elaborating on these cases, I wish to comment first on my decision to become a teacher researcher in my own classes. While some composition scholars have argued that teacher research is not as credible as other types of research (Applebee; Hillocks; North), the teacher-research movement has attained increased acceptance as a legitimate approach to scholarly inquiry. Teacher researchers have demonstrated the potential of this research for offering context-full descriptions, encouraging critical reflection, and achieving change (Cochran-Smith and Lytle; Fleischer; Ray). Cathy Fleischer argues that teacher research provides insights into classrooms and students that outside researchers would have difficulty discerning (92, 94–95). She says, "Present day in and day out, teachers are able to observe classrooms in their fullness: They are able to observe their teaching and their students' learning and to reflect productively on the relationships between that teaching and that learning" (88). Thus, though aware of the limitations of this approach, most stemming from my own insider status, I adopted it for the many insights it promised.

In both of my case studies, I used similar methods for collecting and analyzing data. I interviewed students and clients, used questionnaires to solicit general information from the students about their experiences with the projects, and collected and analyzed all of the documents the students produced, including correspondence and the final deliverables for the projects. I also collected documents and correspondence provided by the clients, such as their initial explanations of the projects and their written responses to the students' work.

In my interviews with the students, which I audio-taped and transcribed, I asked about their perceptions of the projects and of the associated tasks. I also asked how similar those tasks seemed to ones they already had completed or expected to complete in the workplace. In addition, I asked about the purposes and audiences for the assignments, and about the difficulties they had addressing the audiences. I also asked about their roles during the projects, along with their senses of the clients' roles. I questioned students about their level of motivation during the projects, their senses of the projects' instructional usefulness (whether they found them worth doing), and what, generally, they liked and disliked about them. Finally, I also asked them about the feedback they received during the projects.

The student questionnaires solicited similar information, which I used to supplement the information I received from the interviews. I asked the students what they found most valuable about the projects, as well as what they found most frustrating. I also asked them what they learned that they felt would be useful to them in the future, and I asked about their experiences working collaboratively, both with their peers and with the clients. Finally, I asked what they might do differently if they were to work on projects like these in the future.

When I spoke to the clients, I asked many of the same questions, primarily to see if their perceptions of the projects and of the students' experiences with them were similar to the students' perceptions. In other words, I was interested in exploring whether the clients' descriptions of the projects matched the students' interpretations of what the clients wanted them to do. I also wished to examine whether the clients' sense of the feedback they provided matched the students' sense, and whether their definitions of the purposes and audiences for the projects were similar. Also, I was interested in seeing how much value the clients admitted attaching to the projects. I also interviewed two clients and two students with whom I had worked in other collaborations. In analyzing my data, I looked for evidence addressing the four issues—exposure, authenticity, transition, and response.

In both of the case studies, the classroom-workplace projects lasted approximately two-thirds of the semester. At Univ A, the client, three technical writers from a large computer and electronics company, asked the students to develop a set of icons for the hard copy and online Unix documentation they were writing. This documentation would have a multinational audience, so the client wanted the icons to appeal to and be usable in all of the cultures addressed by it. The client asked the students for five deliverables: an initial project proposal; an annotated bibliography of sources; a preliminary design report presenting initial ideas for the icons, along with test results; an oral presentation to be delivered at the company; and a final recommendation report. My students, whom I divided into three groups of four and one group of three, worked on the project for seven weeks (I gave them at least 20 minutes during each class meeting to work on the project). All of the groups completed the same tasks (they did so knowing that the client would select the best set of icons) and submitted deliverables to both me and the client. Generally, I collected the documents and gave them to the client, who then reviewed them and responded to the students by e-mail. This process usually took two or three days. The client also visited the class periodically to provide additional direction. While the client reviewed and gave feedback on each of the deliverables, I evaluated and assigned grades to them.

At Univ B, the client, two linguists who had founded and who administered a large Web-based listserv for their discipline, asked the students to document the administrators' and editors' tasks for this listserv. Because of its scope, the listserv is staffed by several editors, who monitor postings; one programmer; and three site administrators (the two linguists who were the client and a third at another university). For this project, the 18 students worked in teams of four or five, with each team responsible for a different part of the documentation.

These students worked on the project from the fifth week to the end of the semester. Since each group completed a different part of the larger document, the groups coordinated their efforts to arrive at a consistent style for all of the parts. In addition to a style guide, the written deliverables for the project included an information plan, a project plan, content specifications, a progress report, and the final manuals. The client visited the class three times during the semester to review these documents. The client and other subject matter experts (the programmer and three of the editors) also met with the students several times outside of class for research, testing, and reviewing. In addition, students met in their groups during each class period to work on the project. The students delivered the final documents (five 15- to 20-page instructional manuals) the last week of class. The client, who attended the final class, offered their general impressions of the documents, while I evaluated and assigned grades to them.

Teaching and Learning Professional Genres

My findings from these cases shed light on what students may learn from classroom-workplace collaborations and how they learn it. They also begin to address the question of whether we can effectively use such assignments to teach professional genres. I acknowledge, however, that in studies like this one, students' reactions may be as much a response to the particular projects and/or to how those projects are implemented in a particular course. However, I also believe that such studies still can shed light on these activities and on their usefulness for teaching professional genres. Below I explore my findings as they relate to the four issues that I identified earlier.

Exposure

Concerning the ways in which classroom-workplace collaborations may expose students to workplace practices and genres, my research led me to make three observations. First, students, although not totally immersed in workplace cultures in such activities, gain exposure through these projects to workplace writing and general workplace practices. Such activities, while perhaps not replicating the social realities of the workplace exactly, at least give students an understanding of those realities (Freedman, Adam, and Smart; Knoblauch). My second observation is that through this exposure students begin to develop the history of interactions with the activity system that Russell says they need; they also seem to realize the value of the exposure. And finally, my third observation, which I support later, is that the context of school in these projects may support students' encounters with the new activity systems.

Meaningful Exposure to Workplace Practices. Client projects carried out in the classroom can hardly provide the kind of immersion that scholars say is needed to learn professional genres. However, my findings suggest that such projects still may provide a certain amount of it, especially since they usually give students contact with some community outside of the classroom. In particular, though these projects certainly fall short on the immersion criteria suggested by genre scholarship, they still can *expose* students to workplace writing practices, as well as to the activity systems of particular workplaces. Russell characterizes the process by which newcomers learn genres as a problem of expanding one's involvement with activity systems (516). He defines activity system as any ongoing, object-directed, historically conditioned, dialectically structured, tool-mediated human interaction (510). He also addresses how newcomers typically lack a sufficient history of interactions with unfamiliar activity systems to have much agency in them; therefore, he stresses the importance of developing this history. My findings suggest that workplace projects may help our students accomplish this (538, 541).

Stephen Doheny-Farina also presents ideas that relate to these concerns. In distinguishing writing as techne and writing as praxis, he says, in a move that is consistent with recent perspectives on genre,

> Learning to write as praxis means learning the boundaries, customs, and languages of a community, learning what counts as knowledge, learning what counts as appropriate forms, appropriate styles, and valid lines of reasoning, and deliberating on the means and goals of a community. Techne involves producing a clear document. Praxis involves living and contributing to an enterprise. (222)

He believes students may begin being socialized to workplace practices during their academic training. In other words, learning to write as praxis can occur, at least in part, in the classroom. Classrooms can also be productive sites for questioning workplace practices (229).

By their very nature, classroom-workplace collaborations expose students, at least to some extent, to the activities that are carried out and/or considered important in the workplace. They teach writing as praxis. These collaborations also may help students develop histories of interaction, and they may encourage the critical stances that Doheny-Farina and other scholars call for. As an example of this exposure, the students who participated in the icon project at Univ A were introduced to the project at the client's company. After being informed about the project by the technical writers, they were given a tour of the company and introduced to some of the engineers and programmers who worked there. These professionals told the students about their work and about the company. At the end of the project, the students returned to the company to present their recommendations. Their audiences included both the technical communicators who had been their contacts, as well as the engineers and programmers. The latter groups challenged the students by questioning the procedures they had used to arrive at their recommendations. Since the students had not been informed that these individuals would be attending the presentation, they were caught off guard by their questions. However, most of the students acknowledged later that hearing these alternative viewpoints was valuable. In general, this project exposed the students to several professional communities.

The listserv project also exposed the students to new professional communities. This project differed somewhat from the icon project since it originated and was carried out in the university setting. However, it exposed the students not only to a new professional culture but also to the genres that play a central role in that culture. The students became almost as familiar with the listserv as the editors who worked on it. They learned both the editorial and technical processes required to maintain the listserv, and they also gained exposure to the academic conversations that take place through it.

Students' Valuing of This Exposure. My research also provided evidence that the students valued this exposure to these professional cultures and activities. Alison (all names are pseudonyms), who participated in the listserv project, anticipated being able to apply this exposure in her career:

> Everything I learned about the whole documentation process from this project I will be able to apply to my future job—the information gathering, the group work, the style guides/templates, the actual writing, the user testing. What was cool was that when I interviewed . . . they talked about information plans and content specs, and I knew what they were talking about.

Jim, who participated in the same project, said the exposure helped him understand what occurs in such projects prior to writing:

> Definitely they're instructionally useful. I think [the listserv project] was particularly useful in learning the front end of the job. . . . I thought you

> just sat down and started writing. I was completely unaware of all of the planning and research. That was extremely useful . . . because I didn't know how much goes into the front end.

Jim, who had worked as a magazine editor for several years, added, "the projects have been really valuable in helping me see the whole picture rather than just focusing on the writing of the document—the whole process of documentation."

The clients also addressed the value of this exposure for students. Catherine, the owner of a small company specializing in online help and Web development, said, "They [the students] get their hands dirty, and they get a feel for what it's actually like to work on a technical communication project and have deliverables. It's concrete and not abstract." Catherine, who has worked on several of these projects, also addressed the value of these experiences for mentoring students:

> I think the students get a couple of things from the projects. They get experience working with a real client or with peer technical communicators, and they get mentoring. . . . With me it's a mentoring thing, and it happens either by their observing me or by osmosis. I walk them through what they need to do. They also get a taste for what the field is like. . . . They make contacts in the field and are able to network.

Not all clients perceive the mentoring potential of the projects like Catherine, but many do. In general, my experience has been that clients enjoy sharing their tricks of the trade with students.

Sonya, who worked on the listserv project, articulated explicitly the value of these experiences: "They're a real good start in terms of exposing students to these cultures. I think it's a really good point that to serve a community you have to understand it and to understand it you have to be involved in it." Sonya also expressed her sense of how the projects had exposed her to new aspects of the field: "I've liked the idea that it's introduced me to new areas. Last year I had to go looking for something, so I had to think about what contacts I have. It's broadened my areas of interest and knowledge." Her comments, in addition to illustrating her sense of how the projects are similar to those in the workplace, also suggest their potential for broadening students' perspectives.

Authenticity

The second issue I explored concerned students' perceptions of the authenticity of these activities, or, how similar they perceived them to be to actual workplace projects. Most research emphasizes the differences between classroom and workplace contexts, calling into question the ability of any classroom project to convey the rhetorical contexts and social actions of the workplace (Freedman, Adam, and Smart). In my case studies, I wished to look beyond these differences to consider the ways in which such activities may be similar to those in the workplace, and the potential significance of those similarities.

My findings suggest that students still may view such projects as artificial, but that they also may discern some authenticity in them. The students in my studies also tended to value the classroom-workplace collaborations more highly than traditional assignments. They found the audiences they addressed with these projects to be more concrete than those they typically address in more traditional assignments. Finally, my students also seemed motivated and challenged by the projects. However, to be motivated, the students wanted to know that the clients also valued and were invested in the projects.

Students' Perceptions of the Projects as Artificial. My findings suggest that, similar to cases, classroom-workplace collaborations do not fully replicate workplace contexts. The students still viewed the projects as artificial, even though they were provided by actual clients. In other words, despite the fact that the projects were from the workplace and not case studies, the students, and even the clients, still considered them as more like school projects. For example, Tim, who worked on the icon project, said, "As we started we definitely saw it as a school assignment. Then we thought of it not as a professional or business-type thing because it's not, but something that stood on its own." The clients seemed to share this perception. Catherine, quoted above, said,

> The projects are somewhat real, but not totally real. We're not giving them actual client work. I could see doing it for a client maybe if they didn't have a lot of money, and they wanted something done. This might provide one alternative for them. . . . Generally, though, the students don't get as realistic sense of what a client would be like to work for. Certainly, though, they get something for their portfolio and resume.

Catherine addresses here how the projects she asks students to complete typically are not the projects her own clients would give her. She said she defines the projects "more in terms of a noncritical path for the company. These aren't flagship projects. They're more of an ancillary or sideline project."

For the students, the projects seem similar to workplace projects, but also seem to be less demanding. For example, commenting on why she thought I assigned it, Terri, who worked on the icon project, said,

> I think that your goal was to give us a taste of what it was like—not exactly, but close to what it would be like to go through a real project like this with an employer. You held our hand a lot more than a real employer ever would. . . . I don't think that it was as stressful as it would be if we had been doing it for a real client.

Jim, the former magazine editor, also distinguished these assignments from workplace projects:

> I don't think it duplicates the intensity of the work you'd do in the workplace. The documentation project was a nice, easy, relaxed, and

> comfortable pace. . . . It still feels that these are sort of fun things we do together for practice, but it's not that sort of structured work environment we'll end up in. . . . Doing these projects it feels like we're one big happy family in there doing this together. That wasn't my experience previously in a corporate setting where it was more each individual for himself.

Jim also stated that the projects do not entail some of the less glamorous tasks that writers inevitably encounter in everyday work: "I think that there are a lot of trivial, painful details of this job that we don't get. For example, things we might do that are deadly dull and how do you cope with doing things that you can't bear to look at? So these are more interesting." He even described the projects as fictional: "In a certain respect I think these real-world clients are fictional in a sense. This has to do with the fact that they're getting things for free. . . . " Since Jim, like many nontraditional students at Univ B, had previous professional experience, he brought to the projects an awareness of workplace practice. Thus, for Jim, the projects seemed idealized.

These students' perceptions of the projects as artificial may be unavoidable. In other words, the context of the classroom may constrain such projects just enough to encourage such perceptions. In addition, the projects seldom are ones that are critical for the client. More often, they are projects clients wish to have completed but have little time for. Nonetheless, they still are workplace projects, and the students still value them; therefore, this perception of artificiality may not be an insurmountable obstacle, as the next section also suggests.

Students' Valuing of the Projects. Despite their characterizations of the projects as artificial, the students also said that they valued the projects. Many also acknowledged that the projects seemed like real workplace projects at least to some extent. For example, Tim, the student quoted previously, also said, "It's not that this is part of our job, but neither was it just an assignment for class." Andrew, a student from Univ B, said,

> I don't have any real-world experience, but some things seemed very real to me. For example, for two weeks we were stopped in our work because we couldn't use some of the comments. It turned out to be very simple. I think things like that come up on the job all the time. What's artificial . . . or contrived was the fact that when we couldn't figure that out, our wheels were spinning. . . .

Andrew also said, "I know motivationally I got more out of this and more work done than if you had given us work out of a book." And Sonya, the former attorney quoted above, said that one of the projects in which she participated seemed contrived at first, but that she and her classmates ended up feeling that it was less contrived when they learned the client had made changes as a result of their recommendations: "But then you said we found things and they're making changes, which made us feel better about it."

A number of the students were similar to Andrew and Sonya in that they both valued the projects and found them motivating. For some students, the motivation came from the trust and accountability the projects engendered; for example, Pat, a student at Univ B, said, "I liked it because it was a real experience. It made me feel important as a student that you trusted us enough to do this. It made it more challenging, exciting. It was an honor to do it." For others, it was simply the projects themselves and what they allowed the students to accomplish. For example, Sonya said,

> These exercises feel like real-world exercises, so I think that makes them more appealing. Because it's more appealing you think about it more and [you approach it] more creatively. . . . I think I'm more motivated by these, and I think the fact that someone would use your work in an actual workplace situation is a definite motivation.

Students Finding the Audiences for the Projects More Concrete. Students who participate in projects like these also may value the senses of audience they provide. For Rozumalski and Graves, awareness of audience was an important factor in students' valuing of the case studies and in their viewing them as authentic—students completing the cases in their study exhibited a greater sensitivity to their audiences (77, 88, 92). In the classroom-workplace collaborations I studied, students also seemed to exhibit a heightened sensitivity to audience. Several students indicated that the audiences for these projects seemed much more concrete than those for more traditional assignments. For example, Pat, who participated in the listserv project, said, "The audience did feel more concrete. Sometimes I'd even visualize a graduate student sitting down with my document in front of the computer. I thought of that a lot." She also said,

> I definitely think the audience was more real. I thought it was very valuable to work with real . . . clients versus a made-up project. I was more careful because I knew this was going to real people. I think in some ways it was harder too, but I appreciate that because this is what I'm going into. It didn't just feel like an exercise. . . .

Pat found that the realness of the project and the concrete audiences for it made her care more: "In [English] 324 all of the projects were fictitious, and I took it less seriously and was less careful."

Sonya, quoted above, said that as a result of these projects she also thinks more about audiences now:

> These projects have certainly been exercises in thinking about how your audience will use your work. . . . In the editing class we talked about not stepping on the toes of the writer and encouraging them. One of the students I edited was writing in a legal environment and used a phrase that's inappropriate. I decided that was something you wouldn't comment on right away, so I went about it differently. The editing project is another example—the fact that they most appreciated the positive at the start.

Sonya's last comment refers to specific feedback the students received from an editing client. This client appreciated the positive comments about the document that the students had included with their edits.

The Importance of Client Investment. Sonya's comments above, and really the comments of all of the students, support a final important observation regarding the authenticity of classroom-workplace projects: students want to know that clients value and are invested in the projects, that they view them as important and intend to use them. This observation resembles Freedman and Adam's finding that the criterion of success in internships is that learners must see their tasks as authentic and as having consequences (411). The students in my classes generally shared this perspective. For example, Jeremy, from Univ A, said that even though the engineers intimidated them at the presentations, they also made them feel like the company valued the project:

> After they invited in the other engineers, it made it more real. If they weren't there I would have felt that it was just for you and the grade. This made it seem more relevant and that you're working for a company that values this and is willing to let people take work time out for this. It was important to me. They spent the time to come up—took man-hours off to see this.

Jeremy's classmate, Terri, expressed a different perception of this client's valuing of the project: "I do feel they took our work seriously, but I don't think it was at the top of their list, and I don't expect it to be. But technically they are getting this for free. But if they want the same quality as from their employees, maybe they should put more effort into guiding our work." According to Terri, this client had not devoted sufficient energy to the project, a perception that significantly impacted her experiences with the project.

Transition

The third issue I identified as important led me to investigate the ways in which these projects may facilitate students' transitions to the workplace. Existing research tells us that students have difficulties with such transitions, and we have begun to understand some of the reasons for these difficulties (Anson and Forsberg; Freedman and Adam; Winsor); however, we have not determined yet how to lessen them. My research suggested that classroom-workplace projects may act as a bridge between school and work; classroom and workplace activity systems may overlap with the projects since students get a taste of workplace practices while still experiencing the structure, support, and familiarity of the academic learning environment (a kind of guided legitimate peripheral participation) (Lave and Wegner). Students participate in workplace activities, but those activities are undertaken for the express purpose of learning (Freedman and Adam 402–03). They become socialized, at least partially, and are exposed to the cultural knowledge that Winsor identifies as being so important in writing ("Writing Well" 160). However, despite this structure and support, the students I studied still seemed to experience frustrations.

My findings here are supported also by Russell. For example, he says that the genre system of a classroom, or the activity system of a course, "forms a complex, stabilized-for-now site of *boundary work* [his emphasis] . . . between the activity system of a discipline/profession . . . and that of the educational University" (530). Classrooms exist on the boundaries of activity systems (541), which is where these kinds of collaborative activities also seem to be situated. He also says that intertextual links between professional and classroom genres lead to similarities in the two genres (531). In other words, the genres the students write in their classes can resemble the professional genres (they certainly do in these situations). And, perhaps most important, he conveys a sense that the closer courses and assignments get to the boundary of the activity system, the more context students discern; also, the more they see the relevance of their writing to the discipline and to other social practices (539). Students start out at the edge of a discipline's collective life and gradually move toward its center, a conception that also resembles Jean Lave and Etienne Wegner's notion of legitimate peripheral participation (Russell 540). This conception also relates to Winsor's ideas about the tacit and socially based nature of knowledge about writing ("Writing Well" 158–59).

Bridging Classroom and Workplace Activity Systems. My students' comments suggest that classroom-workplace collaborations may begin to provide the types of experiences that scholars like Russell and Winsor describe. For example, Pat, who worked on the listserv project, specifically addressed transitional issues:

> I don't know yet how important these experiences will be since I haven't graduated, but I can't imagine they won't be extremely valuable. I think the transition from the cocoon of college to the real-life world would be much harder without these experiences. I can't imagine what it'd be like if I didn't have your classes and these experiences. I see it as a perfect stepping stone, a kind of halfway point. We're not completely on our own; we still have you, and they're not getting completely professional work. . . .

Pat's comments suggest that students may experience less pressure with these kinds of experiences than if they simply are left on their own in a new setting. In other words, the projects allow students to carry out tasks they will be asked to carry out in the workplace, but they also provide a supportive environment. They allow students to experience workplace practices without the usual accountability of the workplace.

This lack of accountability may have a downside, however. For example, Jim, the former magazine editor, said,

> I think the big difficulty is that we know we have a safety net. . . . We know we can send an email to you and you'll sort it out. I don't think it gives us as complete [a] sense of responsibility. I think that's what leads

> to people not attending completely to everything because they know they're not the ones who are ultimately responsible.

Jim makes a valid point. Students conceivably make compromises in their work because they ultimately do not feel responsible. As facilitators of these experiences, we may need to take measures to guard against this. One way may be to allow students to experience consequences when they do not meet their responsibilities. This occurred with the icon project. All of the groups failed to take the second deliverable seriously, and the client was very dissatisfied with the outcomes, which they let students know during a class meeting. Because of a professional conference, I missed this meeting. When I returned, students were lined up to apologize for what had happened. All of their remaining documents met the client's expectations.

Fortunately, most of my students have recognized that the experiences are valuable, and, therefore, have taken them seriously. For example, Jim also said,

> They're definitely worth doing. I can't imagine how you would teach this in a non-work situation. It wouldn't have any value to teach it that way, where you don't get any feedback. . . . I agree with the value of doing client projects with outsiders—the value of going to meetings at the client site. It gives you a sense of doing a real job. So I think the outside stuff is the way to go. Everyone in class likes the sense of having a real client.

Jim's comments again suggest that a beneficial outcome of these projects is the exposure they offer to workplace cultures and practices.

Andrew, who also worked on the listserv project, said that the projects not only provide a useful transitional experience but also help students apply and make sense of course content. They provide structured and meaningful ways for students to apply their knowledge:

> Initially I was turned off by the fact we were doing these projects—slave labor was my first impression. I was coming from a liberal arts background, so I was concerned about that initially. Once I got into it it emphasized things that were emphasized in the Hackos' text, like the planning. You can emphasize this all you want, but it didn't make sense to me until we were in the middle of it with a real client. . . It gave me a chance to learn as I went [along].

Andrew added, "I find a lot of the readings for technical writing very dry and difficult to stay with. The projects helped me to go back and pick up things. Also, it seems like this is good job experience. This is just added experience to bring to an employer." Thus, the meaningfulness of the projects, and the opportunities they provide for applying classroom knowledge, help make them beneficial learning experiences.

Students' Frustrations with the Projects. Some other aspects of transitions that rhetorical scholars address also are evident in my findings—in particular, the disorientation, frustration, and double binds that scholars say students experience when they encounter new contexts and genres (Anson and Forsberg 214; Russell 534, 541). Such disorientation seems to occur most often at the outset of the projects: students feel overwhelmed and unsure of how to proceed (Burnett). Jen's comment about the icon project is characteristic of the kinds of comments I often hear at this stage:

> When we went out there we came back with this, "Oh my gosh, what are we going to do now?" It seemed huge. It seemed like an incredibly huge thing at first that we'd never be able to finish—or especially be able to get started. Then when we got into it and saw the stages it got a lot more reasonable.

Dianne, another student who participated in this project, ended up feeling that instead of being easier, the project was actually more complex than the client portrayed it:

> In the first sheet they gave us . . . , it didn't seem as complicated as what it's turned out to be. There's been a lot more work than anticipated. From what they gave us it just seemed. . . . There was a lot more that they weren't overly specific about. I think more input from their side would have helped.

Last year, students in my technical communication graduate course expressed relief when experts in online help development told them they also feel overwhelmed often when they start new projects. The writers also told the students that their anxieties usually subside once they begin the projects, another experience some of my students acknowledged. For example, Kerry, who did the icon project, said,

> Right in the beginning it was very unclear to me what the project was. I didn't understand what they meant or what they wanted. . . . It was initially overwhelming, but now it's clearer and doesn't seem as bad. . . . Once we got the first thing in it got better. . . . I didn't know what they were talking about at first. . . . I thought in the beginning they should've made it clearer and more basic. Sometimes you would tell us something, but we'd want to hear it from the client because they were who we were really doing this for.

Kerry's comments also suggest how quickly students become accountable to clients.

Since most students have never participated in this kind of activity, a factor that itself can be disorienting, it also may be that they simply need to become more familiar with the projects and with what they entail. Also, most students are accustomed to more traditional assignments; therefore, they may be unfamiliar with the more implicit learning that tends to occur with these projects. In such cases, experience may be the only, and best, remedy, as Andrew says,

> I feel better this semester than I did last semester just because I think. . . . There's almost that holding pattern at the start of the project that tends to

> be stressful. Now I know that's OK and you'll probably feel you're behind your entire project. I don't see any way of getting around that.

For Andrew, and for other students who have worked on multiple classroom-workplace projects, dealing with the disorientation inherent in these activities seems to become easier with practice, even if the disorientation itself never goes away. Students benefit from having time to reflect on, understand, and work through their uncertainties.

In addition, it also may be, as Rebecca Burnett's and Mike Rose's work suggests, that we may need to provide more explicit instructional cues during activities such as these—rather than relying on students to discern and interpret our implicit instructional strategies, which they may not have the skills to do. In other words, by keeping the learning so implicit, we may be asking too much of our students. Rose says,

> To move into authentic practice does not rule out along the way a host of traditional teacherly devices, from the pep talk, to direct instruction, to the quick quiz. In fact, for some, full participation may require it; otherwise one gets a shadow involvement never leading to true participation and competence. (154)

Rose also says, "I would simply suggest that pedagogic strategies not normally found in work sites and social groups could facilitate transparency and access—and without compromising the conceptual power of practice theory" (154–55). These points may be especially important with assignments like client projects.

Response

Finally, the last issue that I investigated suggested considering how both clients and instructors respond to students' work, along with how useful students find this response, and what value they assign to it. My findings suggested that feedback and response often are problem areas in these types of projects. The students in my studies generally were dissatisfied with the feedback they received from the clients. My findings also seemed consistent with the findings of other scholars who have explored this issue (Anson and Forsberg; Burnett; Freedman and Adam; Freedman, Adam, and Smart). Specifically, these scholars suggest that there are differences in the nature of responding in the two settings. They attribute these differences, at least in part, to differences in the concerns in each setting, a finding my data also support. However, my findings also suggest that clients, who are acting outside of their familiar workplace contexts, may not always know or understand how best to respond to students' work. I have observed that, as a result of this uncertainty, the clients may not respond at all or may respond in an extreme manner—being overly critical or overly complimentary. In all of these cases, the students I studied were dissatisfied, and sometimes even angry, with the responses from the clients. This dissatisfaction, in turn, usually led them to value my response more highly. However, despite this valuing, and despite often having less than realistic expectations of what this response should be like, the students still expressed a desire to receive feedback from the client.

Student's General Dissatisfaction with Client Feedback. Generally, the students I interviewed said the feedback they received from the clients during these collaborations was in some way deficient—e.g., it was not enough to give them direction for revising the document or to help them determine whether they were on the right track. Many also indicated that they ultimately got more from my feedback than the client's. This seemed to be the case, especially with the students who participated in the icon project. Jen said,

> I don't think we got much feedback, so I was disappointed. And some of the things they wrote, it was like, "What do you mean by this?" So if they would've been a lot more explicit. In terms of feedback, what we got from you was a lot more helpful . . .

Terri, another student who worked with Jen, expressed similar views:

> The feedback was not helpful—we didn't get much. And Jen wrote lots of email to the client, but the responses weren't very informative. You gave us good feedback. We knew what to do from what you said. [The clients] sent the stuff about it being sloppy, but we needed more specifics. We also assumed we were on the right track because [they] didn't mention or say they were looking for "this."

Students are most familiar with the response they usually receive in the classroom; therefore, they may expect a similar kind of response from clients and be frustrated if they do not receive it.

I should note, too, that in my own experiences with these projects, students often start out being very concerned, and even anxious, about their final grades. However, as the students become more involved, they often end up worrying much less about my expectations and evaluations than about completing the projects in a manner acceptable to the client. This greater concern with the client's expectations may be a result, at least in part, of the classroom culture I cultivate, which does not overemphasize grading and which acknowledges that mistakes are bound to occur. I tell my students repeatedly that my primary concerns are with their learning from their experiences and with the quality of their work relative to the client's expectations. In turn, my students seem to figure out quickly that if they do their best to meet those expectations, they also will do fine in my class. In addition, I give students ample feedback throughout the projects, and my evaluation of their work is not limited to their final deliverables.

Overly Critical and Overly Complimentary Feedback. The students in my studies also expressed frustration when the client's feedback was overly critical. Some clients, when they review students' work, focus primarily on what is wrong with it. This is where the different motivations in responding may come into play. In other words, clients may focus on what's wrong, not with the intention of being overly critical, but with the intention of pointing out weaknesses so that the students can fix them—the idea of helping students shape the drafts (Freedman and Adam). Freedman and Adam also note how students tend to view response as evaluative and final (because of their experiences as students); therefore, they may see a supervisor's or client's critical comments as negative evaluation and end up resisting the evaluation (418). Some of this, I believe, occurred with the students in the icon project. Throughout this project the client's response tended to be very critical (perhaps a little too critical, but, again, not intentionally to discourage the students). The client wanted to help the students do their best work. For this reason the client spent a great deal of time reviewing and commenting on all of the students' drafts. The students' perceptions of the responses, however, were very different from what the client intended. Rather than viewing the responses as attempts to help them improve their work, the students perceived the responses as unnecessarily harsh.

When the students discussed this client's response, they often made comments like this one from Greg, which expresses surprise at the harsh tone of the feedback:

> When we turned in our initial proposal, some of the comments, if they had said them verbally, would have seemed kind of rude. I think that they took it seriously, but they were kind of harsh about it. They have all these professional standards they work by, and they applied them to us. It was just kind of surprising.

In his next comment, Greg compared this client's critical feedback with the more suggestive comments professors usually make: "Most professors make comments like, 'Maybe you could expand,' or, 'This is nice,' but they were more like, 'No, this isn't going to do,' that's it." Greg was more familiar with the kind of constructive feedback his professors usually gave him, and he preferred it. Dianne's comments suggest the potentially negative effects of such critical feedback: "I would say, at first, I felt like this was a great opportunity. Then we'd write something, and they'd tear it apart. It didn't seem like they realized we were trying our hardest. . . . " Again, the intentions of the client, and the student's perceptions of those intentions, were very different. Dianne found the client's criticisms discouraging. They impacted both her motivation and her confidence as she worked on the project. (I should note that situations like these could possibly be avoided if instructors monitor client feedback. In this case, I might have tried to redirect the client's response. I realized too late that the students were finding it overly critical.)

In the listserv project, the client took a very different approach to response, offering mostly praise. However, the students in this project still seemed to be frustrated. Jim, for example, said,

> One of my biggest difficulties is that I didn't get a sense that Judy had a lot of critical distance. It would have been more helpful if she had given more criticism. When everything is great I wonder if you're making the necessary connection with the client. I wonder if everything was really

> that great, or if she was just so happy to be getting things that anything was sufficient.

Jim continued, "I was actually frustrated by the fact that Judy consistently said everything was 'wonderful.' I'm always suspicious of people who give you kudos for everything from your writing to the way you tie your shoes. I would have been more comfortable if she had shown a bit more critical distance." (Again, in this case I could have monitored the feedback and encouraged the client to offer constructive criticism, although clients still may have difficulty doing this. For example, this client was so grateful just to have the documentation that she seemed hesitant to criticize it.) Jim also added that his motivation for these projects comes more from my response than the client's:

> My motivation comes from producing a project that you approve of. I'm much more interested in producing something you think is good. That's the value of the course for me and what motivates me. It means less to me if Judy finds it good. . . . So I'm motivated by my sense of responsibility to you and to the other students.

Jim's comments suggest again that students often place a higher value on the instructor's feedback. Of course, this may be because of their greater familiarity and comfort with it.

Students Still Wanting Client Feedback. Despite expressing their comfort with and preference for instructor feedback, most students indicated that they still want feedback from the clients. Some even want it to be fairly formal. For example, Roger, who received critical feedback on the icon project, said, "My only complaint is that I'd have liked more formal documents with feedback. . . . like a memo or something. . . . They could've developed their ideas more if they'd have addressed us maybe in a more formal sense." Dianne, one of his classmates, expressed a similar interest: "Maybe more elaboration from them would have been better. Maybe a memo or letter back from them—full comments—rather than being . . . critical." It may be that what the students really want is a detailed response similar to what they get from teachers, although I am not certain that this is the case, or even the best option. Given the value of these projects as transitional experiences and their potential for exposing students to workplace practices, students might prefer to receive responses similar to what the client would provide to a writer in the workplace. What may be needed for this to occur and be productive is education, both for the students—about the nature of this response—and for the clients—about effective ways to respond (clients may not know how to respond effectively; therefore, instructors may need to take an active role, guiding clients in this respect).

Conclusion

My examination of classroom-workplace collaborations suggests that, despite their practical limitations, these activities still may have a number of benefits.

For example, my research suggests that they can be valuable experiences for our students, exposing them to the cultures and activities of the workplace and gradually introducing them to the genres that both arise from and support those cultures and activities. Thus, we can use these assignments to begin teaching professional genres. These projects also can act as useful transitional experiences for our students: students can get a taste of workplace writing practices while still having the guidance and support of their instructor and classmates. Such activities also may provide productive occasions for students to reflect on and apply their classroom and theoretical knowledge, and even to question the conventional nature of the genres they end up generating. There may be lessons from these projects that students can take with them and use in their future professional roles, a factor we also should consider in our research.

My research also suggests the importance of continuing to assess these projects. Such assessments can serve the dual purpose of shedding light on how successful they are in our classes as well as on their value as strategies for teaching professional genres. What I hope my own research suggests is the value of considering a range of factors when we carry out such assessments. In this article I have considered four of these factors. There certainly are others, and identifying and considering these will allow us to draw more substantial and productive conclusions about the value of these kinds of assignments.

Finally, we also should be concerned with structuring and carrying out such collaborations in ways that make them more productive experiences for our students. My research, and my experiences with carrying out such collaborations more generally, has suggested to me several questions that instructors should pose in planning such activities. For example, with respect to exposure, instructors should ask,

- Who will the client be? What is the nature of the client's work? What genres does the client typically produce?
- How much and what kind of exposure will the students get to the client's workplace practices and genres?

Relating to the issue of authenticity, instructors should ask,

- What kinds of tasks will the students be asked to undertake? Are the tasks ones they will likely be called upon to complete in the workplace and/or in their careers?
- Where will they complete these tasks?
- What resources will the students need to carry out these tasks and what kind of access will they have to those resources?

And relating to transition and response, instructors should ask,

- How much structure and support will the students receive from their instructor, from their classmates, and from the client?
- How accountable will the students be to the instructor, to the client, and to their classmates? In what ways will they be accountable?

- How will the students' work be evaluated? To what extent and how will the client be involved in evaluating the project? How often and when will the client visit the class, meet with the students, and review the students' work?

Thinking through these questions will help instructors, in collaboration with workplace clients, to construct more productive experiences for exposing and introducing students, if only gradually, to the professional activity systems they seek to enter.

WORKS CITED

Anson, Chris M., and L. Lee Forsberg. "Moving beyond the Academic Community: Transitional Stages in Professional Writing." WC 7 (1990): 200–31.

Applebee, Arthur. "Musings." *RTE* 21 (1987): 5–7.

Bazerman, Charles. "Editor's Introduction." *Reality by Design: The Rhetoric and Technology of Authenticity in Education*. By Joseph Petraglia. Mahwah, NJ: Lawrence Erlbaum, 1998. ix–x.

Berkenkotter, Carol, and Thomas N. Huckin. *Genre Knowledge in Disciplinary Communication: Cognition/Culture/Power*. Hillsdale, NJ: Lawrence Erlbaum, 1995.

Berkenkotter, Carol, Thomas N. Huckin, and John Ackerman. "Social Context and Socially Constructed Texts: The Initiation of a Graduate Student into a Writing Community." *Textual Dynamics of the Professions: Historical and Contemporary Studies of Writing in Professional Communities*. Ed. Charles Bazerman and James Paradis. Madison: U of Wisconsin P, 1991. 191–215.

Blakeslee, Ann M. "Activity, Context, Interaction, and Authority: Learning to Write Scientific Papers in Situ." *JBTC* 11 (1997): 125–69.

Burnett, Rebecca E. "Some People Weren't Able to Contribute Anything but Their Technical Knowledge': The Anatomy of a Dysfunctional Team." *Nonacademic Writing: Social Theory and Technology*. Ed. Ann H. Duin and Craig J. Hansen. Mahwah, NJ: Lawrence Erlbaum, 1996. 123–56.

Cochran-Smith, Marilyn, and Susan L. Lytle. "The Teacher Research Movement: A Decade Later." *Educational Researcher* 28 (1999): 15–25.

Doheny-Farina, Stephen. *Rhetoric, Innovation, Technology: Case Studies of Technical Communication in Technology Transfers*. Cambridge, MA: MIT P, 1992.

Engeström, Yrjo. *Learning by Expanding: An Activity Theoretical Approach to Developmental Research*. Helsinki: Orienta-Konsultit Oy, 1987.

Fleischer, Cathy. "Researching Teacher-Research: A Practitioner's Retrospective." *English Education* 26 (1994): 86–124.

Freedman, Aviva, and Christine Adam. "Learning to Write Professionally: 'Situated Learning' and the Transition from University to Professional Discourse." *JBTC* 10 (1996): 395–427.

Freedman, Aviva, Christine Adam, and Graham Smart. "Wearing Suits to Class: Simulating Genres and Simulations as Genre." *WC* 11 (1994): 193–226.

Freedman, Aviva, and Peter Medway, eds. *Genre and the New Rhetoric*. London: Taylor & Francis, 1994.

Haas, Christina. "Reading Biology: One Student's Rhetorical Development in College." *WC* 11 (1994): 43–84.

Hillocks, George. *Research on Written Composition*. Urbana, IL: NCTE, 1986.

Knoblauch, Cyril H. "The Teaching and Practice of 'Professional Writing." *Writing in the Business Professions*. Ed. Myra Kogen. Urbana, IL: NCTE, 1989. 246–66.

Lave, Jean, and Etienne Wegner. *Situated Learning: Legitimate Peripheral Participation*. Cambridge, UK: Cambridge UP, 1991.

Miller, Carolyn R. "Genre as Social Action." *QJS* 70 (1984): 151–67.

North, Stephen M. *The Making of Knowledge in Composition*. Upper Montclair, NJ: Boynton/Cook, 1987.

Petraglia, Joseph. *Reality by Design: The Rhetoric and Technology of Authenticity in Education*. Mahwah, NJ: Lawrence Erlbaum, 1998.

Prior, Paul. *Writing/Disciplinarity: A Sociohistoric Account of Literate Activity in the Academy*. Hillsdale, NJ: Lawrence Erlbaum, 1998.

Ray, Ruth. "Composition from the Teacher-Research Point of View." *Methods and Methodology in Composition Research*. Ed. Gesa Kirsch and Patricia A. Sullivan. Carbondale and Edwardsville, IL: Southern Illinois UP, 1992. 172–89.

Ray, Ruth E. "Afterword: Ethics and Representation in Teacher Research." *Ethics and Representation in Qualitative Studies of Literacy*. Ed. Peter Mortensen and Gesa E. Kirsch. Urbana, IL: NCTE, 1996. 287–300.

Rose, Mike. "'Our Hands Will Know': The Development of Tactile Diagnostic Skill—Teaching, Learning, and Situated Cognition in a Physical Therapy Program." *Anthropology and Education Quarterly* 30 (1999): 133–60.

Rozumalski, Lynn P., and Michael F. Graves. "Effects of Case and Traditional Writing Assignments on Writing Products and Processes." *JBTC* 9 (1995): 77–102.

Russell, David R. "Rethinking Genre in School and Society: An Activity Theory Analysis." *WC* 14 (1997): 504–54.

Spinuzzi, Clay. "Pseudotransactionality, Activity Theory, and Professional Writing Instruction." *TCQ* 5 (1996): 295–308.

Swales, John. *Genre Analysis: English in Academic and Research Settings*. Cambridge, UK: Cambridge UP, 1990.

Wickliff, Gregory A. "Assessing the Value of Client-Based Group Projects in an Introductory Technical Communication Course." *JBTC* 11 (1997): 170–91.

Winsor, Dorothy A. *Writing Like an Engineer: A Rhetorical Education*. Mahwah, NJ: Lawrence Erlbaum, 1996.

———. "Writing Well as a From of Social Knowledge." *Nonacademic Writing: Social Theory and Technology*. Ed. Ann H. Duin and Craig J. Hansen. Mahwah, NJ: Lawrence Erlbaum, 1996. 157–72.

APPLIED THEORY

22 Communicating Across Organizational Boundaries: A Challenge for Workplace Professionals

RACHEL SPILKA

When students enter the workplace, they will face many challenges. Some, such as how to adapt their writing skills to the various genres and activity networks they'll confront, have been addressed in considerable detail by researchers and teachers. Others, however, such as how they will interact and negotiate across *organizational boundaries, have not. In this essay, Spilka presents the results of a longitudinal study of upper-level professionals in a state government, examining and outlining the social and rhetorical strategies that enabled them to carry out and manage "cross-boundary communication" (p. 372 in this volume). Arguing that this kind of communication is becoming more prevalent and essential to success, she provides a summary of the work prior to her study, some of it contradictory; illustrates the benefits, risks, and problems in this work; and concludes by offering useful strategies for those engaged in this work. In addition, she offers some suggestions for educators to consider in order to prepare students for this important and difficult collaborative task.*

In government, business, and other occupational arenas, professionals often need to communicate assertively and effectively outside the social boundaries of their own organization or organizational unit (such as outside their own department, division, or project group). Unfortunately, professionals might discover that engaging in cross-boundary communication can be a baffling and stressful experience that does not always result in a desirable outcome. Although many practitioners need to draw on an array of social and rhetorical strategies to succeed in cross-boundary communication and to avoid or overcome its associative risks, sacrifices, and problems, relatively little is known about how to interact and negotiate across organizational boundaries. This article aims to add to our knowledge of cross-boundary communication by presenting the results of a longitudinal qualitative study of (1) how upper-level professionals in one division of a state government department both benefitted and suffered from communicating with

From *Technical Communication* 42, no. 3 (1995): 436–50.

representatives from other "outside" organizational units and (2) which social and rhetorical strategies helped these professionals cope reasonably well with cross-boundary communication. After describing two cases from this study that illustrate the importance of learning more about cross-boundary communication, I will briefly survey research to date on this topic, describe the study's site and methodology, summarize the study's findings, and then speculate about their implications for practitioners and those who choose in the future to teach, theorize about, or research cross-boundary communication.

Why Should Professionals Learn More about Cross-Boundary Communication?

Although many technical communicators, especially those working within small companies, rarely or never communicate for professional purposes outside the boundaries of their organizations, or even outside their own organizational divisions or departments, a growing number of communicators are discovering that cross-boundary communication is becoming a regular professional activity that is increasingly integral to success in fulfilling key organizational goals (Olsen 1993). As the following cases illustrate, technical communicators would benefit greatly from learning effective strategies for negotiating cross-boundary communication.

Case I: Negotiating a Memorandum of Agreement

Professionals in a small, relatively new division of state government hope to collaborate with other state government agencies to produce a memorandum of agreement that would define federal, state, and district roles and responsibilities in a statewide urban conservation program. However, these division professionals find it difficult even to initiate this project because other agencies remain unfamiliar with the division's functions and goals and initially see no benefit in joining forces with the division to create the memorandum. It takes a long time for the division professionals to explain their purpose and identity to the other agencies and to convince the other agencies that they would benefit, as well, from the proposed collaboration. Furthermore, even after agreeing to collaborate with the division, the other agencies continue to question the division's integrity and aims and threaten to deprive the division of some of its current and potential power and control. As a result, the division professionals worry constantly about both the present (What are their roles, responsibilities, and authority in this project?) and the future (Can they preserve their division's identity and image in this project? Can they build more power and establish more credibility as the project goes on?). The division professionals find themselves constantly debating the social parameters of the collaboration (Who can do what? Who has legal rights and obligations? What needs to happen for certain laws to be changed, so that social roles and responsibilities can also change?). They also doubt their own ability to emerge from this collaboration any closer to fulfilling their environmental goals or realizing their desire to become more visible to other organizations, add to their own credibility, and increase their own authority in future, similar collaborative ventures.

Case II: Negotiating a Long-Term Plan

The upper-level staff of a state government division are eager to produce a long-range plan that would determine which division goals and activities would be given priority in the next 5 years. Toward this end, they decide to form a partnership with both lower-level staff in their own division and representatives of outside agencies with similar environmental goals. Although the upper-level staff have embraced, in spirit, the philosophy and ethics of this type of total quality management collaboration, they resist most suggestions made by the lower-level staff about the plan, especially those that might strip the upper-level staff of some of their power and authority in the division. In particular, they discover from planning meetings that their notions about how to manage and run the division differ dramatically from those of the lower-level staff. Their solution is to continue soliciting the opinions of the lower-level staff during early meetings, but to ignore that type of input in later, private meetings when they work on their own—without outside input—to produce the final draft of the document. As a result of the upper-level staff's decision to give priority to preserving and building on their own authority and power in the division, the lower-level staff end up feeling betrayed when they discover that their early input has had minimal impact on the final draft of the plan. Their increased resentment toward the upper-level staff does not bode well for future relations between the two components of this division, which need to cooperate with each other regularly and effectively to resolve division problems and fulfill division goals.

As these cases suggest, unsuccessful cross-organizational communication can lead to both internal anxiety and tension and territorial battles between multiple organizations or organizational units. These cases also illustrate how social groups can suffer in a variety of ways from shaky or failed attempts to collaborate successfully with other social groups: they can suffer on a practical level, for example, from wasted time and economic loss; but, they can also suffer on a social level, for instance, from a shaken identity due to a tarnished image or reputation, greater insecurity about their present or potential power and authority, and increased doubts about their ability to preserve or build on goals they have worked hard to achieve. Without sufficient analytic tools for understanding more clearly how other social groups operate in terms of functions, goals, and constraints or how various groups prefer to work with each other, workplace professionals are likely to display insensitivity to their "outside collaborators," perhaps to the extent that they interact with them in a clumsy and alienating way, thereby increasing the risks that joint projects will suffer from delays, misunderstandings, painful negotiations, and other such problems.

RESEARCH TO DATE

To any technical communicator aware of the increasing frequency and importance of cross-boundary communication, it might seem odd, at least initially, that most research on this topic was conducted before the 1980s, and that, in general, scholars in a variety of fields have attended to this topic just peripherally in the past 15 years. So far, scholars, not in rhetoric and composition, but rather in organizational communication and related fields (such as organizational culture, intergroup relations/conflict, small group behavior, interpersonal communication, cross-cultural communication, organizational psychology, and sociology) have conducted most of the research on cross-boundary communication. Yet, even over 4 decades, most of these scholars have limited the scope of their investigations to identifying particular attributes that tend to characterize cross-boundary communication. For example, Hage (1974) explored the potential impact of physical distance between organizational subsystems; Klauss and Bass (1982) studied the degree of trust and similarity between professionals; Leblebici and Salancik (1982) examined the influence of environmental uncertainty, or the degree of stability and predictability of cultures; and Van de Ven and Walker (1984) investigated the degree of similarity between cultures, or "domain similarity." Although identifying these attributes is a helpful step, these scholars have not as yet developed a broad, intricate picture of the typical social and cognitive dynamics and relationships that characterize cross-boundary communication. A handful of these researchers have focused on rhetorical and social processes related to interactions across organizational units, but the scope of their examinations also has tended to be relatively restrictive: for example, Assael (1969) looked at different types of conflict in organizations; Boje and Whetten (1981) studied how status hierarchies emerge in interorganizational networks, as opposed to how they emerge in other social configurations; and Roloff (1987) explored how interactions across organizations can influence "boundary spanners," or those individuals representing their own cultures when interacting with those from other cultures.

Logically, one might assume that in the past 15 years, scholars specializing in both professional communication and rhetoric would have chosen to study cross-boundary communication quite closely, especially given the growing popularity of qualitative studies conducted in organizations, but just the opposite has been true. For the most part, perhaps because of the relative recency of qualitative studies conducted at worksites, most rhetoric researchers have deliberately focused on observing how professionals communicate within a single organization or organizational unit (see Selzer 1983; Paradis, Dobrin, and Miller 1985; Doheny-Farina 1986; Mirel 1989; Winsor 1989, 1993). With this approach, scholars have been able to describe single organizational cultures and to identify the unique communication patterns and relationships characterizing those cultures, but they have been unable to observe intensely or at close range how professionals also manage to communicate successfully across organizational boundaries to resolve shared problems or fulfill shared goals.

It is encouraging that at least a handful of rhetoric scholars have deliberately focused theoretical analyses or designed empirical investigations to consider what characterizes communication that crosses multiple worksites. Several of these rhetoricians have reinforced the profession's awareness that cross-boundary communication can have both highly positive[1] and highly negative outcomes. For example, Harrison (1987) speculates that this type of communication can lead to more creativity in organizations; to Debs (1989), it can lead to a healthy diversity of viewpoints; to Sullivan (1991), it can assist professionals in becoming agents of change; and to Burnett (1991), it can open opportunities for professionals to engage in substantive, positive types of conflict. On the other hand, Mathes (1989) notes that technical communicators engaged in this type of communication can confront severe resistance to their needs or requests. In addition, as Sullivan (1991) suggests, technical communicators can be seen as "outsiders" by members of all groups involved in cross-boundary communication, a perspective that can be a problem because technical communicators are often responsible for "capturing all the viewpoints" (Sullivan 1991, p. 491) or for developing "a sense of shared responsibility" (Debs 1989, p. 40) when working on documentation.

Rhetoricians who have conducted qualitative studies have demonstrated that groups that need to collaborate for just a single time need to "gel quickly" (Sullivan 1991, p. 486) and "forge a set of common (group) goals" (Sullivan, 1991, p. 489), and that different organizational units working together either once or multiple times need to establish a common task representation (Debs 1989; Spilka 1990; Sullivan 1991). Although I previously found that involving readers early in a partnership venture can improve chances for a document to be well received later on (Spilka 1990), Karis and Doheny-Farina (1991) observed just the opposite, that involving readers early in the process of this type of communication can lead to delays and destructive conflict.[2]

In recent research reports, some rhetoricians have described cases involving cross-boundary communication (see, for example, Kleimann 1993; Dautermann 1993; Smart 1993; and Cross 1993), but these and other rhetoric scholars have not yet focused research questions, designs, and analyses specifically on the issue of how professionals communicate across organizational boundaries. As a result, the rhetorical perspective remains inadequate of the complex concerns and strategies professionals need to draw on as they attempt to negotiate successfully across organizational boundaries.

Study Site and Methodology

In this longitudinal qualitative study, conducted from January 1992 to January 1994, I was interested in concerns professionals might have when they communicate across organizational boundaries, as well as which social and rhetorical strategies, if any, they might draw on to negotiate cross-boundary communication effectively. More specifically, I observed how professionals in the upper-level component of one division of a state government department interacted with lower-level professionals in the same division, with representatives of other divisions of the same department, and with a wide variety of professionals from other local, state, and federal agencies to move closer to fulfilling both shared and internal goals.

The organizational unit I observed most closely in this study is the upper-level component of a state government division that I am calling the Soil and Water Division (SWD) (see Figure 1). The SWD primarily facilitated successful partnerships between the state's 92 counties (also called districts) and various state and federal government agencies and organizations to obtain the shared goal of preserving natural resources throughout the state. The SWD, which was concerned with conserving state soil and water resources, was situated within a larger department of natural resources and was a relatively new (it originated in 1987) and small one within that department. Within the SWD, at least three organizational groups could be identified on the basis of their primary functions:

- The upper-level managers—and their secretarial, technical, and engineering assistants—who initiated, coordinated, or facilitated SWD programs and partnerships from various locations (most were housed in a suite of offices in a state capital government building, but some were situated in government buildings in the five conservation areas of the state)
- Middle-level urban conservation and educational specialists situated in the five conservation areas of the state who oversaw programs and partnerships in those areas

FIGURE 1 Cross-Boundary Communications between SWD Upper-Level Professional and Other Organizational Units

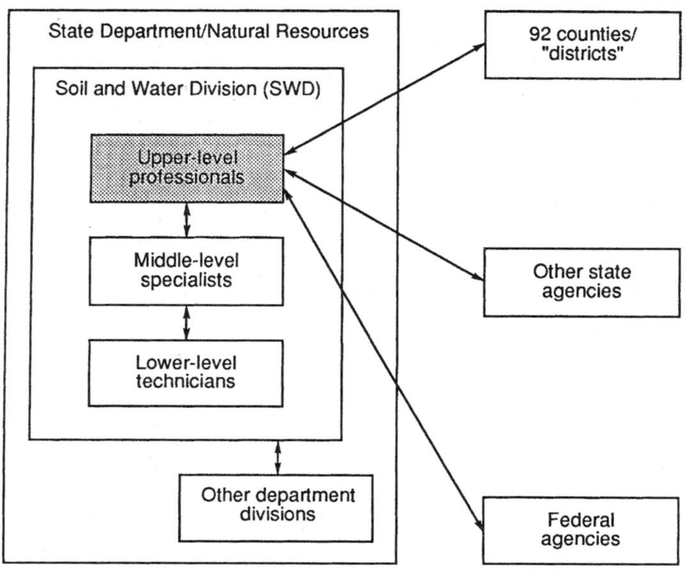

- Lower-level erosion control technicians who worked at the 92 district sites alongside members of other federal and state agencies to ensure successful implementation of primarily agricultural programs and partnerships in those counties

In this study, I observed two rhetorical situations involving the evolution of major documents instrumental in promoting SWD goals. As illustrated in the two case studies described above, in the first rhetorical situation, these professionals initiated and sustained a partnership between SWD and other government, private, and public agencies to produce a memorandum of agreement that would define state- and district-level roles and responsibilities in a statewide urban conservation program. In the second rhetorical situation, the upper-level professionals formed a partnership with both lower-level staff of SWD and representatives of outside agencies to produce a long-range (5-year) plan that would define SWD goals and activities to be given priority in the immediate future. In both situations, my observations focused primarily on the experiences of those upper-level professionals (including the SWD director, five program directors, and the SWD information specialist) responsible for most of the writing and decision making concerned with those documents.

The study consisted of three stages:

- Conducting preliminary observations to learn about SWD culture and writing activities (January 1992 to September 1992)
- Collecting data about interactions between professionals in SWD's upper-level component and others outside that upper-level component who were involved in the two rhetorical situations studied (October 1992 to October 1993)
- Collecting retrospective data about social and rhetorical strategies used by the professionals in SWD's upper-level component to overcome problems in those select situations (November 1993 to January 1994)

To obtain research data, I collected documents produced before, during, and after those rhetorical situations; observed meetings and various other formal and informal social interactions between those involved in the rhetorical situations; conducted preliminary and ongoing open-ended and retrospective-structured interviews about social and rhetorical strategies used to cope with problems resulting from cross-boundary communication; and conducted discourse-based interviews about writing strategies and their relationship to organizational goals. During an early phase of the study, in the summer of 1992, a research assistant also conducted observations and collected data.

FINDINGS

From this study, I discovered that, even under favorable circumstances, any alliance that crosses organizational boundaries can become an uneasy social and rhetorical struggle resulting in some key benefits, but also in numerous internal risks and sacrifices. I also learned that professionals who engage in cross-boundary communication can find the experience mysterious and confusing, especially if they lack knowledge of how to ease tensions and overcome differences between organizational units and simultaneously attend to the sometimes contrastive needs and goals of their own organizational unit. The following sections summarize some benefits and problems that can characterize cross-boundary communication and identify some social and rhetorical strategies used by professionals in the study, who attempted to negotiate cross-boundary communication as successfully as possible.

What Must Be in Place for Cross-Boundary Communication to Work Well?

This study confirms previous research findings (see, for example, Klauss and Bass 1982; Van de Ven and Walker 1984) that, for one organizational unit to communicate successfully with another, the units must be similar in some ways. For example, the units need some similarity in philosophy, goals, or functions; otherwise, it becomes especially difficult for professionals in them to understand, appreciate, and respect one another's needs and to overcome incompatibilities or resolve problems that can serve as potential barriers to smooth and profitable communication. For example, when SWD initiated a collaborative venture with a federal agency, the SWD liaison was confident that similarities between the two agencies would prevail over obvious differences between them. Although the two agencies differed significantly in their reasons for joining the partnership (the state agency primarily wanted to add to its own legitimacy and authority, whereas the federal agency primarily wanted to fulfill a legal mandate), they shared a major goal (establishing a statewide urban conservation program) and agreed that collaborating smoothly with each other was a key ingredient for successfully fulfilling that goal. As one SWD professional put it, SWD and the federal agency "are going to the same end, and just using different means. . . . We're on the same bus, just on different seats."

On the other hand, the study also suggests that organizational units must be dissimilar in some ways if professionals in them are to recognize what would be gained in terms of unique resources or capabilities from working with each other. For instance, at the start of cross-organizational collaborations, professionals in this study typically asked a key question: What can the other units bring to the collaboration that we lack or need? In one case, while attempting to establish a collaborative urban conservation program, the SWD recognized that it required the legal authority of a federal agency. In turn, the federal agency recognized that SWD's vast network of (and close, positive ties with) districts throughout the state could become an indispensable means of gaining statewide cooperation for its federal mandate.

What Are Some Benefits of Cross-Boundary Communication?

The upper-level professionals in SWD benefited from communicating closely with other organizational units in two distinct ways: by supplementing their own arsenal of resources and by determining new ways to enhance their own goals of self-preservation and growth. The SWD professionals profited from access to relatively practical resources, such as an expanded network of personnel that became available from other organizational units to assist in various shared activities or partnerships, but perhaps they benefitted the most from both the social and technical knowledge that "outsiders" and "outside documents" could bring to those ventures. Often, these professionals sought the social and political advice of officials high in the hierarchy of other partnership organizations, and, just as often, they sought the technical (and experiential) advice of lower-level staff from their own division and others. The professionals also routinely consulted written sources from other states for guidance in how to design, write, or revise their own documents.

However, when deciding whether to work with other organizational units, these professionals also had larger social goals in mind beyond supplementing their own resources. For example, a key goal for them was self-preservation, because their own division was relatively new, barely tested in terms of what it could accomplish, and eager to survive (especially in light of rough economic times) in the sometimes fierce competition for resources and prestige between their division and the other, more established divisions of this state government department. They realized that, to preserve what they had worked so hard to achieve, they would need to borrow from the resources of other organizational units if they hoped, at a bare minimum, to fulfill their own basic mission; they also hoped to maintain the respect that they had earned up to that point from various outside organizational units.

Because the SWD professionals wanted their own organizational unit not only to survive, but also to continue growing, they actively initiated partnerships with other organizational units to enhance their positive image and visibility. By associating themselves with other organizational units widely known and respected for their power and prestige, these upper-level professionals felt they could enhance their own status, power, and authority.

What Are Potential Problems with Cross-Boundary Communication?

Previous scholarship has identified a number of problems associated with cross-boundary communication, such as inefficiency and the hazards (e.g., bias and distortion) of transferring information across organizational units (Tushman 1977). As Van de Ven and Walker (1984) point out, these types of problems can be so formidable that many organizational units prefer to avoid becoming involved in interorganizational relationships "unless they are compelled to do so" (p. 601).

In this study, I identified one overriding difficulty associated with forming partnerships that cross organizational boundaries: the professionals routinely experienced tension when attempting to fulfill both internal goals of their own organizational unit and various external goals of the partnership (or of select organizational units involved in the partnership) that conflicted or were incompatible with those internal goals. Adams (1976), who has also recognized this tension, speculates that it results from the need to be sensitive "to two sets of needs, norms, and values," those of one's own organization and those of other organization(s) involved in the collaboration (p. 1179).

The upper-level professionals of SWD encountered the following two tensions when seeking to accomplish their own internal goals and various external goals of their partnership ventures.

Maintaining Independence and Authority in Decision Making versus Confronting the Possibility of Losing Some Power when Relating with Other Partnership Units. The upper-level professionals in the SWD continuously worried that the process of working with "outsiders" from other organizational units would strip them of some of their independence and authority in decision making. They were concerned that working closely with "outsiders" might result in "turf battles," in which some units would compete for shared resources or would attempt to assume greater power and authority than other units. For example, at a staff meeting, the SWD director, referring to another state agency involved in a partnership venture, said, "I don't know why we're getting so irritable with each other; we're biting each other." Another SWD professional replied, "It's survival and who can steal from who." The SWD professionals seemed especially concerned that other units would assume "too much" power, especially if their own unit assumed a reactive instead of a proactive role in partnership ventures. To the SWD professionals, being proactive in cross-boundary communication was a way either to assume control over other units or to prevent other units from assuming control over them. For example, in one verbal exchange, one SWD professional asked, "Why should we be the one to establish the committee?" Another SWD professional replied, "So we can be in control." In another typical exchange, the SWD director noted in a staff meeting that SWD would be "run by the feds" unless they initiated a new program with a federal agency: "To be honest," he added, "I'm getting a little disgusted marching to someone else's drumbeat."

At the same time, the SWD upper-level professionals were hesitant to make any decisions or take any actions that might encroach on others' "territory." For example, they were eager to fulfill an internal goal of ensuring consistency in policy making across the five conservation areas of the state, but simultaneously, they needed to acknowledge that those areas would resist any movement toward statewide conformity, because they had an incompatible goal of emphasizing their own particular strengths.

In some cases, tension can arise when an organizational unit gives more priority to one internal goal than to another, even when the second goal is one shared with "outsiders" in a partnership venture. In this study, for example, a key internal goal of the SWD upper-level professionals was to become indispensable in providing guidance and technical resources to the 92 districts around the state. However, an incompatible second internal goal of theirs, one also shared with most other units in several partnerships to which they belonged, was to increase the districts' own power and individuality and to empower the districts to lead their own political battles. Although some districts had no desire to become further empowered, most wanted increased autonomy in decision making and tended to resent it when the upper-level professionals and others "interfered" with their operations and plans. Therefore, the first goal of becoming indispensable to districts was known at SWD as a "bathroom goal," one that would remain unwritten and (they hoped) unconveyed and unknown to the districts.

Incompatible goals like these seemed to be especially stressful for the upper-level professionals, who repeatedly debated whether they would be willing to give less priority to their first internal goal (to become indispensable to others) and more priority to the second goal, which they shared with "outsiders" (to empower others).

Preserving and Building on a Unit's Own Sense of Identity, while Also Adapting to Continuous Social (and Therefore Identity) Changes Brought on by Partnership Ventures. When the SWD upper-level professionals worked closely with other organizational units, they felt that the integrity of their own unit's identity was almost constantly in flux, in question, and at risk. At the same time that they were attempting deliberately and assertively to enhance their unit's image, increase its visibility and status, and both preserve and build on its powers, they were discovering that the process of communicating regularly with other organizational units brought with it continuous challenges to these goals. Because they hoped to remain strong members of the partnership, they felt enormous pressure to repeatedly reexamine the social roles and responsibilities characterizing their unit and SWD as a whole. During the 2 years of this study, in both informal conversations and formal meetings, the upper-level professionals continually attempted to reach a consensus among themselves about their division's roles and responsibilities and their own roles and responsibilities within the division. For example, they would often ask: What are we supposed to be doing? What are we allowed to do? Should we advise or directly influence other organizational units? How broad or narrow should we be in our roles? How big do we want to become? How small are we willing to become, if necessary? They would also debate the roles and responsibilities of other organizational units in partnership ventures. They would ask: Who's in charge? What do the other units do, and what do they want to do? They seemed especially concerned about possible overlap between SWD functions and those of other organizational units. For example, one SWD professional asked during a staff meeting: "Why are the programs identical for different sources of funding? Why should new programs do what the SWD is doing already? My concern is, will someone lose power?"

In addition, they often talked about confusion that they noticed throughout both their own division and other units belonging to their partnership ventures about who had, wanted to have, or should have authority in any given situation. For example, they would ask, repeatedly: Which organizational unit should do what in this situation? Should or can those roles and responsibilities change given that times and circumstances have changed, and if so, how might we facilitate those changes? They also wondered whether their division would even survive in partnerships with competitive government agencies. They would ask: Should we do more to justify our existence and demonstrate to others more assertively that we are valuable members of the partnership ventures and are worth supporting? How much can we contribute to partnership ventures? How much can we handle, given our resources? How can we survive without giving some goals and activities priority over others? Which goals and activities should be given priority?

Complicating this cross-boundary communication was the constantly changing nature of the social parameters of the partnerships and of select units within the partnerships. In all partnership units, personnel tended to turnover rapidly, a situation that led to new representatives taking part in partnerships at key junctures of joint projects. Adding to the confusion about who or what comprised various social groupings was an ongoing debate at the federal and state levels about whether to reconfigure geographical boundaries, and, if so, how these changes would or should affect other social configurations at various levels of government. For example, government officials were debating whether to change area boundaries in the state to larger, more amorphous watershed boundaries and whether to change county (district) boundaries to cross-district or cross-state (i.e., regional) boundaries. They worried that if the current area or district boundaries became untenable as a result of new geographical configurations, various federal and state agencies and local districts would need to change their social compositions. For example, perhaps some agencies or districts would need to merge to cover a wider geographical area, or perhaps some would need to vanish entirely.

Because the nature, composition, and orientation of the partnership coalitions and individual organizational units within those coalitions tended to be in continuous flux, the upper-level professionals found it difficult to define and acculturate to the social configurations and social agendas of these coalitions. When learning (or contributing to) the unique cultural features of each new social group, these professionals often needed to assume new social roles and responsibilities that, at times, radically differed from those they had held within their own organizational unit. A group leader in one's own unit, for instance, might need to become a follower in a partnership venture. In addition, they sometimes found it quite challenging to negotiate smoothly with representatives from other units whose philosophies, values, and goals differed radically from their own. For example, the SWD upper-level professionals, who saw themselves primarily as advisors encouraging volunteer cooperation, often needed to work closely with representatives from another unit, who saw themselves primarily as regulators enforcing the law. These two groups tended to delay progress in joint ventures while trying to learn about, understand, and accept each other's social roles, goals, and agendas.

What Social and Rhetorical Strategies Can Be Useful for This Type of Rhetoric?

This study suggests that the friction associated with attempting to fulfill conflicting or incompatible goals can be stressful, both temporarily and in the long term, but can also lead to healthy internal debates about which social and rhetorical changes or sacrifices, if any, the professionals are willing to make to ensure that their own organizational units succeed along with the partnerships. Although the upper-level professionals often were confused, worried, and pessimistic about what might happen to their own unit as a result of participating in partnership ventures, these professionals also recognized that maintaining their membership in these partnerships was necessary to ensure a strong, viable future for their own unit and division.

As a liaison between the SWD and other state agencies put it, "People need to learn how to deal on other people's turf." In this study, the SWD professionals attempted to do so by inventing (and using regularly) an array of social and rhetorical strategies that helped them cope adequately with the tensions and difficulties produced by partnership ventures between organizational units.

Social Strategies. The upper-level professionals observed in this study relied on the following social strategies for coping effectively with the difficulties of communicating with other organizational units:

- *Consider or involve other organizational units in decision making.* The professionals found that it was politically astute to avoid considering just their own internal goals during decision making or making decisions entirely on their own. Instead, they routinely (1) considered the needs and goals of other organizational units during decision making and (2) involved other organizational units throughout decision making or deliberately sought their input before finalizing any decisions made on their own.
- *Attempt to fulfill all goals, regardless of their conflictive nature.* The professionals never considered abandoning a goal simply because it conflicted with another goal; instead, they tried to fulfill all goals as much as was possible under the circumstances.
- *Adapt to the reality that it is often impossible to fulfill conflicting or incompatible goals equally well – acknowledge that external goals of partnerships might need to take precedence over internal goals.*
- *Adapt to the reality that some internal goals can be counterproductive.* The professionals needed to abandon some attempts at achieving consistency throughout the five conservation areas of the state to ensure that the unique needs, orientations, and circumstances of each area would be considered and respected during decision making.
- *Work deliberately and without hesitation to protect the interests of other organizational units participating in partnership ventures.* Although the upper-level professionals tended to complain about other organizational units in private meetings and conversations, they consistently defended those units in response

to public criticism and were careful to avoid embarrassing their partners in any public forum. Demonstrating public loyalty to partners was a way to build up good relations between units. Similarly, protecting the interests of other units was a way to protect their own interests and those of the partnerships. One SWD professional said about defending a federal agency in public meetings, "it couldn't hurt to help them out." In an SWD staff meeting, the director admitted that "for political reasons, I don't want to embarrass [the federal agency]."

- *Gather as much knowledge as possible about the rhetorical situation before making final decisions.* The professionals were aware that "knowledge equals power." Before participating actively and vocally in partnership ventures, they routinely researched how other states handled similar situations, as well as the history, goals, and political orientation of other organizational units, to impress the other units and to argue their own positions as forcefully as possible.
- *Delay action until sufficient knowledge about the problem had been collected.* The professionals attempted to know for certain that a problem did exist and was not hearsay before taking action on that problem. This caution helped avoid embarrassment and protect their image in partnerships.
- *Discuss frequently the need to protect the integrity and power of individual units in the partnership.* As a means of self-preservation, the professionals often brought up, in both private and public discussions, the need to prevent too much overlap between units in terms of social roles and responsibilities, along with the possibility that any one unit would usurp the power of any other units. Their concern was to avoid dissolution of their own unit and of the partnerships.
- *Take a proactive versus a reactive role whenever possible.* Although the professionals suffered somewhat from too little time and too few resources, they often initiated new projects in partnerships and assumed leadership roles in those projects. One aim of this strategy was to establish and build an image of power, although perhaps the primary aim was to exercise power to the fullest extent possible, especially when dealing with competitive partners.
- *Participate in partnerships as much as possible, becoming a highly visible partner and volunteering for leadership roles.* The professionals felt that it was important to attend all meetings involving partnership concerns and to participate in partnership activities as much as possible. In their eagerness to be considered full, influential partners with considerable clout and influence, they also volunteered often for leadership responsibilities in partnership ventures.
- *Establish new social parameters in terms of which organizational units would have authority in which circumstances in any given partnership.* The upper-level professionals not only worked hard among themselves to redefine their own social roles and responsibilities in each new partnership (or whenever each partnership underwent social changes), but they also initiated similar discussions with other organizational units in an attempt to reach a consensus about which units would have the ultimate authority in particular types of partnership decisions or activities.
- *Educate other organizational units often about continuing or revised social parameters.* The upper-level professionals considered it a routine daily task to field questions (mostly in phone calls, but also at meetings) about the social roles

and responsibilities of their own division. These questions would come regularly from other units within their own division, as well as those units external to their division.

- *Deliberately blur social distinctions between units in some circumstances.* To bolster unity between units in a partnership, the professionals sometimes decided to de-emphasize or ignore social distinctions between the units. For example, they deemed it important, at times, to identify similarities between their own division and select other units in the partnership to demonstrate solidarity and strength (e.g., power) of those units in the partnership.

Rhetorical Strategies. The SWD upper-level professionals also relied on rhetorical strategies for coping effectively with the difficulties of communicating with other organizational units. To address their concerns about SWD's *image, self-preservation, and survival,* they used the following strategies when producing documents aimed at a multiple audience that included partnership members:

- *To preserve a unit's positive image, check that the content of unit documents is accurate and detailed.* When working on their own documents or revising documents created by other members of the partnership, the professionals tried to avoid embarrassment and to impress other members of the partnership. To obtain these goals, they paid special attention to the accuracy of details and to any phrases and descriptions (i.e., of the division's responsibilities) that needed to reflect well on the division. They also decided that it would be better "to list everything under the sun" and be "foolproof," than to be simple but incomplete in coverage to avoid embarrassing the division.
- *To ensure a unit's continued visibility in a partnership, check that names are positioned advantageously.* The SWD professionals were concerned about the visibility of their division's name on written and video products. They paid special attention to any document features giving high status to some units of the partnership and low status to other units. For example, they were elated to see SWD's name listed at the top of a section in a telephone directory, but dismayed when the name was omitted from the list of partnership units at the end of a promotional video.
- *To demonstrate and justify the value of a unit's services, create a written reporting system.* The professionals were so concerned about their survival and about whether partnership alliances would strip them, eventually, of their authority and power, that they initiated a reporting system in which low- and middle-level staff members would provide details about their daily and monthly accomplishments. This system gave rise to new written documents, including an evaluation checklist, to enable staff members to record and, therefore, justify the work they accomplished for the division. As another protective measure, the professionals also checked carefully to see whether the date was indicated on each document draft as a way to justify how they were thinking at that juncture of the composing process and to ensure that readers would know they were looking at an interim draft (with provisional information) and not at a final draft (with final decisions and policies).

- *Repeatedly clarify a unit's functions, roles, and responsibilities.* As a daily responsibility, the upper-level professionals fielded questions concerning SWD functions, roles, and responsibilities both from others in the SWD and from representatives of other organizations. Therefore, they decided to provide similar explanations in various types of documents, such as brochures and newsletters, for the same diverse group of questioners. To help readers understand their explanations, the professionals used repetition of key terms and concepts.

To address their concerns about *the maintenance and growth of their unit's or their division's power and authority*, the professionals used the following rhetorical strategies when producing documents aimed at least partially at a partnership audience:

- *To clarify a unit's roles and its relationships with other units, use organizational charts and other explanatory documents.* During the study, the upper-level professionals found the visual mapping of their organizational chart especially useful as an argumentative tool to strengthen their proposal (to higher-level department managers) to add more administrators to their staff.
- *To assert a unit's authority, change style and word choice late in the documentation process.* The upper-level staff deliberately waited until late drafts of a long-range plan to alter specific phrases and words previously written by lower-level staff to make them more generic or to omit them entirely. By revising or omitting the written contributions of lower-level staff on earlier drafts, the upper-level staff attempted to silence the voices of those "outsiders," while at the same time asserting (and protecting) their own authority in the SWD. This strategy had negative repercussions in the study: although it protected the interests of upper-level staff, it also alienated and frustrated the lower-level staff who had wanted to participate in a "true" total quality management system of documentation.
- *When preparing unit documents, select content cautiously and time carefully the delivery of information to an audience.* The upper-level professionals were cautious about writing about problems that had not yet been fully documented. Instead, they routinely delayed documents until they knew for certain that a problem existed. Their careful timing of documents and their deliberate omission or inclusion of particular facts (depending on their controversial nature) were strategies aimed at manipulating how quickly their audience would become educated about a problem and how much they would learn about it. For these writers, delays in documentation often had a positive, self-serving impact that increased their power and authority in sensitive situations related to a partnership.
- *Express gratitude to other members of the partnership generously, but check that the unit's important role in a joint venture is indicated clearly.* The upper-level professionals routinely acknowledged the assistance of other partnership members in documents such as brochures, newsletters, and pamphlets as a way of demonstrating solidarity and unity. However, at the same time, they usually located information about the SWD in prominent locations on these documents and emphasized SWD's leadership role in producing the documents, which not only increased their own visibility but also conveyed the sense that

the SWD was assuming a proactive, and not a reactive, role in the partnership endeavors.

- *Gather as much knowledge as possible from documents produced in other states and regions and use that information in a unit's documents.* The upper-level professionals felt strongly that they gained prestige and credibility by citing sources produced in other states or including sections of those sources in SWD documents. They reasoned that, because these other states had developed more experience in particular conservation programs, their expertise and advice assumed special meaning for SWD's readership.

Implications for the Future

This study involved observations of just one relatively new organizational unit actively seeking to use its authority and power as fully as possible to maximize its opportunities to grow and prosper in competitive government partnerships. The social and rhetorical behavior of the SWD upper-level professionals might differ radically from that of professionals in other types of organizational units situated in other occupational arenas, such as corporations and private agencies. However, the study suggests the following strategies for professionals who face the challenges of cross-boundary communication:

1. They might consider trying some of the social and rhetorical strategies outlined in this article.
2. Early in the composing process, they could benefit from expanding their analysis of their external audience of any documents aimed at a partnership readership. For example, professionals might want to analyze how their counterparts in other organizational units typically communicate in partnership ventures or how they react to problems or obstacles during joint projects. They might also analyze their counterparts' internal and external goals, as well as the general functions and orientations of their organizational units: Do their units primarily seek volunteer cooperation, or do they primarily enforce laws? Are their units mostly interested in salvaging the resources they have gathered so far, or are they eager to add to their power and authority? Asking these types of questions about their partnership audience might help professionals in planning a sensitive, tactful strategy for simultaneously communicating with their counterparts effectively to help them fulfill their goals while also fulfilling their own internal goals.
3. Professionals might give more consideration to the ethics of their social and rhetorical behavior in this type of rhetoric. They might benefit from asking: What is the positive but also the negative impact of our communication strategies on other organizational units? Can we minimize tension between the units or the potential harm a partnership might cause to other units? Given that we are interested primarily in fulfilling our own goals, can we still be fair and equitable when communicating with other members of a partnership, regardless of any negative attitudes or behavior they might exhibit?
4. Professionals need to recognize that tension can be a healthy springboard to more careful thought and debate about how best to relate to "outsiders" during the evolution of documents in partnership ventures. With more extensive

consideration of the complexities involved with this type of rhetoric, professionals might discover new opportunities to strengthen bonds between themselves and other organizational units and to promote more profitable future partnerships with those units.

For educators of professional communicators, this study suggests that their student writers might encounter more complex rhetorical situations than most educators focus on in their classroom assignments and exercises. In many, if not most, professional writing courses, students gain practice in analyzing just one organizational culture and in confining their communication efforts to that one culture. Educators could make a stronger effort to diversify and expand the types of rhetorical situations their students encounter in courses, particularly in terms of providing them with the experience of communicating with a varied, complex internal and external audience with different, possibly conflicting, goals. Students might encounter this type of complex audience in internships, but they also could encounter it in courses requiring them to produce documentation for actual clients, reviewers, and multiple audience segments situated in a variety of on- and off-campus settings.

For professional writing scholars, this study calls for more extensive, more focused explorations of the complexities of the type of communication that occurs within the broad universe of partnerships comprised of multiple organizational units that might differ radically from each other in philosophy, orientation, attitude, and behavior. Theorists must depart from the prevalent assumption that social configurations in the workplace are inflexible and static and acknowledge the amorphous, ever-changing nature of the populations and parameters of those social configurations. They would also benefit from seeking new ways to define and discuss "discourse communities," "social contexts," "organizations," "organizational units," and "organizational cultures." Which term or terms would be most effective in describing the complex social configurations that form, change, and dissolve continuously in partnership coalitions? Would theorists prefer to call these configurations "groups," "cultures," "units," "contexts," "communities," or some other term? What might be the best way to examine social and rhetorical behavior both within and across these social configurations?

This study also suggests the need for more research focusing on rhetoric across multiple organizational units, especially in corporate and computer networks. A larger, collaborative research project would be useful in examining more fully the impact of particular social and rhetorical strategies for cross-organizational communication on individual units of the partnership and on the partnership as a whole. For example, how do other organizational units respond to document choices and changes made by other units in a partnership, and why? Researchers should compare how organizational units might approach this type of rhetoric differently depending on their longevity, history, clout, status, and intent in joining the partnership venture (are they mostly eager to salvage resources already accumulated or to accumulate more power and authority from the partnership venture?) They should also study the ethics of organizational units that give more priority to internal goals than to shared goals in a partnership, especially if doing so is at all harmful to other organizational units. By examining the complexities of this type of rhetoric, in particular, the potential impact of social agendas, changes in social parameters, and ethical considerations on rhetorical choices in partnership ventures, scholars can add immeasurably to our understanding of the broad social universe of workplace writing.

NOTES

1. Some scholars in organizational studies have also discovered that professionals have quite a bit to gain from successful cross-boundary communication. As Van de Ven and Walker (1984) point out, organizational units typically initiate such mergers to draw on the resources of other organizations in ways that assist them in fulfilling highly valued goals. For example, one organizational unit might have personnel with experience or expertise that another unit lacks but needs to succeed in a project. Tushman (1977) argues that smooth relations between organizational units are also a requirement for successful innovation. In Adams's view (1976), the ability to interact smoothly with the environment outside one's own organization is critical to an organization's ability to prosper, but also to survive in an increasingly competitive world. For instance, by establishing smooth working relations with "outsiders," organizational units can establish long-term relationships that are economically and socially protective, in both the short and the long run.

2. Doheny-Farina (1992) also reported on a study of technology transfer that involved professionals communicating across organizational boundaries; however, since his research questions focused on other concerns, findings from this study do not address the issue of how to negotiate this type of rhetoric successfully.

REFERENCES

Adams, J. S. 1976. "The structure and dynamics of behavior in organizational boundary roles." In *Handbook of industrial and organizational psychology*. M. D. Dunnette, ed., pp. 1175–1199. Chicago, IL: Rand McNally.

Assael, Henry. 1969. "Constructive role of interorganizational conflict." *Administrative Science Quarterly* 14: 573–581.

Boje, David M., and D. A. Whetten. 1981. "Effects of organizational strategies and contextual constraints on centrality and attributions of influence in interorganizational networks." *Administrative Science Quarterly* 26: 378–395.

Burnett, Rebecca E. 1991. "Substantive conflict in a cooperative context: A way to improve the collaborative planning of workplace documents." *Technical Communication* 38: 532–539.

Cross, Geoffrey. 1993. "The interrelation of genre, context, and process in the collaborative writing of two corporate documents," In *Writing in the workplace: New research perspectives*. R. Spilka, ed., pp. 141–152. Carbondale, IL: Southern Illinois University Press.

Dautermann, Jennie. 1993. "Negotiating meaning in a hospital discourse community." In *Writing in the workplace: New research perspectives*. R. Spilka, ed., pp. 98–110. Carbondale, IL: Southern Illinois University Press.

Debs, Mary Beth. 1989. "Collaborative writing in industry," In *Technical writing: Theory and practice*. B. E. Fearing and W. K. Sparrow, eds., pp. 33–42. New York, NY: Modern Language Association.

Doheny-Farina, Stephen. 1986. "Writing in an emerging organization: An ethnographic study." *Written Communication* 3, no. 2: 158–185.

———. 1992. *Rhetoric, innovation, technology: Case studies of technical communication in technology transfers*. Cambridge, MA: MIT Press.

Hage, J. 1974. *Communication and organizational control: Cybernetics in health and welfare settings*. New York, NY: Wiley.

Harrison, Teresa. 1987. "Frameworks for the study of writing in organizational contexts." *Written Communication* 4: 3–23.

Karis, William, and S. Doheny-Farina. 1991. "Collaboration with readers: Empower them and take the consequences." *Technical Communication* 38: 513–19.

Klauss, R., and B. M. Bass. 1982. *Interpersonal communication in organizations*. New York, NY: Academic Press.

Kleimann, Susan. 1993. "The reciprocal relationship of workplace culture and review." In *Writing in the workplace: New research perspectives*. R. Spilka, ed., pp. 56–70. Carbondale, IL: Southern Illinois University Press.

Leblebici, Huseyin, and G. R. Salancik. 1982. "Stability in interorganizational exchanges: Rulemaking processes of the Chicago Board of Trade." *Administrative Science Quarterly* 27: 227–242.

Mathes, J. C. 1989. "Written communication: The industrial context." In *Worlds of writing*. C. B. Matalene, ed., pp. 222–246. New York, NY: Random House.

Mirel, Barbara. 1989. "The politics of usability: The organizational functions of an in-house manual." In *Effective documentation: What we have learned from research*. S. Doheny-Farina, ed., pp. 277–297. Cambridge, MA: MIT Press.

Oslen, Leslie A. 1993. "Research on discourse communities: An overview." In *Writing in the workplace: New research perspectives*. R. Spilka, ed., pp. 181–194. Carbondale, IL: Southern Illinois University Press.

Paradis, J., D. Dobrin, and R. Miller. 1985. "Writing at Exxon ITD: Notes on the writing environment of an R&D organization." In *Writing in nonacademic settings*. L. Odell and D. Goswami, eds., pp. 281–307. New York, NY: Guilford Press.

Roloff, Michael E. 1987. "Communication and conflict." In *Handbook of communication science*. C. R. Berger and S. H. Chaffee, eds., pp. 484–534. Newbury Park, CA: Sage Publications.

Selzer, Jack. 1983. "The composing processes of an engineer." *College Composition and Communication* 34: 178–187.

Smart, Graham. 1993. "Genre as community invention: A central bank's response to its executives' expectations as readers." In *Writing in the workplace: New research perspectives*. R. Spilka, ed., pp. 124–140. Carbondale, IL: Southern Illinois University Press.

Spilka, Rachel. 1990. "Orality and literacy in the workplace: Process- and text-based strategies for multiple audience adaptation." *Journal of Business and Technical Communication* 4: 44–67.

Sullivan, Patricia. 1991. Collaboration between organizations: Contributions outsiders can make to negotiation and cooperation during composition." *Technical Communication* 38: 485–92.

Tushman, Michael. 1977. "Special boundary roles in the innovation process." *Administrative Science Quarterly* 22: 587–603.

Van de Ven, Andrew, and G. Walker. 1984. "The dynamics of interorganizational coordination." *Administrative Science Quarterly* 29: 598–621.

Winsor, Dorothy A. 1989. "An engineer's writing and the corporate construction of knowledge." *Written Communication* 6: 270–285.

———. 1993. "Owning corporate texts." *Journal of Business and Technical Communication* 7, no. 2; 179–195.

ADDITIONAL READINGS

Anson, Chris M., and Lee L. Forsberg. "Moving Beyond the Academic Community: Transitional Stages in Professional Writing." *Written Communication* 7, no. 2 (1990): 200–31.

Artemeva, Natasha, Susan Logie, and Jennie St-Martin. "From Page to Stage: How Theories of Genre and Situated Learning Help Introduce Engineering Students to Discipline-Specific Communication." *Technical Communication Quarterly* 8, no. 3 (1999): 301–18.

Aschauer, Ann Brady. "Tinkering with Technological Skill: An Examination of the Gendered Uses of Technology." *Computers and Composition* 16 (1999): 7–23.

Baker (Graham), Margaret Ann, and Carol David. "The Rhetoric of Power: Political Issues in Management Writing." *Technical Communication Quarterly* 3, no. 2 (1994): 165–78.

Beaufort, Anne. "Learning the Trade: A Social Apprenticeship Model for Gaining Writing Expertise." *Written Communication* 17, no. 2 (2000): 185–223.

Berkenkotter, Carol, Thomas N. Huckin, and John Ackerman. "Social Context and Socially Constructed Texts: The Initiation of a Graduate Student into a Writing Research Community." In *Textual Dynamics of the Professions: Historical and Contemporary Studies of Writing in Professional Communities*, edited by Charles Bazerman and James Paradis, 191–215. Madison: U of Wisconsin P, 1991.

Blakeslee, Ann M. "Activity, Context, Interaction, and Authority: Learning to Write Scientific Papers in Situ." *Journal of Business and Technical Communication* 11, no. 2 (1997): 125-69.

Bosley, Deborah S. "Collaborative Partnerships: Academia and Industry Working Together." *Technical Communication* 42, no. 4 (1995): 611–19.

Burnett, Rebecca E. "Conflict in Collaborative Decision-Making." In *Professional Communication: The Social Perspective*, edited by Nancy R. Blyler and Charlotte Thralls, 144-62. Newbury Park, CA: Sage, 1993.

Couture, Barbara, and Jone Rymer. "Situational Exigence: Composing Processes on the Job by Writer's Role and Task Value." In *Writing in the Workplace: New Research Perspectives*, edited by Rachel Spilka, 4–20. Carbondale and Edwardsville, IL: Southern Illinois University Press, 1993.

Cross, Geoffrey A. "A Bakhtinian Exploration of Factors Affecting the Collaborative Writing of an Executive Letter of an Annual Report." *Research in the Teaching of English* 24, no. 2 (1990): 173–203.

Dautermann, Jennie. "Negotiating Meaning in a Hospital Discourse Community." In *Writing in the Workplace: New Research Perspectives*, edited by Rachel Spilka, 98–110. Carbondale: Southern Illinois UP, 1993.

Doheny-Farina, Stephen. "Research as Rhetoric: Confronting the Methodological and Ethical Problems of Research in Nonacademic Settings." In *Writing in the Workplace: New Research Perspectives*, edited by Rachel Spilka, 253–67. Carbondale: Southern Illinois UP, 1993.

Driskill, Linda. "Understanding the Writing Context in Organizations." In *Writing in the Business Professions*, edited by Myra Kogen, 125–45. Urbana, IL: NCTE, 1989.

Ecker, Pamela S., and Katherine Staples. "Collaborative Conflict and the Future: Academic-Industrial Alliances and Adaptations." In *Computers and Technical Communication: Pedagogical and Programmatic Perspectives*, edited by Stuart Selber, 375–88. Greenwich, CT: Ablex, 1997.

Faigley, Lester. "Nonacademic Writing: The Social Perspective." In *Writing in Nonacademic Settings*, edited by Lee Odell and Dixie Goswami, 231–48. New York: Guilford, 1985.

Forsberg, Lee. "Who's Out There Anyway? Bringing Awareness of Multiple Audiences into the Business-Writing Class." *Journal of Business and Technical Communication* 1, no. 2 (1987): 45–69.

Freedman, Aviva, Christine Adam, and Graham Smart. "Wearing Suits to Class: Simulating Genres and Simulations as Genre." *Written Communication* 11, no. 2 (1994): 193–226.

Haller, Cynthia R. "Revaluing Women's Work: Report Writing in the North Carolina Canning Clubs, 1912–1916." *Technical Communication Quarterly* 6 (1997): 281–92.

Harrison, Teresa M., and Susan M. Katz. "On Taking Organizations Seriously: Organizations as Social Contexts for Technical Communication." In *Foundations for Teaching Technical Communication: Theory, Practice, and Program Design*, edited by Katherine Staples and Cezar Ornatowski, 17–30. Greenwich, CT: Ablex, 1997.

Henry, Jim. "Teaching Technical Authorship." *Technical Communication Quarterly* 4, no. 3 (1995): 261–82.

———. *Writing Workplace Cultures: An Archaeology of Professional Writing*. Carbondale: Southern Illinois UP, 2000.

Herndl, Carl, Barbara Fennell, and Carolyn Miller. "Understanding Failures in Organizational Discourse: The Accident at Three Mile Island and the Shuttle Challenger Disaster." In *Textual Dynamics of the Professions: Historical and Contemporary Studies of Writing in Professional Communities*, edited by Charles Bazerman and James Paradis, 279–305. Madison: U of Wisconsin P, 1991.

Katz, Susan M. "A Newcomer Gains Power: An Analysis of the Role of Rhetorical Expertise." *Journal of Business Communication*, 35, no. 4 (1998): 419–42.

Kent-Drury, Roxanne. "The Nature of Leadership in Cross-Functional Proposal-Writing Groups." *IEEE Transactions on Professional Communication*, 43, no. 2 (2000): 90–98.

Lutz, Jean. "Understanding Organizational Socialization: The Role of Internships in Helping Students Acquire Strategies for Writing Effectively in Organizations." In *Establishing and Supervising Internships*, edited by William O. Coggin, 78–91. Association of Teachers of Technical Writing, 1989.

Lutz, Jean, and C. Gilbert Storms, eds. *The Practice of Technical and Scientific Communication*. Stamford, CT: Ablex, 1998.

Mackinnon, James. "Becoming a Rhetor: Developing Writing Ability in a Mature Writing Intensive Organization." In *Writing in the Workplace: New Research Perspectives*, edited by Rachel Spilka, 41–55. Carbondale: Southern Illinois UP, 1993.

Ornatowski, Cezar. "The Writing Consultant and the Corporate/Industry Culture." *Journal of Business and Technical Communication*, 9 (1995): 446–60.

Paradis, James, David Dobrin, and Richard Miller. "Writing at Exxon ITD: Notes on the Writing Environment of an R&D Organization." In *Writing in Nonacademic Settings*, edited by Lee Odell and Dixie Goswami, 281–307. New York: Guilford, 1985.

Rozumalski, Lynn P., and Michael F. Graves. "Effects of Case and Traditional Writing Assignments on Writing Products and Processes." *Journal of Business and Technical Communication* 9 (1995): 77–102.

Smart, Graham. "Genre as Community Invention: A Central Banks' Response to Its Executives' Expectations as Readers." In *Writing in the Workplace: New Research Perspectives*, edited by Rachel Spilka, 124-40. Carbondale: Southern Illinois UP: 1993.

Southard, Sherry G. "Protocol and Human Relations in the Corporate World: What Interns Should Know." In *Establishing and Supervising Internships*, edited by William O. Coggin, 65–78. Association of Teachers of Technical Writing, 1989.

Spilka, Rachel. "Collaboration Across Multiple Organizational Cultures." *Technical Communication Quarterly* 2, no. 2 (1993): 125–42.

Subbiah, Mahalingam. "Social Construction Theory and Technical Communication." In *Foundations for Teaching Technical Communication: Theory, Practice, and Program Design*, edited by Katherine Staples and Cezar Ornatowski, 53–66. Greenwich, CT: Ablex, 1997.

Thralls, Charlotte, Nancy Blyler, and Helen Rothschild Ewald. "Real Readers, Implied Readers, and Professional Writers: Suggested Research." *The Journal of Business Communication* 25, no. 2 (1988): 47–65.

Weiss, Timothy. "'Ourselves Among Others': A New Metaphor for Business and Technical Writing." *Technical Communication Quarterly* 1, no. 3 (1992): 23–36.

Winsor, Dorothy. "An Engineer's Writing and the Corporate Construction of Knowledge." *Written Communication* 6 (1989): 270–85.

———. "Rhetorical Practices in Technical Work." *Journal of Business and Technical Communication* 12 (1998): 343–70.

———. *Writing Like an Engineer: A Rhetorical Education*. Mahwah, NJ: Ablex, 1996.

CHAPTER SIX

Working within and across Cultures

Chapter Six: Introduction

In 1987, an influential study commissioned by the U.S. Department of Labor called *Workplace 2000* predicted, quite accurately, that in the new millennium the labor force would change dramatically, with minorities and women, many of them immigrants, constituting larger segments. In addition, the study explained that jobs in high-skilled professions, requiring more education and skills in math, language, and reasoning, would grow rapidly (97).

Our multicultural, diverse society, along with the global economy and global workforce, presents a vast array of new challenges and opportunities for teachers of technical communication. One such opportunity involves helping companies and organizations to recognize and integrate the distinctive values, needs, and cultural backgrounds of their employees, target populations, and collaborators into their communication strategies and plans.

The essays in this chapter will introduce you to the opportunities and changes that are occurring in our field as a result of the changes in society. Beamer's and Thrush's essays provide an overview and foundation for the issue of intercultural/multicultural communication competence and offer frameworks for ways to better analyze diverse audiences and, as a result, create more effective messages. The pieces by Lay and Gurak and Bayer outline changes (both in society and in the discipline) that offer opportunities for feminist perspectives to gain prominence, which, they propose, may lead to improvements in collaborative enterprises and industrial processes. Finally, the applied theory essay, collaboratively written by authors from Japan and the United States, demonstrates that a user-centered approach that is informed by some of these new perspectives can counter some of the problems associated with ethnocentric assumptions (Thatcher).

Ours is a social field, and if we consider the "social roles, group purposes, communal organization, ideology, and finally theories of culture" (Faigley 236) and build them into our pedagogies, we can teach our students to become competent communicators who recognize cultural and gender differences, use their knowledge to effect successful communication, and work for organizational transformations. We can also encourage them to become critical citizens who ask difficult questions in order to avoid mindsets that "exist when groups or individuals look out for their own interests and have little concern for others'" (Gudykunst 5).

WORKS CITED

Faigley, Lester. "Nonacademic Writing: The Social Perspective." In *Writing in Nonacademic Settings,* edited by Lee Odell and Dixie Goswami, 231–48. New York: Guilford, 1985.

Gudykunst, William B. *Bridging Differences: Effective Intergroup Communication.* Newbury Park: Sage, 1991.

Johnson, William B., and Arnold H. Packer. *Workforce 2000: Work and Workers for the 21st Century.* Indianapolis: The Hudson Institute, 1987.

Thatcher, Barry. "Issues of Validity in Intercultural Professional Communication Research." *Journal of Business and Technical Communication* 15, no. 4 (2001): 458–89.

23 Learning Intercultural Communication Competence

LINDA BEAMER

Few would argue that professional communicators—and nearly everyone in the workplace for that matter—would benefit from becoming more competent communicators. Competency, however, is a fluid and dynamic term. In the early part of the twentieth century competence usually meant learning to communicate effectively within the boundaries of one's own corporate culture. Today, however, competency often involves the ability to transcend not only corporate boundaries but also national and cultural ones. Thus, Beamer's essay, which is one of the first in our field to discuss intercultural competence and to present a learning model, is of great value. Beamer explains that models of intercultural communication "must take social and cultural environment into account" (p. 401 in this volume), in addition to the "factors that shape the structuring categories of the receiver's repository. . . . values, attitudes, beliefs, and behaviors" (p. 402). After offering this definition and explaining that individuals must be willing to challenge their own perceptions, she outlines a learning model with five levels leading to the ability to analyze communication episodes and generate "other-culture" messages. Especially important is her acknowledgment that, in her model, learning will be both linear and incremental as well as cyclical and recursive.

Increasingly, as the value of intercultural communication competence is stressed by international organizations, curricula in schools and business reflect that concern. But the process by which intercultural communication competence is learned is not well understood. Without a clear idea of (a) what constitutes competence and (b) the learning process to accomplish that goal, business communicators flounder and business communication educators are left without a basis for a pedagogical posture. This paper offers a learning process model, and prefaces the model with a description of intercultural communication.

From *The Journal of Business Communication* 29, no. 3 (1992): 285–303.

Perception in Intercultural Communication

The best way to understand intercultural communication is to focus on the decoding process and the role of perception in communication. This is because in intercultural communication, decoding by the receiver of signals is subject to social values and cultural variables not necessarily present in the sender. Communication itself can best be understood from the perspective of the receiver, not the sender or the channel or even the encoded message itself. Bowman and Targowski (1987, p. 17) have argued that communication does not occur without the perception that communication is taking place. A sender may transmit unconscious or unintentional signals along with the intended message, which may obscure or enhance it; intended messages may not be picked up at all by the receiver. Transmission by itself is not communication, but the conscious perception of signals at the receiver's end is essential for communication to have taken place.

A communication model such as the Shannon-Weaver model, that represents sender, message, channel, and receiver, is understood as a sequential, linear process in time. Written communication over distance (space) does function in time. In dyadic interpersonal exchanges, however, sender and receiver are simultaneously present in the same person, sending and receiving multiple messages. What does take place sequentially is perception: recognizing, structuring, and attributing meaning to signals. Perception is what gives process to communication. Therefore, any process model of communication should focus on the receiver (who is either party). Models also need to represent meaning, along with intention (Limaye & Victor, 1991).

Perception begins with the recognition that signals are being sent. The initial recognition of signals is not random, but selective. A person chooses to encounter some signals but not others, and to pay attention to some but not others. Recognition does not equal communication, however, because at this point the perceiver may choose to "lose" the signal—not to retain it. Then signals are structured into categories that exist in the receiver's mind, since each human being possesses internal images of the physical and social world (Samovar, Porter, & Jain, 1981, p. 106; Gudykunst & Kim, 1984, chap. 5). Culture itself conditions the categories, so the signal is structured in a way dictated by culture. Finally, meaning is attributed to the structured perceptions. At this point cultural influence is profound. The meaning attached to a signal will derive from a store or repository of meanings that are culturally determined. No two meaning reservoirs are identical, but the differences are pronounced when life experiences come from different cultures.

A perception-based approach differs from the approach shown by a linear sender-receiver model such as the channel-ratio model of Haworth and Savage (1989). That model emphasizes channel, the ratio of intentional message to implied message, and a sequential-exchange pattern; a perception-based approach emphasizes interactions in which perception by each communicator is simultaneous with sending messages. In 1954 the Schramm model suggested communication is not sequential, but is a "continuing interaction between people" (Bowman & Targowski, 1987, p. 26).

Models of intercultural communication must take social and cultural environment into account; several are outlined by Bowman and Targowski in their comprehensive analysis of communication models (1987). The Gudykunst and Kim (1984) model shows the communicator, who is both encoder and decoder, surrounded by four contexts: environmental, cultural, sociocultural, and psychocultural. Yet this model and the Haworth and Savage model suggest cultural "context" is something *outside* the communicator, rather than inside the communicator's consciousness. A problem with the notion of "context," represented by a circle around the sender or receiver, is the inability of the model to show what happens to communication when one party has no knowledge of the other's context, or knowledge of the other's context is very small on one side and very large on the other.

The Semiotic Sign as a Unit of Communication

A vocabulary from semiotics may be helpful in clarifying the nature of received signals. The receiver-decoded signal is a "sign" made up of two parts, the signifier and the signified (Saussure, 1949/1983, part chap. 4; Barthes, 1964/1967, part II). The signifier is the sound or shape of the signal; in other words it is the sensorially perceived signal without meaning yet attached. The signified is the meaning. The relationship between signifier and signified is arbitrary; that is, no logical motivation connects them. Meaning is usually attributed, not inherent, in all verbal and nonverbal communication systems. In this paper, a sign is a signal that is recognized, structured into a category and assigned meaning.

When the communicator, *C*, structures a signal according to previously learned categories, the signal—or at this point, the signifier without a signified—is matched with the signs in the reservoir of the receiver. If the signifier appears identical with a sign in the reservoir, *C* "understands" the signifier and it becomes a complete sign. If the signifier appears very similar, but not identical, to an existing sign, then *C* may decide the new signifier should have the same signified as the previously existing sign—in other words, that the new sign means the same as the sign already in the reservoir. The linkage of new, unattributed signifiers to already-existing signifieds is a large part of the process of decoding communication messages.

Where no match can be found, *C* either discards the signifier as no sign at all, or leaves it a signifier without a known signified. It either does not exist or it exists as a fragment of communication—something waiting for elucidation or simply an unknown. Communication across cultures is dysfunctional when signs are not recognized because they differ from the known signs in the culture-driven repository. The cognitive matching, analyzing process is shown in Figure 1.

The receiver of intercultural messages is constantly adjusting and adapting the incoming signifiers to the existing repository of signs, and adapting

FIGURE 1 The Cognitive Matching Process

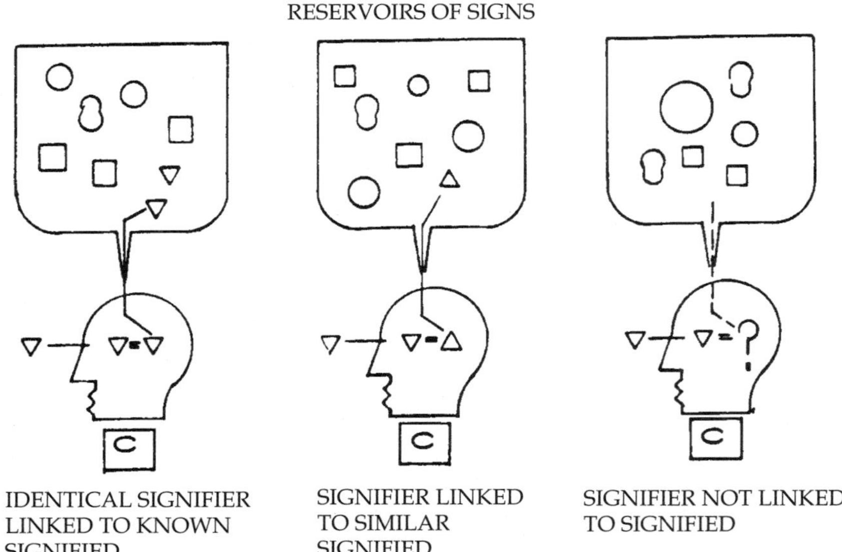

The figure shows identical signs matched, signifiers matched though not identical, or signifiers discarded.

and adjusting the repository of signifieds to create new signs. An interculturally competent receiver will keep challenging his or her own repository of existing signs and expanding the repository, in order to play a part in the matching of signs with the other communicator.

Understanding what happens when intercultural communication takes place enables us to consider how to effect it. In order to communicate across cultures, the encoding and the intentional, conscious directing of signs to a receiver will have to take into account the factors that shape the structuring categories of the receiver's repository. These are cultural factors: values, attitudes, beliefs, and behaviors. Brislin (1981) has identified eight dimensions at work when categories are formed, mostly having to do with the psychocultural orientation of the communicator. Similarly, the decoding and the attribution of signifieds to signifiers will have to take cultural factors into account. That is cognitively learned knowledge of the cultures involved may be the basis for developing communication competence. "The barriers to communication . . . can best be lowered by a knowledge and understanding of cultural factors that are subject to variance, coupled with an honest and sincere desire to communicate successfully across cultural boundaries" (Samovar et al., 1981, p. 32). In summary, intercultural communication competence is the encoding and decoding of attributed signifieds to signifiers in matches that correspond to signs held in the other communicator's repository. This definition means that the personality of the communicatior—as for example empathic, outgoing, sensitive, caring, flexible, which has been stressed by other authors as critical for intercultural success (for example, Kealey, 1990)—is less important for business communicators than a cognitive understanding of another culture.

The next step is to understand how the goal of intercultural communication competence can be acquired—and taught.

Understanding the Process of Learning Intercultural Communication Competence

The learning process by which men and women gain intercultural competence and become "fluent" in more than one culture is the subject of work by various authors with varied applications in mind. A review of some models, both formal and informal, of intercultural learning indicates that not only is the process unclear, but that learning for the specific context of international business has not received particular attention. Finally, the models are not specifically designed to show the learning of intercultural *communication* competence.

Many scholars agree the process of learning intercultural competence is developmental. Brislin, Landis, and Brandt (1984) imply a developmental approach when they suggest six apparently incremental "antecedents" to describe how intercultural behavior arises. The six steps ask the individual to consider (a) past experiences with people of the target culture, (b) role and norm differences, (c) anxiety, (d) the goals of the intercultural training, (e) perceptual and cognitive sets of a world view and, (f) self-image: that is, to see oneself able to "walk in the other's moccasins" (p. 5). This model attempts to describe what intercultural behavior is and to outline a strategy for personal development. Especially valuable in this model is the view that intercultural behavior is successful when seen to be so in the eyes of a person from the target culture. Drawbacks of this model are that the application appears to be culture-specific, and to be limited to sojourners. The antecedents appear to constitute bases for comment on the communication context (metacommunication) but the model does not address communication.

Gudykunst and Hammer (1982) discuss a three-stage approach to learning intercultural competence beginning with (a) the psychological framework of an intercultural perspective followed by (b) interaction with members of another culture and, finally, (c) context-specific training within another country. Again, this model focuses on the "sojourner," rather than communicators who do not necessarily make a sojourn. Even more sojourner-based is a learning model developed by James McCaffery (1986) from his work for the United States Peace Corps; it focuses on training sojourners to be independently effective in their new culture. The model is experiential, and acknowledges a debt to Gudykunst and Hammer. It represents the behavioral learning cycle that moves from experience to analysis to generalization to application to experience again, but it does not focus on communication. A useful phenomenological model created by Milton J. Bennett (1986) outlines the development of an individual's sensitivity. Bennett's approach identifies six stages, beginning from the ethnocentric denial of difference, to defense against difference, to minimization of difference, and then to the "ethnorelative" stages of acceptance, adaptation, and integration of difference. This sequence of changes in the perception of difference and meaning attributed to difference is helpful in describing what should take place for communication competence to occur—communication competence being closely related to the "intercultural sensitivity" that is the goal of training with this model. Rosita Daskal Albert (1983) poses an informal model of culture learning as a "spiral" in which new information or learned cognitively proceeds to (unspecified) experiential and behavioral phases that prepare the individual for further learning.

Two valuable premises in these five developmental models are that learning is incremental and that the individual's internal perceptions, challenged through personal experience, are the starting point of learning intercultural competence. So far, however, and in spite of the excellent work that has been briefly reviewed above, no adequate model exists to explain the process of learning intercultural *communication* competence, let alone its application in world business. Therefore a model is proposed here, the purpose of which is to describe the process of acquiring intercultural communication competence, and by so doing to lay the foundation for a pedagogical posture.

The Intercultural Learning Model

Like those described above, this model is developmental. Principles underlying this model are: culture is learnable (Terpstra & David, 1992); cultures are whole and coherent; all cultures are equally valid in the ways they organize and explain human experience; and the interculturally competent communicator acknowledges that cultural bias always exists. Finally, the relationship of culture and communication, terms used interchangeably in much of the literature following Edward Hall's dictum that "culture is communication" and "communication is culture" (1959; Samovar et al., 1981), is resolved for purposes of this paper by the principle stated by Goodenough (cited in Baxter, 1983): culture governs communication behavior.

This model postulates five levels of learning, which can each be represented by a circle or disc. The discs are stacked, like records in an old jukebox. The five levels are (a) acknowledging diversity, (b) organizing information according to stereotypes, (c) posing questions to challenge the stereotypes, (d) analyzing communication episodes, and (e) generating "other culture" messages (Figure 2).

The aim of the learning process modeled here is to develop the ability to decode effectively signs that come from members of other cultures within a business context, and to encode messages using signs that carry the encoder's intended meaning to members of other cultures. The five levels of learning describe an incremental development, but the model also may describe a *cyclical* process. Therefore, the five levels are connected by cyclical patterns to indicate they are not left behind once achieved, but are constantly revisited in the process of learning. The diversity is always being experienced; even when one has some familiarity with a culture, new differences between that culture and others are constantly being discovered. Stereotyped categories are constantly being formed and constantly being challenged, as long as the

FIGURE 2 Model of Intercultural Communication Learning in Five Levels

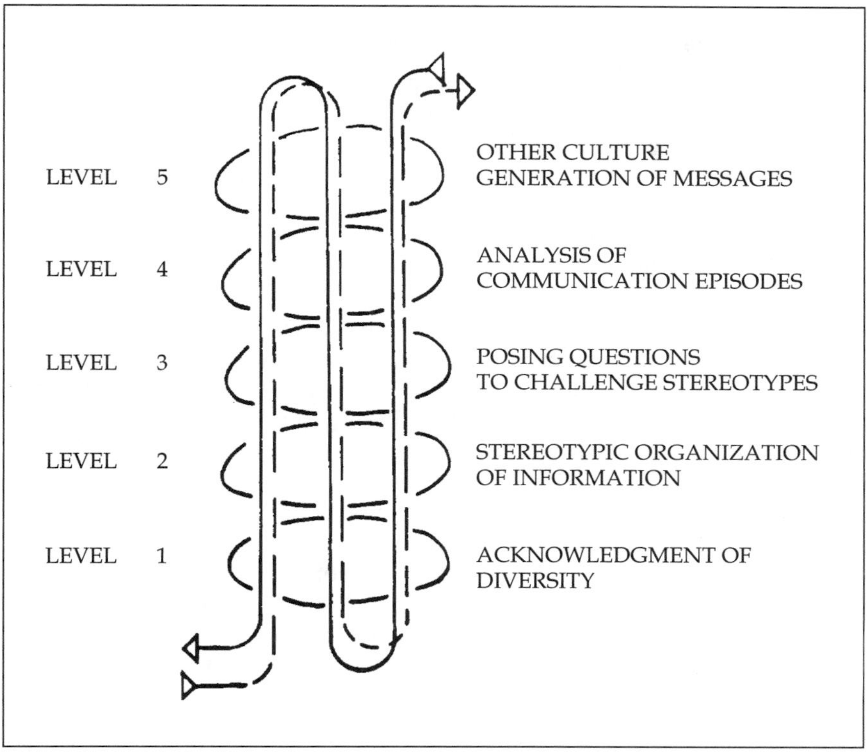

LEVEL 5 OTHER CULTURE GENERATION OF MESSAGES

LEVEL 4 ANALYSIS OF COMMUNICATION EPISODES

LEVEL 3 POSING QUESTIONS TO CHALLENGE STEREOTYPES

LEVEL 2 STEREOTYPIC ORGANIZATION OF INFORMATION

LEVEL 1 ACKNOWLEDGMENT OF DIVERSITY

individual continues to accept new meanings attributed to familiar signs. Past communication acts remain open to analysis, and new communication is being generated as long as one is participating in another culture.

Acknowledging Diversity

The first and most basic level in intercultural learning is an awareness of differences; it may be the "key organizing concept" for intercultural sensitivity to occur (Bennett, 1986, p. 181). At this point, the learner addresses the initial issue of perception: recognition that previously unknown and unrecognized signs are being sent. Members of homogeneous, high-context cultures have a limited experience of cultural diversity. They need to begin by acknowledging the diversity of signifiers—sounds, shapes, gestures, and so on—for signifieds already understood. Then they can become open to the possibility of new signifieds as well. At this level, definitions of basic concepts for discussing diversity are important, such as "bias," "ethnocentricity," "stereotype," "value," and "culture." The most obvious cultural difference, especially when discussing signifiers, is linguistic. Fluency in another language is unarguably valuable, but does not always produce *cultural fluency*—intercultural communication competence does not automatically accompany linguistic skill.

Organizing Information According to Stereotypes

The second level of intercultural learning is developing basic categories of certain selected characteristics that distinguish a particular culture and its members. Thus: Arabs like to stand very near a listener when speaking; Chinese always initially refuse hospitality when offered; Latin Americans only like to do business with people who show consideration for their family affairs. These categories enable us to familiarize an unfamiliar culture, and to make it comprehensible. They demonstrate that Arabs, Chinese, and Latin Americans are not all alike in their difference from, say, Canadians. These examples are stereotypes. Stereotypes are not usually as simple or brief as the examples above; indeed, they are often many-layered, "complex, multidimensional images" (Brislin, 1981, p. 44). They may be helpful and even accurate to some degree, but they are limited insights, revealing only a part of the whole culture. Stereotypes can be obstacles to intercultural communication competence (Kealey & Ruben, 1979; McCaffery, 1986). Two or three stereotypes of one culture, or even a dozen or a score, do not equal an understanding of that culture. For people in business, the danger is that communication with members of the culture may be limited to the inflexible dictates of the stereotypes. The lists of do's and taboos, so beloved of business people, are helpful in categorizing the unfamiliar, but they rarely offer more than stereotypes. Unhappily, some people never progress beyond this level of intercultural communication. They do not challenge the signs within their own repository of meanings; they do not ask if some other signified can be associated with a signifier.

Posing Questions to Challenge the Stereotypes

At the third level of learning, stereotypes are challenged. The intercultural communicator asks questions about other cultures in order to break out of the stereotypes. Put another way, to communicate competently across cultures one needs enthnographic tools as well as business communication tools. One may ask questions, for example, about how members of a business organization describe that organization, about their relationships to one another and to their material environment, about their position in relation to the universe. Questions reveal attitudes that are important for understanding business activities, such as attitudes toward time, status and role, obligations in relationships, responsibility and the decision-making processes, the role of law, and the role of technology. Answers to the questions may be sought from various research sources, published and primary. The function of this step is to expand the possible store of signifieds for the signs reaching the communicator from another culture. Since cognitive understanding of another culture may be the key to intercultural communication competence, this is the strategy for increasing knowledge of a particular culture.

Questions, although admittedly chosen in a "somewhat arbitrary manner" (Glenn & Glenn, 1981, p. 8), can be used to challenge stereotypes. The culturally shaped questions constructed for this model probe what members of another culture value, how they behave in certain circumstances because of their values, what their attitudes are toward institutions in their society and toward events beyond their control. The constructs are derived largely from the work of Condon and Yousef (1975), who owe a debt to the five questions that Kluckhohn and Strodtbeck (1961) said all cultures must answer:

- the character of innate human nature
- the relation of human beings to nature
- the temporal focus of human life
- a model for human activity
- a model for human relationships (p. 11)

Kluckhohn and Strodtbeck found five corresponding areas of "value orientations" with three possible positions in each of the five value orientations. Condon and Yousef expand these five sets of value orientations to 25, and following Kluckhohn and Strodtbeck, they offer three choices in each category, bringing the total number of possible value orientation choices to 75. They describe six areas: Self, Family, Society, Human Nature, Nature, and the Supernatural.

Gudykunst and Kim (1984) define three areas for inquiry into the cultural environment of intercultural communication: postulates (the culture's world view), ends and means. They call these the components of culture. The postulates include: world view, value orientations (for example, human nature, time, activity), and six "pattern variables." These six oppose characteristics such as self-orientation versus the collective, and universalism versus particularism. Gudykunst and Kim are able to ask questions about immediate versus delayed gratification in a culture's values, specific responses to people and events versus diffuse responses, ascription of qualities of people and things versus achievement of qualities, and similar questions.

The model offered here shifts the emphasis to stress the cultural differences in behavior and attitude that affect business communication. It presents five areas of value orientations: Thinking and Knowing, Doing and Achieving, the Self, Social Organization, and the Universe. While this list of value orientations is a start, it does not presume to be exhaustive, and these terms themselves are acknowledged to be culture bound.

Since most cultures are not oriented entirely to one or another value, this model offers a graphic shape, a pair of triangles with adjoining points, to show a culture's value orientation along a dimension, rather than the three categories of Condon and Yousef. The hourglass shape, "filled" more on one end than the other, represents a culture's great tendency toward one extreme than its opposite value orientation. Since absolute measurements of a culture's value orientations are impossible, the shape easily describes "generally," and "rarely" without being forced into one of three unequivocal categories. As familiarity with the culture grows, and as categories and meanings in the communicator's mental repository expand with new insights, the shaded area may change toward one extreme and away from the other, just as sand in an hourglass easily moves from one end to the other.

1. Thinking and Knowing. The first group of questions concerns how members of a culture "acquire, organize, and transmit information" about that culture (Glenn & Glenn, 1981, p. 7). The first question is about ways to know, from abstracts and concepts to specific experience. In some cultures, one only knows something when it is conceptualized and abstracted, while in other cultures, to know something requires firsthand experience. Another dimension concerns the activity that results in knowledge: at one end knowing is achieved by probing, questioning, and atomizing, while at the other end knowing is by mastering a received body of knowledge to the point where it can be reproduced. Yet another variable is the extent of knowledge: everything is knowable on the one hand while on the other hand the ineffable nature of some things prevents their being known completely. The way things may be known is also closely related to the patterns of thinking in a culture. Some cultures use mainly cause-and-effect patterns: these cultures may value planning, and their systems (conceptualizations, language, institutions) reveal linear thinking patterns. Other cultures emphasize context in patterns of thinking: the interconnections and relationships between things are important and a lattice or net pattern emerges. These four questions are shown by the four hourglass shapes making an octagon in Figure 3, with a hypothetical culture's profile indicated.

2. Doing and Achieving. The second value orientation group concerns activity and achievement. Not all cultures share the North American need to identify goals and work toward them; some societies emphasize the present moment and celebrate simply being. Related to this dimension is another: results-oriented cultures seem at a polarity with relationship-oriented cultures. This set of polarities corresponds closely to the cause-and-effect pattern of thinking versus the context pattern. A third set of polarities is a sequential approach to tasks versus a simultaneous approach. For example, in some cultures, one seller who can serve four people at once is viewed as highly efficient, whereas in other cultures it is appropriate to devote attention exclusively to one customer at a time. A fourth dimension concerns uncertainty avoidance at one end, and a tolerance of uncertainty at the other. Finally, some cultures view luck as a significant factor in outcomes including business activities, while other cultures attribute little or no importance to luck.

3. The Self. The third set of value orientations concerns the individual person. One dimension is the relative importance of individualism versus interdependence and interrelatedness. In business cultures where the individual is rewarded, personal competitiveness is high; in cultures towards the other extreme, competitiveness may be abhorrent. Managers may be at a loss to motivate workers who are not interested in individual achievement. In the second dimension, youth is opposed to age; in some business environments age is more important than training or even experience, but this is not true of other cultures. The third dimension involves attitudes towards the sexes: equality versus inequality. Questions can be posed about a culture's preference for one sex over the other for a particular job.

FIGURE 3 Thinking and Knowing

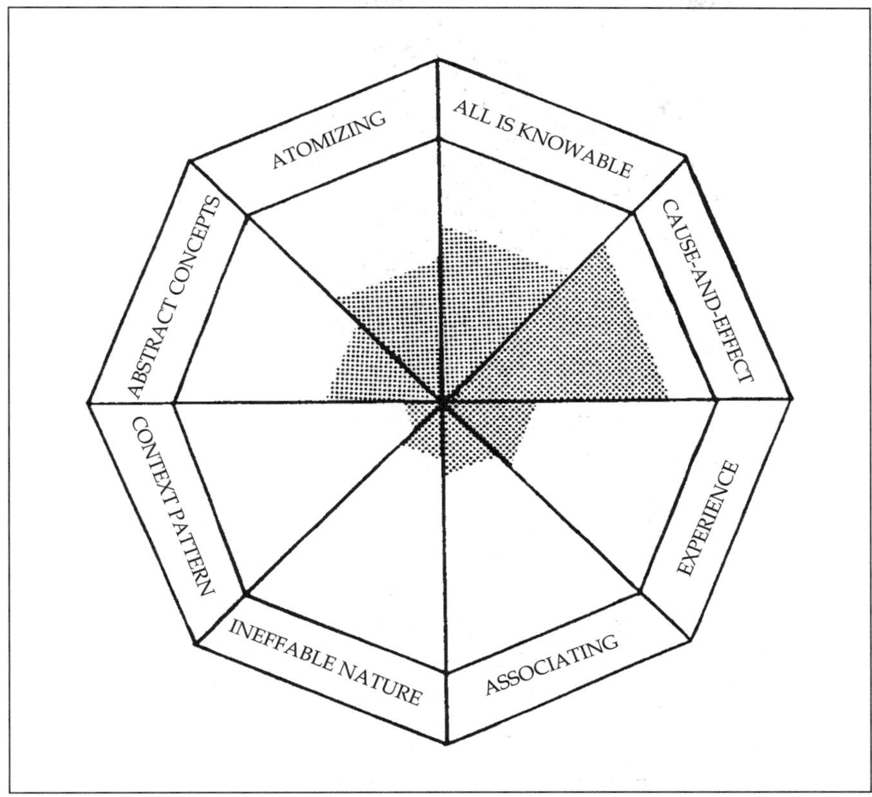

The shaded areas show a culture with value orientations that are more Western than Eastern.

4. The Organization of Society. Social structure is the next general area (see Figure 4). The opposed value orientations include (a) a tendency toward temporary versus permanent group membership; (b) preference for private ownership of material goods versus community ownership; (c) a tendency to distrust form versus a preference for form; (d) more egalitarianism versus more hierarchical structure; and (e) a general practice of approaching authority directly versus using a mediated link to authority. These orientations will affect format, organization, and tone of business communication documents, as well as interpersonal communication. For example, the degree to which a business letter writer speaks for a collective rather than as an individual, can vary greatly and will determine the vocabulary and tone of the letter. An employee who views employment within an organization as a lifelong commitment, which perhaps extends to descendants as well, will frame messages differently from an employee who views the organization as a career-building stepping stone. The degree to which the writer expects the reader to react as an individual with authority to

FIGURE 4 Organization of Society

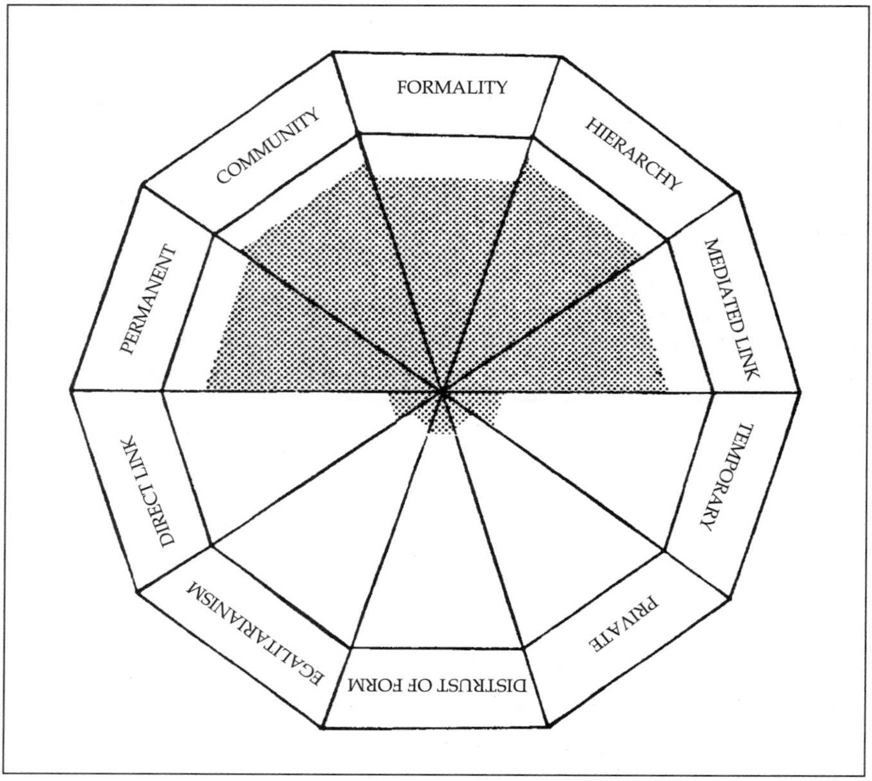

FORMALITY
HIERARCHY
MEDIATED LINK
TEMPORARY
PRIVATE
DISTRUST OF FORM
EGALITARIANISM
DIRECT LINK
PERMANENT
COMMUNITY

The shaded areas show a culture with value orientations similar to Japan's.

respond, or as a representative of a group who must consult the group before responding, will also be important.

The dimension dealing with frequent use of form versus lack of form is useful for communication in business. In the United States, business people observe form rarely and are somewhat suspicious of it; given names rather than family names are used in business and casual dress may be acceptable—men may remove their jackets, for example, while working. By contrast, Japanese never use given names in business and men rarely remove their jackets while at work. To require much attention to form makes United States business people uncomfortable; to dispense with form makes Japanese business people uncomfortable. Both formality and informality assure members in their respective cultures that they are behaving correctly and not risking embarrassment, but the very assumptions about what constitutes comfortable behavior are not universal and can cause discomfort to members of the other culture.

5. The Universe. The relation of the members of the culture to the universe include view of nature: does man dominate nature or does nature dominate man? The perspective about time is another value orientation: time is linear in one view while time is cyclical in another view. Some cultures focus on humans and see human activity at the center of the universe, while in other cultures divine beings are at the center in every activity, including business. Change is always good in some cultures, while in others change is always bad. Obviously, if business people from a "change" culture are attempting to do something new in a "no-change" culture, they need to understand what will make change acceptable before using words like "new," "improved," "different," and "never before." Finally, in the last cultural dimension in this category, death is the end of life for members of some cultures, while for others death is merely a part of life.

One can pose these questions of a new culture (or of one's original culture) and use hourglass-shaped value dimensions to illustrate the preferences of a specific culture. The hexagon, octagon, or decagon shapes that result when the hourglass dimensions are grouped together give a profile of a culture for each of the five value orientation categories. Thus the differences in two or more cultures can be compared at a glance, by looking at the five shapes each culture makes in the five categories of value orientations. Therefore, these figures can be used for a culture-general learning strategy as well as for culture-specific understanding.

Analyzing Communication Episodes

Once the learner has actively sought to understand a culture through posing questions to challenge stereotyped categories, the understanding can be used to analyze communication episodes in actual cases. Episodes may show successful communication, or failed communication, or both. As the episode is analyzed, new meanings for communication behavior can be attributed. At this fourth level of learning intercultural communication competence, emphasis is culture-specific; learning focuses on depth of understanding, and application of the abstractions considered in level three during the plotting of a culture's value orientations. The inventory of questions to pose about the culture is refined and augmented with the addition of new insights from specific communication cases. The vocabulary of behavioral signs for a particular culture is expanded. This increases competence in both encoding and decoding intercultural messages.

Generating "Other-Culture" Messages

The communicator becomes interculturally competent when messages may be encoded and directed as if from within the new culture when messages from the new culture may be decoded and respond successfully. This is similar to the standard suggested by Brislin (1984) in their description of intercultural behavior as an ability to "walk in the other's moccasins," because the communicator's perception is so attuned that he or she has "the ability to 'become' the other."

When communicators achieve this level of intercultural competence they are constantly evaluating messages against the repository of signs they have stored in their mental data bases. They have flexibility to alter the data base or to match incoming signs and messages to those already known. The communicator is able to manipulate information received as well as information stored and to make linkages between levels of understanding. Then in turn messages can be encoded that draw upon this complex matrix of constantly revised signs.

For example, according to the stereotype of the behavior of Arab letter-writers, a letter usually begins with a generalized benediction upon the reader and family. An actual letter will be tested against this expectation and may confirm or contradict or partly confirm the expectation. Meaning will be attributed to the actual communication after *C* (see Figure 1) considers the cultural factors informing the categories that structure the letter writer's set of signs. One category may be a conscious effort on the part of the writer to emulate the letter-writing supposed to be familiar to *C*. *C* may compare the letter with other similiar documents and consider the results of analysis of other cases. At this point, *C* will be understanding the communication in the same way as someone from the letter writer's culture would. This is intercultural communication competence. *C* now can send a message back that will conform to the revised signs in the repository. The other communictor can do the same thing, if competent.

Senders of messages from other cultures may themselves offer evaluations (metacommunication) of their own communication, as well as "typical" communication, and these meanings also will be assessed in the revision of signs. Some success in understanding one formerly unfamiliar culture well enough to communicate with its members usually produces confidence in the communicator about identifying the questions to ask in order to communicate effectively in another unfamiliar culture. At this point, the communicator has a culture-general, rather than a culture specific, competence.

Summary of the Learning Model

Learning intercultural communication competence requires a willingness to acknowledge the frequently unexpected differences in a new culture; it requires a willingness to accept the stereotypical characteristics of the new culture for what they are. Learning competence further includes identifying questions to ask about the culture that will reveal fundamental values and meanings that motivate the way people communicate in particular situations. Next in learning intercultural competence is the development of the ability to analyze communication behavior within the context of the values. Finally, competence means being able to generate and respond to communication messages as if from within another culture, and this competence is transferrable to more than one culture.

Conclusions

Acquiring knowledge and understanding of cultural factors is the key to successful communication across cultures. This is the key also to developing an appropriate pedagogical posture for the teaching of intercultural business communication. If the process by which one acquires intercultural communication competence can be identified, the process for intercultural communication instruction will also have been identified. Trainers and educators can use the model as a rational basis for courses to develop intercultural communication competence in students.

REFERENCES

Albert, R. D. (1983). The intercultural sensitizer or culture assimilator: A cognitive approach. In R. W. Brislin & D. Landis (Eds.), *Handbook of intercultural training* (Vol. 2, pp. 186–217). Toronto: Pergamon.

Barthes, R. (1967). *Elements of semiology*. (A. Lavers & C. Smith, Trans.) New York: Hill and Wang. (Original work published 1964.)

Baxter, J. (1983). English for intercultural competence: An approach to intercultural communication training. In R. W. Brislin & D. Landis (Eds.), *Handbook of intercultural training* (Vol. 2, pp. 290–324). Toronto: Pergamon.

Bennett, M J. (1986). A developmental approach to training for intercultural sensitivity. *International Journal of Intercultural Relations, 10*(2), 179–195.

Bowman, J. P., & Targowski, A.S. (1987). Modeling the communication process: The map is not the territory. *The Journal of Business Communication, 24*(4), 21–34.

Brislin, R. W. (1981). *Cross-cultural encounters*. Toronto: Pergamon.

Brislin, R. W., Landis, D., & Brandt, M.E. (1983). Conceptualization: Cultural behavior and training. In R. Brislin & D. Landis (Eds.), *Handbook of intercultural training* (Vol. 1, pp. 2–26). Toronto: Pergamon.

Condon, J. C., & Yousef, F. (1975). *An introduction to intercultural communication*. New York: Macmillan.

Glenn, E. S., & Glenn, C. (1981). Man and mankind: *Conflict and communication between cultures*. Norwood, NJ: Ablex Publishing Corporation.

Gudykunst, W. B., & Hammer, M.R. (1983). Basic training design: Approaches to intercultural training. In R. W. Brislin & D. Landis (Eds.), *Handbook of intercultural training* (Vol. 1, pp. 118–154.) New York: Pergamon.

Gudykunst, W. B., Hammer, M. R., & Weisman, R. (1977), An analysis of an integrated approach to cross-cultural training. *International Journal of Intercultural Relations, 1*(2), 79–109.

Gudykunst, W. B., & Kim, Y.Y. (1982). *Communicating with strangers*. New York: Random House.

Hall, E. T. (1959). *The silent language*. Garden City, NJ: Anchor.

Haworth, D. A., & Savage, G.T. (1989) A channel-ratio model of intercultural communication: The trains won't sell, fix them please. *The Journal of Business Communication, 26*, 231–254.

Kealey, D. J. (1990). *Cross-cultural effectiveness: A study of Canadian technical advisors overseas*. Hull: Canadian International Development Agency.

Kealey, D. J., & Ruben, D. J. (1979). Behavioral assessment of communication competency and the prediction of cross-cultural adaptation. *International Journal of Intercultural Relations, 3*, 15–47.

Kluckhohn, F., & Strodtbeck, F. L. (1961), *Variations in value orientations*. Evanston, IL: Row, Peterson.

Limaye, M. R., & Victor, DA. (1991). Cross-cultural business communication research: State of the art and hypotheses for the 1990s. *The Journal of Business Communication, 28*, 277–299.

McCaffery, J. A. (1986). Independent effectiveness: A reconsideration of cross-cultural orientation and training. *International Journal of Int Relations, 10*(2), 159–177.

Samovar, L. A., Porter, R. E., & Jain, N. C. (1981). *Understanding intercultural communication*. Belmont, CA: Wadsworth Publishing Company.

Saussure, F. de (1983). *Course in general linguistics*. Edited by Charles Bally and Albert Sechehaye, with the collaboration of Albert Reidlinger; translated and annotated by Roy Harris. London: Duckworth. (Original work published in 1949.)

Terpstra, V., & David, K. (1992). *The cultural environment of international business* (3rd ed.). Cincinnati: South-Western Publishing Company.

24 Multicultural Issues in Technical Communication

EMILY A. THRUSH

In this review essay, Thrush makes it clear that technical communicators, particularly those working in the software industry, need to know more about multicultural and intercultural communication. As she says, "there's no escaping the increasing internationalization of business" (p. 415 in this volume). She outlines "what is known about technical and business writing in other cultures" (p. 416) and then, by relying on concepts from various fields (e.g., linguistics, sociology, and economics), she illustrates strategies that technical communicators can use to analyze diverse audiences to create more effective communication. Her overview provides a foundation for and illustration of many of the issues and problems that technical communicators face now and will continue to face. In addition, the series of questions she poses at the end are valuable for teachers to consider. As our classrooms and the workplaces that our students will enter become more diverse, we would do well to consider strategies that can, at a minimum, introduce these issues and problems. We need to do more than just offer prescriptive rules or stereotypic anecdotes.

INTRODUCTION

Does anyone still doubt the need of today's technical communicator to be aware of cultural differences in reading and writing? Most practitioners have probably encountered cultural differences directly on their jobs—in writing computer documentation for products to be sold worldwide, in designing maintenance manuals to be used by technicians of varying cultural backgrounds, or in working with the managers of their foreign-owned companies.

The numbers have often been recited: more than 35,000 Americans are working for foreign-owned companies overseas (Lathan, 1982, p. 16), 300,000 are working for Japanese-owned companies in the United States (Haight, 1991, p. 1), and more than 30,000 American companies are involved in

From *Foundations for Teaching Technical Communication*, edited by Katherine Staples and Cezar Ornatowski, 161–78. Greenwich, CT. Ablex, 1997.

exporting goods (Lathan p. 16), often equaling 25–50 percent of their total sales (Sprung, 1990, p. 71). According to a 1992 *Newsweek* article (Samuelson, 1992), between 1989 and 1991, United States exports to Mexico increased 62 percent to a total of $33.3 billion a year (p. 48)—and that was before the passage of NAFTA.

The implications for the technical communicator are clear, especially if one looks more closely at the software industry, a major employer of technical writers. In the countries making up the new European Union, for example, 19 of the 30 best selling software packages are American, and American software products account for 60 percent of total sales. Britain's *Economist* magazine ("Europe's Software Debacle," 1994) has recently reported that because of the various advantages (in expertise and financing) enjoyed by high-tech firms in the United States, many of Europe's largest software companies are opening management offices in the United States and transferring much of their operations here, where American and European designers, programmers, and managers will work side by side (pp. 77–78). Design and documentation for all these products, whether American or European produced, will need to take into account audiences on both sides of the Atlantic. The *Economist* reports that when Microsoft, purchaser of the Intuit line of software, wanted to market the very successful personal financial management package *Quicken* in France, the interface had to be redesigned to use an image other than that of a check, familiar to United States users, but much less widely used in France (p. 77).

There's no escaping the increasing internationalization of business. Even in my area, Memphis, Tennessee—not known as a center for international business nor as a destination for immigrants to the United States—we feel the effects of the changing world. One local writer, Steve Gillespie, has recently moved from rewriting installation manuals for Korean-made escalators at Dover Elevator Company to working with Japanese managers and writing user instructions for Brother typewriters. Federal Express, a major employer in the area with its home office here, has gone international in a big way (even changing its name to FedEx, partly because it's more pronounceable for non-English speakers) and regularly trains employees for transfer overseas. We even have an International MBA program, one of many springing up around the country, in which American students take intensive language instruction and do internships abroad while international students study English and intern locally.

The signing of NAFTA, the APEC agreement with Asian countries, and the GATT treaty with Europe mean that new opportunities, and challenges, will open up for many industries all across the country. With increasing exports comes increasing need for documentation, manuals, and instructional materials of all kinds, from the simplest to the most complex. (Remember the story of Kellogg's Corn Flakes in England? Nobody bought any until the company put instructions on the box for adding sugar and milk.) Those who sell their skills in communicating for a living need to be prepared to meet the new challenges and take advantage of the opportunities.

Members of the technical and professional writing community generally agree that there is a need to:

- Raise awareness of the differences in communication styles and strategies across national and cultural boundaries.
- Demonstrate sensitivity to those cultures and avoid implications that we are measuring other cultures by our own or that we are trying to manipulate members of the other cultures.
- Avoid the cultural imperialism implicit even in such statements as "people are really all alike underneath," because this statement often means "people are just like me, want the same things I want, and will eventually learn to get them the same way I do, therefore I can just continue to do things the way I always have."

The question, of course, is how to do that? The danger is falling back on "tips" on international communication ("this is how the Japanese write a business letter" or "here's what a French computer manual looks like"), when those may not be the best models and certainly may reflect only the choices made by one writer in one particular context. What is needed is a framework for looking at cultures, a framework that will help technical communicators make reasonable hypotheses about how members of the culture will communicate and how they will receive and interpret attempts at communication.

In the rest of this chapter, I will review briefly what is known about technical and business writing in other cultures, then attempt to set up a preliminary framework—based on concepts from anthropology, sociology, history, political science, and economics—through which communicators can better analyze culturally diverse audiences to make informed communication choices.

Concepts from Linguistics

Contrastive Rhetoric

Much of what we know about international and intercultural communications comes from an area of linguistic study called contrastive rhetoric. People engaged in contrastive rhetoric research look at how members of various cultures accomplish certain communication tasks. They look at such features of a text as its pattern of organization, length, phrasing, and format. They are also interested in how members of different cultures accomplish specific speech acts such as persuasion or requests.

One problem with contrastive rhetoric is that it deals with individual documents, thereby making generalization difficult and risky. Also, to analyze a text and make reasonable assumptions about what is going on in it, the researcher must have not only a great facility with the language, but also a depth of understanding of the culture that is rare even in linguists. Many of the contrastive rhetoric studies in the literature were done using texts written by nonnative speakers of English in their English classes. While these texts reveal differences from the way native speakers of English would write, it's tricky to separate what features remain from the native language and what is the result of previous learning about English. It's also difficult to make statements about how other members of the culture would handle a similar communication task even in English because individual styles within a culture may vary depending on whether the writer was educated in another country (often Britain, the United States, or France) or whether the country was recently a colony, in which case the writing style typical of the colonizing culture may be found side by side with the native style (Eggington, 1987).

Here's a sampling of what contrastive rhetoric teaches about documents in different cultures:

- In France, business documents such as proposals and reports tend to include more detailed information, statistics, and technical specifications in the body of the text than do American documents. On the other hand, business correspondence may include few details. Business transactions are often based on trust developed through long-term relationships between companies, so correspondence can use the kind of "shorthand" commonly found in communications between individuals who know each other well (Hall & Hall, 1990, p. 23).
- German documents tend to include considerable elaboration on the history of the organizations and their business relations (Hall & Hall, 1990, p. 35).
- Some cultures, including the Japanese, often prefer a narrative organization in business documents, which can place the main point of the text near the end rather than at the beginning, as is preferred in United States business documents (Haneda & Shima, 1982).
- Japanese writing tends to be writer-oriented (that is, designed to express the thoughts and feelings of the writer) while United States writing is reader-oriented (that is, with emphasis placed on the needs and wants of the reader). Chinese writing may be changing from writer-oriented to reader-oriented (Hinds, 1987). Traditional Chinese texts of all kinds use extensive imagery and discourage the intrusion of the individual (Shen, 1989).
- Many cultures, including the French (Hall & Hall, 1990, pp. 103–104) and some African cultures (Boiarsky, 1995), value sophisticated, complex linguistic structures as reflective of a high level of education and competence in their fields. The short, simple sentences often favored by Americans may be viewed in these cultures as the product of carelessness or ignorance.
- Writing in Middle Eastern cultures traditionally does not focus on cause and effect relationships as much as writing in Western cultures (Liebman-Kleine, 1986).
- What counts as evidence to prove a point or to persuade varies from culture to culture: repetition and citation of authority in the Middle East (Liebman-Kleine, 1986), appeals to the emotion in Latin countries (Hall & Hall, 1990).
- Preference for graphics varies; some research indicates that certain types of graphics (three-tone drawings, line drawings, color photographs, etc.) may be processed better by members of some cultures than others (Sukaviriya & Moran, 1990), colors may carry different connotations (red versus green for warnings, for example) or evoke different feelings (del Galdo, 1990, p. 7), and

ambiguity in images may be better tolerated by some cultures than is typical of Americans (Heba, 1994).

For more information on these findings from contrastive rhetoric, the reader should consult the work of researchers such as Ulla Connor, Robert Kaplan, and Ilona Leki. I have also discussed the issues mentioned above at greater length elsewhere (Thrush, 1993). The point I want to make here is that technical communicators can't and shouldn't wait for contrastive rhetoric researchers to examine documents from even the major cultures before the material on communicating across cultures is incorporated into professional writing classes. The texts subjected to contrastive rhetoric research represent a particular communicator in a particular organization at a particular point in time. There are obviously individual differences within cultures as well due, for instance, to the influence of "corporate cultures." Also, communication styles change with time; many English language programs in Asia are beginning to use American business writing texts, and a recent British text, *International Business English* by Leo Jones and Richard Alexander (1989), espouses principles strikingly closer to current American style than to traditional British business writing.

Masculinity versus Femininity

From linguistics, technical communication also got the concepts of masculinity and femininity in communication styles. According to the ways men and women communicate in mainstream United States culture, masculine style is defined as confrontational and assertive while feminine style is consensus-seeking, more intuitive, and emotional. Cross-cultural research shows that in some countries the "feminine" style of communication is widespread and characteristic of business and political negotiations, while in others the "masculine" style is prevalent (Dorfman, 1994). The Netherlands and France, for example, rank on the feminine side of the scale, while the United States and, perhaps surprisingly, Japan fall on the masculine side (Hofstede, 1993). Surprisingly, because the Japanese are known for seeking consensus, but their communication style is certainly not emotional or intuitive. The implications of this for designers and writers of technical and business communications are clear. The direct, unelaborated style of American business writing with its emphasis on facts and statistics is directly related to the dominance of the masculine style in our business environment.

Concepts from Anthropology

High versus Low Context

Anthropologists classify cultures on a continuum from high context to low context. In a high-context culture, the members share a great deal of information because of a common education, religion, ethnic background, and so on. In a high-context culture, writers and speakers do not need to give extensive details or to give much support for their opinions because they can assume that the audience shares their values and attitudes. A low-context culture, on the other hand, is one in which the members have differing religious, ethnic, and educational backgrounds, so the writer must work hard to make sure that analogies are clear, details are inclusive, and sufficient support is included to persuade someone who comes to the text with entirely different assumptions about the world and how it works. The United States is an excellent example of a low-context culture, which explains why good business writing contains all relevant details and is explicit in expressing what the writer wants the reader to do. Take, for example, this letter from an insurance company to an insured individual who has just bought a new car:

> Enclosed is the application on your new Nissan Altima. Please sign this at the bottom where indicated in yellow, and return the form to our office with a check for $60.17. A stamped return envelope is enclosed for your convenience.

Not a word is wasted, and the reader is left with no doubt about what to do next.

Most contrastive rhetoric texts that contrast documents from a high-context culture to documents from a low-context culture point out that members of high-context cultures are irritated by instructions such as those in the example above. They feel that their intelligence is in question and that the writer is being condescending. Because most of the researchers are American and their purpose is often to show Americans how to communicate better with other cultures, less has been written about the reverse effects. One exception is a case study in Andrews and Andrews' *Business Communication* (1992) that describes an interaction between an American and a Japanese company. After a face-to-face meeting where they set a schedule for a number of shipments, the representatives of the two firms returned to their countries. As the time for the first shipment approached, the Americans became concerned because they hadn't heard anything from the Japanese. Eventually they sent a fax that said, in essence, "Do you still plan to ship on time? *Please respond.*" The Japanese were puzzled—why should there be any question about whether they were keeping to the schedule? The problem was that the Japanese assumed there was no need for further communication as long as everything proceeded as planned, while the Americans expected to receive updates and confirmations. The lack of a continual flow of communication caused considerable anxiety among the low-context Americans.

I saw the same principle at work recently when I acted as United States contact for a Summer Institute in languages and the Teaching of English as a Foreign Language to be held in the Czech Republic. I sent out information on the program, but people had to write or fax the administrators of the program directly. Most received an initial confirmation that they were registered for the program. Some received an information packet with a housing request form; other didn't because of the vagaries of international mail. When the applicants called me, I was usually able to confirm that the administrators knew they were coming because I was in e-mail contact with a colleague who was there on a Fulbright fellowship. For many, this was enough. Others, however, became extremely frustrated with the lack of communication and called or wrote me constantly, looking for reassurance. One even mailed a check to the Czech Republic as a deposit, even though the initial information specifically said that they were unable to deal with American checks and preferred people to pay with travelers' checks on arrival. (The check disappeared somewhere—either in the mail or in the hands of a Czech who didn't know what to do with it.)

The degree of frustration and even anger expressed by the (low-context) Americans was surprising and illuminating. These were people who teach students from all over the world—if they were unprepared and unwilling to cope with differences in amount and type of communications, how could others be expected to? I also learned that explaining the basis for the differences satisfied some on the surface, but never really removed the underlying discomfort. My colleague had also tried to explain to the Czechs that the Americans needed more information, but with limited success. The moral of this story seemed to be that advocating change of deep-seated, culturally determined communication patterns is risky and often unproductive, while encouraging understanding may yield only limited results.

Concepts of Time and Space

Two other concepts from anthropology that may be relevant to our study of written documents have to do with time and space. Anthropologists talk about monochronic versus polychrome cultures. In a monochronic culture, such as the mainstream United States, the members are most comfortable doing one task at a time. All of their time and attention are devoted, at least for a short period of time, to that one task. In a polychronic culture, on the other hand, members typically give attention to several activities at once. The classic example of the clash that can result from the meeting of monochronic and polychrome cultures is the business meeting during which the monochronic participants are annoyed and irritated as the polychrome participants take phone calls, talk to visitors, and generally split their attention several different ways.

In written communication, this focus on completion of one task at a time translates into a particular rhetorical style, which influences even academic writing in United States school systems. Composition classes teach that paragraphs, and essays, have one main idea, with supporting details directly related to only that idea. In other words, each essay works to accomplish one, and only one, task. The greater degree of tolerance for discussion of peripherally related ideas in the expository essays of other cultures corresponds to the degree to which members of the culture are willing to divide their time and attention among topics.

Similarly, the advice on writing business letters in American textbooks is to "get to the point quickly" (that is, state the one main idea), then give only information that is directly relevant to what you want to accomplish (do one task at a time). In other cultures, a business letter may be expected to perform social as well as business functions and thus may be more discursive.

Also, when each period of time is devoted to only one task, it becomes important to complete the task quickly to move on to the next item of business. Consequently, conciseness of expression is highly valued in monochronic cultures. A problem encountered by companies selling computer equipment and software internationally is that manuals written in the United States contain very little redundancy of information. Because strategic repetition of important points is often expected in educational materials in other cultures, including most Latin cultures (Mikelonis, 1994), this brevity works against the effectiveness of the documentation when translated.

In addition, cultures treat space differently. It is fairly widely known that members of the mainstream American culture require greater personal space than members of many other cultures. This is expressed in the distances maintained between speakers during conversations, the size of houses and apartments, and the preference for open and uncluttered work spaces. This probably also explains the American preference for large amounts of white space in business and technical documents.

Concepts from Sociology

Group-Orientation versus Individualism

Sociology looks at the behavior of people in groups. The behavior patterns revealed in this research are reflected in, and influence, communication patterns. For example, one continuum on which sociologists place cultures is that of group versus individual orientation. In group-oriented societies, everyone is a part of a group, whether that group be the family or some larger unit. The individual receives rewards from the group and is expected to contribute to the good of the group in return. This translates into loyalty to the employer, emphasis on group decisions, and rewards for conformity. In individualistic societies, individuals may still be members of family and business groups, but they are expected to achieve and survive on their own. This is manifested in "job-hopping" to advance the career, a desire for autonomy, and greater expectation for individual performance (Dorfman, 1994). The United States is placed by most sociologists at the individualistic end of this spectrum. But several of the subcultures within the United States are more group-oriented, which has often resulted in miscommunication between management and workers.

One of the ways in which this difference in orientation manifests itself in business communication is the use of the signature to assign responsibility. In American correspondence, contracts, and other documents, the signature indicates the individual who takes ultimate responsibility for the contents of the document. If an executive, for example, signs a contract containing terms that are unacceptable to the company the executive represents, that executive's job may be at risk. In Japan, on the other hand, contracts are often sealed with the company stamp rather than the signature of an individual, reflecting the fact that the terms of the contract are the result of a group decision-making process. Even though this may seem a minor point, the emphasis on individual responsibility and achievement versus the group affects all phases of business negotiations and conduct.

Competition versus Consensus

Related to the differences in orientation toward the group or the individual is the difference in focus on competition versus consensus. When people strive for individual success, they are likely to be in competition with each other. This increases the emphasis on closing the deal and making the sale. The result is the kind of assertive, self-confident style of expression advocated in American business writing texts. In consensus-seeking, group-oriented cultures, the individual is unlikely to pose as having greater abilities or intellect than others, but will strive to appear humble and self-effacing. This is evident in the samples of Japanese business letters examined by Haneda and Shima (1982) and Chinese correspondence analyzed by Halpern (1983).

It has sometimes been stated, erroneously, that Japanese has no word for "no." What is true is that the Japanese, among other consensus-seeking cultures, are reluctant to say "no" in business negotiations, both for fear of destroying the possibility of reaching consensus and from reluctance to cause another to "lose face." Much anecdotal evidence exists for the problems this causes when correspondence goes unanswered because the answer is "no" or negotiators think an agreement has been reached because no one said "no" during the discussions. However, there is a remedy for this communication problem. English teachers working with students from consensus-seeking cultures have learned not to ask questions that might force the listener into an answer that would embarrass either party. "Do you understand?" is not likely to elicit accurate information, but "Would you like me to repeat?" permits a "yes" answer that insults neither the learner nor the teacher. Even better is "Which part of the lesson would you like to go over?" Similarly, in a business negotiation, training session, or needs analysis, questions that avoid the necessity of "no" responses will be more effective and less awkward.

History, Political Science, and Economics

The political and economic history of a culture has a distinct impact on communication strategies. Think about how American business works: rewards, in the form of promotions and raises, are based on individual performance. If you get the deal signed, you get rewarded. If you don't, eventually you will probably find yourself out of a job. In recent history, this has been particularly true for management personnel as companies "down-sized." In the 1980s, an estimated 3 million managers lost their jobs. It is easy to see how the strong incentives to get the deal signed, partnered with the fear of being unemployed, led to the aggressiveness of the American business style. If time is money, and money is the way success is measured by the society, then time is too precious to waste on developing relationships with business contacts or indeed on any activity that does not directly lead to increased profits.

In many other countries, including Japan and most of Western and Eastern Europe, instability of employment has not been the case. Employees were seldom fired, and promotions came with seniority, not performance. Also, the net of social services in these countries made the specter of unemployment considerably less frightening. Successful business dealings were still a goal, but there was less pressure to conduct business quickly. According to Robert Samuelson (1992, p. 48), a *Newsweek* analyst, "[G]enerous welfare benefits make it easier for people to survive without work. . . . In 1991, about 6 percent of unemployed Americans had been without a job for more than a year; in Europe, the comparable figure was 46 percent."

There are indications that this is changing. Articles in the European press in the past few years have discussed the need for greater flexibility in hiring, firing, and reassigning employees. Still, most attempts to reform employment practices are met with resistance and, at times, demonstrations and strikes.

The Central and Eastern European countries are in the process of change from a heavily socialized system, in which there were few rewards for individual achievement, but also few penalties for inefficiency or incompetence, to a market economy. Most of these nations have not yet reached a final determination on how much social support will be offered. Already, however, employers and managers have had to learn to give more specific information on business transactions and employment conditions than was true in the days when all these items were determined centrally, by the government, and everyone understood what prices could be charged and how much labor was worth (Hall & Thrush, 1992).

The effect of this difference on communication styles is understandable. If your job is not on the line every morning when you report to work, you are more likely to devote time and energy to long-term goals rather than to turning an immediate profit. Considerable anecdotal evidence exists of American companies losing major contracts because they rushed the negotiations or presented a written proposal, with its emphasis on bottom-line costs and profits, without establishing an interpersonal relationship of trust beforehand and without taking into consideration the values and goals of the foreign organization. On the other hand, where international business arrangements have been successfully completed, as in the opening of McDonald's in the Soviet Union (Puffer & Vikhansky, 1994) or Toys 'R Us in Japan and Europe ("The World," 1992), they have usually resulted from years of negotiation and study of local conditions.

Another effect of the political system seems to be the institutionalization of hierarchy. When political systems and business organizations are highly stratified, that structure is reflected in the communication style, especially in the maintenance of distance between reader and writer. It has often been noted that the Japanese language contains a system of particles that, added to words, indicates precise degrees of status between the reader and writer.

Although few other languages have such a finely tuned way of reflecting hierarchy as this, distance is often maintained by formality and impersonality of tone. Or, as an Argentinian commented, "The more closely you approach a dictatorship, the more formal the language becomes" (Boiarsky, 1995). In contrast, the more open, democratic style of American business is reflected in the friendly tone and "you" perspective prevalent in documents, from memos to proposals to operation manuals.

The Multicultural Workforce

As little as we know about technical communication in other countries, it is startling how little research has been done on subcultures within the United States, especially in light of the fact that they are expected to make up 21–25 percent of the workforce by the year 2000. This includes African-Americans, Hispanic-Americans, and Asian-Americans as the largest groups of American-born minorities. The fact that little research has been done on the rhetorical styles of these groups (aside from some discussion of the language of sermons in African-American churches) is probably partly political. Discussion of whether a distinctive Black English vernacular exists has been highly controversial, with objections that the proponent supporting the existence of such a dialect were primarily white (Wolfram, 1990).

However, the problems raised by culturally patterned variances in communication style are widely recognized. The July 1994 issue of the *Journal of Business and Technical Communication* was devoted to articles on workplace diversity, most of them documenting difficulties experienced by companies with increasingly diverse workforces or implementing human resource policies fostering diversity.

Nasreen Rahim (1994) of the Institute for Business and Community Development in the San Jose/Evergreen Community College District teaches courses in workplace English and communication skills for companies in her area. In addition to vocabulary and basic grammar, she has discovered that her students need to learn how to be "politely assertive." That is, they need to be able to communicate with supervisors, particularly about equipment needs and safety concerns, and to learn how to persist until their concerns are heard. She concentrates on the use of expressions such as "could you" and "would you." These expressions moderate questions in English to make them more polite, and they are used much more extensively in English than their equivalents in other languages.

There are programs like Ms. Rahim's all over the United States, but they address almost exclusively the needs of immigrants in low-skill jobs. At the more highly skilled and management levels, many companies provide courses in writing or in making presentations; however, these are seldom focused on the problems caused by cultural differences. Seminars in diversity training address issues of culturally determined behavior and informal, oral communication differences, based on work done by researchers in the field of organizational behavior. But few researchers have looked specifically at differences in writing strategies or the processing of texts in subcultures of the United States. In fact, it is hard to find in the literature any acknowledgment that we need to understand these processes to produce effective technical documents and training materials for workplaces that include members of these subcultures. The need for research in this area is urgent; overcoming the political problems of getting funding and access will not be easy.

Conclusion

At the 1st Annual Conference on International Communications, held in Ames, Iowa, in the summer of 1994, two questions were raised that may be unanswerable at this point. Do certain principles of communication, whether from traditional rhetorical theory or from reading research, cut across cultural, national, and organizational differences? Should they be taught universally? One problem with the principles we normally teach in our classrooms is that they are all based on Western culture, whether we are teaching rhetorical principles from Aristotle to Bruffee, or relating research on how readers process texts. All that research was performed on American readers. Are the writing strategies that were successful with those readers successful because they corresponded with the expectations of Western readers or because all brains process text the same way? For example, cognitive linguists claim that readers of English expect to find some kind of statement of the main idea of a text at the end of the first paragraph in a short text, or by the end of the second or third paragraph in a longer text. Is that because American readers are accustomed to seeing main ideas in those locations? Until research can tell us whether members of other cultures process texts in the same way, we cannot be sure even that what we know about the advantages of headings, white space, and active verbs holds true for all audiences in all environments.

Some evidence has been found for similar argumentative structures across some European and American writing, including problem to solution organization, similar means of asserting and justifying claims, and awareness of audience (Connor & Kaplan, 1987). But this study did not examine more disparate cultures to see if those structures also existed in non-Western texts. Then how do we know what to teach to prepare students for the multicultural and international workplace they will be entering? As Nancy Allen (1994) pointed out recently in *Technical Communication Quarterly*, we need to do more than give students formulaic rules for making decisions in their writing. We can do this by referring to research that "illustrates the interactive nature of reading by describing ways in which readers draw on their own backgrounds, values, and communities to create meaning as they respond to verbal, visual, and cultural cues in the text before them" (p. 351). While most of the currently available workplace-based research does not deal with multicultural and international issues, we can enrich our examination of this research with the framework I've suggested in this essay for identifying the values and communities of a wide variety of possible audiences.

REFERENCES

Allen, N. (1994). Review of four technical writing textbooks. *Technical Communication Quarterly, 3,* 351–356.

Andrews, D. C. & Andrews, W. D. (1992). *Business communication.* (2nd Ed.). New York: Macmillan.

Boiarsky, C. (1995). The relationship between cultural and rhetorical conventions: Engaging in international communication. *Technical Communication Quarterly,* 4, 245–259.

Connor, U. & Kaplan, R. B. (Eds.). (1987). *Writing across languages: Analysis of the L2 text.* Reading, MA: Addison-Wesley.

del Galdo, E. (1990). Internationalization and translation: Some guidelines for the design of human-computer interfaces. In J. Nielson (Ed.), *Designing user interfaces for international use* (pp. 1–10). New York: Elsevier.

Dorfman, P. (1988). *Advances in international comparative management.* (Vol. 3). JAI Press. (Reprinted in D. Marcic & S. M. Puffer [Eds.]. [1994], *Management international: Cases, exercises, and readings* [pp. 151–157]. St.Paul, MN: West Publishing).

Eggington, W. G. (1987). Written academic discourse in Korean: Implications for effective communication. In U. Connor & R. B. Kaplan (Eds.), *Writing across languages: Analysis of the L2 text* (pp. 153–168). Reading, MA: Addison-Wesley.

Europe's software debacle. (1994, November 12–18). *The Economist,* 77–78.

Ferraro, G. P. (1994). *The cultural dimension of international business.* (2nd Ed.). Englewood Cliffs, NJ: Prentice Hall.

Haight, Robert. (1991). *Infusing a global perspective into business communications courses: From rhetorical strategies to cultural awareness.* Unpublished Manuscript.

Hall, C. & Thrush, E. A. (1992, May 10). *Technical communications in eastern Europe.* 39th Annual Conference of the Society for Technical Communication. Atlanta, GA.

Hall, E. T. & Hall, M. R. (1990). *Understanding cultural differences.* Yarmouth, MA: Intercultural Press.

Halpern, J. W. (1983). Business communication in China: A second perspective. *Journal of Business Communication, 20,* 43–54.

Haneda, S. & Shima, H. (1982). Japanese communication behavior as reflected in letter writing. *Journal of Business Communication 19,* 19–32.

Heba, G. (1994, July 30). After words: A rhetoric of international multimedia communication. InterComm, '94, Ames, IA.

Hinds, J. (1987). Reader vs. writer responsibility: A new typology. In U. Connor & R. B. Kaplan (Eds.), *Writing across languages: Analysis of the L2 text* (pp. 141–152). Reading, MA: Addison-Wesley.

Hofstede, G. H. (1993). Cultural constraints in management theories. *The Executive, 7,* 81–94.

Jones, L. & Alexander, R. (1989). *International business English.* Cambridge, UK: Cambridge University Press.

Kaplan, R. B. (1966). Cultural thought patterns in intercultural education. *Language Learning 16,* 1–20.

Lathan, M. G. (1982). Internationalizing business communication. *Mid-South Business Journal, 2,* 16–18.

Leki, I. (1991). Twenty-five years of contrastive rhetoric: Text analysis and writing pedagogies. *TESOL Quarterly, 25* (1), 123–143.

Liebman-Kleine, J. (1986). *Towards a contrastive new rhetoric – A rhetoric of process.* Teachers of English to Speakers of Other Languages. 20th Annual Meeting, Atlanta, GA.

Mikelonis, V. (1994, July 30). Rhetoric of transition in central and eastern Europe. InterCom '94, Ames, IA.

Puffer, S. M. & Vikhansky, O. S. (1993). Management education and employee training at Moscow McDonald's. *European Management Journal, 11,* 102–107. (Reprinted in D. Marcic & S. M. Puffer [Eds.]. [1994], *Management international: Cases, exercises, and readings* [pp. 151–157]. St.Paul, MN: West Publishing).

Rahim, N. (1994, July 30). *Linguistic and cultural diversity on practical, on-the-job problems and changing roles in teaching and training communication skills.* 1st Annual Conference on International Communications, Ames, IA.

Samuelson, R. J, (1992, March 23). The gloom behind the boom. *Newsweek*, 48.
Shen, F. (1989). The classroom and the wider culture: Identity as key to learning English composition. *College Composition and Communication, 40*, 459–466.
Sprung, R. C. (1990). Two faces of America: Polyglot and tongue-tied. In J. Nielson (Ed.), *Designing interfaces for international use* (pp. 71–101). New York: Elsevier.
Sukaviriya, P. & Moran, L. (1990). User interface in Asia. In J. Nielson (Ed.), *Designing interfaces for international use* (pp. 189–218). New York: Elsevier.
Thrush, E. (1993). Bridging the gaps: Technical communication in an international and multicultural society. *Technical Communication Quarterly, 2*, 271–285.
Wolfram, W. (1990). *Dialects and American English.* Englewood Cliffs, NJ: Prentice Hall.
The World "S" Ours. (1992, March 23). *Newsweek*, 46–47.

25 Feminist Theory and the Redefinition of Technical Communication

MARY M. LAY

In her foundational essay, Lay asks and answers the question "How has technical communication been affected by feminist theory and gender studies?" Based on the work of others on the issue of scientific objectivism and the integration and adoption of naturalistic, ethnographic studies, she proposes an important "affiliation for technical communication and feminist theory" (p. 429 in this volume). The essay is valuable reading for anyone, but particularly for those who have little background in feminist theory. Lay explains the characteristics of feminist theory, outlines three important issues of debate among feminists, and then assesses the impact of feminist theory on technical communication. Equally valuable is her discussion about the uses and appropriateness of ethnography to technical communication, particularly because of the collaborative nature of communication in the field. Her discussion of gender roles and the issue of conflict is also useful. Lay believes that the work of feminist theorists "can show how these conflicts may be affected by gender roles" (p. 442), leading to new models of collaboration, which will result in more effective industrial processes and communications.

Technical communication scholars take an interdisciplinary approach to their field. In addition to theories and methodologies from linguistics, speech communication, literature, anthropology, science, and rhetoric, feminist theory and subsequent gender studies now also influence technical communication research, as well as other disciplines. Women's experiences have become legitimate subjects for study: Women researchers acknowledge their distinct interests as they generate knowledge, social structures have been scrutinized for sexual bias, and scholars have identified women's ways of knowing, communicating, and leading (see Gilligan; Belenky et al.; Helgesen, all of which attempt to describe the distinct ways in which women make ethical decisions, determine knowledge, and manage others).

How then has technical communication—either directly or through its affiliation with these other disciplines—been affected by feminist theory and

From *Journal of Business and Technical Communication* 5, no. 4 (October 1991): 348–70.

gender studies? Defined initially as the objective transfer of information, technical communication has long been privileged in its affiliation with science and technology. Now, however, feminist scholars expose the scientific positivist and androcentric bases for scientific objectivity. The studies from these scholars show the need for a redefinition of technical communication.

Moreover, in the 1980s and 1990s, technical communication has adapted ethnography, an anthropological research method, to explore workplace environments. The most recent ethnographic studies in technical communication parallel the concerns of feminist scholars by acknowledging the subjective point of view of the researcher, looking for messages as well as silences and gaps within communities, and emphasizing group values and lived experience.

The subject of these ethnographic studies in technical communication has often been collaborative writing. Again, feminist theory has much to offer technical writing researchers and teachers in analyzing successful collaboration. Particularly, psychological studies and object-relations theory reveal the familial and cultural roots of women's strong psychological connections with others, and scholars describe the strategies that women frequently use to encourage that closeness. These strategies, if made available to all members of a collaborative writing team, should encourage effective collaboration.

In this essay, I explore how current views of scientific objectivism and the adoption of ethnographic studies—particularly those of collaborative writing—necessitate a new and, perhaps, revolutionary affiliation for technical communication and feminist theory. Although many scholars mentioned in this essay would readily call themselves *feminists* – those who recognize and wish to correct the unequal treatment of women in our culture—even those who may not feel comfortable with this feminist label have conducted work that exposes sexual inequality. To frame this exploration, I first discuss six common characteristics of feminist theory, as well as three issues that divide feminists. These characteristics and issues from the work of feminist literary theorists, the object-relations area of psychology, and feminist critiques of science will be evident in new definitions of technical writing.

CHARACTERISTICS OF FEMINIST THEORY

Although feminist theorists resist uniformity of definition and methodology, a survey of their theories reveals six common characteristics:

1. celebration of difference
2. theory activating social change
3. acknowledgment of scholars' backgrounds and values
4. inclusion of women's experiences
5. study of gaps and silences in traditional scholarship
6. new sources of knowledge—perhaps a benefit of the five characteristics above

Discussing the characteristics of feminist theory is difficult. Feminist theorists are often suspicious of traditional studies within history, literature, psychology, and science, because, if these traditional studies address women at all, they portray them as Woman or Other. Feminist theorists then resist a uniform definition of feminist studies to avoid stereotyping women in their roles as scholars or research subjects. According to de Lauretis, feminist studies must be "absolutely flexible and readjustable, from women's own experience of difference, or our difference from Woman and of the difference among women," and this is a shift to the more complex notion that the female subject is a "site of differences," rather than a subject defined by sexual difference (14). Thus feminists see any unified image of women as reductive: "Instead, having been constrained and divided by definitions imposed upon us by others, we tend to value autonomy and individual development. Definitions, whether formulated by feminists or not, threaten to divide us" (Meese 73; see also Delmar 9). Moreover, according to Harding, not only have traditional theories made it "difficult to understand women's participation in social life, or to understand men's activities as gendered," but also traditional theories "systematically exclude the possibility that women could be 'knowers' or *agents of knowledge*" ("Introduction" 3). Thus the first characteristic of feminist theory becomes resistance to definition and a celebration of diversity.

For many feminists, the insistence on diversity consequently becomes a political or activist stance—the second common characteristic of feminist theory. As Harding stated, in resisting a search for "the one, true story of human experience," feminism may avoid replicating the tendency in the patriarchal theories to "police thought by assuming that only the problems of *some* women are reasonable ones" ("Instability" 284–85). For many, this insistence on diversity is consistent with the larger women's movement (see Kolodny 162). Put simply by Weedon, "Feminism is a politics. It is a politics directed at changing existing power relations between women and men in society" (1). Feminist theorists recognize that change will bring positive aspects to women's lives. More specifically, theorists such as Delmar believe that at the

> very least a feminist is someone who holds that women suffer discrimination because of their sex, that they have specific needs which remain negated and unsatisfied, and that the satisfaction of these needs would require a radical change (some would say a revolution even) in the social, economic, and political order. (8)

Most recently, *standpoint* feminist theorists "attempt to move us toward the ideal world by legitimating and empowering the 'subjugated knowledge' of women" (Harding, "Instability" 295–96). Thus the second characteristic of feminist theory is the assumption that new knowledge about women's lives will change and improve those lives—the personal is political.

If feminist criticism and theory are political, the reader should be aware of the feminist writer and feminist critic's beliefs and values. Thus the acknowledgment of scholars' backgrounds and values is the third demand of feminist theory. Moi found this characteristic "one of the fundamental assumptions of any feminist critic to date"; the feminist critic should "supply the reader with all necessary information about the limitations of one's own perspective at the outset" (43–44; see also Kaplan 40). This third feature of feminism places the researcher on the same plane as the subject, particularly within science. According to Harding, "the class, race, culture, and gender assumptions, beliefs, and behaviors of the researcher her/himself must be placed within the frame of the picture that she/he attempts to paint" ("Introduction" 9). This admission comes closer to true, rather than simply asserted, objectivity. As Harding stated,

> We need to avoid the "objectivist" stance that attempts to make the researcher's cultural beliefs and practices invisible while simultaneously skewering the research objects beliefs and practices to the display board. . . . Introducing this "subjective" element into the analysis in fact increases the objectivity of the research and decreases the "objectivism" which hides this kind of evidence from the public. ("Introduction" 9)

Revealing the characteristics of the researcher not only helps eliminate bias, but also places the researcher on a more equal level with the subject of the study.

A unique appreciation of both audience and subject further motivates feminists to reveal their own beliefs and behaviors. Feminist research will be *used* by the audience, because it will "provide for women explanations of social phenomena that they want and need" (Harding, "Introduction" 8). To determine these explanations, the subject matter of feminist research is women's experiences—the fourth characteristic among feminist theorists. Feminists see a definite relation between experience and discourse. "One distinctive feature of feminist research," according to Harding, "is that it generates its problematics from the perspective of women's experience. It also uses these experiences as a significant indicator of the 'reality' against which hypotheses are tested" ("Introduction" 7). The audience of feminist scholarship benefits from linking literature to life, from texts that engage in "nurturing personal growth and raising the individual consciousness" (Moi 43). This encouragement to test text against experience also reveals what is missing within other discourses and theories. "When we begin inquiries with women's experiences instead of men's," said Harding, "we quickly encounter phenomena (such as emotional labor and the positive aspects of 'relational' personality structures) that were made invisible by the concepts and categories of these theories" ("Instability" 284). Thus feminist critics relate to their audiences by acknowledging their own backgrounds, by investigating experiences that their audiences have, and by inviting their audiences to test feminist investigations against their own experience.

Seeking the gaps or silences within traditional scholarship—the fifth characteristic of feminist theory—relates to this appreciation of women's experiences. Gaps or silences have been examined in two ways: the identity of the missing and the potential nature of the study had the missing been included. Feminist critics who seek the identity of the missing must decide if deconstruction is helpful, particularly Derridean *difference*. According to Meese, the deconstructive critic "seeks to temporalize or negate the stasis of 'difference' as a structure of paired opposites inscribed and reinscribed forever in a fixed power relationship within a closed system" (80). The deconstructive process opens the gaps in the structure to reveal what women's natures might be if not defined in terms of the opposite of men. Feminist critics, whether in science, literature, psychology, or other disciplines, also speculate what their disciplines might have studied and what methods and discoveries might be sanctioned if women had been included in these disciplines.

Had women been empowered as critics, as audiences, and as sources of experience throughout the histories of the disciplines, they might have established new theories of knowledge and reality—a sixth common characteristic of feminist theory. Feminists acknowledge that what constitutes self-image is not just a matter of personal experience, but that image is "interpreted or reconstructed by each of us within the horizon of meanings and knowledges available in the culture at given historical moments" (de Lauretis 8). If women's experiences had contributed to those meanings and knowledges, women would have been a source of knowledge, of what culture determines as reality, and of what scholars canonize. Feminists have struggled with the power of the canon. Canonization, said Kolodny, "puts any work beyond questions of establishing its merit and, instead, invites students to offer only increasingly more ingenious readings and interpretations, the purpose of which is to validate the greatness already imputed by canonization" (150). By asserting that women are subjects or sources of knowledge, rather than objects of study as Other or Woman, feminists empower women and change definitions of reality or canonized texts. Feminism, stated Delmar, transforms women "from object of knowledge into a subject capable of appropriating knowledge, to effect a passage from the state of subjection to subjecthood" (25). Feminism then can ultimately initiate changes not only in political, social, and economic structures but also in sources of knowledge.

Issues in Feminist Theory

Before assessing the impact that these six characteristics of feminist theory have on new definitions of technical communication, I must acknowledge three issues of debate among feminists, because technical communication scholars may have to decide where they stand on those issues:

1. Should feminists emphasize similarities or differences among men and women?
2. Should these differences be located in cultural or biological traits?
3. Should these first two issues promote or displace binary opposition?

The first issue of debate involves whether women should emphasize their differences from men or their similarities to men. Should women try to take on traditionally defined masculine traits? For example, should women in the workplace learn the language of power? Or should women celebrate what have been labeled feminine traits? For example, as Rosenthal asked, should women "insist on the 'humaneness' of typical female qualities like compassion, help, nurture, and self-sacrifice—to put these qualities into practice in their professions . . . "(66)? Or should both men and women move toward androgyny, a "non-sex-marked humanity" (66)? The French feminists, such as Cixous, Kristeva, and Irigaray, have chosen the second option to celebrate those traits that have been labeled feminine traits: Moi said that while "extolling women's right to cherish their specifically female values," the French feminists "reject 'equality' as a covert attempt to force women to become like men" (98). Any application of feminist theory to technical communication will have to struggle with the choice of emphasizing similarities or differences between men and women.

The second issue involves controversy about the origins of differences between men and women. Whether or not theorists decide to emphasize the differences or the similarities between gender traits, they recognize traits as biological, social, or a combination of both. Epstein summarized this issue within her definitions of maximalist and minimalist feminist perspectives. The maximalist holds that there are basic differences between the sexes; some proponents ascribe these differences to biology or to social conditioning, whereas others claim the differences are "lodged in the differing psyches of the sexes by the psychoanalytic processes that create identity" (25). "These scholars," said Epstein, "typically believe that differences are deeply rooted and result in different approaches to the world, in some cases creating a distinctive 'culture' of women" (25). Epstein's minimalist position contends that men and women are essentially similar. Gender differences are "superficial" because they are "socially constructed (and elaborated in the culture through myths, law, and folkways) and kept in place by the way each sex is positioned in the social structure" (25). The origin of difference affects the ease with which men or women can assume the traditional traits of the other gender—another issue of importance to the technical communication researcher.

The third issue is whether scholars can and should avoid reinforcing binary opposition in discussions of difference. Moi identified the goal of feminism to "deconstruct the death-dealing binary opposition of masculinity and feminity," for here the feminine is the negative of the masculine, always lower in the hierarchy (13). Feminists such as Epstein warn that by celebrating a woman's culture, feminists may reinforce the opposition and this hierarchy (25). On the other hand, the French feminists emphasize the differences between men and women; for example, they celebrate *jouissance,* a type of sexual and physical joy that can be experienced *only* by women, or as Jones defined it, "the direct re-experience of the physical pleasures of infancy and of later sexuality, repressed but not obliterated by the Law of the Father" (87).

These three issues of debate among feminists are highly related. Although feminist theories promote difference and resist uniform definition of feminist methodology, should they promote difference or stress similarity of experience when studying men and women? Moreover, where should the origin of difference be located, within biology or society? Finally, will the result of exploring difference promote or displace binary opposition? Again, these issues cannot be ignored when applying feminist theory to technical communication.

Redefinition of Technical Communication

These traits and issues of debate within feminist theory inform the pressure to redefine technical communication that comes from exposing the myth of scientific objectivity, adapting ethnographic research techniques, and studying collaborative writing.

The Myth of Objectivity

Traditional definitions of technical communication affiliate it with the quantitative and objective scientific method, calling technical communication a "data retrieval method" for the specialized audience (Harris 137). Redefinitions of technical communication have been influenced by composition scholars who question the classical distinction made between rhetoric and science. For example, Berlin proposed a "New Rhetoric," which acknowledges that truth is "dynamic and dialectic," and that language "creates the 'real world' by organizing it, by determining what will be perceived and not perceived, [and] by indicating what has meaning and what is meaningless" (774–75). He opposed the popular Current-Traditional Rhetoric, with its link to scientific positivism and the myth of objective reality—the assumption that truth could be discovered through the experimental or scientific method if the individual was "freed from the biases of language, society, or history" (770). Berlin, in some sense, defied the Aristotelian binary opposition of rhetoric and science.

Thus technical communication scholars such as Halloran, relating to Kuhn, admit that "in a very fundamental way," science is "argument among scientists," but that technical communication maintains the deceptive ethos of the "dispassionate, disinterested truth-seeker" (85). Miller asserted that technical communication, as commonly taught, is "shot through with positivist assumptions" ("Humanistic Rational" 613); instead, technical communication should be viewed as a matter of "conduct rather than of production, as a matter of arguing in a prudent way toward the good of the community rather than of constructing texts" ("What's Practical" 23). Samuels, reacting to Halloran, Miller, as well as Kuhn, then defined technical communication as a "recreation of reality for special purposes"; rather than transmitting or inventing reality, the communicator "extends" perceptions of truth (11). Finally, Dobrin decided that technical communication simply "accommodates technology to the user," for any claim of objectivity is based on scientific domination (242; see also Goldstein 25). As the distinctions between science and rhetoric disappear, truth is defined as agreement within a community, not as discoverable and describable reality. Technical communication then offers culturally based perceptions to the audience, rather than objective information and data.

Although gender roles are part of culture, few scholars, so far, have examined the impact of these roles on the technical communicator. Sterkel did a quantitative study that suggests that women have adopted the language of power in business writing. Smeltzer and Werbel found that the type of communication required makes more difference than does the gender of the writer, and Tebeaux discovered distinct differences among male and female inexperienced business writers. However, if new definitions of technical communication acknowledge the culturally based perceptions within scientific and technical discourse, gender studies of science and technology must change the way technical communication scholars view their field.

Over the last decade, feminist scholars have identified masculine bias within the discovery and discourse of science and technology. These biases, according to Bleier, are both the source of science's "great strength and value" and of its "oppressive power" (57). For example, in Keller's examination of the genderization of science, she traced the mythology that assigns objectivity, reason, and mind to the male, and subjectivity, feeling, and nature to the female (*Reflections* 6–7). This binary opposition limits women's experiences as valid scientific subjects, as well as prevents women from being sources of scientific knowledge. Keller concluded that in the family structure masculinity is associated with "autonomy, separation, and distance" (*Reflections* 79):

> Thus it is that for all of us—male and female alike—our earliest experiences incline us to associate the affective and cognitive posture of objectification with the masculine, while all processes that involve a blurring of the boundary between subject and object tend to be associated with feminine. (*Reflections* 87)

Keller's study of scientist Barbara McClintock's disregard for the traditional separation from her subject reveals a gender-free approach to science (*Feeling* xvii). Rather than using a static objectivity that distances scientists from their subjects, Keller proposed a dynamic objectivity that "actively draws on the commonality between mind and nature as a resource for understanding" (*Reflections* 117). Keller, Bleier, and other feminist theorists expose the biases of the scientist hidden behind the ethos of objectivity and identify women's experiences within the gaps and silences of traditional science.

The resistance toward including women's experiences and employing women as sources of knowledge is particularly strong in science. Perhaps for this reason, acknowledging the connections between feminist theory and technical communication will be difficult for many. Within science and central to the image of masculinity, according to Harding, is the "rejection of everything that is defined by culture as feminine and its legitimated control of whatever counts as feminine" (*Science* 54). In a sense, science has identified the masculine with the human and so has excluded the feminine. Also, science has tended to define femininity by biological, rather than cultural, traits. In particular, a woman's reproductive capacity is seen by science as "an immense biological burden, condemning her to the world of nature, of the body, of emotions, and subjectivity" (Fee 44). And so, many eminent scientists have concluded, as did nuclear physicist Rabi in 1982, that women are "temperamentally unsuited to science" because of their nervous systems:

> It makes it impossible for them [women] to stay with the thing. I'm afraid there's no use quarreling with it, that's the way it is. Women may go into science, and they will do well enough, but they will never do great science. (qtd. in Gornick 36)

This resistance to women's concerns carries over into technology and the social sciences. For example, Hacker found that engineers often described social sciences as womanly—"soft, inaccurate, lacking in rigor, unpredictable, amorphous" (345). She also found that engineers assign more status to areas that seemed the "cleanest, hardest, most scientific" such as electrical engineering and less status to such fields as civil engineering that were more involved in social sciences (345). In turn, the social sciences, in particular psychology, often assign higher ranking to experimentalists, seen as particularly objective and linked to *hard* science, and lower ranking to developmentalists who might have more *social* concerns. As with engineering, areas in psychology that could take on the appearance of objectivity appear at the top of the hierarchy (Sherif 41–42).

In affiliating with scientific positivism and in defining itself as the objective transfer of data, truth, and reality, traditionally defined technical communication ranks higher than other supposedly *subjective* types of writing, engages in dualistic thinking, and maintains closeness with patriarchal institutions of power. Therefore, to enhance legitimacy for their field, technical communication scholars and teachers may resist redefinition that divorces technical writing from this source of power. However, feminist theorists affect the recent redefinitions of technical communication as made by scholars such as Miller, Samuels, Dobrin, and Halloran. Feminist theorists challenge technical communicators to reevaluate their fields by exposing the masculine bias of science and technology, insisting that women cease to be the object and instead become the subject of science, and defying the dualism of masculine/feminine, objective/subjective, and culture/nature. This revision, I believe, will be most useful as technical communication scholars employ ethnographic studies, particularly those that study collaborative writing.

Ethnographic Studies

With the current emphasis on both the social nature of writing and the ways in which a discourse community produces documents, ethnographic methods have been adopted by technical communication scholars. To use ethnographic methods, technical communicators must study what constitutes a discourse community, what and why interactions take place within that community, what texts are produced, what subjects are considered appropriate within those texts, how genres are evolved, and how methods of inquiry are chosen and approved (Faigley 241). Ethnography is also appropriate because of the interdisciplinary nature of technical communication:

> Because those of us teaching business and technical communication possess a wide range of disciplinary training—from linguistics to literature to business education to computerized-document design, we can bring a multidisciplinary perspective to ethnographic research. (Halpern 30)

The cultures that technical communication ethnographers study within the industrial setting and their respect for subjects "who are, in some ways, far more expert and knowledgeable than are the ethnographers" are most essential to this ethnographic research (Doheny-Farina and Odell 507); in technical communication ethnographies, there is no Other. The technical communication audience tests what the ethnographer says against subjects' own experiences.

Parallels between ethnography and feminism include multiplicity, acknowledgment of the researcher's values and background, appreciation of lived experience and new sources of knowledge, and discovery—rather than testing—of meaning. Kantor's five characteristics of communication ethnography include these parallels: (a) contextuality, (b) researcher as participant-observer, (c) multiple perspectives, (d) hypothesis generating, and (e) meaning making (72–74). Because ethnography stresses that behavior is expressed and influenced by the groups and the cultures to which individuals belong, the ethnographer spends long periods of time within a community to get detailed, concrete records of that community's behavior, including language and communication. The ethnographer's perceptions become part of the record: "Typically researchers begin by assessing their own knowledge, experiences, and biases, and reevaluate those influences as their study proceeds" (73). This stance of being both participant and observer can be called "disciplined subjectivity" (73).

Ethnographers use triangulation or more than one means of record keeping—sometimes a combination of interviews, field notes, and diaries—and seek the reactions from other researchers or community members to enhance their interpretations. Within their observations, ethnographers generate rather than test hypotheses; they may develop more research questions than they answer. The purpose of ethnography is "to look at ways in which individuals construct their own realities and shared meanings" (Kantor, Kirby, and Goetz 298).

In ethnographic thick description, the researcher, much like the feminist scholar, records the daily details of community life. The ethnographer then discovers within this detail the meanings and values that people, not just those with power, attribute to phenomena. By triangulation, the ethnographer seeks multiple impressions; the feminist theorist in turn finds multiplicity essential in integrating women, not Woman, into the world picture. Much like feminist theorists, the ethnographic observer-participants examine and admit their own background and cultural bias, including their gender roles within the observed community and the audience of the ethnographic description.

Ethnographers share with feminist theorists the goal of understanding rather than evaluating a community, seeking new meanings within previous gaps and silences, and finding new sources for that knowledge. "Ethnography attempts to bring stories not yet heard to the attention of the academy," concluded Brodkey (48).

In addition to including women's lives in their studies, female ethnographers have speculated recently about the ways their sex affects their assimilation into a community and their consequent research. Again, ethnographic narratives in general "jeopardize the positivist campaign to deny anyone's lived experience, in the name of objectivity" (Brodkey 41). However, female ethnographers face recurring issues, such as protective behavior triggered by their sex and the great difference between their own life-styles and those of the women they study (Golde; Warren; Whitehead and Conaway).

Feminist traits are inherent in contemporary ethnographic methodology. Ethnographers reject the received view within social science, as Agar defined it, "a view that centers on the systematic test of explicit hypotheses"; ethnography does not claim that anyone using the same methods would come to the same conclusions (11). At the least, ethnographers' varied backgrounds and intended audiences cause different conclusions. The traditional scientific hierarchy between researcher and subject is abolished, and connections are sought:

> Ethnographers set out to show how social action in one world makes sense from the point of view of another. Such work requires an intensive personal involvement, an abandonment of traditional scientific control, an improvisational style to meet situations not of the researcher's making, and an ability to learn from a long series of mistakes. (Agar 12)

Rather than seeking similarities or universals as in traditional science, the ethnographer reacts to breakdowns or differences. These breakdowns are resolved "by changing the knowledge in the ethnographer's tradition" (25), or as in feminist theory, sources of knowledge are not dictated by the power elite. In this way, ethnography has activist characteristics.

In their challenges to the received view within social science, ethnographers question binary opposition or dualistic thinking about qualitative and quantitative research. Firestone characterized ethnographers as pragmatists—as opposed to purists—and believed that ethnographers contrast quantitative researchers who assume that there are "social *facts* with an objective reality apart from the beliefs of individuals" to qualitative researchers who believe that "reality is socially constructed through individuals or collective *definitions of the situation*" (16; see also Howe). In fact, pragmatists like Goetz and LeCompte suggested that ethnography is more objective than quantitative research because ethnographers admit their subjective experiences (9; see also Hymes; Geertz; North)—a conclusion identical to Harding's. Ethnography, then, is rhetorical because ethnographers must understand and influence their audiences (see Kleine). Thus the ethnographer, again like the feminist theorist, attempts to incorporate into the canon research methods and subjects that were excluded by scientific positivism and a quantitative focus, and the ethnographer questions the binary opposition that excluded these research methods and subjects in the first place.

More particularly, the technical communication ethnographer frequently studies how editors, writers, technical developers, potential customers, and graphic artists collaborate to produce a document. Composition specialists, such as Bruffee, have for over a decade stressed the social nature of writing and questioned the image of the solitary writer. According to Bruffee, texts are "constructs generated by communities of like-minded peers" (774). Some composition researchers, in particular LeFevre, assert that the myth of the solitary writer complements a gender-biased social view: "The persistence of such an ideal of individual autonomy in male-centered, capitalistic culture further explains why a Platonic view of invention, which stresses the writer as an isolated unit apart from material and social forces, has been widely accepted" (22). Therefore, technical communication researchers must attend to how gender roles affect industrial collaborative writing.

Ethnographic studies of the workplace reveal that effective collaborators have good interpersonal skills, the ability to connect and maintain connections with collaborators even in times of conflict over ideas (see, for example, Doheny-Farina 181; Debs 3). Researchers do stress that collaborators "should be reassured that conflict over ideas, over *substantive* matters, can be a positive development in the collaborative process" (Karis 121). In addition, feminist scholars Keller and Moglen proposed, "Under certain circumstances, cooperation may actually be facilitated by differentiation and autonomy" (27). However, this substantive conflict is most productive in solid relationships in which people have developed enough trust to self-disclose and to not feel threatened by criticism. Thus Ede and Lunsford profiled effective collaborators as

> flexible; respectful of others; attentive and analytical listeners; able to speak and write clearly and articulately; dependable and able to meet deadlines; able to designate and share responsibility, to lead and to follow; open to criticism but confident in their own abilities; ready to engage in creative conflict. (66)

Feminist theorists, particularly object-relations theorists in psychology, enhance these ethnographic studies of collaborative writing, because these theorists relate how and why males and females connect and cooperate.

Collaborative Writing

Studies reveal that girls and boys in the pre-Oedipal stage of life differ in their urge to connect with or distinguish themselves from others. Because mothers still do so much of the parenting, girls identify with this main parenting figure, whereas boys identify with the father who appears independent and involved in the world outside the home. As Chodorow concluded,

> Girls emerge from this period with a basis for "empathy" built into their primary definition of self in a way that boys do not. Girls emerge with a

> stronger basis for experiencing another's need or feeling as one's own (or of thinking that one is so experiencing another's needs and feelings). (167)

Girls define themselves as "continuous with others," whereas boys define themselves as "more separate and distinct": "The basic feminine sense of self is connected with the world, the basic masculine sense of self is separate" (169). Boys may develop into men who avoid close connections because these connections threaten their sense of self, whereas girls may develop into women who seek close relationships and assume responsibility for cooperation.

Gilligan, in her study of adult ethics, stated that men may see connections as threatening to their place in the competitive work hierarchy, whereas women fear being "too far out on the edge"—too far from connections with others (43). Building on the research of Chodorow and Gilligan, Belenky and her coauthors distinguished the separate knowing of many men from the connected knowing of many women. In groups, authority or knowing for women is commonality of experience, which requires "intimacy and equality between self and object not distance and impersonality" (183). Obviously, gender roles, as established in the family structure, influence how men and women relate to the demands of collaboration—a topic of much interest to technical communicators.

Feminist theorists' elevation of women's experiences and knowledge and the feminist debate over the origin of difference inform studies of collaboration. If women more easily *connect*—a virtue when functioning on a writing team—can men learn these connecting strategies too? Minimalists, as defined by feminist theorist Epstein, would see that change as quite possible, although usually feminists have studied the ease with which women have taken on traditional male traits. Because gender roles are socially constructed—created by nurture rather than nature—they can be changed. According to Flynn, "Women share interpretive frameworks and strategies because they have had common experiences, ones different, for the most part, than those of men. Such a position is optimistic in the sense that it posits that different experiences can produce different interpretations" (4). Thus gender roles are not static.

Whether optimistic about this change or not, feminist theorists at the very least can point out *what* makes it difficult for men to balance competitive impulses with cooperative needs. Again, object-relations theorists stress basic differences in masculine and feminine self-identity and the difficulty in overcoming the effects of the family structure: "The boy's repression of the female aspect of himself is one of the reasons men find it hard to be nurturant as adults" (Flax 178). And feminist theorists, who identify themselves as practicalists—or believe that thinking arises from practices—suggest that "maternal thinking" comes from maternal practice and is accessible to all who practice it (Ruddick 13–14). Knowing why men resist connections and anticipating the effects of men's increasing participation in parenting are the first steps to overcoming this resistance.

Because of these gender roles, men's and women's attitudes toward conflict during collaboration differ. Technical communicators need to learn what feminist theorists say about these different gender roles in order to manage conflict effectively, which helps to ensure the success of collaboration. Women are taught to avoid conflict and may view all conflict as interpersonal and potentially damaging to relationships (Lay 20–22). Men tend to view conflict as healthy competition and as primarily substantive (Hocker and Wilmot 61). In resolving conflict, men and women also use different strategies: "Two males in a conflict typically employ bargaining techniques, logical arguments, and anger to manage the situation. In contrast, two females in a conflict situation focus on understanding each other's feelings" (Putnam 47–48). Again, understanding the cultural and familial origins of these differences through feminist studies is the first step toward effective collaboration.

Finally, feminist theorists can help technical communicators provide new models of effective collaboration—models that help collaborators break out of gender roles. These new models would also help collaborators value women's experiences and strategies, because these strategies include interpersonal skills. Such strategies—well documented in communication and feminist theory—include self-disclosure, sensitivity to nonverbal cues, perception of others' emotions, questioning intonations in responses, acknowledgment of previous speakers, and resolution of conflict in nonpublic ways (Knapp, Ellis, and Williams 275; Baird 192; Hall and Sandler 10; Treichler and Kramarae 120).

One of the most recent new models of collaborative writing comes from Ede and Lunsford, who recognized that a dialogic model is articulated mainly by the female technical writers they interviewed. Ede and Lunsford described the traditional model of collaboration as hierarchal, with productivity and efficiency the goal. In the traditional model, "the realities of multiple voices and shifting *authority* are seen as difficulties to be overcome or resolved" (133). On the other hand, in the dialogic model, roles are fluid, each collaborator may take on "multiple and shifting roles," and "the process of articulating goals is often as important as the goals themselves and sometimes even more important" (133). Ede and Lunsford also said, "Furthermore, those participating in dialogic collaboration generally value the creative tension inherent in multivoiced and multivalent ventures" (133). This dialogic model is predominantly feminine, "so clearly 'other,'" and Ede and Lunsford lamented that there is no "ready language" to describe it (133). However, feminist theorists could supply that language to Ede and Lunsford; Jordan and Surrey label the capacity to move from one perspective to another as "oscillating self-structure" (92). Although Jordan and Surrey applied the term to the mothering process, the term well represents the process that Ede and Lunsford observe in dialogic collaboration. As technical communication scholars explore the collaborative writing process, they can learn much from feminist studies.

Linking technical communication with feminist theory may seem alien to many. However, at the very least, the interdisciplinary nature of technical communication will lead the field in the direction of feminist theory. As feminist theorists attack the last vestiges of scientific positivism within science and technology, technical communication must also let go of the ethos of the objective technical writer who simply transfers information and accept that writers' values, background, and gender influence on the communication produced. As technical communicators convince their audiences to accept a version of reality, they develop persuasion strategies by identifying with their audiences. In many major corporations, technical writers are the customers' representatives and advocates and must discover the fine details of their customers' experiences.

As technical communicators explore collaborative writing through ethnographies, they again adopt stances similar to feminist theorists. Their own backgrounds and values as ethnographers must be admitted to their audiences. They must seek the many voices of those who witness and experience the culture they investigate. These technical communicators also expose the gaps and silences in previous studies and identify new sources of knowledge that may challenge dominant or traditional cultures.

The mission of most technical communication scholars is to prepare future technical writers to enter industry and to improve the industrial processes that produce communications. Because so many documents are collaboratively produced and their effectiveness threatened when collaborative teams suffer interpersonal conflicts, again the work of feminist theorists can show how these conflicts may be affected by gender roles. New models of collaboration, such as those suggested by Ede and Lunsford, recognize the effects of collaborators' gender roles.

In acknowledging these connections with feminist theory, technical communication must wrestle with the issues that confront feminist theorists. In suggesting effective collaborative strategies, should technical communicators stress the similarities or differences between men and women? In doing so, can they avoid the labeling that contributes to dualistic thinking or binary opposition? Should male collaborators know that they are being encouraged to adopt what have been labeled *female* interpersonal traits? Are the sources of these gender traits primarily social or biological? If they are social, collaborators can move more easily toward androgyny. If not, change will be more difficult. How will or how should the industrial setting be affected by these ethnographic studies of gender roles and collaborative traits? Should technical communicators become activists in industrial settings as they explore gender roles within collaboration? The answers to these questions remain for future technical communicators to discover. However, technical communication must be redefined to include these issues.

REFERENCES

Agar, Michael H. *Speaking of Ethnography*. Beverly Hills, CA Sage, 1986. Vol. 2 of *Qualitative Research Methods*. 23 vols.

Baird, John E., Jr. "Sex Differences in Group Communication: A Review of Relevant Research." *Quarterly Journal of Speech* 62.1 (1976): 179–92.

Belenky, Mary Field et al. *Women's Ways of Knowing: The Development of Self, Voice, and Mind*. New York: Basic Books, 1986.

Berlin, James A. "Contemporary Composition: The Major Pedagogical Theories." *College English* 44.8 (1982): 765–77.

Bleier, Ruth. "Lab Coat: Robe of Innocence or Klansman's Sheet. "*Feminist Studies/Critical Studies.* Ed. Teresa de Lauretis. Bloomington: Indiana University Press, 1986. 55–66.

Brodkey, Linda. "Writing Ethnographic Narratives." *Written Communication* 4.1 (1987): 25–50.

Bruffee Kenneth A. "Social Construction, Language, and the Authority of Knowledge: A Bibliographical Essay." *College English* 48.8 (1986): 773–90.

Chodorow, Nancy. *The Reproduction of Mothering: Psychoanalysis and the Sociology of Gender.* Berkeley: University of California Press, 1978.

Debs, Mary Elizabeth. "Collaborative Writing: A Study of Technical Writing in the Computer Industry." *Dissertation Abstracts International* 47 (1986): 2141A. Rensselaer Polytechnic Institute.

de Lauretis, Teresa. "Feminist Studies/Critical Studies: Issues, Terms, and Contexts." *Feminist Studies/Critical Studies.* Ed. Teresa de Lauretis. Bloomington: Indiana University Press, 1986. 1–19.

Delmar, Rosalind. "What Is Feminism?" *What Is Feminism: A Re-Examination.* Ed. Juliet Mitchell and Ann Oakley. New York: Pantheon, 1986. 8–33.

Dobrin, David. "What's Technical about Technical Writing?" *New Essays in Technical and Scientific Communication: Research, Theory, Practice.* Ed. Paul Anderson, R. John Brockmann, and Carolyn R. Miller. Farmingdale, NY: Baywood, 1983. 227–50.

Doheny-Farina, Stephen. "Writing in an Emerging Organization: An Ethnographic Study." *Written Communication* 3.2 (1986): 158–85.

Doheny-Farina, Stephen, and Lee Odell. "Ethnographic Research on Writing: Assumptions and Methodology." *Writing in Nonacademic Settings.* Ed. Lee Odell and Dixie Goswami. New York: Guilford, 1985. 503–35.

Ede, Lisa, and Andrea Lunsford. *Singular Texts/Plural Authors: Perspectives on Collaborative Writing.* Carbondale: Southern Illinois University Press, 1990.

Epstein, Cynthia Fuchs. *Deceptive Distinctions: Sex, Gender, and the Social Order.* New Haven, CT: Yale University Press; New York Russell Sage, 1988.

Faigley, Lester. "Nonacademic Writing: The Social Perspective." *Writing in Nonacademic Settings.* Ed. Lee Odell and Dixie Goswami. New York: Guilford, 1985. 231–48.

Fee, Elizabeth. "Critiques of Modern Science: The Relationship of Feminism to Other Radical Epistemologies." *Feminist Approaches to Science.* Ed. Ruth Bleier. New York: Pergamon, 1986. 42–56.

Firestone, William A. "Meaning in Method: The Rhetoric of Quantitative and Qualitative Research." *Educational Researcher* 16.7 (1987): 16–21.

Flax, Jane. "The Conflict Between Nurturance and Autonomy in Mother-Daughter Relationships and within Feminism." *Feminist Studies* 4.2 (1978): 171–89.

Flynn, Elizabeth A. "Toward a Feminist Social Constructionist Theory of Composition." Conference on College Composition and Communication. Chicago, 22 Mar. 1990.

Geertz, Clifford. *The Interpretation of Cultures: Selected Essays.* New York: Basic Books, 1973.

Gilligan, Carol. *In a Different Voice: Psychological Theory and Women's Development.* Cambridge, MA: Harvard University Press, 1982.

Goetz, Judith Preissle, and Margaret Diane LeCompte. *Ethnography and Qualitative Design in Educational Research.* New York: Academic Press, 1984.

Golde, Peggy. *Women in the Field: Anthropological Experiences.* 1970. 2nd ed. Berkeley: University of California Press, 1986.

Goldstein, Jone Rymer. "Trends in Teaching Technical Writing." *Technical Communication* 31.4 (1984): 25–34.

Gornick, Vivian. *Women in Science: 100 Journeys into the Territory.* 1983. rev. ed. New York: Simon & Schuster, 1990.

Hacker, Sally L. "The Culture of Engineering: Woman, Workplace, and Machine." *Women, Technology, and Innovation.* Ed. Joan Rothschild. New York: Pergamon, 1982. 341–53.

Hall, Roberta A., and Bernice Sandler. "The Classroom Climate: A Chilly One for Women?" Washington, DC: Project on the Status and Education of Women, Association of American Colleges, 1982.

Halloran, S. Michael "Technical Writing and the Rhetoric of Science." *Journal of Technical Writing and Communication* 8.2 (1978): 77–88.

Halpern, Jeanne W. "Getting in Deep: Using Qualitative Research in Business and Technical Communication." *JBTC* 2.2 (1988): 22–43

Harding, Sandra. "The Instability of the Analytical Categories of Feminist Theory." *Sex and Scientific Inquiry.* Ed. Sandra Harding and Jean F. O'Barr. Chicago: University of Chicago Press, 1987. 283–302.

———. "Introduction: Is There a Feminist Method?" *Feminism and Methodology*. Ed. Sandra Harding. Bloomington: Indiana University Press, 1987. 1–13.

———. *The Science Question in Feminism*. Ithaca: Cornell University Press, 1986.

Harris, John S. "On Expanding the Definition of Technical Writing." *Journal of Technical Writing and Communication* 8.2 (1978): 133–38.

Helgesen, Sally. *The Female Advantage: Women's Ways of Leadership*. New York: Doubleday, 1990.

Hocker, Joyce L., and William M. Wilmot. *Interpersonal Conflict*. Dubuque, IA: Brown, 1985.

Howe, Kenneth R. "Against the Quantitative-Qualitative Incompatibility Thesis or Dogmas Die Hard." *Educational Researcher* 17.8 (1988): 10–16.

Hymes, Dell. *Language in Education: Ethnolinguistic Essays*. Language and Ethnography Series. Washington, DC: Center for Applied Linguistics, 1980.

Jones, Ann Rosalind. "Writing the Body: Toward an Understanding of *L'ecriture Feminine*." *Feminist Criticism and Social Change: Sex, Class and Race in Literature and Culture*. Ed. Judith Newton and Deborah Rosenfelt. New York: Methuen, 1985. 86–101.

Jordan, Judith V., and Janet L. Surrey. "The Self-in-Relation: Empathy and the Mother-Daughter Relationship." *The Psychology of Today's Woman: New Psychoanalytical Visions*. Ed. Toni Bernay and Dorothy W. Cantor. Cambridge, MA: Harvard University Press, 1986. 81–104.

Kantor, Kenneth. "Classroom Contexts and the Development of Writing Intuitions: An Ethnographic Case Study." *New Directions in Composition Research*. Ed. Richard Beach and Lillian S. Bridwell. New York: Guilford, 1984. 72–94.

Kantor, Kenneth J., Dan R. Kirby, and Judith P. Goetz. "Research in Content: Ethnographic Studies in English Education." *Research in the Teaching of English* 15.4 (1981): 293–309.

Kaplan, Sydney Janet. "Varieties of Feminist Criticism." *Making a Difference: Feminist Literary Criticism*. Ed. Gayle Greene and Coppelia Kahn. New York: Methuen, 1985. 35–58.

Karis, Bill. "Conflict in Collaboration: A Burkean Perspective." *Rhetoric Review* 8.1 (1989): 113–26.

Keller, Evelyn Fox. *A Feeling for the Organism*. San Francisco: Freeman, 1983.

———. *Reflections on Gender and Science*. New Haven, CT: Yale University Press, 1985.

Keller, Evelyn Fox, and Helene Moglen. "Competition: A Problem for Academic Women." *Competition: A Feminist Taboo?* Ed. Valerie Miner and Helen E. Longino. New York: Feminist Press, 1987.

Kleine, Michael. "Beyond Triangulation: Ethnography, Writing, and Rhetoric." *Journal of Advanced Composition* 10.1 (1990): 117–25.

Knapp, Mark L., Donald G. Ellis, and Barbara A. Williams, "Perceptions of Communication Behavior Associated with Relationship Terms." *Communication Monographs* 47.4 (1980): 262–78.

Kolodny, Annette. "Dancing through the Minefield: Some Observations on the Theory, Practice, and Politics of a Feminist Literary Criticism." *The New Feminist Criticism: Essays on Women, Literature and Theory*. Ed. Elaine Showalter. New York: Pantheon, 1985. 144–67.

Kuhn, Thomas. *The Structure of Scientific Revolution*. 1962. Chicago: University of Chicago Press, 1970.

Lay, Mary M. "Interpersonal Conflict in Collaborative Writing: What We Can Learn from Gender Studies." *JBTC* 3.2 (1989): 5–28.

LeFevre, Karen Burke. *Invention as a Social Act*. Carbondale: Southern Illinois University Press, 1987.

Meese, Elizabeth. *Crossing the Double-Cross: The Practice of Feminist Criticism*. Chapel Hill: University of North Carolina Press, 1986.

Miller, Carolyn. "A Humanistic Rationale for Technical Writing." *College English* 40.6 (1979): 610–17.

———. "What's Practical about Technical Writing?" *Technical Writing: Theory and Practice*. Ed. Bertie E. Fearing and W. Keats Sparrow. New York: Modern Language Association, 1989. 14–24.

Moi, Toril. *Sexual/Textual Politics: Feminist Literary Theory*. New York: Methuen, 1985.

North, Stephen M. *The Making of Knowledge in Composition: Portrait of an Emerging Field*. Upper Montclair, NJ: Boynton/Cook, 1987.

Putnam, Linda L. "Lady You're Trapped: Breaking out of Conflict Cycles." *Women in Organizations: Barriers and Breakthroughs*. Ed. Joseph J. Pilotta. Prospect Heights, IL: Waveland, 1983. 39–53.

Rosenthal, Peggy. "Feminist Criticism: What Difference Does It Make?" *Women's Language and Style*. Ed. Douglas Buturff and Edmund L. Epstein. Proceeding of a Conference on Language and Style. 1977. Akron, OH: Department of English, University of Akron, 1987. 62–74.

Ruddick, Sara. *Maternal Thinking: Toward a Politics of Peace*. Boston: Beacon, 1989.

Samuels, Marilyn S. "Technical Writing and the Recreation of Reality." *Journal of Technical Writing and Communication* 15.1 (1985): 3–13.

Sherif, Carolyn Wood. "Bias in Psychology." *Feminism and Methodology*. Ed Sandra Harding. Bloomington: Indiana University Press, 1987. 37–56.

Smeltzer, Larry R., and James D. Werbel. "Gender Differences in Managerial Communication: Fact or Folk-Linguistics?" *Journal of Business Communication* 23.2 (1986): 41–50.

Sterkel, Karen S. "The Relationship between Gender and Writing Style in Business Communication." *Journal of Business Communication* 25.4 (1988): 17–38.

Tebeaux, Elizabeth. "Toward an Understanding of Gender Differences in Written Business Communication: A Suggested Perspective for Future Research." *JBTC* 4.1 (1990): 23–43.

Treichler, Paula A., and Cheris Kramarae. "Women's Talk in the Ivory Tower." *Communication Quarterly* 31.2 (1983): 118–32.

Warren, Carol A. B. *Gender Issues in Field Research*. Beverly Hills, CA: Sage, 1988. Vol 9 of *Qualitative Research Methods*. 23 vols.

Weedon, Chris. *Feminist Practice and Poststructuralist Theory*. New York: Basil Blackwell, 1987.

Whitehead, Tony Larry, and Mary Ellen Conaway. *Self, Sex and Gender in Cross-Cultural Fieldwork*. Urbana: University of Illinois Press, 1986.

26 *Making Gender Visible: Extending Feminist Critiques of Technology to Technical Communication*

LAURA J. GURAK AND NANCY L. BAYER

Gurak and Bayer begin their essay by presenting an opportunity for change caused by the fact that the field of technical communication, a field comprised predominantly of women, is now positioned to have an impact on the domains of science and engineering, fields with historic masculine biases. They argue that technical communicators are in a position to "make gender visible," (p. 447 in this volume) and, as a result, "encourage the incorporation of feminist approaches [such as participatory design] into engineering and product design" (p. 445). Their essay, valuable for its overview of the ways in which technology studies and feminist criticism have merged, summarizes four categories of feminist critiques and focuses on demonstrating how recent feminist theories of technology relate to technical communication. Teachers hoping to engage their students with questions of ethics and power dynamics will benefit from both the background information Gurak and Bayer provide and the questions they pose about the implications of a feminist approach.

In the late 1970s, the field of technical writing shifted to a new paradigm. A change in nomenclature from technical *writing* to technical *communication* signaled a move from the positivist model that had dominated the field since its inception (noted by Halloran; C. Miller, "Humanistic Rationale"). Once, technical writers simply "wrote up" what engineers and scientists had already developed or invented. Yet a post-Kuhnian perspective on the rhetorical nature of science and technology has provided a sense of communication as part of the process of invention and development, not just a way of reporting outcomes.

This conceptual shift was paralleled by changes in industry. Many technical communicators began to function not only as writers but also as part of product development teams. At the software company where one of us is employed, for example, this change has become evident. Technical communicators work closely with product developers, attending weekly status meetings and participating in online conversations about product development

From *Technical Communication Quarterly* 3, no. 3 (1994): 257–70.

issues. In addition to producing documentation, many technical communicators play a role in developing integral parts of the product, such as user interfaces or online help screens, which require close collaboration with programmers and engineers.

Yet by moving into the domains of science and engineering, technical communicators are entering a world with a historic masculinist bias. The male perspective has dominated science and technology for centuries (see for example Noble; Pacey) and has regularly produced technologies with a masculine focus. Technical communication, on the other hand, is a field comprising predominantly women (as noted by the Society for Technical Communication's *Profile* 92) and is concerned with issues such as the needs of the user or how best to collaborate with other writers. For both authors of this paper, the early days of working with product developers raised many issues of gender bias in product design that were often not evident to our engineering colleagues. For example, early computer software often used error messages such as "abort" or "kill," which we and other women computer users have found offensive (Turkle and Papert, "Styles and Voices").

Now that technical communicators are directly involved in product design processes that lead to such uses of language and other masculinist design choices, they are in a position to make gender visible, and we suggest that one approach is to employ feminist critiques based in interdisciplinary areas such as science and technology studies. In doing so, we join others who have called for feminist approaches to technical communication (Allen; Lay; C. Miller, "What's Practical"). Thus, we seek to advance the discussion about feminism, technology, and technical communication by presenting a range of feminist critical perspectives on technology. We also, however, build on the work of others such as Cynthia Selfe, who have made clear the pragmatic importance of connecting feminist thought with technology.

Of course, applications and theories relevant to technical communication that might arise from feminist critiques of technology are likely to be varied and diverse, as diverse as the feminist theories that inform them; so in this paper we organize feminist critiques of technology both chronologically and in relation to several perspectives. We begin with a brief overview of how feminist criticism and technology studies merged. We go on to summarize four categories of feminist critiques: women as technologists; women's technologies; women, technology, and the workplace; and technology, cyberspace, and the body. We then discuss liberal, radical, and postmodern feminist theories of technology and show how they relate to technical communication. Finally, we conclude by calling for further exploration, suggesting participatory design as one possible feminist approach to product design.

Background: Feminist Critiques of Technology

Historically, the merging of technology studies and feminist theories began in the late 1970s. Joan Rothschild surveys early feminist critiques of technology and notes that the academic programs in technology studies that began to develop in the 1970s were interdisciplinary in nature (*Machina Ex Dea*). Out of these programs came critiques that examined various relationships among technology, culture, and society; however, these works rarely addressed technology and gender directly. At the same time, feminist critics were beginning to explore women's roles in society and culture. Drawing from much the same disciplines as those informing technology studies (history, anthropology, sociology, psychology, and literature), feminists in the late 1970s began to look at technology and critically examine the relationship of technology and gender.

Noting that feminist critiques range widely, Judy Wajcman provides a good overview of this scholarship. Relying on Wajcman's interpretations as well as Rothschild's, we find the following framework useful:

- *Rewriting the history of technology to include women as technologists.* These studies uncover the accomplishments and contributions of individual women as inventors and developers of technologies.
- *Redefining technology to include women's technologies.* Tending to focus on household and reproductive technologies, these critiques challenge the history of technology by "extending the range of subject matter to include woman-associated activities and . . . [to] redefin[e] what is significant technology" (Rothschild; *Teaching Technology* 6).
- *Studying the ways technology affects women in the workplace; studying the effects of new technologies on organizational structures.* More recent studies focus on women and computers, word processing, and the effects of workplace technologies on women's roles in organizational and management hierarchies.
- *Analyzing the relationship of the human body to technology, especially new electronic communication technologies such as electronic mail, virtual reality, and other "cyberspace" forums.* This area presents exciting possibilities for feminist action because some have claimed that these technologies provide features that make gender invisible and therefore allow more participatory and democratic communication.

These categories hint at broader questions about institutions of technology and the ways in which feminist concerns and female voices can be brought into the study and design of all technologies. They also span a range of feminist ideologies, from liberal feminist perspectives, which view technologies themselves as neutral but male-dominated; to cultural feminist perspectives, which recognize institutions themselves as gender-biased; to postmodern perspectives, which bring into question dichotomous notions of gender and how these have become part of the underlying structure of institutions.

One can see also that feminist critiques have moved chronologically from revising history, to including women and women's technologies, to questioning why women are not well-represented in technology, to considering alternatives, and finally to challenging gender roles and the specialization of disciplines and institutional structures that create gender bias as a social phenomenon.

Approaches to Feminist Critiques of Technology

Women as Technologists

A number of studies rewrite the history of technology by documenting women inventors and technologists. By bringing women inventors and technologists into the traditional male-dominated canon of technologists, these studies push the limits of what counts as technology. As Wajcman notes, although it is not usually mentioned among the contributions of feminism to technology, the early work of Lewis Mumford recognized the central role women played in early domestication technology (Wajcman 18). Other studies that open up the canon of "the inventor" include Autumn Stanley's general essay on revising the history of technology, Martha Moore Trescott's paper on Lillian Moller Gilbreth and industrial engineering, and Helen Deiss Irvin's paper on Shaker women and technology. Edith Vare and Greg Ptack's book, *Mothers of Invention*, re-"her"storicizes women inventors, bringing them into the canon of technologists, and Wajcman reminds us that "during the industrial era, women invented or contributed to the invention of such crucial machines as the cotton gin, the sewing machine, the small electric motor, the McCormick reaper, and the Jacquard loom" (16).

Although there have been women inventors, women have traditionally constituted a minority among engineers. Thus, there are many current efforts that examine why women are so underrepresented in technology fields. Lilli Hornig asks, "women in science and engineering: why so few?" Her answer reveals the historical reasons for women's relative absence from engineering. Sherry Turkle and Seymour Papert also examine the question of why women are kept out of engineering, specifically computer science, and argue that "equal access to even the most basic elements of computation requires an epistemological pluralism accepting the validity of multiple ways of knowing and thinking" ("Reevaluation" 3).

As these studies make clear, underrepresentation is a major source of gender bias in technology: with only half the population doing the designing, women's perspectives have not been voiced. Turkle and Papert have documented this problem in the area of computer software: the predominance of male engineers has produced male-oriented software products. Their suggestion that computer science would benefit from an "epistemological pluralism" that includes women's perspectives can easily be extended to all fields of engineering ("Styles and Voices").

Women's Technologies

Evaluating household technologies is another approach taken by feminists to redefine the history of technology. Ruth Schwartz Cowan's various works on women and household technologies ("Industrial"; "Virginia": *More Work*) are joined by those of Rothschild (*Machina Ex Dea; Teaching Technology;* "Technology, Housework"); Christine Bose, Philip Bereano, Mary Malloy; and Jan Zimmerman.

In some cases the purpose of the scholarship is not only to open up technology to include traditional women's technologies, but also to challenge "popular beliefs about the positive effects [of household technologies on women]" (Bose, Bereano, and Malloy 53) by showing that such beliefs are not based in research, but are based in broad cultural beliefs that household technologies will free up women from their traditional roles and tasks. Looking closely at language like "laborsaving devices" (Bose, Bereano, and Malloy 53) and keywords like "efficiency" (Altman 98), these scholars challenge current scholarship and common misperceptions.

Reproductive technology is another heavily researched area. From 1984 through the present, feminist critiques of reproductive technology have maintained a similar focus as those of household technologies: to problematize what we label and study as technology, and to challenge and question cultural biases, political views, and power structures underlying these technologies (Arditti, Klein, and Minden; Zimmerman; Wajcman). Finally, work exists that links particular women with efforts to create particular technological devices, such as the typewriter (Davies), printing press (Schulman), and electric power (Hinton). In addition, these studies ask us to look at what counts as technology and the amount of funding provided for the development of technologies. For example, military equipment has traditionally received far more financial support than research in reproductive or household technologies. Again, technical communicators working in product development have the potential to influence what counts and what gets funded.

Women, Technology, and the Workplace

Office automation, especially the word processor, figures centrally in a number of works that investigate how these technologies affect women in the workplace. Although too numerous to explore in depth here, some examples include work by Erik Arnold; Roslyn Feldberg and Evelyn Glenn; Zimmerman; and a large number of empirical studies in industrial psychology, management, and organizational communication. Many of the latter are based on field work and detailed analysis, such as Shoshana Zuboff's and Sally Hacker's ground-breaking studies of automation and technology, respectively.

Studying the impact of office automation in the early 1980s, when organizations were first moving from manual record-keeping systems to electronic information technology, Zuboff argues that electronic technology provides organizations with two choices: to *automate* or to *informate.* Automating involves using electronic information systems to reinforce existing hierarchical and gender-based standards; informating means using the technology to change the hierarchy by allowing workers to access and use information traditionally available only to managers. Theoretically, clerical workers, many of whom are women, should benefit from a shift toward informating because their positions would be enhanced and empowered through an increased involvement in understanding and managing information. Hacker's study, on the other hand, focuses on the idea of technological displacement. She observes that at AT&T, women's occupations were most drastically impacted by new technologies. Her study also challenges Marxist analyses and suggests that analysis of workplace and technology be expanded to include gender issues along with economic ones.

Both studies analyze the impact of new technologies on women's jobs, and challenge the popular belief that technologies are designed and chosen from value-neutral positions. Technologies, they argue, are often designed to reinforce traditional organizational and gender structures. Even when a technology offers the potential to change existing structures (Zuboff's *informate* option), designers and managers usually opt for systems that continue traditional, often biased, social roles. Informed by such studies, the technical communicator can become more aware of how various products impact women and other marginalized groups; and of how systems can be designed to either reinforce oppressive or inequitable roles, or to change these roles and the social structures that reinforce them.

Technology, Cyberspace, and the Body

Finally, the idea of *cyberspace* raises new possibilities for feminist theory. Cyberspace is generally conceived of as the entire electronic forum where communication takes place in bits and bytes, where our relations are not face to face, but byte to byte. E-mail, Internet and other networks, and virtual reality are examples of cyberspace "places" where we go to communicate, share information, and learn from each other. In these places—the rhetorical "*poli*" or forums of the next century—gender awareness is skewed. By their very nature, these forums alter our perceptions of our bodies, of gender, and of other social constructions, creating what has been called a "virtual landscape" where writing, thinking, and social action can potentially become more egalitarian and democratic (Selfe and Selfe).

Donna Haraway uses the image of the cyborg, a creature "simultaneously animal and machine," to discuss the idea that feminist thinking should "[take] pleasure in the confusion of boundaries" that results in part from electronic communication technologies (66). For Haraway, the boundaries between nature and technology are not as clear as they might have once seemed. Using such blurred boundaries as a model, feminists are directed to take a hybrid approach, one which defines feminist objectivity as "situated knowledge" (188) and moves beyond dichotomous discussions of technology as either evil and deterministic on the one hand, and wondrous and savior-like on the other.

Allucquere Rosanne Stone describes virtual reality, electronic bulletin boards, and e-mail as places that "instantiate the collapse of the boundaries between the social and technological" (85). Anne Balsamo's work on the culture of virtual reality illustrates another such boundary-confusing technology. Virtual reality, defined as simulation through which people enter three-dimensional computer-generated worlds, is a concept that urges the reexamination of gender roles, because participants in virtual reality can assume a different sex and try to sense another gender experience. Balsamo's study shows, however, how virtual reality culture is filled with sexist stereotypes and how cyberspace reinforces "conventional inscription of the gendered, race marked body" (26).

As do the studies on women, technology, and the workplace, these studies ask those involved in product development to take a hard look at how their product will impact women and other marginalized groups. These studies also make clear the potential of these technologies to change our social reality—including gender roles—and thus show that design decisions may have broad-reaching implications. In another direction, many observers of computer networks have suggested that new technologies have the potential to democratize communication because they make social cues such as status, gender, and rank less visible (Kiesler, Siegel, and McGuire). Computer networks can be used to flatten hierarchy (Zuboff) and to create new "social spaces" (Harasim 15) and "virtual landscapes" (Selfe and Selfe) where "communities" can meet, socialize, and create social action in an open, bottom-up rhetorical structure (Gurak; Rheingold). Yet Susan Herring among others has noticed that despite these claims, gender still creeps in and makes its face known and its power obvious.

Feminist Theory: Technology and Gender

By relating the studies above to broader themes in feminist thinking, educators and practitioners can identify the ideological implications of working with various feminist critiques. Scholarship in the first three categories suggests that the problem with technology from a feminist perspective is that women have been underrepresented: in terms of technologies that traditionally affect women, in terms of women themselves as inventors and engineers, and in terms of the impact that technologies have on traditional women's roles in the home and office. Typical of early feminist critiques of technology that center around equality for women, an underlying assumption of these feminist critiques is that technology itself is value-neutral; and the problem lies in the fact that technology institutions are male-dominated. The solution, according to these critiques, lies in equal access for women to education, credentials, and job opportunities. Taking a "generic human" approach and minimizing gender differences between women and men, this position is sometimes categorized as "liberal feminism" (Eisenstein).

Although there is no doubt that demands made by liberal feminists were instrumental in initiating the informal and formal programs of the 1970s that gave many women access to education and jobs in technology institutions, some critics point out that access by women has not changed the nature of the institutions, and certainly hasn't changed the nature of technology. Sandra Harding asks if women would have struggled so hard to gain access if "they had understood how little equity would be produced by eliminating the formal barriers against women's participation" (21). Thus, critics of this position assert that simply bringing women into the arena of product development may not induce any significant change.

At the same time, other feminists began moving beyond a conception of the problem as a matter of the exclusion of women. Challenging the assumption of a neutral technology, a "radical" feminist would likely view technology as inherently gender-biased. Reappropriating the female nature, radical feminists celebrate qualities traditionally associated with the feminine (e.g., nurturance, pacifism, humanism, gentleness, and intuitiveness). In emphasizing biological and psychological gender differences, radical feminists emphasize dichotomies on several dimensions that traditionally map to the male/female dichotomy: culture/nature, mind/body, reason/emotion, objectivity/subjectivity, and public realm/private realm (Wajcman 3–4).

A radical feminist approach envisions a technology based on values often assumed to be inherent to women: that is, feminist technology embracing feminine subjectivity and intuition. For example, Wajcman describes how "feminist analysis has sought to show how the subjective, intuitive, and irrational can and do play a key role in our science and technology" (18). Furthermore, radical feminist thought suggests that women would contribute needed ethical points of view to technological decision making: decision making that, according to Pacey, usually focuses only on economic/management concerns, or on technique and innovation (101).

Several criticisms have been aimed at radical feminism's emphasis on a female essence. First, this emphasis which, according to Linda Alcoff, "hovers near the edge of biologism," reflects traditional cultural assumptions about women and assumes a universal conception of "woman." However, women's experiences are not universal; they are divided by culture, class, and race. Second, radical feminist thought reinforces qualities that have developed under the historical oppression of women, and although many of these qualities are positive, it is important to see them in the historical context within which they developed, and to recognize that masculinity and femininity are socially constructed; they are not ahistorical and are not necessarily immutable (Wajcman). Finally, because the concept of dichotomies itself may be gender-biased, radical feminist thought may insufficiently challenge the underlying structure of institutions themselves. Critics of this position would argue that more women technical communicators in product development does not necessarily lead to a more collaborative or non-violent environment (Eisenstein).

Attempting to overcome the limitations of radical feminism, "postmodern" feminism proposes to "transform the fundamental character of [technological] institutions in contemporary society and the forms of political power that [technology] bestows on specific social groups" (Wajcman 12). Postmodern feminism calls for eliminating binary thinking and identifies gender, along with class and race, as a historical construct. Examples from our fourth category, technology, cyberspace, and the body, best illustrate postmodern ideology. For example, using technology as a way to critique the underlying structure of institutions through the metaphor of the cyborg,

Donna Haraway reveals the binary thinking that dichotomizes male/female and culture/nature. When women and men participate on computer networks and in "virtual spaces," will gender fall away as a distinguishing factor? Do the designs of these technologies truly make gender disappear? Such are the questions postmodern feminist positions prompt.

One criticism of postmodern approaches is that they threaten, once again, to make gender invisible. If we cannot use the category of "woman" as a focal point, how can we speak about gender biases in our culture and in our technology institutions? How can we begin to bring theory to practice? Several feminist critics, notably Alcoff, Mary Poovey, and Theresa de Lauretis, offer perspectives that respond to this paradox. As well, challenging the notion that technologies such as computer-mediated communication can actually make gender invisible, linguist Herring has illustrated what she calls the "sex-based differences" of discourse from a computer conference, noting that even without the physical cues of face-to-face conversation, "it is often possible to tell whether a given message [is] written by a man or woman, solely on the basis of the rhetorical and linguistic strategies employed" (7).

The questions posed by postmodern feminist thinking move us from concerns about how women can be more equitably treated in technology and about how women's values might reform the nature of technology to asking whether technology and its underlying epistemologies and practices are redeemable or in need of radical reconstruction. Each position necessarily brings with it a different set of implications for technical communicators. Is it enough to get more women into product design positions? Or does a feminist approach mean that some products should not be developed, or that the entire structure of technological decision-making needs reform? Those of us who teach technical communication need to help students identify how certain critical approaches to technology bring with them specific ideological and practical questions. We should also be familiar enough with feminist theory to identify the ideologies underlying the feminist critiques we introduce into technical communication curricula or into the workplace.

Conclusion

In this paper, we have suggested that the role technical communicators now play in the product development process has brought into focus the issue of gender bias and the need to make gender visible by challenging this bias, and we have suggested that feminist critiques of technology can provide needed critical perspectives from which to approach this issue.

This stance presents new challenges and opportunities. First we encourage technical communicators to become aware of feminist critiques of technology and recognize that these critiques speak to technical communication. Second, we urge incorporating feminist critiques of technology into technical communication curricula. Finally, we argue for the use of feminist theory as a framework for critically evaluating the existing product development process and working for changes not only in this process but also in the structures that underlie it.

Modeling the Future

A number of models encourage the incorporation of feminist approaches into engineering and product design. One suggestion is that participatory design allows for voices from various disciplines, including anthropology, sociology, computer science, psychology, and graphic design (Williams and Begg). Another suggestion is that feminist theories have in fact informed the participatory design model (S. Miller); participatory design does mirror elements of feminist approaches, including dialogue and collaboration.

Other models for feminist technology, however, could be based on computer-mediated communication and "virtual space." These technologies, still undergoing development and change, offer potential for open participation, non-hierarchical structure, and increased collaboration among participants.

Models employing participatory design, computer-mediated communication, and virtual reality are certain to be joined by other alternative approaches to technology as feminist voices are increasingly represented in the development of technology. Thus, we find ourselves at the end of this essay but also at the beginning of a stage where we must explore at length the actual applications and potentials of blending feminist thought with technical communication and the development of new technologies. For now, we end our part of this conversation and urge on-going discussion in which technical communication practitioners, researchers, and instructors continue to explore and articulate these exciting alternatives.

WORKS CITED

Alcoff, Linda. "Cultural Feminism versus Post-structuralism: The Identity Crisis in Feminist Theory." *Signs* 13.3 (1988): 405–36.

Allen, Jo. "Gender Issues in Technical Communication: An Overview of the Implications for the Profession, Research, and Pedagogy." *Journal of Business and Technical Communication* 5.4 (1991): 371–92.

Altman, Karen E. "Modern Discourse on American Home Technologies." *Communication and the Culture of Technology*. Ed. Martin J. Medhurst, Alberto Gonzalez, and Tarla Rai Peterson. Pullman: Washington State UP, 1991. 95–111.

Arditti, Rita, Renate Duelli Klein, and Shelley Minden, eds. *Test-tube Women: What Future for Motherhood?* London: Pandora, 1984.

Arnold, Erik. "Women and Microelectronics: The Case of the Word Processor." *Women, Technology and Innovation*. Ed. Joan Rothschild. New York: Pergamon, 1982. 321–40.

Balsamo, Anne. "The Virtual Body in Cyberspace." *Journal of Research in Philosophy and Technology* 13 (1992): 119–40.

Bose, Christine, Philip Bereano, and Mary Malloy. "Household Technology and the Social Construction of Housework." *Technology and Culture* 25.1 (1984): 53–82.

Cowan, Ruth Schwartz. "The 'Industrial Revolution' in the Home: Household Technology and Social Change in the 20th Century." *Technology and Culture* 17.1 (1976): 1–23.

———. "From Virginia Dare to Virginia Slims: Women and Technology in American Life." *Technology and Culture* 20.1 (1979): 51–63.

———. *More Work for Mother: The Ironies of Household Technology from the Open Hearth to the Microwave*. New York: Basic Books, 1983.

Davies, Margery W. "Women Clerical Workers and the Typewriter: The Writing Machine." *Technology and Women's Voices*. Ed. Cheris Kramarae. New York: Routledge, 1988. 29–40.

de Lauretis, Theresa. *Alice Doesn't*. Bloomington: Indiana UP, 1984.

Eisenstein, Hester. *Contemporary Feminist Thought*. Boston: G. K. Hall, 1983.

Feldberg, Roslyn L., and Evelyn Nakano Glenn. "Technology and Work Degradation: Effects of Office Automation on Women Clerical Workers." *Machina Ex Dea: Feminist Perspectives on Technology*. Ed. Joan Rothschild. New York: Pergamon, 1983. 59–78.

Gurak, Laura J. "The Rhetorical Dynamics of a Community Protest in Cyberspace: The Case of Lotus Marketplace." Diss. Rensselaer Polytechnic Institute, 1994.

Hacker, Sally L. *Doing It the Hard Way: Investigations of Gender and Technology*. Boston: Unwin Hyman, 1990.

Halloran, S. Michael. "Technical Writing and the Rhetoric of Science." *Journal of Technical Writing and Communication* 8.2 (1978): 77–88.

Harasim, Linda M. "Networlds: Networks as Social Space." *Global Networks: Computers and International Communication*. Ed. Linda M. Harasim. Cambridge: MIT P, 1993. 15–34.

Haraway, Donna. "A Manifesto for Cyborgs." *Socialist Review* 15.2 (1985): 65–107.

Harding, Sandra. *The Science Question in Feminism*. Ithaca: Cornell UP, 1986.

Herring, Susan C. "Gender and Democracy in Computer-Mediated Communication." *Electronic Journal of Communication* 3.2. Available through Comserve computer network: send email to Comserve@vm.its.rpi.edu with message Get Herring V3N293. 1993.

Hinton, Leanne. "Oral Traditions and the Advent of Electric Power." *Technology and Women's Voices*. Ed. Cheris Kramarae. New York: Routledge, 1988. 29–40.

Hornig, Lilli S. "Women in Technology." *Technology Review* 92 (Nov./Dec. 1989): 29–41.

Irvin, Helen Deiss. "The Machine in Utopia: Shaker Women and Technology." *Women, Technology, and Innovation*. Ed. Joan Rothschild. New York: Pergamon, 1982.

Kiesler, Sara, Jane Siegel, and Timothy W. McGuire. "Social Psychological Aspects of Computer-Mediated Communication." *Computerization and Controversy: Value Conflicts and Social Choices*. Ed. Charles Dunlop and Rob Kling. San Diego: Academic P, 1991. 330–49.

Lay, Mary M. "Feminist Theory and the Redefinition of Technical Communication." *Journal of Business and Technical Communication* 5.4 (1991): 371–92.

Miller, Carolyn R. "A Humanistic Rationale for Technical Writing." *College English* 40.6 (1979): 610–17.

———. "What's Practical about Technical Writing?" *Technical Writing*. Ed. Bertie E. Fearing and W. Keats Sparrow. New York: MLA, 1989. 14–24.

Miller, Steven E. "From System Design to Democracy." *Communications of the ACM* 36.4 (1993): 38.

Noble, David F. *A World Without Women: The Christian Clerical Culture of Western Science*. New York: Knopf, 1992.

Pacey, Arnold. *The Culture of Technology*. Cambridge: MIT, 1983.

Poovey, Mary. "Feminism and Deconstruction." *Feminist Studies* 14.1 (1988): 51–65.

Rheingold, Howard. "A Slice of Life in My Virtual Community." *Global Networks: Computers and International Communication*. Ed. Linda M. Harasim. Cambridge: MIT P, 1993. 57–80.

Rothschild, Joan, ed. *Machina Ex Dea: Feminist Perspectives on Technology*. New York: Pergamon, 1983.

———. *Teaching Technology from a Feminist Perspective: A Practical Guide*. New York: Pergamon, 1988.

———. "Technology, Housework, and Women's Liberation: A Theoretical Analysis." *Machina Ex Dea: Feminist Perspectives on Technology*. Ed. Joan Rothschild. New York: Pergamon, 1983. 79–93.

Schulman, Mark. "Gender and Typographic Culture: Beginning to Unravel the 500-year Mystery." *Technology and Women's Voices*. Ed. Cheris Kramarae. New York: Routledge, 1988. 98–115.

Selfe, Cynthia L. "Technology in the English Classroom: Computers through the Lens of Feminist Theory." *Computers and Community: Teaching Composition in the Twenty-First Century*. Ed. Carolyn Handa. Portsmouth: Boyton/Cook, 1990. 118–39.

Selfe, Cynthia L., and Richard J. Selfe. "Writing as Democratic Social Action in a Technological World: Politicizing and Inhabiting Virtual Landscapes." *Nonacademic Writing: Social Theory and Technology*. Ed. Ann Hill Duin and Craig J. Hansen. Hillsdale: Erlbaum, 1996. 325–58.

Society for Technical Communication. *Profile 92*. Arlington: STC, 1991.

Stanley, Autumn. "Women Hold up Two-thirds of the Sky: Notes for a Revised History of Technology." *Machina Ex Dea: Feminist Perspectives on Technology*. Ed. Joan Rothschild. New York: Pergamon, 1983. 5–22.

Stone, Allucquere Rosanne. "Will the Real Body Please Stand Up? Boundary Stories about Virtual Cultures." *Cyberspace: First Steps*. Ed. Michael Benedikt. Cambridge: MIT, 1991. 81–118.

Trescott, Martha Moore. "Lillian Moller Gilbreth and the Founding of Modern Industrial Engineering." *Machina Ex Dea: Feminist Perspectives on Technology*. Ed. Joan Rothschild. New York: Pergamon, 1983. 23–35.

Turkle, Sherry, and Seymour Papert. "Epistemological Pluralism and the Reevaluation of the Concrete." *Journal of Mathematical Behavior* 11 (1992): 3–33.

———. "Epistemological Pluralism: Styles and Voices within the Computer Culture." *Signs* 16.1 (1990): 128–57.

Vare, Edith, and Greg Ptack. *Mothers of Invention from the Bra to the Bomb: Forgotten Women and Their Unforgettable Ideas*. New York: Morrow, 1988.

Wajcman, Judy. *Feminism Confronts Technology*. University Park: Penn State UP. 1991. 1–26.

Williams, Marian, and Vivienne Begg. "Translation between Software Designers and Users." *Communications of the ACM* 36.4 (1993): 102–3.

Zimmerman, Jan, ed. *The Technological Woman: Interfacing with Tomorrow*. New York: Praeger, 1983.

Zuboff, Shoshana. *In the Age of the Smart Machine*. New York: Basic, 1988.

27 Illustrations in User Manuals: Preference and Effectiveness with Japanese and American Readers

WAKA FUKUOKA, YUKIKO KOJIMA, AND JAN H. SPYRIDAKIS

In their collaboratively researched and written article, Fukuoka, Kojima, and Spyridakis conduct a usability study of the attitudes of both Japanese and American readers of user manuals. The most interesting finding was that there were "no significant differences between American and Japanese subjects" (p. 471 in this volume), at least in terms of their preferences for the integration of text and illustrations. This finding worked against preconceptions of designers from both cultures. This study points to the effects of globalization, highlighting the need for information/document designers in all cultures to have a more complete understanding of their users. In addition, it points out that assumptions, even those based on some cultural knowledge, may be incorrect, a finding that challenges stereotypes, illustrates the need for intercultural communication competence, and calls for a more user-centered approach to design and collaboration.

INTRODUCTION

With the increasing globalization of business, document designers are being required to localize user manuals. Many American companies that export their products to Japan and vice versa are localizing the manuals that accompany the products. In the localization process, texts are translated into target languages, yet in most cases, the manual format and the illustrations often remain the same. The use of a static format may be caused by document designers not knowing how different people from different cultures use and comprehend illustrations.

Although much has been written about how to design the "look" of illustrations for different cultures to ensure that the use of colors and symbols is appropriate for a given culture (for example, Horton 1993, 1994; Forslund 1996), we still do not know much about whether people from different cultures have similar attitudes about the use of illustrations in instruction manuals. Specifically, we do not know whether Japanese and American users have

From *Technical Communication* 46 (1999): 167–76.

the same attitudes about the number and type of illustrations that make a manual most usable. Several studies have pointed out that Japanese users appreciate the generous use of graphics in user manuals, and other studies have revealed that American users perform tasks better when procedures are accompanied by illustrations. Despite such findings, Japanese and American manuals differ in their use of illustrations. Japanese manuals often include an illustration with each procedural step, but American manuals include fewer illustrations with procedural steps. Japanese manuals also use cartoon graphics to convey concepts, yet few American manuals do so.

We do not know, however, whether these document design tendencies reflect differences between audiences in these cultures or simply the difference in assumptions of document designers in these cultures. To appropriately localize manuals for each other's culture, we need to understand whether these two cultures differ in their views on these issues. Therefore, we conducted a study to investigate Japanese and American users' preference on first impression and perceived effectiveness for instructional formats that varied in their use of illustrations that accompany instructional steps. We were concerned with people's first impressions because impressions can heavily influence their permanent perceptions of a manual. Another part of our study included the assessment of Japanese and American users' attitudes about the use of cartoon graphics in manuals. After a brief review of the literature on the subject, we present our study.

Relevant Literature

Several researchers have found that illustrations enhance the comprehensibility of instructions for American readers. In an investigation of different instructional formats, Stone and Glock (1981) had subjects assemble a loading cart while referring to one of three instructional formats. They found that subjects who viewed the format with both illustrations and text made fewer assembly errors than subjects who viewed the illustration-only or text-only formats. By conveying 3-dimensional information, illustrations showed a significant advantage in preventing subjects from making errors in orienting parts. Booher (1975) found that illustrations were effective in facilitating the performance of operational tasks. In his study, subjects who used the formats with text and illustrations performed tasks faster and more accurately than those who used text- or illustration-only formats. His results indicate that illustrations facilitate operational tasks—especially when the illustrations convey spatial information about the location of the objects to be manipulated.

Another study assessed the effectiveness of illustrations in a chemistry laboratory manual. In a test of a written manual with and without the addition of pictures and diagrams, Dechsri, Jones, and Heikkinen (1997) found that text accompanied by graphics led to higher scores on achievement and psychomotor skill tests and more positive attitudes toward laboratory activities. Devlin and Bernstein (1995) assessed the effectiveness of text and graphics with a "wayfinding" task, in which subjects were instructed to navigate their way on a computer simulation of a college campus. Using one of seven types of instructional aids, which consisted of various combinations of text, photographs, or maps, with or without landmarks noted in the text or labeled on the graphic, subjects made the fewest errors with text accompanied by photos or with the maps that had labeled landmarks. Further, subjects performed the fastest with the text accompanied by photos. Regardless of task, these studies have shown that instructional text accompanied by illustrations positively affects comprehension, performance, and task attitude.

Maitra and Goswami (1995) mentioned that American and Japanese readers differed in terms of expectations for the roles of visuals. In their study, American subjects, who were document designers and engineers, were confused by illustrations and graphics in the annual report of a Japanese company. They found it difficult to comprehend the relationship between the text and graphics. The Japanese president of the company explained that some of the graphics sought to give readers a good impression and did not necessarily relate to the text. But his intentions seemed contrary to the expectations of the American subjects who expected the visuals to convey or clarify information and to act as reference tools. Whereas the company report was probably quite appropriate for its original Japanese readers, it fell short with the American readers.

In contrast with these studies with American subjects, few researchers have examined the effects of illustrations on task operation with Japanese subjects. A study conducted by Hiruma and Kaiho (1991) implies that illustrations that show the results of actions may enhance the quality of user manuals. In their study, native Japanese college students and technical writers were asked to imagine that they were using a word processor and to evaluate nine instructional formats. In a comparison of formats that had either written descriptions of the results of actions or no descriptions of the results of actions with formats that also included a screen shot of the results, both subject groups gave higher evaluations to the formats with the added screen shots. Subjects also evaluated the formats on four criteria for defining good user manuals. The student subjects regarded degree of confidence as the second most important of four criteria (comprehensibility, degree of confidence, facilitation of manipulation, and ease of learning, in order of importance). In contrast, the technical writers regarded degree of confidence as the least important criterion (comprehensibility, facilitation of manipulation, ease of learning, and degree of confidence, in order of importance). These results reveal that the students and the writers gave different emphasis to their criteria for defining good user manuals, thus suggesting a possible perceptual gap between users and designers.

The studies reviewed here clearly herald the positive effects of illustrations that accompany instructional text. American document designers, however, tend to use fewer illustrations to support verbal context than Japanese document designers. This tendency is apparent in various kinds of documents. Moriguchi (1998) points out that books in the *Dummies* series, some of the most popular computer primers in the U.S., in general contain one illustration per two pages, whereas Japanese primers use two to four illustrations per page. Beniger and Westney (1981) found that the *Asahi shimbun*, a Japanese newspaper, contained 3.2 times as many illustrations as the *New York Times*. Our brief comparison of two sets of user manuals revealed the same trend. The Japanese version of the manual for the Sony DCR-TRV9 digital camcorder contains 50 percent more illustrations than the Japanese-designed English version. The Japanese-designed user manual for the Vivace 330 copier (made by Fuji Xerox Co., Ltd., in Japan) also contains more illustrations for the same functions than the American-designed user manual for a similar copier—the Xerox 5343 copier (made by the Xerox Corporation in the U.S.).

These design tendencies may be based on assumptions that Japanese readers have a stronger preference for illustrations than American readers, in addition to the financial constraints of using more illustrations. Kohl, Barclay, Pinelli, Keene, and Kennedy (1993) point out the Japanese emphasis on visual communication. Lombard (1992) reported the reluctance of Japanese customers to read technical manuals with few illustrations. The Japanese subjects she interviewed wanted more "graphics, white space, conceptual images conveying tasks," and "icons in the books to help the readers navigate" (p. 690). She also mentioned that comic characters (that is, cartoons) were used in all kinds of Japanese reading material, including technical manuals, to help make difficult tasks seem like fun.

Some Japanese technical writers use cartoons to motivate readers to read manuals. Aizu and Amemiya (1985) added cartoon-type illustrations to their Japanese computer manual that was localized from an American manual; they believed that the illustrations would create a friendly appearance. They reported that the localized manual received favorable responses from Japanese readers. Such cartoon graphics are not commonly found in American user manuals, although one study with American college students found that subjects preferred a "flashier" textbook with cartoons to a traditional textbook with few illustrations (Ramsey 1983). Relying on their first impressions, the majority of subjects thought the flashier format would help them learn more than the traditional format, which they saw as being more scholarly, more difficult, and more likely to be used in a graduate course by an older teacher. It is impossible to determine whether these students liked the flashier textbook simply because it contained illustrations or because the illustrations were cartoons.

In summary, previous studies have found that users comprehend more information and perform better with instructional materials that contain illustrations. However, previous research still does not tell us what combination of text and illustrations users prefer on first impression or believe to be most effective with step-by-step instructions, nor does the research compare the views of Japanese and American users on this topic. Previous research also has not compared Japanese and American users' attitudes about the use of cartoon graphics in manuals.

Therefore, using American and Japanese subjects, we conducted an experiment to investigate both the perceived effectiveness of and preference for instructional formats that vary in their use of illustrations in an instruction manual. For the study, American and Japanese subjects examined four different page formats that provided instructions about setting an alarm function on a CD/radio cassette player. They also stated their opinions about the use of cartoon graphics in user manuals.

The literature review led us to the following three hypotheses:

- Japanese subjects will prefer the formats with illustrations more than American subjects.
- Both American and Japanese subjects will believe that formats with some illustrations will help them complete tasks more easily and more quickly.
- Japanese subjects will have more positive attitudes about cartoons than American subjects.

METHOD

Design

This study was a two-way design that included two independent variables: nationality with two levels (American and Japanese) and format with four levels (full, half, overview, and text-only). Four dependent variables were analyzed:

1. The most preferred format
2. The least preferred format
3. Format effectiveness in terms of subjects' beliefs about the ease of following procedures and speed of finishing tasks
4. Subjects' attitudes about the use of cartoons in a user manual

The reasons for subjects' format preferences were also examined.

Subjects

Thirteen American and 16 Japanese volunteers were secured in Seattle, WA, through advertisements on University of Washington bulletin boards and two different newsletters for international students, and by word-of-mouth. The American subject group included eight females and five males, and the Japanese subject group included eight females and eight males. The mean ages of the American and Japanese subjects were 27 and 26 years old, respectively. The majority of subjects were students at the University of Washington, majoring in various fields (for example, computer science, library science, geography, law). To qualify for the subject pool, American subjects had to have grown up in the U.S. and Japanese subjects had to have grown up in Japan and had to have been living in the U.S. for less than five years.

Materials

The test packets contained five parts:

1. A cover page with demographic questions
2. Four experimental manual formats
3. A full-page illustration of a CD/radio cassette player
4. Two questionnaires to examine format preference and effectiveness
5. A page with two cartoon graphics from a Japanese manual followed by a preference question

Test packets for the two groups were identical except that the text in the four experimental formats was written in either English or Japanese for the related subject group. All other parts of the test packet were in English.

Experimental Formats. The four experimental formats were created by modifying an instructional procedure excerpted from the English user manual for the Sony CFD-370 CD/radio cassette player (1996). This procedure contained six written steps about how to set the wake-up timer of the CD/radio cassette player. For the Japanese subjects, the instructional content was translated to Japanese by one of the Japanese researchers and checked for accuracy by another researcher and a professional Japanese translator. The Japanese and English instructions contained exactly the same written information. Each format was printed on a sheet of 11″ × 14″ (21.5 × 35.5 cm) legal paper.

The experimental formats differed in the amount, location, and detail of the illustrations that accompanied the six written, instructional steps:

- The full format used a single-step illustration beside each of the six steps.
- The half format used a single-step illustration beside three of six steps.
- The overview format had one generalized illustration at the top of the page.
- The text-only format contained only the written steps.

All illustrations, adapted from the original manual, showed the front of the CD radio/cassette player, but the labeling and detail level differed between the overview and the full and half formats. The overview illustration used labels and flow lines to provide spatial information regarding the location of four controls on the front of the cassette player (Figure 1). The illustrations for the full and half formats also showed the front of the cassette player, but they also contained a superimposed small blown-up diagram of a control on the front of the cassette player to highlight the control needed for a given step. Labels and flow lines provided spatial information about the location of the control, and a superimposed hand provided operational information about using that control (that is, the action of pressing the control), the latter of which might enable users to understand what actions to perform without reading the text. There was a total of three differently labeled illustrations (showing three different controls) in the half and full formats (Figure 2). The

FIGURE 1 Overview Format

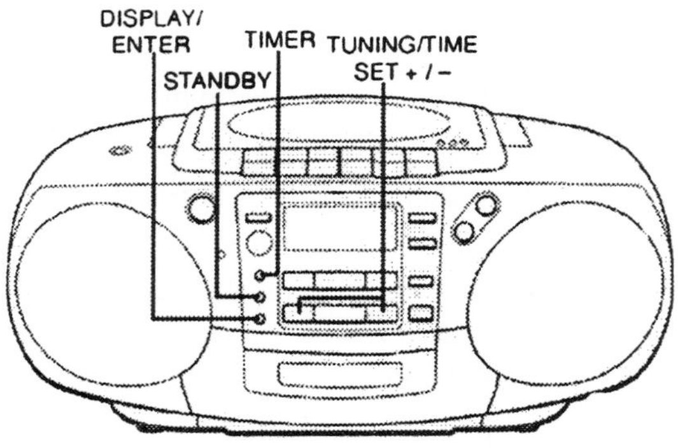

FIGURE 2 Used in Full and Half Formats

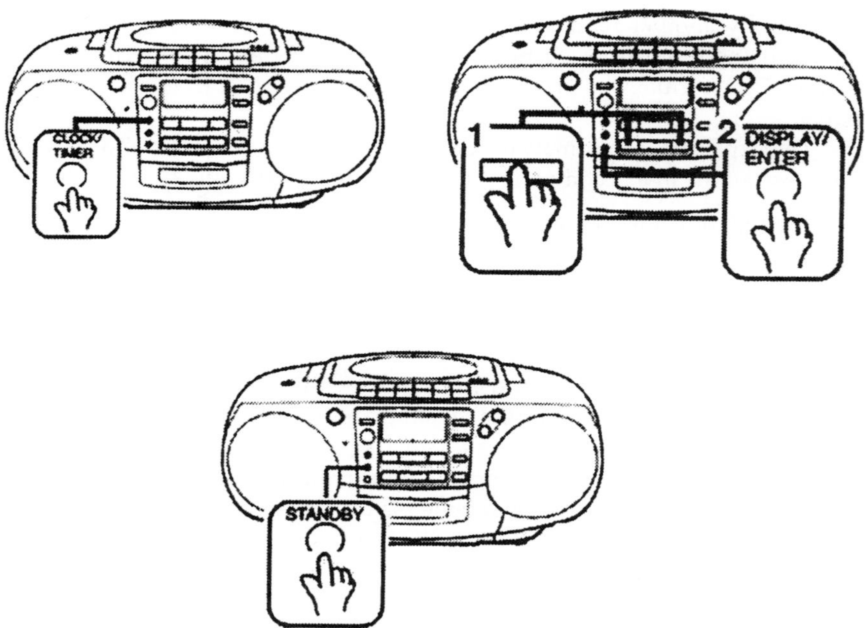

full format contained six illustrations, using some of the illustrations more than once (one illustration three times, another illustration twice, and another illustration once). Although we realized that the differences between the detail level and labels on the overview versus the full and half formats would make our results more difficult to interpret (that is, a nonfactorial design with regard to illustration type), we wanted to use the two types of illustration formats that are common in user manuals, yet limit the number of conditions in this first experiment. The appearance of the English and Japanese instructional texts ensured equivalent quality (for example, the character size and line spacing).

Throughout the test packets, the formats were indicated by letters (A, B, C, or D) instead of by format names (such as "full format"). The letters were randomly assigned to the formats in different test packets so that subjects could not consistently rely on alphabetic preference in answering questions about the formats.

Besides the four experimental formats, a larger view of the front of the CD/radio cassette player (landscape orientation on 8 ½″ × 11″ [21.5 × 28 cm] paper) was provided for use with the effectiveness questionnaire. The figure was excerpted from the original user manual and resized to half the size of the cassette player with the names of controls added.

Questionnaires. Two questionnaires accompanied the experimental formats: one examined format preference and the other examined formal effectiveness. The preference questionnaire directed subjects to spread out the four experimental formats on a table so that they could look at them simultaneously. It further instructed them not to read the content of the pages but to rely on their first impression. The questionnaire then asked subjects to select which formats they would most and least prefer to use if a 30-page user manual consistently followed the formats. Subjects were also asked to select the reasons for their preferences from a list of options or to write down their own reasons. Finally, subjects were asked whether they would want to use a manual that followed their least preferred format.

The effectiveness questionnaire instructed subjects to look at the full-page figure of the CD/radio cassette player and imagine that they were reading a user manual to do a task with the cassette player shown in the figure. The questionnaire then asked subjects to rate (on 5-point scales) how easy it would be to follow the steps with the different formats and how fast they would finish the steps with the different formats. Although this method may not replicate situations in which subjects actually perform a task with a real product in the fullest sense, a similar method has been used in several studies (for example, Hiruma and Kaiho 1991).

Cartoons. The final page of the test packet showed two cartoons, one of an unhappy computer and one of a man flexing his biceps muscle (Figure 3), and then asked subjects how they would feel about a manual that used these illustrations to emphasize written information in the manual. The cartoons were excerpted from a Toshiba computer manual where they were used to emphasize cautions such as not turning off the computer before saving data and taking an occasional break from the computer while working for long periods to avoid eye strain and stiff muscles.

FIGURE 3 Cartoon Graphics

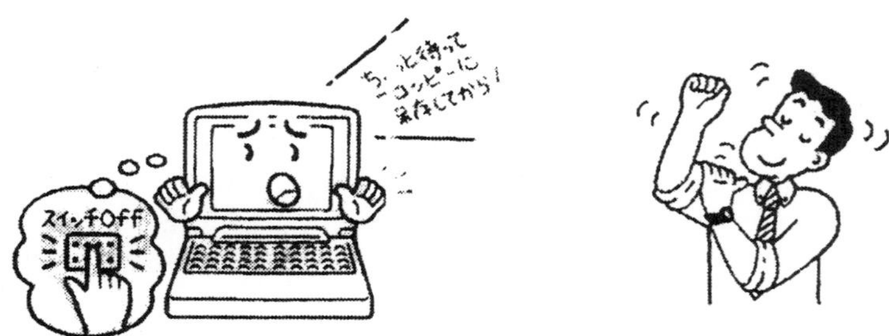

Procedure

Test packets were randomly handed out to subjects to ensure the random distribution of the different, alphabetically labeled test formats. Some subjects answered the test packets at a place where the researchers were present, and others answered them at home and then returned the packets. The testing site differences were not deemed to be significant because the test packets were designed to be used by subjects on their own. All subjects followed written test instructions, proceeded through the test packet at their own pace, and were allowed to ask questions in person, by phone, or by e-mail, although none did. The data was analyzed using *Statview* 4.5 and *SPSS* 6.1.1.

RESULTS AND DISCUSSION

After a brief discussion of the demographic results, the results are discussed in the following three subsections: format preferences, format effectiveness, and attitudes toward cartoons. With statistical tests, only results with a p value $\leq .05$ are considered significant. In other words, a statistical test must show that there is at least a 95 percent probability that the results are due to the experimental conditions, and only a 5 percent probability or less that the results are due to chance.

The results of the demographic questions confirmed that the two subjects groups did not differ in gender or age. A Chi-square test was used to assess the gender variable, and a t test was used to assess the age variable; the tests were nonsignificant. As stated earlier, there were eight females and five males in the American subject group and eight females and eight males in the Japanese subject group. The mean ages of American and Japanese subjects were 27 and 26 years old, respectively. Although Japanese subjects qualified to participate if they had been living in the U.S. for less than 5 years, as it turned out, the majority of Japanese subjects (81 percent) had been living in the U.S. for less than 1.5 years.

Format Preferences

Contrary to the hypotheses that expected differences between the nationality groups, there were no clear differences between Japanese and American subjects regarding preference for formats that varied in the use of illustrations. But the results of subjects' views format preference are noteworthy.

Regarding the most preferred format, because a Chi-square test revealed no significant difference between the two nationality groups on this variable, the two groups' ratings were collapsed for further analysis. A Chi-square test revealed a significant difference across the four formats, $\chi^2(3) = 10.31$, $p = .0161$. As shown in the Total row in Table 1, all subjects preferred to use a format with illustrations (the full, half, or overview format) and no one preferred to use the text-only format.

Even though the two subject groups did not significantly differ in terms of their most preferred format, it is interesting to note that a preponderance of American subjects (46.2 percent) preferred the overview format, whereas a preponderance of Japanese subjects (43.8 percent) preferred the full format. One issue to consider is that all the illustrations in the full format looked identical at a quick glance, and subjects had been told to judge their preference on first impression. One American subject, who pointed out the similarity of the illustrations, did not select the full format as preferred because the format gave him the impression of redundancy. If the full format had used illustrations that show six distinctly different views, perhaps more American subjects would have preferred it.

As for the reasons for their choices, most subjects in both groups selected "the format looks more organized," "the procedure steps look easier," or "I would feel more confident with this format." There was no clear difference between the reasons that each group selected.

Regarding the least preferred format, because a Chi-square test revealed no significant difference between the two nationality groups on this variable, the two groups' ratings were collapsed for further analysis. A Chi-square test revealed a significant difference across the four formats, $\chi^2(3) = 52.24$, $p<.0000$. As shown in the Total row in Table 2, the majority of subjects least preferred to use the text-only format.

As for the reasons for their choices, most American subjects selected "the format looks less friendly" and "I would feel less confident with this format." Moreover, three American subjects explicitly stated that they preferred to see illustrations. On the other hand, most Japanese subjects selected "the procedure steps look more difficult" as well as the reasons selected by American subjects. This difference implies that Japanese readers might be more intimidated by texts without illustrations.

Further, a Chi-square test found no difference between the groups on their responses to whether they would want to use a manual that used their least preferred format. Most subjects stated that they would not mind using a manual with their least preferred format but that they would not like using it. However, four subjects (two Japanese and two Americans) stated that they

TABLE 1 Most Preferred Formats

	Formats			
Nationality	*Full*	*Half*	*Overview*	*Text-only*
American (n = 13)	30.8% (n = 4)	23.0% (n = 3)	46.2% (n = 6)	0% (n = 0)
Japanese (n = 16)	43.8% (n = 7)	31.2% (n = 5)	25.0% (n = 4)	0% (n = 0)
Total (n = 29)	37.9% (n = 11)	27.6% (n = 8)	34.5% (n = 10)	0% (n = 0)

TABLE 2 Least Preferred Formats

	Formats			
Nationality	*Full*	*Half*	*Overview*	*Text-only*
American (n = 13)	7.7% (n = 1)	15.4% (n = 2)	0% (n = 0)	76.9% (n = 10)
Japanese (n = 16)	12.5% (n = 2)	0% (n = 0)	0% (n = 0)	87.5% (n = 14)
Total (n = 29)	10.3% (n = 3)	6.9% (n = 2)	0% (n = 0)	82.8% (n = 24)

would never want to use a manual with such a format. It is noteworthy that these four subjects selected the text-only format as their least preferred format.

The preference results overall show that both American and Japanese subjects preferred to use a format with illustrations and equally disliked a format without illustrations, at least when judged by subjects' first impressions of a manual. These results imply that the assumption that Japanese readers like illustrations more than American readers is incorrect when it comes to the design of user manuals.

Format Effectiveness

As hypothesized, both American and Japanese subjects believed that the formats with both text and illustrations would help them follow procedures more easily. A repeated-measures analysis of variance (ANOVA) (nationality × format) on the perceived ease of following procedures revealed a significant effect for formats, $F(3, 27) = 19.28$, $p < .0001$, and no significant effect for nationality or any interaction. Figure 4 contains a bar graph of the results of subjects' ratings on the four formats. On the questionnaire scale, 1 was hardest, 2 was harder, 3 was normal, 4 was easier, and 5 was easiest.

Given that the ANOVA revealed a significant difference for formats, the next question is which formats significantly differed from each other. We answered this question by using a statistical method appropriate for a within-subjects design—that is, a design in which subjects rate more than one format (in this case all formats). This method reveals how much the means need to differ mathematically to represent a significant difference (Loftus and Masson 1994). The critical difference was .83 (that is, the means for the format ratings needed to differ by at least .83 to be significant). The full, half, and overview formats were rated significantly higher than the text-only format, and the full format was also rated significantly higher than the overview format (Table 3).

FIGURE 4 Ratings on Perceived Ease of Following Steps

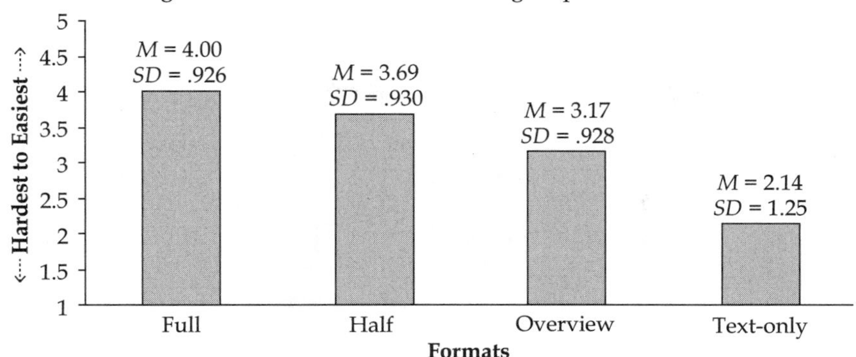

TABLE 3 Mean Differences on Ease Ratings

Format Comparison	*Mean Differences*
Full—half	.31
Full—overview	.83*
Full—text-only	1.86*
Half—overview	.52
Half—text-only	1.55*
Overview—text-only	1.03*
(Critical differences = .83)	

◆ *$p \leq .05$.

Clearly, subjects thought that any format with illustrations would make the instructions easier to follow than a format with text alone. But they also thought that instructions with an illustration beside each step would be easier to follow than a format with one illustration at the top of the page. It is difficult to be certain whether their preference for the full format resulted from the help provided by an illustration accompanying each step or the help provided by the highlighted control in the illustration. We suspect that the answer leans more toward the use of the step-by-step illustrations. If the higher ratings for the full format (M = 4.00) versus the overview format (M = 3.17) were due solely to difference in illustrations between the two formats, then it is likely that the half format would also have significantly differed from the overview format in that the half and full formats used the same type of illustrations.

As we had hypothesized, formats with both text and illustrations positively affected subjects' ratings of task speed. A repeated-measures ANOVA (nationality × format) on the perceived speed of following procedures revealed a significant effect for formats, $F(3, 27) = 11.27$, $p < .0001$, and no significant effect for nationality or any interaction. Figure 5 shows a bar graph of the results of subjects' ratings on the four formats. On the questionnaire scale, 1 was slowest, 2 was slower, 3 was normal, 4 was faster, and 5 was fastest.

FIGURE 5 Ratings on Perceived Speed of Following Steps

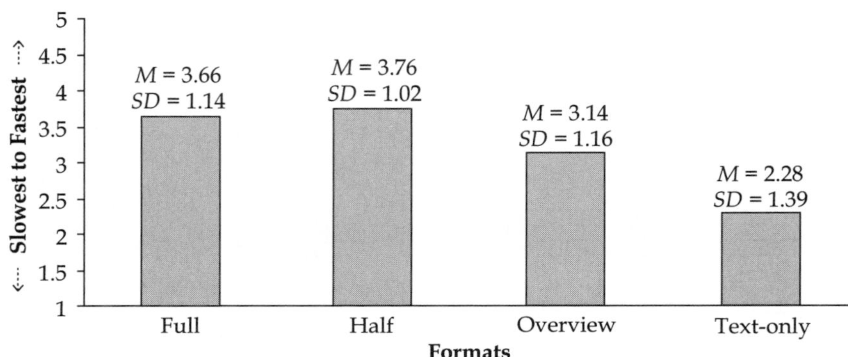

To evaluate which formats significantly differed from each other, we again calculated how much the means needed to differ mathematically to be considered a significant difference. The critical difference for the speed ratings was .99. The full and half formats were both rated significantly higher than the text-only format; subjects believed that the formats with the step-by-step illustrations would help them complete the task faster (Table 4). Interestingly, the overview format did not significantly differ from the text-only format on the speed ratings as it had with the ease ratings.

At this point, it is interesting to think about the results for the four dependent measures all together. For the type of hands-on task assessed in this experiment, subjects most preferred formats with illustrations and least preferred a text-only format. They believed that any format with illustrations would make instructions easier to follow than text alone; they also believed that an instructional format with step-by-step illustrations would be easier to follow than a format with one overview illustration at the top of the page. Further, they believed that a format with step-by-step illustrations would help them complete a task more quickly.

This hierarchy of "the more illustrations the better" is quite logical when one thinks about how users would interact with the different formats. If a format has an illustration for each step (that is, our full format), that illustration will most likely highlight details relating to the step. Users can easily rely on this illustration for help in understanding the written instructions—or perhaps in ignoring the written instructions all together. If a format has an illustration for some steps (such as our half format), users can rely on the illustrations for some steps and, in doing so, reduce their reliance on the written instructions to some degree. If a format has one illustration at the top of the page that attempts to make itself useful for all steps (such as our overview format), then by its very nature the illustration will probably offer less instructional information than step-by-step illustrations do. Users will also have to continually shift their gaze from the text up to the illustration, back again, and then to the mechanism. The tight visual connection of text and graphics that occurs with the step-by-step illustrations is lost. Finally, if a

TABLE 4 Mean Differences (Absolutes) on Speed Ratings

Format Comparison	*Mean Differences*
Full—half	|.10|
Full—overview	.52
Full—text-only	1.38*
Half—overview	.62
Half—text-only	1.48*
Overview—text-only	.86
(Critical differences = 99)	

◆ $^*p \leq .05$.

format contains no illustrations (such as our text-only format), users will have to read all steps in detail, search for the appropriate controls on the machine, and then perhaps reread the text to remember what to do with the control.

Attitudes toward Cartoons

Contrary to our hypothesis, both American and Japanese subjects had similar attitudes toward the cartoon graphics: a Chi-square test found no difference between the two groups. We, therefore, combined the data from both groups for another Chi-square analysis of the three response categories. This Chi-square revealed a significant difference, $\chi^2(2) = 6.28$, $p = .0434$. The majority of subjects (52 percent) stated that they would not care whether such cartoons were used in a manual to emphasize the contents of texts, 34 percent would like to see such cartoons, and only 14 percent would dislike such cartoons. Apparently cartoon graphics, which are so commonly used in Japanese manuals, would be equally acceptable in English manuals for American users.

CONCLUSION

Existing research suggests that illustrations are effective adjuncts to text in instructional manuals. But American manuals typically contain fewer illustrations than Japanese manuals. These document design practices may be based on different assumptions about the views that Japanese and American users have toward illustrations in manuals. Our study revealed no significant differences between American and Japanese subjects in terms of their preferences for and perceived effectiveness of illustrations in user manuals.

American and Japanese subjects found the formats that contained both text and illustrations more preferable and believed they would be more effective in terms of ease of following instructions. They did believe, however, that illustrations accompanying each instructional step would make instructions easier to follow than a format with a single illustration at the top. Similarly, they believed that formats with step-by-step illustrations would facilitate task speed more than a text-only format. These results suggest that preference and perception of effectiveness are not necessarily one and the same. Although users may, on first impression, prefer a manual with any amount of illustrations relevant to the tasks to be performed over a manual without illustrations, their perception of ease of following instructions and speed of completing tasks is somewhat more discriminating. Document designers should realize that a user's first impression of a document may not necessarily reveal how effective a user would find a document.

These results provide some implications for the localization of user manuals. Although document designers may include overview illustrations in manuals to help orient users to a device or portion of a device, the designer should also provide step-by-step illustrations as often as possible beside individual instructions. Further, when preparing English manuals, Japanese document designers need not believe in the myth that Americans prefer fewer visuals than Japanese. In other words, they need not reduce the number of illustrations on the assumption that American readers will be annoyed by the inclusion of many illustrations. Second, American document designers should consider using more illustrations in manuals to help illustrate instructional steps.

The results of subjects' attitudes toward the use of cartoon graphics in manuals also have implications for document designers. Because regardless of nationality, half of the subjects would not mind such graphics and one-third of the subjects would like such graphics, Japanese document designers should spend less time worrying about deleting cartoon graphics from manuals localized for American users. And perhaps designers of English manuals should consider using cartoon graphics to emphasize content.

As an initial investigation, this study has provided helpful information for document designers, but more work is needed. Another study should separate the variables of the number of illustrations from the amount and type of information shown and labeled. Further, a future study should reinforce our results by using Japanese subjects who have been living in Japan and have little experience abroad. Because this study used college students as subjects, it would be interesting to examine the views of other audiences in terms of age, gender, education, occupation, and native country. It would be extremely interesting to examine subjects' perceptions of the formats used in this study if these formats were part of much longer manuals (for example, more than 100 pages). Finally, it would be informative to examine format preference and effectiveness with subjects actually conducting the assigned tasks.

WORKS CITED

Aizu, I., and H. Amemiya. 1985. "The cultural implications of manual writing and design." *32nd International Technical Communication Conference proceedings*, pp. WE33-WE35. Washington, DC: Society for Technical Communication.

Beniger, J. R., and D. E. Westney. 1981. "Japanese and U.S. media: Graphics as a reflection of newspapers' social role." *Journal of communication* 31, no. 2:14–27.

Booher, H. R. 1975. "Relative comprehensibility of pictorial information and printed words in proceduralized instructions." *Human factors* 17, no. 3:266–277.

CFD-370 *CD radio cassette-corder operating instructions*. 1996. Tokyo, Japan: Sony Corporation, pp. 20–21.

Dechsri, P., L. L. Jones, and H. W. Heikkinen. 1997. "Effect of a laboratory manual design incorporating visual information-processing aids on student learning and attitudes." *Journal of research in science teaching* 34, no. 9:891–904.

Devlin, A. S., and J. Bernstein. 1995. "Interactive wayfinding: Use of cues by men and women." *Journal of environmental psychology* 15:23–38.

DynaBook GT-R590 *Toriatsukai setsumeisho* [user's guide]. 1995. Tokyo, Japan: Toshiba Corporation, p. 5.

Forslund, C. 1996. "Analyzing pictorial messages across cultures. In Deborah C. Andrews, ed., *International dimensions of technical communication*, pp. 45–58. Arlington, VA: Society for Technical Communication.

Hiruma, F., and H. Kaiho. 1991. "*Manyuaru ni okeru sousa setsumei no saiteki sekkei* [Optimal design for a presentation of action-sequences in a user manual]." *Japanese Journal of educational psychology* 39, no. 4:461–466.

Horton, W. 1993. "The almost universal language: Graphics for international documents." *Technical communication* 40:682–693.

Horton, W. 1994. *The icon book*. New York, NY: John Wiley & Sons, Inc.

Kohl, J. R., R. O. Barclay, T. E. Pinelli, M. L. Keene, and J. M. Kennedy. 1993. "The impact of language and culture on technical communication in Japan." *Technical communication* 40:62–73

Loftus, G. R., and M. E. J. Masson. 1994. "Using confidence intervals in within-subjects designs." *Psychonomic bulletins and review* 1, no. 4:476–490.

Lombard, C. 1992. "Let's get visual: Revelations after six days with Japanese customers." *Technical communication* 39:689-691.

Maitra, K., and D. Goswami. 1995. "Responses of American readers to visual aspects of a mid-sized Japanese company's annual report: A case study." *IEEE transactions on professional communication* 38, no. 4:197–203.

Moriguchi, M. 1998. "Visualization in technical communication and its cultural differences." In *45th STC Annual Conference proceedings*, p. 191. Arlington, VA: Society for Technical Communication.

Ramsey, R. D. 1983. "Audience reactions to two visual formats." In *35th International Technical Communication Conference proceedings*, pp. G&P39-G&P42. Washington, DC: Society for Technical Communication.

Stone, D. E., and M. D. Glock. 1981. "How do young adults read directions with and without pictures?" *Journal of educational psychology* 73, no. 3:419–426.

ADDITIONAL READINGS

Allen, Jo. "Women and Authority in Business/Technical Communication Scholarship: An Analysis of Writing Features, Methods, and Strategic." *Technical Communication Quarterly* 3, no. 3 (1994): 271–92.

Artemeva, Natasha. "The Writing Consultant as Cultural Interpreter: Bridging Cultural Perspectives on the Genre of the Periodic Engineering Report." *Technical Communication Quarterly* 7, no. 3 (1997): 285–300.

Beamer, Linda. "The Imperative of Culture." *Journal of Business and Technical Communication* 13, no. 4 (1999): 457–62.

Boiarsky, Carolyn. "The Relationship between Cultural and Rhetorical Conventions." *Technical Communication Quarterly* 4, no. 3 (1995): 245–59.

Chu, Steve W. "Using Chopsticks and a Fork Together: Challenges and Strategies of Developing a Chinese/English Bilingual Web Site." *Technical Communication* 46, no. 2 (1999): 206–19.

Constantinides, Helen, Kirk St. Amant, and Connie Kampf. "Organizational and Intercultural Communication: An Annotated Bibliography." *Technical Communication Quarterly* 10, no. 1 (2001): 31–58.

Cook, Kelli Cargile. "Writers and Their Maps: The Construction of a GAO Report on Sexual Harassment." *Technical Communication Quarterly* 9, no. 1 (2000): 53–76.

Cronn-Mills, Kirstin. "A Visible Ideology: A Document Series in a Women's Clothing Company." *Journal of Technical Writing and Communication* 30 (2000): 125–41.

Dell, Sherry A. "Promoting Equality of the Sexes Through Technical Writing." *Technical Communication* 37 (1990): 248–51.

DeVoss, Danielle, Julia Jasken, and Dawn Hayden. "Teaching Intracultural and Intercultural Communication: A Critique and Suggested Method." *Journal of Business and Technical Communication* 16, no. 1 (2002): 69–94.

Goby, Valerie Priscilla. "Teaching Business Communication in Singapore." *Journal of Business and Technical Communication* 14, no. 1 (2000): 92–102.

Hansen, Craig. "Writing the Project Team: Authority and Intertextuality in a Corporate Setting." *Journal of Business Communication* 32, no. 2 (1995): 103–22.

Herndl, Carl G. "Teaching Discourse and Reproducing Culture: A Critique of Research and Pedagogy in Professional and Non-Academic Writings." *College Composition and Communication* 44 (1993): 349–63.

Huettman, Elizabeth. "Writing for Multiple Audiences: An Examination of Audience Concerns in a Hospitality Consulting Firm." *The Journal of Business Communication* 33, no. 3 (1996): 257–73.

Kleimann, Susan. "The Reciprocal Relationship of Workplace Culture and Review." In *Writing in the Workplace: New Research Perspectives*, edited by Rachel Spilka, 56–70. Carbondale, IL: U of Southern Illinois P, 1993.

Koltay, Tobor. "Writing Globally." *Journal of Business and Technical Communication* 13, no. 1 (1999): 86–96.

Kostelnick, Charles. "Cultural Adaptation and Information Design: Two Contrasting Views." *IEEE Transactions on Professional Communication* 38 (1995): 182–96.

LaDuc, Linda. "From Schroesinger's Cat to Flaming on the Internet: Exploring Gender's Relevance for Technical/Professional Communication." In *Foundations for Teaching Technical Communication: Theory, Practice, and Program Design*, edited by Katherine Staples and Cezar Ornatowski, 119–32. Greenwich, CT: Ablex, 1997.

Lay, Mary. "The Law and Traditional Midwifery: A Rhetorical Analysis of the Legal Status of Midwives in the United States in the 1990s." In *Body Talk: Rhetoric, Technology, Reproduction,* edited with Laura Gurak, Clare Gravon, and Cynthia Myntti, 226–43. Madison: Wisconsin UP, 2000.

———. "The Value of Gender Studies to Professional Communication Research." *Journal of Business and Technical Communication* 8 (1994): 58–90.

Miles, Libby. "Globalizing Professional Writing Curricula: Positioning Students and Re-Positioning Textbooks." *Technical Communication Quarterly* 6, no. 2 (1997): 179–200.

Raign, Kathryn Rosser, and Brenda R. Sims. "Gender, Persuasion Techniques, and Collaboration." *Technical Communication Quarterly* 2, no. 1 (1993): 89–104.

Ranney, Frances. "Beyond Foucault: Toward a User-Centered Approach to Sexual Harassment Policy," *Technical Communication Quarterly* 9, no. 1 (2000): 9–28.

Sauer, Beverly A. "Communicating Risk in a Cross-Cultural Context: A Cross-Cultural Comparison of Rhetorical and Social Understandings in U.S. and British Mine Safety Training Programs." *Journal of Business and Technical Communication* 10 (1996): 306–29.

———. "Sense and Sensibility in Technical Documentation: How Feminist Interpretation Strategies Can Save Lives in the Nation's Mines." *Journal of Business and Technical Communication* 7, no. 1 (1993): 63–83.

Shenk, Robert. "Gender Bias in Naval Fitness Reports? A Case Study on Gender and Rhetorical Credibility." *Journal of Technical Writing and Communication* 24 (1994): 367–87.

Smith, Elizabeth Overman, and Isabelle Thompson. "Feminist Theory in Technical Communication." *Journal of Business and Technical Communication* 16, no. 4 (2002): 441–77.

Spain, Daphne. "The Contemporary Workplace." In *Gendered Spaces*. Chapel Hill: U of North Carolina P, 1992. 199–230.

Tebeaux, Elizabeth. "Toward an Understanding of Differences in Written Business Communications: A Suggested Perspective for Research." *Journal of Business and Technical Communications* 4, no. 1 (1990): 25–43.

Thatcher, Barry. "Cultural and Rhetorical Adaptations for South American Audiences." *Technical Communication* 46, no. 2 (1999): 177–95.

———. "Issues of Validity in Intercultural Professional Communication Research." *Journal of Business and Technical Communication* 15, no. 4 (2001): 458–89.

Thrush, Emily A. "Bridging the Gaps: Technical Communication in an International and Multicultural Society." *Technical Communication Quarterly* 2, no. 3 (1993): 271–83.

Tumminello, Joanna and Pär Carlshamre. "An International Internet Collaboration." *Technical Communication* 43, no. 4 (1996): 413–18.

Ulijn, Jan M. and Kirk R. St. Amant, "Mutual Intercultural Perception: How Does It Affect Technical Communication? Some Data from China, the Netherlands, Germany, France, and Italy." *Technical Communication* 47, no. 2 (2000): 220–37.

Weiss, Edmond H. "Technical Communication across Cultures." *Journal of Business and Technical Communication* 12, no. 2 (1998): 253–70.

Zak, Michele Wender. "'It's Like a Prison in There': Organizational Fragmentation in a Demographically Diversified Workplaces." *Journal of Business and Technical Communication* 8 (1994): 281–98.

CHAPTER SEVEN

Writing and Working in Digital Environments

Chapter Seven: Introduction

In the introduction to *Computers and Technical Communication*, his 1997 groundbreaking collection of essays on specific ways teachers and program directors in technical communication might make "informed decisions about the curricular integration of computer hardware and software" (1), Stuart Selber offered four important reasons why teachers need a "critical, contexualized view of computers and technical communication," which included the fact that much of the then current pedagogy did not take into account the "social, cultural, and ethical perspectives" and the ways that "computer technologies might. . . challenge traditional norms of nonacademic writing processes and products" (2). The essays in Selber's collection addressed those issues by providing some "key directions" for faculty to use to consider "ideological perspectives," "identifying legal and ethical issues in the production of online texts," and demonstrating the kinds of power structures inherent in technological systems (3–4), along with a range of other useful perspectives.

The essays in this chapter build on the fine work that Selber and his contributors began. Breuch's essay actually addresses those four reasons Selber listed and narrows the focus to look at pedagogical implications in terms of student learning objectives. The collaborative piece by Selber, Johnson-Eilola, and Selfe, actually written earlier than the Selber collection, focuses on some of those key issues from a programmatic perspective. Teachers can learn much from extrapolating from that perspective. Selfe and Hawisher's ethnographic research study helps to put the questions into a historical perspective and use that perspective to look forward to the twenty-first century to determine what teachers of technical communication need to know and consider as they prepare their students for the many tasks they'll face. The final piece, by Robey, Khoo, and Powers, outlines some of those tasks, demonstrating that the workplace our students will enter is already complex, requiring problem-solving skills that assume a high level of electronic literacy, the ability to collaborate with people across a variety of boundaries (not the least of which is culture), and the ability to learn on the job.

Teaching technical communication is a complex task, and teachers need to have a broad perspective of the roles and responsibilities their students will face. One of our duties is to understand and think critically about technological and electronic literacy, as well as understand the problems embedded in communicating via technology. As Breuch points out, "the agenda of a technical communication class is already packed with theory and practice about oral, written, and visual communication genres, collaboration, intercultural communication, and ethics" (p. 492 in this volume). As teachers, we need to consider carefully how and why we integrate or add anything else. One of the essential points that these writers make is that we cannot ignore the issues of technological and electronic literacy if we want to prepare our students for the workplaces of the twenty-first century. These workplaces, which will be quite similar to the one outlined in the article by Robey, Khoo, and Powers, require us to consider the issue of computers, literacy, and communication simultaneously and recognize that technology, "especially when it networks writers to other writers, is more than a mere scribal tool" (Dautermann and Sullivan vii). To function, workers must take on new roles such as product designer, information architect, process facilitator, interpersonal communication advisor, and usability specialist (Shirk). These roles entail new literacies, and, in order to prepare students for these roles and help them become literate, we need to recognize the complexity of the problem and integrate solutions to it into our pedagogy.

WORKS CITED

Dautermann, Jennie, and Patricia Sullivan. "Introduction: Issues of Written Literacy and Electronic Literacy in Workplace Settings." In *Electronic Literacies in the Workplace: Technologies of Writing*, edited by Patricia Sullivan and Jennie Dautermann, vii–xxxiii. Urbana, IL: NCTE, 1996.

Selber, Stuart. Introduction to *Computers and Technical Communication*, edited by Stuart Selber, 1–16. Greenwich, CT: Ablex, 1997.

Shirk, Henrietta. "New Roles for Technical Communicators in the Computer Age." In *Computers and Technical Communication*, edited by Stuart Selber, 353–74. Greenwich, CT: Ablex, 1997.

28 Thinking Critically about Technological Literacy: Developing a Framework to Guide Computer Pedagogy in Technical Communication

LEE-ANN KASTMAN BREUCH

In this article, Kastman Breuch, frustrated by the multitude of voices and lack of common ground about teaching with computers, seeks to lay a foundational framework to help technical communication teachers formulate useful computer pedagogy. She outlines a set of three issues about technological literacy, discusses each of them in detail, puts her position in context with others' in the field, and presents its pedagogical implications. Central to her argument are her beliefs that "pedagogy must drive technology *[italics in original]" (p. 491 in this volume) and that "we view technological literacy in a fully integrated manner" (p. 491). Kastman Breuch's article is useful from many perspectives, not the least of which is the concise literature review she offers. More important, she focuses on student learning, going so far as to offer a table of learning objectives (performance, contextual, and linguistic) tied to specific activities such as conducting Web research. As you read her article, consider it as she does, a "starting point" (p. 496), one you can use as you work within the circumstances at your own institution.*

In May 2001, I witnessed a lively discussion about the role of technology in technical communication instruction. This discussion took place in an annual colloquium for the Industrial Affiliates Program at the University of Minnesota, in which members from partner industries, faculty from the Scientific and Technical Communication program, and undergraduate and graduate students gathered to discuss industry-academic partnerships in technical communication. Participants raised the issue of computer "tools" and the degree to which students should be responsible for learning various computer technologies. The discussion arose because many of our industry partners provide internships and full-time employment for graduates of our programs, and they sought guidance about expectations of our students regarding the use of computer technology. At the heart of this conversation, industry partners were asking the following questions: "What do we want students to know about technology?" and "How are students being prepared

From *Technical Communication Quarterly* 11, no. 3 (2002): 267–88.

to work with technologies in the workplace?" Interestingly enough, after some discussion industry partners unanimously agreed that there were no specific "tools" that students should learn, for they acknowledged that tools vary widely from workplace to workplace. However, they collectively voiced the expectation that students understand technologies and have the aptitude to learn them quickly; thus, they implied that students be very familiar with common and emerging technologies in their academic programs. What our industry partners were asking, in other words, was that students be technologically literate.

Naturally, the response to this discussion was "What does it mean to be technologically literate?" and "How should technological literacy be integrated in technical communication classes?" These questions are certainly not new to technical communication instructors, as evidenced by growing scholarship on computers and pedagogy. Scholars interested in this area have given careful thought to the integration of computer technology in writing classrooms (Selber; Selfe and Hilligoss; Hawisher and Selfe; Galin and Latchaw). Many of these studies yield useful suggestions for assignments and activities on anything from evaluating Web resources to engaging in asynchronous discussions about course material. Similarly, scholars interested in nonacademic writing have discussed the increasing role of technology in workplace activities such as online editing and composing (Farkas and Poltrock; Dautermann; Henderson; Wieringa et al.); database management (Mirel; Day); hypertext (Charney; Selber et al.); and e-mail correspondence (Hansen; Sims).

These areas provide helpful starting points for instructors of technical communication who wish to integrate computers; however, they do not explicitly address issues of technological literacy. That is, they do not present central objectives that we could communicate, for example, to industry partners who want and need to know how students are being prepared to use technology. Nor does any central framework exist that drives our pedagogical decisions about using computers in technical communication instruction. Rather, current literature provides an array of suggestions for how computers can be integrated in both workplace and academic environments. These suggestions are often contextualized within specific university programs or workplaces (e.g., Palmquist et al.; Cohen and Lanham; Henderson; Sims; Zappen, Gurak, and Doheny-Farina) and more recently, within specific theoretical frameworks. For example, scholars have discussed computer pedagogy in the context of current-traditional, expressive, cognitive, and social theories (Hawisher); postmodern theory (Barker and Kemp; Cooper); feminist and ideological theory (Flores; Lay; Selfe, "English Classroom"; Wahlstrom, "Communication"; Haynes); social theories (Duin and Hansen, "Reading"; Johnson-Eilola; Skubikowski and Elder); and collaborative theory (Burnett and Clark; Forman).

Although I appreciate the multiple perspectives presented in scholarship about computer pedagogy, I have personally been frustrated by the lack of common ground for teaching with computers. For guidance, I have turned to computer-assisted instruction, composition pedagogy, technical communication pedagogy, scholarship on nonacademic writing, computer-mediated communication, and distance education to construct a basis for computer pedagogy. Yet when addressing questions about goals for teaching with technology, this diverse scholarship offers scattered answers, and I have found the variety of approaches in these fields overwhelming. For me, this frustration has raised the following question, which is central to this article: How can computer pedagogy be made more meaningful for technical communication?

Reflecting on my discussions with workplace professionals, I have begun to consider whether technological literacy could be a framework for pedagogy in technical communication—a framework that would make sense of the multiple perspectives in computer pedagogy. By "technological literacy," I mean scholarship that addresses the ability to use technology; the ability to read, write, and communicate using technology; and the ability to think critically about technology. By "framework" I mean a *set of issues* about technology and literacy that would be useful to students preparing for the workplace as well as for teachers forming everyday lesson plans. This framework could draw from cross-disciplinary definitions of technological literacy such as "cyberliteracy," "digital literacy," "electronic literacy," and "computer literacy" (Gurak, *Cyberliteracy*; Tyner; Welch; Warshauer; Selfe, *Technology and Literacy*; Haas; Faigley; Dautermann and Sullivan; Costanzo; Hilligoss and Selfe) as well as multiple perspectives of issues related to technology and literacy. The strength of this framework would not be in finding consensus about key issues of technological literacy or in forwarding any specific theoretical position with regard to technology and literacy, but rather in *identifying* key issues presented in this literature. Thus, I consider this article only a small starting point in the larger quest to explore technological literacy for technical communication pedagogy. My purpose is to identify issues and review cross-disciplinary literature about these issues. Future examinations may move toward a firmer theoretical stance with regard to these issues in technical communication pedagogy.

To begin, I assert that the following set of issues is central in scholarship about technological literacy and would be very useful for computer pedagogy in technical communication:

1. How important is technological performance, or the ability to use a computer?
2. To what degree should we consider contextual aspects of technology, such as political, economic, social, or cultural factors?
3. How does technology influence linguistic activities such as reading, writing, and communicating?

As I explain in the following sections, I propose that this set of issues be adopted collectively as a pedagogical guide for technical communication instructors. As a framework, this set of issues neither prescribes a particular pedagogical approach, nor does it forward a specific definition of technological literacy. Rather, this framework provides a consistent structure for thinking critically about pedagogy specific to technical communication—a structure that, in my opinion, is desperately needed. In the following sections, I explain each issue in more detail, and then I conclude by emphasizing the collective adoption of these issues as a pedagogical framework.

How Important Is Technological Performance, or the Ability to Use a Computer?

As Laura Gurak explains in *Cyberliteracy*, performance addresses one's ability to use computer technology, or, as she explains, "to learn how to use a computer and keyboard" (13). She suggests that performance-based definitions of literacy are ultimately limited. Cynthia Selfe also reports that some definitions of technological literacy simply advocate the use of technology on a functional level (*Technology and Literacy*). Nevertheless, performance has often been emphasized in early definitions of technological literacy. For example, the 1996 government publication titled "Getting America's Students Ready for the Twenty-First Century: Meeting the Technology Literacy Challenge" clearly notes this emphasis:

> Technological literacy—meaning computer skills and the ability to use computers and other technology to improve learning, productivity, and performance—has become as fundamental to a person's ability to navigate through society as traditional skills like reading, writing, and arithmetic.

Not only can performance relate to basic computing and navigation skills, but it can also refer to the operation of software programs. It is in this sense in which the word "tools" often surfaces—that is, describing software programs as "tools" for technical communicators. Scholars in both computers and writing and in technical communication report on such tools and suggest how they can be implemented in the classroom. For example, edited collections, such as *The Computer in Composition Instruction: A Writer's Tool* (Wresch), illustrate what students can do with computer-based editing and grammar programs (Southwell; Kiefer and Smith; Cohen and Lanham) and word-processing programs (Bridwell and Ross; Marcus). Other scholarship addresses software that enables synchronous and asynchronous chats, hypertext programs such as Storyspace and Hypercard, collaborative software like groupware, and server technologies like gopher (see Hawisher; Forman; Burnett and Clark; Day; Gillespie; Venable and Vik; Felter and Schultz).

Although the word "tools" is commonly used to describe computers and software programs, its relation to the issue of performance is hotly debated in technical communication. On one hand, it is easy to understand that employers—as well as technical communication students—expect familiarity and competence with various computer programs. As one industry partner told me: "Students can easily pick up programs unique to our workplaces, but it helps them to have a general knowledge of the types of programs available." For students, this ability translates into familiarity with at least one version of the following programs: word processing, database management, desktop publishing, and Web authoring. On the other hand, technical communication instructors are careful not to stress performance and tools too much since the tools are always changing. For example, an instructor might argue that rhetorical principles of audience and purpose should take precedence over knowledge of any particular tools or the ability to use them. Furthermore, ensuring exposure to the latest and greatest software programs is difficult in academia, for compared to the workplace, the academic world updates its software at a glacial pace due to limited budgets and administrative red tape.

In addition to these concerns, several scholars have noted the dangers of emphasizing "tools"—and consequently technological performance—too much (Warshauer; Haas; Johnson-Eilola; Wahlstrom, "Teaching"; Selfe, *Technology and Literacy*; Gurak, *Cyberliteracy*). The primary criticism here is the suggestion that technology is neutral and does not influence our literacy practices. For example, Christina Haas suggests that a tools-based perspective creates the myth that technology is separate and transparent—an "instrument" with little to no impact on communication practices: "Such an instrumentalist view sees technology as a mere tool—a neutral and transparent means to produce written language, which is somehow imagined to exist independent of that means" (21). Mark Warshauer shares this criticism when he states: ". . . the computer becomes a vehicle for literacy (albeit of a limited scope) but does not itself become a medium of literacy practices" (15–16). Ultimately, many scholars argue that a tools-based stance is dangerous because it suggests that technology is not problematic and does not require the involvement of instructors, students, or communicators employing the technology (Haas; Wahlstrom, "Teaching"; Selfe, *Technology and Literacy*; Gurak, *Cyberliteracy*; Warshauer; Johnson-Eilola).

Thus, in considering technological performance, technical communication instructors must be aware that students need exposure to basic computing and software programs but that they also need to develop an awareness that computers are not neutral tools.

To What Degree Should We Consider Contextual Aspects of Technology, Such as Political, Economic, Social, or Cultural Factors?

While technological performance forms the basis of earlier definitions of technological literacy, recent definitions reflect a more complicated view of technological literacy—one that advocates a critical perspective and an understanding of context surrounding technology. By context, I mean the political, economic, social, and cultural factors that may impact the creation, design, access, and use of technology. Deborah Brandt champions this perspective in *Literacy as Involvement*, in which she argues that "language and context mutually and inextricably constitute each other" (30). Brandt suggests that literacy not be defined by products but by process. As she explains, this type of literacy "places one's involvement with other people—rather than with texts—at the center of literate interpretation and development" (32). Several scholars have begun to describe a more complex view of technology and literacy as well. For example, in *Technology and Literacy in the Twenty-First Century*, Selfe offers the following definition:

> Technological literacy refers to a complex set of socially and culturally situated values, practices, and skills involved in operating linguistically within the context of electronic environments, including reading, writing, and communicating. The term further refers to the linking of technology and literacy at fundamental levels of both conception and social practice. (11)

The definition offered by Selfe suggests a critical perspective of technology that goes well beyond conceptualizing the computer as a tool. William Dugger offers another definition that involves not only an ability to use technology but also an understanding of the technology from cultural and political perspectives:

> Technological literacy is the ability of a person to use, manage, assess, and understand technology. A person who is technologically literate understands, in increasingly sophisticated ways that evolve over time, what technology is, how it is created, and how it shapes and is shaped by society. (514)

Other scholars acknowledge contextual factors as well. For example, Gurak uses the term "cyberliteracy" to describe a critical perspective of technology that requires us to "not just [know] how to use the technology but how to live with it, participate in it, and take control of it" (*Cyberliteracy* 11). Like Selfe and Dugger, Gurak argues that we must "become familiar with the social, rhetorical, and political features of digital communication" (11), and she suggests that a literacy based on performance is inadequate as technology becomes a greater part of our lives. Speaking of "electronic literacy," Warshauer agrees that "literacies are not context-free, value-neutral sets of skills" (374); he carefully examines "struggles for social and cultural equality" in regard to computer technology (176). Similarly, Kathleen Welch acknowledges contextual factors in her explanation of literacy: "literacy has to do with consciousness: how we know what we know and a recognition of the historical, ideological, and technological forces that inevitably operate in all human beings" (67).

Scholars in technical communication have also recognized contextual factors of technology. Stuart Selber notes, for example, in his 1997 edited collection *Computers and Technical Communication*, the need for increased research on technology in terms of political, social, and cultural factors (see also Selfe and Hilligoss; Haas; Johnson-Eilola). Indeed, we can learn from scholarship that describes how technology can profoundly influence work environments (Kaufer and Carley; Zuboff; Hiltz and Turoff). For example, in *In the Age of the Smart Machine*, Shoshana Zuboff explains how the introduction of technology into a workplace can fundamentally change human relationships, organizational schemas, and work systems (389). In another contextual perspective,

Haas explores the political and social factors involved in the creation of a technology for a university campus. In her particular case study, she concluded that technology development is "vastly more complicated" than what we might expect, involving factors such as "issues of power and politics, matters of timing and cost, and rival theories about software design" (163). These studies illustrate in a powerful way how technology cannot be separated from its context.

Considering the contextual aspects of technology can help technical communication instructors think more critically about their teaching environments. For example, Billie Wahlstrom powerfully argues that technical communication curricula have endorsed a literacy concerned with performance through "production courses" ("Teaching" 130). She suggests that instructors look beyond this simplistic literacy toward a "literacy of agency" that would examine the "relationship between technological change and cultural change" (131). With further regard to the teaching in computer-enhanced classrooms, Brad Mehlenbacher offers a sobering picture of designing online environments for teaching technical communication. He argues that technical communication instructors must be aware that problems in establishing such environments result from contextual factors such as "departmental, institutional, political, and extraorganizational factors" (219–20), rather than problems stemming from technology alone. Such strong support for recognizing contextual factors has thus begun to shape specific learning objectives in technical communication. For example, Johndan Johnson-Eilola asserts that "students understand their responsibilities toward users and society in broad, political ways. . . . Students must begin by recognizing that technologies are always political in development and use, even if they appear neutral at an abstract level" (124). Similar learning objectives appear in current technical communication literature (Warshauer; Hawisher and Selfe; Faigley; Selfe and Selfe).

So in answer to the question "To what extent should we consider contextual factors of technology?," scholarship suggests we should consider context a great deal. In doing so, we must also recognize that context is complex (Hansen 306). For technical communication instructors, this complexity might mean not only requiring students to use technology that will be useful to them in the workplace but also reflecting critically on their experience of and with that technology. One suggestion might be a "contextual analysis" of technology that considers political, economic, social, or cultural factors. Perhaps such analysis would address why certain programs have been chosen, who had the power to choose them, and whether and how the technology facilitates visual or written communication.

How Does Technology Influence Linguistic Activities Such as Reading, Writing, and Communicating?

So far, I have reviewed perspectives of technological literacy that have emphasized either performance or contextual aspects of technology. In addition, we must consider the ways that technology influences activities such as reading, writing, and communicating. Entering this arena requires caveats, for as Warshauer suggests, our understanding of literacy may constantly change due to technological, economic, and social changes (11). However, we might begin by returning to Selfe's assertion that technological literacy involves "operating linguistically within the context of electronic environments, including reading, writing, and communicating"(*Technology and Literacy* 11). It is important to recognize these fundamental literacy activities, for as Kathleen Tyner suggests in *Literacy in a Digital World*, reading and writing have traditionally formed the basis of definitions of literacy (25). Gurak also emphasizes specific literacy activities when she suggests that the Internet "is a technology of reading, writing, and speaking, and it brings with it changes for all things affected by human communication" (*Cyberliteracy* 26). In addition to literacy acts of reading, writing, and communicating, some scholars have posited that technology enforces multiple literacies or layered literacies, which may include visual, ethical, oral, written, social, or critical (Brasseur; Cargile Cook; Wahlstrom, "Teaching and Learning"). Considering the impact of technology on literacy activities, then, is quite a complex task.

In considering this complexity, in *Technology and Literacy in the Twenty-First Century*, Selfe offers useful guidance in thinking about literacy by making a distinction between literacy *events* and literacy *practices*. Events can be applications, as Selfe explains,

> understanding and valuing the uses of common computer applications for generating, organizing, manipulating, researching, producing, and distributing information, discourse, and texts . . . ; and using such tools as databases, word-processing packages, multimedia production packages, e-mail, listserv software, bulletin boards, and graphics and line-art packages. (11–12)

Selfe suggests that literacy events can also be activities like "navigating on-line communication environments such as the World Wide Web (WWW), the Internet, activities that require, for example, the use of browsers and search engines in order to locate information and engage in online conversations" (12). According to this explanation, literacy events could include a plethora of instructional activities, such as the use of "E-journals" (Gillespie; Wolffe), networked discussions (Felter and Schultz; Hardcastle and Hardcastle; Shamoon), and computer-supported collaboration (Venable and Vik; Forman; Burnett and Clark).

Certainly, we could identify any number of literacy events that technology facilitates. However, in considering literacy events, we must also consider the influence of technology on linguistic acts within these events. Jennie Dautermann and Patricia Sullivan illustrate this point as well when they argue that we have many studies about technology applications and new literacies, but that "few subsequent studies have developed the issues related to how technology shapes, and is shaped by, writing practices in actual workplaces" (xiii). In understanding the influence of technology on literacy events, we might review, for example, works like *Writing Technology: Studies on the Materiality of Literacy*, in which Haas reports findings of studies about technology on reading and writing practices. Specifically, Haas suggests that reading on a computer screen produces difficulty in spatial recall and "sense of text" (61, 67); of writing, she suggests that writers plan less when using word-processing software (95). In a similar fashion, Curtis Bonk, Thomas Reynolds, and Padma Medury discuss the effects of technologies on nonacademic writing; they suggest that technologies facilitate the *reprocessing* of a writer's thoughts rather than mere transcription through word processing (298). We need more research that demonstrates how linguistic activities are influenced and shaped by technology. This research could extend to multiple literacies, not only describing how these literacies emerge through technology but also how technology alters our linguistic acts.

In addition to reading and writing with technology, we must also consider how we communicate via technology (what Selfe calls literacy *practices*), and scholarship in computer-mediated communication (CMC) is enormously helpful in this regard. (CMC research is relevant to technical communication because workplace communication increasingly occurs online.) For example, Susan Herring suggests that computer-mediated communication is a growing area of research among linguists (155), in part because computer-mediated communication resembles both spoken and written language (158) ranging from "public text [to] ephemeral private communication" (165). Herring also asserts that because online communication is so diverse, no single set of guidelines exists that reflects all online interaction (165). Brenda Sims, for example, describes e-mail use in two workplace settings, suggesting that e-mail correspondence reflects aspects of oral and written communication, and differs in formality depending on the hierarchy of e-mail systems (41). In addition, Craig Hansen suggests that uses of technology for communication in workplaces are enormously complex, as well as motivated by factors such as individual preferences and workplace culture (321). Computer-mediated communication is also of interest to technical communication regarding the formation of online communities (Gurak, "Technology"; Doheny-Farina) and online learning communities (Duin and Hansen, "Reading"; Zappen, Gurak, and Doheny-Farina). Because of the strong social implications of online communication for technical communication, scholars have begun to relate these practices to social theories. For example, Ann Hill Duin and Craig Hansen relate the social aspects of online communication to workplace environments in suggesting a "sociotechnological" perspective, which invokes social theories to demonstrate how

> social context shapes the use of any new technology . . . Patterns of interaction, formal and informal power hierarchies, and priorities embedded in organizational culture affect the adoption and use of that technology. In turn, characteristics of new technology, access to that technology, and interaction with others via the new technology change the existing social context. ("Setting" 5)

In considering issues of linguistic activities, then, technical communication instructors may encourage students to think about how technology affects their reading, writing, and communication practices. One pedagogical suggestion is to have students keep a journal in which they reflect on how technology has affected their coursework in a technical communication class. For example, they could document uses of computer technology for activities such as reading online, conducting Internet research, working with groups in electronic spaces, writing documents, participating in a listserv, or creating computer-generated graphics. In documenting these activities, students can reflect on how technology may have influenced their linguistic activities.

Applying Technological Literacy to Technical Communication

I have thus far identified a framework for technical communication pedagogy based on a set of issues addressing technological literacy. In applying this framework of technological literacy to technical communication, I advocate the *collective* adoption of these issues discussed in literature about technological literacy, for I believe it can provide many benefits to technical communication instructors, students, and professionals.

In advocating a collective adoption of issues about technological literacy, to some degree I break with scholars who promote one issue of technological literacy over others. For example, several scholars note the inadequacy of performance as a basis for technological literacy (see also Gurak, *Cyberliteracy;* Tyner). Stuart Blythe suggests that an instrumental or tools-based perspective of technology is incompatible with a substantive (or critical) view of technology; thus, he suggests the instrumental perspective be rejected entirely (98). Haas similarly rejects the instrumental perspective in favor of a more critical approach to understanding technology. While I agree with the idea that technology is not neutral, I argue that technical communication instructors need to discuss each of the issues to better prepare students for technology literacy. For example, by being introduced to performance issues of technology, students would be better equipped to identify limitations of performance in actual practice. Similarly, addressing contextual issues of technology would encourage students to ask questions about aspects of history, power, access, and culture that may otherwise remain ignored. Collectively adopting the set of issues of technological literacy would benefit students by providing a broad spectrum of perspectives that would inform their practice and study of technical communication and perhaps encourage them to become active agents of change.

In addition, adopting the technological literacy framework I have proposed would centrally promote issues of performance, context, and linguistic activities without privileging one over others. In relation to technical communication, I maintain that each of these issues is equally important. This point becomes important, for example, if one were to endorse contextual issues of technology over linguistic or performance issues of technology. To illustrate this point, I would argue that although technological performance presents a limited view of technology, it is critical for students to develop a level of technological performance, and for two reasons. First, as many scholars report, technical communication workplaces demand that our graduates have skills in using technology (Dautermann and Sullivan; Selber; Shirk). For evidence that students need to be prepared for technological performance, we might note publications like *Intercom* and *Technical Communication* that regularly highlight emerging tools for technical communicators. (See the September/October 2001 issue of *Intercom,* which highlights illustration software.) Second, in order to develop a critical understanding of technology, students must also be experienced in the use of technology. Furthermore, the connection between technology and linguistic activities is especially relevant to technical communication because of its inclusion of oral, written, and visual communication. Technologies that address these linguistic activities appear regularly in workplace contexts—such as online composing and collaboration, Internet correspondence, video conferencing, and desktop publishing. Thus, I believe it is critical to adopt the set of issues related to technological literacy collectively. In discussing these issues with students, instructors can use them as springboards for discussing the various perspectives associated with them.

In addition to these benefits, using the framework I am proposing may provide a touchstone that helps make sense of literature about computers and pedagogy that otherwise may seem fragmented. I mentioned earlier that computers and writing has been addressed from multiple theoretical and practical perspectives. Collectively, these discussions present a rich tapestry through which computer technology is woven; however, they also represent inconsistent rationales and objectives for implementing technology in technical communication instruction. When we view these multiple perspectives in terms of technological literacy, we may find that common issues about technology emerge. For instance, feminist, ideological, and postmodern theory might view technology through a critical/contextual lens; cognitive, social, network, and collaborative theories may highlight linguistic practices among communities. In addition, as my brief review of the literature demonstrates, considering central issues of technological literacy is advantageous because it borrows from several disciplines. Technological literacy seems to provide an umbrella, if you will, under which research from these various fields can thrive.

Pedagogical Implications

In discussing pedagogical implications of technological literacy for technical communication, I reinforce the idea that *pedagogy must drive technology.* There is no doubt that this sentiment has become increasingly important to technical communication pedagogy. For example, in *Computers and Technical Communication: Pedagogical and Programmatic Perspectives,* editor Selber suggests four reasons why integrating computer technology is important to technical communication instruction (in sum): (1) experience with technology prepares students for the workplace, (2) computer software and hardware are not current and prevent pedagogical effectiveness, (3) computer spaces are inadequate, and (4) the number of technical communication programs is increasing nationally. While these reasons are critically important, what struck me about them is the absence of clear learning objectives for students. I return, once more, to the question my industry colleagues asked me: "What do we want students to learn about technology?" I argue that we need to address this question, not to provide industry with answers, but to guide our instruction more purposefully with regard to technology.

Certainly, we have *many* answers to this question, as evidenced by scholarship on theoretical perspectives of computers, activities and assignments, and practices involving technology in technical communication workplaces. But we have no central answer to this question that could guide pedagogical decisions about integrating computers. Interestingly, Lester Faigley has articulated collective learning objectives for technology in relation to composition instruction—they could just as well apply to technical communication:

> What do we want students to learn? I believe we have good answers to this question. We want students to recognize and value the breadth of information available and to evaluate, analyze, and synthesize that information. We want students to construct new meaning and knowledge with technology. We want students to be able to communicate in a variety of media for different audiences and purposes. And we want students to become responsible citizens and community members. We want them to understand the ethical, cultural, environmental, and societal implications of technology and telecommunications, and develop a sense of stewardship and responsibility regarding the use of technology. (137)

This list is impressive because it nicely summarizes issues of importance with regard to technology. However, it raises the question of how we should approach learning objectives regarding technology. The agenda of a technical communication class is already packed with theory and practice about oral, written, and visual communication genres, collaboration, intercultural communication, and ethics. Is technological literacy simply another topic to add to a technical communication class?

In integrating technological literacy into technical communication instruction, I propose that we view technological literacy in a fully integrated manner—similar, really, to the way writing is viewed in writing-across-the-curriculum movements in composition. A full integration of technological literacy in this manner would require that central issues of technological literacy serve as the basis for pedagogical objectives. That is, applying critical questions associated with central issues of technological literacy could help generate objectives for specific assignments, activities, or practices involving technology (see Table 1). Although separated for purposes of illustration in Table 1, I argue that issues of technological literacy are fully integrated with one another, like overlapping circles. The combination of performance, contextual factors, and linguistic activities provides a consistent framework

TABLE 1 Critical Questions for Technological Literacy Learning Objectives

Technological Literacy Issues	*Critical Questions*
Performance	What tools (hardware and software) must students know? What level of proficiency with tools is needed? What actions must students be able to complete?
Contextual Factors	What social, political, cultural, and historical factors exist that influence the technology necessary to complete the task at hand? What issues of access surround the communication task?
Linguistic Activities	What literacy events and practices are involved in the task? Does technology alter linguistic acts in any way?

through which to view technology. Yet it provides flexibility when applied to individual activities involving technology.

For an example, we might apply this framework to the popular assignment of evaluating Web resources. This assignment typically asks students to find sources using the Internet but also to think critically about source credibility. In terms of performance, students must have access to the Web, know how to locate a browser, conduct keyword searches, and select appropriate sources that address the topic they are researching. In terms of contextual aspects, students may be asked to consider the author, source, or professional organization sponsoring the information and think critically about the accuracy of the message. In terms of linguistic activities, conducting research on the Web involves reading and navigating hypertext, scanning, and Web module design. This short exercise reminds us to think comprehensively about issues related to technological literacy. It can be applied to several assignments and/or activities, as Table 2 illustrates.

Applying technological literacy in this integrated manner provides a structure for thinking about technological literacy while also providing the flexibility for multiple teaching possibilities. Most importantly, it provides a consistent framework to think critically about technological literacy through a spectrum of perspectives.

CONCLUSION

Although a wealth of scholarship exists about computers and instruction, I have suggested that central issues related to technological literacy provide a useful frame for thinking critically about our pedagogical decisions. By examining performance, contextual factors, and linguistic activities, students can identify breadth and depth of issues associated with technological activities. In response to the question "What do we want students to know about technology?" we can suggest that we want students to be capable users of technology who understand broader implications and the potential influence of technology on linguistic activities. These objectives can be applied

TABLE 2 Learning Objectives Generated by Technological Literacy Issues

Activities/Assignments	*Performance Objectives*	*Contextual Factors Objectives*	*Linguistic Activities Objectives*
Conducting Web Research	Access Internet; Use Web browsers; Navigate the Web through hypertext links	Critically evaluate sources of information; Consider issues of authorship; Evaluate organizations sponsoring information; Review issues of access to Internet resources	Read online; Scan text online
Creating Visual Displays of Information	Use spreadsheet or statistical analysis tools; Understand tools for generating charts and graphs	Evaluate usefulness of statistical data; Evaluate persuasiveness of visual displays; Recognize limitations of computer programs to display data	Communicate verbal message through nonverbal means
Publishing Web Pages	Write HTML; Use Web editors; Understand servers; Integrate visuals with text	Review issues of access to server; Explore social conventions for Web sites; Analyze organizational structure and design; Consider international reach and ethical implications of messages; Examine regulation for publication on Web	Read and write in linear and nonlinear patterns; Consider audio and visual supplements
Participating in Asynchronous Discussions	Use e-mail; Use Internet chat functions	Review issues of access to Internet; Analyze roles of power in discussion environment; Understand larger context of discussion	Write online; Interact via Internet
Writing Collaboratively via Distance	Use collaborative software like groupware; Use word-processing editing tools; Use Internet attachments	Review expectations for Internet access in professional publishing; Consider issues of plagiarism and authorship generated by electronic collaboration	Correspond with others; Edit collaborative text; Provide written commentary

TABLE 2 (cont'd)

Activities/Assignments	*Performance Objectives*	*Contextual Factors Objectives*	*Linguistic Activities Objectives*
Creation of Online Courses	Write HTML; Use Web editors; Understand servers; Integrate visuals; Use Web course programs	Review issues of access to servers and necessary equipment; Analyze political or organizational support for online courses; Review implications of learning online vs. face-to-face	Write "chunks" or modules; Supplement text with visuals; Consider nonlinear reading patterns
Document Design	Use desktop publishing tools such as PageMaker, Quark Xpress, Framemaker	Consider cultural reading patterns; Consider cultural implications of color, images; Recognize attitudes about computer-generated templates	Understand visual communication including text, space, and graphics

consistently to a variety of contexts, theoretical perspectives, and activities in technical communication instruction.

I pose this framework only as a starting point for further examination of technological literacy in technical communication. That is, my purpose has been to identify key issues related to technological literacy and review literature that specifically addresses these issues; I have also suggested ways these collective issues might be introduced in technical communication classrooms. Given this starting point, future research might apply this framework to pedagogical settings and report results from such application. Future research might also begin to develop stronger theoretical stances with regard to the collective issues I have identified. As a starting point, however, identifying central issues of technological literacy as they specifically relate to technical communication pedagogy seems an important step. Perhaps the framework I have proposed may serve as a springboard for further examination, as well as a structure for helping us think critically about the important connections between technological literacy and technical communication pedagogy.

WORKS CITED

Barker, Thomas T., and Fred O. Kemp. "Network Theory: A Postmodern Pedagogy for the Writing Classroom." *Computers and Community: Teaching Composition in the Twenty-First Century*. Ed. Carolyn Handa. Portsmouth, NH: Boynton/Cook, 1990, 1–27.

Blythe, Stuart. "Networked Computers + Writing Centers = ? Thinking about Networked Computers in Writing Center Practice." *Writing Center Journal* 17.2 (1997): 89–110.

Bonk, Curtis Jay, Thomas H. Reynolds, and Padma V. Medury. "Technology Enhanced Nonacademic Writing: A Social and Cognitive Transformation." *Nonacademic Writing: Social Theory and Technology*. Ed. Ann Hill Duin and Craig Hansen. Mahwah: NJ: Erlbaum, 1996. 281–304.

Brandt, Deborah. *Literacy as Involvement: The Acts of Writers, Readers, and Texts*. Carbondale, IL: Southern Illinois UP. 1990.

Brasseur, Lee. "Visual Literacy in the Computer Age: A Complex Perceptual Landscape." *Computers and Technical Communication: Pedagogical and Programmatic Perspectives*. Ed. Stuart Selber. London: Ablex, 1997. 45–74.

Bridwell, Lillian S., and Donald Ross. "Integrating Computers into a Writing Curriculum; Or, Buying, Begging, and Building." *The Computer in Composition Instruction: A Writer's Tool*. Ed. William Wresch. Urbana, IL: NCTE, 1984. 107–19.

Burnett, Rebecca E., and David Clark. "Shaping Technologies: The Complexity of Electronic Collaborative Interaction." *Computers and Technical Communication: Pedagogical and Programmatic Perspectives*. Ed. Stuart Selber. London: Ablex, 1997. 171–200.

Cargile Cook, Kelli. "Online Technical Communication: Pedagogy, Instructional Design, and Student Preference in Internet-Based Distance Education." Diss. Abstract. Texas Tech Univ. 20 Sep 2001. <http://english.ttu.edu/grad/cargilecook/home/kccdiss.pdf>.

Charney, Davida. "The Effect of Hypertext on Processes of Reading and Writing." *Literacy and Computers: The Complications of Teaching and Learning with Technology*. Ed. Cynthia L. Selfe and Susan Hilligoss. New York: MLA, 1994. 238–63.

Cohen, Michael E., and Richard A. Lanham. "HOMER: Teaching Style with a Microcomputer." *The Computer in Composition Instruction: A Writer's Tool*. Ed. William Wresch. Urbana, IL: NCTE, 1984. 83–90.

Cooper, Marilyn. "Postmodern Pedagogy in Electronic Conversations." *Passions, Pedagogies, and 21st Century Technologies*. Ed. Gail E. Hawisher and Cynthia L. Selfe. Logan, UT: Utah State UP, 1999. 140–60.

Costanzo, William. "Reading, Writing, and Thinking in an Age of Electronic Literacy." *Literacy and Computers: The Complications of Teaching and Learning with Technology*. Ed. Cynthia L. Selfe and Susan Hilligoss. New York: MLA, 1994. 11–21.

Dautermann, Jennie. "Writing with Electronic Tools in Midwestern Businesses." *Electronic Literacies in the Workplace: Technologies of Writing*. Ed. Patricia Sullivan and Jennie Dautermann. Urbana, IL: NCTE, 1996. 3–22.

Dautermann, Jennie, and Patricia Sullivan. "Introduction: Issues of Written Literacy and Electronic Literacy in Workplace Settings." *Electronic Literacies in the Workplace: Technologies of Writing*. Ed. Patricia Sullivan and Jennie Dautermann. Urbana, IL: NCTE, 1996. vii–xxxiii.

Day, Michael. "Writing in the Matrix: Students Tapping the Living Database on the Computer Network." *The Dialogic Classroom: Teachers Integrating Computer Technology, Pedagogy, and Research*. Ed. Jeffrey R. Galin and Joan Latchaw. Urbana, IL: NCTE, 1998. 151–73.

Doheny-Farina, Stephen. *The Wired Neighborhood*. New Haven: Yale UP, 1996.

Dugger, William. "Standards for Technological Literacy." *Phi Delta Kappan* 82.7 (2001): 513–17.

Duin, Ann Hill, and Craig Hansen. "Reading and Writing on Computer Networks as Social Construction and Social Interaction." *Literacy and Computers: The Complications of Teaching and Learning with Technology*. Ed. Cynthia L. Selfe and Susan Hilligoss. New York: MLA, 1994. 89–112.

———. "Setting a Sociotechnological Agenda in Nonacademic Writing." *Nonacademic Writing: Social Theory and Technology*. Ed. Ann Hill Duin and Craig Hansen. Mahwah, NJ: Erlbaum, 1996. 1–16.

Faigley, Lester. "Beyond Imagination: The Internet and Global Digital Literacy." *Passions, Pedagogies, and 21st Century Technologies*. Ed. Gail E. Hawisher and Cynthia L. Selfe. Logan, UT: Utah State UP, 1999. 129–39.

Farkas, David K., and Steven E. Poltrock. "Online Editing, Mark-Up Models, and the Workplace Lives of Editors and Writers." *Electronic Literacies in the Workplace: Technologies of Writing*. Ed. Patricia Sullivan and Jennie Dautermann. Urbana, IL: NCTE, 1996. 154–76.

Felter, Maryanne, and Daniel F. Schultz. "Network Discussions for Teaching Western Civilization." *Electronic Communication across the Curriculum*. Ed. Donna Reiss, Dickie Selfe, and Art Young. Urbana, IL: NCTE. 1998. 263–72.

Flores, Mary J. "Computer Conferencing: Composing a Feminist Community of Writers." *Computers and Community: Teaching Composition in the Twenty-First Century*. Ed. Carolyn Handa. Portsmouth, NH: Boynton/Cook, 1990. 106–17.

Forman, Janis. "Literacy, Collaboration, and Technology: New Connections and Challenges." *Literacy and Computers: The Complication of Teaching and Learning with Technology*. Ed. Cynthia L. Selfe and Susan Hilligoss. New York: MLA, 1994. 130–43.

Galin, Jeffrey R., and Joan Latchaw, eds. *The Dialogic Classroom. Teachers Integrating Computer Technology, Pedagogy, and Research*. Urbana, IL: NCTE, 1998.

Gillespie, Paula. "E-Journals: Writing to Learn in the Literature Classroom." *Electronic Communication across the Curriculum*. Ed. Donna Reiss, Dickie Selfe, and Art Young. Urbana, IL: NCTE, 1998. 221–30.

Gurak, Laura J. *Cyberliteracy: Navigating the Internet with Awareness*. London: Yale UP, 2001.

———. "Technology, Community, and Technical Communication on the Internet: The Lotus MarketPlace and ClipperChip Controversies." *JBTC* 10 (1996): 81–99.

Haas, Christina. *Writing Technology: Studies on the Materiality of Literacy*. Mahwah, NJ: Erlbaum, 1996.

Hansen, Craig. "Contextualizing Technology and Communication in a Corporate Setting." *Nonacademic Writing: Social Theory and Technology*. Ed. Ann Hill Duin and Craig Hansen. Mahwah, NJ: Erlbaum, 1996. 305–24.

Hardcastle, Gary L., and Valerie Gray Hardcastle. "Electronic Communities in Philosophy Classrooms." *Electronic Communication across the Curriculum*. Ed. Donna Reiss, Dickie Selfe, and Art Young. Urbana, IL: NCTE, 1998. 282–95.

Hawisher, Gail E. "Blinding Insights: Classification Schemes and Software for Literacy Instruction." *Literacy and Computers: The Complications of Teaching and Learning with Technology*. Ed. Cynthia Selfe and Susan Hilligoss. New York: MLA, 1994. 37–55.

Hawisher, Gail E., and Cynthia L. Selfe, eds. *Passions, Pedagogies, and 21st Century Technologies*. Logan, UT: Utah State UP, 1999.

Haynes, Cynthia. "Response: Virtual Diffusion: Ethics, Techne, and Feminism at the End of the Cold Millennium." *Passions, Pedagogies, and 21st Century Technologies*. Ed. Gail E. Hawisher and Cynthia L. Selfe. Logan, UT: Utah State UP, 1999. 337–48.

Henderson, Powell G. "Writing Technologies at White Sands." *Electronic Literacies in the Workplace: Technologies of Writing*. Ed. Patricia Sullivan and Jennie Dautermann. Urbana, IL: NCTE, 1996. 65–88.

Herring, Susan. "Linguistic and Critical Analysis of Computer-Mediated Communication: Some Ethical and Scholarly Considerations." *The Information Society* 12.2 (1996): 153–68.

Hilligoss, Susan, and Cynthia L. Selfe. "Studying Literacy with Computers." *Literacy and Computers: The Complications of Teaching and Learning with Technology*. Ed. Cynthia L. Selfe and Susan Hilligoss. New York: MLA, 1994. 336–40.

Hiltz, Starr Roxanne, and Murray Turoff. *The Network Nation: Human Communication via Computer*. London: Addison-Wesley, 1978.

Intercom: The Magazine of the Society for Technical Communication. "An Introduction to Illustration Software." September/October 2001.

Johnson-Eilola, Johndan. "Wild Technologies: Computer Use and Social Possibility." *Computers and Technical Communication: Pedagogical and Programmatic Perspectives*. Ed. Stuart Selber. London: Ablex, 1997. 97–28.

Kaufer, David S., and Kathleen M. Carley. *Communication at a Distance: The Influence of Print on Sociocultural Organization and Change*. Hillsdale, NJ: Erlbaum, 1993.

Kiefer, Kathleen, and Charles R. Smith. "Improving Students' Revising and Editing: The Writer's Workbench System." *The Computer in Composition Instruction: A Writer's Tool*. Ed. William Wresch. Urbana, IL: NCTE, 1984. 65–82.

Lay, Mary M. "The Computer Culture, Gender, and Nonacademic Writing: An Interdisciplinary Critique." *Nonacademic Writing: Social Theory and Technology*. Ed. Ann Hill Duin and Craig Hansen. Mahwah, NJ: Erlbaum, 1996. 57–80.

Marcus, Stephen. "Real-Time Gadgets with Feedback: Special Effects in Computer-Assisted Writing." *The Computer in Composition Instruction: A Writer's Tool*. Ed. William Wresch. Urbana, IL: NCTE, 1984. 120–30.

Mehlenbacher, Brad. Technologies and Tensions: Designing Online Environments for Teaching Technical Communication." *Computer and Technical Communication: Pedagogical and Programmatic Perspectives*. Ed. Stuart Selber. London: Ablex, 1997. 201–18.

Mirel, Barbara. "Writing and Database Technology: Extending the Definition of Writing in the Workplace." *Electronic Literacies in the Workplace: Technologies of Writing*. Ed. Patricia Sullivan and Jennie Dautermann. Urbana, IL: NCTE, 1996. 91–114.

Palmquist, Mike, Kate Keifer, James Hartvigsen, and Barbara Goodlew. *Transitions: Teaching Writing in Computer-Supported and Traditional Classrooms*. London: Ablex, 1998.

Selber, Stuart A. Introduction. *Computers and Technical Communication: Pedagogical and Programmatic Perspectives*. Ed. Stuart Selber. London: Ablex, 1997. 1–16.

Selber, Stuart A., Dan McGavin, William Klein, and Johndan Johnson-Eilola. "Issues of Hypertext-Supported Collaborative Writing." *Nonacademic Writing: Social Theory and Technology*. Ed. Ann Hill Duin and Craig Hansen. Mahwah, NJ: Erlbaum, 1996. 257–80.

Selfe, Cynthia L. *Technology and Literacy in the Twenty-First Century*. Carbondale: Southern Illinois UP, 1999.

———. "Technology in the English Classroom: Computers through the Lens of Feminist Theory." *Computers and Community: Teaching Composition in the Twenty-First Century*. Ed. Carolyn Handa. Portsmouth, NH: Boynton/Cook, 1990. 118–39.

Selfe, Cynthia L., and Richard J. Selfe, Jr. "Writing as Democratic Social Action in a Technological World: Politicizing and Inhabiting Virtual Landscapes." *Nonacademic Writing: Social Theory and Technology*. Ed. Ann Hill Duin and Craig Hansen. Mahwah, NJ: Erlbaum, 1996. 325–58.

Selfe, Cynthia L., and Susan Hilligoss. *Literacy and Computers: The Complications of Teaching and Learning with Technology*. New York: MLA, 1994.

Shamoon, Linda K. "International E-mail Debate." *Electronic Communication across the Curriculum*. Ed. Donna Reiss, Dickie Selfe, and Art Young. Urbana, IL: NCTE, 1998. 151–61.

Shirk, Henrietta Nickels. "The Impact of New Technologies on Technical Communication." *Foundations for Teaching Technical Communication: Theory, Practice, and Program Design*. Ed. Katherine Staples and Cezar Ornatowski. London: Ablex, 1997. 179–92.

Sims, Brenda R. "Electronic Mail in Two Corporate Workplaces." *Electronic Literacies in the Workplace: Technologies of Writing*. Ed. Patricia Sullivan and Jennie Dautermann. Urbana, IL: NCTE, 1996. 41–64.

Skubikowski, Kathleen, and John Elder. "Computers and the Social Contexts of Writing." *Computers and Community: Teaching Composition in the Twenty-First Century*. Ed. Carolyn Handa. Portsmouth, NH: Boynton/Cook, 1990. 89–105.

Southwell, Michael G. "The COMP-LAB Writing Modules: Computer-Assisted Grammar Instruction." *The Computer in Composition Instruction: A Writer's Tool*. Ed. William Wresch. Urbana, IL: NCTE, 1984. 91–104.

Tyner, Kathleen. *Literacy in a Digital World: Teaching and Learning in the Age of Information*. Mahwah, NJ: Erlbaum, 1998.

U.S. Department of Education. "Getting America's Students Ready for the Twenty-First Century: Meeting the Technology Literacy Challenge: A Report to the Nation on Technology and Education." Washington, D.C., 1996. 20 Sep 2001. <http://www.ed.gov/Technology/Plan/NatTechPlan/execsum.html>.

Venable, Carol F., and Gretchen N. Vik. "Computer-Supported Collaboration in an Accounting Class." *Electronic Communication across the Curriculum*. Ed. Donna Reiss Dickie Selfe, and Art Young. Urbana, IL: NCTE, 1998. 242–54.

Wahlstrom, Billie J. "Communication and Technology: Defining a Feminist Presence in Research and Practice." *Literacy and Computers: The Complications of Teaching and Learning with Technology*. Ed. Cynthia L. Selfe and Susan Hilligoss. New York: MLA, 1994. 171–85.

———. "Teaching and Learning Communities: Locating Literacy, Agency, and Authority in a Digital Domain." *Computers and Technical Communication: Pedagogical and Programmatic Perspectives*. Ed. Stuart Selber. London: Ablex, 1997. 129–48.

Warshauer, Mark. *Electronic Literacies: Language, Culture, and Power in Online Education*. Mahwah, NJ: Erlbaum, 1999.

Welch, Kathleen. *Electric Rhetoric: Classical Rhetoric, Oralism, and a New Literacy*. Cambridge, MA: MIT P, 1999.

Wieringa, Marvin, C. McCallum, Jennifer Morgan, Joseph Y. Yasutake, Hachiro Isoda, and Robert M. Schumacher, Jr. "Automating the Writing Process: Two Case Studies." *Electronic Literacies in the Workplace: Technologies of Writing*. Ed. Patricia Sullivan and Jennie Dautermann. Urbana, IL: NCTE, 1996. 142–53.

Wolffe, Robert. "Math Learning through Electronic Journaling." *Electronic Communication across the Curriculum*. Ed. Donna Reiss, Dickie Selfe, and Art Young. Urbana, IL: NCTE, 1998. 273–81.

Wresch, William, ed. *The Computer in Composition Instruction: A Writer's Tool*. Urbana, IL: NCTE, 1984.

Zappen, James, P., Laura J. Gurak, and Stephen Doheny-Farina. "Rhetoric, Community, and Cyberspace." *Rhetoric Review* 15.2 (1997): 400–19.

Zuboff, Shoshana. *In the Age of the Smart Machine: The Future of Work and Power*. New York: Basic, 1984.

29 Contexts for Faculty Professional Development in the Age of Electronic Writing and Communication

STUART A. SELBER, JOHNDAN JOHNSON-EILOLA, AND CYNTHIA L. SELFE

In this synopsis from a symposium, three of the most prominent scholars in the field outline contexts for faculty development to enable a stronger program in professional communication. While the audience for this piece is program administrators, everyone who teaches in the discipline would benefit from an exposure to and understanding of these contexts. Essential points include 1) seeing technical communication "as a complex set of social practices" involving a number of key groups (e.g., writers, readers, educated citizens) who address issues that include "ownership, ethics, and control in online information space and the collaborative dimensions of writing and reading" (p. 501 in this volume), and 2) learning to use computer technologies "in innovative and contextual ways that support . . . instructional needs and objectives and the goals of . . . students" (p. 501). Much of what these authors say about preparing teachers can be used to help prepare students, who also must gain an appreciation for the complexity of working with digital technologies, which requires much more than learning a set of skills or strategies.

At least three broad contexts might inform a comprehensive program of faculty professional development in terms of computer technologies. The scope of these contexts is necessarily broad because preparing teachers for the age of electronic writing and communication must occur differently within specific technical communication programs. Such specialized preparation is constrained by a wide range of factors, including institutional policies and politics, the kinds and ranges of available resources, and the levels of enthusiasm and interest of faculty. Local constraints, however, cannot be the only considerations. In fact, learning and using computer technologies such as hypertext, the Internet and its resources, multimedia authoring environments, and electronic publishing systems may be most productive when located within the following overlapping and constantly evolving contexts:

- An expanded sense of technical communication as a profession
- An appreciation for the literacy expertise of technical communication teachers
- A robust, interdisciplinary knowledge of technology criticism

From *Technical Communication* 42 (1995): 581–84.

Context 1: An Expanded Sense of Technical Communication as a Profession

Strong connections exist between how the profession defines, understands, and shapes technical communication practice and theory and the ways teachers and students approach technology development and use. In classroom settings where the functions and features of technical communication are represented in narrow terms—by outmoded textbooks, underprepared teachers, or both—computer technologies are often treated naively: they support, but do not centrally influence, writing and communication practices. For example, in instructional contexts where the goal of technical writing and communication is "to transfer discrete bits of information with minimum distortion, to decrease entropy" (Mitchell and Smith 1989, p. 118), computer technologies are often viewed as neutral carriers of information—apolitical tools that simply facilitate the process of creating and delivering technical information (Selber 1994). Faculty professional development, from this perspective, would primarily emphasize isolated training in the use of operating systems, applications software, and hardware.

Although teachers need opportunities in which to develop these important skills, such work may occur more productively within an expanded sense of technical communication as a profession—one that locates writing and its associated activities within the richly textured cultural contexts of a technological society. If technical communication is viewed in more robust ways as a complex set of social practices through which meaning is made collaboratively among groups of writers, subject-matter experts, readers of technical discourse, and educated citizens, then an expanded set of issues is necessarily discussed (Redish 1993; Blyler and Thralls 1993; Bazerman and Paradis 1991). These issues include ownership, ethics, and control in online information space and the collaborative dimensions of writing and reading in computer-supported work environments. Faculty professional development that is predicated on this expanded sense of technical communication locates computer-based skill building within larger organizational, rhetorical, social, and ideological contexts, thereby encouraging teachers to consider the perils as well as the promises of computer technologies, and the many levels at which online writing environments influence the processes and products of technical communication.

Context 2: An Appreciation for the Literacy Expertise of Technical Communication Teachers

Limited perspectives on technical communication not only submerge the rhetorical, social, and ethical dimensions of working with computers, but mask the literacy expertise of faculty that should inform the teaching and learning of computer technologies in central ways. By separating technology development and use from the specializations of teachers, the profession significantly reduces the contributions that these individuals might make to enrich technical communication practice and theory. In fact, perhaps the most pressing issues facing the field require interdisciplinary lines of inquiry that primarily address complex literacy issues, or how individuals make meaning with texts in a wide range of social environments and across media. These issues include

- Effective ways of representing tasks and navigating in online information space
- Testing the usability of products used by multiple and heterogeneous audiences
- Making explicit to management the contributions of technical communicators to product development teams
- Identifying the social responsibilities that technical communicators have in relation to technology development and use

Researching these issues demands a strong grounding in theories of discourse, models of human-computer interaction, and systematic approaches to research, including theoretical, rhetorical, empirical, and historical methods. In short, by valuing functional over literacy expertise within technological contexts, the profession risks reducing teachers to skilled technicians who ignore the rhetorical and humanistic traditions that inform technical communication studies at the most essential levels.

An important task during faculty professional development sessions, therefore, is to help teachers learn and use computer technologies in innovative and contextual ways that support their instructional needs and objectives and the goals of their students and programs. In developing such an integrated program of faculty professional development, individuals charged with the computer-related education of technical communication teachers, often computer specialists or other faculty support staff, might initially consider these five strategies:

1. Recruit enthusiastic teachers who can help shape the pedagogical, practical, and critical dimensions of these programs, as well as convince other faculty that participating can be valuable to them both professionally and personally
2. Provide teachers with the technical and educational support they need to work productively within computer-based communication contexts and courses
3. Identify the instructional goals of teachers through personal interviews and course-related materials grounded in approaches that demonstrate sound practice and theory
4. Develop specific ways of supporting the instructional goals of teachers, because even experienced individuals can be overwhelmed by the complexities of computer hardware and software
5. Provide practice sessions before (and after) teachers enter classroom settings, because the complications of teaching about—and with—computer technologies are difficult to predict outside the instructional context, and, even within these spaces, there are often unforeseen events and activities that can challenge the most committed teachers

Context 3: A Robust Interdisciplinary Knowledge of Technology Criticism

A comprehensive program of faculty professional development in terms of computer technologies should encourage technical communication teachers to become technology critics as well as technology consumers and users. Recently, with the help of such technology theorists such as Langdon Winner (1986), Andrew Feenberg (1991), John Street (1992), and Theodore Roszak (1994), technical communication teachers have come to recognize the ideological dimensions of computer technologies and the need to examine the particular forms of power and authority that they embody (Hawisher and Selfe 1991; Johnson-Eilola and Selber in press). Unfortunately, such examinations remain rare, particularly in preparatory programs that stress a limited sense of technology application and practice (Selfe 1992; Selber 1994).

Although technical communication students often possess more advanced machine skills than do many teachers, those skills may be primarily functional. Students will, for example, know how to work across many different platforms and applications, cruise the Internet and its resources with great aplomb, and communicate with each other in a variety of ways over local area networks (LANs) and wide area networks (WANs). However, they seldom have experience in tracing and understanding the complex ways in which their online activities are both productively and unproductively mediated by the hardware and software that they employ, including how "productively" and "unproductively" might be defined in various contexts. This situation is all the more disturbing when we realize that these technical communication students will be among the next generation of media designers—the individuals responsible for constructing and shaping the virtual spaces that professionals will inhabit during much of their work lives. Because teachers will help students develop the critical sensitivities needed to make social and ethical judgments about the design and use of online information space, we should prepare them as both technology critics and consumers.

Conclusion

These three contexts—an expanded sense of technical communication as a profession, an appreciation for the literacy expertise of technical communication teachers, and a robust, interdisciplinary knowledge of technology criticism—represent starting places for a comprehensive program of faculty professional development enriched rather than limited by computer technologies. Although the specifics of any particular program must be considered within the contexts of individual institutions and departments, these broad suggestions should help teachers and students work both productively and responsibly with computing systems and applications.

References

Bazerman, Charles, and James Paradis, eds. 1991. *Textual dynamics of the profession*. Madison, WI: The University of Wisconsin Press.

Blyler, Nancy Roundy, and Charlotte Thralls, eds. 1993. *Professional communication: The social perspective*. Newbury Park, CA: Sage.

Feenberg, Andrew. 1991. *Critical theory of technology*. New York, NY: Oxford University Press.

Hawisher, Gail E., and Cynthia L. Selfe. 1991. "The rhetoric of technology and the electronic writing class." *College Composition and Communication* 42: 55–65.

Johnson-Eilola, Johndan, and Stuart A. Selber. 1996. "After automation: Hypertext, and corporate structures." In *Electronic literacies in the workplace: Technologies of writing*. Patricia Sullivan and Jennie Dautermann, eds., pp. 115–41. Urbana, IL: National Council of Teachers of English.

Mitchell, John H., and Marion K. Smith. 1989. "The prescriptive versus the heuristic approach in technical communication." In *Technical writing: Theory and practice*. Bertie E. Fearing and W. Keats Sparrow, eds., pp. 117–127. New York, NY: Modern Language Association.

Redish, Janice C. 1993. "Understanding readers." In *Techniques for technical communicators*. Carol M. Barnum and Saul Carliner, eds., pp. 14–41. New York, NY: Macmillan Publishing Company.

Roszak, Theodore. 1994. *The cult of information: A neo-luddite treatise on high-tech, artificial intelligence, and the true art of thinking*. Berkeley, CA: University of California Press.

Selber, Stuart A. 1994. "Beyond skill building: Challenges facing technical communication teachers in the computer age." *Technical Communication Quarterly* 4: 365–390.

Selfe, Cynthia L. 1992. "Preparing English teachers for the virtual age: The case for technology critics." In *Re-imagining computers and composition: Teaching and research in the virtual Age*. Gail E. Hawisher and Paul LeBlanc, eds., pp. 24–42. Portsmouth, NH: Boynton/Cook Publishers, Inc.

Street, John. 1992. *Politics & technology*. New York, NY: Guilford Press.

Winner, Langdon. 1986. *The whale and the reactor: A search for limits in an age of high technology*. Chicago, IL: The University of Chicago Press.

30 A Historical Look at Electronic Literacy: Implications for the Education of Technical Communicators

CYNTHIA L. SELFE AND GAIL E. HAWISHER

Selfe and Hawisher's article, which "informs the profession's current approaches to teaching electronic literacy" (p. 506 in this volume) is valuable for many reasons. First, they define electronic literacy, differentiating it, for example, from computer literacy, because they argue for an increased emphasis on "literacy," *which means more attention to "communication skills and values" (p. 506). Second, they trace the history of the ways in which computer technology has entered the world of technical communication, demonstrating the value of a historical perspective. Third, they offer, by presenting their findings, a description of the demographics of the field of technical communication. However, this preliminary work merely sets the stage for their discussion of their qualitative study, which leads them to offer some hypotheses "about the literacy skills and values technical communicators need to succeed in the twenty-first century and about the field of technical communication itself" (p. 527–28). Anyone teaching in this field will benefit from reflecting on their observations and considering their hypotheses.*

Finding a technical communication classroom or workplace that does not depend—in fundamental ways—on communication in electronic environments is unusual (cf. United States, *Digest 1996*; United States, *Economic* 1997, 1998; United States, *Getting*; Selber, *Computers*; Sullivan and Dautermann; Duin and Hansen; Lutz and Storms). Technical communication instructors and workplace supervisors now expect both students and professionals to acquire electronic-literacy skills. Yet, despite the ubiquitous presence of electronic environments, the profession itself knows less than it might about the social, economic, political, and educational factors that affect the acquisition and practice of electronic literacy, in either preprofessional or professional environments, and the nature of the support systems that technical communicators need—at home, at school, and at the workplace—to develop electronic literacy.

From *Journal of Business and Technical Communication* 16, no. 3 (2002): 231–76.

Unfortunately, to date, the profession of technical communication has lacked specific information about how and why individuals gain access to technology and instruction in electronic literacy—at home, in school, and in the workplace. As a result, we continue to have a limited understanding of how the specific social factors associated with the acquisition of electronic literacy work within our culture. Nor do we know how such factors serve to limit access to the academic programs of technical communication that feed into and, ultimately, comprise our profession. In an effort to address this situation, we have collected literacy autobiographies[1] from 55 participants on the Techwr-l listserv. In reading and reporting on these personal narratives, we have focused on the following central research questions:

- How and why have technical communicators in the period from 1978 to 2000 acquired electronic literacy?
- What factors (e.g., social, economic, cultural, educational, political) influenced this acquisition?
- What patterns or trends are evident in these data that can assist technical communication instructors, program directors, and workplace supervisors in identifying increasingly effective approaches to teaching electronic literacy and in setting professional policy concerning such literacies?

The research reported here is intended to inform the profession's current approaches to teaching electronic literacy in technical communication classrooms and workplaces and to shed some light on how the teaching of electronic literacy has evolved over the years.

Electronic Literacy in Twentieth-Century America and in the Profession of Technical Communication

To provide a context for the current project, we first define electronic literacy and then provide readers with a brief historical review of the multiple routes by which such literacy found its way into the profession of technical communication and became valuable to practitioners and the American public at large.

By *electronic literacy*, we mean the practices involved in reading, writing, and exchanging information in online environments as well as the values associated with such practices—social, cultural, political, educational. For us, the term differs from *computer literacy* in that it focuses primarily on the word *literacy*—and, thus, on communication skills and values—rather than on the skills required to use a computer. To distinguish electronic literacy from computer literacy, literacy scholars have also used the related terms *technological literacy* (Selfe; Hawisher) or *digital literacy* (Tyner); both terms are synonymous with our use of electronic literacy. These terms also focus on literacy practices in online environments—and the social, cultural, political, and educational values associated with these practices—rather than on the skills required to use the computers themselves.

In the last two decades of the twentieth century, electronic literacy became increasingly important as a social construction. During this period, for teachers and employers of technical communicators—for the American population at large—literacy instruction of all kinds became fundamentally and inextricably linked with technological environments. These changes were due, in part, to the increasingly rapid pace of technological change and to the social dynamics associated with this change. In 1993, the Clinton administration—inspired by the economic potential of computers—issued the President's Technology Literacy Challenge to schools across the country. This program, perhaps more than any other single piece of government legislation, fueled the country's ability to graduate large numbers of computer-savvy students. It also helped to show both educators and the publics they served the value of electronic literacy; thus, it had direct bearing on the work that technical communication specialists did, both in the classroom and in the workplace. However, if the goal of the Technology Literacy Challenge was to provide all school-age children with instruction in electronic literacy, the effort proved less than even in its effects. In the American school system as a whole, and in the culture that this system reflected, computers continued to be distributed differentially along the related axes of race and socioeconomic status. This distribution contributed, moreover, to ongoing patterns of racism and to the continuation of poverty. The poorer and less educated individuals were (conditions closely correlated with race), the less likely they were to have access to computers in their classrooms and their schools and the less likely they were to develop skills with multiple computer applications that were required by high-tech, high-paying jobs in fields such as technical communication (cf. United States, *Condition 1997* 212; United States, *Digest 1996* 458; United States, *Getting 36*; Coley, Crandler, and Engle 3). This situation, too, had an impact on the profession of technical communication.

The widespread marketing of relatively cheap personal computers in the early 1980s led rapidly, in that decade, to an increasingly technological workplace for the American corporate sector. By the end of the decade, a growing number of digital environments had been established in workplace environments, and a growing number of technical communicators were using them on a daily basis. On the heels of that first influx of personal computers into American workplace environments came early publications that chronicled the changes associated with electronic communication, including, for example, Roxanne Hiltz and Murray Turoff's examination of networked computer-based communication across time and distance, Shoshana Zuboff's landmark study of technology's integration in the workplace, and Lee Sproull and Sara Kiesler's study about how technological environments differed from traditional print and face-to-face environments.

Quickly, technical communicators became caught up in the new technological environments: as authors of software and hardware documentation (e.g., Sides; Horton; Price; Price and Korman; Weiss), as trainers and the authors of training materials in computer-based environments (e.g., Kearsley, *Computer-Based, Training*; Heines), as layout and design specialists (e.g., Beach; White), and as employees working in, and programming for, computer-based environments (e.g., Greenberg; Dumas). By 1997, as Henrietta Shirk pointed out, "no disagreement that computer technologies are important 'tools of the trade' for technical communicators" existed (353).

As computers were becoming essential for technical communication, their presence was also increasing in academic programs that aimed to educate technical communicators for the workplace and for teaching college-level programs of technical communication. As early as 1984, for example, Gilbert Storms noted the criticality of computers:

> The growing importance of computers in every aspect of industry, including technical communication, suggests that technical communication programs could help their graduates by adding one or more courses in computer science to their requirements. Such courses should show students how computers work, how they perform business functions, and how they are used in communication, particularly word processing, information storage and retrieval, and information management. (19)

Articles by Elizabeth Tebeaux, in 1989, and by Sherry Little, in 1990, acknowledged the enormous role of technology in the workplace and the need for technical communication students and instructors to learn computer-based literacies of all kinds. In 1994, Stuart Selber (*Hypertext*) discussed the ways in which 39 different colleges had integrated technology into their technical communication programs at various levels and in various ways. And by 1997, the third volume of the Association of Teachers of Technical Writing (ATTW) Contemporary Studies in Technical Communication series was dedicated to computers and technical communication (Selber, *Computers*).

In some ways, this cataloging of the ways in which computer technology entered the professional world of technical communication during the last part of the twentieth century may seem superfluous. After all, we all know that the technology is with us today and that our jobs—either as students, as instructors, or as professional communicators—have become virtually impossible without the new information technologies. However, we should not forget how these technologies made, and continue to make, their way through our culture in general and our profession in particular. Without documenting such large-scale social movements, the profession of technical communication will be hard put to trace and understand the context within which electronic literacies developed in the last century and to anticipate the context within which they will develop in the next century.

Approaches to the Study of Electronic Literacy

After obtaining approval to conduct human-subjects research from both Michigan Technological University and the University of Illinois, Urbana-Champaign, we asked participants on the Techwr-l listserv to volunteer for the task of completing literacy autobiographies, self-told personal histories focused around a standard set of questions about family literacy practices and values, individual literacy practices and values, and the processes through which they learned to use computers to read and write in computer-based contexts. Techwr-l, a nonacademic listserv with more than 4,900 subscribers, was founded in 1993 for the express purpose of providing a forum for any and all technical writing issues (see http://www.raycomm.com/techwhirl/sitemap.html). The list is aimed primarily at practicing technical communicators and, in general, includes discussions of various software programs, methods for creating various kinds of technical publications, and various conferences that might be useful to technical communicators (Johnson-Eilola and Selber).

Of the 4,900 subscribers to Techwr-l, 55 individuals—46 women and 9 men—chose to complete the online form, which was stored on a Web site and password protected. This activity was completed between April 15 and June 30, 2000. The questions comprising this form (see Appendix) were derived from the project's central research questions; they had also been field-tested and refined in a series of preliminary interviews as part of a larger literacy project we were undertaking during the same period. Individuals from 20 different states were represented in this self-selected sample as well as individuals from four different Canadian cities and one technical communicator, an American, who was working abroad in Europe. By far, the greatest number of participants who volunteered for this study classified themselves as technical writers—other occupations participants mentioned included project manager, senior editor, consultant, self-help author, training specialist, software company president, and documentation specialist. Several respondents had had military careers and, when they retired, entered the computer industry. Not surprisingly, the military seemed to provide better computer-skills training than colleges did, especially in the early years of computers. The autobiographies completed by these volunteers provided a robust set of situated data about individuals' literacy practices and values; they also provided the background for relating these data to home life, schooling environments, and workplace cultures as well as to cultural, geographic, and social contexts.

Although the online autobiographies proved exceedingly valuable, they did not provide the immediate opportunity to follow up on questions or to probe further. Thus, to supplement the 55 online autobiographies, we also conducted oral, face-to-face interviews with four additional people. These four constituted a sample of convenience. Like the online participants, all four volunteered in response to a call for participants and were associated with the profession of technical communication: a faculty member who taught technical communication courses, a professional communicator, and two students of different backgrounds majoring in technical communication. These face-to-face interviews were audiotaped, and the tapes were later transcribed for analysis and summary in responding to the research questions. All literacy autobiographies, once obtained, were coded for confidentiality, purged of information that might identify the participants, and—through the process of multiple readings—analyzed for details, patterns, and trends that might shed light on the project's central questions. Specifically, we were looking for details, patterns, and trends related to the acquisition of electronic literacy and to social, economic, cultural, educational, and political factors that might have influenced this acquisition.

All analyses were collaboratively authored by both of us. In conducting these analyses, moreover, we also attempted to situate the events mentioned by participants, whenever possible, within the context of large-scale historical events. In this way, we sought to identify salient relationships between individuals, their collective practices, and sociohistorical change. With this particular qualitative-methodology approach, we patterned our efforts on the strategies employed by literacy researchers, such as Deborah Brandt ("Accumulating," "Sponsors," "Literacy," *Literacy*), and David Barton and Mary Hamilton, whose own work is, in turn, grounded in oral history and life history research practices developed by scholars such as Daniel Bertaux and Paul Thompson (*Between*, *Pathways*), Paul Thompson (*Edwardians*, *Voice*), and Paul Thompson, Catherine Itzin, and Michele Abendstern. The strategies we found most useful included conducting in-depth interviews with participants, paying close attention to the personal narratives that people told about their lives, and focusing on the large-scale historical events that people mentioned in their autobiographies.

Brandt's oral-history and life-history methodology is also congruent with an ecological model of electronic-literacy studies outlined by Bertram Bruce and Maureen Hogan. As these researchers point out, electronic-literacy practices and values can be understood only as

> constituent parts of life, elements of an ecological system . . . that gives us a basis for understanding the interpenetration between machines, humans, and the natural world. . . . Literacies, and the technologies of literacy, can only be understood in relation to larger systems of practice. Most technologies become so enmeshed in daily experience that they disappear. (272)

For this project, then, we also tried to compile a rich sense of the specific *cultural ecology*[2]—the "existing stock of social forces and ideas" (Deibert 31), political and economic formations, and available communication environments—within which the participants acquired electronic literacy. In using this term and this approach, we emphasize the importance of context in the study of electronic literacy—how particular historical periods, cultural milieus, and material conditions affected technical communicators' acquisition of electronic literacy.

The strengths of this combination of qualitative methodological approaches lie in its ability to capture the life stories of individuals inhabiting a particular period of history—in rich detail and in personal terms. This approach does not purport to identify generalizable results. In this article, therefore, we have been primarily concerned with preserving both the tone and the content of the participants' personal stories while ensuring their privacy and making their stories accessible to readers. Because the questions asked within the autobiography protocol are not strictly chronological and because we want to provide readers with a concise and coherent discussion, we have excerpted and sometimes reordered the comments taken from these autobiographies. Ellipses in the texts that follow mark the removal of conversational markers, interruptions, and asides (in the case of face-to-face interviews) as well as obvious digressions, backtracking, and information that might identify participants or their place of work (in the case of both face-to-face and online interviews). Brackets indicate explanatory additions by the researchers.

The following unusual features of this particular self-selected sample illustrate the limitations of the data with which we worked. First, although the population of technical communicators subscribed to Techwr-l represents a range of ages, educational levels, and socioeconomic classes, the technical communication professionals who chose to complete the online protocol of questions included a surprisingly high proportion of women. Of the 55 autobiographies collected, 46 were completed by women and only 9 by men. Although the owner of the discussion group, Eric Ray, could not provide specific statistics about the genders of the list's subscribers, he did express the belief, in a follow-up conversation, that its membership reflected the general population of technical communicators, which has a slightly higher proportion of women than men. To provide a comparative statistic, we note that the Society for Technical Communication (STC) reports its membership as approximately 65 percent to 70 percent female. Within this context, we can only speculate about why the self-selected sample for this study contained such a high proportion of women; perhaps women are more likely to respond to online requests for surveys than men are, especially in a survey being sent out by two women, or they may perceive themselves as having a higher stake in being in a survey involving their acquisition and use of electronic literacies. Second, only 1 of the 55 online interviews was completed by a person of color, an African American woman. Third, of the 55 individuals completing autobiographies, the vast majority classified their current socioeconomic status as middle-class or upper-middle-class, although they were evenly divided between those who said they had been raised in economically disadvantaged households and those who considered themselves raised in middle-class homes. A few individuals, whose fathers were engineers or lawyers, considered themselves as always having been part of the upper middle class. And fourth, we should note that the respondents' mean age was 40, with their birth dates ranging from 1939 to 1976. In a self-selected sample, this factor, too, might indicate a limitation, although we have no systematic information about the population of professional communicators on Techwr-l that we can use to determine whether that is so. Demographic data from STC indicate the mean age of its members to be about 42.

Electronic-Literacy Autobiographies from the Techwr-l Sample

The written autobiographies that we collected for this project provided a rich tracing of the routes through which computers, in general, and personal computers, in particular, came to shape the profession of technical communication and the literacy practices of technical communicators within the changing cultural ecologies of the 1970s, 1980s, and 1990s. These autobiographies contributed a great deal of information about how and why 55 technical communicators living from 1978 to 2000 have acquired electronic literacy, and about some of the social, economic, cultural, educational, and political factors that influenced this acquisition. These narratives indicated that the opportunities participants had to learn the new technologies varied tremendously from 1980 to 2000; these opportunities, however, seemed most dependent on the age of the individuals and on the sociohistorical contexts that shaped their early exposure to computers.

For a time, in the early age of personal computers—the late 1970s and first half of the 1980s—being computer literate meant being able to program computers. Even individuals who planned to become technical communicators had to become quasi-computer scientists: professionals able to name the parts of a computer—sometimes to assemble the machine itself—and, finally, to make it work (Dennis and Kansky). Not surprising, then, is that among those future technical communicators who entered college in the late 1960s, 1970s, and early 1980s, a pattern of early involvement in computer science courses emerged. Usually, these individuals enrolled in a language course involving FORTRAN or COBOL. One of the technical communicators, for example, noted that in her "third year of college, 1977, at age 27," her college adviser recommended "COBOL/FORTRAN courses as necessary for future success in any field. I took his advice." Another stated,

> My first contact with computers was when I was in college—approximately 1968. I was 20 years old and took a class in FORTRAN programming. The computer used was a mainframe, so our contact consisted of writing the program, which was then given to the punch key operators who created the cards that went into the computer.

More often than not, the participants' tales of these first experiences with computers were horror stories. One technical writer described his early experience with computers, a programming class in FORTRAN:

> Stand in line for access to one of the two keypunches. Type furiously to get the code entered in the allotted time, usually 15 or 30 minutes, depending on the length of the line waiting, hoping not to run out of cards. Loading fresh cards wasn't difficult; one just had to wait for the administrator from hell to break out a new lot. Pray (and this is why the computer center, I think, was located in the basement of the chapel) that none of the cards would be rejected. If so, get back in line for the keypunch. Hope that you don't drop your cards (some would jostle others in line, and the victim would then have to collect the scattered cards and resort, losing the cherished place in line). Under the guidance of the administrator from hell, load the program cards into the input hopper and start the program. Collect cards and program printout and exit smartly. Then spend (n) hours studying the program results, trying to figure out what went wrong. Go to the beginning.

This description was typical of those contributed by many other participants in this project—right down to the use of such words as "administrator from hell." Anxiety, frustration, and sheer desperation all seemed to characterize many of the older respondents' early computer programming experiences. Fortunately, as computer science programs matured and adapted to the growing number of students taking programming courses, some of these conditions improved. Respondents who had attended college in the mid-1980s, for example, were writing about more convenient access:

> My motivation in taking programming courses was to get a piece of paper that said I knew the theory behind my work. These courses were mainly in FORTRAN and COBOL. I had 24-hour a day access and used it nearly every day during this phase of college, about one year.

Another respondent attending college during this period wrote:

> As a college freshman in 1984, I took a FORTRAN class. The professor taught us computer basics and was available in class, in his office, and in the lab for help. Access was available to the computer lab 24 hours a day, 7 days a week. For my journalism classes, I used the computers 3 to 4 days a week.

Yet, despite improved access for these students attending college in the mid-1980s and the fact that their experiences were no longer consistently marked by hostility, the education of many technical communication students was still constrained by impoverished notions of electronic literacy. To prepare themselves for succeeding in the workplace, these individuals wanted and needed less course work in programming and more instruction that focused on computing abilities easily transported and applied to their professional responsibilities as technical communicators. Thus, although the usual course of study in college during the mid-1980s may have served to introduce a number of the participants in this study to computers, the focus of the instruction they received did not prove to be the most effective one for educating them for their chosen profession. Typically, respondents from this generation of technical communicators attributed whatever mastery they acquired with electronic literacy not to their schooling but to their own resourcefulness, to learning from a friend or family member, or to learning on the job.

For those technical communicators who entered college during the late 1980s and early 1990s, the profile differed dramatically. Many of these individuals acquired electronic literacy informally and at home even as they were being introduced to computers at school. Moreover, when they did use computers in more formal educational settings, they were exposed to a broader range of skills associated with electronic literacy—reading, composing, and researching in electronic contexts—as often as to the skills of programming. One participant wrote about getting her first computer:

> I was a kid, about 9 or 10, and begged my parents to buy one. *Everyone* has one! I *have* to have one! So they brought home a Commodore 64, ostensibly for the family, but I used it constantly. It nearly supplanted books as my recreation of choice.

Another participant with a similar profile commented about her early Internet access:

> As I became a teenager, I did all my homework and personal writing on computers and when I entered college in 1993, I got my first e-mail account and was on the Internet by 1994. I was confused more than anything else when people said that 1998 was the year that the Internet "really took off."

And still another respondent attending school during the late 1980s and early 1990s suggested that tutorials were fun:

> My Dad bought one of the first Macintosh computers. We didn't have a computer table in the house, so we set it on the living room floor. My sister and I ran through all the tutorials and thought it was fun.

Computers were part of everyday life in the cultural ecology of participants from this generation, and respondents consistently remarked about how much fun computers were and how natural they felt learning about the ways in which computers worked—especially in self-sponsored settings.

Positive school experiences, however, still seemed relatively rare for these participants. Comments like the following—about teachers' early level of expertise with, and attitudes about, computers—were common:

> The teachers were skeptical about the new technology. Most didn't know anything about the computers.
>
> None of the teachers seemed to know or care about computers until much later. My 11th-grade English teacher was the one who ran the journalism class, where we put together the school paper. We were taught how to paste up the paper on boards with T-squares and rubber cement. No one could run the *PAGEMAKER* program properly, so we'd print out the stories from it and paste them onto the boards.

Although this generation of technical communicators were quick to learn on their own, parents and teachers, for the most part, could not pass on to the new generation electronic-literacy abilities that they themselves did not possess. Fortunately, students had other ways of learning—from their friends, from younger family members, and even on their own. Typical remarks in the autobiographies from this group included comments about sources of help:

> My support includes my friend Mike, the one who helped me put this computer together, and anyone else I interact with.
>
> My younger sister is very computer literate, and she helps me out a lot.
>
> The *PAINTSHOPPRO* and *DREAMWEAVER* manuals are essential to my learning. I also have an HTML reference book. I use these three books constantly.

These individuals seemed to know intuitively that in the twenty-first century, computers, the Internet, and the Web would be every bit as critical a medium for their professional literacy activities as books, paper, pens, and pencils were in the twentieth century.

Having sketched the general historical patterns that characterized technical communicators' acquisition of electronic literacy during the cultural ecologies of the 1970s, 1980s, and 1990s, we turn in the next two sections to four case studies developed from the face-to-face interviews conducted for this project. These personal narratives provide a more nuanced understanding of the social, economic, educational, and political conditions that may have encouraged—or not—the acquisition of electronic literacy for four individuals who were associated with technical communication as a profession.

Two Case Studies of Individuals Who Came of Age in the Cultural Ecology of the 1960s and 1970s

We situate the first two case studies primarily within the cultural ecology of the 1960s and 1970s to give a historical sense of the social, political, and economic times within which these two technical communicators acquired electronic literacy. Much turmoil marked these radical times. The 1968 assassinations of Martin Luther King and then Robert Kennedy, the civil rights marches and riots, the American massacre of villagers at My Lai, draft-card burning, prison rebellions, protests of Native Americans, and the first attempts of state legislative acts to legalize abortion were only a few of the events to occur during the 1960s and their reverberations continued well into the 1970s. As Howard Zinn observed, never before were so many movements for change concentrated during so short a stretch of time. At a women's antiwar meeting in Washington, in 1968, women marched to Arlington National Cemetery and symbolically buried "traditional womanhood," and in New York, to protest the Miss America pageant, women "threw bras, girdles, curlers, false eyelashes, and wigs . . . into a Freedom Trash Can" (260). While these events were being carried out by ordinary Americans, in this same year, the cultural ecology of the times was also to be affected dramatically by the concept of a decentralized communication network that the RAND Corporation presented to the Advanced Research Projects Agency (ARPA)—the first plans for ArpaNet and what would eventually become the Internet.

The two professionals whose narratives we highlight in this section were born in the 1950s and were 19 and 13 years of age in the turbulent transition year of 1969. Interestingly, however, whereas Barbara Evans, born in 1950, became caught up in the antiwar movements that marked the times, Doug Williams, born in 1956, proceeded doggedly through college, just missing the draft and attending a high school and university sheltered from the uprisings. Although Barbara's early attempts at education and life after high school were fraught with the difficulties some young hippies faced during the 1960s and early 1970s, Doug's choices stuck to the straight and narrow. Despite these differences, however, the cases of both these established technical communicators hint at some of the technological and social transformations that have occurred during their lifetimes in the last 50 years of the twentieth century. Neither of these individuals had extensive early support for the acquisition of electronic literacy, as we have defined that term in this article, yet each of them managed, eventually, to create conditions that later allowed them to develop extensive electronic literacy as technical communicators. And despite sometimes tremendous obstacles—social, political, economic—they managed very well indeed. The same resourcefulness and persistence they applied in their everyday lives, they brought to their literacy work with computers. They were not the recipients of concerted efforts to provide electronic literacy in school-based environments; instead, they are among the technical communicators who led—and continue to lead—the way in terms of acquiring electronic literacy on the job or at home. They were also part of the first wave of middle-class Americans who considered a college education as one of their rights as Americans. During these times, more young people began attending college than ever before in the history of the United States (Rudolph), and both Barbara Evans and Doug Williams were among the huge demographic wave of baby boomers (those born between 1946 and 1964) who moved through state systems of higher education. Their autobiographies help answer our research questions about how and why professional communicators living during this period acquired electronic literacy and about the social, economic, cultural, educational, and political factors that influenced their acquisition of such literacy.

Barbara Evans: A College Teacher of Technical Communication

When we encountered Barbara Evans (all names used in this article are pseudonyms), she was a 50-year-old beginning assistant professor of technical communication at a state college in the southern part of the United States.

Like many who came of age during the 1960s, Barbara's career path zigzagged through the difficult times that marked her childhood as well as her adult life in the Southeast: enduring her parents' divorce, attending 11 schools in six years between the 7th and 12th grade, going through several relationships and a divorce of her own, starting and stopping taking classes in a variety of community colleges and four-year schools, living in a commune in the early 1970s, giving birth to a child with severe health problems, experiencing a long stint of political activism, and obtaining a successful career in marketing and management within a national corporation to have the bottom drop out of it in the early 1990s' recession, which suddenly placed her and her son below the poverty line. Although various levels of poverty were not new to Barbara, this was the first time that her difficult and shabby circumstances qualified her and her son for fully financed college educations through Pell Grants and other available means of financial aid.

During the next six years, Barbara earned first a BA in professional and technical writing and then a PhD in English with a specialization in technical communication before, finally, becoming a professor of professional writing at a well-respected university in the Southeast. Although Barbara moved from state to state in her first 50 years, she remained within the rural and urban areas of the American Southeast.

In many respects, this brief review of Barbara's life neglects the many accomplishments she achieved along the way, and, unsurprisingly, her achievements were intimately connected to her formal education, to her conventional literacy practices and values, and, eventually, to her acquisition of electronic literacy as well. Despite her many moves—or perhaps because of them—Barbara was always a "voracious" reader, as she noted, as well as a writer. She prided herself especially on her writing abilities, relating, for example, her literacy expertise to her success as a secretary and finally to her work as a corporate executive. She noted that even when she was a beginning secretary, the president of the particular company for which she was working sent out a memo to all management personnel instructing them that no letter was ever to leave the company without Barbara's looking it over. During her interview, she summed up her conventional literacy abilities:

> I had a facility with language. So, I had it made—that's why I made good grades in school . . . because . . . you give me an essay exam and I'm going to make an A. I don't care what it is in. I don't need to know anything about it. It just needs to be something that I write. And anyway, so, uh, I had always gone around the workplace calling myself a frustrated writer.

Barbara attributed some of her expertise to a very fine early education system in which she was placed in "special resource classes" between the third and sixth grades. A select group of students attended these special classes in which trigonometry, binary codes, and linguistics were taught. Although she did not return to this school system until her senior year in high school, she regarded her experiences within it as the best she received throughout her public education.

In addition to Barbara's school-honed literacy abilities, her family had a history of technological expertise. Her grandfather was part of a team that worked on developing the first televisions in the 1940s; her father was similarly involved in electronics in the next generation, and Barbara remembers always being able to fix any mechanical device she laid her hands on in much the same way that she was later able to program and work with computers. She joked, "Mechanical devices like me. Computers like me, too. When people are having problems, I don't have to do anything—I just walk near them and the computers start working." But Barbara was also very serious about the technological abilities she acquired. The knowledge she came by in the many diverse and sometimes painful workplace settings was often achieved at the expense of time she might have spent with her son or devoted to classes that promised to bring her standard of living above the poverty line.

During the course of Barbara's varied jobs, sporadic courses, and at-home recreation, she managed to accumulate a working knowledge of the many different kinds of electronic machines that populate the workplace. She also acquired the multiple literacy skills needed to operate them. From learning to run a telex machine in her first job at 18 years of age, to mastering databases and entering information in local and national crime centers for a police department, to working with electronic ordering machines that communicate with suppliers' mainframe computers for a supermarket chain, Barbara acquired electronic literacy on the job within the workplaces she inhabited.

Some of the electronic skills she acquired built on skills she learned at school: In high school, for instance, she learned to type 70 words a minute on manual typewriters, and she learned how to program BASIC at a community college. Her formal schooling, however, seemed less important than her actual work experience, at least as far as her development of electronic literacies was concerned. Her recreation at home was likewise important. Whether she was playing early computer games, such as *Pong*, with her son or building a microcomputer out of spare parts with a friend, Barbara was becoming part of a small cadre of computer experts of the 1980s. By the time she received a PhD in technical communication at age 49, Barbara had managed to develop the kind of electronic literacy that few women of her age had acquired.

Doug Williams: A Professional Communicator

When we turn to Doug Williams, a 44-year-old professional writer and public relations coordinator at a midsize, midwestern state university, we encounter a very different kind of career path—one that, in the 1970s and 1980s, had few detours along the way. In 1974, Doug's first year of college, the antiwar movement had peaked, and Saigon fell the following year. Doug told us that the antiwar movement had little visibility at his institution although he was against the war. Doug attended college, first as an undergraduate engineering major and then as a professional communication major. As a junior, he dropped out of engineering courses, which he disliked, and enrolled in his school's professional writing program, newly established in the late 1970s. He became an editor of the school's newspaper and, eventually, after graduating and working briefly in the Southeast as the communication director for his fraternity's national headquarters, returned to the Midwest to attend graduate school at a large state research institution. Two years later, after earning a master's degree in journalism, Doug secured a position at his undergraduate institution in public relations and professional writing for the alumni office. He has worked successfully in this position since 1985.

Like his uninterrupted career path, Doug's early life seems typical for a boy growing up in a white, middle-class family during the late 1950s and 1960s. He had parents who were both teachers and a twin brother whom he regards as abler than he in all respects. His brother acquired a computer a year before Doug. Unlike Barbara Evans, Doug does not remember having a particular talent for writing; he does, however, remember learning to read in kindergarten. His father had Doug show off his reading abilities in front of the third-grade class he was teaching. As children, he and his brother often borrowed similar books from the library and were expected to read for half an hour in bed before going to sleep. The first time Doug ever regarded himself as a writer by profession occurred when he became an editor of the college newspaper.

At first glance, few similarities seem prevalent in the lives of Doug and Barbara. Certainly none of the roller-coaster ups and downs that characterized

Barbara's life were evident in the account of Doug's home life, school experiences, and professional positions. Nor, when growing up, did Doug possess the same extraordinary technological capabilities Barbara did. He appears, on all counts, to be what some would call a regular, middle-of-the-road guy, and a successful one at that. Unlike Barbara, Doug avoided much of the turmoil that often accompanied the activist movements of the times. Also unlike Barbara, he was able to rely on financial support from first his parents and then his spouse in earning his BA and MA degrees. But, on closer examination, strong similarities become apparent in the lives of these two professionals, especially in their experiences with acquiring expertise in electronic literacy.

As was the case with Barbara and many of the respondents, schooling contributed to Doug's education with computers, but it was not responsible for the enthusiasm for or direct expertise in electronic literacy he was later to develop. Doug's first exposure to computers came in his first year at college during the early 1970s when he took a course on FORTRAN. In the course, he remembered coding stacks of punched cards, running the stacks of 80 or so cards through a reader, and then waiting to find out whether the program would compile. More often than not, he would need to start all over again, checking for minor mistakes he made in entering the data. At the time, a limited number of card readers existed on campus, so students waited for hours just to have their punched cards read. In this course, Doug did not have easy or direct access to the mainframe computer to which his card data were sent—it resided behind locked doors in an air-conditioned space, safe from the hands of most curious and untrained college students. Doug became the school's newspaper editor in his senior year, but in the 1970s, writing for the newspaper was still done on machines that more closely resembled typewriters than computers. He recalled that his early computer experiences had been frustrating and time consuming:

> [By the time] I entered grad school, I finally began viewing [computers] as this sort of nice work-saving device after having been used to, well, when I was working at the [newspaper], you know, we had this, uh, thing that looked like an IBM Selectric, but you, it had this little dial on it that you had to use to justify the columns, and every line had to be done separately to get the right number of pages so it would be justified. So I'm thinking about that and how long it took to get the newspaper done every week with that thing.

Doug did not work directly on mainframe computers until he took a programming course while working as a professional communicator for his national fraternal organization in the South. In these early days of computers, concepts of computer literacy were tied intimately to being able to program, and Doug set about learning BASIC. By the late 1970s, he was able to enter his programs on a mainframe rather than going through the punched-card routine. But still, computers did not become an integral part of his literacy practices and values until 1983, when his wife helped him buy the family's first personal computer so that he could use it to complete papers for his master's degree. Word processing—with *Wordstar*—became Doug's main mode of writing as a graduate student and, two years later, as a professional writer. As Doug recalls it:

> And then here I am, you know, five, five and a half years later, and I've got this machine with a screen on it, and if you want to justify, you can type in a code, you know control-J or whatever it was, and boom, it's justified. Don't like it, type control-L and undo it. And there was this little, um, foldout card that came with it with frequently used commands. So I taped that on the wall next to the computer at home in our apartment and used that frequently, especially at the beginning.

Over the years, and after assuming his current position as a professional communicator at a midsize university in the Midwest, Doug continued to learn programs that, like the early *Wordstar*, were essential to his writing and to his responsibilities for producing professional-quality publications for the university. He came to rely on *Word, Page Mill, Photoshop*, and *Quark*, oftentimes because the designers with whom he worked used them. He explains his acquisition of software skills:

> I write the magazine, they design it, and then I have to get into their file to do the final edits before it goes to the press, so I had to learn at least enough of [*Quark*] to do that. As long as it's learning the basics, you know, I'm pretty comfortable with learning enough to do what I need to do. I mean, I don't dig into programs and try to do everything they can do, but more, okay, what do I have to know to make this thing do what I want it do? I don't know; this may go back with being sort of an early adopter, I guess, because 1983 was pretty much the Stone Age in terms of the PCs.

Thus, Doug acquired—and continues to acquire—electronic-literacy skills and values that undergird his successful performance within his workplace environment. In this way, his experience is much like Barbara's. She, too, acquired most of her electronic-literacy skills on the job, as she explained in an interview:

> The reason that I had always believed that I was able to move up in the workplace was because of my literacy skills, as well as my keyboarding skills, and facility with [learning] computer technologies when they came into the workplace.

If the 1960s and 1970s marked a time of radical political transition, the 1970s and 1980s marked a time of radical literacy transition. Sophisticated digital communication environments were developed, and these inventions provided a fertile ground for the emergence of electronic-literacy practices that began to compete with more conventional print literacy practices. In this transitional cultural ecology, Barbara and Doug attended secondary school and college. As a result, they really accumulated two sets of literacy skills and values, one for conventional print literacy and one for the newer electronic literacy. Their conventional literacy was acquired from formal schooling and supported in the home. And, although schools also provided their first exposure to computers, these experiences were focused on programming rather than on electronic-literacy practices. Both individuals, therefore, developed their electronic-literacy skills primarily at home or on the job, as the computer hardware and software that supported such literacy practices—desktop publishing and page-layout software, photo-manipulation software, Web-publishing software—came on the market and were integrated into workplace settings. Their experiences as early adopters of technology, even when painful, have given them a high level of confidence both about the electronic-literacy skills they currently practice in digital environments and about their ability to continue acquiring new literacy skills within these environments.

Two Case Studies of Individuals Who Came of Age in the Cultural Ecology of the 1980s and 1990s

When we turn to today's preprofessional communicators—individuals who developed electronic literacy in the cultural ecology of the 1980s and 1990s—we see a very different pattern. Barbara and Doug, and the online respondents in their general age-group, had few of the educational opportunities to learn electronic literacy that we map out here. In addition, the requirements for learning to create communication in digital environments during the 1970s and early 1980s demonstrate only the initial elements of electronic-literacy expertise required of today's students. The students we present next—Angela and Pauline—encountered electronic technologies one generation after Barbara and Doug, but the cultural ecology of Angela and Pauline's generation, as far as information technologies are concerned, had changed dramatically over 25 years. As a result, the autobiographies of these two individuals contributed additional information about how and why professional communicators living from 1978 to 2000 acquired electronic literacy and about the social, economic, cultural, educational, and political factors that influenced their acquisition of such literacy.

The lives of these two students—both women majoring in technical communication, one at the undergraduate level and one at the graduate level—are roughly contemporaneous with the invention of the microcomputer. Thus, they provide two cultural tracings of how and when personal computers, mass-produced and mass-marketed beginning in 1977, initially found their way into the lives of individuals and families. Moreover, the period during which these two individuals first attended public schools—entering first grade in 1978 (Pauline) and 1983 (Angela)—witnessed public school educators in many areas of the country making some of the first significant efforts to integrate personal computers into public education, even when, as the online respondents pointed out, these efforts were insufficient.

During this period of time, handheld computer games—*Home Pong, Chuck E. Cheese, Space Invaders, Lunar Lander, Asteroids*—became increasingly popular and commercially viable, and educators were quick to catch on to the productive connections between learning and computers. For instance, Seymour

Papert's *LOGO*, initiated as a development project in 1967, became increasingly popular as a computer game/programming language/learning environment designed to stimulate children's creative thinking. And educational computer games were only the first tentative step of integrating technology into education. The use of microcomputers in public schools increased from 18 percent to 85 percent from 1981 to 1984. By 1984, approximately 82 percent of American elementary schools, 94 percent of junior high schools, and 95 percent of high schools reported using microcomputers for instruction. Even more important, perhaps, the personal computers that were entering American schoolrooms were being used as environments to teach literacy skills as well as programming skills. From 1984 to 1994, for instance, the number of schoolchildren who used computers as a literacy tool increased dramatically from 23.4 percent to 68.3 percent (United States, *Condition 1997* 56). And by 1994, 87 percent of students in grade 11 used computers at home and at school for writing stories and papers, 71 percent used computers to learn things, and 61 percent used computers in a library setting (Coley, Crandler, and Engle 27).

Unfortunately, despite the fact that computers were being rapidly deployed in American schools as literacy tools during this period, their distribution was far from equitable across the population. A 1987 report authored by Cole and Griffin, for instance, indicated unfortunate inequities:

- More computers are being placed in the hands of middle- and upper-class children than poor children.
- When computers are placed in the schools of poor children, they are used for rote drill and practice instead of the cognitive enrichment that they provide for middle- and upper-class students. (43–44)

By the end of the 1980s, then, although computers were increasingly present in many schools, they were being used in ways that sustained educational problems aligned along the axes of race and poverty. In 1984, for example—when Pauline was in seventh grade—14.3 percent of American students in grades 7 to 12 reported using computers in their homes, and 30.7 percent reported using computers at school (United States, *Condition 1998* 189). However, students' access to these machines in both homes and schools differed significantly for students in high- and low-income families. Unsurprisingly, computers were much more common in high-income families. Similarly, whereas 35.8 percent of high-income students reported using a computer at school, only 21.8 percent of low-income students were able to do so (United States, *Condition 1998* 189). This situation, moreover, was mirrored in schools with high populations of students of color. Whereas 30 percent of white students reported using computers at school, only 17 percent of black students reported doing so (United States, *Digest 1995* Table 415).

Within the rapidly changing cultural ecology of the 1980s and the 1990s, Angela's and Pauline's cases represent a historically situated study of how two young people were exposed to the new technology of microcomputers as these machines first became a regular part of the literacy instruction future technical communicators were receiving. These cases are also intriguing because they help bracket the processes of acquiring electronic literacy within two very different kinds of cultural, material, educational, and familial contexts. Angela—white and from a middle-class background—grew up in a context that provided extensive, varied, and sustained support for both literacy and electronic-literacy efforts. Pauline—black and from a working-class background—grew up in a family that had to struggle to support literacy and electronic-literacy efforts. In this sense, these cases provide some beginning clues about the fundamental ways in which factors within a cultural ecology shape the electronic literacy that technical communicators are able to acquire.

The decade of the 1980s marked the beginning of the Reagan presidency in January of 1981. Approximately a year and a half after that date—in September of 1982—Angela entered kindergarten in a midsize city in the Midwest, and Pauline entered fifth grade in a midsize city in the South.

Angela Ashton: Acquiring Electronic Literacy in a White, Middle-Class Family

Angela, like many technical communication students of her generation, remembered using educational computer games as her very first experiences with technology in elementary school:

> In the third grade . . . we would use a computer program on Apple computers to help learn math facts, such as the multiplication tables. It would ask us problems, and we'd have to type in the answers. . . . I first learned to use the computer in the fourth grade; we started playing games such as the *Oregon Trail*, and we also began typing in word-processing programs. . . . I was probably about 9 years old. . . . We had maybe two hours a week access to the computers. It was usually in the afternoon . . . , and the other students and the teacher were there. I never used a computer by myself. . . . We were allowed to talk, but it wasn't rowdy.

Although Angela could not remember any specific content matter from these programs—and did not mention that the games she played were challenging in an intellectual sense—we cannot argue, based on her perspective, that the early use of educational games was wholly ineffective. Unlike Barbara and Doug, or the other technical communicators in their general age cadre who responded online, Angela began early in her schooling experience to associate computers with fun, privilege, and a sense of accomplishment. And these positive game-playing experiences were linked to electronic-literacy practices as well:

> In fourth grade, we started playing games . . . , and we also began typing in word-processing programs. This was all done on the Apple IIe computers with the green screens. With this [word processing], we started to have to learn to turn on and off the machines and be able to get to the program we wanted by typing various commands.

The instruction Angela received in school, however, was only one of many factors affecting her acquisition and development of electronic literacy. She lived, as well, in a home environment that offered robust systems of support.

Among the most important circumstances that contributed to Angela's eventual acquisition of electronic literacy at home was a set of related factors that had little to do—at least directly—with computer hardware or software: the high value that her parents placed on conventional print-literacy activities in general, the ability of her parents to provide sustained economic support for such values and activities, and the degree to which her parents believed a formal education to be the key to their children's and their own prosperity.

Not surprisingly, when the time came to choose the college she would attend, Angela sought out institutions and academic majors that took advantage of her electronic-literacy practices and strengths. She became an undergraduate scientific and technical communication major at a midsize, midwestern university that emphasized technology in most of its major areas of study. As a scientific and technical communication major, Angela noted, she was expected to have considerable knowledge of computers and to be proficient in literacy practices within digital environments:

> I use the Web for a lot of research-type things. I also use it to find images and graphics I need. I use the Web to buy tickets for concerts, to buy CDs and books and other shopping things, and I use the Web to get free e-mail when I'm home. I also use the Web to put up my Web page to show off my résumé to employers. Just recently, I used the Web to research a Web site I made about backcountry downhill skiing. . . . I use the computer to type papers and memos; I use the computer for e-mail, the Internet, and creating various desktop publishing things, posters, table tents, and so on; and I use the scanner and software like *Photoshop*, and Macromedia [*Director*], [and] *Freehand*/Adobe *Illustrator* to create graphics for various things like papers, projects, and Web sites.

Pauline Patterson: Acquiring Electronic Literacy in a Black, Working-Class Family

Another technical communication student we interviewed, Pauline Patterson, an African American who grew up in an economically disadvantaged family, inhabited a different cultural ecology than did Angela, and followed a different route to acquiring electronic literacies as well. Although Pauline's working-class mother, Jean, placed a high value on education and literacy, she had to struggle against economic odds to provide her daughter the support she needed to succeed: "My mother and I were always avid readers. As a child, I was encouraged to read and write. It was my primary source of entertainment throughout my childhood and teen years."

Pauline's first exposure to computer technology came in 1980 when an expert on mainframe computers came to talk to her third-grade class. At that point in history, relatively few public school teachers were familiar with computers—given that the access to the large mainframes was limited within colleges and universities and that the mainframes themselves were so expensive as to be out of reach for most public schools. Nevertheless, the general enthusiasm for computers ran high among educators, if not always among students. As Pauline recalled: "What I remember about computers . . . was that they were enormous in size and were mostly for businesses and the government. I know that some people in my school had the personal computers that they played games on."

Pauline, like many other students of color, continued to have limited access to computers through the decade of the 1980s—even though Americans in general were increasingly aware of the power that these new machines had to change the nature of learning and the need to prepare students for an increasingly technological workplace. At the time Pauline entered ninth grade in 1986, her high school, in which 40 percent of the enrollees were students of color, was not yet integrating computers into a wide range of courses or providing all students a robust program of access to technology. Given these circumstances, in the summer before Pauline entered the ninth grade, her mother took the practical step of encouraging her daughter to seek access to computers outside of the regular school environment in a summer computer course. To support her daughter's work in computer-based communication environments, Pauline's mother also bought a $300 word processor from Sears—a purchase that, although not as expensive as a fully functional personal computer, represented a major expenditure of family resources. As Pauline remembered it: "I thought . . . [computers were] something that rich people and spoiled kids had. I knew that I would never have one. Not even a question."

Computers were good news for education, but not necessarily for all students. In 1989, for instance, when Pauline was a senior in high school, 65.5 percent of high-income students reported using a computer at school, whereas only 53.3 percent of low-income students were able to do so (United States, *Condition 1998* 189). Similarly, 40.6 percent of white students in grades 9 to 12 reported using computers at school, whereas only 33.6 percent of black students reported doing so (United States, *Digest 1995* Table 415). As Pauline remembers the situation at her own high school, computers may have been present, but they were not integrated systematically into the courses she took—even in her senior year.

Pauline, however, understood that an increasing number of American workers were using computers for work in communication contexts (United States, *Digest 1992*). To prepare for this new environment, she enrolled in college in 1989 and signed up immediately for the university's introductory course on computer applications. By the time Pauline had finished a second university-level course in computer applications, she had become accustomed to learning computer-based literacies on her own or with the help of other students in the university computer labs. And she had also grown accustomed to the value that the university community put on computer-based literacies:

> I began to use computers to type papers and to complete the assignments that required computer usage. Mostly *Word* and *Excel* stuff. I started using *Powerpoint* my junior/senior year, around 1994. . . . It was exciting.

> I know that students received higher grades if they gave a presentation using *Powerpoint* rather than just doing posters and such.

In 1995, Pauline graduated from the university with a bachelor of science degree in marketing and a minor in speech communication. During the next four years, she became a buying assistant for a shoe company, a freelance writer, a transcriptionist for a video producer, an assistant to a record producer, and a reporter for a large publishing firm. In each of these jobs, Pauline used computers for reading and writing and communicating on a routine basis.

By 1999, however, motivated by a desire to find a job that went beyond conventional writing and editing and branch out into computer-assisted design work, Pauline returned to her alma mater to begin a master's-level graduate program in professional communication. And though she knew graduate school would strain her financial resources severely, Pauline began her graduate career by purchasing a computer of her own as an investment in her academic success:

> I purchased my computer online. When I decided to return for graduate school in August of 1999, I knew that I had to have a computer. I started researching by reading technology and computer magazine like *PC World* and *PC Shopper*. I looked at price and value comparisons, in mags and on the Web.
>
> My computer cost me just under $1,500. I pay $38 a month. I was afraid to make the investment because I knew that I would live like a pauper in grad school. But it was imperative that I have one, so I made the sacrifice.

At the time of her interview in the spring of 2001, Pauline was employed as the graduate assistant editor at the university's publication office. Her duties, as she noted, involved "writing/editing/proofing copy for brochures, posters, catalogs, the alumni magazine, ads, and so on . . . work[ing] with the designers to create the visual images . . . reformatting and redesigning of existing documents . . . us[ing] *Word, Photoshop, Illustrator, Pagemaker*."

Pauline currently relies on her computer to support many of her academic and leisure-time activities and is confident of her electronic-literacy abilities:

> I think I have an above-average skill level [with computers]. I find that I grasp new technology quickly. I am very comfortable with computers and technology. I am proficient with Microsoft Office programs, except *Access*. (I'm familiar but not good.) I know Adobe *Pagemaker* and *Photoshop*. I'm comfortable with Macromedia [*Director*], *Dreamweaver*. I am still trying to learn *Flash*. I learn best when I just sit down and play. I've been introduced to MOOing. I want to learn Quark [*Xpress*] and *Illustrator*.

Given the rapid rate of technological and social change occurring from the 1960s to the 1990s, the cultural ecologies that Angela and Pauline inhabited were very different from those that shaped the electronic literacies of

Barbara and Doug. As a result of the different social, political, economic, and technological factors characterizing these ecologies, the computing sophistication that Angela and Pauline have acquired while in college—although they came to it along very different routes—was on a par with that which Barbara, Doug, and the early adopters in our online sample achieved only after years in the workplace. And what is every bit as striking is that Angela and Pauline are not atypical. In one generation, the advanced literacies of electronic environments have become commonplace among members of this succeeding age group.

Observations about the Development of Communication Instruction in the Twenty-First Century

The firsthand accounts that we have presented in this article can help us trace the ways in which 59 technical communicators acquired electronic literacy with computers during a particularly dynamic period in our nation's history. Deborah Brandt argues persuasively:

> The history of literacy at any moment involves a complex, sometimes cacophonous mix of fading and ascending materials, practices, and ideologies. Literacy is always in flux. Learning to read and write necessitates an engagement with this flux, with the layers of literacy's past, present, and future, often embodied in materials and tools and just as often embodied in the social relationships we have with the people who are teaching us to read and write. ("Accumulating" 666)

To this thought, we might add "learning to read and write on and off computers," for information technologies today clearly are engrained in our notions of what being fully literate in the twenty-first century means.

We do not mean to suggest that the few stories we present here comprise any kind of a complete history. Clearly, they represent only a small portion of some larger narratives that link electronic literacy with the profession of technical communication: how different groups of technical communicators adapted their literacy values and practices to computer-supported environments; how technical communicators gained access to computers; how race, class, and gender affected this access; how and why electronic literacy has thrived within the American workplace and the global marketplace; how technical communicators have employed electronic literacy within the workplace.

We recognize, in other words, that no one story—and certainly not this collection of stories—can be considered indicative or representative of any larger population. Far too many stories remain uncollected, unheard, unappreciated for such larger narratives to be considered completely, or even accurately, rendered. This recognition, however, does not diminish the value of these firsthand accounts themselves. They are richly sown with information that we can use to construct some tentative observations—hypotheses really—about the literacy skills and values technical communicators need to succeed in the twenty-first century and about the field of technical communication itself. These can then be tested further through additional study.

We know the observations that follow will speak differently to individual readers about patterns or trends in these data—and about how the data can assist technical communication instructors, program directors, and workplace supervisors in identifying increasingly effective approaches to teaching electronic literacy or setting professional policy concerning electronic literacy. The resonance of autobiographies always varies according to the personal experiences of readers who, themselves, grew up in particular cultural ecologies. Hence, observations we identify do not represent the only instruction that readers can or should draw from the cases we have provided nor have the observations been somehow scientifically derived from the cases themselves. Moreover, our articulation of these observations may change as we learn more about how technical communicators acquired electronic literacy in the last three to four decades of the twentieth century. These particular observations have come to us, as teachers of technical communication, because of our own background and gender; the ways we learned to use technology ourselves; the schools and workplaces we have inhabited; and, finally, our own connections with, and understanding of, the individuals with whom we worked. These observations, in other words, make sense to us.

Observation 1: To be considered fully literate at the beginning of the twenty-first century, technical communicators must be able to read, write, and navigate in technological contexts. This new definition of literacy now constitutes a de facto standard within the profession of technical communication.

During the last two decades of the twentieth century, literacy and technology became inextricably connected in the consciousness of Americans and in the social fabric of this country (Selfe). This study suggests that the new definition of literacy emerging from this period—which includes the ability to read, write, and navigate in technological contexts, or electronic literacy—has also changed the profession of technical communication in fundamental ways. The online personal histories of technical communicators—the two case studies of communication professionals and the two case studies of students majoring in technical communication—suggest a pattern of shifting educational and professional values within the dynamic cultural ecology of the computer revolution. We believe this revolution, especially that part of it that coincides with the commercial production and marketing of personal computers, has resulted not only in an important change in society's basic definition of literacy but also in our profession's definition of literacy and in the skills that citizens need to succeed as technical communicators in the workplace.

During the early years in which these changes were taking place, as the autobiographies in this project suggest, those individuals responsible for the education of technical communicators initially understood computers as calculating machines—not as writing or communication systems—and were unaware of how radically the practice of electronic literacy would change the world around them. Educators did, however, recognize the growing importance of computers in the American culture. Future technical communicators also understood that knowing how to communicate with, on, and about computers would be indispensable to their professional aspirations, and they acted on this tacit understanding. In the autobiographies collected for this project, evidence of such foresight appears again and again: in stories of an adviser recommending a programming course, a parent buying a computer that she knew little about, or a future technical communication specialist slogging through a tortuous course of computer programming to glean as much information as possible about the new machines. Each of these stories provides a tracing of how microcomputers came to lodge themselves in the professional experiences and consciousness of technical communicators.

Observation 2: Literacy exists within a complex cultural ecology of social, historical, and economic effects. Within this cultural ecology, literacies have life spans.

The autobiographies we collected for this project suggest the dynamic, culturally determined nature of electronic-literacy activities as they are practiced and valued in any given historical period. And the data here may support a revision of what Brandt has referred to as "accumulating" literacies: the "piling up and extending out of literacy and its technologies" that "give a complex flavor even to elementary acts of reading and writing . . . creating new and hybrid forms of literacy where once there might have been fewer and more circumscribed forms." The "rapid proliferation and diversification of literacy," Brandt argues, places increasing pressure on individuals, whose ultimate success may be "best measured by a person's capacity to amalgamate new reading and writing practices in response to rapid social change" ("Accumulating" 651).

Based on what we have learned from this project, however, we would also argue the possibility that forms of literacy—different sets of communication practices and values—may have *life spans*, half-lives determined by their fitness with, and influence on, the cultural ecology within which they exist. This finding helps explain how multiple forms of literacy emerge, compete and accumulate, flourish, and fade over time, depending on their general fitness with, and influence on, a broader cultural ecology. Literacies accumulate, we suspect, when a culture is undergoing a particularly dramatic or radical transition—for instance, during the computer revolution. We also believe, as Brandt suggests ("Accumulating"), that in our contemporary culture, which is making the transition from print-based literacies to digitally based literacies, multiple literacies are accumulating and competing. During such a period, we believe that professional communicators and people in general succeed best when they value and practice both emerging and competing forms of literacy, like Barbara, Doug, Angela, and Pauline: print and digital literacies, alphabetic literacies, visual literacies, and intertextual forms of media literacies (George and Shoos). Eventually, however, we suspect that this accumulation reaches a limit—humans can only cope with so many literacies at once, and the cultural distribution of literacies takes time to unfold. And so we see evidence that a process of selection occurs. Sets of literacy practices and values that fit less well with changing cultural ecologies fade while other literacy practices that fit more robustly with those contexts flourish.

Within the context of this finding, we can understand how more experienced technical communicators like Barbara and Doug felt when faced with the prospect of learning the emerging communication practices associated with mainframe computer programming and, later in their lives, the even newer communication practices associated with microcomputer and networked computer environments. During the transition period of the past 20 years, these individuals have had to cope not only with the demands of more conventional literacy practices (e.g., composing a memo on a typewriter, drafting a report by hand, calling contacts on the telephone) valued in traditional corporate cultures and, sometimes, the culture at large, but they have also had to learn the digitally based literacies associated with word processing, e-mail, and network navigation. Understanding that literacies emerge, compete, and fade within the context of a particular cultural ecology also helps explain why computer-based communication practices—which fit well within the increasingly global activities of corporate workplaces and the technological environments of educational institutions—have become more important to today's technical communicators within the context of their careers. It also helps explain why the conventional print-based literacy practices in which these same individuals used to engage (e.g., handwritten letters or typed memos) have faded in their importance.

The model further suggests in what ways literacy practices might be accumulating in the academic lives of younger technical communication students and in the cultural ecology that they inhabit. The literacy practices in which these students engage involve their using several word-processing packages, several e-mail and page-layout programs, graphics and photo-manipulation programs, Web- and multimedia-design software, rendering and animation software, video- and audio-capture software, HTML, stand-alone computers, networked computers, and the World Wide Web. In their technical communication programs, these students complete many of their class projects and much of their peer-group communication entirely online.

Data from these autobiographies suggest that technical communicators need to be able to deal flexibly with both emerging and fading forms of literacy as communication systems continue to undergo rapid change in the cultural ecology of twenty-first-century America. Lending weight to this suggestion are the dynamic communication situations resulting from the increasing influence of globalization, the emergence of transnational financial and political entities, the formulation of new online interest groups, and America's growing dependence on electronic information services—all of these factors and more contribute to a milieu in which change is the only real constant and flexibility the only effective response.

Observation 3: Although a complex of factors have affected technical communicators' acquisition of digital literacy, race and class—and sometimes gender and age – can assume all too important a role in the lives of some individuals because these factors are linked with other social formations at numerous levels and because their effects were multiplied and magnified by these linkages.

A number of the autobiographies we collected for this project indicate that race and class, and sometimes gender and age—because they are articulated with so many other social, cultural, and material formations—have been key factors in shaping the cultural ecologies within which individual technical communicators acquired electonic literacy during the end of the twentieth century. Pauline's narrative, for example, details the substantial role that both race and class can exert on individuals' opportunities to acquire and develop technological literacy—and, indeed, literacy in general. Race exerted a major influence on Pauline's educational experience in a school enrolling a high population of students of color, determining, at least in part, the opportunities she had to develop electronic literacy.

The effects of race and class manifested themselves in the lives of technical communicators throughout the end of the twentieth century. Families of color, for instance, continued to be less likely than were white families to have computers in their homes, in part because race and poverty also continued to be closely aligned in this country:

- In 1998, "73% of white students owned home computers, only 32% of African American students owned one," a difference that correlated with students' reported household income (Hoffman and Novak 390).
- In 1998, "White households continued to own computers at a rate roughly twice that of Black and Hispanic households" (United States, *Falling* 84).
- These substantial inequities increased rather than decreased at the end of the century. From October 1997 to December 1998, the gap between white and black households that reported having a computer "increased 5.1 percentage points from a 13.5 percentage point difference in 1997 to an 18.6 percentage point difference in 1998." From December 1998 to August 2000, the divide between white and black households increased 4 percentage points, "resulting in a difference of 22.6 points between white and black households" (United States, *Falling* 16).

Race and class also affected people's access to computers, and thus their digital literacy, in US workplaces from 1978 to the end of the twentieth century. A great deal of evidence corroborates this claim:

- In 1993, for example, 48.7 percent of white workers (18 years and older) used computers at work, whereas only 36.2 percent of black workers did (United States, *Digest 1999* ch. 7, Table 430).
- In 1997, 53.8 percent of white workers (18 years and older) used computers at work, whereas only 40.0 percent of black workers did (United States, *Digest 1999* ch. 7, Table 430).
- In 2000, 14.1 percent of white workers had access to the Internet at work, whereas only 8.1 percent of black workers and 5.6 percent of Hispanics did (United States, *Falling* 47).

If, however, the cases presented here have convinced us that race and poverty are key factors that often shape the digital literacy of individuals, they also indicate that race and class alone do not always fully determine the lives and the electronic literacies of individuals. Pauline, for instance, although limited by her education and economic situation, managed to create the conditions under which she could develop electronic literacy, go to college, and become a technical communicator—working against the prevailing grain of poverty, race, and education that structured her life.

Similarly, gender and age, especially when they are articulated with other social, cultural, and material factors such as race and poverty, can be key factors in determining whether, how, and when individuals acquire (or fail to acquire) digital literacy. Barbara's autobiography, for instance, indicated how the cultural ecology inhabited by women—especially those who are single parents in economically disadvantaged situations—can affect their acquisition of electronic literacy. In this country, for example, two-parent households are "nearly twice as likely to have Internet access as single-parent households" (60.6 percent for two-parent households versus 32.8 percent for single-parent households). Even more important, however, single male-headed households are also more likely than are single female-headed households to have such access (36 percent for single male-headed house holds and 30 percent for single female-headed households) ("Native" 18). Barbara's case has also convinced us, however, that economically disadvantaged women whose access to technology is constrained early in their lives can often still acquire and develop electronic literacies later, given that appropriate access, sponsors, timing, motivation, and other conditions are in place.

Recognizing the effects of race, class, gender, and age on the electronic literacy of technical communicators, we can see not only the importance of providing all children and college students with access to an equitable education fully supported by computer technology but also of establishing continuing education programs within workplaces and professional organizations. These programs would serve to ameliorate the effects of race, poverty, gender, and age by providing equitable opportunities for all technical communicators to expand their electronic literacy.

Observation 4: Technical communication programs – and the faculty who teach within them – may need to be increasingly active in learning to value and teach both emerging and fading literacy practices.

Unfortunately, as these autobiographies indicated, the educational environments that young technical communication students inhabit are still not uniform in their predisposition toward the new digital communication practices. Although most academic programs of technical communication, for instance, now value computer-based literacies, they also, understandably, continue to value the traditional and conventional literacies that have shaped faculty members' educational experiences, their grading and evaluation standards, the hiring decisions of many employers, the expectations of parents, the degree requirements of universities, and the historically defined literacy ideals of the culture at large.

In this context, technical communication programs may be particularly vulnerable to contested literacy practices. Such programs typically employ a volatile mixture of English composition teachers who may value print-based systems of communication and conventional literacy practices and multimedia/design specialists who may value digitally based communication practices and unconventional standards of composition. Clearly, this transitional context can make for a contested landscape in which literacies accumulate and compete. As a result, technical communication students in many programs must not only develop a robust set of online communication practices, the ability to work effectively with visual images and arguments, and a full complement of skills in Web-based and multimedia design but also an equally impressive set of print-based skills, linear text-based arguments, and facility with alphabetic communication practices. Moreover, these students must determine, within each course and sometimes from assignment to assignment, which of these skills and complex understandings will be valued and assessed positively by a particular instructor.

This situation suggests that faculty within technical communication programs—especially during this time of rapid and dramatic social and cultural transformation—may need to be much more active in recognizing, studying, and addressing a range of literacies and in understanding how such literacies are operating within historical periods and cultural ecologies. These faculty members need to make this effort so that they can help students successfully negotiate and reconcile contested literacy values and practices. The effort may also help technical communication faculty understand why many conventional print-based literacy standards—and the more traditional curricular practices and standards they engender—seem to hold a declining relevance for younger technical communication students and for the public at large. It may also provide technical communication faculty with motivation for studying a larger range of the literacy practices now emerging in electronic environments as individuals read and compose images and animations, multimedia creations, and assemblages of graphics and text and communicate on the Web and in chat rooms, in combinations of moving images, still graphics, text, and voice.

Observation 5: Individual technical communicators may need to be increasingly active in teaching both themselves and their peers emerging forms of electronic literacy.

The online responses and cases also indicated that not always did the adviser, parent, or instructor necessarily teach the emerging, digital-literacy practices. In fact, more often than not, a friend or sometimes a younger family member came to the rescue. In many of the cases we encountered in this project, teachers and parents lacked the knowledge to transmit the requisite computer expertise to students and children.

As early as 1970, Margaret Mead described the unsettling sense of functioning within a culture in which adults lack the necessary knowledge and abilities to pass on to the next generation. She called cultures of this kind "prefigurative." The prefigurative learning culture occurs in a society where change is so rapid that adults are trying to prepare children for experiences the adults themselves have never had. The prefigurative cultural style, Mead argued, prevails in a world where the "past, the culture that had shaped [young adults'] understanding—their thoughts, their feelings, and their conceptions of the world—[is] no sure guide to the present. And the elders among them, bound to the past, [can] provide no models for the future" (70). Mead traced these broad patterns of cultural change particularly in terms of American culture, all the while setting her analysis within a global context. She claimed that the prefigurative culture that is characteristic of America in the 1960s and ensuing years—and, we maintain, in the new millennium—is symptomatic of a world changing so fast that it exists "without models and without precedent," a culture in which "neither parents nor teachers, lawyers, doctors, skilled workers, inventors, preachers, or prophets" (xx) can teach children what they need to know about the world. Mead noted that the immediate and dramatic needs that our prefigurative culture faces—fueled by increasing world hunger, the continuing population explosion, the rapid explosion of technological knowledge, the threat of continued war, global communication—demand a new kind of social and educational response that privileges participatory input, ecological sensitivity, appreciation for cultural diversity, and intelligent use of technology, among other themes. In the prefigurative society, Mead argued, students must—at least to some extent—learn important lessons from each other, together finding their way through an unfamiliar thicket of issues and situations about which elder members of the society are uncertain. Unlike previous generations, adults cannot promise to provide students with a stable and unchanging body of knowledge—especially in connection with the acquisition of electronic literacy. Within such a context, technical communication students must be willing to experiment with emerging forms of digital—and even nonalphabetic—literacies and to help each other master the skills needed to succeed with these forms.

The autobiographies that we have collected suggest, however, that individuals are not simply victims caught in a web of circumstances. In some circumstances, they can—and do—affect the cultural ecology within which they live. Thus, personal motivation and interest, we believe, can play a substantial role in the development of electronic literacy. Barbara, for example, managed to complete her graduate studies, against significant economic and personal odds, because of her personal confidence in her literacy skills and her interest in technology. Pauline honed her electronic-literacy skills—both in college courses and on her own time—because she wanted access to jobs that required such skills. As these two cases suggest, some individuals, under the right combination of circumstances, may find ways to develop or support their electronic-literacy activities even when conditions are far from ideal. Timing may also play an important role in how and when individuals acquire electronic literacy. As Barbara's and Pauline's case studies, and many of the other autobiographies, indicated, individuals who were not able to gain access to computers—or to the right kinds of computers—at one point in their lives, found ways, at other points, to improve considerably their access to appropriate technology.

> *Observation 6: The digital divide characterizing the end of the twentieth century—and affecting the prospects of some technical communicators—will never be fully addressed until access to computers and to the acquisition and development of electronic literacy is understood as a vital, multidimensional part of a larger cultural ecology.*

The preceding discussion of case studies from this project illustrates only a portion of the complexity associated with access to computers—and, thus, to digital literacy—as well as the specific conditions characterizing this access. Given both the complexity and the overdetermined nature of cultural ecologies, no one action or set of solutions is going to address the entire range of access and literacy issues associated with the digital divide in this country or the future prospects of all technical communicators. Nor will this situation improve with statements such as the one President Clinton made in the 1996 report *Getting America's Students Ready for the 21st Century* (United States), which only began to hint at the multiple dimensions of access as an important feature of the digital divide:

> We know, purely and simply, that every single child must have access to a computer, must understand it, must have access to good software and good teachers and to the Internet, so that every person will have the opportunity to make the most of his or her own life. (4)

The autobiographies on which we have focused this project indicate that closing the gaps associated with the digital divide in this country will depend not on providing individuals access to computers through one technology gateway (e.g., home, school, community centers, workplace) but on providing them access through several such gateways.

In addition, the autobiographies indicate that equitable access, by itself, is only a starting point, especially for citizens in poverty and citizens of color. The specific conditions of access must also be addressed to assure individuals productive environments within which access can make a real difference. One necessary, but insufficient, element of these conditions must be a broad understanding and valuing of multiple literacies—emerging, competing, and fading—in home, school, and workplace environments.

None of these considerations, of course, can be addressed in isolation from the cultural ecology within which access to computers and the acquisition and development of digital literacies make a difference for technical communication students and professionals.

Conclusion

What does this study have to say about the education technical communicators will need to face the challenges of electronic literacy in the initial decades of the twenty-first century? Because we cannot generalize the findings from this series of case studies, we can offer only speculative answers to this question, but readers may find that these speculations fit well with their own personal experiences in the rapidly changing world of the twenty-first century.

To us, the study suggests the need for increased flexibility and expanded ways of thinking about electronic literacy. The profession of technical communication, for example, needs to extend its thinking about what literacy—and technical communication—now entails in digital environments and how new electronic-literacy skills and values can best be taught in preprofessional programs and in on-the-job contexts. The profession also needs to look beyond the boundaries of the workplace to consider how critical social factors—including socioeconomic status, gender, race, and past access to computers—affect the electronic-literacy skills and values that practitioners bring to the workplace. Armed with this information, professional communicators might be more effective in designing and offering on-the-job educational opportunities for a whole range of technical communicators who bring less than a full set of electronic-literacy skills into the workplace or for those who want to extend their electronic literacies in new and productive directions. The autobiographies we have collected also point to a new level of responsibility for students of professional communication. These individuals must be willing to experiment with new forms of digital and visual literacies and be active in teaching themselves and their peers how to employ these skills effectively, with appropriate concern for audience, purpose, the nature of information, and the context of the communication task.

Given the rapid and far-reaching changes that continue to characterize communication contexts in the twenty-first century, these recommendations should neither surprise nor dismay us. Indeed, if we take them as a collective challenge, they represent an exciting direction and future for the profession of technical communication.

APPENDIX

Interviewer ____________________
Time, date, and city ____________
*Setting*________________________

Protocol on Electronic Literacy

The purpose of this study is to identify how Americans born during this century learned to be literate—either with print or with computers, or with both. We will be interviewing people of different ages, genders, races, and socioeconomic status in various parts of the country about their experiences reading and writing in print and/or on computer. We will ask you questions about your first use of computers and about your experiences over the years with computers. We hope the results of this study will be used to improve literacy instruction and to understand, historically, how computer literacy developed in the United States during the latter half of the twentieth century.

Name:
Current occupation:
Academic major (if applicable):
Previous occupations:

Intended occupation (if applicable):
Nationality:
Race:
Ethnic heritage:
Sexual/gender orientation (e.g., heterosexual, gay, lesbian, bisexual, transgendered, other—only if participant is comfortable answering):
Religion/denomination (only if participant is comfortable answering):
Immediate family members and ages:
How would you describe your family circumstances? (your income level)
  Growing up?
  Now?
Parents'/guardians' literacy histories (e.g., the value they placed on reading/writing at home/at school, their thoughts about education, their reading/writing/computing activities, their stories about reading/writing):
Parents'/guardians' education and professions:
Your place and date of birth:
Where did you live?
  Growing up?
  Now?
Schooling history
  Elementary
  Secondary
  College
  Other
Can you tell us how/when/why you learned to read and write?
Can you tell us the story(ies) about when, where, how you *first* came in contact with computers (including mainframe computers, personal computers, computer games)?
Can you tell us the story(ies) about when, where, how you *first learned* to use computers? Did anyone help or encourage you?
Do you remember what the prevailing images/representations of computers were when you were growing up (e.g., movies, television, magazines, books)?
Can you tell us how you felt about computers/and used computers when you were growing up?
Can you tell the story(ies) of how you first learned to use the computer at school: What was your motivation? Age? Who helped? How did they help? What kind of support did you have? In what classes did you learn to use the computer? How much access did you have to a computer per day/week/month? How often did you actually use the computer per day/week/month?
Are there any stories/incidents that you can remember about this?
Do you (or your family) own a computer(s) *now*? If so, please describe it (them).
For what purposes do you use this computer (e.g., what kinds of work, what applications)?
For what purposes do your siblings/parents/children use the computer?
  Who taught them? Who provides support? (e-mail?)
Do you access the Web? What do you use it for?
Do you currently have access to a computer someplace other than at home? Where (workplace, school)? When? For how long? How often? How do you get there? How much does it cost to use this computer? How do you get that money to pay for access?
How important would you say computers are in your life?
Anything more you'd like to say about your relationship with computers?

NOTES

1. This study of technical communicators is part of a larger study of electronic literacy in the United States. For the larger study, which focuses on a general history of how citizens in this country have acquired the literacies of technology, we have gathered more than 350 literacy autobiographies. The report of the findings from this larger study can be found in *Literate Lives in the Information Age: Stories from the United States* (Mahwah, NJ: Lawrence Erlbaum, forthcoming).

2. In using this term, we borrow in part from Ronald Deibert's work in communication and from other scholars' work with the emergence and fitness of communication media in historical contexts. To us, however, an ecological model also suggests a duality of structuring between social systems and literacy practices (Giddens) that comes through more clearly in the work of Anthony Giddens and Manuel Castells (*Rise, Power, End*). In combination, the work of these scholars suggests to us that literacies in general—and electronic literacies in particular—emerge, compete, flourish, and fade because they share a "fitness" (Deibert 31) with the cultural ecology of a given era. This ecology structures, and is structured by, human beings who use literacy as a means of social action.

REFERENCES

Barton, David, and Mary Hamilton. *Local Literacies: Reading and Writing in One Community*. London: Routledge, 1998.

Beach, Mark. *Getting It Printed*. Cincinnati, OH: North Light Books, 1986.

Bertaux, Daniel, and Paul Thompson. *Between Generations: The Life History Approach*. Newbury Park, CA: Sage, 1993.

———. *Pathways to Social Class: A Qualitative Approach to Social Mobility*. Oxford, Eng.: Clarendon, 1997.

Brandt, Deborah. "Accumulating Literacy: Writing and Learning to Write in the Twentieth Century." *College English* 57 (1995): 649–68.

———. *Literacy in American Lives*. New York: Cambridge University Press, 2001.

———. "Literacy Learning and Economic Change." *Harvard Educational Review* 69 (1999): 373–94.

———. "Sponsors of Literacy." *College Composition and Communication* 49 (1998): 165–85.

Bruce, Bertram, and Maureen P. Hogan. "The Disappearance of Technology: Toward an Ecological Model of Literacy." *Handbook of Literacy and Technology: Transformations in a Post-Typographic World*. Ed. David Reinking, Michael C. McKenna, Linda D. Labbo, and Ronald D. Kieffer. Mahwah, NJ: Lawrence Erlbaum, 1998. 269–81.

Castells, Manuel. *End of the Millennium*. Malden, MA: Blackwell, 1998. Vol. 3 of *The Information Age: Economy, Society, and Culture*.

———. *The Power of Identity*. Malden, MA: Blackwell 1997. Vol. 2 of *The Information Age: Economy, Society, and Culture*.

———. *The Rise of the Network Society*. Maiden, MA: Blackwell, 1996. Vol. 1 of *The Information Age: Economy, Society, and Culture*.

Cole, Michael, and Peg Griffin. *Contextual Factors in Education: Improving Science and Mathematics Education for Minorities and Women*. Madison: Wisconsin Center for Education Research, University of Wisconsin–Madison, 1987.

Coley, Richard J., J. Crandler, and P. Engle. *Computers and Classrooms: The Status of Technology in U.S. Schools*. Princeton, NJ: Educational Testing Service, 1997.

Deibert, Ronald J. *Parchment, Printing, and Hypermedia: Communication in World Order Transformation*. New York: Columbia University Press, 1997.

Dennis, J. Richard, and Robert J. Kansky. *Instructional Computing: An Action Guide for Educators*. Glenview, IL: Scott Foresman, 1984.

Duin, Ann H., and Craig Hansen, eds. *Nonacademic Writing: Social Theory and Technology*. Mahwah, NJ: Lawrence Erlbaum, 1996.

Dumas, Joseph S. *Designing User Interfaces for Software*. Englewood Cliffs, NJ: Prentice Hall, 1988.

George, Diana, and Diane Shoos. "Dropping Bread Crumbs in the Intertextual Forest: Critical Literacy in a Postmodern Age." *Passions, Pedagogies and 21st Century Technologies*. Ed. Gail E. Hawisher and Cynthia L. Selfe. Logan: Utah State University Press, 1999. 115–26.

Giddens, Anthony. *Central Problems in Social Theory: Action, Structure and Contradiction in Social Analysis*. Berkeley: University of California Press, 1979.

Greenberg, Saul. *Computer-Supported Cooperative Work and Groupware*. London: Harcourt Brace Jovanovich, 1991.

Hawisher, Gail E. "Accessing the Virtual Worlds of Cyberspace." *Journal of Electronic Publishing* 6 (2000). 8 Jan. 2002. http://www.press.umich.edu/jep/06-01/hawisher.html.

Heines, Jesse M. *Screen Design Strategies for Computer-Assisted Instruction*. Bedford, MA: Digital Press, 1984.

Hiltz, Star Roxanne, and Murray Turoff. *The Network Nation*. New York: Addison-Wesley, 1978.

Hoffman, Donna L., and Thomas P. Novak. "Bridging the Racial Divide on the Internet." *Science* 17 Apr. 1998: 280, 390–91.

Horton, William K. *Designing & Writing Online Documentation: Help Files to Hypertext*. New York: John Wiley, 1990.

Johnson-Eilola, Johndan, and Stuart Selber. "Policing Ourselves: Defining the Boundaries of Appropriate Discussion in Online Forums." *Computers and Composition* 13 (1996): 293–302.

Kearsley, Greg: *Computer-Based Training: A Guide to Selection and Implementation*. Reading, MA: Addison-Wesley, 1983.

———. *Training for Tomorrow: Distributed Learning through Computer and Communications Technology*. Reading, MA: Addison-Wesley, 1985.

Little, Sherry Burgus. "Preparing the Technical Communicator of the Future." *IEEE Transactions on Professional Communication* 33 (1990): 28–30.

Lutz, Jean A., and C. Gilbert Storms, eds. *The Practice of Technical and Scientific Communication: Writing in Professional Contexts*. Stamford, CT: Ablex, 1998.

Mead, Margaret. *Culture and Commitment: The New Relationships between the Generations in the 1970s*. New York: Doubleday, 1970.

"Native Americans and the Digital Divide." *The Digital Beat*. Benton Foundation Web site. 30 Oct. 2001. http://www.benton.org/DigitalBeat/db101499.html.

Papert, Seymour. *Mindstorms: Children, Computers and Powerful Ideas*. New York: Basic Books, 1980.

Price, Jonathan. *How to Write a Computer Manual: A Handbook of Software Documentation*. Menlo Park, CA: Benjamin/Cummings, 1984.

Price, Jonathan, and Henry Korman. *How to Communicate Technical Information*. Redwood City, CA: Benjamin/Cummings, 1993.

Ray, Eric. Personal communication. 29 Jan. 2001.

Rudolph, Frederick. *The American College and University: A History*. New York: Vintage, 1972.

Selber, Stuart A. *Computers and Technical Communication: Pedagogical and Programmatic Perspectives*. Greenwich, CT: Ablex, 1997.

———. *Hypertext and Technical Communication: The Case for Critical Perspectives*. Diss. Michigan Technological University. Ann Arbor, MI: University Microfilms International, 1994. 95138653.

Selfe, Cynthia. *Technology and Literacy in the Twenty-First Century: The Importance of Paying Attention*. Carbondale: Southern Illinois University Press, 1999.

Shirk, Henrietta N. "New Roles for Technical Communicators in the Computer Age." *Computers and Technical Communication: Pedagogical and Programmatic Perspectives*. Ed. Stuart A. Selber. Greenwich, CT: Ablex, 1997. 353–74.

Sides, Charles H. *How to Write Papers about Computer Technology*. Philadelphia: ISI, 1984.

Sproull, Lee, and Sara Kiesler. *Connections: New Ways of Working within the Networked Organization*. Cambridge, MA: MIT Press, 1991.

Storms, Gilbert C. "Programs in Scientific and Technical Communication." *Technical Communication* 31.4 (1984): 13–20.

Sullivan, Patricia, and Jennie Dautermann, eds. *Electronic Literacy in the Workplace: Technologies of Writing*. Urbana, IL: National Council of Teachers of English, 1996.

Tebeaux, Elizabeth. "The High-Tech Workplace: Implications for Technical Communication Instruction." *Technical Writing: Theory and Practice*. Ed. Bertie Fearing and W. Keats Sparrow. New York: Modern Language Association, 1989. 136–44.

Thompson, Paul. *The Edwardians: The Remaking of British Society*. Bloomington: Indiana University Press, 1975.

———. *The Voice of the Past: Oral History*. Oxford, Eng.: Oxford University Press, 1988.

Thompson, Paul, Catherine Itzin, and Michele Abendstern. *I Don't Feel Old: The Experience of Later Life*. Oxford, Eng.: Oxford University Press, 1990.

Tyner, Kathleen. *Literacy in a Digital World: Teaching and Learning in the Age of Information*. Mahwah, NJ: Lawrence Erlbaum, 1998.

United States. Council of Economic Advisors. *Economic Report of the President*. Washington, DC: GPO, 1997

———. ———. *Economic Report of the President*. Washington, DC: GPO, 1998.

———. Dept. of Commerce. *Falling through the Net: Defining the Digital Divide.* Economic and Statistics Administration and National Telecommunication and Information Administration. Washington, DC: GPO, 1999.

———. ———. *Falling through the Net: Toward Digital Inclusion, A Report on Americans' Access to Technology Tools.* Economic and Statistics Administration and National Telecommunication and Information Administration. Washington, DC: GPO, 2000.

———. Dept. of Education. *Getting America's Students Ready for the 21st Century: Meeting the Technology Literacy Challenge, A Report to the Nation on Technology and Education.* Washington, DC: GPO, 1996.

———. ———. Natl. Center for Education Statistics. *The Condition of Education 1997.* NCES 98-013. Washington, DC: GPO, 1997.

———. ———. ———. *The Condition of Education 1998.* NCES 97-388. Washington, DC: GPO, 1998.

———. ———. ———. Office of Educational Research and Improvement. *Digest of Educational Statistics 1992.* NCES 92097. 20 Feb. 2001. http://nces.ed.gov/spider/webspider/92097.shtml

———. ———. ———. ———. *Digest of Educational Statistics 1995.* NCES, 1995. 20 Feb. 2001. http://nces.ed.gov./pubsold/D95

———. ———. ———. ———. *Digest of Educational Statistics 1996.* Washington, DC: GPO, 1996.

———. ———. ———. ———. *Digest of Education Statistics 1999.* NCES, 2000. 20 Feb. 2001. http://nces.ed.gov./pubsearch/pubsinfo.asp? pubid=2000031.

Weiss, Edmund H. *How to Write a Usable User Manual.* Philadelphia: ISI, 1985.

White, Jan V. *Editing by Design: A Guide to Effective Word-and-Picture Communication for Editors and Designers.* New York: R. R. Bowker, 1982.

Zinn, Howard. *The Twentieth Century: A People's History.* New York: Harper Perennial, 1998.

Zuboff, Shoshana. *In the Age of the Smart Machine: The Future of Work and Power.* New York: Basic Books, 1988.

APPLIED THEORY

31 Situated Learning in Cross-Functional Virtual Teams

DANIEL ROBEY, HUOY MIN KHOO,
AND CAROLYN POWERS

In this study of virtual, cross-functional teams from the largest division of a U.S. soft goods manufacturer and importer, Robey, Khoo, and Powers examine the ways in which the team members learn work practices that help them meet the challenges posed by cultural and geographic boundaries. While the study is valuable from the perspective that it focuses on a virtual environment and on the variety of communication technologies used to meet the communication needs, it is also valuable in that it demonstrates the importance of situated learning and the effects of temporal, cultural, and geographic boundaries (and the need to learn to bridge those boundaries to succeed). Finally, it highlights teams that were extremely diverse, consisting of personnel from sales and/or merchandising, product development, production, administration, and customer service. For teachers, this article raises useful questions about our pedagogy, and asks us to think through the value of teamwork and collaborative projects and wrestle with the kinds of communication problems involved, including the types of communication skills needed for success. This essay illustrates, quite conclusively, that communication skills are essential for students in nearly every field and that what we teach will add value to nearly every organization.

With the advent of worldwide connectivity through the Internet and other telecommunications technologies, organizations are increasingly adopting virtual organizational forms that operate more independently of time and space than traditional organizations. As a result, more professional workers are finding themselves as members of virtual teams, consisting of members in remote locations who work together primarily through computer-mediated communication (Grenier and Metes 1995; Townsend, DeMarie, and Henrickson 1998; Lipnack and Stamps 1997). In many cases, virtual teams include members from different functional areas of an organization, thereby increasing the team's coordination requirements.

From *IEEE Transactions on Technical Communication* 43 (2000): 51–66.

Customers, vendors, and other business partners may also contribute members to virtual teams, further increasing their diversity and their communication and coordination requirements. Although they typically operate in multiple remote locations, members of virtual teams must execute a large number of intricate and interrelated tasks for their work to be effective. Frequently, members of virtual teams are not closely supervised. Rather, they function as empowered professionals who are expected to use their own initiative and resources to contribute value to customers and other stakeholders (Hammer 1996).

This study investigates the ways in which members of cross-functional teams learn work practices that allow them to meet the challenges that their virtual status poses. The study conceives of virtual teams as communities of practice (Wegner 1998; Brown and Duguid 1991; Brown 1998) and focuses on learning that is situated in work practice rather than on knowledge acquired outside the context of actual work. According to this theoretical perspective, participants in a community of practice learn work practices that satisfy their local needs, and they often ignore or neglect formally prescribed practices that are seen as less relevant to performance (Orr 1996). Understanding how such learning occurs and how it affects team performance is important, especially in the context of virtual cross-functional teams.

To investigate this issue, we interviewed 22 workers and managers in three cross-functional teams in a single large company. The teams bridged not only functional divides but also geographic and cultural ones, and members used a variety of media to manage the production and delivery of products to serve their customers. Our findings reveal how team members responded to the demands of the team arrangement, how they communicated both remotely and face-to-face, and how their learning was situated in virtual communities of practice. The results extend the theoretical concept of situated learning to virtual teams and generate several practical implications for managing virtual cross-functional teams.

Virtual Cross-Functional Teams

Traditional organizations are designed around work functions, wherein specialists from a particular occupational category are grouped together. The functional organization structure is frequently criticized because it increases the communication and coordination requirements across functions. Managing conflicts across functional boundaries in organizations is a research concern that spans at least 30 years (Walton and Dutton 1969; Walton, Dutton, and Cafferty 1969; Kusunoki and Numagami 1998).

To facilitate cross-functional coordination, many organizations have created teams in which members of various functions work together to bring their respective skills and perspectives to a common work output (Wynn and Novick 1995). For example, process re-engineering and supply-chain management efforts undertaken throughout the 1990s resulted in the creation of many teams focused on customers instead of functions (Grenier and Metes

1995; Greis and Kasarda 1997). These teams often become microcosms of the larger functional organization and must develop internal means for managing inter-functional conflicts.

Perhaps the most commonly prescribed and least controversial means for overcoming cross-functional differences is communication (Kusunoki and Numagami 1998). Although an obvious solution, ensuring effective communication within cross-functional teams has always been difficult. Even in high-performing teams, communication across functional divides presents a constant challenge for members who must simultaneously represent their trained specialization and subordinate their interests to the shared goals of their teams (Pinto and Pinto 1990).

Contributing to the challenge of effective cross-functional communication is the fact that an increasing number of cross-functional teams span geographic and temporal boundaries. These virtual teams may include members of a single organization working in different locations around the world, members of different organizations with shared business interests, and customers (Lipnack and Stamps, 1997).

Virtual organizational forms have become popular, and the professional management literature consistently promotes the virtues of going virtual (Boudreau and others 1998; Davidow and Malone 1992; Grenier and Metes 1995; Townsend and others 1998). Much of the academic and professional interest in virtual teams so far has been on the quality of supporting technologies and their contribution to knowledge generation and knowledge sharing (for example, Gorton and Motwani 1996; Marshall, Shipman, and McCall 1995; Osterlund 1997). However, deploying those technologies in an organization does not determine how they will be used.

In practice, teams appropriate specific features of available technologies and employ them to support their particular work needs. Some uses of enabling technologies in virtual teams may conform to the expectations of managers or researchers (DeSanctis and Poole 1997). Others uses, however, may develop out of unique and unanticipated needs of a team members and represent contradictory or paradoxical uses of technology (Robey and Boudreau 1999). One of the objectives in this study is to shed light on the ways members of cross-functional virtual teams actually communicate and learn to adjust to their task requirements.

Research on Learning and Communication in Virtual Teams

Researchers have studied virtual teams using a variety of theoretical concepts and research methods, but no general framework has yet been produced to guide research on situated learning in virtual teams. Reviews of virtual organizations (Robey, Boudreau, and Storey 1998), virtual teams (DeSanctis and Poole 1997), and related concepts such as remote work (Belanger and Collins 1998) have begun to appear. However, none of these previous studies focuses on the processes whereby members of virtual teams learn as they participate in practice.

In the absence of such an organizing theoretical framework, the research we present in this article relies on related empirical studies to illuminate topics that we believe to be relevant to the study of learning in virtual teams. Collectively, these earlier studies provide findings about work demands and learning in virtual teams, and about communication and media use. We also review research relevant to learning situated in communities of practice.

Work Demands and Learning in Virtual Teams

A common presumption about virtual teams is that most workers will experience them as novel forms. This will probably not be the case in the near future, but it is a safe presumption today. Thus, Townsend and his colleagues (1998) argued that virtual team members must learn to "rebuild interpersonal interaction" because traditional, face-to-face interactions will be replaced to a great degree by remote communication. The novelty of virtual teams thus poses a significant demand on members to learn new ways to behave and interact.

Virtual teams are also demanding because they frequently empower members to act more independently from direct supervision (Grenier and Metes 1995). Unlike traditional novelty effects, which are transitory in nature (Robey and Bakr 1978), the demands imposed by empowering team members represent ongoing challenges. Cross-functional teams in particular are unlikely to settle into routine problem-solving under the direction of watchful supervision. To the contrary, cross-functional teams are formed to resolve nonrecurring problems. Because cross-functional teams are often focused on satisfying customers, whose expectations may change frequently, teams may face a steady flow of new demands rather than transitory novelty effects.

Research studies confirm these expectations about the demands facing members of cross-functional virtual teams. In one of the few studies to investigate the novelty of virtual work, Whiting and Reardon (1998) surveyed employees from 10 regional offices of a *Fortune* 500 firm. Of 373 sales and systems engineering employees, 186 moved to the virtual office and the remaining 187 remained in traditional work settings in regional offices. Two surveys were conducted: the first mailed to participants during the transition to virtual work, and the second administered one year after the transition. Whiting and Reardon showed that, during the transition, virtual office members were less committed to the organization than were their colleagues in the traditional office. The researchers explained this result in terms of the insecurity that members experienced regarding their future in the organization. Following the transition, however, no significant differences were found in the level of commitment between employees in virtual and traditional offices. This result suggests that novelty effects had been overcome and that virtual workers had adjusted to the change.

Several studies have emphasized the importance of learning as a response to the demands of virtual teamwork. Staples, Hulland, and Higgins (1998) gathered responses from 376 workers who worked remotely from their managers in 18 North American organizations. The employees with greater experience and training at working remotely had higher levels of remote-work self-efficacy, which led to better job performance and more positive job attitudes. Also, those with superior information technology skills had greater remote-work self-efficacy. Workers learned their communication practices by modeling their managers' behaviors, and this practice in turn led to greater self-efficacy, better performance, and more positive job attitudes.

In a study of three global virtual teams, Maznevski and Chudoba (in press) also found communication patterns to be associated with team effectiveness. Communication incidents that fit the teams' structures and processes were judged to make teams more effective. These results support the conclusion of Belanger and Collins (1998) regarding the importance of self-sufficiency, reliability, and communication skills in remote work.

Communication and Media Use

Most studies of virtual teams emphasize the importance of communication to accomplishing team requirements for coordination and efficient task execution (DeSanctis and Poole 1997). Effective teams need to find ways to fulfill task expectations while meeting other social outcomes like satisfaction, organizational commitment, organizational identity, cultural understanding, and trust. However, because virtual teams typically span functional, geographic, and cultural boundaries, the volume of communication within teams may increase and be transmitted via a wider assortment of media.

Empirical studies support the important role that communication plays in virtual teams. In Whiting and Reardon's study (1998), the impact of formal and informal communication on organizational commitment was greater for virtual office employees than for those who worked in traditional offices. Communication thus played a more important role in virtual organizations than it did in traditional offices. Grabowski and Roberts (1998) argued that communication is essential to mitigating safety risks by helping to clarify potential threats to worker safety and by opening dialog on improved work practices.

When virtual teams span the boundaries of individual organizations, communication between them allows different cultures to be melded into a cohesive whole. However, attention must also be given to the design of control systems that promote safe behavior. Jarvenpaa and Leidner (1998) also found that communication was an important factor contributing to trust in virtual teams composed of students from different universities. They found that social communication complemented task communication: members who explicitly verbalized their commitment, excitement, and support were seen as more trustworthy. Kraut and his colleagues (1998) also found the use of electronic networks and personal relationships to be complementary. Finally, Wiesenfeld, Raghuram, and Garud (1998) found that communication was instrumental to increasing organizational identification in virtual teams through the sharing of norms, values, and culture.

It is difficult to understand communication in virtual teams without appreciating the variety of communication media and technologies used by team members. It is widely acknowledged that advanced applications of information technology have enabled the creation and spread of virtual organizations, virtual teams, and other form of distributed work. Technologies such as videoconferencing, groupware (software that facilitates collaborative work), and Internet/intranet systems now supplement earlier technologies such as electronic mail, telephone/voice mail, and facsimile transmission (Townsend and others 1998).

Technology-enabled communication may not completely replace face-to-face meetings or the mailing of printed documents, however. Thus, members of virtual teams are typically faced with more choices of media, protocols, and formats. Greater variety may lead to more flexibility, creativity, and responsiveness to both internal and external demands, but it may also lead to confusion and reluctance to use technologies like electronic mail that jeopardize personal privacy (DeSanctis, Staudenmayer, and Wong in press).

In the face of this wider range of choices, team members must learn to mix old and new technologies. A recent study (Sarbaugh-Thompson and Feldman 1998) showed that electronic media use tends to reduce the incidence of casual conversations and greetings, thereby reducing overall communication. To compensate for such effects, teams may be designed so that social greetings can be restored through periodic face-to-face meetings. Kraut and his colleagues (1998) found that the uses of electronic media and personal relationships complemented each other in dealings with external suppliers. Maznevski and Chudoba (in press) also found that face-to-face meetings in global virtual teams provided a "deep rhythm," which permitted intense focus during short intervals and less intense focus during longer intervals of remote communication using electronic media. Thus, it appears that face-to-face communication may be an important ingredient in making virtual teams more effective.

Learning Situated in Communities of Practice

Virtual teams constitute a variation on what Wegner (1998) described as a "community of practice." According to Wegner, the idea of community provides

> . . . a way of talking about the social configurations in which our enterprises are defined as worth pursuing and our participation is recognizable as competence. . . . Practice refers to the shared historical and social resources, frameworks, and perspectives that can sustain mutual engagement in action.
>
> . . . These practices are thus the property of a kind of community created over time by the sustained pursuit of a shared enterprise. (pp. 5, 45)

Learning within such communities is situated in practice. New members assume roles as peripheral participants, initially performing a limited range of activities under the guidance of more experienced community members (Lave and Wegner 1991). As peripheral members gain experience, they become more complete participants. Their learning is thus situated in practice, rather than formulated and delivered outside of the context of practice.

Situated learning thus differs from formal training, in which knowledge is codified and transferred to learners in special training sessions. Situated learning occurs within communities of practice as members adjust to each other's needs. In some corporations, such as Xerox, awareness of situated learning has led to revisions in training programs so that members of teams may learn together within a shared work space (Stamps 1997). Such practices are undertaken with the full recognition that communities of practice rarely follow "corporate doctrine" or implement "canonical knowledge." Rather, communities of practice establish idiosyncratic knowledge that reflects local experience and meets local requirements. Tacit knowledge is generated and transferred by members as they work together (Nonaka 1994).

Most examples of situated learning involve communities of practice that are geographically proximate—that is, communities that share space and time. In proximate settings, the elements of social interaction, physical activity, and physical setting assume central importance in situated learning. For example, workers in traditional offices, production plants, and research laboratories share space and interact frequently, making it possible for peripheral participants to learn through direct communication with more experienced colleagues (Brown and Duguid 1991; George, Iacono, and Kling 1995; Tyre and von Hippel 1997; Wynn and Novick 1995). Their learning includes visual, tactile, and verbal communication, and may result in such outcomes as psychological safety for team members and effective team performance (Edmondson 1999).

In virtual teams, where the community of practice is geographically distributed and temporally disconnected, opportunities for visual, tactile, and verbal communication are significantly limited. Virtual arrangements potentially threaten the process of situated learning because members are not located together. As a community of practice, a virtual team must generate local knowledge when its members are not local. Its situated learning must occur outside of a physical situation and be generated by persons who may never meet face to face.

These requirements pose serious challenges to members of teams, to designers of support technologies, and to managers and customers who depend on teams to perform effectively. While members may be trained in the principles and procedures of the technologies that bind them together, virtual teams may decide to appropriate some features and to ignore others, despite their apparent advantages. Moreover, teams may "reinvent" technologies to work in ways that satisfy locally understood team requirements, regardless of the intended uses of the technology. These effects are well established in the literature on traditional teams, and they are likely to be more pronounced in virtual teams, which depend even more on information technologies (Robey and Boudreau 1999).

Beyond their understanding of tools and technologies, virtual team members must also develop communication practices that operate across time and space. They may develop electronically mediated substitutes for the visual and nonverbal cues that operate in teams that meet face-to-face. They may create rules of conduct, social structure, and temporal rhythms that enable them to perform their work effectively. And they may learn to manage conflicts and disagreements in ways that make members feel psychologically safe. They may even form social and emotional bonds through their electronic interactions. All these practices are situated within the virtual cross-functional team, and this study seeks to understand how such learning occurs.

Method

Our research uses an interpretive methodology. This methodology makes the fundamental assumption that social reality is constructed and interpreted by actors rather than being objectively definable (Deetz 1996; Orlikowski and Baroudi 1991; Walsham 1995; Mason 1996). The research methods that fit this assumption seek access to social actors' subjective knowledge. Accordingly, the methodology used in this study relies on interview data and qualitative data analysis. This methodology is appropriate because learning that is situated within a community of practice is likely to occur in ways other than those imposed by a deductive research framework. Thus, an interpretive methodology is designed to inductively generate constructs relevant to individuals and their work, which can be assessed through responses to open-ended questions about aspects of practice. Respondents' interpretations of their own experience in cross-functional virtual teams are likely to be a valuable foundation for building knowledge about situated learning within them.

Interpretive methodology requires that the researchers' own subjectivity be acknowledged (Mason 1996). In this study, we are motivated to produce knowledge that will be useful in making cross-functional virtual teams more effective for a variety of stakeholders, including managers and team members.

The site chosen for this research is the largest division of a U.S. soft goods manufacturer and importer, here given the pseudonym SoftCo. SoftCo had sales of approximately $300 million USD in 1998, when the study was conducted, and competes in an industry that has undergone significant changes over the last decade. Faced with the demands of more globally distributed manufacturing and increased customer demands for more timely fulfillment of their orders, many firms in SoftCo's industry failed to survive. SoftCo coped with these pressures by forming closer alliances with both customers and suppliers to coordinate inventory, shipping, and manufacturing schedules more tightly.

A process re-engineering project conducted in 1995 emphasized better management of the supply chain and created three teams focused on specific customer groups. Each team was both virtual and cross-functional. Each team included sales and/or merchandising personnel from one cosmopolitan northern U.S. city (hereafter referred to as North) and administration, product development, production, and customer service personnel from the division headquarters, located in a small town in the southern U.S. (hereafter referred to as South).

Each virtual team also included people located in other places, such as geographically remote sales personnel, customers, and suppliers. The teams were also permanently established, a fact which enabled access to retrospective accounts of work within the teams by members who had experienced the transition to teams 3 years earlier. Figure 1 shows the teams schematically.

SoftCo was selected as the research site because its virtual teams spanned corporate functions as well as culturally and demographically diverse regions of the U.S., thereby increasing their coordination and communication requirements. The origin of cultural differences between North and South locations is embedded in historical circumstances that once separated northern and southern states politically. Although the U.S. Civil War ended 135 years ago, regional differences in dialect and customs prevail. Moreover, North-South cultural differences are related to the cosmopolitan character of the Northern city and the more local or traditional character of the Southern town.

Data was generated (Mason 1996) using face-to-face, in-depth, semi-structured interviews with 22 individuals. Two interviewers working together conducted most interviews, but either one or three interviewers conducted some of them. All interviews were tape-recorded after interviewers assured confidentiality and obtained permission from the respondents. The interview

FIGURE 1 Configuration of Virtual Teams at SoftCo

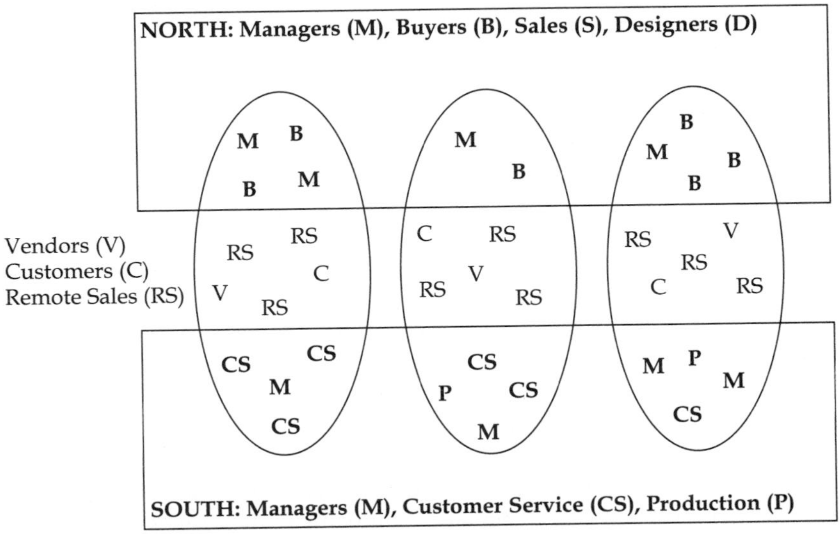

protocol included six broad topic areas, but most interviews followed a natural course, wandering to topics of interest to the respondent. Interviews lasted between 40 and 60 minutes, and were conducted at either the South location or the North location. The manager and at least two team members were interviewed in each location; interviewees are identified by bold type in Figure 1.

During the data generation period, the research team recorded and shared their preliminary impressions. These field notes included casual observations of office layout, dress and physical appearance of employees, and other considerations. However, prolonged systematic observation of people at work was not possible. The interviews were primarily conducted in a room reserved for that purpose.

Following transcription of the interviews, two of the researchers coded segments of the transcripts using the following five categories:

- Demands of virtual work
- Process of situated learning
- Use of technology
- Role of face-to-face meetings
- Management

These codes were not tied to a specific theoretical framework but rather treated as a starting position for analyzing the data. Coding categories were based on the interests of the researchers, the nascent literature on situated learning, and impressions gained during the interviews themselves. After both coders had coded the same 10 interviews, they compared their results to modify coding categories. Disagreements were discussed, and the coding scheme was expanded to include two additional categories:

- Communication
- Effectiveness

These categories thus arose out of the data itself (Mason 1996). All transcripts were then coded or re-coded to include these new categories where appropriate. The coders divided the set of transcripts, each coding half of the total. One of the coders had participated in 19 of the 22 interviews, and the other coder had not conducted any interviews. No computer-aided analysis tools were used in the coding process.

The analysis continued by examining the statements made under each coding category and abstracting a framework that described the overall pattern of results. The coding category of effectiveness was not included in the framework because all respondents considered their teams to be effective, so our analysis was unable to distinguish factors accounting for differences in effectiveness. The category of management was not treated separately in the framework because managers were included along with team members. Finally, we found the three teams to be relatively similar to each other, so we did not include a comparative analysis of teams in the results.

RESULTS

Figure 2 presents a preliminary theoretical framework abstracted from the analysis of the interview data. Consistent with the research methodology, the framework was derived inductively from the coded data and is supported by specific quotations from the interviews, as presented below. The framework shows that the demands of the virtual cross-functional team led to a variety of communication practices, including face-to-face communication and remote communication using a variety of technologies. Through communication, team members learned various aspects of practice. They developed means for choosing and using appropriate technologies, for adjusting to differences in work pace and timing, and for meeting customers' needs. Collectively, their learning was situated in a community that was largely virtual but nevertheless capable of developing practices that its members found useful. New members were socialized to these practices over time.

We now present the evidence supporting the framework in Figure 2, using the main elements in the figure as an outline for organizing the results. To identify quotations from respondent interviews, a first letter (N or S) designates the location (North or South), and a second letter (M or T) designates the respondent's role as a Manager or a Team member.

The Demands of Virtual Teamwork

We expected that both workers and managers would regard virtual teamwork as a novel experience, and that fact in turn would produce the need for learning. For most participants, virtual work was seen as a change from their normal work, but for some it was the only work arrangement that they had known. Without more traditional work arrangements as a basis for comparison, one younger worker did not consider virtual teamwork unusual.

FIGURE 2 Framework for Situated Learning in Virtual Teams

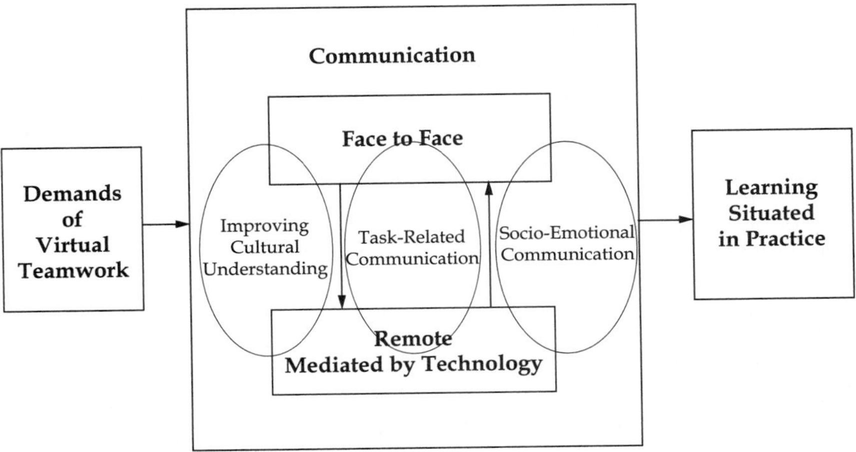

However, both older and younger workers acknowledged the demands posed by virtual work.

One North manager considered the need for cross-functional coordination to be more demanding than the novelty of the teams. That need had existed even before the people from different functions were organized into virtual teams:

> I have always thought that it was nothing that revolutionary . . . . We were set up this way already with sales and administration. That is sales support functions here and operations and customer services [in the South]. . . . I mean, you still have, obviously, on this side a sales person with a set department, a certain set of accounts, his or her support here in the North, and then down South you have an operations manager who basically mirrored your accounts, and your point of business and customer services, and production planners who just about do the same thing. (NM)

Managers did, however, describe differences in how they managed, needing to trust the team members more than in the past. For example, a South manager remarked:

> Traditionally all those years, especially for longer term employees, [it is difficult to come to terms with the fact] . . . that this is for real and you need to step outside what you were used to. They used to be told, and now we are asking them to think and the old statement of thinking outside the box. You are asked to be innovative. (SM)

A South team member confirmed this greater responsibility:

> We pretty much are our own boss as far as our time and what goes on in our areas. (ST)

The changing nature of work was also demanding for team members. A North team member remarked:

> The team is very exciting because it changes from day to day. You don't ever know what is going to happen next. (ST)

Demands were clearly related to the distance between team members located in North and South. A North team member who was relatively new to the company commented on her adjustment to working with remote South members:

> It was kind of strange at first because I had been talking to them a lot on the phone, but I hadn't seen anyone or met anyone yet. So it was good once we were able to meet each other, connect faces to voices. (NT)

A South team member agreed:

> Yeah, it is really interesting having half of your office in a totally different state and the other half here. . . . The functions are related, but they are totally different. (ST)

In sum, both managers and workers felt new challenges: the need to communicate over distance and the need to take more initiative in solving problems rather than turning to managers for direction. Most respondents generally viewed these challenges in a positive way, but collectively they represent demands on the team and its members. How they met those demands was the primary focus of other questions in the interviews, and the following comments about communication show the extent and nature of its importance.

Communication

Both team members and managers mentioned communication as a primary means of meeting the demands of working in virtual cross-functional teams. Managers spoke abstractly yet fervently about the need for communication. Workers found ways to improve communication on their own, setting up specific arrangements with remote counterparts. We sorted communication into three types:

- Improving cultural understanding
- Task-related communication
- Socio-emotional communication

Under communication, we also present results about

- Remote communication technologies
- The role of face-to-face meetings

Improving Cultural Understanding. At a superficial level, team members from the North had to learn literally how to comprehend the accents of their Southern counterparts. A North team member explained:

> It was a different accent. You know, because they have a down-South accent. And then I picked that up, and I had to get used to hearing it. And some of the slang and stuff like that. So, I have never lived down South. I have lived in New York most of my life. (NT)

This superficial problem was symptomatic of a perception on the part of many that there were differences in the abilities of North and South workers. A South manager explained:

> There was a perception that if you were from south of the Mason-Dixon line that your IQ was about 50 points below everybody from above just because of the mannerisms and the way we speak and the grammar, those type things. That was something that was thrown out at one of the team meetings that the folks in the South said that they felt like those from the North acted like we were not capable of doing some of the stuff. Yet all the administrative functions fall on the South to do, so if you don't think we're capable why do you keep asking us to do it? What it is is that we are not smart enough to tell you no. So there was some growing on both sides. To give you another example, the folk in the South say "no, sir" and "yes, ma'am." That's the way we were raised. It doesn't matter whether you were 50 years old or what. They looked at that as if we were trying to be subservient. But it's not. That's just manners. (SM)

Thus, communication among team members needed to respect linguistic conventions and overcome the stereotypical expectations often associated with cultural differences.

Improved cultural understanding allowed workers to coordinate their activities more effectively. A North manager explained how cultural differences affected the coordination of work schedules between North and South:

> I have to realize that they are on a much more structured schedule. They come in, there is a lunchtime, and they leave at a reasonable hour. And our day is much longer. But I have a tendency to look for people at lunch hour, cause I sit at my desk, you know, most of the day. I have to be aware that they are entitled to that time spot. Because sometimes I am looking for people at the wrong times, you know, in the evenings. For the most part, if you call down and they are not at their desk, they are calling you right back. (NM)

In this example, the appreciation of cultural differences was not simply a matter of greater understanding. It also led directly to practices affecting work scheduling and performance. Other workers described systems that they had developed with their remote counterparts to improve communication, such as the making of checklists or the scheduling of regular phone calls.

Task-Related Communication. One important example of task-related communication was a Southern manager's realization that he needed to request more resources from his superior in the North.

> I reckon I wasn't vocal enough, that I wasn't sure one operations manager could handle all the responsibilities of the group. But anyway, once I made the point to him that maybe there wasn't enough of me to go around and that was affecting my performance level, within three days he had gotten approval for us to hire another operations manager. That helped a lot. Just the fact that we had opened that dialog. I started realizing then, and I later even told him, that for me to get what I need I had to tell him what I need. (SM)

In this case, communication was important to his future success at SoftCo because without resources, he could not perform.

In another case, a Southern worker explained how her better communication skills made her more influential than other workers on the team. She said:

> . . . it is kind of split between the North and here. Sometimes our boss knows things that he doesn't really tell us about. He assumes, OK, well they will know this. But unless he tells us, a lot of things we don't know. And with the North, my communication would be a lot better, I guess, if I made more trips to the North. But, I don't want to do that. . . . I guess I am a good communicator. I guess that is probably it. Between me and Carol, we probably inform the team as a whole, including sales men and the North, better than anyone else. Because we know the repercussions if we don't inform them. It causes us problems in the very end. (ST)

This comment shows that in an empowered team, which receives relatively less direction from its manager, communication channels must be opened and used effectively for the team to perform. Clearly, this worker and others we spoke to realized the importance of clear communication to task performance.

Socio-Emotional Communication. Communication also improved the social and emotional relationships among workers in remote locations. We were told several stories about workers extending social and emotional support across geographic and cultural boundaries. The best example was reported by a female team member in the North who had assumed a mentoring role with workers in the South. She explained:

> Like with the people down South, it is like every time you pick up the phone, somebody is usually depressed because they are overloaded. And I just feel that since I have been working with this department and with my team, no one has been happy, honestly. I have to honestly tell you that. No one is happy. . . . No one is listening to these little people. Maybe they are and there is nothing else they can do for them down there. I don't know. I don't know what I can do because I am overloaded myself. . . . I mean, I try to cheer them up. I try to ask them, you know, "Is there anything I can do to help from up here?"
>
> And then there are times when people are stressed and you just tell them like anyone else, you know, "What is going on?" And then they tell you. Either they are sick or, you know, their husband, or I am dating this guy. And I am like, "Oh, yeah." You can tell in people's voices once you get to know them whether are happy. And I am like, "Oh, what happened?" I have very good relations. I am really friendly, honestly, I get along with like everyone. I really don't have a problem with anyone. (NT)

This description conveys the degree of intimacy achieved with remote communication that spanned functional, geographic, and cultural divides. This worker explained that she did not have time to visit the South location as often as she wanted to, but she clearly stayed in touch with her counterparts through other means.

Remote Communication Media. Communication within virtual teams at SoftCo relied on a variety of media including telephone, voice mail, fax, e-mail, videoconferencing, and face-to-face meetings. There was no dedicated collaborative technology or groupware in place, so team members and managers mixed the available media to satisfy their needs. Choices among media were based on numerous considerations: urgency, individual preference, need for documentation, and ease of use. Each respondent, however, seemed to apply these criteria in different ways, supporting our expectation that communication practices would develop to meet locally understood needs. For example, a Northern manager explained his preference for e-mail when communicating with someone he described as a particularly difficult employee:

> I have a tendency to communicate with him by e-mail. I have no problem picking up the phone and calling anybody else. It is because I don't want to deal with the issue of him getting upset. (NM)

Several other practices illustrate the creativity and complexity of media choices. In one case, a Southern team member described how she used the telephone when she was away to contact another worker who would read her e-mail.

> I have a [woman] that works for me, and she can get into my e-mail and she can check my e-mail to see if there is anything real important. If you don't have a laptop, you can't just go to another office and check your e-mail or make sure, unless you are set up on their computer. And I am set up on the computer in the North also. So I could check my e-mail while in the North. If I was in Atlanta, though, like I am going to be tomorrow, I couldn't check my e-mail. So the [woman] that works for me, she checks it. She has my password and she can get in and check it. And usually, she and I are getting the same e-mail. (ST)

In another case, a Southern team member explained how data was shared. Rather than accessing a shared database, which was available on the company's mainframe in a public folder, workers called each other or attached spreadsheet files to their e-mail messages.

> We have different drives where there are public folders, and you can go in and look and see. Like I do a report, it is a blanket, where we actually purchase material and we purchase it like six months at a time and they give us a certain price, a certain delivery. And that is out there on . . . [what] we call the H-drive. And anybody can go in and look at that. (ST)

When asked if the shared databases were consulted, this same respondent admitted:

> No. Uh-uh. Not for my stuff. I am sure they do for other things. They probably do for, you know, for other stuff that really relates to them. This relates to them too, but they usually just pick up the phone and call me. I remind them about it every time they do that. That it's there and how to get there. But, I guess they just feel like it is easier just to pick up the phone and call and ask. (ST)

These explanations show that different technologies were used in inelegant yet innovative ways, often to compensate for difficulties in accessing or using available media. A team member from the North explained one reason for the practice of avoiding shared databases:

> [The mainframe] is a good system in some respects, but it is fragmented. I mean, you can go from this screen to that one and it kind of like drives you crazy. And then you take the information and you wind up putting it on an Excel spreadsheet. This is OK, but this takes a lot of time. But I

> think that one of the other great things is that we pretty much all have our own laptops. You find yourself taking it home. You take it home on the weekends. (NT)

A North manager confirmed the practice of producing spreadsheets from mainframe data, attaching them to e-mail messages, and updating and returning them:

> When I send out monthly statements, I do it on an attachment from Excel. And everybody has Excel. . . . And that is how I send it out in e-mail. I hardly send out paper anymore. They are all attachments. (NM)

In addition, videoconferencing was used frequently. In one North manager's assessment, videoconferencing added personal presence to remote communication:

> [Videoconferencing] would be used to kind of bridge the gap and somewhat make it a little bit more personal interaction, but it is not used as broadly as or as often as we probably should and we like. (NM)

In both the North and South locations, rooms equipped with videoconference facilities were available, although we did not have the opportunity to observe them in use. In fact, the room used in the North for our interviews was a room normally reserved for videoconferences.

Although many of the communication practices described may appear to be inefficient, and perhaps a threat to data integrity or security, they had evolved over time in the teams and seemed to satisfy people's needs to communicate remotely.

Face-to-Face Communication. Face-to-face communication occurred through two primary means: business meetings involving travel by individual workers in both directions between North and South, and quarterly team meetings involving all team members from both locations. Although business travel was time-consuming, several workers commented on its value. A South manager noted:

> It's just better to let people meet face-to-face. When you just talk to somebody on the phone, it's just fine, we just feel it's effective, but it doesn't really have a big impact. I mean, because our North staff is not that big compared with some of the other areas—we only have about five people up there—and they don't mind coming down here. They kind of like it, and the people down here don't mind going up there so. That's one good thing. They enjoy going up there. (SM)

A South team member described what business travel was like.

> Yeah, when they come, they come over and sit at our desks and use our phone, or whatever. And we go to dinner, lunch, or whatever. You know, we are pretty close when it comes to going out. When the girls go up there, they all spend time together. It's a real togetherness thing. It's not like you go up, you go to a meeting, you go to your room, you never see

> them again. Everybody gets along well. And we have fun on those kinds of going-out-of-town things. You know, we all go to dinner and everybody, you know, cuts loose, and has fun, or whatever. It's not just all work. And you have gotta have that or you wouldn't get along with anybody. (ST)

The other form of face-to-face meetings were periodic business meetings, usually held at locations such as golf courses, beaches, or mountain resorts. The normal format was to mix business with social activities over the course of two or three days, but the exact format varied across teams. A new North team member described the experience.

> So with the three or four meetings, we accomplish more in those two days than we can accomplish here in like two weeks. So then it pays. Like we are having the same issue back and forth. And if we just bring those copies that we have and resolve them there, then it goes quicker while we are there. Maybe something is getting lost from the time [it takes to go from] . . . here to there, when we are e-mailing or on the phone. But when we are face to face, it is quite simpler. . . . That's because, there you see them in a different environment than normally, not in the office. It is outside. And it was in a resort so people were more relaxed. They were eating dinner with some people that [they] normally would not . . . eat with. So it was different. (NT)

Remote and face-to-face communications were frequently combined in ways that satisfied individual preferences and task needs. By traveling to each other's sites and to the quarterly meetings, workers at SoftCo gained respect for each other as people. The closer interpersonal relationships helped them to devise mutually compatible procedures for using remote communication technologies to accomplish their shared work so that customers were satisfied and performance goals were met. Communication in its various forms both produces and reflects the practices that the teams learned.

Learning Situated in Practice

We use the active verb form "learning" here instead of the noun "knowledge" because we understood knowledge generation to be ongoing and dynamic. Thus, what was learned through the complex communication practices described earlier was not static. Because it was situated in practice, learning continued to evolve. We invited everyone we interviewed to provide examples of practices that they had learned, and most reports included descriptions of how that learning continued. Some of these accounts pertained to learning between co-located workers, sometimes from different teams. Others involved learning between remote members.

Co-located learning was important to virtual teamwork because it oriented new workers to the special demands of remote work. For example, a South team member explained how she taught her skills to the most recently hired customer services person.

> She sat with both Donna and I and caught on really quick. I mean we went over everything, but she pretty much watched us do the work and then just caught on like that. To me that is the only way that you can learn what we are doing. It helps to know, like when I would get off the phone, I would say, "Well, he called and wanted to place a personal use order and this is, you know, how you give a discount and these are the screens that I went into." So you try to sort of walk them through it, let them know what the customer wanted. (ST)

Managers appreciated this mode of learning through watching experienced workers and explaining what was done. A South manager explained:

> You know, they will always try to ask a neighbor. And that is something that our team does. Instead of just calling to me every time, they will ask the person sitting by them. "Well, what do you think? Do you think that we should give them this?" And there's a lot of communication going on within customer services. (SM)

These accounts of learning include the visual, tactile, and verbal communication processes that co-located workers enjoy. For both managers and workers learning across locations, different processes were engaged. One South manager described the challenge of getting more resources from his boss, who was located in the North:

> In the case of somebody being in the office a lot of the time, I was used to him knowing what I wanted just from visually seeing what's wrong. But when you are 1,000 miles away, they can only go by what they hear, and you have to be more verbal about what you need and what you don't need. In this case I needed help and didn't have it, and I was expecting him to know without telling him. . . . Now I have learned . . . that if you deal effectively with your boss as well as your subordinates, you've got to tell them what you expect. That's not a concept I'm used to, and maybe that's my Southern raising. I'm used to my boss telling me what to expect and knowing what I need and telling me "Here's where we go." It was more that I had to take a proactive role in directing the actions. This was something I had to adjust to, so that was not all his adjusting. (SM)

Although it may seem obvious that a remote boss cannot see the distant employee's needs, the manager was quite candid about the difficulty in making this discovery.

In our earlier descriptions of communication practices, we mentioned cases where workers learned to appreciate the differences in work pace between the North and South locations. To illustrate how such differences were recognized and resolved, we include comments from an extremely animated Northern team member:

> It is not hard for me to want to go 75 and 90 miles an hour. And I think that I had a hard time coming to grips with the fact that maybe those people really aren't going to go but 45 miles an hour. And I had no problem just jumping right down their throats. And all a sudden, it was like, this

> is not the way to win friends and influence them.' Cause, you know what? I am going to get nothing out of it. So, you just have to take a step back, and then I realized that there are times that I just have to take a big deep breath, and make the phone call and say, "Let's work our way through it." (NT)

When asked whether the people in the South had made adjustment to her, the North team member replied:

> No. I have made adjustments to them. I will admit that, you know. It has been more one way than the other. I know that they know that there isn't anything that I would . . . ask them to do that I wouldn't do myself. And they know that if it takes staying until 7 o'clock, 10 o'clock, coming in at 5 o'clock in the morning, seven days a week, I am right there. So it is like, they know that I would never ask them to go any extra that I wouldn't be there going the extra too. (NT)

Another North team member, who described a difficult relationship with her Southern counterpart, confessed that she had come on too strong:

> I used to haunt her to death. That could have had a lot to do with the way our relationship developed. I used to haunt her to death. I used to call her 50 times a day. "How do I do this? What do I do?" (NT)

This worker continued by explaining a recent incident:

> You know, sometimes I guess my sense of urgency, sometimes, isn't like her sense of urgency. You know, I had a problem the other day, and I said that when she finds that information, she has got to tell me. Because we are able to fix it up here sometimes better than in the South. . . . And I asked when did she find out the information. And this just happened when I got in Monday. She said she found out on Thursday. And I said to her: "You have to let me know something happened on Thursday when you are discussing it with somebody else. I have got to know that day." (NT)

Situated learning was also illustrated by the relationship between customer service people located in the South and remote sales people, who traveled regularly and were hard to reach. A customer service person explained:

> Well, we have a salesman that I will be seeing tomorrow, and I can't wait to get there. I have a few things to discuss with him. A problem . . . is that he travels a lot. And we get a lot of his phone calls that we know nothing about. I mean, I will take any call, but I want to know some up front information. I don't want somebody to call me and say, "Hey, Jake Harper told me to call you regarding blah blah blah." And I am like, "OK." And I don't have a clue. If somebody tells someone to call me, they should at least say, "OK, you are probably going to get some phone calls regarding this, this, this." But, you know? I get blind-sided a lot when it comes to him. But I deal with it. I am going to say to him, "You know, I need a little help here. I don't think that is fair to me just to drop your work on me and not even let me know it going to come." He and I

> sort of have a love-hate thing going on. We let each other have it. But it works out. (ST)

The customer service worker explained how hard it was to "train" a salesman:

> It is hard to train a salesman that is not here and doesn't know what you are looking at. I mean, he may send in an order and expect you to ship tomorrow. Well, that's not going to happen. I mean, you have got to do a lot of day-to-day training with your salesmen. You know, "This will work better for me and I think it will help you too if you fax it in. You know? And we can't turn an embroidery order in 24 hours." Those types of things that you have to learn as you go. (ST)

These excerpts show that adjustments to work schedules and expectations were made after workers experienced difficulty establishing mutually acceptable work practices. In each case, the resolution was produced directly by the persons involved, rather than imposed from the outside. By situating their learning in a virtual community of practice, the workers both resolved specific problems and laid the groundwork for continued learning.

Finally, one incident described by a South manager revealed how the virtual teams exercised social control over team members who violated practices that the team had learned. In this case, the issue involved a team member who used e-mail to expose a fellow team member's mistakes to everyone, including higher-level managers. The manager used this story to illustrate how teamwork was different from traditionally organized work, and how such behavior could not be tolerated.

> We have one person in there that has been there a long time, who last week showed highly visible signs of being a little more for their own interest and taking advantage of the situation to make themselves look better. Now, that person was severely chastised. And I say chastised. What happened was, they were in this situation where another member of the team had made a decision for the benefit of the company and the e-mail consisted of pointing a finger at that person: "Somebody needs to go down and bust their ass, bust their butt." I said "Whoa, whoa, watch it. What do you mean there?" And this was to the higher-ups. And I can't tolerate that. Because that is a clear sign then of saying: "Hey, look at me. I am doing great. But that dummy done wrong." And that was not tolerated. (SM)

Discussion and Conclusions

By using an interpretive approach, we have drawn ourselves closer to the experience of work in cross-functional virtual teams. We have reported personal accounts of how members adjusted to demands of a virtual team environment, how they communicated both remotely and face-to-face, and how they learned new practices to accomplish their work and satisfy their social needs. By extending the concept of community of practice to include virtual communities, we are able to focus on communication and learning practices and the consequences they bring to team members.

Although working in virtual teams permits infrequent face-to-face communication, learning can be effectively situated in virtual space. The framework describing our results may guide further research, which would be expected to produce useful elaborations of the concepts that comprise the framework and greater understanding of the relationships among concepts.

A number of implications can be drawn from this study. The teams at SoftCo demonstrated great resourcefulness in solving problems and finding a mixture of communication media to support the learning of work practices. The creative accommodations and adjustments described in this article are evidence of how work practices can emerge as a product of community interaction. The practices devised to coordinate work pace and work schedules succeed because they respond to local needs. Learning how to work virtually is indeed situated in practice rather than imposed from above or from the outside. Managers of virtual cross-functional teams need to understand this phenomenon and use a "hands-off" style that empowers team members. SoftCo's workers responded to their greater responsibility by improvising work practices that met their needs. It is doubtful that managers could anticipate every team need and develop formal work practices to guide team members.

Managers do, however, need to support virtual teams with appropriate rhetoric, reward systems, and technologies. They also need to stage opportunities for face-to-face meetings. Respondents were overwhelmingly positive about the quarterly meetings that gave them chances to meet each other. The fact that these were held in attractive locations, and that no team members were excluded contributed to their value. Workers also seemed able to manage their own level of business travel so that Southern workers who enjoyed trips to the North could go more frequently. Team members felt empowered to mix remote and face-to-face communication using their own recipes. Incentives were also used to motivate team performance, and team members were well aware of the sizeable bonuses that came from satisfying customers.

The role played by information technology in SoftCo's virtual teams is consistent with our conclusions about situated learning and empowerment. SoftCo's team members relied on a variety of communication technologies: telephone, fax, electronic mail, and videoconferencing. These rudimentary technologies were used in creative ways to satisfy communication needs. By contrast, much attention is currently placed on the design of special collaborative technologies to support virtual teams (Rittenbruch, Kahler, and Cremers 1998). From the theoretical perspective of learning situated in virtual communities of practice, the imposition of a special collaborative technology effectively restricts members' choices of media.

Virtual teams, as communities of practice, may be more effective if they are not constrained by technology, no matter how elegant or powerful it might be. While both team members and managers were aware of the limitations of the technologies available to them, they creatively overcame many of those limitations by combining media, even though such practices introduced redundancy and security and privacy concerns.

Our findings clearly show the value of face-to-face meetings in establishing a greater social connection among team members. Workers frequently mentioned the value of "putting a face" on their remote counterparts, and they used this knowledge to greater advantage when communicating remotely. Socio-emotional communication typically began during face-to-face visits connected with business travel or at quarterly business meetings, and was sustained electronically after these meetings. Members appreciated these opportunities to meet their counterparts in person, partly because such meetings were instrumental to accomplishing their mutual tasks and partly because of the social benefits of getting together. Designers of virtual cross-functional teams should try to devise means for both remote and face-to-face communication to occur.

Because our approach was interpretive, we are limited in our ability to generalize to other settings. Our findings incorporate the subjective responses of participants in one particular, socially constructed world of work that may differ from the worlds of other workers. However, a benefit of the interpretive methodology is that it extracts detail that might be masked in a survey targeted at a larger sample. Our respondents talked at length about learning and communication, bringing these abstractions to life in their own words. We imagine that other virtual cross-functional teams would be similar in some ways while sustaining distinctive characteristics of their own.

The implications developed here reflect an awareness of virtual teams as distinct communities, capable of learning their own particular practices. However, we expect that the processes of teaming and communication described here would occur in some fashion in every virtual team faced with the need to coordinate across business functions. Consequently, the framework describing our results (illustrated in Figure 2) has general value beyond the case of SoftCo managers and workers.

In conclusion, we have presented, mostly in the voices of team members and managers themselves, how learning occurs in virtual cross-functional teams. Like co-located teams, members of a virtual team comprise a community of practice. Using available resources, they develop practices that reflect their unique needs, both task-oriented and social. They create and share knowledge and socialize new members to team practices. Their learning is situated in practice even though their situation is one that spans geographic boundaries and cultural divides. Not only do these findings provide implications for the management of work in virtual teams, but they also reinforce the value of viewing work, even virtual work, as a community of practice in which learning is situated.

REFERENCES

Belanger, F., and R. W. Collins. 1998. 'Distributed work arrangements: a research framework." *The information society* 14:137–152.

Boudreau, M.-C., K. D. Loch, D. Robey, and D. Straub. 1998. "Going global: Using information technology to advance the competitiveness of the virtual transnational organization." *Academy of management executives* 12, no. 4:120–128.

Brown, J. S. 1998. "Internet technology in support of the concept of 'communities-of-practice': The case of Xerox." *Accounting, management and information technologies* 8:227–236.

Brown, J. S., and P. Duguid. 1991. "Organizational learning and communities-of-practice: Toward a unified view of working, learning, and innovation." *Organization science* 2, no. 1:40–57.

Davidow, W. H., and M. S. Malone. 1992. *The virtual corporation: Structuring and revitalizing the corporation for the 21st century*. New York, NY: Harper Business.

Deetz, S. 1996. "Describing differences in approaches to organization science: Rethinking Burrell and Morgan and their legacy." *Organization science* 7, no. 2:191–207.

DeSanctis, G., and M. S. Poole. 1997. "Transitions in teamwork in new organizational forms." *Advances in group processes* 14: 157–176.

DeSanctis, G., N. Staudenmayer, and S.-S. Wong. 2000. "Interdependence in virtual organizations." In *Trends in organizational behavior*, ed. C. Cooper and D. Rousseau. New York, NY: John Wiley & Sons.

Edmondson, A. 1999. "Psychological safety and learning behavior in work teams." *Administrative science quarterly* 44, no. 2:350–383.

George, J. F., S. Iacono, and R. Kling. 1995. "Learning in context: Extensively computerized work groups as communities-of-practice," *Accounting, management and information technologies* 5, no. 3/4:185–202.

Gorton, I., and S. Motwani. 1996. "Issues in cooperative software engineering using globally distributed teams." *Information & software technology* 38, no. 10:647–655.

Grabowski, M., and K. H. Roberts. 1998. "Risk mitigation in virtual organizations." *Journal of computer-mediated communication* 3, no. 4. http://www.ascusc.org/jcmc/vol3/issue4/grabowski.html

Greis, N. P., and J. D. Kasarda. 1997. "Enterprise logistics in the information era." *California management review* 39, no. 3:55–78.

Grenier, R., and G. Metes. 1995. *Going virtual: Moving your organization into the 21st century*. Englewood Cliffs, NJ: Prentice Hall.

Hammer, M. 1996. *Beyond reengineering: How the process-centered organization is changing our work and our lives*. New York, NY: Harper Business.

Jarvenpaa, S. L., and D. E. Leidner. 1998. "Communication and trust in global virtual teams." *Journal of computer-mediated communication* 3, no. 4. http://www.ascusc.org/jcmc/vol3/issue4/jarvenpaa.html.

Kraut, R., C. Steinfield, A. Chan, B. Butler, and A. Hoag. 1998. "Coordination and virtualization: The role of electronic networks and personal relationships." *Journal of computer-mediated communication* 3, no. 4. http://www.ascusc.org/jcmc/vol3/issue4/kraut.html.

Kusunoki, K., and T. Numagami, 1998. "Interfunctional transfers of engineers in Japan: Empirical findings and implications for cross-functional integration." *IEEE transactions on engineering management* 45, no. 3:250.

Lave, J., and E. Wegner. 1991. *Situated learning: Legitimate peripheral participation*. Cambridge, UK: Cambridge University Press.

Lipnack, J., and J. Stamps. 1997. *Virtual teams: Reaching across space, time, and organizations with technology*. John Wiley & Sons.

Marshall, C. C., F. M. Shipman, and R. J. McCall. 1995. "Making large-scale information resources serve communities of practice." *Journal of management information systems* 11, no. 4:65–86.

Mason, J. 1996. *Qualitative researching*. Thousand Oaks, CA: Sage.

Maznevski, M. L., and K. M. Chudoba. 2000. "Bridging space over time: Global virtual team dynamics and effectiveness." *Organization science* 11, no. 5: 473–92.

Nonaka, I. 1994. "A dynamic theory of organizational knowledge creation." *Organization science* 5, no. 1:14–37.

Orlikowski, W. J., and J. J. Baroudi. 1991. "Studying information technology in organizations: Research approaches and assumptions." *Information systems research* 2, no. 1:1–28.

Orr, J. E. 1996. *Talking about machines: An ethnography of a modern job*. Ithaca, NY: ILR Press.

Osterlund, J. 1997. "Competence management by informatics in R&D: The corporate level." *IEEE transactions on engineering management* 44, no. 2:135–145.

Pinto, M. B., and J. K. Pinto. 1990. "Project team communication and cross-functional cooperation in new program development." *Journal of product innovation management* 7, no. 3:200–212.

Ritttenbruch, M., H. Kahler, and A. B. Cremers. 1998. "Supporting cooperation in a virtual organization." In R. Hirschheim (Ed.), *Proceedings of the nineteenth international conference on information systems: Dec.* 13–16 (pp. 30–38). Atlanta: ICIS Administrative office.

Robey, D., and M. M. Bakr. 1978. "Task redesign: Individual moderating and novelty effects." *Human relations* 31, no. 8:689–701.

Robey, D., and M, -C. Boudreau. 1999. "Accounting for the contradictory organizational consequences of information technology: Theoretical directions and methodological implications." *Information system research* 10, no. 2:167–185.

Robey, D., M. -C. Boudreau, and V. C. Storey. 1998. "Looking before we leap: Foundations for a research program on virtual organizations." In *Electronic commerce: Papers from the third international conference on the management of networked organizations*, ed. G. St. -Amant and M. Amami, pp. 275–290.

Sarbaugh-Thompson, M., and M. S. Feldman. 1998. "Electronic mail and organizational communication: Does saying 'Hi' really matter?" *Organization science* 9, no. 6:685–698.

Stamps, D. 1997. "Communities of practice: Learning is social. Training is irrelevant?" *Training* 34, no. 2:34–42.

Staples, D. S., J. S. Hulland, and C. A. Higgins. 1998. "A self-efficacy theory explanation for the management of remote workers in virtual organizations." *Journal of computer-mediated communication* 3, no. 4. http://www.ascusc.org/jcmc/vol3/issue4/staples.html.

Townsend, A. M., S. M. DeMarie, and A. R. Henrickson. 1998. "Virtual teams: Technology and the workplace of the future." *Academy of management executives* 12, no. 3:17–29.

Tyre, M. J., and E. von Hippel. 1997. "The situated nature of adaptive learning in organizations." *Organization science* 8, no. 1:71–81.

Walsham, G. 1995. "The emergence of interpretivism in IS research." *Information systems research* 6, no. 4:376–394.

Walton, R. E., and J. M. Dutton. 1969. "The management of interdepartmental conflict." *Administrative science quarterly* 14: 73–84.

Walton, R. E., J. M. Dutton, and T. P. Cafferty. 1969. "Organizational context and interdepartmental conflict." *Administrative science quarterly* 14:522–542.

Wegner, E. 1998. *Communities of practice: Learning, meaning and identity*. Cambridge, UK: Cambridge University Press.

Whiting, V. R., and K. K. Reardon. 1998. "Communicating from a distance: Establishing commitment in a virtual office environment." Paper presented to the Academy of Management.

Wiesenfeld, B. M., S. Raghuram, and R. Garud. 1998. "Communication patterns as determinants of organizational identification in a virtual organization." *Journal of computer-mediated communication* 3, no. 4. http://www.ascusc.org/jcmc/vol3/issue4/wiesenfeld.html.

Wynn, E., and D. G. Novick. 1995. "Relevance conventions and problem boundaries in work redesign teams." *Information technology & people* 9:61–80.

ADDITIONAL READINGS

Beason, Gary. "Redefining Written Products with WWW Documentation: A Study of the Publication Process at a Computer Company." *Technical Communication* 43, no. 4 (1996): 339–48.

Blythe, Stuart. "Designing Online Courses: User-Centered Practices." *Computers and Composition* 18 (2001): 329–46.

Bolter, Jay David. "Ekphrasis, Virtual Reality, and the Future of Writing." In *The Future of the Book*, edited by Geoffrey Nunberg, 253–72. Berkeley: U of California P, 1996.

Brasseur, Lee. "Visual Literacy in the Computer Age: A Complex Perceptual Landscape." In *Computers and Technical Communication: Pedagogical and Programmatic Perspectives*, edited by Stuart A. Selber, 75–96. Greenwich, CT: Ablex, 1997.

Brown, John Seely, and Paul Duguid. *The Social Life of Information*. Boston: Harvard Business School Press, 2000.

Dautermann, Jennie, and Patricia Sullivan. "Issues of Written Literacy and Electronic Literacy in Workplace Settings." In *Electronic Literacy in the Workplace: Technologies of Writing*. Eds. Jennie Dautermann and Patricia Sullivan. Urbana, IL: NCTE, 1996. vii–xxxiii.

Dayton, David. "Electronic Editing in Technical Communication: A Survey of Practices and Attitudes." *Technical Communication* 50, no. 2 (2003): 192–205.

Doheny-Farina, Stephen. *The Wired Neighborhood*. New Haven: Yale UP, 1996.

Duin, Ann Hill, and Ray Archee. "Collaboration via E-mail and Internet Relay Chat: Understanding Time and Technology." *Technical Communication* 43, no. 4 (1996): 402–12.

Duin, Ann Hill, Lisa D. Mason, and Linda A. Jorn. "Structuring Distance-Meeting Environments" *Technical Communication* 41, no. 4 (1994): 695–708.

Farkas, David K., and Steven E. Poltrock. "Online Editing, Mark-Up Models, and the Workplace Lives of Editors and Writers." In *Electronic Literacies in the Workplace: Technologies of Writing*, edited by Patricia Sullivan and Jennie Dautermann, 154–76. Urbana, IL: NCTE, 1996.

Gillette, David. "Pedagogy, Architecture, and the Virtual Classroom." *Technical Communication Quarterly* 8, no. 1 (1999): 21–36.

Grabil, Jeffrey T. "Utoptic Visions, The Technopoor, and Public Access: Writing Technologies in a Community Literacy Program." *Computers and Composition* 15 (1998): 297–315.

Graves, Heather Brodie, and Roger Graves. "Masters, Slaves, and Infant Mortality: Language Challenges for Technical Editing." *Technical Communication Quarterly* 7, no. 4 (1998): 389–414.

Gurak, Laura. "Technology, Community, and Technical Communication on the Internet: The Lotus *MarketPlace* and Clipper Chip Controversies." *Journal of Business and Technical Communication* 10, 1 (1996): 81–99.

Hansen, Craig J. "Contextualizing Technology and Communication in a Corporate Setting." In *Nonacademic Writing: Social Theory and Technology*, edited by Ann Hill Duin and Craig Hansen, 305–24. Mahwah, NJ: Erlbaum, 1996.

———. "Networking Technology in the Classroom: Whose Interests Are We Serving?" In *Electronic Literacies in the Workplace: Technologies of Writing*, edited by Patricia Sullivan and Jennie Dautermann, 201–15. Urbana, IL: NCTE, 1996.

Howard, Tharon. *A Rhetoric of Electronic Communities*. Greenwich, CT: Ablex, 1997.

Johnson-Eilola, Johndan. *Nostalgic Angels: Rearticulating Hypertext Writing*. Norwood, NJ: Ablex, 1996.

———. "Wild Technologies: Computer Use and Social Possibility." In *Computer and Technical Communication*, edited by Stuart Selber, 97–128. Greenwich, CT: Ablex, 1997.

Lupton, Ellen, and J. Abbott Miller. *Design Writing Research: Writing on Graphic Design*. London: Phaidon Press, 1999.

Mirel, Barbara. "Analyzing Electronic Help Exchanges: An Inquiry into Instructions for Complex Tasks." *Technical Communication* 41, no. 2 (1994): 210–23.

National Telecommunications Information Administration. "Executive Summary". In *Falling through the Net: Toward Digital Inclusion*. Washington, DC: US Department of Commerce, October 2000. http://www.ntia.doc.gov/ntiahome/digitaldivide/execsumfttn00.htm (accessed Dec. 7, 2002).

Rea, Alan, and Doug White. "The Changing Nature of Writing: Prose or Code in the Classroom." *Computers and Composition* 16 (1999): 421–36.

Rubens, Philip. "Interactive Media and Technical Communication: Incorporating Emerging Technologies into the Information Domain." In *Technical Communication Frontiers: Essays in Theory*, edited by Charles H. Sides, 117–46. St. Paul, MN: ATTW, 1994.

Selber, Stuart A. "Beyond Skill Building: Challenges Facing Technical Communication Teachers in the Computer Age." *Technical Communication Quarterly* 3, no. 4 (1994): 365–90.

———. "The Politics and Practice of Media Design." In *Foundations for Teaching Technical Communication: Theory, Practice, and Program Design*, edited by Katherine Staples and Cezar Ornatowski, 193–208. Greenwich, CT: Ablex, 1997.

Selfe, Cynthia. *Technology and Literacy in the Twenty-First Century: The Importance of Paying Attention*. Carbondale: Southern Illinois UP, 1999.

Selfe, Cynthia L., and Richard J. Selfe. "Writing as Democratic Social Action in a Technological World: Politicizing and Inhabiting Virtual Landscape." In *Nonacademic Writing: Social Theory and Technology*, edited by Ann Hill Duin and Craig J. Hansen, 325–58. Mahwah, NJ: Lawrence Erlbaum, 1996.

Smith, Catherine F. "Nobody, Which Means Anybody: Audience on the World Wide Web." In *Weaving a Virtual Web: Practical Approaches to New Information Technologies*, edited by Sibylle Gruber. Urbana: NCTE, 2000.

Smith, Douglass K., and Barbara J. Minnick. "Electronic Teacher-Student Communication." *Business Communication Quarterly* 59, no. 1 (1996): 74–85.

Sullivan, Patricia, and Jennie Dautermann, eds. *Electronic Literacies in the Workplace: Technologies of Writing*. Urbana, IL: NCTE, 1996.

VanHoosier-Carey, Gregory. "Rhetoric by Design: Using Web Development Projects in the Technical Communication Classroom." *Computer and Composition* 14 (1997): 395–407.

Wahlstrom, Billie J. "Communication and Technology: Defining a Feminist Presence in Research and Practice." In *Literacy and Computers: The Complications of Teaching and Learning with Technology*, edited by Cynthia L. Selfe and Susan Hilligoss, 171–85. New York: The Modern Language Association of America, 1994.

Wickliff, Gregory, and Janice Tovey. "Hypertext in a Professional Writing Course." *Technical Communication Quarterly* 4, no. 1 (1995): 47–61.

CHAPTER EIGHT

Looking to the Future

Chapter Eight: Introduction

In the foreword to the recently published *Reshaping Technical Communication: New Directions and Challenges for the 21st Century*, Janice Redish begins by proclaiming that it is "an exciting time for technical communicators." Indeed it is. With membership in the Society for Technical Communicators up in the past decade from 13,778 members in twenty-four countries to more than 21,789 members in forty-eight countries (Redish vii) and an increase in graduate programs in the field, technical communication is quickly becoming a respectable and respected discipline. However, as evidenced by the fact that Redish also explains that many people in the field still feel isolated or undervalued, it is clear that we're not there yet.

In this chapter, three prominent scholars in the field present their ideas about what technical communicators and technical communication teachers need to do to succeed in the postindustrial twenty-first century. Their emphases are on the classroom and on representation, and they highlight the fact that, if technical communication wants to be taken seriously, members of the field need to recognize both the changes that are taking place in society and how their roles, current and future, need to shift to take advantage of those changes. Johnson-Eilola encourages us to revision our sense of ourselves and shift the emphasis from *technical* to *communication* in order to highlight the positive impact we have as "symbolic analysts," people who can positively affect the way knowledge is organized, transmitted, shared, and understood. Ornatowski and Bernhardt also agree that we need to see ourselves differently, and they emphasize that education is a key component in the kinds of transition that Johnson-Eilola proposes.

While some years have passed since these articles were written, the points that these authors make about technical communicators as "symbolic-analytic workers" (Johnson-Eilola, p. 574 in this volume), "agent[s] of change" (Bernhardt, p. 599, and decision makers who stand at the critical "intersection of technology and its various producers, users, and publics" (Ornatowski, p. 605) remain valid. Most important, their suggestions for us to consider will help us develop the kinds of communities—of teaching, practice, research, and users—that Redish advocates (viii–xii). Communities focus on communication and participation; they encourage interactivity and a sharing of knowledge and expertise. In essence, by joining together to demonstrate the ways in which we improve communication, help others cultivate goals and values, and have an impact on information technology and knowledge transfer, we can both take steps to diminish feelings of isolation and inadequacy and construct new identities as creators of knowledge.

WORK CITED

Redish, Janice. Foreword *to Reshaping Technical Communication: New Directions and Challenges for the 21st Century,* edited by Barbara Mirel and Rachel Spilka, vii–xiii. Mahwah, NJ: Lawrence Erlbaum, 2002.

32 Relocating the Value of Work: Technical Communication in a Post-Industrial Age

JOHNDAN JOHNSON-EILOLA

Johnson-Eilola argues that technical communicators should shed their personas as long-suffering servants in an industrial age and take their place alongside members of other occupations such as management consulting who have embraced the designation of "symbolic-analytic work" in the postindustrial age (p. 575 in this volume). These workers have come to understand that "knowledge does work" (p. 580), and they recognize that communication is at the nexus of organization and not just a set of skills or tools. By putting the emphasis on "communication" rather than "technical" and pointing out that technical communicators "identify, rearrange, circulate, abstract, and broker information" (p. 582), Johnson-Eilola makes his case for seeing them as symbolic analysts who add value to organizations. As you read, consider his tactics for rearticulating and reinventing technical communication education: "collaboration, experimentation, abstraction, and system thinking" (p. 582) and his five key projects for educators (e.g., "connect education to work," and "build metaknowledge, network knowledge, and self-reflective practices" [p. 589]). Consider ways in which we might use these tactics to better prepare our students and to represent ourselves to others in the academy and the workplace.

As we enter the post-industrial age, we enter a time of great potential for revising the relationship between technology and communication. Fifty years ago, at the tail end of the industrial age, technological products generated income. Factories produced concrete goods—washers, automobiles, clothing, televisions—that consumers purchased. In that climate, information was subordinate to industry. Information may have supported products, but the highest value was typically in the industrial product. Today, however, we live and work in an increasingly post-industrial age, where information is fast becoming the more valuable product. Products are still manufactured and purchased, but, in a growing number of markets, primary value is located in information itself.

From *Technical Communication Quarterly* 5, no. 3 (1996): 245–70.

In this article, I argue that rearticulating technical communication in post-industrial terms provides a common ground between academic and corporate models of technical communication, which are notoriously disparate (Scanlon and Coon; Carliner). Robert B. Reich's definition of "symbolic-analytic work" offers a way to relocate value in technical communication contexts, from an industrial to post-industrial relationship. Symbolic-analytic workers rely on skills in abstraction, experimentation, collaboration, and system thinking to work with information across a variety of disciplines and markets. Importantly, symbolic-analytic work mediates between the functional necessities of usability and efficiency while not losing sight of the larger rhetorical and social contexts in which users work and live.

This article begins by exploring some of the problems of technical communication's current service orientation as it affects professional and users and, recursively, educators and students. Next, I describe other disciplines that have been able to define their work in post-industrial ways. The second half of the article starts by defining symbolic-analytic work in relation to other occupational classes. In the midst of this definitional work, I provide a more productive framework for technical communication by positioning current research and practice in technical communication within specific aspects of symbolic-analytic work. Finally, I describe five key educational projects that might help educators begin better educating students for new occupational positions.

Technical Communication as Service

Technical communication has traditionally occupied a support position in both academic and corporate spheres. In general, this model encourages communicators to focus on either technologies or on the limited aspects of a user's overall project that require technologies. Although the tendencies are present in varying degrees in most areas of technical communication, they are most visible in documentation, the primary genre discussed below. By relocating the value of documentation into a post-industrial relationship, we can work to rearticulate technical communication as a post-industrial discipline, with documentation blurring into other areas of our work.

Currently, most technical communication projects enhance other processes and products: well-written software documentation allows users to complete their primary work (writing a report on a word processor, compiling a business productivity chart in a spreadsheet). Technical communication, as support, occupies a secondary position to the users' main objective, their "real work" (see e.g., Carroll; Horton; Bowie; Weiss, "Retreat"). The difficulty here is that real work easily becomes defined in reductive, context-independent ways: small, decontextualized functional tasks rather than large, messy, "real world" projects. Telling a user the menu command for placing a graphic on a page is typically much easier than teaching the user both that functional task and the broader, more complicated basics of rhetoric and page design. Although in one sense the general "task" orientation of technical manuals appears to be a movement away from technology and toward the user's context, that movement is a deceptive one, because the user's tasks are defined almost completely in relation to the technology: the user's contexts are typically invisible.

This service orientation is multiplied, fractal-like, in academia, where technical communication educators frequently find themselves called upon to fulfill wish-lists of skills to industry. This position is readily apparent in a recent issue of *Technical Communication* on education. "The role of industry" in academic/industry collaboration, argue three technical communicators, "is to lend the structure and services of the institution to a design and content shaped by industry" (Krestas, Fisher, and Hackos). Another author cites a 1969 textbook in technical communication (his only bibliographic source) to argue for technical communication as "the presentation of verifiable data" and a renewed emphasis on providing hands-on, skills-based learning in "the latest automated word processing applications" (Merola). I've frequently found myself on the pointy end of such arguments, in virulent disagreements over whether I should be teaching basic rhetorical, usability, and visual design techniques or if I should be concentrating on teaching students application-specific skills in programs such as FrameMaker® 4.0 or Doc2Help®. I even see *typing speed* listed as a job qualification in want ads for technical writers. These things, as you might expect, trouble me greatly.

Focusing primarily on teaching skills places technical communication in a relatively powerless position: technical trainers rather than educators. Responding to the demands of industry, almost by definition, disempowers technical communicators, relegating them to secondary roles in education, industry, and larger social spheres of importance (see laments in Kreppel 603; Zimmerman and Muraski; Jones; Steve and Bigelow). A number of theorists have suggested the need to move beyond our current, limited status by methods such as integrating technical writing earlier into the design process (Doheny-Farina; Conklin; Horton) or by broadening our goals beyond simple skills (Selber; Southard and Reaves). These calls are useful but they do not go far enough. Although there are obvious (and financial) benefits to describing education in terms of what employees will need to do, there are also values—extremely important values—in taking a broader view, and talking about what technical communication *should be.*

If we truly wish to effect change in our positions, we need to rethink our mission in more fundamental ways than how to make our current practices more efficient. As I argue in the second half of this article, symbolic-analytic work provides a systematic framework for re-understanding the value of technical communication (both current and potential value). This framework is doubly valuable because it can help connect research and practice in useful ways. Prior to exploring this possibility, however, I want to lay out in more detail some of the negative consequences of our current service orientation.

Consequences of the Support Model for Professionals

The support model of technical communication encourages corporations to view technical communication as something to be added on to a primary product. Because the value is located in a discrete, technological product such as a piece of software, support becomes easily devalued, added at the end of the project (with too little time or too few staff members), or perhaps omitted entirely. This explains why technical communicators struggle to make documentation a part of the software development process rather than an afterthought (Horton; Doheny-Farina; P. Sullivan; Weiss, "Usability"). Although current textbooks do a good job of teaching rhetorical analysis, task analysis, information organization, and page layout, they do little to help students or professionals learn how to work on teams writing or revising product specifications or how to design a documentation project around rapidly changing and frequently unstable alpha products.

In addition, the workplace power structures implicated in this model downplay the authority of technical communicators even in areas they are qualified to speak to. In an ethnographic study of the document review process of two writers in an organization, Mary Elizabeth Raven discovered that over fifty percent of the revisions each writer made were, at least in part, to "maintain good interpersonal relations with one or more of the reviewers" (406). For comparison, the next most frequently cited reason for revision was for accuracy, safety, or completeness with a frequency of nineteen and twenty-six percent for each writer (Table 1). Overall,

> [w]riters had little control over reviewers who wanted to include content simply because they thought it should be in the book. These reviewers did not listen to arguments about what was appropriate for the audience of the book and they forced the writers to make certain changes that were not beneficial—and may have even been detrimental—to the audience. (406)

Most writers have struggled with reviewers who misunderstand their responsibilities or work at cross purposes, but the interactions described here are symptomatic of the current problems of technical communication's relation to technological products.

Practicing technical communicators themselves also tend to downplay the complexity of their discipline. In a recent survey of practicing technical communicators (Scanlon and Coon) on the content of a college technical communication course, respondents systematically preferred an emphasis on teaching writing as a static, linear process of mechanical discovery and reporting with emphases on audience analysis, outlining, clarity, and mechanics. In other words, the technical communicators in the study emphasized relatively mechanical writing skills that have been, over the last three decades, systematically revised and augmented by theorists and practitioners in not only composition but also communication, rhetoric, management theory, and nearly every other field that studies and practices situated communication. As illustrated below, work in these broader fields is being taken up by technical communicators in both academia and industry. But without a fundamental rethinking of the relationship between technology and communication, that work will remain marginalized or co-opted by other fields.

As the next section argues, the subordination of technical communication to technological support limits possibilities for not only technical communicators but also users. In a recursive fashion, the absence of discussions about larger, social projects tends to also encourage some users to limit their own thinking and use of technologies to those aspects explicitly allowed and described by technologies and documentation.

Consequences of the Support Model for Users

Ironically, in carefully limiting technical communication to a support role, we may also end in disempowering users, the group that most technical communicators would claim to be helping. Users, in turn, may be disempowered when technical communication prioritizes its supportive role. Thinking of communication as an auxiliary tool ignores the constructive role that users play in the process. In addition, the support model frequently becomes articulated around the technology (and technical systems), with the user subordinated to an external part (Johnson; Johnson-Eilola, "Wild"; D. Sullivan). The common practice of instructing users in functional but not conceptual aspects of technologies, for example, can adversely or even fatally affect users, as James Paradis has argued in his study of documentation written for construction equipment operators. In a more extreme case, Stephen Katz suggests that the rhetorical emphasis on expediency and decontextualization inherent in technical communication allowed Nazi administrators and engineers to sidestep ethical issues involved in the construction of vehicles for transporting prisoners to death camps and mass executions. But even more everyday instances of technical communication such as interface design (Laurel; Selfe and Selfe) and cartography (Barton and Barton; Wood; Soja) contribute in fundamental ways to how a user thinks, communicates, and acts in the world.

Consider a person using a word processor to write a resume in response to a job advertisement. Computer documentation would traditionally treat the problem by analyzing users' experience with the software in question, their educational level, and their job function. A technical communicator would choose whether to design a tutorial, a user guide, a reference guide, or some other genre of documentation, perhaps even a range of these. Although the ordering and depth of discussion would vary for each genre, the technical communicator's work would invariably begin with the program functions: creating a new document; inserting text; changing margins, spacing, and font styles; and previewing and printing a document. Some programs might even automate this process by allowing users to fill in the blanks on a pre-designed resume template.

Here, however, the technical communication usually stalls, failing to consider the broader, social purposes and contexts of the user's work. In this way, the primary task is fragmented and decontextualized so that it can be documented as a set of formal functions. As business writing teachers (and personnel managers) know, the primary task here—creating a resume in order to find employment—is difficult to learn, certainly requiring more than a template for any but the most artificial situations. The complexities of rhetorical purpose, audience analysis, the user's personal and professional qualifications, the resume reader's personal and professional experiences and motivations, the specific line of work being sought, and so on all combine in ways that make writing an effective resume an extremely difficult task to teach or learn. One would expect that documentation about how to write a resume would either attempt to deal with those issues with some complex algorithm (a task not currently computationally feasible) or help users learn how to understand the complexity of those issues so that they could make intelligent, informed decisions about how to use the program. But such an approach would shift the focus of computer use from the computer to the user's communicative situation: the computer would become a secondary component to the process (taking the role that was currently occupied by technical communication). The limiting aspects of the genre of the instructional manual are so strong that it is difficult to envision a manual that successfully de-emphasized technology use and instead focused on broader issues. So the traditional support role for technical communication—in other words, education—participates in (or is the scapegoat for) broader reductions that disempower not only the technical communicator but also the user.

This narrow focus may begin to broaden in contexts where documentation is produced as the primary rather than secondary product, such as in companies that produce third-party manuals. In a detailed discourse analysis of manufacturer-developed and third-party documentation for software (Walters and Beck), researchers found that manuals included with software concentrated on helping users learn specific software functions; successful third-party books on the same products attempted to cover not only local program functions but also broader issues. For a word-processing program, for example, the third-party book included discussions of writing processes and design guidelines, the qualifications and experiences of the writer of the manual, and more detailed examples of contexts in which the software might be used. Writers of the third-party manuals were positioned less as inhouse support for technology use, so could act as teachers rather than technology cheerleaders. In other words, writers were allowed to understand the location of value differently: the user's broader tasks come into focus. Rather than a manual supporting the use of a tool, the manual helps a user create conditions in which he or she undertakes more general forms of work. Technologies are still involved, but they are not the primary focus.

Relocating the Value of Work: From Technical to Communication

If this shift from efficiency and speed to connection and selection has been largely ignored by technical communication, it has been successfully adopted and adapted in numerous other areas, including such diverse occupations as management consulting and literary theory. In particular, two key shifts can aid our work here: the transformation from an industrial economy to an information economy, and the flattening of corporate hierarchies.

Even corporations that one might commonly think of as producing technological products are in many ways now in the business of producing and selling information. The rapid growth of the computer industry, for example, now relies on the demands made by new software releases in order to drive hardware purchases. Twenty years ago, companies such as IBM and Wang provided customers with "big iron" computing systems as their primary product; support systems such as software and technical assistance were considered valuable by customers, but were clearly subordinated to the hard technology. Today, software companies like Microsoft explicitly dictate standards for major sections of the computer hardware industry. Similarly, software companies now exploit lucrative markets by selling streams of information in one form or another; by providing "tiered" support (higher-paying customers gaining faster and more personalized support); by offering software "subscriptions" (scheduled software updates prepaid with a flat, yearly or quarterly fee); and by negotiating site and enterprise licenses for large, corporate customers (who are offered slightly lower per-copy fees essentially in exchange for requiring every user to adopt the same package). In fact, software itself is rarely purchased outright by customers, because "shrink wrap" agreements (small-print contracts on the outside of the sealed envelopes containing program disks) explicitly state that the software companies continue to own the software; the user has merely purchased the right to run the programs on a specific number of machines. In a growing number of cases, software is explicitly purchased on a short-term or per-use basis. This capability is one of the interesting features of programs written in Java and designed to be distributed to users on the fly over the Internet or an intranet, potentially even to diskless computers which cannot even store programs—users pay for and download programs each time they use them. Many companies have shifted portions of their revenue streams to providing information rather than technological products. In addition, some organizations work specifically in information and produce little or no products of the industrial type. High-profile, Web-based companies such as Yahoo, Alta Vista, and eXcite, for example, excel at arranging, condensing, indexing, and reorganizing information according to the needs of different customers. In one way of thinking, these companies are realizing a possibility hinted at by print-bound indices and encyclopedias. In these Web-based ventures, the index moves out from the back of the book, becomes fluid, customized, and of primary rather than secondary value.

At the same time, we find a shift in workplace structures that flattens traditional organizational hierarchies. Companies such as Ford Motor Corporation re-engineer key processes to minimize the amount of times information changes hands (Hammer and Champy 39–44). Such re-engineerings, almost as a rule, insist that hierarchy and departments act as barriers to the efficient flow of information in an organization (50–64). The focus on processes rather than products does not abandon the value of concrete goods—many corporations are still much involved in the production of concrete goods. But in these post-industrial corporations, traditional, industrial economies of scale are no longer seen as adequate and can in fact be damaging when they prevent a company from reacting quickly to changing technologies and markets.

But, as with capital itself, it is no longer so much the physical instantiation of money (coins and bills) as the movement of money (stocks and bonds)—moving from corporation to employee then back into other corporations—that has value: knowledge *about* the movement of capital rather than simply static capital. Peter Drucker identifies the roots of the emphasis on knowledge all the way back to the beginning of the industrial revolution itself, as *technê*—practical knowledge—is transferred from the minds and bodies of craft laborers into what Shoshana Zuboff calls "externalized knowledge": training materials and mechanical assemblages capable of either automating or semi-automating what previously took a skilled laborer. For Drucker, contemporary capitalism (what he terms "post-capitalism") is the era in which knowledge does work (50)—in other words, communication. Reengineering guru Michael Hammer likewise places communication processes at the nexus of contemporary organizations (Hammer and Champy; Hammer and Stanton).

But, while the shift to information economies and flattened organizational structures has received much attention in both popular press and management and labor theory, it has been largely ignored by technical communication practice or theory: technical communication still defines itself as an industrial rather than post-industrial enterprise. The following sections begin to sketch the outlines of a model of technical communication suited to the post-industrial age, under the job description "symbolic-analytic worker."

From Support to Symbolic-Analytic Work

In addition to participating in (if not causing) changes in workplace structures and international economies, information technology provides the backdrop for a new class of service work, one inherently rooted in information space. Symbolic-analytic work, a new classification proposed by U.S. Secretary of Labor Robert B. Reich, involves working within and across information spaces. Such workers are highly skilled in information manipulation and abstraction, critical and much sought-after skills in an age where information overtakes industry in terms of social and economic value. As the analysis below illustrates, many of the key abilities possessed by symbolic-analytic workers are the same skills now possessed, in varying degrees, by technical communicators. However, we will need to redefine our practices and images, both to ourselves and to the public, to make those connections (and their value) clear.

To make the differences in classes of service work apparent, the following sections work through three primary areas of service work analyzed by Reich: Routine Production, In-Person Service, and Symbolic-Analytic Work. Importantly, the current broad definitions of technical communication position the discipline partially in every class described below. This ambiguity, although often a vexing problem when it comes time to write job descriptions or tenure statements, has worked to keep the borders between service classifications open, making the move into symbolic-analytic work feasible in theory and practice, provided we are willing to make that movement.

Routine Production "entail[s] the kinds of repetitive tasks performed by the old foot soldiers of American capitalism in the high-volume enterprise" (Reich 174). These jobs include traditional blue-collar positions and also a number of white-collar jobs—"foremen, line managers, clerical supervisors, section chiefs—involving repetitive checks on subordinates' work and the enforcement of standard operating procedures" (174). These workers are valued for their ability to follow rules, remain loyal to a company, and work accurately and quickly.

Technical communicators fall into routine production in cases where their work becomes defined solely in terms of routine manual writing for large, homogeneous software products (the writers, for example, who must produce the definitions for four hundred technical procedures following a predetermined template, vocabulary, and readability level). As Reich points out, "contrary to prophets of the 'information age' who buoyantly predicted an abundance of high-paying jobs even for people with the most basic of skills, the sobering truth is that may information-processing jobs fit easily into this category" (175).

Job advertisements for technical communicators that list familiarity with specific brands of word-processing and page-layout software but do not discuss more complex skills, for example (and these ads are legion), offer visible reminders of the tendencies toward thinking of technical communication as routine production. There are, of course, elements of such work in the practices of many technical communicators, although this job classification prioritizes (and often restricts activity to) such types of work.

Furthermore, the prevalent tendency for the general public to believe that complex rhetorical tasks such as resume writing or Web page design can be easily automated by templates or software wizards illustrates how routine and repetitious some people consider technical communication to be. Although most technical communicators would argue to the contrary, we have done little to convince the public otherwise. And once public perception brackets technical communication in this manner, technical communicators will have a difficult time arguing that they are capable of more complex and valuable (non-routine) activities.

In-Person Service Workers, like those in routine production, complete routine, repetitive tasks and are usually closely supervised. The primary difference between routine production workers and in-person workers is that in-person service workers deal with people directly. So in addition to the skills of routine production, in-person workers must possess what Reich calls "a pleasant demeanor. They most smile and exude confidence and good cheer, even when they feel morose. They must be courteous and helpful, even to the most obnoxious of patrons. Above all, they must make others feel happy and at ease." (176). In-person service workers have replaced much of the historical emphasis on routine production work. There were more in-person service jobs created during the 1980s than there are total workers in the steel, textile, and automobile job classes *combined* (177).

Technical communicators, especially those working freelance or in large companies, may frequently find themselves doing in-person service work. The common activity of interviewing technological content-area experts to document software or other products sometimes falls under in-person service work, especially in cases where the status differential between technical communicator and resource person are laid bare (Raven). In addition, technical communicators acting as in-person service workers are increasingly located in help desk or help line departments, where they answer questions for users over the phone or on the Internet. As most technical communicators have discovered, many users refuse to read printed or online documentation. Because of the routine nature of the bulk of users' calls to help desks or help lines, operators in many organizations find they can answer most questions with a small set of stock responses (frequently assembled into a database for easy reference by staffers). In essence, these workers read documentation to users unwilling to do so on their own. In some cases, however, help line operators act as symbolic-analytic workers. If the problems are of sufficient complexity or uniqueness to prevent a corporation from easily setting up a "knowledge base" that matches common problems to routine, pre-scripted answers, these operators may begin to work as symbolic analysts.

Symbolic-Analytic Workers possess the abilities to identify, rearrange, circulate, abstract, and broker information. Their principal work materials are information and symbols, their principal products are reports, plans, and proposals. They frequently work online, either communicating with peers (they rarely have direct organizational supervision) or manipulating symbols with the help of various computer resources. Symbolic analysts go by a wide variety of job titles, including investment banker, research scientist, lawyer, management consultant, strategic planner, and architect.

In most ways, symbolic analysts differ from the other job classifications in terms of status, responsibility, geographic mobility, and pay. Unlike routine production workers, they are more able to move from place to place because of their higher disposable incomes and because companies will often pay moving expenses for their services. They can also frequently telecommute, uploading and downloading information over the World Wide Web, Internet, and intranets; faxing reports to clients; and conference calling on the telephone. And unlike in-person service workers (who may communicate with customers via phone, fax, or computer network as well as face to face), symbolic-analytic workers deal with situations not easily addressed by routine solutions.

Although the discipline does not yet stress this point, technical communicators do frequently work as symbolic analysts. The ability to manipulate, abstract, revise, and rearrange information is itself one version of the classic task of the technical communicator: someone who takes pre-existing knowledge about technology and explains it to others. In an industrial economy, such a job description prioritizes the technology (and technologist) and subordinates the technical communication (and communicator). But post-industrial work inverts the relationship between technical product and knowledge product: symbolic analysts make it clear—to themselves, to their employers, to the public—that in an age of ubiquitous technology and information, knowledge attains primary value. Refocusing on communication also authorizes an expansion of technical communication. If technology use is replaced with broader conceptions of work, then users' "tasks" are no longer simply low-level, machine-reliant functions, but contextualized, real-world projects.

Instances of technical communication as symbolic-analytic work provide some leverage points for rethinking our current disciplinary definitions. Consider the general occupation of developing and maintaining sites on the World Wide Web. Although this role is currently filled by workers in diverse areas of expertise—from computer science and technical communication through advertising, graphic design, and individuals working in their spare time—the work (at least when it is done well) is clearly technical communication, much as writing product specifications or feasibility studies is technical communication done by a wide range of professions. Of particular interest in Web design is the focus on communication (rather than technology) as a primary product and process. In a postmodern sense, these communications are sometimes valued for their collection and arrangement of pre-existing information rather than new content creation. In Figure 1, Web site designers at Sun Microsystems offer users connections to other sites on the Web with relevant information, and also broad rather than simply functional advice about designing Web pages. This site acts as an instructional manual for a technology (the computer being used to design and serve Web pages) but focuses on broader issues. "Manuals" such as this (which are increasingly common on the World Wide Web) succeed at making technology subordinate to communication. The typical decontexualized focus of print documentation is replaced by broad-based teaching and learning.

Even though it is certainly possible to translate traditional, decontextualized technical documentation over to the Web, good Web design draws on a wider range of skills and concerns to make it a form of symbolic-analytic work. Unlike industrial models of technical communication (which would prioritize efficient technology use), such forms of Web design blur the boundary between "technology" and "communication" in important ways, without necessarily downplaying the richness of communication contexts. In fact, current forms of Web design provide only a limited view of the ways that technical communicators might reinvent their work. The rapid adoption of communicative links in technologies (from networked computers in home and workplace to cellular telephone links in automobiles, airplanes, and purses) offers the potential to integrate communication into a much broader range of technological contexts. And although most Web sites offer one-way communication (a print distribution model), sites are now beginning to offer better facilities for interpersonal communication, a feature that makes clearer the emphasis on communication over technology. If the printing press engendered a massive increase in the

FIGURE 1 Subsection of Web Style Guide from Sun Microsystems

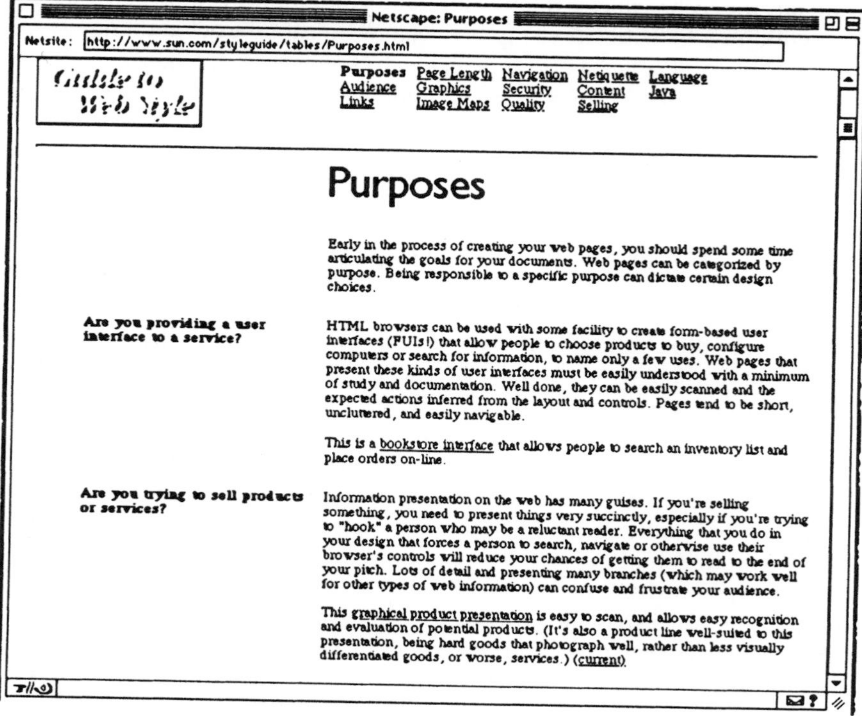

distribution of information, the Web can square that revolution, making literate communication recursive rather than linear.

TACTICS FOR REARTICULATING TECHNICAL COMMUNICATION

Reich outlines four key areas of education for symbolic analysts that we can use to reinvent technical communication education in a post-industrial age: collaboration, experimentation, abstraction, and system thinking. Like the symbolic analysts Reich evaluates, technical communicators need to illustrate both to themselves and to the rest of the world that technology is easy to come by, but understanding and strategic use are both rare and valuable. In each of the areas listed below, I note the ways that the area can be seen to describe existing work in technical communication. By seeing these activities as instances of symbolic-analytic work, we can begin the process of relocating value in a post-industrial age.

Experimentation involves forming and testing hypotheses about information and communication. For symbolic analysts, this experimentation is sometimes formally scientific but also sometimes intuitive. Because of the unique nature of most work done by symbolic analysts, preconceived approaches are, at best, only starting points. If a class of problems becomes so common that it can be answered by reference to a rule book, then the problem moves into the domain of routine production workers. But in order to broaden our work beyond isolated technical functions, we'll also need to expand on our common use of the term "usability." Even though, as with all four of the areas covered here, technical communicators currently do something similar to symbolic-analytic work, traditional notions of instructional documentation tend to orient those skills toward functionalism, decontextualized uses of technology rather than broader, contextualized communication processes.

For technical communicators, usability studies constitute a primary area for experimentation, a place to try out different approaches to problems. Technical communication often limits usability studies to straightforward checks for accuracy and ease of use (P. Sullivan), a fact reflective of the common focus on functionalism over critical interpretation in technical communication (Selber; Blyler). Lee Brasseur, for example, has described the negative effects of default fill patterns in computer programs for drawing graphs and charts. Users took advantage of fill patterns for charts automatically, resisting the possibility of either omitting patterns when they were not necessary or changing patterns used in a chart to avoid similar patterns in adjacent areas. The goals of the program and documentation were defined in terms of basic program functions ("Can the user construct a chart?") rather than more difficult but very important critical perspectives of the user's broader projects ("Is the chart effective?"). In other words, the software was *usable* in an instrumental, technocentric sense: users could successfully construct charts. But at the broader level, the default settings automated the selection of chart fill patterns in ways that actually damaged the overall quality and success of the charts. But this distinction becomes apparent only when users—on their own or with encouragement—learn to step back and think about the broad, contextual purpose of the program rather than the narrow, functional use.

Technical communicators must continue to investigate broader forms of usability studies, such as workplace ethnographies. The growing popularity of such work is a positive sign. In such work, researchers are less concerned with discovering universal, static truths about users than constructing shared accounts of situated understanding and social action (Blyler 340–42) and maps that can help both technical communicators and users negotiate and navigate social realms (Sullivan and Porter). Rather than emphasizing program logic, contextually situated research methods help technical communicators understand and assist users in ways consistent with their existing work and to help them re-invent that work in helpful ways (Beabes and Flanders 411). Contexualized research and practice make it clear that communicators cannot focus simply on applying simple, universal principles to documents but must instead begin a recursive project of expansion and contraction, in which they investigate concrete local contexts and, in doing so, think about the broad projects in which those users are engaged.

Beverly Sauer's study of risk communication in mine construction provides a striking example of the value of such broad, situated inquiry. Comparing commonly used texts on roof control between British and U.S.

mining professions, Sauer notes the ways different rhetorical maneuvers are used in each. In texts for miners in the United States, discussions of roof control methods are presented as a straightforward, relatively uncontested decision in favor of roof bolting due to both economic and technological superiority. The text then deals unproblematically with the proper procedure for installing roof bolts. In British texts, however, the discussion is much more complex, admitting that different methods may be applicable in different situations, attempting to lay out a broader range of situations and possibilities without selecting a single, universal solution. As Sauer notes, one likely reason for the richer (if less easy) approach of the British manual can be traced to political and social concerns of miners who worry about the tradeoffs between cost cutting and safety as well as the U.S. origination of the roof-bolting method. Because of the political, economic, and social aspects of all technologies, technical communication should not limit itself to simple functionalism, but must also include broader and more complicated concerns.

Clearly, the types of experimentation afforded by narrow versions of usability studies—accuracy, speed of use, and so on—are only a limited (and perhaps limiting) version of what Reich suggests as a core skill for symbolic analysts. Insisting on broader forms of usability serves a double purpose for technical communicators: it helps us produce documentation and assistance more attuned to a user's broader needs, and it also shifts the focus of value away from a discrete technology and toward communication and learning.

Collaboration helps symbolic analysts work together to solve problems while crossing complex disciplinary domains. Software projects, for example, typically require not only programmers but user interface designers, marketing experts, usability testers, technical communicators, and graphic artists. Team members brainstorm ideas and solutions, critique each other's work, and provide support and feedback to the teammates. Collaboration marks one area that technical communication has entered into relatively quickly, both responding to and critiquing workplace processes and structures for writing (see e.g., Paradis, Dobrin, and Miller; Burnett; Thralls and Blyler; Doheny-Farina). By attempting to both learn from and change existing collaborative practices, we position ourselves and our students as socially responsible experts—in other words, we help students learn to be both effective participants and responsible community members (Rymer). Such skills are valuable not only within the confines of the classroom and workplace but in re-envisioning users as fuller participants in communication processes.

In terms of rearticulating technical communication as symbolic-analytic work, it is crucial that we increase our research and teaching into issues of power in group dynamics. As numerous accounts have illustrated, technical communicators are frequently in positions of low power in workplace teams (see, among others discussed above, Raven; Doheny-Farina). With better understandings of these situations, students can learn to negotiate these difficult situations and develop tactics for avoiding the nearly automatic subordination of communication to technological values. Continuing the emphasis on collaborative work—and strengthening current approaches and emphases—is important in the quest to rearticulate technical communication as symbolic-analytic work. Furthermore, we must strengthen our current work in computer-supported collaboration such as e-mail, synchronous and asynchronous conferencing, and World Wide Web development.

Abstraction requires students not merely to memorize information but also to learn to discern patterns, relationships, and hierarchies in large masses of information. A paradigmatic example of this skill can be found in one of the most common tasks in software documentation: rethinking a series of system commands so that it coincides with a user's task representation and context. Current approaches to this activity, however, tend to oversimplify the task to one of straightforward audience analysis. Textbooks such as Woolever and Loeb's *Writing for the Computer Industry* provide chapters on defining audiences and objectives, on getting information, and on organizing information—each crucial aspects of writing software documentation—but do not explicitly attempt to bridge the gap between *getting* information about either program or users and *structuring* that information in ways appropriate for specific types of users in certain contexts. In practice, most technical communicators develop skills in abstraction based on modeling existing documentation, frequently under the guidance of more experienced technical communicators (who themselves probably learned abstraction through similar methods).

As with other aspects of symbolic-analytic work, the low profile of abstraction relates partially to notions of authorship that prioritize the creation of "original" content and subordinate work that seems derivative and functional (Foucault). As cultural theorist Jean-François Lyotard among others has argued, originality in a postmodern era is of declining value. Technical communication theorists have recently begun applying this worldview to technical communication theory and practice (Porter; Freed). In order to validate our work as symbolic-analytic work, we can make such concerns and approaches commonplace in our teaching and research.

System thinking works at a level above abstraction, requiring symbolic analysts to recognize and construct relationships and connections in extremely broad, often apparently unrelated domains. System thinking works *beyond* problem-solving approaches in order to understand (and remake) systemic conditions. In other words, where traditional approaches to technical communication rely heavily on breaking a problem into small, manageable parts to be solved by short, simple help texts, a symbolic analyst would step back to took at larger issues in the system to determine how the problem develops and in what contexts it is considered a problem.

Such work is rare in technical communication because we systematically define our work in limited ways. (Contributing in fundamental ways to this absence is the narrow conception of usability discussed above.) Although many aspects of our work do involve high-level system thinking, they are not addressed formally in our education or research; in many cases, these difficult activities occur unseen and unvalued. As long as technical communication is defined in decontextualized, functional ways, thinking in terms of broad systems is virtually prohibited. In the academic world, however, researchers and theorists possess the freedom (some would say the ivory tower atmosphere) to attempt thinking at the system level. Recent work in issues of gender and technology (see e.g., LaDuc and Goldrick-Jones; Lay) offers one useful starting point. Researchers have begun to question masculinist assumptions not merely in technical communication but in technological development itself. As Laura Gurak and Nancy Bayer's survey of feminist technology critique argues, the high percentage of women working as technical communicators constitutes both a problem and an opportunity: a problem for women working to overcome masculinist assumptions and processes; an opportunity for women, as technical communicators, now increasingly involved in the design process for technologies, a position in which they can contribute in positive ways to developing technologies accessible to women. This critical insight relies on the ability of technical communicators not only to construct abstract representations of complex data sets (the overwhelmingly limiting technological contexts in which many women work) but also to bring together abstractions and key concepts across other areas (technological development, changing roles for technical communicators, social perceptions of gender roles in general, the statistical makeup of engineering teams, etc.).

Because of the complexity and broad reach of system thinking, this skill has proven extremely difficult to carry over into technical communication practice—such concerns are external to models that prioritize technology over communication and learning. In fact, advocates of minimalist documentation argue that computer documentation should abandon the attempt to provide broad, conceptual materials for users (Carroll; Weiss, "Retreat"). But such a position, while it may certainly increase accuracy and speed in the short-term, disempowers users by assuming as a rule that they already know how to complete their general tasks (writing a memo, composing a presentation, etc.) (Brasseur; Redish; Johnson-Eilola, "Wild"). Furthermore, the decontexualized, functionalist position prevents consideration of sociopolitical terms. A model of communication that presents technology as neutral and discrete makes invisible the social reproduction of gender bias inherent in technological development and use. As we shift the value of technical communication away from discrete technological products and toward contextualized communication, the social aspects of technological use are more amenable to critique and change.

The shift into symbolic-analytic work will not be an automatic one; it will probably be extremely difficult to make given the cultural and economic capital involved. But without a concerted effort on the part of our field, our positions will certainly be entrenched in routine production or in-person service. Despite frequent and loud announcements by futurists of the coming leisure age and by management theorists about empowering workers to take responsibility, the workplace continues to increase the distance between upper-level and lower-level workers. As Reich notes, in-person service work has increased at an astounding rate over the last decade. The largest employer in the United States today is Manpower, which specializes in providing companies with temporary employees, primarily in the clerical classes. If technical communicators do not take action to change their current situation, they will find their work increasingly contingent, devalued, outsourced, and automated. It is not impossible for technical communicators to do well in contract and freelance situations; in fact, symbolic-analytic workers are frequently in such positions. But a major distinction between symbolic-analytic work and other service work lies in the location of value.

Recent initiatives in organizations like the Society for Technical Communication to standardize technical communication by providing certification procedures as well as academic program guidelines will probably do little to change our status—they may in fact entrench the discipline in the support model. The reason is simple but forceful: because these studies are often based on surveys of existing technical communication practice, they are primarily descriptive, defining the status of a job classification that currently places itself in increasingly devalued service areas. And such studies quickly become prescriptive, because they provide a highly visible record of what a technical communicator does. If the discipline wants to enact broad changes in the discipline, improving the status and the areas of work open to technical communicators, it must take a critical stance and use gathered data to illustrate the problems and limitations of current definitions and practices.

Technical Communication Education: Five Key Projects

Technical communication must begin by making it clear that its work is not secondary to the product, but sometimes primary. Studies of the value added by technical communicators such as those described in Redish and Ramey provide a useful beginning to this rearticulation. But such studies, although important, fail to rethink the project in the fundamental ways necessary to shift technical communication into the realm of symbolic-analytic work. The position of "value added" necessarily posits an original object that the technical communication somehow relates to—it is this original object that holds primary value. At best, in such situations, technical communication can show that it enhances value or provides a return on investment. At worst, the "support" position limits the potential value of technical communication by encouraging both customers and managers to focus on the technology rather than the transformative knowledge potentially contained in the communication.

If we truly wish to effect change in our positions, we need to rethink our mission in more fundamental ways than how to make our current practices more efficient. As a method for strengthening the symbolic-analytic skills discussed in the previous section, educators can address five key projects that might help our students become better educated for their new roles:

1. Connect education to work
2. Question educational goals
3. Question educational processes and infrastructures
4. Build metaknowledge, network knowledge, and self-reflective practices
5. Rethink interdisciplinarity

1. Connect Education to Work

I mean connect education to work in a critical rather than accommodating way. Not only do we need to investigate how to fulfill the traditional roles of technical communicators, but we also need to look to the types of research going on in management theory, information management, interface design, and labor theory. Some of the most advanced and powerful work in such areas is actually technical communication: Hammer and Champy's "re-engineering," one of the latest fads in the corporate world, is at its lowest level a critical focus on the processes of communication within corporations. We need to investigate such movements and participate in them rather than be acted on by them. Hammer and Champy's work is groundbreaking precisely because most companies do not understand communication, information, and knowledge. Technical communicators do.

2. Question Educational Goals

Similarly, we need to take on the difficult task of questioning educational goals at a variety of levels. These are questions many technical communication educators have already begun asking: Should we be filling job and skill slots determined by industry? For that matter, are more corporate-oriented organizations such as the Society for Technical Communication shaping roles for technical communicators, or are they themselves filling slots dictated by industry? A more productive position (but a more difficult one) would be to take the tack described in the first project and apply it to education. Educating students as symbolic-analytic workers is an important step in this direction.

3. Question Educational Processes and Infrastructures

This is one project that many of us are already beginning to undertake, albeit in a sometimes haphazard way. Computer networks provide the opportunity for nonstandard teaching, learning, and working situations. Such situations provide students, teachers, and professionals with the opportunity to work together despite geographical and temporal differences. At the same time, this is one area in which we must exercise the most care: in the long run, some forms of distance learning may tend to isolate learners by physically separating them from their peers and mentor. Paying for college is always a burden; given the opportunity, many families faced with the choice between sending their offspring 500 miles away and having them stay at home may choose the distance education route. We need to make it clear what the benefits are of residence learning; we need to insist on defining education in broad terms that must include more than just seat time and test scores. At the same time, we need to understand ways that networked communication can positively affect education and work and to create additional positive environments.

4. Build Metaknowledge, Network Knowledge, and Self-Reflective Practices

Perhaps more importantly, we must move beyond the idea that the network is a medium for transmitting knowledge. A more radical notion is that the network is also an environment for learning, working, and living. Put in a different way, we need to think about new formations for knowledge that rely on network organization, metaknowledge and metawork that act at a level above current knowledge structures. This is another way of saying we need to redefine technical communication in broader terms than functional skills: we should be *teaching* rather than *training*. We have already begun to research the dynamics of learning and working as a way of improving those activities in areas such as critical literacies (Selber), usability (P. Sullivan), and economics (Johnson-Eilola, "Accumulation"). Now we can take the next step: collapsing distinctions between teacher/student/user in an attempt to help all of us understand the potential richness of crossing over those functional roles in broad communication contexts.

5. Rethink Interdisciplinarity

Finally, we must struggle to overcome disciplinary boundaries. Many of the things I've suggested here are drawn from other fields, work I've discovered by backtracking threads from popular accounts back to professional journals and publications. Too frequently, we merely take what we're given. The task of software documentation, for example, typically starts with the end product, a piece of late-beta or even golden master software. We build our documentation on what we're given. We are blocked out of the formative stages—where we might make productive changes in the dynamics and the form of software in order to increase usability and efficiency—because we are not able to speak the discourse of software development. It is crucial that we encourage, even require, our students to gain the fundamentals of their respective specialty fields, perhaps multiple fields. Furthermore, we may wish to require classes in rapid field learning that help students develop strategies and tactics for picking up the basics of new fields quickly so that they can enter into the formative stages of those conversations.

Conclusions

Technical communication has long suffered from an accepted emphasis on the "technical" portion of the disciplinary title. As we enter the information age, we face the possibility of rearticulating the value of what we do to emphasize the "communication" half of our work.

Technical communication can begin transforming the location of value by rethinking what it means to teach, to practice, and to research technical communication. Symbolic-analytic work offers a potential common ground between the broad, conceptual and social issues frequently espoused by academics and the pragmatic, functional concerns of practitioners. As I argued earlier, the industrial model of technical communication is outmoded in terms of value, but it continues to work as long as technologies and techocentric corporations are allowed to redefine users' tasks. If "good writing" is cast as template filling, for example, then automation is a viable solution. Technical communicators will find their work increasingly devalued as industrial labor, even as other disciplines learn to take on the roles of communicators in the post-industrial workplace.

If we wish to shift that value to the post-industrial emphasis on communication, we'll need to make it clearer why this model must be rejected even though it works. In effect, we can argue that the symbolic-analytic or post-industrial model subsumes the functional or industrial model: the technology does not disappear but is now organized under broader, more valuable concerns.

Technical communication education has traditionally centered on teaching practical, immediately useful skills at the expense of broader forms of learning (Selber). While certainly such skills assist technical communicators in gaining ready employment, this limited focus traps the discipline in the very support positions critiqued above: useful but only infrequently valued. Reich's descriptions or symbolic-analytic work offer one strategy that technical communicators and educators might adopt in rearticulating our shared (and publicized) visions of what technical communicators do.

By rearticulating technical communication as symbolic-analytic work, we might use our professional diversity and flexibility to empower ourselves and technology users. The examples provided here are admittedly sketchy, at best. But the general model provided should suggest numerous points for rethinking technical communication in fundamental ways: shifting the focus on communication beyond the technology and toward social contexts and processes, coupled with an emphasis on considering technical communication as one form of symbolic-analytic work, provide a general strategy for not merely critiquing current practices but also for changing them. This disciplinary movement will not be an easy one, given our diversity and size. But failure to attempt this rearticulation will likely move technical communication into the realm of two, less attractive types of service work—routine production and in-person (areas we have already begun to occupy, if somewhat unwillingly). By centering our teaching and research on primary skills for symbolic analysis—collaboration, experimentation, abstraction, and system thinking—we can make it clear to ourselves, to our students, and to the world at large the true value of technical communication in the twenty-first century.

WORKS CITED

Barton, Ben F., and Marthalee Barton. "Ideology and the Map: Toward a Postmodern Visual Design Practice." *Professional Communication: The Social Perspective.* Ed. Nancy Roundy Blyler and Charlotte Thralls. Newbury Park, CA: Sage, 1993. 49–78.

Beabes, Minette A., and Alicia Flanders. "Experiences with Using Contextual Inquiry to Design Information." *Technical Communication* 42 (1995): 409–20.

Blyler, Nancy Roundy. "Narrative and Research in Professional Communication." *Journal of Business and Technical Communication* 10 (1996): 330–51.

Bowie, John S. "Information Engineering: Using Information to Drive Design." *Intercom* May 1996: 6–9, 43.

Brasseur, Lee E. "How Computer Graphing Programs Change the Graph Design Process: Results of Research on the Fill Pattern Feature." *Journal of Computer Documentation* 18.4 (1994): 4–20.

Burnett, Rebecca E. "Conflict in Collaborative Decision Making." *Professional Communication: The Social Perspective*. Ed. Nancy Roundy Blyler and Charlotte Thralls. Newbury Park, CA: Sage, 1993. 144–62.

Carliner, Saul. "Finding a Common Ground: What STC Is, and Should Be, Doing to Advance Education in Information Design and Development." *Technical Communication* 42.4 (1995): 546–54.

Carroll, John. *The Nurnberg Funnel*. Cambridge, MA: MIT P, 1990.

Conklin, James. "The Next Step: An Integrated Approach to Computer Documentation." *Technical Communication* 40.1 (1993): 89–96.

Doheny-Farina, Stephen. *Rhetoric, Innovation, Technology: Case Studies of Technical Communication in Technology Transfers*. Cambridge, MA: MIT P, 1992.

Drucker, Peter F. *Post-Capitalist Society*. New York: HarperBusiness, 1993.

Foucault, Michel. "What Is an Author?" *Language, Counter-Memory, Practice: Selected Essays and Interviews*. Ed. Donald F. Bouchard. Trans. Donald F. Bouchard and Sherry Simon. Ithaca, NY: Cornell UP, 1977. 113–38.

Freed, Richard C. "Postmodern Practice: Perspectives and Prospects." *Professional Communication: The Social Perspective*. Ed. Nancy Roundy Blyler and Charlotte Thralls. Newbury Park, CA: Sage, 1993. 196–214.

Gurak, Laura J., and Nancy L. Bayer. "Making Gender Visible: Extending Feminist Critiques of Technology to Technical Communication." *Technical Communication Quarterly* 3 (1994): 257–70.

Hammer, Michael, and James Champy. *Reengineering the Corporation: A Manifesto for Business Revolution*. New York: HarperBusiness, 1993.

Hammer, Michael, and Steven A. Stanton. *The Reengineering Revolution*. New York: HarperBusiness, 1995.

Horton, William. "Let's Do Away with Manuals . . . Before They Do Away with Us." *Technical Communication* 40.1 (1993): 26–34.

Johnson, Robert R. "The Unfortunate Human Factor: A Selective History of Human Factors for Technical Communicators." *Technical Communication Quarterly* 3.2 (1994): 195–212.

Johnson-Eilola, Johndan. "Accumulation, Circulation, and Association: Economies of Text in Online Research Spaces." *IEEE Transactions on Professional Communication* 38.4 (1995): 228–38.

———. "Wild Technologies: Computer Use and Social Possibilities." *Computers and Technical Communication: Pedagogical and Programmatic Perspectives*. Ed. Stuart A. Selber. Norwood, NJ: Ablex, 1997. 97–128.

Jones, Dan. "A Question of Identity." *Technical Communication* 42.4 (1995): 567–69.

Katz, Stephen B. "The Ethic of Expediency: Classical Rhetoric, Technology, and the Holocaust." *College English* 54 (1992): 255–75.

Kreppel, Maria Curro. "Wanted: Tenure and Promotion for Technical Communication Faculty." *Technical Communication* 42.4 (1995): 603–06.

Krestas, Shirley A., Lori H. Fisher, and JoAnn T. Hackos. "Future Directions for Continuing Education in Technical Communication." *Technical Communication* 42.4 (1995): 642–45.

LaDuc, Linda, and Amanda Goldrick-Jones, eds. *Technical Communication Quarterly* 3.3 (1994). Special issue on gender and technical communication.

Laurel, Brenda. *Computers as Theatre*. Reading, MA: Addison-Wesley, 1993.

Lay, Mary M. "Gender Studies: Implications for the Professional Communication Classroom." *Professional Communication: The Social Perspective*. Ed. Nancy Roundy Blyler and Charlotte Thralls. Newbury Park: Sage, 1993. 215–29.

Lyotard, Jean-François. *The Postmodern Condition: A Report on Knowledge*. Trans. Geoff Bennington and Brian Massumi. Minneapolis: U of Minnesota P, 1984.

Merola, Paul. "Putting the Technical in Technical Communication." *Technical Communication* 42.4: (1995): 585–86.

Paradis, James. "Text and Action: The Operator's Manual in Context and in Court." *Textual Dynamics of the Professions: Historical and Contemporary Studies of Writing in Professional Communities*. Ed. Charles Bazerman and James Paradis. Madison: U of Wisconsin P, 1991. 266–78.

Paradis, James, David Dobrin, and Richard Miller. "Writing at Exxon ITD." *Writing in Nonacademic Settings*. Ed. Lee Odell and Dixie Goswami. New York: Guilford, 1985. 281–307.

Porter, James E. "Professional Writing as Postmodern Work: Toward a Postmodern/Critical Rhetoric." 1996 Business and Technical Writing Lecture. Department of English, University of Wisconsin-Milwaukee. Milwaukee, WI. 24 February 1996.

Raven, Mary Elizabeth. "What Kind of Quality Are We Ensuring with Document Draft Reviews?" *Technical Communication* 42.3 (1995): 399–408.

Redish, Janice. "Are We Entering a Post-Usability Era?" *Journal of Computer Documentation* 19.1 (1995): 18–23.

Redish, Janice, and Judith A. Ramey, eds. "Special Section: Measuring the Value Added by Professional Technical Communicators." *Technical Communication* 42.1 (1995): 23–83.

Reich, Robert B. *The Work of Nations: Preparing Ourselves for 21st-Century Capitalism*. New York: Alfred A. Knopf, 1991.

Rymer, Jone. "Collaboration and Conversation in Learning Communities: The Discipline and the Classroom." *Professional Communication: The Social Perspective*, Ed. Nancy Roundy Blyler and Charlotte Thralls. Newbury Park: Sage, 1993. 179–95.

Sauer, Beverly A. "Communicating Risk in a Cross-Cultural Context: A Cross-Cultural Comparison of Rhetorical and Social Understandings in U.S. and British Mine Safety Training Programs." *Journal of Business and Technical Communication* 10.3 (1996): 306–29.

Scanlon, Patrick M., and Anne C. Coon. "Attitudes of Professional Technical Communicators Regarding the Content of an Undergraduate Course in Technical Communication: A Survey." *Technical Communication* 41.3 (1994): 439–46.

Selber, Stuart A. "Beyond Skill Building: Challenges Facing Technical Communication Teachers in the Computer Age." *Technical Communication Quarterly* 3 (1995): 365–90.

Selfe, Cynthia L., and Richard J. Selfe. "The Politics of the Interface: Power and Its Exercise in Electronic Contact Zones." *College Composition and Communication* 45 (1994): 480–504.

Soja, Edward. *Postmodern Geographies: The Reassertion of Space in Critical Social Theory*. London: Verso, 1989.

Southard, Sherry G., and Rita Reaves. "Tough Questions and Straight Answers: Educating Technical Communicators in the Next Decade." *Technical Communication* 42 (1995): 555–65.

Steve, Mike, and Tom Bigelow. "Coping with Downsizing as a Writing and Editing Group." *Technical Communication* 40.1 (1993): 20–25.

Sullivan, Dale. "Political-Ethical Implications of Defining Technical Communication as a Practice." *Journal of Advanced Composition* 10 (1990): 375–86.

Sullivan, Patricia A. "Beyond a Narrow Conception of Usability Testing." *IEEE Transactions on Professional Communication* 32.4 (1989): 256–64.

Sullivan, Patricia A., and James E. Porter. *Writing Technologies and Critical Research Practices*. Norwood, NJ: Ablex, 1997.

Thralls, Charlotte, and Nancy Roundy Blyler. "The Social Perspective and Pedagogy in Technical Communication." *Technical Communication Quarterly* 2.3 (1993): 249–70.

Walters, Nancy James, and Charles E. Beck. "A Discourse Analysis of Software Documentation: Implications for the Profession." *IEEE Transactions on Professional Communication* 35.3 (1992): 156–67.

Weiss, Edmond H. "Usability: Stereotypes and Traps." *Text, Context, and Hypertext: Writing with and for the Computer*. Ed. Edward Barrett. Cambridge, MA: MIT P, 1988. 175–85.

———. "The Retreat from Usability: User Documentation in the Post-Usability Era." *Journal of Computer Documentation* 19.1 (1995): 3–17.

Wood, Denis. *The Power of Maps*. New York: Guilford, 1992.

Woolever, Kristin R., and Helen M. Loeb. *Writing for the Computer Industry*. Englewood Cliffs: Prentice Hall, 1994.

Zimmerman, Donald E., and Michel Muraski. "Reflecting on the Technical Communicator's Image." *Technical Communication* 42.4 (1995): 621–23.

Zuboff, Shoshana. *In the Age of the Smart Machine: The Future of Work and Power*. New York: Basic Books, 1988.

33 *Educating Technical Communicators to Make Better Decisions*

CEZAR M. ORNATOWSKI

In this essay, Ornatowski, drawing on his work as both consultant and educator, argues that technical communicators are decision makers who have expertise in areas far beyond the scope of writing or computer skills. With knowledge and experience in such areas as team work and project management (p. 596 in this volume), technical communicators play a central role in shaping perceptions, "'diffusing conflict, and socializing readers into the knowledge and values' of a new technology or system" (Mirel, qtd. on p. 597). As teachers, if we accept his argument, we have to consider the impact on our pedagogy. We cannot simply train; we have to educate, and those we educate will possess more than skills; they will have the knowledge and qualifications to enter a profession, with the attendant responsibilities to society.

Several years ago, I found myself in the dual role of researcher and communication consultant at a large aerospace company in southern California. As a researcher, I was examining the generation and circulation of technical information in the company: who communicates what to whom, how, why, and with what results (Ornatowski 1991). As a consultant, I was asked to note major communication problems and advise management how to solve them. Somewhere in the middle of my almost two-year stint with the company, I experienced a kind of epiphany when one of the engineering managers concluded a team discussion of what constitutes good engineering reports with an insight: good communication means making better decisions.

In what follows, I want to argue that looking at technical communication in terms of making decisions, that is, looking at what decisions technical communicators make, what the scope is of those decisions, and what their implications are, provides a new and critical dimension to technical communication education.

From *Technical Communication* 42 (1995): 576–80.

Technical Communicators as Decision Makers

Technical communicators function in many decision-making capacities, some more and some less directly related to their responsibilities as communicators. As Deborah Bosley (1992) notes, technical communicators do many things in addition to writing: they function in interpersonal and intrapersonal contexts; negotiate workplace politics; collaborate with technicians, programmers, and engineers; achieve competence on a variety of computer systems; and manage team projects (Bosley 1992, p. 43). Green and Nolan (1984) report that technical communication positions above the entry level often involve communicators in project management and other management-level decision making. In all these capacities, technical communicators must make decisions that call for expertise and savvy in interpersonal relations, organizational politics, oral communication, teamwork, and project management.

In this discussion, however, I want to focus on the potential scope and significance of decisions technical communicators make *as communicators*. These decisions, I would argue, are no less—and perhaps even are more—complex than the ones made in nonwriting capacities but are less apparent and, therefore, often made unconsciously or by default—and thus, not really made at all. Yet, it is the capacity of technical communicators to make these sorts of decisions that constitutes the specificity of their professionalism. These decisions go beyond the "technical" aspects of preparing rhetorically successful documents (although they are implicit in the latter) and have technological, cultural, and political implications. In what follows, I will discuss these decisions briefly, assigning them to three categories.

Decisions Related to Technology

Technologies are not only products of esoteric, specialized "technical" knowledge. As research in the sociology of technology has begun to show, technologies are shaped by people working within social collectives and influenced by a multitude of cultural, political, and ideological factors (Bijker, Hughes, and Pinch 1987; MacKenzie and Wajcman 1985; Pinch and Bijker 1987). Technologies are shaped through the process of technology development. This process begins with front-end marketing and continues through product design and manufacturing to installation, training, and after-sale service. The process involves diverse groups and interests, often having different needs and objectives, such as different groups within the company (marketing, design engineering, manufacturing, and project management) and different stakeholders in the emerging technology (the producer, the government, regulatory agencies, contractors, and the customer). The factors that influence technology development include political and physical exigencies, market needs and conditions, institutional dynamics, established procedures and conventions, industry practices, and cultural beliefs and values.

The process of technology development is largely a process of negotiation and adjustment. As Stephen Doheny-Farina (1992) has recently argued, the entire range of activities involved in developing new technologies and their applications for the marketplace *"at their core . . .* involve individuals and groups *negotiating* their visions of technologies and applications, markets and users in what they all hope is a common enterprise" (p. 4). This enterprise is largely document and communication driven. Communication of information through different documents helps to create different representations of the emerging technology and to adjudicate between the different, often competing, interests and needs. Through this "interpretation, negotiation, and adjustment" (Doheny-Farina 1992, p. 6), both the emerging technology and its potential users are changed and adapted. In this process, technical communicators play a central role.

Of course, it may be argued that technical communicators do not really make any decisions in this process; they just do what they are told. I think, however, that it is the condition of their professionalism that they should know what they do. I will argue that point at more length at the end of this discussion.

Decisions Related to Culture

As sociologists of technology have demonstrated, technologies are also society shaping, that is, they influence, sometimes profoundly, the societies into which they are inserted (Winner 1980; Pacey 1983; Bijker, Hughes, and Pinch 1987). Think how our lives and our world have been changed by such technologies as the telephone, electric light, the automobile, and the computer.

A critical moment in this process of change is technology insertion: the adaptation of technology to perceived social needs as well as the adaptation of potential users to technology (Dobrin 1989). The critical moment in technology insertion is shaping the perceptions of potential users, as well as mutual adaptation of the technology, the needs and capabilities of the users, and the surrounding culture. In this shaping, technical communicators again play a central role. Barbara Mirel (1988) has shown, for example, how even a relatively "local" document, such as an office computer manual, may fulfill, in addition to its ostensible training function, "more subtle communication purposes of reducing uncertainty, diffusing conflict, and socializing readers into the knowledge and values" of a new technology or system (p. 287).

In addition, in a society increasingly driven by technology, the technical communicator is becoming an important voice in determining how the issues involving technology, as well as particular technologies, are framed and approached. In our culture, technical expertise and technical information constitute, along with science, primary discourses of authority on many matters. This authority is invoked to buttress claims and to support agendas, many of them not necessarily in and of themselves "technical." As Dorothy Nelkin (1992) notes, controversies over technologies often also reflect other issues and broader tensions in society: disagreements over the appropriate role of government in public life, the use of resources, and the impact of technology and technical expertise on the democratic process; struggles between different visions of technology and its role in society; and disagreements over the shape of society itself. Therefore, technical documents often become statements in wider debates and arenas.

Decisions Related to Public Policy

Finally, technology is not individual pieces of equipment, just as a company is not an isolated enterprise, separate from its customers, contractors, investors, and the market. Technology comprises interlocking systems made up of hardware, software, institutions, and constituencies (Hughes 1987). These systems may be local (encompassing an office or a single community), regional, national, or even international in scope. Consider, for instance, the light bulb. The light bulb implies a larger technological system of power generation and transmission. This system, in turn, implies issues associated with the development and management of such large systems (i.e., issues of control, centralization vs. decentralization, and development policy). In addition, there are social and political issues related to the process of electrification and to choice of desirable power (i.e., coal, solar, or nuclear and issues of energy policy, public safety, and others) (Hughes 1983). Technological systems include both physical artifacts (for example, computers, coaxial cables, and data storage devices) and organizations (hardware and software manufacturers, data managers, financial institutions, and investors), networks, users, scientific and research components (R&D programs, universities, and professional associations and publications), and legislative artifacts (regulatory and proprietary laws, data protection laws, and rules and protocols for communication and data transmittal) (MacKenzie and Wajcman 1985; Pinch and Bijker 1987).

Viewed from the perspective of the technological system, the roles of technical communicators transcend mere transmission of information, just as the decisions they make go far beyond the "technical" in their scope and potential consequences. Technical communicators work at the intersection of the various components and impacts of the system: the technology; the organizations involved in its implementation and management; the various interests vested in the system or arrayed against it; and the various publics which the system impacts (Killingsworth and Steffens 1989; Bryan 1992; Nelkin 1992). It is from their position at this intersection that both the complexity of the technical communicators' task and the burden of their professional responsibility arise.

Communication of technical information helps to harmonize the various factors that make up the system into a working whole. In the course of this harmonization, technical communicators not only adjudicate conflicting interests and goals, create representations of emerging technologies, and shape the perception and reception of technologies, they also make judgments of value and decisions that involve uncertainty and risk. Although not all their daily decisions have the magnitude of the Challenger, the Three Mile Island, or the Exxon Valdez cases (Farrell and Goodnight 1981; Winsor 1988,

1990; Dombrowski 1991; Herndl, Fennell, and Miller 1991), most form links in a chain of relationships and consequences that reach far beyond the communicator's office door. As James Paradis (1991) has shown even a user manual for a power tool may have consequences unforeseen by its creator.

Conclusion

As Charles Bazerman (1988) notes, texts are meaningful only in context; it is difficult to understand what any text means without understanding the context within which the text serves as a significant activity. The contexts in which texts created by technical communicators serve as significant activities extend beyond the immediate circumstances of their writing. More important, the communicative decisions made by technical communicators have implications that go far beyond the physical considerations of document design, wording, or presentation. Not that these considerations are not critical; they are. However, they are critical precisely *because* their implications are so extensive and important. After all, that is precisely what technical communication as an organized profession has been trying to convince potential employers of for years.

The technical communicator, as I have argued, stands at the intersection of technology and its various producers, users, and publics. The communicator's decisions, just as the documents the communicator designs, are shaped by, and, in turn, shape, diverse needs and interests and have implications in the realms of technology, culture, and public policy. By virtue of their positions, the technical communicators have tremendous power in a technological society. To understand and use that power, communicators must be aware of the diversity of interests and stakes involved, of the purpose of the communication in regard to those interests, and of the implications of different communicative choices. As Carolyn Miller (1979) puts it, "to write well is to understand the conditions of one's own participation" in the social context in which one acts (p. 617). If technical communicators are not aware of these "conditions of their participation," they may unwittingly adopt what Steven Katz (1992) has called the "ethics of expediency," in which technical and instrumental imperatives override the human and social implications of decisions, and their communicative expertise may become, as Nelkin warns, merely "reduced to a weapon in the political arsenal of competing groups" (p. xix).

Thinking of technical communication in terms of "making better decisions" (however one may want to interpret this phrase in any concrete instance) complements and extends the usual way of approaching the subject of technical communication education. Typically, discussions of technical communication education take as their point of departure the tasks technical communicators perform and the skills they need to perform these tasks. From these, educators deduce the appropriate curriculum (for a review of various surveys of what technical communicators do and their implications for technical communication education, see Zimmerman and Long 1993). I call this way of thinking about education "intensive," because it focuses on elaborating the number and specificity of areas of concrete "technical" expertise.

However, educators need to consider both what technical communicators *do* and the *meaning* of what they do. To get at this meaning, educators should consider the scope, effects, and implications of the decisions technical communicators are called on to make. Such a perspective involves discussions of technical communication education with issues of responsibility and ethics. That involvement, I would argue, marks the difference between education and training, just as it defines the distinction between being a professional and simply having a set of skills. I would call such an approach to education "extensive," because it engages judgments of value and quality. A more extensive education in this sense does not come merely from taking more courses; neither does it amount to simply another call for more liberal education. Rather, it is a matter of designing a curriculum that is extended along the lines outlined in this discussion and that deals with the full dimensions of what technical communicators do and the implications of what they do. It is, put simply, a curriculum that helps technical communicators make better decisions.

REFERENCES

Bazerman, Charles. 1988. *Shaping written knowledge: The genre and activity of the experimental article in science*. Madison, WI: The University of Wisconsin Press.

Bazerman, Charles, and James Paradis, eds. 1991. *Textual dynamics of the professions: Historical and contemporary studies of writing in professional communities*. Madison, WI: The University of Wisconsin Press.

Bijker, Wiebe E., Thomas E. Hughes, and Trevor J. Pinch, eds. 1987. *The social construction of technological systems: New directions in the sociology and history of technology*. Cambridge, MA: The MIT Press.

Bosley, Deborah S. 1992. "Broadening the base of a technical communication program: An industrial/academic alliance." *Technical Communication* 1: 41–56.

Bryan, John. 1992. "Down the slippery slope: Ethics and the technical writer as marketer." *Technical Communication* 1: 73–90.

Dobrin, David N. 1989. *Writing and technique*. Urbana, IL: National Council of Teachers of English.

Doheny-Farina, Stephen, ed. 1988. *Effective documentation: What we have learned from research*. Cambridge, MA: The MIT Press.

———. 1992. *Rhetoric, innovation, technology: Case studies of technical communication in technology transfers*. Cambridge, MA: The MIT Press.

Dombrowski, Paul. 1991. "The lessons of the Challenger investigations." *IEEE Transactions on Professional Communication* 34: 211–216.

Ellul, Jacques. 1964. *The technological society*. Translated by John Wilkinson. New York, NY: Vintage.

Farrell, Thomas, and Thomas Goodnight. 1981. "Accidental rhetoric: The root metaphors of Three Mile Island." *Communication Monographs* 48: 271–300.

Green, Marcus M., and Timothy D. Nolan. 1984. "A systematic analysis of the technical communicator's job: A guide for educators." *Technical Communication* 31: 9–12.

Herndl, Carl, Barbara Fennell, and Carolyn Miller. 1991. "Understanding failures in organizational discourse: The accident at Three Mile Island and the shuttle *Challenger* disaster." In *Textual dynamics of the professions: Historical and contemporary studies of writing in professional communities*. Charles Bazerman and James Paradis, eds., pp. 279–305. Madison, WI: The University of Wisconsin Press.

Hughes, Thomas P. 1983. *Networks of power: Electrification in western society: 1880–1930*. Baltimore, MD: Johns Hopkins University Press.

———. 1987. "The evolution of large technological systems." In *The social construction of technological systems: New directions in the sociology and history of technology*. Wiebe E. Bijker, Thomas E. Hughes, and Trevor J. Pinch, eds., pp. 51–82. Cambridge, MA: The MIT Press.

Katz, Steven B. 1992. "The ethics of expediency: Classical rhetoric, technology, and the holocaust." *College English* 54: 255–275.

Killingsworth, M. Jimmie, and Dean Steffens. 1989. "Effectiveness in the environmental impact statement: A study in public rhetoric." *Written Communication* 6: 155–180.

MacKenzie, Donald, and Judy Wajcman, eds. 1985. *The social shaping of technology: How the refrigerator got its hum.* Milton Keynes, PA: Open University Press.

Miller, Carolyn R. 1979. "A humanistic rationale for technical writing." *College English* 40: 610–617.

Mirel, Barbara. 1988. "The politics of usability: The organizational functions of an in-house manual." In *Effective documentation: What we have learned from research.* Stephen Doheny-Farina, ed., pp. 277–297. Cambridge, MA: The MIT Press.

Nelkin, Dorothy, ed. 1992. *Controversy: Politics of technical decisions.* 3rd ed. Newbury Park, CA: Sage.

Ornatowski, Cezar M. 1991. *Between efficiency and politics: Technical communication and rhetoric in an aerospace firm.* Ph.D. dissertation, University of California, San Diego.

Pacey, Arnold. 1983. *The culture of technology.* Oxford, England: Blackwell.

Paradis, James. 1991. "Text and action: The operator's manual in context and in court." In *Textual dynamics of the professions: Historical and contemporary studies of writing in professional communities.* Charles Bazerman and James Paradis, eds., pp. 256–278. Madison, WI: The University of Wisconsin Press.

Pinch, Trevor J., and Wiebe E. Bijker. 1987. "The social construction of facts and artifacts: Or how the sociology of science and the sociology of technology might benefit each other." In *The social construction of technological systems: New directions in the sociology and history of technology.* Wiebe E. Bijker, Thomas E. Hughes, and Trevor J. Pinch, eds., pp. 17–50. Cambridge, MA: The MIT Press.

Winner, Langdon. 1980. "Do artifacts have politics?" *Daedalus* 109: 121–36.

Winsor, Dorothy A. 1988. "Communication failures contributing to the Challenger accident: An example for technical communicators." *IEEE Transactions on Professional Communication* 31: 101–107.

———. 1990. "The construction of knowledge in organizations: Asking the right questions about the Challenger." *Journal of Business and Technical Communication* 4: 7–21.

Zimmerman, Donald E., and Marilee Long. 1993. "Exploring the technical communicator's roles: Implications for program design." *Technical Communication Quarterly* 2: 301–318.

34 Teaching for Change, Vision, and Responsibility

STEPHEN A. BERNHARDT

Linking technical communication and rhetoric and calling the convergence "fortuitous" (p. 604 in this volume), Bernhardt, a past president of two of the major organizations in the discipline (ATTW—Association of Teachers of Technical Writing and CPTSC—Council of Programs of Technical and Scientific Communication), argues that, as a result of the "'information age'" and "'knowledge economy'" (p. 603) technical communicators have much to offer society. Not only do we offer specialized disciplinary emphases in such areas as risk and environmental communication, we also can act as "agent[s] of change" (p. 605) because we teach students how to learn in a technological world and encourage "informed practice" that takes into account the common good. The key to success lies in the classroom, depending on how we, as teachers, see not only ourselves but also our students and our profession.

Technical communication, as a field of study and as a career, needs to go beyond anticipating and responding to change. Technical communication needs to discover the opportunities created by change and lend its expertise to creating a society that fosters full individual development within appropriate social structures.

Everywhere we look, we see transforming changes in the social structures of both work and community. Corporations are flattening their hierarchies, encouraging workers to work smarter in a leaner environment. Work is being reengineered, with workers expected to perform on cross-functional teams under the fleeting structures of temporary alliances within virtual corporations. Benefits are disappearing and unions atrophying further with the traditional voices of worker advocacy silenced in a buyer's labor market. Experiencing less and less organizational commitment to their individual careers, workers are adrift as individual agents with portfolios of varying relevance. Those who embrace change see opportunities for selling the right skills; those who fear change or whose skills lag perceptibly suffer uncertainty and live in anxiety.

From *Technical Communication* 42 (1995): 600–02.

Change in the Structures of Social Lives

Although it is hard to separate real social change from its projection through the filters and frames of the media, we at least sense change in the structures of our social lives. We sense failure or dysfunction in some of the large organizing structures of society: in our large cities, in local and national government, in the healthcare system, and the welfare state. We sense alienation from the *polis*, with declining participation in civic affairs, whether measured by voting, by participation in PTA meetings, or by active engagement in civic affairs. Cynicism has largely replaced a unifying belief expressed through shared values and language.

The academy struggles with change: students are older and nontraditional; programs look more vocational or technologically specialized than liberal or humanistic; and persistent, nay, perennial underfunding cripples efforts at improvement. Students are educated through a series of courses offered with little overall integration, and students are graduated with diplomas that attest to little more than their having sat through a collection of courses. Many more students graduate than there are jobs. Although students may receive begrudging admission that they have some command over specific subject matter, it is offered in the midst of withering criticism that they cannot communicate, solve problems, think critically, or manage resources and projects.

Amidst the gloom such generalizations provoke, where is there room to embrace change?

Changes and Convergences

I believe the current scene can be reframed in ways that recognize and take advantage of identifiable convergences. Technical communication as a discipline and practice is uniquely positioned to help people understand current changes and to take advantage of the convergences. The nature of work and the growth of technology converge in the phenomenon of the "information age" or the "knowledge economy." Academic programs can help students understand information and command its technologies. Universities are hubs of the information network as intelligence (artificial and human), libraries, and computer centers converge into knowledge nets. Schools are positioned to take advantage of these coalescing knowledge nets to create a new generation of students and workers who are comfortable in cyberspace, familiar with information protocols, conversant within the new media, and at home in virtual environments. The individual with such skills possesses a key adaptive ability: the ability to learn new behaviors within new technological environments. Nothing is more fundamental in an age of change than is knowing how to learn, and the current contexts for learning are technological.

Technology and text are converging in ways that open many new opportunities for those who manage or teach about information technology. Texts are changing shape with shifting media and suddenly, there are manifold opportunities to design new types of books, new teaching and training materials, and new forms of literate entertainment. There is a blooming epistolary culture on the Internet, with an incredible growth of new communities, new forms of political engagement, and new patterns of work, all mediated by e-mail and its progeny. For those keyed into information technologies, opportunities are just beginning to show in the telecommunications industries, software development, direct sales, and networking services.

There is a fortuitous convergence of rhetoric and technical communication as a coalescing discipline for disparate areas of inquiry. Rhetorical study, the traditional centerpiece of humanistic education, is reasserting itself as a unifying discipline. On an individual level, technical communication helps students develop skills in writing and self-expression, interpersonal interaction, and the use and design of information (what used to be called reading and writing). Rhetoric encourages students to think analytically about complex situations, to understand the diversity of human motives, and to learn to act strategically in delicate situations.

Rhetorical study also encourages the convergence of individual skills with an excellence in character that finds expression in civic virtue. Rhetoric encourages students to develop strong individual communication skills while taking into consideration the implications of individual behavior for the common good. Rhetoric continues to encourage, as it always has, the development of the good person speaking (and writing) well. Rhetoric encourages an informed practice, a theoretically and practically informed praxis that serves the common good. Rhetoric encourages the development of ethical character, and ethical character serves the corporation well.

Convergence of Specialized Disciplinary Understandings

The power of rhetorical studies for understanding and organizing life in a changing culture is evidenced within the academy by the emergence of new fields that reflect a convergence of specialized disciplinary understandings.

Risk communication asks how the costs and benefits of various technological and scientific endeavors can be weighed; considers the balance of corporate, individual, and common good; and suggests how public opinion can be engaged through informed consent.

Environmental communication asks how a public ethic can inform scientific understanding of ecosystems to encourage the reestablishment of a shared environmental ethic based on the commons or on sustainable systems.

Business communication addresses issues of how to encourage teamwork, how to change corporate cultures, and how to create cultures that embrace the differences of age, gender, language, and ethnicity that make up the new workforce.

Human factors and usability studies ask how technology can be adapted to users, how genuinely helpful systems can be created, and how we know whether systems are designed in ways that are "natural" to people and that support worthy social and business goals.

Scientific rhetoric asks how we can gauge progress, where society should invest its resources, how far we can trust "facts," and to what extent all knowledge is subjective.

CONCLUSION

Technical communication, broadly construed, thus has much to offer a society in change. To the individual, it offers usable skills because the ability to communicate is foundational to success in all other pursuits. There is much work to be done to create a society that encourages technical literacy in the interest of broad economic participation. We are threatened by a schism separating the skilled worker from the unskilled, with a growing gap between those who are perceived as being valuable in the workplace and those who are consigned to low wage, low skill, meaningless work. Technical communication has been fixated as a field on those who write technical documentation as a profession, but there is much to be done to understand and foster the more basic kinds of technical literacy necessary to adapt to the current workplace. Because technical communication welcomes technological change and works to understand it, the field can help students become comfortable in an information age and help them develop those literacies that are valued in work settings. Technology and literacy converge here in a notion of information literacy that can contribute to economic success.

Beyond the individual level, the rhetoric of technical communication encourages individuals to consider those imperatives for acting in the common good entailed in the pursuit of individual or corporate goals. Rhetoric reframes all issues of technological expediency, complicating notions of pure efficiency with consideration of the public good. Rhetoric helps us recall our social obligations in the midst of change. The changes we see in social structures, in the academy, in technology, and in the workplace all create convergences that technical communicators are uniquely equipped to understand and take advantage of. We have only to think broadly of what kinds of expertise we might genuinely claim, what human and technological values we are interested in promoting, and what sort of society we are interested in creating. We can then claim a rightful place as an agent of change.

ADDITIONAL READINGS

Hackos, JoAnn T. "Trends for 2000: Moving Beyond the Cottage." *Intercom* (2000): 6–10.

Hart-Davidson, William. "On Writing, Technical Communication, and Information Technology: The Core Competencies of Technical Communication." *Technical Communication* 48, no. 2 (2001): 145–55.

Hughes, Michael. "Moving from Information Transfer to Knowledge Creation: A New Value Proposition for Technical Communicators." *Technical Communication* 49, no. 3 (2002): 275–85.

Meyer, Paul R., and Stephen A. Bernhardt. "Workplace Realities and the Technical Writing Curriculum: A Call for Change." In *Foundations for Teaching Technical Communication: Theory, Practice, and Program Design*, edited by Katherine Staples and Cezer Ornatowski, 85–98. Greenwich, CT: Ablex, 1997.

Redish, Janice. "Adding Value as a Professional Technical Communicator." *Technical Communication* 4, no. 1 (1995): 26–39.

Spilka, Rachel. "Becoming a Profession." In *Reshaping Technical Communication: New Directions and Challenges for the 21st Century*, edited by Barbara Mirel and Rachel Spilka, 97–109. Mahwah, NJ: Lawrence Erlbaum, 2002.

Sullivan, Patricia. "Technology, Education, and Workplaces of the Future: A Parent's View." In *Expanding Literacies*, edited by Mary Sue Garay and Stephen A. Bernhardt, 81–96. Albany: SUNY P, 1998.

Zachry, Mark, et al. "The Changing Face of Technical Communication: New Directions for the Field in a New Millennium." *Proceedings of the 19th Annual International Conference on Computer Documentation*. Santa Fe, New Mexico, USA, 2001. 248–60.

ANNOTATED BIBLIOGRAPHY OF PEDAGOGICAL WORK

As I have argued elsewhere, teaching technical communication is a complex activity, a *technê* not a knack. It requires a fundamental understanding of the subject matter, the rhetorical situation (which includes not only the institution and its values and needs but also the students and theirs), and an understanding of the act of teaching, of trying to communicate with others to encourage and assist them to learn. As a result, it would be impractical of me to provide a standard syllabus, consisting of a single methodology, and suggest that anyone reading this book would do well to follow or emulate it. Doing so would not take into account the many diverse situations teachers will encounter. Teachers at a two-year college will have different considerations than those at either a four-year liberal college or a four-year technological institution.

However, there are a number of pedagogical topics that most teachers of technical communication will have to consider regardless of their situation or level of experience: which genres of documents to teach in their class; whether or not and, if so, how to integrate collaborative projects; which method(s) of evaluation to use on student papers; and whether or not to try their hand at experiential learning strategies. In addition, most teachers will have to consider whether or not and, if so, how to incorporate online components (and perhaps even whether or not to teach their class entirely online), and they will need strategies for teaching the basics of audience, style, and organization, which are rooted in the canons of classical rhetorical theory.

Fortunately, because our field is a pedagogical one, there is much published advice on these topics. In this bibliography, I include a wide range of sources where you might find answers to your questions, ideas that may help you create and evaluate assignments, and stories that will help you realize that you are part of a larger community. I present a range of articles—from the earliest issues of the field's journals to the most recent—and offer what I hope will be succinct, useful annotations. Many of these articles will be familiar to those of you who have been members of the field for some time, but I suspect that some won't.

This bibliography is by no means a "best of" list, and the fact that an article is not included does not mean that it is not worth reading. Instead this list is an attempt to provide you with a variety of perspectives on the field and strategies you might use in your classroom. This list of articles is, in effect, a collection of starting places that may encourage you to research further into the field's rich historical, theoretical, and practical resources in order to become a practitioner who is truly user-centered and reflective.

WORK CITED

Dubinsky, James M. "More than a Knack: *Techê* and Teaching Technical Writing." *Technical Communication Quarterly* 11, no. 2 (2002): 131–47.

Teaching Tips and Strategies

Grant-Davie, Keith. "Teaching Technical Writing with Only Academic Experience." *Journal of Technical Writing and Communication* 26, no. 3 (1996): 291–306.
Grant-Davie outlines the essential knowledge that teachers who have only an academic background need to teach technical communication to nonmajors (e.g., a command of research in the field). He also offers suggestions about how those same teachers can get experience in the workplace.

Morgan, Meg, et al., eds. *Strategies for Technical Communication: A Collection of Teaching Tips.* Arlington, VA: Society for Technical Communication, 1994.
This collection of short articles describes strategies and suggestions for teaching technical communication. The articles range from teaching the résumé as a technical document to using spreadsheets as a method of invention. Especially useful are the chapters on collaboration and editing.

Reynolds, John Frederick. "Classical Rhetoric and the Teaching of Technical Writing." *Technical Communication Quarterly* 1, no. 2 (1992): 63–76.
Reynolds argues that many textbooks have ignored the value of classical rhetorical principles, and he offers three key concepts (rhetoric and dialectic; ethos, pathos, and logos; the five canons) to help teachers create more effective courses.

Thompson, Isabelle. "An Educational Philosophy of Technical Writing." *Technical Communication Quarterly* 1, no. 2 (1992): 33–46.
Thompson examines both John Dewey's and Louise Rosenblatt's transactional approaches to learning and literacy and arrives at four maxims for teachers to consider in order to create a classroom environment that facilitates learning through "immersion."

Audience and the Writing Process

Beaufort, Anne. "Operationalizing the Concept of Discourse Community: A Case Study of One Institutional Site of Composing." *Research in the Teaching of English* 31, no. 4 (1997): 486–529.
Using a case study that focuses on writing activities in a nonprofit organization, Beaufort provides insight about audience expectations and the problems writers confront and adaptations they make related to audience and genre when they face writing tasks involving several discourse communities. She also argues for the notion of discourse community as a useful heuristic in teaching.

Coney, Mary B. "Contemporary Views of Audience: A Rhetorical Perspective." *The Technical Writing Teacher* 14 (1987): 319–36.
In this overview, Coney examines the influence of work of Perelman, Burke, Booth, and Ong, and outlines the implications of their work for technical writing.

Couture, Barbara. "Categorizing Professional Discourse: Engineering, Administrative, and Technical/ Professional Writing." *Journal of Business and Technical Communication* 6 (1992): 5–37.

Couture offers a useful taxonomy of three important categories of discourse to illustrate the constraints of communal values and reveal both textual and contextual elements inherent within a community.

Faigley, Lester. "Competing Theories of Process: A Critique and a Proposal." *College English* 48 (1986): 527–42.

Faigley offers a valuable discussion/critique of three theories of the composing process—expressive, cognitive, and social—giving the nod to the social.

Flower, Linda S., and John R. Hayes. "A Cognitive Process Theory of Writing." *College Composition and Communication* 32 (1981): 365–87.

In this classic article, Flower and Hayes describe what teachers can learn about the writing process through "protocol analysis"—asking writers to think aloud while writing and then analyzing the writers' narratives.

Hart, Geoff. "The Five W's: An Old Tool for the New Task of Audience Analysis," *Technical Communication* 43, no. 2 (1996): 139–45.

A short but useful piece that commends using the journalist's five *W*'s heuristic to ensure that information products meet users' and readers' needs.

Johnson, Robert R. "Audience Involved: Toward a Participatory Model of Writing." *Computers and Composition* 14 (1997): 361–77.

In this award-winning article, Johnson discusses the implications of and rationale for adding a third model of audience (audience involved) to those outlined by Lunsford and Ede (audience invoked and audience addressed).

Killingsworth, M. Jimmie, and Preston Lynn Waller. "A Grammar of Person for Technical Writing." *The Technical Writing Teacher* 17 (1990): 26–40.

In this award-winning article, Killingsworth and Waller explain how teachers can use grammatical relations between audience and author to model rhetorical relations and represent major genres (e.g., manual, proposal).

Pomerenke, Paula J. "Process: More than a Fad for the Business Writer." *Journal of Business Communication* 24, no. 1 (1987): 37–39.

Pomerenke makes a case for the process method and outlines a strategy for using it to teach a course in business communications.

Redish, Janice C. "Understanding Readers." In *Techniques for Technical Communicators*, edited by Carol M. Barnum and Saul Carliner, 14–42. New York: Macmillan, 1993.

Informed by her research as director of the Document Design Center of American Institutes for Research, Redish provides a comprehensive overview of an essential principle: understanding readers' actions and motivations.

Roundy, Nancy. "Audience Analysis: A Guide to Revision in Technical Writing." *The Technical Writing Teacher* 10 (1983): 94–100.

Roundy presents a clear, organized discussion of a teacher-research project that illustrates the connection of audience to the entire writing process.

Souther, James. "What to Report." *IEEE Transactions on Professional Communication* 28, no. 3 (1985): 5–8.

In this short but oft-cited article, Souther describes the results of a study of the reading habits of a group of Westinghouse managers that demonstrates how and what they read.

Spilka, Rachel. "Studying Writer-Reader Interactions in the Workplace." *The Technical Writing Teacher* 15 (1988): 208–21.

Relying on her study of engineers' composing processes, Spilka offers a rationale for workplace ethnographies, describes how the findings challenged assumptions about the ways writers in the workplace compose documents, and outlines some pedagogical applications.

Sullivan, Patricia. "Teaching the Writing Process in Scientific and Technical Writing Classes." *The Technical Writing Teacher* 8 (1980): 10–16.

Sullivan presents a strategy for teaching the writing process that is adaptable to various assignments (e.g., instructions and résumés).

Warren, Thomas L. "Style in Technical Writing. "*The Technical Writing Teacher* 6 (1979): 47–49.
In this short, informative piece, Warren describes connections between content and style, audience and style, and the writer's purpose and style.

———. "Three Approaches to Reader Analysis." *Technical Communication* 40 (1993): 81–88.

Relying on a survey of textbooks, Warren reviews and categorizes ways to analyze readers (demographic, organization, and psychological) in order to help writers develop more effective audience assessment techniques.

Whitburn, Merrill D. "The First Day in Technical Communication: An Approach to Audience Adaptation." *Technical Writing Teacher* 3 (1976): 115–18.
Although nearly thirty years old, this article offers sound advice to build community and introduce a key concept on the first day of class.

Style, Editing, and Grammar

Campbell, Charles P. "Engineering Style: Striving for Efficiency." *IEEE Transactions on Professional Communication* 35, no. 3 (1992): 130–37.
Campbell examines style as a problem in "user-interface engineering" (132), and, by relying on linguistic research, he presents some strategies (e.g., "always contextualize") that may help writers meet reader expectations.

Dragga, Sam, and Gwendolyn Gong. *Editing: The Design of Rhetoric*. Amityville: Baywood, 1989.
In this award-winning book, Dragga and Gong provide a comprehensive overview of the editing process by examining the rhetorical canons (invention, arrangement, style, and delivery) and the corresponding rhetorical objectives of editing (accuracy, clarity, propriety, and artistry).

Gerich, Carol. "How Technical Editors Enrich the Revision Process." *Technical Communication* 41, no. 1 (1994): 59–70.
By relying on a case study, Gerich offers insight into ways to create a more collaborative approach to editing that involves editors in the process of document creation/production earlier and leads to more substantive revisions and, as a result, better documents.

Graves, Heather Brodie, and Roger Graves. "Masters, Slaves, and Infant Mortality: Language Challenges for Technical Editing." *Technical Communication Quarterly* 7, no. 4 (1998): 389–414.
Relying on scholarship from critical linguistics and the rhetoric of science, the authors highlight the need for technical editors to be capable of challenging writers' uses of language, looking for underlying values or ambiguity.

Graves, Richard L. "A Primer for Teaching Style." *College Composition and Communication* 25, no. 2 (1974): 186–90.
Graves discusses techniques for teaching style to demonstrate the importance of this classical canon of rhetoric in writing instruction.

Horner, Bruce. "Rethinking the 'Sociality' of Error: Teaching Editing as Negotiation." *Rhetoric Review* 11, no. 1 (1992): 172–99.
Horner offers an argument that errors are instances of writers and readers failure to negotiate an agreement on how their relationship is to be achieved in the text and some pedagogical suggestions to help writers, particularly those teachers label "basic."

Lybbert, E. K., and D. W. Cummings. "On Repetition and Coherence." *College Composition and Communication* 20, no. 1 (1969): 35–38.
The authors explain differences between unity and coherence and consider ways to use repetition and parallelism to make writing more coherent.

Messer, Donald K. "Six Common Causes of Ambiguity." *The Technical Writing Teacher* 7 (1980): 50–52.
In a succinct discussion with useful illustrations, Messer explains grammatical issues that create confusion for readers.

Ohmann, Richard. "Use Definite, Specific, Concrete Language." *College English* 41 (1979): 390–97.

Ohmann critiques an oft-used comment by teachers by explaining that offering students such advice infantilizes them, denies them the power of abstraction, and fosters an ideology privileging ahistoricism, empiricism, fragmentation, solipsism, and denial of conflict.

Rosner, Mary. "Sentence-Combining in Technical Writing: An Editing Tool." *The Technical Writing Teacher* 9 (1982): 100–07.
Relying on a strategy that, while not often discussed, still may be useful, Rosner outlines an entire learning module to teach editing skills.

Rude, Carolyn. *Technical Editing*. 3rd ed. Boston: Allyn & Bacon, 2002.
Rude's comprehensive overview of the editing process includes chapters on electronic editing and editing for global contexts.

———, ed. *Teaching Technical Editing*. Lubbock, TX: Association of Teachers of Technical Writing, 1985.

An early but still useful collection of eighteen articles that covers course theory, as well as editing topics and exercises, and also includes a bibliography.

Schleppegrell, Mary J. "Grammar as Resource: Writing a Description." *Research in the Teaching of English* 32, no. 2 (1998): 182–211.
Although primarily directed toward ESL and nonstandard dialect speakers, this study of the writing produced by 128 middle school students demonstrates that functional grammar analysis has value. Teachers can provide explicit instruction in the grammatical structures present in specific writing genres to focus on sociocultural expectations of academic writing.

Selzer, Jack. "What Constitutes a 'Readable' Technical Style?" In *New Essays in Technical and Scientific Communication: Research, Theory, Practice*, edited by Paul V. Anderson, R. John Brockmann, and Carolyn R. Miller, 71–89. Farmingdale, NY: Baywood, 1983.
Selzer reviews research in psycholinguistics and comprehension to argue against relying upon readability formulas as guides to produce technical documents.

Witte, Stephen P., and Lester Faigley. "Coherence, Cohesion, and Writing Quality." *College Composition and Communication* 32 (1981): 189–204.
Relying on the work of Halliday and Hasan, the authors outline the difference between cohesion and coherence, and discuss the connection to style and writing quality.

GENRES

Battalio, John. "The Formal Report Project as Shared-Document Collaboration: A Plan for Co-Authorship." *Technical Communication Quarterly* 2, no. 2 (1992): 147–60.
To prepare students to be competent members of teams who can collaborate on projects, Battalio outlines a four-phase project for a formal report project and discusses the student feedback he received.

Blyler, Nancy Roundy. "Rhetorical Theory and Newsletter Writing." *Journal of Technical Writing and Communication* 20 (1990): 139–52.
By applying rhetorical theory to newsletters (an often overlooked but ubiquitous genre) produced by two political-activist organizations, Blyler illustrates the value/uses of three aspects of rhetorical theory (schema, social construction, and theories of audience).

Charney, Davida H., and Jack R. Rayman. "The Role of Writing Quality in Effective Student Résumés." *Journal of Business and Technical Communication* 3, no. 1 (1989): 36–53.
Charney and Rayman present findings from a study that involved eighteen recruiters analyzing and rating seventy-two student résumés. They conclude that writers need to highlight work experience and present a clear, correct persona by eliminating mechanical errors.

Coletta, W. John. "The Ideologically Biased Use of Language in Scientific and Technical Writing." *Technical Communication Quarterly* 1, no. 1 (1992): 59–70.
Relying on technical descriptions from a number of sources (e.g., biology and engineering), Coletta argues that instructors should make ideology more visible to demonstrate how language use shapes our understanding of the world.

Curry, Jerome M. "Technical Instruction and Definition Assignments: A Realistic Approach." *Journal of Business and Technical Communication* 6 (1992): 116–22.

In this piece, Curry explains ways to approach two standard assignments in a service course to help students prepare for their workplace tasks.

Debs, Mary Beth, and Lia Brillhart. "Technical Listening/Technical Writing." *The Technical Writing Teacher* 8 (1981): 83–84.

Debs and Brillhart offer a strategy to integrate listening into a course by relying on the genre of abstracts, which is useful given recent emphasis on communication across the curriculum.

Devitt, Amy J. "Generalizing about Genre: New Conceptions of an Old Concept." *College Composition and Communication* 44 (1993): 573–86.

In this foundational article, Devitt explains the implications of rethinking the concept of genre from a formal concept to a rhetorical and semiotic one, and outlines the relationships of reader expectations within discourse communities to writing.

Devitt, Amy J., Anis Bawarshi, and Mary Jo Reiff. "Materiality and Genre in the Study of Discourse Communities." *College English* 65, no. 5 (2003): 541–58.

In this series of three short, interconnected essays, the authors examine how genre theory may yield valuable insights about teaching and research regarding legal practice, medical practice, and classroom teaching.

Freed, Richard C., and Glenn J. Broadhead. "Using High-Affect Goals in Teaching Proposal Writing." *Journal of Advanced Composition* 7 (1987): 131–38.

The authors explain six subgoals embedded in writing proposals (e.g., feeding a wish, avoiding a threat) that can help teach students to affect their readers emotionally.

Gould, Jay, "Improving Technical Writing." In *Technical and Professional Writing*, edited by Herman A. Estrin, 221–24. New York: Preston, 1976.

In this short, informative piece, Gould, one of the field's founders, outlines definition, description, and directive writing.

Greenly, Robert. "How to Write a Resume." *Technical Communication* 40 (1993): 42–48.

Based on firsthand experience in the aerospace industry, the author offers practical advice and tips by addressing issues of style, content, and format.

Inkster, Robert. "Rhetoric of the Classroom: The Exigencies of the Technical Writing Class as Topics for Memos." *Technical Communication Quarterly* 3, no. 2 (1994): 213–25.

Based on Bitzer's "Rhetorical Situation," Inkster proposes using the exigencies of the classroom to create rich, real technical writing problems that students respond to using memos.

LaDuc, Linda. "Infusing Practical Wisdom into Persuasive Performance: Hermeneutics and the Teaching of the Sales Proposal." *Journal of Technical Writing and Communication* 21, no. 2 (1991): 155–64.

LaDuc argues for using hermeneutic theory as a basis for teaching by focusing on the genre of sales proposals, which, according to her, can be vehicles for building and maintaining long-term relationships if the underlying ethical principles involved in transactions are emphasized.

Lay, Mary M. "Teaching Narrative in Technical Writing Classes." *The Technical Writing Teacher* 9 (1982): 156–58.

Lay outlines a heuristic for teaching narrative, an issue often overlooked in our field, in order to help students understand their audience's needs and interests.

Locker, Kitty O. "What Do Writers in Industry Write?" *The Technical Writing Teacher* 9 (1982): 122–27.

Locker provides an overview of why and what writers in industry write as a means to demonstrate to students the amount and importance of writing in the workplace.

Norman, Rose, and Marynell Young. "Using Peer Review to Teach Proposal Writing." *Technical Writing Teacher* 12 (1985): 1–9.

Norman and Young outlines a sequence of assignments to teach students the grant proposal and review process inductively.

Orr, Thomas. "Genre in the Field of Computer Science and Computer Engineering." *IEEE Transactions on Professional Communication* 42, no. 1 (1999): 32–37.

Orr identifies nearly ninety written genres in the field of computer engineering and classifies them according to five central aims. His study illustrates how, by focusing on the character of texts within a field and the contexts in which texts are situated, we can learn much about the nature of work in that field.

Pinelli, Thomas, et al. "Report Format Preferences of Technical Managers and Nonmanagers." *Technical Communication* 31, no. 2 (1984): 20–24.

By relying on survey data, these authors document the review and reading practices of a broad group of professionals, highlighting the value they place on summaries, abstracts, introductions, and conclusions.

Popken, Randall. "The Pedagogical Dissemination of a Genre: The Resume in American Business Discourse Textbooks, 1914–1939." *Journal of Advanced Composition* 19, no. 1 (1999): 91–116.

In this article, Popken describes how authors of business-writing textbooks stabilized and disseminated the résumé genre; his study is useful for historical background and to demonstrate how genres are formed/change over time.

Rice, H. William. "Teaching the Art of the Memo: Politics and Precision." *Business Communication Quarterly* 58, no. 1 (1995): 31–34.

Rice advocates a teaching strategy that turns a class into a company and uses memos to simulate a corporate environment with the goal of enabling students to discover and emulate complex writer-reader relationships.

Roberts, David. "Teaching Abstracts in Technical Writing: Early and Often." *Technical Writing Teacher* X (1982): 12–16.

Roberts outlines a method for teaching abstracts, a genre that students, particularly those in the sciences, need to understand.

Rude, Carolyn. "The Report for Decision Making: Genre and Inquiry." *Journal of Business and Technical Communication* 9, no. 2 (1995): 170–205.

In this award-winning article, Rude outlines essential characteristics of the decision-making report and explains differences between it, the proposal, the report of scientific experiment, and the persuasive essay, focusing on assumptions about the nature of inquiry and problem solving.

Ryan, Charlton. "Using Environmental Impact Statements as an Introduction to Technical Writing." *Technical Communication Quarterly* 2, no. 2 (1993): 205–13.

Ryan explains how environmental impact statements can be an effective means of introducing students to technical writing, arguing that these documents are accessible and useful as illustrations in courses with students from a variety of backgrounds, and who have a range of expertise and writing ability.

Souther, James. "Design That Report!" In *Technical and Professional Writing,* edited by Herman A. Estrin, 225–28. New York: Preston, 1976.

Relying on lessons learned as a consultant and teacher, Souther argues for creating writing situations based on problems students would encounter in the workplace.

Wahlstrom, Ralph. "Teaching the Proposal in the Professional Writing Course." *Technical Communication*." 49, no. 1 (2001): 81–88.

Wahlstrom suggests that proposals can be taught using a variety of document forms (e.g., memo, letter, report), and argues for using proposals as the basis and motivation for a course.

Walzer, Arthur E. "Ethos, Technical Writing, and the Liberal Arts." *The Technical Writing Teacher* 8 (1981): 50–53.

Walzer presents an assignment that focuses on ethos to help students learn to examine arguments, strategies, and tone in a trade journal.

COLLABORATION, TEAMWORK, AND PEER-REVIEW STRATEGIES

Barker, Randolph T., and Frank J. Franzak. "Team Building in the Classroom: Preparing Students for Their Organizational Future." *Journal of Technical Writing and Communication* 27, no. 3 (1997): 303–15.

Barker and Franzak offer a brief survey of team-building literature, and suggest team-building exercises that are based on studies they conducted of team formation and team building in organizational behavior and marketing classes.

Barnum, Carol. "Working with People." In *Techniques for Technical Communicators*, edited by Carol M. Barnum and Saul Carliner, 108–36. New York: Macmillan, 1993.

Barnum presents an overview of project teams and their characteristics, and outlines the challenges of collaborative writing. Her article includes a particularly useful section on group building and individual roles in groups.

Belanger, Kelly, and Jane Greer. "Beyond the Group Project: A Blueprint for a Collaborative Writing Course." *Journal of Business and Technical Communication* 6 (1992): 99–115.

The authors describe a course that revolves completely around collaborative activities, focusing on teaching students to become "self-reflexive, flexible writers." Equally valuable is the explicit discussion of methods that teachers can use to address problems they might encounter in the classroom.

Bishop, Wendy. "Revising the Technical Writing Class: Peer Critiques, Self-Evaluation, and Portfolio Grading." *The Technical Writing Teacher* 16 (1989): 13–26.

Bishop offers an interesting approach that emphasizes students' growth and development as writers/editors. Some of these assignments, such as the interview and literary autobiography, can be adapted easily to nearly any introductory-level class.

Bosley, Deborah S. "Cross-Cultural Collaboration: Whose Culture Is It, Anyway?" *Technical Communication Quarterly* 2, no. 1 (1993): 51–62.

Bosley explains how teachers can help students enhance cross-cultural collaboration by focusing on cultural differences that influence ways different group members function.

Burnett, Rebecca E. "Conflict in Collaborative Decision-Making." In *Professional Communication: The Social Perspective*, edited by Nancy R. Blyler and Charlotte Thralls, 144–62. Newbury Park, CA: Sage, 1993.

Burnett examines the issue of conflict, and, by relying on a case study of an upper-level writing class, she offers observations about collaborative work, conflict, and decision making, concluding with some implications for pedagogy and practice.

Morgan, Meg. "The Group Writing Task: A Schema for Collaborative Assignment Making." In *Professional Communication: The Social Perspective*, edited by Nancy Blyler and Charlotte Thralls, 230–42. Thousand Oaks, CA: Sage Publications, 1993.

Morgan's piece is valuable because she creates a schema or plan to help teachers design more effective group/collaborative assignments.

Renshaw, D. A. "In-class Collaborative Cases." *Bulletin of the Association for Business Communication* 53, no. 2 (1990): 63–65.

In this short piece, Renshaw describes a collaborative classroom process and offers six teaching tips to build cohesion among group members.

Roever, Carol, and Diane Mullen. "Teamwork: Preparing Students for the New Reality." *Journal of Business and Technical Communication* 8, no. 4 (1994). 462–74.

The authors present a model of collaboration that focuses on working in teams, writing collaboratively, peer review, and participating in meetings.

Walvoord, Barbara E. Fassler. "Using Student Peer Groups." In *Helping Students Write Well: A Guide for Teachers in All Disciplines*, 111–22. New York: Modern Language Association, 1986.

In this discussion of peer-group work, the author defines two types of peer groups (the response group and task groups) and describes techniques for setting up groups and dealing with problems in each type of group.

Evaluation and Assessment

Allen, Jo. "A Machiavellian Approach to Grading Writing Assignments." *The Technical Writing Teacher* 15 (1988): 158–60.

Allen offers insights about creating grading standards in class with students and provides some examples of paragraphs to elicit student responses.

Beard, John D., Jone Rymer, and David L. Williams. "An Assessment System for Collaborative Writing Groups: Theory and Empirical Evaluation." *Journal of Business and Technical Communication* 3 (1989): 29–51.

This collaborative piece outlines a system for evaluating group/collaborative writing that proved highly satisfactory to students studied.

Charney, Davida. "The Validity of Using Holistic Scoring to Evaluate Writing: A Critical Overview." *Research in the Teaching of English* 18 (1984): 65–81.

By focusing on issues of reliability and validity, Charney questions our field's emphasis on holistic scoring, arguing that scorers are often influenced by legibility, length, and unusual diction.

Dragga, Sam, ed. *Technical Writing: Student Samples and Teacher Responses*. St. Paul: ATTW, 1992.

In this very useful book published by the Association of Teachers of Technical Writing, the editors bring together nine experienced teachers and papers from thirty-four of their students to identify commenting practices that teachers might wish to adopt or adapt.

Haswell, Richard H. "Minimal Marking." *College English* 45 (1983): 600–04.

Haswell demonstrates that a "minimal marking" approach to grammatical/mechanical mistakes in student writing leads to students pinpointing and correcting them.

Quible, Zane K. "The Efficacy of Several Writing Feedback Systems." *Business Communication Quarterly* 6, no. 2 (1997): 109–25.

Quible outlines advantages and disadvantages of three different methods of providing feedback to students: written comments, conferences, and peer editing.

Robertson, Michael. "Writing and Responding." In *Writer's Craft, Teacher's Art: Teaching What We Know*, edited by Mimi Schwartz, 115–24. Portsmouth, NH: Boynton/Cook, 1991.

Relying on experiences with an editor at a New York magazine and on a medical/diagnosis analogy, Robertson offers four principles to use in responding to students' prose.

Rogers, Priscilla S. "Analytic Measures for Evaluating Managerial Writing." *Journal of Business and Technical Communication* 8 (1994): 380–407.

Arguing that holistic evaluation does not provide a useful tool for identifying persuasiveness, and is not useful for teaching or research, Rogers offers two assessment tools (the Analysis of Argument Measure and the Persuasiveness Adaptiveness Measure) to identify important elements of persuasive writing and sensitize writers to rhetorical considerations.

Shay, Suellen. "Portfolio Assessment: A Catalyst for Staff and Curricular Reform." *Assessing Writing* 4, no. 1 (1997): 29–51.

The author describes how a portfolio-assessment project at the University of Cape Town (UCT) led to both a staff dialogue on the nature of written competence within the discipline and curricular reform that focused on teaching writing conventions and strategies for particular tasks.

Smith, Summer. "The Genre of the End Comment: Conventions in Teacher Responses to Student Writing." *College Composition and Communication* 48, no. 2 (1997): 249–68.

Using a representative sample of papers, Smith categorizes sixteen primary genres of end comments and contends that although the end comment may be easy to generate, it may also be ineffective.

Sommers, Nancy. "Responding to Student Writing." *College Composition and Communication* 32 (1982): 148–56.

By studying professors' comments on student papers, the author finds that many are not text specific, and offers suggestions about commenting on different drafts and ways to encourage students to rethink or clarify their position on an issue.

Online/Electronic Classroom Strategies

Carbone, Nick. "Trying to Create a Community: A First-Day Lesson Plan." *Computers and Composition* 10, no. 4 (1993): 81–88.

Although outdated in terms of technologies highlighted, this article provides a very useful discussion of first-day strategies for teaching in an electronic environment, with emphases on the value of electronic discussion and peer feedback.

Gillette, David. "Pedagogy, Architecture, and the Virtual Classroom." *Technical Communication Quarterly* 8, no. 1 (1999): 21–36.

Gillette discusses the structuring of an online course, and offers insight into the issues a teacher may face when trying to start and maintain an online course.

Goubil-Gambrell, Patricia. "Designing Effective Internet Assignments in Introductory Technical Communication Courses." *IEEE Transactions on Professional Communication* 39, no. 4 (1996): 224–31.

Goubil-Gambrell offers useful advice on how to create a range of assignments (e.g., evaluating Web sites and conducting literature reviews) teachers in an introductory course might include.

Johnson-Eilola, Johndan, and Stuart A. Selber. "Policing Ourselves: Defining the Boundaries of Appropriate Discussion in Online Forums." *Computers and Composition* 13 (1996): 269–91.

By analyzing a debate over appropriate topics in a public Listserv for technical writers, the authors demonstrate the range and limits of discourses and how those discourses "write us" (270). They then recommend that students learn to "recognize the mechanisms through which these rules operate so that they might negotiate a variety of positions within online forums and possibly enact change" (271).

Klemm, W. R. "Computer Conferencing as a Cooperative Learning Environment." *Cooperative Learning and College Teaching* 5 (1995): 11–13.

In this article, Klemm explains why instructional designs suitable for typical classroom settings are not necessarily suitable for computer-conferencing situations and outlines four basic principles for success.

Mabrito, Mark. "Real-Time Computer Network Collaboration: Case Studies of Business Writing Students." *Journal of Business and Technical Communication* 6, no. 3 (1992): 316–36.

In this early discussion of computer collaboration, Mabrito presents results of a case study comparing experiences of student groups who met both in traditional classrooms and online, using synchronous (real-time) software. This piece would be useful for a literature review.

Miles, Thomas H. "Teaching Technical Writing through E-mail: Making Hyperspace Personal." *Technical Communication* 42 (1995): 658–60.

Miles discusses two potential problems ("hypertext—or surrealistic—consciousness" and "the impersonality factors" [659]) that can occur when teaching online.

Spooner, Michael, and Kathleen Yancey. "Postings on a Genre of Email." *College Composition and Communication* 47, no. 2 (1996): 252–78.

Using a dialogic presentation, the authors examine e-mail, considering questions of genre, rhetorical situation, and voice, while also considering the strategies necessary for effective pedagogy.

Tannacito, Terry. "Teaching Professional Writing Online with Electronic Peer Response." *Kairos* 6, no. 2 (Fall 2001–January 2003). http://english.ttu.edu/kairos/6.2/coverweb/de/tannacito/Index.htm.

Based on his own experiences, the author argues for the advantages of electronic peer response (as well as electronic instructor response).

Literacy Issues

Brandt, Deborah. "Accumulating Literacy: Writing and Learning to Write in the Twentieth Century." *College English* 57, no. 6 (1995): 649–68.

Brandt offers a fascinating discussion of literacy practices that draws upon two extended examples to illustrate ways in which individuals adapt or transform practices they learned.

Cushman, Ellen. "The Rhetorician as an Agent of Social Change." *College Composition and Communication* 47 (1996): 7–28.

In this Braddock Award–winning article, Cushman pushes the contact zone to a new level, and by focusing on the importance of literacy in a civic-minded classroom, she argues that academics can work collaboratively with community members to help bring about change if they share resources, provide tutoring services, or integrate service-learning projects into their courses.

Flower, Linda. "Negotiating Academic Discourse." In *Reading to Write: Exploring a Social and Cognitive Process*, edited by Linda Flower, et al., 221–61. New York: Oxford UP, 1990.

Although the study described the transition of first-year students entering the academic community, much of what the author explains has value for students negotiating the challenges of entering the workplace (e.g., the author's discussion of "strategic knowledge" [222–23], "transformation of knowledge" [225–27], and "building a theory of the task" [250–52]).

Peck, Wayne Campbell, Linda Flower, and Lorraine Higgins, "Community Literacy." *College Composition and Communication* 46 (May 1995): 199–222.

In this essay, the authors demonstrate the successful approach taken by the Community Literacy Center in Pittsburgh to promote community action through enabling community members to respond collaboratively to conflicts and negotiate problems by using writing as a tool.

Case-Based Approaches

Couture, Barbara, and Jone Rymer Goldstein. *Cases for Technical and Professional Writing*. Boston: Little Brown, 1985.

In this collection, Couture and Rymer provide cases that mirror issues and problems that entry-level professionals might face. Part one offers a method of analyzing contexts for writing, model responses, and procedures students might follow to work with cases, and part two offers more than thirty cases. While a bit outdated, there is much of value here for teachers who find this pedagogical strategy useful.

Gale, Fredric G. "Teaching Professional Writing Rhetorically: The Unified Case Approach." *Journal of Business and Technical Communication* 7, no. 2 (1993): 256–66.

Gale describes a unified case method for teaching professional writing in which all writing assignments for a semester were constrained and shaped by the context of one particular situation.

Jameson, Daphne A. "Using a Simulation to Teach Intercultural Communication in Business Communication Courses." *Bulletin of the Association for Business Communication* 56 (1993): 3–11.

Jameson discusses a game in which students simulate three cultures coming together in a business venture in order to sensitize students to cultural differences, reveal assumptions, and help them think about successful interactions.

Malone, E. L. "More than One Way to Skin a Cat—Divergent Approaches to the Same Writing Case." *Technical Writing Teacher* 16 (1989): 27–32.

Malone examines four different approaches to a communication case, emphasizing that there can be several "right" answers to situational and communication problems.

Raven, Mary Beth. "New Venture Techniques in a Communication Class," *Technical Writing Teacher* 17 (1990): 124–31.

Raven explains and argues for a case-based approach focusing on creating entrepreneurial ventures for small groups. Especially useful is her focus on teaching interpersonal and written communication and effective techniques for small group interaction.

Experiential Learning (Client-Based and Service Learning)

Anson, Chris. "On Reflection: The Role of Logs and Journals in Service-Learning Courses." In *Writing the Community: Concepts and Models for Service-Learning in Composition*, edited by Linda Adler-Kassner, Robert Crooks, and Ann Watters, 167–80. Washington, DC: AAHE, 1997.

In this theoretically and practically informed article, Anson advocates the use of journal writing to encourage and elicit reflection. He provides suggestions for integrating outside readings and class discussion to enrich or deepen reflection on social practices, as well as for how teachers can respond to journal entries.

Cooper, David D., and Laura Julier. "Democratic Conversations: Civic Literacy and Service-Learning in the American Grains." In *Writing the Community: Concepts and Models for Service-Learning in Composition*, edited by Linda Adler-Kassner, Robert Crooks, and Ann Walters, 79–94. Washington, DC: AAHE, 1997.

These authors outline a rationale for service-learning. Although they focus on composition classrooms, their discussion of research projects that ask students to examine their places as members of a community and as citizens in a democracy can be easily applied or adapted to technical communication classes.

Dubinsky, James. "Service-Learning as a Path to Virtue: The Ideal Orator in Professional Communication." *Michigan Journal of Community Service Learning* 8, no. 2 (2002): 61–74.

Based upon classical rhetorical theory and relying on cases studies, the author suggests both a rationale and strategy for using service-learning pedagogy and outlines distinctions between client-based and service-learning-based pedagogies.

Huckin, Thomas N. "Technical Writing and Community Service." *Journal of Business and Technical Communication* 11 (1997): 49–59.

In this introduction to service-learning pedagogy that focuses on small-group collaboration, Huckin advocates and explains procedures for building a course around service-learning projects.

Kastman Breuch, Lee-Ann M. "The Overruled Dust Mite: Preparing Technical Communication Students to Interact with Clients." *Technical Communication Quarterly* 10, no. 2 (2001): 193–210.

Relying on a qualitative case study, the author outlines problems students have when interacting with a client, argues that teachers need to prepare students for these interactions, and suggests ways to do so.

McEachern, Robert. "Problems in Service Learning and Technical/Professional Writing: Incorporating the Perspective of Nonprofit Management." *Technical Communication Quarterly* 10, no. 2 (2001): 211–24.

McEachern outlines potential problems when working with nonprofit agencies and suggests a possible solution based upon nonprofit management theory.

Thomas, Susan G. "Preparing Business Students More Effectively for Real-World Communication." *Journal of Business and Technical Communication* 9, no. 4 (1995): 461–74.

Thomas argues that many courses in the discipline do not effectively prepare students for their real-world tasks, and she offers strategies and techniques to help teachers reframe their courses to focus on communication tasks students will face in corporate settings.

Overview of Field's Practitioners

Lutz, Jean, and C. Gilbert Storms. *The Practice of Technical and Scientific Communication: Writing in Professional Contexts*. Greenwich, CT: Ablex, 1998.

To provide an overview of the field, its tasks, and its challenges, Lutz and Storms offer a collection of twelve articles written by technical and scientific communicators in twelve different professional areas.

Savage, Gerald J., and Dale L. Sullivan, eds. *Writing a Professional Life: Stories of Technical Communicators On and Off the Job*. Boston: Allyn and Bacon, 2001.

Savage and Sullivan collect and present stories from writers new to the field. The stories describe the authors' work in it and their lives beyond it. This collection provides useful examples to bring to class or cull from to teach strategies and rationales.

Anthologies

Allen, O. Jane, and Lynn H. Deming, eds. *Publications Management: Essays for Professional Communicators*. Amityville. NY: Baywood, 1994.

Anderson, Paul V., R. John Brockmann, and Carolyn R. Miller, eds. *New Essays in Technical and Scientific Communication: Research, Theory, Practice*. Farmingdale, NY: Baywood, 1983.

Barnum, Carol, and Saul Carliner, eds. *Techniques for Technical Communicators*. NY: Macmillan, 1993.

Beene, Lynn, and Peter White, eds. *Solving Problems in Technical Writing*. New York: Oxford UP, 1988.

Blyler, Nancy Roundy, and Charlotte Thralls, eds. *Professional Communication: The Social Perspective*. Newbury Park, CA: Sage, 1993.

Cunningham, Donald H., and Herman A. Estrin, eds. *The Teaching of Technical Writing*. Urbana, IL: NCTE, 1975.

Estrin, Herman A., ed. *Technical and Professional Writing: A Practical Anthology*. New York: Preston Publishing, 1976.

Gruber, Sibylle, ed. *Weaving a Virtual Web: Practical Approaches to New Information Technologies*. Urbana, IL: NCTE, 2000.

Hawisher, Gail E., and Cynthia L. Selfe, eds. *Passions, Pedagogies, and 21st Century Technologies*. Logan: Utah State UP and NCTE, 1999.

Johns, Ann M., ed. *Genre in the Classroom*. Mahwah, NJ: Lawrence Erlbaum, 2002.

Kirsch, Gesa, and Duane H. Roen, eds. *A Sense of Audience in Written Communication*. Newbury Park, CA: Sage, 1990.

Kynell, Teresa C., and Michael G. Moran, eds. *Three Keys to the Past: The History of Technical Communication*. Stamford, CT: Ablex, 1999.

Lay, Mary M., and William M. Karis, eds. *Collaborative Writing in Industry: Investigations in Theory and Practice*. Amityville, NY: Baywood, 1991.

Lovitt, Carl R., and Dixie Goswami, eds. *Exploring the Rhetoric of International Communication: An Agenda for Teachers and Researchers*. Thousand Oaks, CA: Sage, 2000.

Lutz, Jean, and C. Gilbert Storms, eds. *The Practice of Technical and Scientific Communication: Writing in Professional Contexts*. Greenwich, CT: Ablex, 1998.

Matalene, Carolyn B., ed. *Worlds of Writing: Teaching and Learning in Discourse Communities of Work*. New York: Random House, 1989.

Mirel, Barbara, and Rachel Spilka, eds. *Reshaping Technical Communication: New Directions and Challenges for the 21st Century*. Mahwah, NJ: Lawrence Erlbaum, 2002.

Odell, Lee, and Dixie Goswami, eds. *Writing in Nonacademic Settings*. New York and London: Guilford Press, 1985.

Reiss, Donna, Dickie Selfe, and Art Young, eds. *Electronic Communication across the Curriculum*. Urbana, IL.: NCTE, 1998.

Savage, Gerald J., and Dale L. Sullivan, eds. *Writing a Professional Life: Stories of Technical Communicators On and Off the Job*. Boston: Allyn and Bacon, 2001.

Selber, Stuart, ed. *Computers and Technical Communication: Pedagogical and Programmatic Perspectives*. Greenwich, CT: Ablex, 1997.

Selfe, Cynthia L., and Susan Hilligoss, eds. *Literacy and Computers: The Complications of Teaching and Learning with Technology*. New York: MLA, 1994.

Spilka, Rachel, ed. *Writing in the Workplace: New Research Perspectives*. Carbondale: Southern Illinois U Press, 1993.

Staples, Katherine, and Cezar Ornatowski, eds. *Foundations for Teaching Technical Communication: Theory, Practice, and Program Design*. Greenwich, CT: Ablex, 1997.

Sullivan, Patricia, and Jennie Dautermann, eds. *Electronic Literacies in the Workplace: Technologies of Writing*. Urbana, IL: NCTE, 1996.

Relevant Journals

Business Communication Quarterly

EDUCAUSE Quarterly

IEEE Transaction on Professional Communication

Journal of Advanced Composition

Journal of Business and Technical Communication

Journal of Computer Documentation

Journal of Writing and Technical Communication

Kairos

Syllabus

Technical Communication

Technical Communication Quarterly

The Writing Instructor

NOTES ON THE AUTHORS

Carolyn R. Miller is professor in the Department of English at North Carolina State University and co-director of the Center for Information Society Studies. She currently serves on the editorial boards of *Issues in Writing* and *College Composition and Communication*.

Robert R. Johnson is the Chair of the Humanities Department at Michigan Technological University where he is coordinating the Michigan Tech Department of Humanities Preparing Future Faculty Initiative to develop innovative approaches to help graduate students meet the changing needs of academia.

Patrick Moore is an Associate Professor at the University of Arkansas, Little Rock where he teaches instrumental discourse, technical communication, and world literature. Moore is author of numerous articles on technical communication as well as literary criticism.

Jo Allen, a tenured professor in the English Department at North Carolina State University is currently interim vice provost for the Division of Undergraduate Affairs at NCSU. She is also president of the Association of Teachers of Technical Writing.

Robert J. Connors was a professor of English and Director of the Writing Center at the University of New Hampshire. He was awarded the Richard Braddock Award by the CCCC in 1982 and was co-recipient of the Mina P. Shaughnessy Award from the Modern Language Association in 1985. Connors passed away in June, 2000.

Katherine T. Durack is an Assistant Professor at Miami University of Ohio in Technical and Scientific Communication. Before joining the faculty as an Assistant Professor at Miami, she worked as a writer, editor, and consultant in the computer industry. She is faculty advisor to Miami's student chapter of STC and also remains active in the Association of Teachers of Technical Writing.

Charlotte Thralls teaches undergraduate and graduate courses in rhetorical theory, professional communication pedagogy, ethical and cultural issues in the workplace, and media analysis. She was founding co-editor of the *Journal of Business and Technical Communication* and co-editor of the collection, *Professional Communication: The Social Perspective.* She is now at Utah State and is currently co-editor of *TCQ.*

Nancy R. Blyler is Professor Emeritus at Iowa State University where she taught for twenty years. Besides numerous publications, Blyler has also won three NCTE awards for her work on technical communication.

Henrietta Nickels Shirk is the department head and professor of Professional and Technical Communications at Montana Tech. She has authored or co-authored more than 60 publications and is a member of the Modern Language Association, the American Medical Writers Association, the Society for Technical Communication, and the Association for Teachers of Technical Writing, among others.

Marcus Fabius Quintilian, c.AD 35–c.AD 95, was an orator, author and teacher who taught rhetoric in Rome to such pupils as Pliny the Younger and possibly Tacitus. Quintilian, who believed that rhetoric is "the good man speaking well" and who is most famous for his *Institutio oratoria,* a survey on rhetoric in which he demonstrated his belief that good taste, moderation, and an in-depth knowledge of subject matter are necessary for successful speaking.

David R. Russell is a Professor in Rhetoric and Professional Communication at Iowa State University. He has published numerous articles and book chapters and his book, *Writing in the Academic Disciplines: A Curricular History,* which examines the history of American writing instruction outside of composition courses, is now in its second edition.

James Porter is a professor and the Director of Rhetoric and Writing at Michigan State University and has authored or co-authored four books. His book *Rhetorical Ethics and Internetworked Writing* (1998) won the *Computers and Composition* Best Book award. He has also won the NCTE book award for Excellence in Technical and Scientific Communication.

Janice C. (Ginny) Redish is president of Redish & Associates, Inc. in Bethesda, MD where she helps companies and agencies bring user-centered design into their processes. She is co-author of *A Practical Guide to Usablity Testing* (2nd ed., 1999) and her *User and Task Analysis for Interface Design,* was the 2001 Goldsmith Award winner from the IEEE.

Barbara Mirel is a visiting associate professor and research investigator in the School of Information at the University of Michigan. Mirel has worked for the VHA National Center for Patient Safety, Lucent Technologies, and has taught seminars to IBM information developers and Caterpillar managers, project leaders, and design engineers. She is the author of *Interaction Design for Complex Problem Solving: Designing Useful and Usable Software* (Elsevier/ Morgan Kaufmann, 2003).

Stephen A. Bernhardt is the first holder of the Andrew B. Kirkpatrick Chair in Writing and Professor of English at the University of Delaware and is a fellow of the Association of Teachers of Technical Writing (ATTW). He consults with major pharmaceutical clients in the U.S. and E.U. and works with McCulley/Cuppan consultants.

Lisa Ann Jackson is the managing editor of Diabetes Website.com, based in Sunnyvale, CA. She is also a contributor to a variety of publications, both consumer and technical.

Carol A. Berkenkotter is a professor in the Department of Rhetoric at the University of Minnesota. She is winner (with co-author Thomas N. Huckin) of the NCTE Best Book Award for *Genre Knowledge in Disciplinary Communication: Cognition/Culture/Power.*

Thomas N. Huckin is a professor and Director of the Writing Program at the University of Utah who, with co-author Carol A. Berkenkotter, was awarded the NCTE Best Book Award in 1996 for Genre Knowledge in Disciplinary Communication: Cognition/Culture/Power.

Aviva Freedman is a professor in the School of Linguistics and Applied Language Studies Carleton College. She is also co-founder of Carleton's Enriched Support Program and served as Dean of the Faculty of Arts and Social Sciences. Freedman received a prestigious 3M Teaching Award in 1996.

Christine Adam is associate director of the Centre for Initiatives in Education and Enriched Support Program at Carleton University.

Clay Spinuzzi is an assistant professor of Rhetoric and Associate Director of Computer Writing and Research Lab at the University of Texas. He has received several grants for his research on technology and received the 2000 Outstanding Dissertation Award from the CCCC Committee on Technical Communication. His book *Tracing Genres Through Organizations: A Sociocultural Approach to Information Design* was published by MIT Press in October 2003. http://www.cwrl.utexas.edu/~spinuzzi/

Ann M. Blakeslee is a professor in the Department of English and Director of Undergraduate Studies at Eastern Michigan University. Her recent book, *Interacting with Audiences: Social Influences on the Production of Scientific Writing,* reports her study of a group of physicists writing for an interdisciplinary audience.

Rachel Spilka is a professor at the University of Wisconsin-Milwaukee. Recently, she served as a Senior Information Design specialist at the American Institutes for Research, a Technical Editor at MicroSim Corporation, and a Communications Analyst for health and military research programs at the RAND Corporation. She is editor of *Writing in the Workplace: New Research Perspectives* (Southern Illinois University Press), winner of the NCTE Award for Excellence in Technical and Scientific Writing.

Linda Beamer is a professor in the Department of Marketing at California State University, Los Angeles. She is the author of many articles and is the co-author of a textbook on the subject. Dr. Beamer is also an adjunct professor at UNITEC in Auckland, New Zealand, and she has taught at the Universidad Nacional del Centro in Argentina, and at universities in China.

Emily A. Thrush is a professor of English who teaches in both the Applied Linguistics and Professional Writing programs at The University of Memphis. She has been an Academic Specialist for the USIA in the Czech Republic, Slovakia, Italy, and Germany, and served as a Senior Fulbright Fellow in Mexico in 2000-2001.

Mary M. Lay is the Director of Graduate Studies in the Rhetoric and Scientific and Technological Communication Program at the University of Minnesota as well as an affiliated faculty member of the graduate program in feminist studies. She was co-Editor and Manuscript Review Editor of *Technical Communication Quarterly* for many years.

Laura J. Gurak is professor and Head of the Rhetoric Department at the University of Minnesota as well as co-director of the Internet Studies Center. Gurak has authored several textbooks, including *Persuasion and Privacy in Cyberspace: The Online Protests over Lotus MarketPlace and the Clipper Chip* (Yale, 1997; to be reissued in 2003), the first book-length study to document the rhetorical dynamics of online communication and one of the first to look at how protests form in cyberspace.

Waka Fukuoka is in charge of localizing user manuals for foreign countries including Asian Pacific countries and U.S. at Fuji Xerox in Tokyo, Japan. She acquired her M.S. degree in Technical Communication from the University of Washington. Her studies focused on cultural differences in text and its influence on comprehension.

Yukiko Kojima is an editor/technical writer at Sony Corporation in Toyko, Japan. She develops templates for user manuals to maximize their usability and production effectiveness. She received her M.S. in technical communication at the University of Washington.

Jan H. Spyridakis is a professor in the department of Technical Communication at the University of Washington, where she teaches courses on technical writing style, research methodology, and international and advanced technical communication. Her research and consulting focus on the effect of document and screen design variables on comprehension and usability. She has received teaching and publication awards, and is a Fellow of the Society for Technical Communication.

Lee-Ann Kastman Breuch is an assistant professor in the Department of Rhetoric at the University of Minnesota, where she has coordinated the undergraduate major in Scientific and Technical Communication. She currently directs the Online Writing Center.

Stuart A. Selber is an assistant professor of English and Director of Technical Writing at Penn State University. The recipient of three national publication awards, he chairs the Conference on College Composition and Communication Committee on Technical Communication and is a past president of the Council for Programs in Technical and Scientific Communication. Selber also holds a faculty position in distance education in the World Campus.

Johndan Johnson-Eilola is a professor and Director of the Eastman Kodak Center for Excellence in Communication in the Department of Technical Communications at Clarkson University. He has co-authored numerous articles and books, and is co-editor with Stuart Selber of *Central Works: Landmark Essays in Technical Communication* (Oxford UP).

Cynthia L. Selfe is a professor of humanities at Michigan Technological University and founder, with Kathleen Kiefer, of *Computers and Composition,* a journal site she co-edits with Gail E. Hawisher. In 1996 Selfe became the first woman and first English teacher to win EDUCOM Medal for innovative computer use in higher education. She has served as chair of both the Conference on College Composition and Communication and College Section of the National Council of Teachers of English.

Gail E. Hawisher is Professor of English and founding Director of the Center for Writing Studies at the University of Illinois, Urbana-Champaign. She has served on the Conference on College Composition and Communication's Executive Committee, NCTE's Executive Committee and as a member of the Modern Language Association's Advisory Committee on the MLA International Bibliography, as well as its Committee on Information Technology. She is co-editor, with Cynthia Selfe, of *Passions, Pedagogies, and 21st Century Technologies,* which won the Distinguished Book Award at Computer and Writing 2000.

Daniel Robey is the John B. Zellars Professor of Computer Information Systems at Georgia State University. He holds a joint appointment in the Departments of Computer Information Systems and Management. Robey is Editor-in-Chief of *Information and Organization* and also serves on the editorial boards of *Organization Science, Information Technology and Management,* and *Information Technology & People.*

Huoy Min Khoo is completing her doctorate in computer information systems from Georgia State University. She holds a master of business administration degree from Mississippi State University and a bachelor of science in computer science degree from the University of Mississippi.

Carolyn Powers is an independent consultant specializing in business process re-engineering and website development. Previously she worked as a director of applicatioin development for a *Fortune* 1000 manufacturer and importer. She has also worked as a manager for Anderson Consulting.

Cezar M. Ornatowski is an associate professor and graduate director in the Department of Rhetoric and Writing Studies at San Diego State University. His articles have been published in such journals as *Technical Communication, Technical Communication Quarterly, Journal of Business and Technical Communication, Journal for the Study of Religion, The European Legacy, Relazioni Internazionali, and Readerly/Writerly Texts.* He has also co-edited the collection *Foundations for Teaching Technical Communication: Theory, Practice, and Program Design,* with Katherine Staples.

NOTE ON THE EDITOR

James M. Dubinsky directs the Professional Writing Program at Virginia Tech and teaches a variety of courses, including Grant Proposal and Report Writing, the senior seminar on Issues in Public and Professional Discourse, and a graduate pedagogy course. His research interests include the scholarship of teaching, civic engagement, and the history of rhetoric. His articles have been published in such journals as the *Michigan Journal of Community Service Learning, TCQ,* and *BCQ,* and he is editing a special issue of *TCQ* on Civic Engagement (with Harrison Carpenter) and co-editing a special issue of *Reflections* on Professional Writing and Service-Learning with Melody Bowdon, both due out in 2004. In 2000, he was awarded Virginia Tech's Student Leadership Award as the Outstanding Service-Learning Educator, and in 2002, he was awarded a College of Arts and Sciences Certificate of Teaching Excellence.

Acknowledgments *(continued from page iv)*

Jo Allen. "The Case Against Defining Technical Writing." From the *Journal of Business and Technical Communication.* Copyright © 1990. Reprinted by permission of Sage Publications, Inc.

Linda Beamer. "Learning International Communication Competence." From the *Journal of Business and Technical Communication.* Copyright © 1992. Reprinted by permission of Sage Publications, Inc.

Carol Berkenkotter and Thomas Huckin. "Rethinking Genre from a Sociocognitive Perspective." From *Genre Knowledge in Disciplinary Communication.* Copyright © 1995 by Lawrence Erlbaum Associates, Inc. Reprinted by permission of the publisher.

Stephen A. Bernhardt. "Teaching for Change, Vision and Responsibility." From *Technical Communication* 42 (1995) pp. 600–02. Copyright © 1995 by the Society for Technical Communication. Arlington, VA, U.S.A. Reprinted by permission of the publisher.

Ann M. Blakeslee. "Bridging the Workplace and the Academy: Teaching Professional Genres Through Classroom Workplace Collaboration." From *Technical Communication Quarterly* 10.2, pp. 169–92. Copyright © 2001. Reprinted by permission of the Association of Teachers of Technical Writing.

Robert J. Connors. "The Rise of Technical Writing Instruction in America." From *Journal of Technical Writing and Communication,* Volume 12 (4), pp. 329–52. Copyright © 1982 by the Baywood Publishing Co., Inc. Reprinted by permission of the publisher.

Katherine R. Durack. "Gender, Technology, and the History of Technical Communication." From *Technical Communication Quarterly* 6.3, pp. 249–60. Copyright © 1997. Reprinted by permission of the Association of Teachers of Technical Writing.

Aviva Freedman and Christine Adam. "Learning to Write Professionally: 'Situated Learning' and the Transition from University to Professional Discourse." From the *Journal of Business and Technical Communication.* Copyright © 1996. Reprinted by permission of Sage Publications, Inc.

Waka Fukoka, Yukiko Kojima, and Jan H. Spyridakis. "Illustrations in User Manuals: Preference and Effectiveness with Japanese and American Audiences." From *Technical Communication* 46 (1999) pp. 167–76. Copyright © 1999 by the Society for Technical Communication. Arlington, VA, U.S.A. Reprinted by permission of the publisher.

Laura J. Gurak and Nancy L. Bayer. "Making Gender Visible: Extending Feminist Critiques of Technology to Technical Communication." From *Technical Communication Quarterly* 3.3, pp. 257–70. Copyright © 1994. Reprinted by permission of the Association of Teachers of Technical Writing.

Lisa Ann Jackson. "The Rhetoric of Design: Implications for Corporate Intranets." From *Technical Communication* 47.2 (2000) pp. 212–19. Copyright © 2000 by the Society for Technical Communication. Arlington, VA, U.S.A. Reprinted by permission of the publisher.

Johndan Johnson-Eilola. "Relocating the Value of Work: Technical Cummunication in a Post-Industrial Age." From *Technical Communication Quarterly* 5.3, pp. 245–70. Copyright © 1996. Reprinted by permission of the Association of Teachers of Technical Writing.

Robert R. Johnson. "Complicating Technology: Interdisciplinary Method, the Burden of Comprehension, and the Ethical Space of the Technical Communicator." From *Technical Communication Quarterly* 7.1, pp. 1–25. Copyright © 1998. Reprinted by permission of the Association of Teachers of Technical Writing.

Robert R. Johnson. "Johnson Responds." From *Technical Communication Quarterly* 8.2, pp. 224–26. Copyright © 1999. Reprinted by permission of the Association of Teachers of Technical Writing.

Lee-Ann Kastmann Breuch. "Thinking Critically about Technological Literacy: Developing a Framework to Guide Computer Pedagogy in Technical Communication." From *Technical Communication Quarterly* 11.3, pp. 267–88. Copyright © 2002. Reprinted by permission of the Association of Teachers of Technical Writing.

Robert Kramer and Stephen A. Bernhardt. "Teaching Text Design." From *Technical Communication Quarterly* 5.1, pp. 35–60. Copyright © 1996. Reprinted by permission of the Association of Teachers of Technical Writing.

Mary M. Lay "Feminist Theory and the Redefinition of Technical Communication." From the *Journal of Business and Technical Communication.* Copyright © 1991. Reprinted by permission of Sage Publications, Inc.

Carolyn R. Miller. "A Humanistic Rationale for Technical Writing." From *College English* 40.6 (1979) pp. 610–17. Copyright © 1979 by the National Council of Teachers of English. Reprinted by permission of the publisher.

Carolyn R. Miller. "What's Practical About Technical Communication?" From *Technical Writing: Theory and Practice,* edited by Bertie E. Fearing and W. Keats Sparrow. Copyright © 1989. Reprinted by permission of the Modern Language Association of America.

Barbara Mirel. "Advancing a Vision of Usability." From *Reshaping Technical Communication,* edited by Barbara Mirel and Rachel Spilka. Copyright © 2002 by Lawrence Erlbaum Associates, Inc. Reprinted by permission of the publisher.

Patrick Moore. "Myths about Instrumental Discourse: A Response to Robert R. Johnson." From *Technical Communication Quarterly* 8.2, pp. 210–23. Copyright © 1999. Reprinted by permission of the Association of Teachers of Technical Writing.

Cezar M. Ornatowski. "Educating Technical Communicators to Make Better Decisions." From *Technical Communication* 42 (1995) pp. 576–80. Copyright © 1995 by the Society for Technical Communication. Arlington, VA, U.S.A. Reprinted by permission of the publisher.

James Porter. "The Exercise of Critical Rhetorical Ethics." From pp. 133–47 in *Rhetorical Ethics and Internetworked Writing* by James Porter. Copyright © 1998. Reproduced with permission of Greenwood Publishing Group, Inc., Westport, CT.

Janice Redish. "What is Information Design?" From *Technical Communication* 47.2 (2000) pp. 561–76. Copyright © 2000 by the Society for Technical Communication. Arlington, VA, U.S.A. Reprinted by permission of the publisher.

Daniel Robey, Huoy Min Khoo, and Carolyn Powers. "Situated Learning in Cross-functional Virtual Teams." From *IEEE Transactions on Technical Communication* 43, pp. 67–76. Copyright © 2000 IEEE. Reprinted by permission of the publisher and the author.

David R Russell. "The Ethics of Teaching Ethics in Professional Communication: The Case of Engineering Publicity at MIT in the 1920's." From the *Journal of Business and Technical Communication.* Copyright © 1993. Reprinted by permission of Sage Publications, Inc.

Stuart A. Selber, Johndan Johnson-Eilola, and Cynthia L. Selfe. "Contexts for Faculty Professional Development in the Age of Electronic Writing and Communication." From *Technical Communication* 42 (1995) pp. 581–84. Copyright © 1995 by the Society for Technical Communication. Arlington, VA, U.S.A. Reprinted by permission of the publisher.

Cynthia L. Selfe and Gail E. Hawisher. "A Historical Look at the Electronic Literacy: Implications for the Education of Technical Communicators." From the *Journal of Business and Technical Communication.* Copyright © 2002. Reprinted by permission of Sage Publications, Inc.

Henrietta Nickels Shirk. "Researching the History of Technical Communication: Assessing and Analyzing Corporate Archives." From *STC's 50th Annual Conference Proceedings.* Copyright © 2003 by the Society for Technical Communication. Arlington, VA, U.S.A. Reprinted by permission of the publisher.

Rachel Spilka. "Communicating Across Organization Boundaries: A Challenge for Workplace Professionals." From *Technical Communication* 42.3 (1995) pp. 436–50. Copyright © 1995 by the Society for Technical Communication. Arlington, VA, U.S.A. Reprinted by permission of the publisher.

Clay Spinuzzi. "Pseudotransactionality, Activity Theory, and Professional Writing Instruction." From *Technical Communication Quarterly* 5, pp. 295–308. Copyright © 1996. Reprinted by permission of the Association of Teachers of Technical Writing.

Charlotte Thralls and Nancy R. Blyler. "The Social Perspective and Pedagogy in Technical Communication." From *Technical Communication Quarterly* 2.3. Copyright © 1993. Reprinted by permission of the Association of Teachers of Technical Writing.

Emily A. Thrush. "Multicultural Issues in Technical Communication." From pages 161–78 in *Foundations for Teaching Technical Communication,* edited by Katherine Staples and Cezar Ornatowski. Copyright © 1997. Reproduced with permission of Greenwood Publishing Group, Inc., Westport, CT.

Quintilian Trans. Rev. John Selby Watson. From the "Institutio Oratorio" Book XII, Chapter 1. From *The Rhetorical Tradition,* edited by Patricia Bizzell and Bruce Herzberg. Copyright © 2001 by Bedford/St. Martin's. Reprinted by permission of the publisher.

INDEX